Critical Issues in the Lives of People with Severe Disabilities

Critical Issues in the Lives of People with Severe Disabilities

edited by

Luanna H. Meyer, Ph.D.

Syracuse University
Syracuse, New York

Charles A. Peck, Ph.D.

Washington State University
Vancouver, Washington

and

Lou Brown, Ph.D.
University of Wisconsin
Madison, Wisconsin

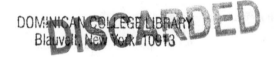
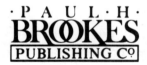
·P·A·U·L·H·
BROOKES
PUBLISHING C^o

Baltimore · London · Toronto · Sydney

Paul H. Brookes Publishing Co.
P.O. Box 10624
Baltimore, Maryland 21285-0624

Typeset by Brushwood Graphics, Inc., Baltimore, Maryland.
Manufactured in the United States of America by
The Maple Press Company, York, Pennsylvania.

Library of Congress Cataloging-in-Publication Data

Critical issues in the lives of people with severe disabilities /
edited by Luanna Meyer, Charles Peck, and Lou Brown.
    p.   cm.
    Contents: Includes bibliographical references.
    ISBN 1-55766-048-4
    1. Handicapped—United States. 2. Handicapped—Deinstitutionalization—
United States. 3. Handicapped—Services for—United States. 4. Handicapped—
Legal status, laws, etc.—United States. I. Meyer, Luanna H. II. Peck, Charles
A. III. Brown, Lou.
HV1553.C75   1990
362.4'048'0973—dc20   90-32081
                                                CIP

Contents

Contributors ix
Editorial Advisory Board xiii
Foreword   *Martha E. Snell* xv
Preface xxi
Introduction   Who Are They and What Do They Want? An Essay on TASH
                Lou Brown xxv

CHAPTER 1   Linking Values and Science in Social Policy Decisions Affecting
             Citizens with Severe Disabilities
             Charles A. Peck 1

SECTION I   DEFINITIONS AND DIAGNOSES
Introduction to Section I 17
DOCUMENT I.1   Definition of the People TASH Serves (Originally Adopted
                December 1985; Revised November 1986) 19
DOCUMENT I.2   Resolution on People with Mental Retardation Who Are Also
                Diagnosed as Mentally Ill (Adopted March 1988) 20
DOCUMENT I.3   Cultural Sensitivity Resolution (Adopted March 1988) 21
DOCUMENT I.4   Resolution Urging Repudiation of States on Friend of the Court
                Brief in *Romeo vs. Youngberg* (Adopted November 1981) 22
DOCUMENT I.5   Immigration Resolution (Adopted October 1987) 23
CHAPTER 2   Testing and Diagnosis: A Review and Evaluation
             Ian M. Evans 25
CHAPTER 3   Functional Assessment: Dynamic and Domain Properties
             Robert Gaylord-Ross and Diane Browder 45
CHAPTER 4   Educating All Students: The Future is Now
             Fred P. Orelove 67
CHAPTER 5   Telling New Stories: The Search for Capacity Among People with
             Severe Handicaps
             John O'Brien and Beth Mount 89
CHAPTER 6   Evaluating Evaluation: A "Fictional" Play
             Mary Ulrich 93
CHAPTER 7   Assessment: Current Concerns and Future Directions
             Adriana L. Schuler and Linda Perez 101

SECTION II   DEINSTITUTIONALIZATION AND COMMUNITY SERVICES
Introduction to Section II 107
DOCUMENT II.1   Deinstitutionalization Policy (Originally Adopted October 1979;
                 Revised November 1986) 109
DOCUMENT II.2   Resolution Opposing Capital Investment in Institutional Settings
                 in the State of New York (Adopted December 1985) 110
DOCUMENT II.3   Gramm Rudman Resolution (Adopted November 1985) 111
DOCUMENT II.4   Policy Statement for Cessation of Capital Investment in
                 Segregated Settings (Originally Adopted October 1981;
                 Revised October 1987) 113
CHAPTER 8   Living It Up! An Analysis of Research on Community Living
             Jan Nisbet, Marsha Clark, and Susan Covert 115
CHAPTER 9   Supported Employment: Emerging Opportunities for
             Employment Integration
             Frank R. Rusch, Janis Chadsey-Rusch, and John R. Johnson 145

CHAPTER 10   Recreation and Leisure: A Review of the Literature and
                      Recommendations for Future Directions
                           John Dattilo 171
CHAPTER 11   Social Relationships
                           Thomas G. Haring 195
CHAPTER 12   Integrated Work: A Rejection of Segregated Enclaves and Mobile
                      Work Crews
                           Lou Brown, Alice Udvari-Solner, Elise Frattura-Kampschroer,
                           Louanne Davis, Charlotte Ahlgren, Patricia Van Deventer,
                           and Jack Jorgensen 219
CHAPTER 13   What's Wrong with the Continuum? A Metaphorical Analysis
                           Colleen Wieck and Jeffrey L. Strully 229
CHAPTER 14   Community Living: Lessons for Today
                           Steven J. Taylor and Julie Ann Racino 235

SECTION III   A REDEFINITION OF THE CONTINUUM OF SERVICES—
                      ZERO EXCLUSION MODELS AND SUPPORTS
Introduction to Section III 239
DOCUMENT III.1   Resolution on the Redefinition of the Continuum of Services
                           (Original Resolution "I.Q. Tests" Adopted October 1979;
                           Revised November 1986) 241
DOCUMENT III.2   Position Statement of the Related Services Subcommittee of the
                           TASH Critical Issues Committee (Adopted November 1986) 243
DOCUMENT III.3   Supported Education Resolution (Adopted December 1988) 244
CHAPTER 15   Supporting the Education of Students with Severe Disabilities in
                      Regular Education Environments
                           Michael F. Giangreco and Joanne W. Putnam 245
CHAPTER 16   Supporting Families of Persons with Severe Disabilities: Emerging
                      Findings, Practices, and Questions
                           George H. S. Singer and Larry K. Irvin 271
CHAPTER 17   Personnel Preparation: Directions for the Next Decade
                           Diane Baumgart and Dianne L. Ferguson 313
CHAPTER 18   Integrated Related Services
                           Winnie Dunn 353
CHAPTER 19   Community School: An Essay
                           Wayne Sailor 379
CHAPTER 20   Social Policy, Social Systems, and Educational Practices
                           Douglas P. Biklen 387
CHAPTER 21   Preparation of Personnel to Educate Students with Severe and
                      Multiple Disabilities: A Time for Change?
                           Doug Guess and Barbara Thompson 391
CHAPTER 22   It's About Relationships
                           Marsha Forest 399
CHAPTER 23   Achieving Integration during the Second Revolution
                           Frank J. Laski 409

SECTION IV   EXTENSIONS OF THE PUBLIC LAW AND EDUCATIONAL
                      SERVICES
Introduction to Section IV 423
DOCUMENT IV.1   Resolution in Support of the Education of the Handicapped Act
                           and Section 504 of the Rehabilitation Act of 1973 (Originally
                           Adopted October 1981; Revised October 1987) 425
DOCUMENT IV.2   Resolution on Extended School Year (Adopted November 1986) 427
CHAPTER 24   Early Childhood Services for Children with Severe Disabilities:
                      Research, Values, Policy, and Practice
                           Carol R. Westlake and Ann P. Kaiser 429

CHAPTER 25   Extended Year Special Education Programming: A Legal Analysis
Carroll L. Lucht and Sondra B. Kaska 459

CHAPTER 26   Extended Year Special Education Programming: Educational Planning
Diane Browder 467

CHAPTER 27   An Essay on Preschool Integration
Philippa H. Campbell 473

CHAPTER 28   Ensuring Quality of Early Intervention for Children with Severe Disabilities
Phillip S. Strain 479

CHAPTER 29   Family Assessment and Family Empowerment: An Ethical Analysis
Ann P. Turnbull and H. Rutherford Turnbull 485

SECTION V   ADULT SERVICES REFORM AND OMNIBUS LEGISLATION ISSUES
Introduction to Section V 489
DOCUMENT V.1   TASH Calls for Adult Service Reform (Adopted November 1983) 491
DOCUMENT V.2   Social Security Resolution (Adopted October 1987) 493
DOCUMENT V.3   Resolution on Choices (Adopted December 1988) 494
CHAPTER 30   A Comprehensive Analysis of Federal Statutes and Programs for Persons with Severe Disabilities
Martin H. Gerry and Celane M. McWhorter 495

CHAPTER 31   Community Services for Adults with Disabilities: Policy Challenges in the Emerging Support Paradigm
Michael W. Smull and G. Thomas Bellamy 527

CHAPTER 32   An Exchange on Personal Futures and Community Participation: An Interview with John McKnight and Ronald Melzer
Susan Brody Hasazi 537

CHAPTER 33   Choices, Communication, and Control: A Call for Expanding Them in the Lives of People with Severe Disabilities
Robert K. Williams 543

SECTION VI   LIFE AND DEATH ISSUES
Introduction to Section VI 545
DOCUMENT VI.1   Resolution on Infant Care (Originally Adopted April 1983; Amended April 1989) 547
DOCUMENT VI.2   Nutrition and Hydration Resolution (Adopted November 1986) 548
DOCUMENT VI.3   Organ Transplant Unit (Adopted March 1988) 549
DOCUMENT VI.4   Resolution on the Cessation of Intrusive Interventions (Originally Adopted October 1981; Revised November 1986) 550
DOCUMENT VI.5   SIBIS Resolution (Adopted March 1988) 551
CHAPTER 34   Medical Treatment
David L. Coulter 553

CHAPTER 35   Nonaversive Interventions for Severe Behavior Problems
Edwin Helmstetter and V. Mark Durand 559

CHAPTER 36   A Dialogue on Medical Responsibility
James Schaffer and Dick Sobsey 601

CHAPTER 37   The Future of Applied Behavior Analysis for People with Severe Disabilities: Commentary I
Robert H. Horner 607

CHAPTER 38   The Future of Applied Behavior Analysis for People with Severe Disabilities: Commentary II
Donald M. Baer 613

CHAPTER 39   A Dialogue on Power Relationships and Aversive Control
Anne M. Donnellan and Barbara C. Cutler 617

CHAPTER 40   Empowerment and Choices
             Herbert Lovett 625

SUMMARY   **POLICY AND PRACTICES**
CHAPTER 41   Advocacy, Research, and Typical Practices: A Call for the Reduction
             of Discrepancies between What Is and What Ought To Be, and How
             To Get There
             Luanna H. Meyer 629

Index 651

Contributors

Charlotte Ahlgren, Ph.D.
Department of Special Education
5700 College Road
Illinois Benedictine College
Lisle, Illinois 60532-0900

Donald M. Baer, Ph.D.
Department of Human Development
University of Kansas
Lawrence, Kansas 66045

Diane Baumgart, Ph.D.
Department of Counseling and Special Education
College of Education
University of Idaho
Moscow, Idaho 83843

G. Thomas Bellamy, Ph.D.
Office of Educational Research and Improvement
U.S. Department of Education
Washington, D.C. 20208-2405

Douglas P. Biklen, Ph.D.
School of Education
Syracuse University
Syracuse, New York 13244-2280

Diane Browder, Ph.D.
111 Research Drive, Building F
College of Education
Lehigh University
Bethlehem, Pennsylvania 18015

Lou Brown, Ph.D.
Department of Rehabilitation Psychology and
   Special Education
432 North Murray Street, Room 305
University of Wisconsin-Madison
Madison, Wisconsin 53706

Philippa H. Campbell, Ph.D.
Family Child Learning Center
Children's Hospital Medical Center of Akron
281 Locust Street
Akron, Ohio 44308

Janis Chadsey-Rusch, Ph.D.
Department of Special Education
110 Education Building
1310 South Sixth Street
University of Illinois
Champaign, Illinois 61820

Marsha Clark, M.Ed.
Institute on Disability
312 Morrill Hall
University of New Hampshire
Durham, New Hampshire 03824

David L. Coulter, M.D.
Pediatric Neurology
Boston City Hospital
818 Harrison Avenue
Boston, Massachusetts 02118

Susan Covert, M.Ed.
RR #1 Box 26
Contoocook, New Hampshire 03229

Barbara C. Cutler, Ed.D.
Boston University School of Education
Boston, Massachusetts 02215

John Dattilo, Ph.D.
Department of Leisure Studies
203 Henderson Building South
Pennsylvania State University
University Park, Pennsylvania 16802

Louanne Davis, M.S.
1400 Oakhill Drive, #421
Escondito, California 92027

Anne M. Donnellan, Ph.D.
Department of Rehabilitation Psychology and
   Special Education
432 North Murray Street
University of Wisconsin-Madison
Madison, Wisconsin 53706

Winnie Dunn, Ph.D. OTR, FAOTA
Occupational Therapy Curriculum
4013 Hinch Hall
Kansas University Medical Center
39th and Rainbow Boulevards
Kansas City, Kansas 66103

V. Mark Durand, Ph.D.
Department of Psychology
1400 Washington Avenue
State University of New York at Albany
Albany, New York 12222

Ian M. Evans, Ph.D.
Psychology Department
State University of New York at Binghamton
Binghamton, New York 13901

Dianne L. Ferguson, Ph.D.
Division of Special Education and Rehabilitation
Specialized Training Program
135 College of Education
University of Oregon
Eugene, Oregon 97403

Marsha Forest, Ed.D.
Centre for Integrated Education and Community
35 Jackes Avenue
Frontier College
Toronto, Ontario M6H 2S5
CANADA

Elise Frattura-Kampschroer, M.S.
Department of Rehabilitation Psychology and
    Special Education
432 North Murray Street, Room 307
University of Wisconsin–Madison
Madison, Wisconsin 53706

Martin H. Gerry, J.D.
8308 Carderock Drive
Bethesda, Maryland 20817

Robert Gaylord-Ross, Ph.D.
Department of Special Education
1600 Holloway Avenue
San Francisco State University
San Francisco, California 94132

Michael F. Giangreco, Ph.D.
Center for Developmental Disabilities
499C Waterman Building
University of Vermont
Burlington, Vermont 05405

Doug Guess, Ed.D.
Department of Special Education
University of Kansas
Lawrence, Kansas 66045

Thomas G. Haring, Ph.D.
Special Education Program
Graduate School of Education
University of California
Santa Barbara, California 93106

Susan Brody Hasazi, Ed.D.
Department of Special Education
405 Waterman Building
University of Vermont
Burlington, Vermont 05405

Edwin Helmstetter, Ph.D.
Department of Counseling Psychology
Washington State University
Pullman, Washington 99164-2131

Robert H. Horner, Ph.D.
Specialized Training Program
135 Education Building
University of Oregon
Eugene, Oregon 97403

Larry K. Irvin, Ph.D.
Oregon Research Institute
1899 Willamette Avenue
Eugene, Oregon 97401-4015

John R. Johnson, M.Ed.
Department of Special Education
110 Education Building
1310 South Sixth Street
University of Illinois
Champaign, Illinois 61820

Jack Jorgensen, M.Ed.
545 West Dayton Street
Madison Metropolitan School District
Madison, Wisconsin 53703

Ann P. Kaiser, Ph.D.
Department of Special Education
Peabody College of Vanderbilt University
Nashville, Tennessee 37203

Sondra B. Kaska, J.D.
Iowa Protection and Advocacy Services, Inc.
DD/MI Clinical Law Project
University of Iowa College of Law
Iowa City, Iowa 52242

Frank J. Laski, J.D.
Public Interest Law Center of Philadelphia
125 South 9th Street, Suite 700
Philadelphia, Pennsylvania 19107

Herbert Lovett, Ph.D.
76 G Street
Boston, Massachusetts 02127

Carroll L. Lucht, M.S.W., J.D.
401A Yale Station
Yale Law School
New Haven, Connecticut 06520

Celane M. McWhorter, M.Ed.
The Association for Persons with Severe Handicaps
1511 King Street
Alexandria, Virginia 22314

Luanna H. Meyer, Ph.D.
School of Education
805 South Crouse Avenue
Syracuse University
Syracuse, New York 13244-2280

Beth Mount, D.P.A.
Graphic Futures
25 Stanley Avenue-B1
Hartford, Connecticut 06107

Jan Nisbet, Ph.D.
Institute on Disability
312 Morrill Hall
University of New Hampshire
Durham, New Hampshire 03824

John O'Brien
Responsive Systems Associates
58 Willowick Drive
Lithonia, Georgia 30038

Fred P. Orelove, Ph.D.
Box 2020
Division of Educational Services
Virginia Commonwealth University
Richmond, Virginia 23284

Charles A. Peck, Ph.D.
1812 East McLoughlin Boulevard
Washington State University–Vancouver
Vancouver, Washington 98663

Linda Perez, Ph.D.
Department of Special Education
1600 Holloway Avenue
San Francisco State University
San Francisco, California 94132

JoAnne W. Putnam, Ph.D.
Department of Teacher Education
University of Montana
Missoula, Montana 59812

Julie Ann Racino, M.A.
Center on Human Policy
200 Huntington Hall
Syracuse University
Syracuse, New York 13244-2340

Frank R. Rusch, Ph.D.
Transition Institute
110 Education Building
1310 South Sixth Street
University of Illinois
Champaign, Illinois 61820

Wayne Sailor, Ph.D.
612 Font Boulevard
San Francisco State University
San Francisco, California 94132

James Schaffer, M.D.
717 West 1st Street
Bloomington, Indiana 47401

Adriana L. Schuler, Ph.D.
Department of Special Education
1600 Holloway Avenue
San Francisco State University
San Francisco, California 94132

George H. S. Singer, Ph.D.
Oregon Research Institute
1899 Willamette Avenue
Eugene, Oregon 97401-4015

Michael W. Smull, B.A.
Applied Research and Evaluation Unit
School of Medicine
630 West Fayette Street
University of Maryland
Baltimore, Maryland 21201-1585

Dick Sobsey, Ed.D.
6-102 Education North
University of Alberta
Edmonton, Alberta T6G 2G5
CANADA

Phillip S. Strain, Ph.D.
Department of Psychiatry
3600 Forbes Avenue, Suite 508
University of Pittsburgh
Pittsburgh, Pennsylvania 15213

Jeffrey L. Strully, Ed.D.
ARC/Colorado
4155 East Jewell Avenue, Suite 916
Denver, Colorado 80222

Steven J. Taylor, Ph.D.
Center on Human Policy
200 Huntington Hall
Syracuse University
Syracuse, New York 13244

Barbara Thompson, Ph.D.
Department of Special Education
University of Kansas
Lawrence, Kansas 66045

Ann P. Turnbull, Ed.D.
Beach Center on Families and Disability
Bureau of Child Research
University of Kansas
Lawrence, Kansas 66045

H. Rutherford Turnbull, III, LL.B., LL.M.
School of Law
Department of Special Education
Beach Center on Families and Disability
University of Kansas
Lawrence, Kansas 66045

Alice Udvari-Solner, M.S.
Department of Special Education and
    Rehabilitation Psychology
432 North Murray Street, Room 302
University of Wisconsin–Madison
Madison, Wisconsin 53706

Mary Ulrich, B.S.
9155 Sunderland Way
West Chester, Ohio 45069

Patricia Van Deventer, M.S.
545 West Dayton Street
Madison Metropolitan School District
Madison, Wisconsin 53703

Carol R. Westlake, M.Ed.
Department of Special Education
Peabody College of Vanderbilt University
Nashville, Tennessee 37203

Colleen Wieck, Ph.D.
Governor's Planning Council on Developmental
   Disabilities
300 Centennial Office Building
658 Cedar Street
St. Paul, Minnesota 55155

Robert R. Williams
Governmental Activities Office
United Cerebral Palsy Associations
1522 K Street, N.W.
Suite 1112
Washington, D.C. 20005

Editorial Advisory Board

Foreword

SAD VOICES FROM THE TWENTIETH CENTURY

Resolutions are statements of beliefs. They can be used to motivate program development or improvement, political action, and social change. This book is about The Association for Persons with Severe Handicaps (TASH), a young organization of people banded together to influence the prevailing practices of society toward their citizens with severe disabilities. TASH has been writing and using resolutions to guide policy and practices for about a decade.

People with severe disabilities are probably the most vulnerable people of all. Throughout time they have had to wait until we understood them and saw their talents and their untapped potentials. It is 1990, the last decade before the twenty-first century, and people with severe disabilities are still waiting.

Listen to the following voices:

One woman at church to another: "What a tragedy, the baby had some awful brain problem. Not enough oxygen at birth, I think. So it [*sic*] ended up with cerebral palsy and will never be normal. They couldn't keep it at home."

The assistant librarian to a library user: "Well, she brings him in the library and he just drools and makes noises that don't mean anything. He doesn't belong here, but she brings him anyway. I don't know how she has so much patience."

Pool staff to a man waiting in line: "Oh! You are here on the wrong night. The special swim is on Thursday nights. Tonight is the family swim. Come back on Thursday at 7:00."

The special education director to the parent of a student with disabilities whose family is moving: "Being a TMR here, she will probably go to their new center program in Standardsville. It's a good program. Brand new building; I saw it last year, it's beautiful: accessible with ramps, special toilets, wheelchair buses, and all those things. She's lucky, the center program will take her till she's 21."

From the Homeward Bound, Inc., et al., v. Hissom Memorial Center, et al. *(No. 85-C-437-E) (N.D. Oklahoma 1987) Findings of Fact and Conclusions of Law (pp. 4–5):* Michael who is 18 and "lives in building no. 12 . . . has little residual hearing and can see only peripherally."

"Michael has developed severe behavior problems at Hissom. These include fits of screaming, fighting and insomnia. There has been no programming provided to correct these behavior problems."

"Michael has suffered abuse and injury. These include bruises, bites on his arms, hands and back. He has been put under restraints on several occasions, without his parents' knowledge, causing bruises on his arms."

"Most of his time is spent in idleness. He had substantial sign language skills before being admitted to Hissom, but these skills have now been lost. He is receiving no real active treatment."

One professional to another: "But it's only a little shock: 80 volts for 80/1000s of a second to be exact. Not anything like the cattle prods. It's more humane than letting them bang their heads for years and years. It's based on research. See, the [Human Technologies] brochure says: 'The SIBIS STIMULUS unit delivers an electrical stimulation that has been engineered to be safe, humane and effective, it is the result of over four years of research and can be more accurately described as a hard pinch rather than a shock' (undated, p. 3).

"I think it would be ideal for kids like Belinda."

School superintendent overheard at a PTA meeting: "Those kids will never hold a job or pay taxes, so I say we don't bother sinking money into their programs."

Two college sophomores joking with each other over a roommate's mistake: "What an absolute idiot!" "No question, she really is brain dead!"

A paragraph from the Brief of the Rochester School District submitted to the U.S. Court of Appeals for the First Circuit (Appeal No. 88-1847), in the case Timothy W. v. Rochester, NH, School District (1989): "Despite all this, finding that Tim does not qualify under the special education laws is still emotionally difficult, because it implies that all humans are not equal, and that some may always function at an infantile, animal, or vegetative level" (p. 50).

"The court emphasized that Tim's case is 'rare.' Dr. Andrews testified that, out of approximately 15,000 handicapped children in New Hampshire, only 15 function at the brain stem level, and that some of these have more brain tissue than Tim. The court emphasized the need for 'extensive' evaluations before initially determining that a child cannot benefit" (p. 49).

THE PREVAILING PRACTICE OF SEPARATION

We have one decade left in the twentieth century. Why do we still hear so many derogatory comments made about people with disabilities? Why do so many people still question the human rights and the basic capabilities of people with severe disabilities? The fact is that most adolescents and adults today have never had an opportunity to come to know a person with disabilities. Most people do not recognize people with disabilities as people first, who are more like them than different. While many adults may voice their beliefs that "people with disabilities have rights too" and "should not be made fun of," or "stared at," and surely "must have a hard life," these people without disabilities base their comments more on beliefs about what they *should say* rather than what they have learned from firsthand experience. But when these same nondisabled persons come face to face with a person having severe disabilities, they rarely feel comfortable and are likely to look for a way out of the situation.

The prevailing practices of segregating people with disabilities in every phase of their lives has created the fears, the insensitivity, and even the repulsion and estrangement that many nondisabled persons express toward other humans who happen to be born with or acquire serious disabilities in life. Lack of familiarity in turn breeds prejudice and the development of different rules and standards for people with disabilities. This promotes a vicious cycle that is not easily stopped and can affect almost every aspect of a person's life and death.

DUAL FOUNDATION OF VALUES AND RESEARCH

TASH aligns itself with the position that "best practices" or "state-of-the-art" procedures should rest solidly on a foundation of research and values. The research findings tell us what happens when the methods of interest are carefully applied to people in certain learning situations. We are able to learn whether the methods work to yield learning, and whether the learning is faster, retained longer, or generalized further than with other methods. The values part of the foundation addresses standards, rules, or principles that are considered important in life. Value statements are often simple and usually more impervious to time and change than are research findings alone.

Value statements can work in synchrony with research. For example, consider Wisconsin TASH's statement: "Every person is capable of growth and development" (G. Jacobs, personal communication, April, 1989). Once such a value is accepted, the task becomes one of discovering some of the facilitating conditions under which this growth toward increased independence best occurs. Time that might be lost to debates over educability is saved and invested instead in demonstrating effective learning conditions and methods.

What follows is a statement of some current research findings on the integration of people with disabilities. By way of contrast, these research statements are followed with an attempt at stating the value support for integration.

Research: Students with severe disabilities have both more positive and more frequent opportunities to interact with nonhandicapped peers when they participate in settings that are integrated. In segregated settings, friendships with nondisabled peers typically cannot be formed by students with severe handicaps nor can meaningful social skills be learned that will generalize into the real world. This is primarily because of the rare and/or unnatural nature of the interactions between persons with disabilities and their nondisabled peers when they are segregated from each other.

Value: Human beings are diverse by nature; thus, understanding and appreciating diversity is dependent upon having positive experiences with many types of people, including people with various disabilities. When integration of people with disabilities into the mainstream is typical and not extraordinary, prejudice and unreasoned opinions in adults can be replaced by reasoned opinions, and young children can learn that the presence or absence of a disability is not predictive of interpersonal compatibility.

Both statements together provide a more accurate rationale for the practice of integration. Next, consider the following summaries of the current research support and values statements about the use of nonaversive approaches for handling problem behaviors in students with severe disabilities.

Research: The use of intrusive, painful, or dehumanizing techniques to eliminate problem behaviors is likely to have undesirable outcomes such as an increase in other problem behaviors, poor maintenance or generalization of effects, little or no improvement in the person's skills, anxiety and physical pain in the person being "treated," and discomfort by family members and by those who apply the "treatment." When programs designed to treat the behavior problems of students address both the skills students are missing and the purpose or purposes that the problem behavior serves for each student, behavior problems are less likely to be maintained by unintentional reinforcement. This approach of teaching meaningful replacement skills is more logical and appears more successful than a behavior reduction approach. Also, this functional analysis approach to treatment is more likely to suggest intervention procedures that are both nonaversive and that assure generalization and maintenance of reductions in serious behavior problems.

Value: The use of intrusive, painful, or dehumanizing techniques to eliminate the problem behaviors of people is judged as being a violation of human rights. Human beings should treat others in compassionate and reasoned ways, and as they would have others treat them. "What is right is what we want for ourselves and for others; we want only that which works; and we do not want that which does not work, particularly if the procedure is deliberately painful and imposed on especially vulnerable people" (Turnbull & Guess, 1986, p. 202).

CONSISTENCY OF VALUES OVER TIME

Best practices will change over time as old practices are replaced with better practices. For each practice, the value basis will have consistency, while the research basis will change as researchers refine and improve existing methods. It is interesting how the citation of the values is less in vogue among scientists and professionals than it is among "ordinary" people in everyday life. Identification of the values basis for professional actions often is viewed as unnecessary and sometimes as ridiculous. Ironically, it is more acceptable for professionals (and others) to rely on a value base when they deal with both the routine events and the extraordinary issues of their personal lives and the current events of society.

Not *every* combination of research and values will create a defensible foundation for guiding decisions in service provision. A recent case in Virginia, *Cullum v. Faith Mission Home Inc.* (1987) illustrates this point well. This case concerned whether or not spanking and slapping should be used to teach people with mental retardation who lived in a large facility run by a religious group. The religious beliefs of those who administered Faith Mission Home included the value "spare the rod and spoil the child," and the lower court approved this practice for two reasons:

1. Faith Mission Home's basis for using corporal punishment as child discipline was legal under an existing Virginia statute exempting licensing requirements for religious groups operating homes for the treatment of persons "by the practice of the religious tenets of any church . . . by spiritual means without the use of any drug or material remedy" (Code of Virginia § 37.1–88).
2. An expert witness testified that there was at least one published study showing that spanking and slapping were effective in eliminating some problem behaviors of people with mental retardation. The judge ruled that "under very limited situations, physical punishment is an indispensable and effective treatment for behavior management of mentally retarded children and adults" (Cullum, 1989, p. 4).

The staff of the home cited their religious values to support their actions; the lower court conceded that a spiritual basis for their practices meant that they could operate without state license. The *atypical values* of a small religious sect were allowed by the court as the basis for defining acceptable practices for teaching anyone living in that setting. Further, the court used publication in a refereed research journal as a second criterion for best practices. Thus the lower court's decision was also grounded in *research findings,* not professional consensus or research combined with values—a single study was viewed as adequate to tip the scale in favor of spanking as a method that *might* be needed and therefore should *not* be banned. In 1989, the Supreme Court of Virginia upheld the decision (*Cullum v. Faith Mission Home Inc.*, 1989).

BARRIERS

The basic values of normalization, integration, lives that reflect dignity and personal fulfillment, and equality of opportunity are more evident in our society now than in the past. But both inside and outside professional circles there are barriers to the application of these basic values to shape services for persons with needs for lifelong support. Fear, a lack of knowledge or skill, and the absence of heartfelt belief in the value are probably the primary barriers.

In the film, *The Elephant Man*, John Merrick states: "People are afraid of what they do not know" (Lynch, 1980). Merrick, born in England around 1880 and called the "Elephant Man" because of his extensive congenital deformities, understood the greatest barrier to disability: fear of the unknown (Howell & Ford, 1980). His words were a simple statement of truth about human beings. Conversations about people with severe disabilities are not popular among individuals who are not disabled. Severe disabilities are described as "tragic," "deviant," and certainly not normal. In fact, most people know very little about severe disabilities; some have sympathetic reactions, many more do not know how to react to a person who has disabilities or even to the topic of disability. It is commonplace to teach children to respect their elders, to avoid teasing others who are different from them, and to practice simple manners—but the typical theme of most "jokes" is that people with lesser intelligence are laughable.

In the typical, everyday interactions in the grocery store, at work and school, at the library, or with your neighbor, it is rare that the topic of conversation concerns people who have quadriplegic cerebral palsy, who are deaf *and* blind, who cannot talk and have severe mental retardation, who have lived most of their lives in institutional settings, who have very few skills, or who injure themselves repeatedly. People with these more serious disabilities are not usually part of our lives, now or in the past. Thus, these people are often feared, pitied, and pushed away. Isolation of people having severe disabilities has only reinforced these misconceptions.

NEW VOICES

Often a lack of knowledge accompanies fear and serves to fuel the emotion. When accurate information is available, fears may weaken and fade. But probably the best antidote to fear is positive, direct experience, rather than simply gaining facts.

Meaningful integration engenders a "genuine involvement of children in a friendship, caring, and support role with their peers" (Forest & Lusthaus, 1989, p. 46). Listen to the real voices of upper elementary kids talking about May and Richard and other peers who used to be in the Life Skills special class, but who now are part of their classes at St. Francis School in Skitchnerer, Ontario (Waterloo Region Roman Catholic Separate School Board, 1988). These are new voices, a sign of the future:

"Last year when May was in our class like for some of the time and then she'd go back to the Life Skills [Class]. Then this year she came [and was part of our class]; she was in here and she changed, really changed. And sometimes for the better and sometimes for the worse! I mean like she had really changed us and she tells you to shut up now and "Get outta town," and all this. She goes "Shhhhh!"

"Well, I figure that they're trying to change her to be good and be nice and act like everyone else. But not everyone else is good and not everyone else is nice. So she has to act like everyone else, so she fools around because she's learning to be normal!"

"Ever since I became friends with Richard, we're always talking and fooling around. So like they're no different than . . . the rest of us; just maybe on the outside."

"May has feelings."

"She's a lot smarter than I thought she was."

"She's a person."

"She can cope with her problems."

"She has feelings like everyone else. . . . If she gets hurt, she'll tell people. She won't just keep it bottled up inside. She'll act like everyone else. And she's a person, not just a thing that you're supposed to be nice to, but an actual person like everyone else."

Martha E. Snell, Ph.D.
Department of Special Education
University of Virginia

REFERENCES

Code of Virginia, Code Ann. §§ 37. 1–188 (1983).

Cullum v. Faith Mission Home Inc., Albemarle Country Circuit Court, Charlottesville, VA, Docket N. 5337–C, Judge Tremblay, February 17, 1987.

Cullum v. Faith Mission Home Inc., 237 Va. 473, 379 S.E. 2d 445 (1989).

Forest, M., & Lusthaus, E. (1989). Promoting educational equality for all students: Circles and maps. In S. Stainback, W. Stainback, & M. Forest (Eds.),

Educating all students in the mainstream of regular education (pp. 43–57). Baltimore: Paul H. Brookes Publishing Co.

Homeward Bound, Inc., et al., vs. Hissom Memorial Center, et al., No. 85-C-437-E (N.D. Okla. 1987).

Howell, M., & Ford, P. (1980). *The true history of the Elephant Man.* London: Allison and Busby.

Human Technologies, Inc. (undated). [Brochure on SIBIS (Self-Injurious Behavior Inhibiting System)]. St. Petersburg, FL: Author.

Lynch, D. (Director). (1980). *The elephant man* [Film].

Timothy W. v. Rochester, NH, School District, Brief of the Rochester School District, Appeal No. 88-1847 (1989).

Turnbull, H.R., & Guess, D. (1987). A model for analyzing the moral aspects of special education and behavioral interventions. In P.R. Dokecki & R.M. Zaner (Eds.), *Ethics of dealing with persons with severe handicaps: Toward a research agenda* (pp. 167–210). Baltimore: Paul H. Brookes Publishing Co.

Waterloo Region Roman Catholic Separate School Board, the Ontario Association for Community Living, Centre for Integrated Education (Producer), & Forest, M., & de Sousa, V. (Directors). (1988). *With a little help from my friends* [Videotape]. Skitchnerer, Ontario: Video Magic Concepts and Production.

Preface

The publication of this book is officially sponsored by The Association for Persons with Severe Handicaps (TASH), through a process that included review of focus and content by two TASH committees—the Publications and the Federal Research, Model Development, and Training Committees—and approval by the Executive Board. The purpose of this project was to provide an analysis of contemporary values, research, and practice as these affect the lives of people with severe intellectual disabilities.

Each of six major sections of the book begins with a series of value statements—the TASH resolutions that have been passed by the Association on specific critical issues of consequence for people with severe disabilities. In response to those values statements, contributions were invited from more than 70 experts and advocates who were given either one of two challenges. Authors of the empirical review chapters were charged to develop a state-of-the-practice review of the existing data base relevant to specific topics addressed by each of the TASH resolutions. Further, these authors were asked to end their chapters with a set of recommendations regarding future directions for research in the area based upon gaps in the existing knowledge base. Authors of the essay and dialogue chapters were asked to pose further directions for the future. These chapters are intended to be uniquely personal statements by distinguished contributors whose lives and professional careers have touched upon those of persons with severe disabilities. The Introduction and Chapter 1 set the stage for the book, and Chapter 41 provides a summary analysis.

In some ways, this book could be viewed as a history of TASH. Our purpose, however, encompasses a great deal more: It is the history of TASH that can be viewed as merely one facet of a far broader social movement. This social movement is, of course, the empowerment of people with severe disabilities as fully participating members of their communities.

The complete picture of this social reform was not nearly as clear in November, 1974, when TASH began as the American Association for the Education of the Severely/Profoundly Handicapped (AAESPH) with fewer than three dozen members. Nor was it fully developed by the time of the first major TASH conference in 1975 in Kansas City, with over a thousand people in attendance. These earlier days of TASH emphasized educational issues: curriculum development, teacher education, interdisciplinary services in the schools, paraprofessional training, parent involvement, and the dissemination of research results. This "school years" focus shifted fairly rapidly to concerns across the life span and in all environments, and so the organization changed its name to TASH to reflect this expanded purpose in 1979. Throughout its history, however, TASH has continued to be the only organization in existence consisting of a working alliance of advocates, policymakers, consumers, families, and professionals whose activities and accomplishments are exclusively dedicated to meeting the needs of people with severe intellectual disabilities.

Much has been accomplished in the decade and a half since TASH began, but it would be immodest to attribute more than a portion of this success to the organization or even to the thousands of members who now belong to the organization. Indeed, TASH exists because of, and continues to contribute to, a rapidly expanding and perhaps inevitable social reform movement granting long-overdue rights to people with disabilities throughout the world. Thus, TASH has acted in concert with many other disability rights and professional associations, joining together to shape public policies and new legislation that would be truly supportive of these new rights to live, work, go to school, and recreate as part of one's family, neighborhood, and community. In addition, TASH as an organization and its members as individuals have provided direct support to the many people with severe intellectual disabilities and their families as they struggled to achieve the rights and services to which they are entitled. This has never been a guild association, concerned with the needs and status of the membership, but has always kept its attention sharply focused upon those individuals who had not had a voice in the much too recent past. To this end, the TASH Executive Board passed its first two resolutions in 1979, and thus began a process of clarification and communication of the values base for TASH activities and future goals. Since then, the passage of approximately two dozen such resolutions chronicled our growing awareness of the critical issues surrounding the achievement of community lifestyles for people with severe disabilities.

Passage of these resolutions has not been without controversy, but each is intended as a statement of values. Collectively, they point to directions for the future as important first steps to educate ourselves and our society about everyday practices that can either violate or support the principles of liberty and justice for everyone, including those who present significant challenges to the implementation of those ideals. TASH has also been an organization of "doers." Resolutions have helped to clarify our goals, but actions accomplish them. TASH membership has always included advocates and professionals alike who were involved daily in the achievement of those goals in schools, in the workplace, at home, and in the community. Because of these collaborative efforts, no textbook or media report should ever again be able to tell readers and the lay public that people with "severe to profound mental retardation" cannot work, live in real homes, enjoy meaningful personal and family relationships, and be a part of their communities. Those failures were our failures, and we have learned that limitations are imposed by those who control resources, expertise, and opportunities. Again, TASH has been part of an international coalition attempting to ensure that the necessary services and supports are available to provide all people with a chance for a decent life.

Finally, TASH has always been an organization supportive of research and scholarship. Its *Journal of The Association for Persons with Severe Handicaps (JASH)* has evolved as a scholarly, peer-reviewed "data base" of effective strategies to articulate and guide the implementation of values and principles. *JASH* has valued both scientific integrity and ecological validity, and provides a major forum for the development of a science that can translate good ideas into validated practices in support of meaningful outcomes. TASH also publishes a monograph series and a newsletter, and participates actively in the dissemination of information through the media regarding promising practices.

Yet, for many people with severe disabilities, neither resolutions nor science has had an impact upon daily life. Tremendous discrepancies in quality of life are widespread, so that one's birthrights are now compromised more by where one happens to live than by the nature of one's disabilities. The purpose of this book is to gather together, in one source, our goals for the future, some of our best thinking about how we might achieve those goals based upon the knowledge we already have, and promising directions for our future efforts to ensure that our values are translated into a better way of life for real people.

ORGANIZATION OF THE BOOK

Each of the six topical sections begins with a listing of the relevant TASH resolutions addressing components of that topic. In each section, the resolutions are then followed by one or more review chapters providing comprehensive summaries of empirical research and theory regarding strategies to achieve the goals they describe. Authors of these chapters (2–4, 8–11, 15–18, 24–26, 30, and 34–35) were identified based upon their own active professional activities in these areas, and peer reviews by members of an Editorial Advisory Board selected for their expertise in relevant areas were carried out to further enhance their authoritativeness. Each of these chapters concludes with recommendations for future research and policy to fill in existing gaps in our knowledge base and resolve discrepancies in practices that fail to reflect the knowledge base we already have. It was our intention that these chapters provide an up-to-date overview of our state-of-the-practice based upon intervention research with individuals, support networks, and systems, and that, where appropriate, they include a review of ethical, legal, and policy guidelines affecting practices.

The essay and dialogue chapters that follow the reviews in each section are quite different in purpose and format. As we have already indicated, these contributions were not structured. The authors were selected based upon their contributions to the lives of people with severe disabilities as consumer, advocate, professional, and/or parent, and were invited to write what seemed most important to them within the framework of topical areas of research and practice. We believe that these chapters succeed in capturing the richness of the provocative new ideas that have brought us as far as this and promise to take us even further. We hope that the readers enjoy the rather unconventional format of these chapters as well, proving that interesting ideas need not always be written in traditional style for texts of this sort.

INTENDED AUDIENCE

Critical Issues in the Lives of People with Severe Disabilities is directed to a wide readership. The collection is designed to provide, first of all, an authoritative, scholarly, and up-to-date review of current knowledge on issues of critical importance to the field. Thus, it should appeal to all disciplines working in related areas, including psychology, education, sociology, social work, communications sciences, physical and occupational therapy, vocational rehabilitation, administration, law, medicine, public health, and policy or political science. Its authors, in fact, include professionals from the majority of these disciplines. The recommendation sections at the conclusion of each of the review chapters and in Chapter 41 are designed to be of particular interest to policymakers. The essay and dialogue chapters are directed to the various professionals as well as parents, advocates, journalists, and the lay public. It is our hope that this book serve as a major forum for the discussion of issues and provide guidance for future work needed to address those issues in the coming years.

ACKNOWLEDGMENTS

For a project such as this, the list of those to be thanked is lengthy. It goes without saying that members of the TASH Publications Committee, the Federal Research, Model Development, and Training Committee, and the Executive Board deserve grateful thanks for their guidance and input. The members of the Editorial Advisory Board gave most generously of their time, and their reviews of individual chapters and overall feedback have contributed greatly to the quality of the final product. Liz Lindley, the Executive Director of TASH, reliably and conscientiously provided the necessary assistance and information whenever we called upon her, as did Celane McWhorter, the TASH Director of Government Relations in the Washington, D.C. office.

Our own universities and departmental office support staff contributed resources, time, and expertise at all stages of production. This project was not supported by any funds from the TASH organization itself, but by contributions of time and resources from our "home bases." We are grateful for the values of higher education and the service delivery community that continue to support work such as this even without external funding to do so. Similarly, each of the chapter authors has waived any royalty payment and absorbed his or her own production costs so that the royalties from this book can go, in total, to TASH activities on behalf of persons with severe intellectual disabilities. We are grateful to them for their fine contributions that have made this project possible.

Finally, many thanks are due to both Susan Hughes Gray, Copy Editor, and Roslyn Udris, Production Manager, at Paul H. Brookes Publishing Co. They were tolerant of the inevitable complications that could only arise in a project of this magnitude and with more than 70 contributors and 3 editors. Yet, their standards of quality were never compromised, and their efforts have contributed greatly to the clarity of style and format that readers have come to expect from Brookes Publishing Co. And a very special thanks is extended to Melissa Behm and Paul Brookes in particular, not only for being the publisher of this particular TASH book, but for their longstanding support of TASH itself. In a very real sense, TASH as an organization and Brookes Publishing as a company have traveled together for the past decade, and many of the authors in this book have worked with them again and again over those years. It is a tribute to their dedication that this partnership has endured and has been responsible for so many good products.

Who Are They and What Do They Want?

An Essay on TASH

LOU BROWN

University of Wisconsin–Madison, Madison, Wisconsin

Some come—sell their kits—make their money—leave.
Some come—tire—find something less demanding.
Some come—lose interest—try something else.
Some come—never grow—just hang around.
Some come—have no agenda—won't step aside.
Some come—take a break—return to fight again.
Some come—want to stay—but are taken.
Some come—fight—realize they can never leave—keep going.

People often ask why we have TASH. Don't we have enough organizations? Is there really a need for a separate group of people to represent the lowest intellectually functioning 1% of our population? Why are TASH people so ideological and demanding? Don't they realize they are running into windmills? Do they really believe those folks can amount to anything? Aren't they wasting their careers and lives? Why don't we put our resources behind those with more potential? Why don't we just join CEC, ARC, AAMD, QRAB? Why . . .

We have TASH because in the late 1960s and early 1970s it was abundantly clear to a few parents and professionals that no other organization was addressing the ideological, research, financial, and programmatic rights and needs of the lowest intellectually functioning 1% of our population: the most vulnerable, segregated, abused, neglected, and denied people in our society. The people who were quarantined in horrible institution wards that were justified and endorsed by AAMD; who were excluded and rejected from public schools by too many of the continuum tolerators of CEC; who were confined to segregated activity centers and workshops that were owned and operated by ARCs; and who were quarantined in nursing homes and other unnatural living environments that were certified as acceptable by the ruling professionals.

In the early days of TASH we often wondered, if professionals are going to devote their careers to people with severe intellectual disabilities; if mothers, fathers, brothers, and sisters are going to spend enormous energies and resources over long periods of time fighting for basic services; and if legislators are going to be pressured to pass much needed legislation and to secure extremely important tax dollars, what is it that we want? Initially, we wanted a ramp, more speech or physical therapy, someone to clean a catheter, money for research, service delivery model development and personnel preparation, a summer school program, and other isolated components. It soon became obvious that we should want the highest possible quality of integrated life for 24 hours a day, 7 days a week, 365 days a year for as long as possible. We started to dream that our lowest intellectually functioning citizens should have all the resources, longitudinal support, respect, dignity, legal protections, and other phenomena necessary to be the most that they can be, to experience a humane existence, and to make meaningful contributions to their communities in accordance with their abilities.

Specifically, we started to strive for the healthiest possible bodies; opportunities for all children to grow up with nondisabled friends, neighbors, brothers, and sisters; a society in which all people lived in decent, family-style homes; the resources and support necessary to perform real work in the real world; and access to the richness and variety of heterogeneous local communities, including becoming involved in the same recreation/leisure environments and activities utilized by nondisabled others. In short, we wanted integration and the resources necessary to realize and enjoy it.

Conversely, we also realized we did not want aversive conditioning, denial of medical treatment, handicapped-only schools, institutions, organ harvesting, workshops, enclaves, group homes, retarded camps, Special Olympics, and other manifestations of segregation and de facto inferiority.

If that was the dream, what was necessary to approximate realizations? Several factors were considered critical at the time and seem at least as important today. *First*, we needed a penetrating, thought-provoking, constantly evolving cluster of values that would show us where to go and guide our way, get us through the rough spots, keep us focused on our targets, and be totally independent of individuals. Values are too important to be ascribed to Blatt, Gold, Haring, Sontag, Sailor, Guess, Bricker, or Gilhool. Individuals become out of date, have clay feet, have lines they will not cross, can sleep with blatant contradictions, become too sensitive to criticism, engender loyalty to person not mission, and die. Values transcend individuals. They must be abstract, ideal, and pure. They must be scrutinized and evaluated in relation to their real and potential effects on the lives of people with disabilities, not on the people who expound them. Values should be enthusiastically discarded when they are no longer healthy or helpful and we should demand more and better from their replacements.

Second, we realized that the individuals we were attempting to serve were the most difficult to teach, the most challenging to render autonomous, and the ones who needed extraordinary assistance and support to realize reasonable personal fulfillment. The extant intellectual wasteland was unacceptable. Thus, one of the more consuming and enduring activities of TASH was, and still is, to use all the energies and resources necessary to convince talented, productive, effective, committed, and ideologically sound young people to pursue a wide variety of careers serving individuals with severe intellectual disabilities.

TASH never has been, and hopefully never will be, an organization that exists for its members. We are not a trade union. We are not interested in a group life insurance policy, a deferred annuity program, a tax-avoiding getaway vacation attached to the conference, or any other divisive, diluting, or distracting irrelevance. We can get all the above and more elsewhere. TASH exists to help people with severe intellectual disabilities and their families live the best possible lives. All we do should be referenced against that quest and anything that interferes should be resisted and resented.

Third, we knew that if we operationalized the best possible services conceivable in 1970, they would be embarrassingly inadequate. Thus, while we should always revere and respect the past and those who created it, we realized that we had a moral obligation to relentlessly pursue a better future. This commitment to new and better values, concepts, and practices often put professional against professional, put family member against family member, and converted friends and colleagues to enemies. It still does. Some said let them die; we said no. Some said harvest their organs; we said no. Some said lock them up; we said no. Some said shock, beat, squirt, and tie them; we said no. Some said activity; we said work. Some said custody; we said access.

Fourth, and perhaps most important, we knew that we needed to join those few parents who were outraged by professional acts of commission and omission; who truly believed their children deserved more; who had the courage, will, and tenacity to challenge existing authorities; and who had the intelligence and insight to see through the mush and get to the heart of what was good for their children.

Who are Mary Ann and Bob Roncker, Mary and Tom Ulrich, Pat Merchant, and Eva and Matt Reddick of Ohio; Leona and Marion Failkowski and Audrey Coccia of Philadelphia; Vern and Frieda Heinrichs, Rose and Don Galati, Silvana and John Porto, and Linda Dionne of Ontario; Bob and Charlotte Alghren, Marge and John Lee, and Lynda and Bob Atherton of Illinois; Peg and Ward Olsen, Marcy Brost, and Karen Roots of Wisconsin; Mary and Bob Yaris, Sue Warner, and Pat Pionke of St. Louis; Arlene Garrity of New Hampshire; and Connie and Harvey Lapin, Willa Lindsay, Beverly Bertiana, and Joyce and Charlie Schleininger of California? They are only some of the many mothers and fathers who did not plan to have a child with severe disabilities, but did. They were told to send them away, lock them up or accept what was. They did not. They devoted unbelievable amounts of energy, creativity, sweat, money, time, and love to the betterment of their children. In most instances it was not their children who benefited from their efforts, but all those like them who followed. We all owe tremendous debts of gratitude, continuous expressions of appreciation, and unbounded respect to these relentless, fantastically effective and creative mothers and fathers.

Who were Burt Blatt, Bill Bricker, and Marc Gold? They were some of the great early professionals of TASH who made wonderful differences in the lives of people with severe intellectual disabilities. They were people of vision, intensity, intelligence, wit, commitment, and charm. They were some of the rare geniuses who guided us in the early days—who made us believe that all people could learn, that all people had the right to live in decent homes, that no one should be abused, and that inclusion is better than exclusion. We cannot call them anymore and we cannot see them at the conference, but their spirits still move us.

Who are Tom Gilhool, Dick Cohen, David Shaw, John MacIntosh, Reed Martin, Frank Laski, Stan Eichner, Bill Dussault, David Baker, Orville Endicott, and Harvey Savage? They are some of the many lawyers who have expended substantial proportions of their professional lives trying to ensure that one third of the government of the United States and a major portion of the government of Canada—the judicial system—work for the most legally denied. They made Pennsylvania stop excluding children from public schools and start closing its institutions. They convinced the courts of the United States and Canada that all means all and that a person with disabilities is not one half, three fifths, or seven eighths of a citizen. It is hard to imagine where we would be without these tough, brilliant, and remarkably effective legal Don Quixotes.

Who are Judge Ellerson of Oklahoma, Judge Broderick and Judge Becker of Philadelphia, Judge Mehredge of Virginia, and Judge Vance of Alabama? They are some of the critically important federal jurists with wisdom, compassion, insight, and sensitivity. We call them spiritual members of TASH. They affirmed that citizens, including those with intellectual disabilities, should live in integrated communities, not in horrible, rotten, degrading, and immoral institution wards; should go to schools with their brothers, sisters, friends, and neighbors and not to segregated playpens that prepare them for nothing but other segregated environments; and have the inherent rights to be free from harm, to be respected and treated with dignity, and to have reasonable access to all public environments.

Consider the power, excitement, inspiration, and spirit in the room when great parents, brilliant and tenacious lawyers, committed and forward-thinking professionals, and a judge who understands the ideals of our society act on behalf of one child who is severely intellectually disabled.

Finally, if we have learned anything at all over the past 20 years, it is that there are some aspects of a person's life that we have no right to compromise. We cannot negotiate the size of an institution; *no one* should live in one. We cannot function on a committee to determine who does and who does not get medical treatment; *everyone* does. We cannot debate who should get an integrated education; *all* must. Just because we are overwhelmed, frustrated, and at a loss for something to do, we cannot tolerate shocks, slaps, pinches, or any other obnoxious violation of dignity. Let the moderates, compromisers, and data worshippers go elsewhere. Let the people of TASH be value based, unbending, tough, aggressive, assertive, graceful, compassionate, and effective.

Have no doubt that the people, allies, values, and experiences of TASH have accomplished much over the past 20 years. Have no doubt that much more must and will be done. Twenty years from now cars will be safer, cancer and AIDS will be cured, racism and sexism will be in our past, acid rain will be conquered, and, if we do our jobs, people with severe intellectual disabilities will live productive, safe, healthy, happy, and integrated lives.

Critical Issues in the Lives of People with Severe Disabilities

Linking Values and Science in Social Policy Decisions Affecting Citizens with Severe Disabilities

CHARLES A. PECK
*Washington State University–Vancouver,
Vancouver, Washington*

I'll believe that integration is a good thing when I see the data, and not before.

— a special education director in
Washington state.

The fate of an epoch which has eaten of the tree of knowledge is that it must know that we cannot learn the *meaning* of the world from the results of its analysis. . . .

—Max Weber (1949, p. 57)

One of the most important and unique developments over the past several years among advocates for people with severe disabilities has been the emergence of a strong and clearly articulated set of values that have guided decisions about policy and practice (Taylor, 1987; Wolfensberger, 1972). This development has been important, both in directing attention to critical policy issues (e.g., social exclusion via segregation, use of aversive intervention, withholding of medical treatment) and also in broadening the sources of knowledge upon which such policy issues are debated. The explicit consideration of values in decisions about policy and practice contrasts sharply with traditional sources of formal knowledge in human services fields, which have reflected an uncritical reliance on social science as a "model of knowing." Moreover, the movement of values onto center stage in policy development by many advocates for individuals with severe disabilities, most notably The Associa-

tion for Persons with Severe Handicaps (TASH), has been a point of acrimonious debate among professionals and researchers. Perhaps most important, policy decisions at the local level that powerfully affect the lives of children and adults with severe disabilities continue to be made on the basis of limited understanding about what guidance science can and cannot offer for social policy development. Too often, we are told that we must wait until research data have been collected and analyzed before we can know what policies to support and what practices to implement. The most important point of the present chapter is that such a view seriously underrepresents the sources of knowledge that are relevant to decisions about policy and practice, and particularly the role that human values play in shaping both research and social policy.

The broad purpose of the chapter is to explore the relationships between values and science as these affect social policy decisions. While acknowledging the critical role data can and should play in social policy development, it is clear that the fields of special education and developmental disabilities have been dominated by a narrowly technical and empirical view of what constitutes "valid" knowledge (Guess & Siegel-Causey, 1985; Skrtic, 1987). Because of this history, emphasis in the present chapter is devoted to explicating the limitations of a purely scientific view in addressing questions of social policy. A brief review is offered of some of the philosophical ar-

Appreciation is expressed to Doug Guess, Rob Horner, and Dick Hansis for their critical comments on an earlier draft of this chapter.

guments that suggest that values are inextricable from both social policy decisions and the research process itself. This is followed by a review of some values implicit in current debates on critical policy issues, and a conceptual framework that considers the general relationships between values, science, and social policy development. Finally, a program of values-relevant research is proposed, with specific reference to the critical issue of enhancing opportunities for people with severe disabilities to participate fully in the mainstream of community life.

PHILOSOPHICAL ISSUES

Before proceeding toward a more focused discussion of the relationship between values, science, and social policy, it is useful to identify several basic assumptions that underlie the positions to be taken. Primary among these is a utilitarian view of science as a *means* of contributing to a rich and multidimensional human knowledge base. This view may be contrasted with a view of science as a higher order source of knowledge or truth itself. Thus, it is expected that knowledge gained through scientific research should affect and be affected by knowledge from other sources, including personal and cultural values. As with any other act of "meaning making," this view of science is informed by intentions for its use. That is, what science is considered to *be* is affected by what one wishes to *do* with it. The functional context of the present view is that of commitment to concrete action toward improving the conditions of life experienced by people with severe disabilities, and by necessary extension all disenfranchised members of the society. This suggests a critical posture toward models of science that claim to proceed independently of human values or feelings, or in a manner that is unaccountable to pressing human needs. This position implies a number of additional assertions about the nature of science and its relation to advocacy and action. Specifically, science may be seen to be essentially value laden, political, and conservative. These characteristics must be acknowledged and clearly understood if science is to play its proper role in policy decisions.

Science is Value Laden

The enormous strength of a scientific approach to human inquiry is that extraordinary efforts are made to define explicitly the conditions under which research questions are asked and answered. This, however, does *not* imply that cultural and personal values are not reflected in the research process. Several points make this clear.

First, it is obvious that all scientific activity is embedded in cultural and historical context. A broad conceptualization of the nature of this context has been advanced by Karl Popper (1979), who notes that all human inquiry takes place in the midst of a cumulative body of human knowledge, including scientific, artistic, philosophical, and technical domains, which is codified in records of human intellectual achievement and synthesized in extant theoretical systems and worldviews. Eccles (1979) has observed that this world of objective knowledge that we have inherited constitutes a source of values and beliefs about the world that permeates all human activity. Our scientific endeavors, no less than any other human activity, reflect our values and beliefs about who we are and what is important for us to do.

Second, it is clear that acts of research have a profoundly *creative* dimension. That is, the selection of a program of research does not simply emerge reactively from analysis of the existing scientific evidence, but reflects a powerful act of choosing that affects the features of the world we may observe. Often it has been suggested that the process of scientific observation is best viewed as a "lens" through which we observe the world, with accompanying restrictions of view due to our choices about subject, filter, focus, and framing. Such choices are made on the basis of one's values and beliefs about what is important, useful, and necessary for human inquiry and action.

Importantly, choices about what shall be researched create direction for scientific activity and social policy not only for the present, but also for the future. No clearer or more compelling example of the creative effects of scientific decisions can be offered than the choice of possible futures entailed in the decision to undertake research on the development of the atomic bomb.

Jungk's (1956) account of the social-political history of the development of the bomb is remarkable in its description of the intertwinement of values and science involved in this momentous scientific and social policy choice.

Although the cultural and historical contexts in which scientific activity are embedded represent the deepest level at which values affect scientific choices, additional value-laden choices are involved throughout the research process. These include choices about measurement, experimental design, data analysis, and interpretation. The basic dilemma is that one cannot measure all phenomena, manipulate all possible experimental variables, or utilize all possible analytic models for the data. The choices that are made about these issues reflect implicit theories about the phenomena under study, as well as beliefs about what is important and valuable to focus upon at each stage of the research process (Hesse, 1980). This is not an argument that research is inevitably biased, but that values drive the purpose of the research, which in turn makes some strategies and decisions more sensible than others.

Science is Political

The very possibility of using science to inform social policy identifies its political dimension. While political meanings are inextricably tied to scientific activity, they are seldom acknowledged, and perhaps are often even unrecognized by researchers. The political agendas motivating research can be ideological, personal, or pecuniary. Indeed, Jerome Bruner (1986) has recently commented that many of the ostensibly theoretical conflicts among researchers are better understood as conflicts for resources, power, and prestige than as unresolvable theoretical differences. Ravetz (1971) has described political consequences of the "industrialization" of science through expansion of the scope and costs of most research projects, which increases reliance on public and private research contracts and grants as a source of support. Although his arguments are made in the context of natural science, the same factors may be seen to operate in the human sciences, and particularly in the fields of developmental disabilities and special educa-

tion, where grant resources support a large portion of research activity. These factors can be expected to produce the same impregnation of research programs with political and entrepreneurial interests that has characterized natural science research.

The important point of the foregoing is that, far from being impervious to political influence, the process and products of research should be understood as having political causes and consequences. To deny this is to ignore the political meaning of one's acts, or to hide that meaning. Jungk's (1956) description of the social process related to the development of the bomb at Los Alamos suggests that the full range of these motivations operated there.

Science is Conservative

Kuhn (1970) and other scholars reviewing the history of science have noted that most science is conducted within the framework of existing conventions and practices, and that major shifts in conceptualization and approach to problems are resisted by scientific communities. This conservatism operates not only at the grand scale, maintaining consistency of thinking within dominant paradigms as Kuhn has argued, but also on the scale of daily practice, favoring incrementalism over radical revision. This is perhaps inevitable in light of the heavy procedural emphasis within traditional scientific method on theory testing, rather than theory generation (Glaser & Strauss, 1967; Kaplan, 1964). However, it seems equally likely that much of this conservative quality stems from the social and political pressures that operate to restrict imaginative work (see Mills, 1959, for a particularly strong indictment of academic social science in this regard). In our field, the ability of science to *generate* innovative social policy is further restricted by the theoretically narrow and procedurally oriented nature of many research training programs (see Chapter 21, this volume).

The conservative and incrementalist character of social science as it has been practiced makes it more useful for the evaluation of social policy than for its invention. It is better suited to tell us what we have achieved, than what we are capable of achieving. Indeed, the ability of science to provide an unblinking reflection of some of the facts of what we have and have not accomplished is a critical contribution to social policy development. However, in addition to being unable to inform us about what is good, the conservative character of science restricts its usefulness in envisioning what is possible. For such ideas, we routinely draw less upon data, and more upon values and philosophy.

This point is illustrated by two particularly noteworthy achievements from our recent history in human services for people with severe disabilities. The first is the tremendous improvement in models for residential services achieved over the past 2 decades (see Chapter 8, this volume, for a review). Although we have a substantial data base comparing and contrasting characteristics of residential arrangements, including institutions, intermediate care facilities (ICFs), and group homes, the sources of *innovation* (i.e., the ideas and visions for improvements in practice) have been drawn almost exclusively from the values embodied in the philosophy of normalization (Nirje, 1969; Wolfensberger, 1972, 1983). This is not to argue that research has not been important, particularly in reflecting the limitations of specific variables, such as downsizing or community placement alone, in accomplishing valued outcomes (Landesman-Dwyer, 1981). However, science alone could never have led us to support people with severe multiple disabilities in buying their own condominiums, hiring their own attendants, and creating circles of friendship and support in the community (Chapter 32, this volume; Snow & Forest, 1987).

A second achievement is equally important, and surprisingly, no less an example of the use of a values base as a source of direction for our work. I refer to the application of the principles of systematic behavioral psychology toward demonstrating the learning potential of people with severe intellectual disabilities. One can hardly identify a more values-inspired position than that articulated by Lindsley (1964) in asserting that retarded behavior is due not to inherent limitations in people, but to inadequacies in the environments we have created. Indeed, the behaviorists' unflinching placement of responsibility for learning outcomes for individuals with disabilities on the shoulders of the teacher rather than of the student must be one of the strongest

statements of egalitarian values in all of social science. These values, rather than any empirical imperative, inspired the vigorous program of research, undertaken initially through the experimental analysis of behavior and later through applied behavior analysis, toward identifying environmental variables controlling "retarded" behavior.

VALUES AND RESEARCH RELATED TO THE LIVES OF PEOPLE WITH SEVERE DISABILITIES

The relationships of values, science, and social policy may be explicated in another fashion by reviewing some of the values reflected in research and debate on several current policy issues. As just argued, the choice of research questions reflects a values-based set of priorities about which issues merit investment of time and resources for research. In our own field, investment of resources in research clearly reflects commitment to a set of values regarding the importance of the lives of individuals with severe disabilities. This commitment has relatively clear meaning at the interpersonal level, but it also reflects values about the desired form and functions of social institutions, and about the desired characteristics of our society. Because these meanings are often unrecognized, and perhaps even accepted uncritically by researchers, practitioners, and parents caught up in the "dailiness" of service and advocacy, it is worthwhile to reflect on some examples of the connections between values and specific policy issues that underlie several areas of research related to the lives of people with severe disabilities.

Social Integration

Much research on social integration, mainstreaming, and related issues has been based on a relatively narrow conceptualization of the meaning of this policy. For example, in the literature related to school policy, most studies that have been carried out reflect the assumption that school integration should be judged on the basis of differences in social or academic outcomes for students in segregated versus integrated settings (see Semmel, Lieber, & Peck, 1986, for an extended review and discussion). In the residential literature, this perspective has been reflected in voluminous research on changes in adaptive behavior accompanying movement into community settings. Developmental outcomes and adaptive behavior changes are undeniably important, but they do not represent the fullest expression of values related to social integration.

The deeper values underlying the integration movement are based in the egalitarian social philosophy expressed in the modern history of Western civilization, particularly since the Magna Carta, and further articulated in the Constitution of the United States, the Fourteenth Amendment, the *Brown v. Board of Education* decision, and the Civil Rights Act of 1964. The normalization principle and related legal enactments such as PL 94-142 and Section 504 of the Vocational Rehabilitation Act of 1973 are extensions of this social philosophy to policy issues affecting people who have been particularly devalued and disenfranchised within our society. At the core of such policy issues is the notion that the *inclusion and participation* of all people in the social and political life of the community is at once a fundamental value of democratic societies, and the principal means by which such societies are sustained. The values underlying the integration movement thus include, but go substantially beyond, maximizing developmental or behavioral outcomes for individuals with disabilities. In the context of school policies, these values suggest the importance of transforming not only instructional practices and placements, but also the general characteristics of schools as social institutions in a fashion that more clearly reflects priorities for expanding inclusion and participation of all children. Even more basically, these values indicate the importance of acting to change cultural myths, attitudes, and fears about the nature of human differences associated with severe disability. Importantly, clarifying the values underlying the integration movement identifies its crucial meaning for *all* citizens as a test of society's willingness and ability to ensure the rights of its members to full inclusion and participation in community life.

Educability

The issue of educability serves as an important example of the confusion of values and science in social policy debates. Indeed, the question "Are all children educable?" (Kauffman, 1981)

has been commonly interpreted as if it were synonymous with the question "Should we attempt to educate all students?" Responses to the former can be evidenced with scientific data, with the crucial caveat that a negative answer must be fallacious on purely logical grounds. That is, simply because we have not yet demonstrated compelling evidence of developmental gains for some students as a result of our interventions, it does not follow that we will not achieve these outcomes in the future (unless, of course we cease the attempt).

"*Should* we attempt to educate all students?" is not a scientific question, but a question of values. At issue here is the meaning and value we attach to providing social support to all people, regardless of what we may expect to gain in return. Education is certainly a most fundamental form of such support, not only because of its central place in any notion of the achievement of human potential, but also because of its symbolic and political meaning as a means of participation in one's community.

Alternative views certainly exist, and are often presented in language reflecting the values of capital investment. The suggestion is that we will get a better "return" on our educational dollars if we invest them in the "best and the brightest." The meaning of such a set of values is manifested not only in policies for exclusion of children with severe disabilities from schooling, but through exclusion of the majority of children from college-preparation "tracks" in high schools (Oakes, 1985), through the exclusion of most children from the advantages and opportunities commonly associated with classrooms for "the gifted and talented [*sic*]," and through the de facto exclusion of minority and other disenfranchised groups from access to higher education through reduction in student assistance programs.

Supported Work

A particularly strong policy initiative at the federal and state levels over the past several years has involved development of support systems for people with severe disabilities in integrated employment settings (see Chapter 9, this volume). The values base underlying this initiative contrasts sharply with the capital-investment values reflected in traditional vocational rehabilitation policy. Specifically, the traditional values orientation has emphasized the potential "employability" of the individual as a criterion for service, with job placement services judged on how quickly people could be placed and services withdrawn.

The values base underlying the supported work movement is broader, emphasizing the social importance of work and work settings in our culture as a means of establishing one's self as an adult and as a means of building social networks with other community members. This is viewed as particularly important for individuals who have routinely been restricted to marginal and child-like roles in our culture. Thus, accepting traditional policies and values functions as an indirect way of excluding people with disabilities from access to adult life. This is equivalent to judging the merit of an individual for participation in the human community on the basis of productivity. Consistent with the values articulated by Lindsley (1964), the phenomenon of low wages often earned by workers with severe disabilities is viewed by supported work professionals as an indication that the quality of work opportunities must be improved, not as an indication of any inherent limitations in the productivity of individuals (Gold, 1973).

Summary

To summarize arguments to this point, the notion that science can or should be conducted outside a values base is both naive and dangerous. Such a position is naive in ignoring the historical and political context in which science is conducted. It is dangerous in ignoring the impact of scientific choices on possible futures we may enjoy. Values must be recognized to pervade scientific activity at all levels, and thus constitute critical foci for explicit discussion and criticism. This position does not deny the importance and usefulness of science to social policy development, but emphasizes the need for careful reflection about its proper role in this process.

INTEGRATING SCIENCE AND VALUES: A CONCEPTUAL FRAMEWORK

Recognizing the basic role values play in shaping scientific decisions, what should be the role

of science in decisions about social policy? How can these two sources of knowledge be linked? An analysis of these issues is represented schematically in Figure 1.1. Several assumptions are implicit in this conceptualization. The first is that the basis on which we take actions that affect people's lives must reflect an integrative use of the full range of available knowledge bases relevant to that action. That is, whatever the merit or feasibility of conducting human inquiry on a purely scientific or purely ideological basis, the limits manifest (and, I believe, inherent) in either of these sources of knowledge at present demand an integrative view. The specific form of this integration, and the roles and valences assigned to science and values may of course vary. The following framework assumes that the relative power of values and science for explicating questions of social policy depends on the type and level of the question under consideration. Specifically, the present analysis follows Weber's (1949) assertion:

> The more "general" the problem involved, i.e., in this case, the broader its cultural *significance,* the less subject it is to a single unambiguous answer on the basis of the data of empirical science and the greater the role played by value-ideas and the ultimate and highest personal axioms of belief. (p. 56)

A second assumption in the present framework for considering the relationship between values and science is that each of these sources of knowledge has changed, and will continue to change over time. That science has evolved over the past centuries (and, indeed, the past decade) is easily appreciated. Less evident, perhaps, is the evolutionary quality of our cultural values. Eccles (1979) has argued that values may be viewed as cultural achievement. Certainly the values implicit in our increased commitment to support and enhancement of the lives of people who have been the most profoundly disenfranchised individuals within our society represent a major achievement. The important point is that these changes in social values and related policies have important historical roots, and should be expected to continue to evolve in the future (Scheerenberger, 1983; Taylor, 1987).

A third assumption for the framework depicted in Figure 1.1 is that the process of developing, implementing, and evaluating social

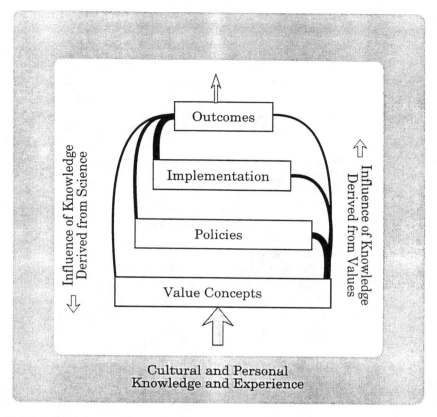

Figure 1.1. Relationships between values and science as sources of knowledge informing policy development.

policy is inescapably reductionist. That is, the conceptual and communicative processes involved in moving from abstract reflection on values and principles toward specific actions involve underrepresenting many issues that are important at each level of the analysis. For example, the process of articulating values underrepresents the background of cultural and personal knowledge and experience that contribute to those values. At a more concrete level, the measurement of outcomes always underrepresents what actually happened to individuals involved in social policy implementation. The importance of this point is that it underscores the indeterminancy of the relationships between what is valued, what is implemented, and what is measured. This means that while data are useful and relevant, they cannot fully capture the outcomes of social policy or the meaning of social values.

Figure 1.1 is intended to map the relationships between values and science in policy formation. I think it is essential to analyze these relation-

ships in the functional context of their actual *use*, since the nature of their relationship is shaped by exigencies in the world of action. In other words, in a world in which actions must be taken immediately, it is pointless to argue that the role of science or values would be different if we had better science or more ideal values. The contributions of each of these sources of knowledge are considered at several levels of policy analysis below.

Cultural and Personal Knowledge and Experience

Figure 1.1 is intended to suggest that values are not given (or received) a priori, but are informed by a wealth of cultural and personal knowledge and experience. This includes the world of "objective knowledge" preserved in records of human cultural and technical achievement as described by Popper (1979). It also includes the interpreted body of direct experiences one has had that have cognitive and/or affective relevance to the issues under consideration. Science, among many sources, contributes to this cultural and personal knowledge base.

Value Concepts

The values that we articulate through concepts such as "democracy" and "egalitarianism" are drawn most strongly from our base of cultural and personal knowledge. They may also be affected by findings of empirical science, although history suggests the direction of this influence tends almost wholly toward buttressing existing values and worldviews rather than "debunking" them (Gould, 1981). However, one example of such debunking is believed by many contemporary participant-observers to be occurring today in the form of a "paradigm shift" from atomistic and mechanistic worldviews toward more systems-oriented and holistic views (Bateson, 1979; Heshusius, 1982; Polkinghorne, 1988; Poplin, 1988). It is further arguable that a change in values may accompany this shift, characterized by a movement from highly materialistic and individualistic values toward increased appreciation of the facts of interdependence and values of interpersonal and geopolitical cooperation (Schumacher, 1973).

Policies

Major social policy initiatives, such as the least restrictive environment (LRE) mandate, are drawn primarily from values rather than from empirical knowledge (Blatt, 1977; Bricker, 1978). Although these also may be affected by scientific findings, the difficulty of effectively using science to evaluate questions of social policy is well known (Weber, 1949). As the civil rights movement demonstrated, changes in social policy are much more likely to reflect changes in public values and attitudes than any findings of empirical science.

Implementation

Choices about strategies for implementation of social policy are affected by both values and science (as well as other factors, of course). It is at this level that empirical science can most directly and clearly guide action. For example, reviews of research on mainstreaming have shown clearly that implementing the LRE mandate by simply placing children with disabilities in regular classes does not ensure that the valued outcomes of social integration will be achieved (Gaylord-Ross & Peck, 1985; Odom & McEvoy, 1989). Moreover, a number of useful strategies for mediating the integration process have been developed through research (e.g., Haring & Lovinger, 1989; Jenkins, Odom, & Speltz, 1989; Voeltz, 1982). Of course, values must also affect choices about implementation, and the means of policy implementation must be as acceptable to our values as the goals. This notion is explicit in the emphasis on the choice of nonstigmatizing, culturally typical means of implementing social policy embodied in the normalization principle (Wolfensberger, 1972).

Outcomes

Choices of outcome measures should be strongly affected by scientific considerations, including those related to psychometric qualities of instruments (reliability, validity, etc.), theoretical relevance, and others. These choices are also driven strongly, if sometimes uncritically, by prevailing values and assumptions about the importance of particular outcomes for measurement. An important limitation to any empirical approach to policy evaluation is that such an approach tends to reduce what is important to what is measured, or worse, to what is measurable. Thus, values cannot be abandoned or held in abeyance in evaluating implementation outcomes, but must be critically and explicitly incorporated in interpreting the significance of the measures that have been chosen and the data that have been collected.

SOME EXAMPLES AND DIRECTIONS FOR VALUES-BASED RESEARCH

The model just presented, together with the arguments made earlier, clarifies how values and science are deeply intertwined and how they contribute jointly to priorities and decisions in the policy development and evaluation process. This section outlines some implications for research that derive from a more explicit consideration of social values than has been traditional in research in special education and developmental disabilities.

What does it mean to use values more explicitly as a source of direction and evaluation for research? A few ideas for such an approach are presented here in the context of the critical issue of public school integration of students with severe disabilities. These ideas are organized in terms of three nested levels of focus: 1) the interpersonal level, referring to interactions between individuals with severe disabilities and peers, teachers, and others; 2) the institutional level, referring to policies and practices for running the schools; and 3) the cultural level, referring to attitudes, beliefs, and values related to disability, education, and equity issues. Core values at each of these levels center on the importance of ensuring the inclusion and participation of *all* children in school and community life.

Interpersonal Issues

Values at this level emphasize the importance of working to expand opportunities for all children to participate in a full range of rewarding human relationships in the context of their schooling experience. A number of research directions are implied. Without negating the contribution of peer modeling, social skills training, and other strategies for inducting children with disabilities into school and community life, values are presently driving inquiry beyond these issues toward increased attention to building social relationships and enriching social networks in which children with disabilities participate (see Chapter 11, this volume). Considering these values, we need increased research that focuses directly on outcomes that reflect more than frequencies of interaction between children in integrated settings (Strully & Strully, 1985). Promising examples of intervention-oriented work that may have an impact on the quality of children's social relationships are now emerging (e.g., Forest & Lusthaus, 1987; Haring & Lovinger, 1989).

Despite the clear implication that the values we hold for integration apply to all children, research on the effects of integrated programs on nondisabled children has been sparse (Esposito, 1987). Moreover, the conceptual scope of most of this work has been very limited, reflecting the apparent assumption that the research agenda for these children simply involves demonstrating that they are not *harmed* by integrated programs. However, qualitative studies conducted in integrated school settings have suggested that the integration experience may have important meaning to nonhandicapped students (Biklen, Corrigan, & Quick, 1989; Murray-Seegert, 1989). For example, Peck, Donaldson, and Pezzoli (1988) conducted a preliminary investigation of the benefits to themselves nondisabled students attributed to their relationships with peers with severe disabilities, and found that these students consistently described changes in their self-concept, social cognition, and personal principles of moral action, which they associated with this experience. Expanding the focus of research on social integration to appraise more carefully the experiences of *all* of the children involved is highly consistent with the values underlying the integration movement.

A final example of how values may affect research at this level involves research methodology. Specifically, it may be argued that many of the social phenomena that are of central importance to values related to social integration demand a broader and more flexible unit of analysis than what has pervaded the vast majority of research in the field of special education. The focus on operational definition of specific behaviors (or clusters of behavior) that has dominated work in our field has been based on the assumption that feelings, cognitions, and other intrapsychic phenomena are irrelevant to the understanding of human behavior (Skinner, 1953). Importantly, within this framework, understanding is considered to be isomorphic with *control*. Consistent with its own theoretical assumptions, this orientation has denied the importance of phenomenological contexts of behavior, and instead has sought to explain human behavior in terms of directly observable and measurable events.

If research is to play a more meaningful part in attaining the valued interpersonal outcomes of the social integration movement, it is essential that we develop strategies for analyzing behavior that do not strip it of its phenomenological meaning. This position does not deny the usefulness and importance of contributions made by behavioral research, and particularly applied behavior analysis, in developing a technology relevant to control of the "elementary" aspects of behavior (Whaley & Malott, 1971). However, our evolving values are driving research focus away from an analysis of elementary phenomena, and toward issues in which meaning is deeply embedded in human perceptions, cognitions, and interpretations about the world. While the problems of analysis and measurement related to these issues are most substantial, some rich theoretical frameworks exist for addressing them (e.g., Bruner, 1986; Wertsch, 1985), as well as useful methodological strategies from fields such as anthropology, sociolinguistics, and semiotics (Gumperz, 1986). As others have argued (e.g., Blatt, 1977), at the core of these suggestions is the assertion that we must seek methods of research that contribute to achievement of valued outcomes, rather than allow our research methods to constrain our goals and practices.

Institutional Issues

The values of inclusion and participation suggest some research agenda focused on the school as a social institution. For example, attaining the valued outcomes of social integration will necessitate research and development work related to curriculum and instructional strategies for heterogeneous groups of students, and to social/political processes for implementing innovation and change. Some directions for value-based research may be delineated in each of these areas.

Curriculum and Instruction

Although wholesale revision of curriculum and instructional practices is clearly not a necessary precondition for social integration, few would argue with the observation that traditional classroom practices are not well suited for responding to the needs of students with diverse backgrounds. Importantly, this issue is central to several research initiatives in the broader field of education (Au & Mason, 1981; Bredekamp, 1987; Goodman, 1986; Johnson & Johnson, 1975; Palinscar & Brown, 1984). Although representing diverse theoretical orientations, in practice these initiatives have two important characteristics in common with innovative work in our own field. First, each of these programs of research and development has focused on human diversity as a centrally important reality of classroom teaching, and has proposed curriculum and instructional strategies that reflect valuation of human

differences. For example, current work in literacy development (Edelsky, 1986; Goodman, 1986) focuses explicitly on strategies for incorporating differences in student background and knowledge into their educational experience and on facilitating students' communication of ideas and experiences that have personal meaning and importance to them. The language and values base of this approach to literacy is notably congruent with innovative work in analysis of communicative intent of children with autism (Prizant & Duchan, 1981), functional approaches to language intervention (Warren & Rogers-Warren, 1985), and approaches to curriculum that emphasize function over the form of behavior (Brown et al., 1979; Peck et al., 1986; White, 1980).

A second common characteristic of these programs is that each of them abandons the limiting traditional assumption that the teacher is the only important source of instruction, and instead recognizes the child's own problem solving, as well as interactions with other students, to constitute valuable sources of learning. Although the value of peer-mediated instruction has been recognized for some time in our field (Apolloni & Cooke, 1975; Strain, 1981), the research and development programs noted above reflect a broader and more reciprocal conceptualization of the learning process.

We are just beginning to explore the resources that these perspectives open as they pertain to the learning experiences of children with and without disabilities. An important research agenda for our field is to begin to identify the links between values and practice that underlie innovative responses to diverse learning needs within general and special education. Particularly promising would be model demonstration efforts focused on the integration of students with severe disabilities into regular classrooms reflecting the innovative educational practices referenced above.

Implementation of Change

Values are relevant to the process as well as to the content of school innovation and reform. Indeed, the same social values of inclusion and participation are reflected by current policy implementation research in shifts toward increased teacher involvement in school change efforts

(Lieberman & Miller, 1986), as well as broader concepts of change emphasizing teacher empowerment and autonomy (Giroux, 1983). Several research needs are indicated.

First, investigations are needed that clarify factors affecting actual implementation of practices that support social integration. The extant research on social integration, which focuses almost exclusively on pedagogical issues and strategies, exemplifies the naiveté of our research efforts in ignoring the social/political contexts in which we attempt to develop and maintain innovative programs. In an important commentary on current "best practices" in our field, Baer (1986) has noted that many of the issues that consume our attention may matter little to the broader constituencies from which we seek support. Consistent with this concern, one recent study (Peck, Hayden, Wandschneider, Peterson, & Richarz, 1989) has suggested that concerns about maintaining social/political control, rather than objections to mainstreaming per se, are at the base of resistance to integration shown by many parents, teachers, and administrators involved in segregated programs. Research directed to improving our understanding of these and other social/political issues is likely to produce important knowledge that is highly relevant to program development efforts.

A second research need is for intervention-oriented work that yields social/political strategies for developing and maintaining innovative programs. For example, Biklen (1985) and his colleagues have reported the results of two qualitative research projects as they contribute to understanding and action in achieving school integration. The work of my colleagues and myself in this area has been focused on developing strategies for broadening the political base of support for integrated programs in local communities (Peck, Richarz, Peterson, Hayden, Mineur, & Wandschneider, 1989). The term *strategies* rather than the term *procedures* reflects the notion that flexibility and adaptability are important characteristics for approaches to system change in which the contexts of implementation are likely to vary greatly (O'Brien, 1987). Research in this area may draw profitably on extensive work in broader fields concerned with public administration (Levin & Ferman, 1986) and

school improvement (Lieberman, 1986; Weick, 1985). Important values-based themes within this literature emphasize administrative support and teacher participation through collaborative, rather than coercive, approaches in school-change efforts (Jacullo-Noto, 1986), and a focus on creativity, rather than compliance, in developing innovations (Lilly, 1988).

Cultural Issues

A third major area in which we may conduct values-relevant research is through inquiry regarding the sources and effects of cultural attitudes and beliefs about human differences. Although we have a plethora of survey and sociometric studies of attitudes toward individuals with disabilities (Gottlieb, 1978), the predominance of this work has been conceptualized in a fashion that has not addressed the broader relationships between cultural beliefs, institutional practice, and interpersonal interactions. However, the feasibility of investigating these kinds of relationships is demonstrated by related ethnographic work from several fields. For example, Goffman (1961) has described the influence of cultural beliefs and values on organizational practices and interpersonal interactions experienced by people who have been devalued and segregated. MacLaren (1989) has investigated the relationships between cultural values and classroom practices as they teach children about roles they are expected to play in adult life. Erickson and Mohat (1982) and Au and Mason (1981) have used microanalytic methods to identify processes by which cultural differences may interfere with learning, and may lead to conflict between students and adults. Each of these issues is enormously relevant to the problems we face in better understanding the challenges and in achieving the outcomes of the social integration movement.

SUMMARY AND CONCLUSIONS: VALUES, SCIENCE, AND ACTION

Perhaps the most important point of the present discussion, which I hope to have made throughout in several forms, is that issues about the appropriate roles of science and values in social policy development can only be clarified by considering them in the contexts of human action in which they are *necessarily* embedded (Mishler, 1979). I have assumed that a defining characteristic of common interests of parents, professionals, and researchers is that of commitment to social action toward enhancing the lives of people with severe disabilities. Within this context, the manifestly incomplete state of our knowledge of the world, including both definitions of the "good" and how that good may be attained, clarifies the need for *both* values and science in making decisions about policy and practice.

An integrative and historical view of these issues suggests that both values and science may be considered as cultural "tools" that have been (and are still being) developed for addressing the problems and dilemmas inherent in human activity (Vygotsky, 1978). Extending this notion, we may think of the instrumental or tool function of values as somewhat analogous to that of *conscience*. The concept of conscience (from the Latin, *conscire*: *con* = [with; together] + *scire* [to know]) suggests knowledge that stands apart from, but connected to, the formal knowledge of science. Values, then, may be considered as a tool for constructing understanding and making decisions that stands apart and does not emerge directly from formal knowledge.

Science, considered in functional context, may perhaps be thought of as a tool of *metacognition,* in the sense that it is a means for thinking about the quality of our thinking. It provides little direct guidance regarding what it is important to think about, but it allows us to evaluate the consistency of our interpretations of the world with such facts as may be observed. Such a tool is obviously a tremendous cultural achievement

that can be enormously useful in evaluating our policy decisions and actions, and in supporting our progress toward outcomes we value.

Ultimately, the common ground of knowledge from values and science must be defined in the contexts of specific action. This does not by any means suggest that answers will emerge easily or crisply from such an analysis, but rather that neither science nor values have much meaning outside specific contexts of their use in addressing the dilemmas of human action.

The importance of adopting a more integrative view of values, science, and action is underscored by the common assertion of parents and professionals that research is simply irrelevant to their needs. While it is common for university researchers to dismiss such a view as underinformed, a more "sense-making" interpretation might be useful. Specifically, combining the assertion (by parents and professionals) that research has not been useful and the assertion (by researchers) that research has not been used, it is clear that science as we have practiced it has been of less value in the lives of people with disabilities than we would like. Reshaping our science in a fashion that is more responsive to our values, as well as more closely grounded in the problems and dilemmas of social action, is a key challenge that will demand serious collaboration among researchers, practitioners, and advocates. For the fields of special education and developmental disabilities, this will also require a substantial broadening in our methodologies, in our theories about human behavior, and in the domains of human experience into which we inquire.

REFERENCES

Apolloni, T., & Cooke, T.P. (1975). Peer behavior conceptualized as a variable influencing infant and toddler development. *American Journal of Orthopsychiatry, 45,* 4–17.

Au, K.H., & Mason, J. (1981). Social organizational factors in learning to read: The balance of rights hypothesis. *Reading Research Quarterly, 17*(1), 115–152.

Baer, D. (1986). "Exemplary service to what outcome?" [Review of *Education of learners with severe handicaps: Exemplary service strategies*]. *Journal of The Association for Persons with Severe Handicaps, 11,* 145–147.

Bateson, G. (1979). *Mind and nature: A necessary unity.* New York: Bantam Books.

Biklen, D. (1985). *Achieving the complete school: Strategies for effective mainstreaming.* New York: Teachers College Press.

Biklen, D., Corrigan, C., & Quick, D. (1989). Beyond obligation: Students' relations with each other in integrated classes. In D.K. Lipsky & A. Gartner (Eds.), *Beyond separate education: Quality education for all* (pp. 207–221). Baltimore: Paul H. Brookes Publishing Co.

Blatt, B. (1977). Research orientations in special education. In B. Blatt, D. Biklen, & R. Bogdan (Eds.),

An alternative textbook in special education: People, schools, and other institutions (pp. 185–191). Denver: Love Publishing.

Bredekamp, S. (Ed.). (1987). *Developmentally appropriate practice in early childhood programs serving children from birth through age 8.* Washington, DC: National Association for the Education of Young Children.

Bricker, D. (1978). A rationale for the integration of handicapped and nonhandicapped preschool children. In M.J. Guralnick (Ed.), *Early intervention and the integration of handicapped and nonhandicapped children* (pp. 3–26). Baltimore: University Park Press.

Brown, v. Board of Education, 347 U.S. 283, 74 S.Ct. 686, 98 L.Ed. 873 (1954).

Brown, L., Branston-McClean, M.B., Baumgart, D., Vincent, L., Falvey, M., & Schroeder, J. (1979). Using the characteristics of current and subsequent least restrictive environments in the development of curricular content for severely handicapped students. *AAESPH Review, 4,* 407–424.

Bruner, J. (1986). *Actual minds, possible worlds.* Cambridge, MA: Harvard University Press.

Eccles, J.C. (1979). *The human mystery* (Gifford Lecture 9: The quest for values and meaning). New York: Springer-Verlag.

Edelsky, C. (1989). *Writing in a bilingual program: Habla una vez.* Norwood, NJ: Ablex.

Erickson, F., & Mohat, G. (1982). The cultural organization of participation structures in two classrooms of Indian students. In G. Spindler (Ed.), *Doing the ethnography of schooling* (pp. 132–174). New York: Holt, Reinhart & Winston.

Esposito, B.G. (1987). The effects of preschool integration on nonhandicapped children. *Journal of the Division for Early Childhood, 12*(1), 31–46.

Forest, M., & Lusthaus, E. (1987). *The kaleidoscope: Each belongs—quality education for all.* Unpublished manuscript, Frontier College, Centre for Integrated Education, Toronto, Canada.

Gaylord-Ross, R., & Peck, C.A. (1985). A social integration of students with severe mental retardation. In D. Bricker & J. Filler (Eds.), *Serving students with severe retardation: From research to practice* (pp. 185–207). Reston, VA: Council for Exceptional Children.

Giroux, H. (1983). Theories of reproduction and resistance in the new sociology of education. *Harvard Educational Review, 53*(3), 257–293.

Glaser, B.G., & Strauss, A.L. (1967). *The discovery of grounded theory: Strategies for qualitative research.* Chicago: Aldine Press.

Goffman, E. (1961). *Asylums: Essays on the social situation of mental patients and other inmates.* New York: Doubleday.

Gold, M. (1973). Research on the vocational rehabilitation of the retarded: The present, the future. In N. Ellis (Ed.), *International review of research in mental retardation* (Vol. 6, pp. 97–147). New York: Academic Press.

Goodman, K. (1986). *What's whole in whole language.* Portsmouth, NH: Heineman.

Gottlieb, J. (1978). Public, peer & professional attitudes toward mentally retarded persons. In M. Begab & S. Richardson (Eds.), *The mentally retarded and society: A social science perspective* (pp. 99–125). Baltimore: University Park Press.

Gould, S.J. (1981). *The mismeasure of man.* New York: Norton.

Guess, D., & Siegel-Causey, E. (1985). Behavioral control and education of severely handicapped students: Who's doing what to whom? and why? In D. Bricker & J. Filler (Eds.), *Serving students with severe mental retardation: From research to practice* (pp. 230–244). Reston, VA: Council for Exceptional Children.

Gumperz, J.J. (1986). Interactional sociolinguistics in the study of schooling. In J. Cook-Gumperz (Eds.), *The social construction of literacy* (pp. 45–68). London: Cambridge University Press.

Haring, T.G., & Lovinger, L. (1989). Promoting social interaction through teaching generalized play initiation responses to preschool children with autism. *Journal of The Association for Persons with Severe Handicaps, 14,* 580–587.

Heshusius, L. (1982). At the heart of the advocacy dilemma: A mechanistic world view. *Exceptional Children, 49*(1), 6–11.

Hesse, M. (1980). *Revolutions and reconstructions in the philosophy of science.* Bloomington: Indiana University Press.

Jacullo-Noto, J. (1986). Interactive research and development—partners in craft. In A. Lieberman (Ed.), *Rethinking school improvement: Research, craft, and concept* (pp. 176–190). New York: Teachers College Press.

Jenkins, J.R., Odom, S.L., & Speltz, M.L. (1989). Effects of social integration on preschool children with handicaps. *Exceptional Children, 55,* 420–428.

Johnson, D., & Johnson, R. (1975). *Learning together and alone: Cooperation, competition, and individualization.* Englewood Cliffs, NJ: Prentice-Hall.

Jungk, R. (1956). *Brighter than a thousand suns: A personal history of the atomic scientists.* New York: Harcourt Brace Jovanovich.

Kaplan, A. (1964). *The conduct of inquiry: Methodology for behavioral science.* Scranton, PA: Chandler.

Kauffman, J.M. (Ed.). (1981). Are all children educable? [Special issue]. *Analysis and Intervention in Developmental Disabilities, 1.*

Kuhn, T.S. (1970). *The structure of scientific revolutions.* Chicago: University of Chicago Press.

Landesman-Dwyer, S. (1981). Living in the community. *American Journal of Mental Deficiency, 86,* 223–224.

Levin, M.A., & Ferman, B. (1986). The political hand: Conditions for effective implementation. In S.S. Nagel (Ed.), *Research in public policy anal-*

ysis and management (pp. 141–169). Greenwich, CT: JAI Press.

Lieberman, A. (Ed.). (1986). *Rethinking school improvement: Research, craft, and concept.* New York: Teachers College Press.

Lieberman, A., & Miller, L. (1986). School improvement: Themes and variations. In A. Lieberman (Ed.), *Rethinking school improvement: Research, craft and concept* (pp. 96–114). New York: Teachers College Press.

Lilly, M.S. (1988). The regular education initiative: A force for change in general and special education. *Education and Training in Mental Retardation, 23,* 253–260.

Lindsley, O.R. (1964). Direct measurement and prosthesis of retarded behavior. *Journal of Education, 147,* 62–81.

MacLaren, P. (1989). *Life in schools: An introduction to critical pedagogy in the foundations of education.* New York: Longman.

Mills, C.W. (1959). *The sociological imagination.* London: Oxford University Press.

Mishler, E. (1979). Meaning in context: Is there any other kind? *Harvard Educational Review, 49,* 1–19.

Murray-Seegert, C. (1989). *Nasty girls, thugs, and humans like us: Social relations between severely disabled and nondisabled students in high school.* Baltimore: Paul H. Brookes Publishing Co.

Nirje, B. (1969). The normalization principle and its human management implications. In R. Kugel & W. Wolfensberger (Eds.), *Changing patterns in residential services for the mentally retarded* (pp. 179–195). Washington, DC: President's Committee on Mental Retardation.

Oakes, J. (1985). *Keeping track: How schools structure inequality.* New Haven, CT: Yale University Press.

O'Brien, J. (1987). Embracing ignorance, error, and fallibility: Competencies for leadership of effective services. In S.J. Taylor, D. Biklen, & J. Knoll (Eds.), *Community integration for people with severe disabilities* (pp. 85–108). New York: Teachers College Press.

Odom, S.L., & McEvoy, M.A. (1989). Integration of young children with handicaps and normally developing children. In S.L. Odom & M.B. Karnes (Eds.), *Early intervention for infants and children with handicaps: An empirical base* (pp. 241–267). Baltimore: Paul H. Brookes Publishing Co.

Palincsar, A.S., & Brown, A.L. (1984). Reciprocal teaching of comprehension-fostering and monitoring activities. *Cognition and Instruction, 1,* 117–175.

Peck, C.A., Donaldson, J., & Pezzoli, M. (1988). *Social contact with students who have severe handicaps: Self-benefits identified by nonhandicapped adolescents.* Paper presented at the annual meeting of The Association for Persons with Severe Handicaps, Washington, DC.

Peck, C.A., Hayden, L., Wandschneider, M., Peterson, K., & Richarz, S.A. (1989). Development of

integrated preschools: A qualitative inquiry into sources of resistance among parents, administrators, and teachers. *Journal of Early Intervention, 13,* 353–364.

Peck, C.A., Richarz, S.A., Peterson, K., Hayden, L., Mineur, L., & Wandschneider, M. (1989). An ecological process model for implementing the least restrictive environment mandate in early childhood programs. In R. Gaylord-Ross (Ed.), *Integration strategies for persons with handicaps* (pp. 281–298). Baltimore: Paul H. Brookes Publishing Co.

Peck, C.A. Schuler, A.L., Haring, T.G., Willard, C., Theimer, R.K., & Semmel, M.I. (1986). Teaching social/communicative skills to children with autism and severe handicaps: Issues in assessment and curriculum selection. *Child Study Journal, 16,* 297–313.

Polkinghorne, D.E. (1988). *Narrative knowing and the human sciences.* Albany: State University of New York Press.

Poplin, M.S. (1988). Holistic/constructivist principles of the teaching/learning process: Implications for the field of learning disabilities. *Journal of Learning Disabilities, 21,* 401–416.

Popper, K.R. (1979). *Objective knowledge.* London: Oxford University Press.

Prizant, B., & Duchan, J. (1981). The functions of immediate echolalia in autistic children. *Journal of Speech and Hearing Disorders, 46,* 24–249.

Ravetz, J.R. (1971). *Scientific knowledge & its social problems.* London: Clarendon Press.

Scheerenberger, R.C. (1983). *A history of mental retardation.* Baltimore: Paul H. Brookes Publishing Co.

Schumacher, E.F. (1973). *Small is beautiful.* New York: Harper & Row.

Semmel, M.I., Lieber, J., & Peck, C.A. (1986). Effects of special education environments: Beyond mainstreaming. In C.J. Meisels (Ed.)., *Mainstreaming handicapped children* (pp. 165–192). Hillsdale, NJ: Lawrence Erlbaum Associates.

Skinner, B.F. (1953). *Science and human behavior.* New York: Free Press.

Skrtic, T.M. (1987). An organizational analysis of special education reform. *Counterpoint, 8*(2), 15–19.

Snow, J., & Forest, M. (1987). *Support circles: Building a vision.* Unpublished manuscript, Frontier College, Centre for Integrated Education, Toronto, Canada.

Strain, P.S. (Ed.). (1981). *The utilization of classroom peers as behavior change agents.* New York: Plenum.

Strully, J., & Strully, C. (1985). Friendships and our children. *Journal of The Association for Persons with Severe Handicaps, 10*(4), 224–227.

Taylor, S.J. (1987). Continuum traps. In S.J. Taylor, D. Biklen, & J. Knoll (Eds.), *Community integration for people with severe disabilities* (pp. 25–35). New York: Teachers College Press.

Voeltz, L. (1982). Effects of structured interactions with severely handicapped peers on children's attitudes. *American Journal of Mental Deficiency, 86,* 380–390.

Vygotsky, L.S. (1978). *Mind in society: The development of higher psychological processes.* Cambridge, MA: Harvard University Press.

Warren, S.F., & Rogers-Warren, A.K. (Eds.). (1985). *Teaching functional language.* Baltimore: University Park Press.

Weber, M. (1949). *The methodology of the social sciences* [E. Shils & H. Finch, Eds. and Trans.]. New York: Free Press of Glencoe.

Weick, K.E. (1985). Sources of order in underorganized systems: Themes in recent organizational theory. In Y.S. Lincoln (Ed.), *Organizational theory and inquiry: The paradigm revolution* (pp. 106–136). Beverly Hills: Sage Publications.

Wertsch, J.V. (1985). *Vygotsky and the social forma-tion of mind.* Cambridge, MA: Harvard University Press.

Whaley, D.L., & Malott, R.W. (1971). *Elementary principles of behavior.* Englewood Cliffs, NJ: Prentice-Hall.

White, O. (1980). Adaptive performance objectives: Form versus function. In W. Sailor, B. Wilcox, & L. Brown (Eds.), *Methods of instruction for severely handicapped students* (pp. 47–69). Baltimore: Paul H. Brookes Publishing Co.

Wolfensberger, W. (1972). *The principle of normalization in human services.* Toronto, Canada: National Institute on Mental Retardation.

Wolfensberger, W. (1983). Social role valorization: A proposed new term for the principle of normalization. *Mental Retardation, 21,* 234–239.

DEFINITIONS AND DIAGNOSES

If you had a severe disability, the very first thing that others would most likely be told about you would be a summary of your "deficits." Chances are, wherever you were, there would be a file containing a lengthy description of your intellectual shortcomings, your physical impairments, and your behavior problems. Even the most rudimentary personal information included on a driver's license—your eye color, hair color, height, and weight—might remain a mystery throughout hundreds of pages of written records. Nowhere would someone learn that you had a lovely smile, a strong sense of identity, and a family that cared about you. Instead, we might read about your "inappropriate affect," your "non-compliance," and the "overprotectiveness" of your "difficult" parents. And although you might like to think of yourself as an active teenager interested in the "top 40" hits and the latest fashion in dress, hairstyle, and make-up, you may find yourself listening to nursery rhymes, dressed in a shapeless sweatsuit, your hair cropped short and straight, and with no access to even acne medication much less make-up. Why? Because an assumption has been made that your *disability* tells all there is to know about you, and from the moment you were diagnosed (or even *dually* diagnosed), you ceased being regarded as a person and became a "subject," a "client," or—worse yet—a "case." Your personality, your identity, and your lifestyle have become minor and even hidden details in a clinical history that tells the world about your weaknesses, faults, and deficits.

Even today, introductory textbooks in required liberal arts courses continue to tell virtually all of today's undergraduate university students that people with severe disabilities have "mental ages" that prevent them from living and working in their communities or even being part of a network of family and friends. And indeed, people with severe disabilities are still denied such opportunities in most parts of the world. Instead, they may be given IQ tests (or judged "untestable") that lead to spending the rest of their lives segregated from others—expected to participate in the kinds of activities most people would find boring, useless, and demeaning. Yet, in other areas, as the material throughout this book makes clear, people with severe disabilities *are* living and working in their communities and *are* valued as friends and family members.

The process of making decisions about the kinds of opportunities that will be made available to individual people with severe disabilities begins with that very first contact with professionals, agencies, and services. From the moment that a person is identified with labels such as autistic, severely retarded, multiply handicapped, or dually sensory impaired, prescriptions for the future are made based upon both professional knowledge and personal beliefs about the capabilities of that individual. Should professional practices continue to emphasize clinical diagnoses and normative assessments that contrast likely accomplishments with those of a typical life history? Or can these practices be altered in significant ways that will lead to the identification of the supports needed by each individual to participate in a meaningful lifestyle?

TASH has often been called upon to define the population we mean by the rather broad phrase "severe disabilities." Traditional definitions of severely handicapping conditions are a chronicle of negative characteristics and the many labels that might be applied to various configurations of those characteristics. In contrast, the TASH definition (see Document I.1, this volume) refers to the level of support needed for full participation in community life as the critical feature. Similarly, each of the other resolutions introduced in this section emphasizes strategies to identify individual needs without sacrificing that person's individual rights to being part of the community. The chapters that follow provide comprehensive reviews of various aspects of the assessment process and illustrate how these dimensions have affected the lives of people with severe disabilities. In addition, alternative diagnosis and assessment practices are explored that might better identify needed services and supports without the use of labels, stereotypes, and activities that devalue, depersonalize, and isolate persons with severe disabilities from their family, friends, and communities.

DOCUMENT I.1

Definition of the
People TASH Serves

The Association for Persons with Severe Handicaps addresses the interests of persons with severe handicaps who have traditionally been labelled as severely intellectually disabled. These people include individuals of all ages who require extensive ongoing support in more than one major life activity in order to participate in integrated community settings and to enjoy a quality of life that is available to citizens with fewer or no disabilities. Support may be required for life activities such as mobility, communication, self-care, and learning as necessary for independent living, employment, and self-sufficiency.

ORIGINAL BEH DEFINITION—APRIL 1985
REVISED AND ADOPTED BY TASH—DECEMBER 1985
REVISED NOVEMBER 1986

*　*　*　*　*

Resolution on People with Mental Retardation Who Are Also Diagnosed as Mentally Ill

TASH recognizes that psychiatric disorders may co-occur with other disabling conditions, including severe disabilities. Mental illness should not be confused with other types of disabilities where an individual's response to other diagnoses, environmental circumstances, or past history may resemble behavior typically associated with mental illness.

TASH is concerned about the growing use of the concept "dual diagnosis," the potential overuse of this new category, and the possible misapplications of the term including:

- The stigma of another label;
- Improper institutionalization of people who are "dually diagnosed";
- Creation of new in-patient units based upon presumed mental illness;
- Use of aversive procedures, punishments, and psychotropic medications as acceptable treatments; and
- The lack of lead responsibility in either the mental health or mental retardation systems which results in some individuals receiving no assistance.

TASH strongly supports the following positions:

- The standard for diagnosis of mental illness for people with mental retardation should be as stringent as for people who are not disabled;
- Programming principles should support individualized, personalized services and non-aversive methods;
- Additional research is necessary to determine the influence of environmental factors affecting the increase in behaviors associated with mental illness;
- TASH publications should not use the term "dual diagnosis," but continue to encourage the use of functional definitions of the behaviors of the individuals, in addition to any medical diagnosis that has been given by a qualified psychiatrist;
- Continued prohibition of aversive procedures regardless of any label; and
- Support and assistance should be based on need rather than labels.

ORIGINALLY ADOPTED MARCH 1988

* * * * *

DOCUMENT I.3

Cultural Sensitivity Resolution

WHEREAS, Individuals with severe handicaps who are also culturally and linguistically diverse may be disadvantaged in educational assessment, placement, and instructional processes because of the potentially discriminatory effects of language and culturally biased testing procedures and instruments.

WHEREAS, The unique linguistic and cultural backgrounds of individuals with severe handicaps and their families are not well recognized and utilized in education and habilitation programs designed to serve individuals with severe handicaps.

WHEREAS, The recognition of unique linguistic and cultural characteristics is fundamental to good school/home cooperation and to the design of programs that promote the maximum individual development and learning.

THEREFORE BE IT RESOLVED, THAT The Association for Persons with Severe Handicaps encourages all service providers to implement culturally and linguistically nondiscriminatory procedures in their work with individuals who have severe handicaps. Because of the central role familial/cultural factors play in development, planning for individual programs must take into account familial preferences and linguistic origins of the individual with severe handicaps.

ORIGINALLY ADOPTED MARCH 1988

* * * * *

DOCUMENT I.4

Resolution Urging Repudiation of States on Friend of the Court Brief in *Romeo vs. Youngberg*

WHEREAS, A brief has been submitted to the Supreme Court of the United States in re: *Youngberg vs. Romeo* listing as friends of the court of the states of Connecticut, Alabama, Arkansas, Florida, Indiana, Kansas, Louisiana, Maine, Michigan, Nebraska, New Hampshire, New Jersey, North Dakota, Ohio, Oregon, Rhode Island, South Carolina, Virginia, Washington, and West Virginia by their respective Attorneys General; and

WHEREAS, This brief submits to the Supreme Court references to recent professional literature in support of the contention that earlier findings that all persons experiencing retardation can respond to education are erroneous; and

WHEREAS, This brief submits to the Supreme Court that the district courts' findings that "all of the residents of the state facility had a constitutional right to treatment in the least restrictive setting" was erroneous; and

WHEREAS, This brief submits references to literature to show that there exists "tremendous controversy and conflict within the profession concerning the suitability of community living arrangements for many of the residents of state facilities, especially those profoundly and severely retarded, residents who are aggressive/assaultive, self-abusive, non-ambulatory, moderately handicapped—multiply handicapped, medically fragile or aged and resistant to leaving"; and

WHEREAS, These contentions by the Attorneys General of the 21 above named states are clearly contradicted by experience gained in numerous state supported programs as well as by an increasing body of professional literature and administrative reports; and

WHEREAS, The position taken by the Attorneys General is in direct contradiction to the TASH stated objective to work toward the "rapid termination of living environments and educational/ vocational/recreational services that segregate, regiment and isolate persons from the individualized attention and sustained normalized community interactions necessary for maximal growth, development and the enjoyment of life"; and

WHEREAS, TASH has previously submitted to the Supreme Court an amicus brief stating clearly its position;

NOW THEREFORE BE IT RESOLVED, THAT TASH call on its members in the above named states:

1. To make known to professionals, parents, legislators, and public officials the position taken by the Attorneys General;
2. To work toward a repudiation of the Attorneys General position in each of the 21 states by appointed or elected officials, by professional organizations, and by parents and other advocacy groups.

ORIGINALLY ADOPTED NOVEMBER 1981

* * * * *

Immigration Resolution

BE IT RESOLVED, THAT The Association for Persons with Severe Handicaps finds unacceptable the manner in which representatives of the United States Immigration and Naturalization Service sometimes conduct inspectional interrogation of persons who are suspected to have a developmental handicap and who seek entry into the United States;

AND BE IT FURTHER RESOLVED, THAT this Association lodge a complaint with the Immigration and Naturalization Service in relation to an incident which took place on October 6, 1987, in which Patrick Worth of Toronto, the President of People First in Ontario, was detained and questioned by U.S. Immigration officials at the Toronto airport in a manner which was unnecessarily lengthy and demeaning because Mr. Worth was perceived as a person who had a developmental handicap and would therefore be excludable;

AND BE IT FURTHER RESOLVED, THAT even though this Association is aware that immigration inspectors must implement the exclusion provision of the Immigration and Nationality Act, this Association urges the Immigration and Naturalization Service to examine its policies with regard to the treatment of individuals who present themselves for admission to the United States, whether as visitors or as persons seeking immigrant status, to insure that inspections of persons who may have developmental disabilities are conducted in a humane and respectful manner;

AND BE IT FURTHER RESOLVED, THAT the Association, being aware that exclusion of persons who have developmental disabilities was put into the Immigration Law at a time when the national awareness of the appropriate manner of responding to persons with developmental disabilities would now be called very backward and uninformed, urge that Immigration inspectors be appropriately trained so that they do not perform their inspectional services in a backward and uninformed manner, and that Immigration policy thus reflect the understanding of developmental disabilities as contained in other federal legislation;

AND BE IT FURTHER RESOLVED, THAT the Association urge Congress to repeal laws which permit exclusion of persons seeking non-immigrant or immigrant status in the United States on the sole basis of having a developmental handicap.

ORIGINALLY ADOPTED OCTOBER 1987

*   *   *   *   *

CHAPTER 2

Testing and Diagnosis
A Review and Evaluation

IAN M. EVANS
*State University of New York at Binghamton,
Binghamton, New York*

When evaluating the literature on definition and classification, one cannot help but be struck by the many incongruities that must be tolerated. For example, a major value that would be expressed by members of an advocacy organization such as TASH is the philosophical opposition to any classification and labeling of people with disabilities. Lapel buttons worn by TASH conventioneers read "Severely Normal"; posters encourage us to "Label jars, not people." And yet if some individuals were not at some point in time identified as needing special requirements because of severe handicaps, there could be no justification for having an organization, a journal, or a book such as this one. Similarly, a behavioral perspective is antithetical to assigning people an IQ score. And yet, if a behavioral rehabilitation program for people with disabilities resulted in all of the clients holding jobs, we would be singularly less impressed if told that the range of IQ scores for the group was 83 to 116. Rightly or wrongly, there is information conveyed by an IQ score that influences our expectations. As a final instance, many question the utility of formal diagnostic criteria for severe handicaps, yet when TASH's president described to the executive board a number of hypothetical individuals, there was less than 50% agreement as to whether they should be considered members of the population served by TASH. In this chapter, empirical findings are presented that might help to resolve some of these ambiguities.

Approximately 2% of the school-age population is identified as severely handicapped for purposes of educational programming. The original federal definition utilized in the language of PL 94-142 identified "severe language and/or perceptual cognitive deprivations" as the critical attribute. Certain excess or abnormal behaviors were identified as being characteristic: 1) failure to respond to pronounced social stimuli, 2) self-mutilation, 3) self-stimulation, 4) manifestations of intense and prolonged temper tantrums, and 5) absence of rudimentary forms of verbal control. Children evidencing such characteristics include those with profound and severe mental retardation, those with two or more serious handicapping conditions (e.g., a student with mental retardation who is also blind, a deaf child with cerebral palsy), and those seriously emotionally disturbed children diagnosed as autistic or schizophrenic.

Clearly this categorization is broad and inclusive, in that it identifies those students whose educational needs most challenge the traditional pedagogical structure and who have been most often excluded from the academic mainstream. The TASH definition is somewhat narrower, since the focus is on severe intellectual disability, and by that standard might be thought to exclude those with severe emotional disorders who are not intellectually disabled. However, by emphasizing the supports that might be needed in more than one life activity, no individual would be excluded from the goal, which is quality of life in the natural community. Thus, a person disabled as a result of a major head injury, as a result of a psychiatric disorder interfering with independent functioning, or as a result of neurological deterioration (e.g., dementia) would clearly be represented by TASH's goals as an organization. But as the focus has traditionally

This chapter was prepared while I was Visiting Fellow in the Department of Psychology at the University of Otago, Dunedin, New Zealand, and I would like to acknowledge with thanks the support and facilities provided.

been on *developmental* disabilities, the special needs of people in the above categories have been attended to less than the general principles of normalization and equity and acceptance. This point is important since any form of identification would then contradict TASH's objectives unless it were to specify clearly the special supports required by the identification of an area of disability. The principles would also apply equally to someone who is very physically disabled but who has no intellectual disability. But again, the general assumption of TASH is that it is intellectual disabilities that interfere with functioning and that require external advocacy. Thus, this chapter begins by considering the relationship between the construct of mental retardation and the measurement of intellectual capabilities.

MENTAL RETARDATION AND PSYCHOLOGICAL TESTING

Mental retardation and IQ testing have long shared social histories, both symbiotic and deeply conflicting. Although "mental tests" (Cattell, 1890) arose from experimental psychology's interest in the wide individual differences that are apparent in basic psychological processes such as sensation, attention, and memory, the first practical "IQ" test developed by Binet and Simon (1905) was, as everyone knows, specifically designed as a selection instrument in an attempt to rationalize admission criteria to special education in Paris. Today, more than 80 years later, the legal, medical, and educational criteria for designating an individual as mentally retarded are almost exclusively contained in obtaining a score more than two standard deviations below the mean on an individual test of "general intelligence" (American Psychiatric Association [APA], 1987; Grossman, 1977).

In response to repeated criticism of the IQ criterion, the American Association on Mental Deficiency (AAMD) did add to its definition of mental retardation a concomitant deficit in adaptive functioning (Heber, 1961). Determination of adaptive behavior, however, was left to clinical judgment. Further, as Baumeister and Muma (1975) noted, since it is a deficit in adaptive behavior that brings most children to clinical atten-

tion in the first place, it is the IQ score that effectively provides the official designation of mental retardation. Thus, intelligence and adaptive functioning were conceptualized as independent constructs, with IQ score clearly dominant as the measure of interest.

It is, then, small wonder that Adams (1973) found psychologists relied almost totally on IQ scores when diagnosing mental retardation, as did physicians—whenever a psychological report was available. As instruments for making clinical and educational decisions, individually administered IQ tests have little function except for assessing persons with suspected handicaps. So it is particularly ironic that they are developed and normed on children considered nonhandicapped, with the resultant data forming the basis for most theories of intelligence. From their first introduction, however, IQ tests and their diagnostic use have been extensively criticized and hotly debated (Block & Dworkin, 1976). As Scarr (1981) commented, IQ tests have been represented either as one of psychology's greatest achievements (e.g., Herrnstein, 1973) or as one of its most shameful (e.g., Kamin, 1974). Some of the most misguided policies of this century for the treatment of those with intellectual handicaps have been justified by social Darwinian philosophies that have also permeated the metatheory of the psychological testing movement (see Gould, 1981).

The purpose of this chapter is not to reiterate the case against tests and their misuse, but to examine the unique problems that pertain when testing and classifying persons with the most severe disabilities. There are three major reasons why this group might represent a special issue when considering the problems of assessment, diagnosis, and judging intellectual potential. First, it is clear that IQ tests, despite their supposedly measuring fundamental cognitive abilities, actually necessitate (and thus gauge) the sorts of academic knowledge and skills traditionally taught in school and fostered in the home environments of the dominant culture (cf. Jencks, 1972). It is this prerequisite repertoire of formal academic knowledge of words, numbers, abstract pictorial symbols, and verbally encoded constructs that children with very severe intellectual handicaps are least likely to have acquired at the time of testing. Second, accepting for the moment the conventional categories of mental retardation, those designated as severely or profoundly mentally handicapped are most likely to have concurrent, sometimes multiple, central neural, sensory, or physical impediments that interfere directly with test performance.

A third reason for severe disabilities representing a special complication in the IQ testing debate is more controversial. It refers to the possibility that IQ tests per se may have had different consequences for persons with severe handicaps than they have had for those labeled as mildly mentally retarded. Individuals in the latter category (which represents about 75%–90% of the total population of people designated as mentally retarded) will typically be diagnosed solely on the basis of their score on an IQ test. Such children generally have no clinically detected pathology, come from socially and economically disadvantaged homes, are not diagnosed until they first enter school, and may not be viewed as mentally handicapped outside the school setting. Certainly one of the great travesties of testing has been the well-documented instances of children being labeled as mentally retarded because of linguistic and cultural factors (Mercer, 1973), but the point being made here goes beyond such instances. Even if the IQ score is perfectly "accurate" and reflects the individual's academic "potential," it is still a totally arbitrary decision that having an IQ score more than two standard deviations below the mean indicates that one should be labeled, educated, and treated differently. This can be seen most clearly in the period when the AAMD cutoff for mental retardation was changed to an IQ score of 85 (Heber, 1961), increasing the number of people in the United States labeled as mentally retarded from about 6 million to 32 million! But when normative comparisons indicate an individual's development is more than *four* standard deviations below the mean (about 5% of all those labeled as mentally retarded fit this criterion), his or her special needs are much more obvious. Some confirmation of this difference in capriciousness can be seen in incidence figures showing that cross-nationally the prevalence of mild mental retardation varies greatly, whereas the prevalence of severe and profound mental retardation is generally consistent (Abramowicz & Richardson, 1975).

Making this distinction in terms of de facto versus inferred disabilities does not necessarily constitute agreement with the view (Zigler, Balla, & Hodapp, 1984) that there are two different distributions, with mild mental retardation representing the lower end of the normal distribution of intelligence and severe to profound mental retardation reflecting organic pathology. In fact, the importance of emphasizing commonalities rather than differences is discussed later in this chapter. But the circumstances of having severe intellectual handicaps does seem to challenge the strictly relativistic interpretation of mental retardation. Conceptions of intelligence are certainly culturally determined (Lutz & Levine, 1983). However, it does not follow, as some would have it (e.g., Turnbull & Wheat, 1983), that all mental retardation is created through the process of classification. While society decides what to do with its least capable members and—far less consciously—on what dimensions competence will be decreed, one of the characteristics of severe mental retardation may be that the same individuals would be judged severely handicapped regardless of the domains on which the judgment is made.

DEFINITION AND CLASSIFICATION

It has already been pointed out how the distinction between mental retardation and non–mental retardation has been based on arbitrary (though not necessarily capricious) criteria. A similar observation can be made regarding the categories or "levels of severity" within the designation of mental retardation. Just because a category is socially determined does not mean that it is without usefulness. Classification within fields such as psychiatry and education is usually justified on the grounds that classification in the *natural* sciences is one of the precursors to understanding. This argument is specious since in the natural sciences there is much greater consensus on the nosological principles. An alternative justification for classification within the applied social services realm is the belief that it helps plan for appropriate services, and, if treatments are differentially effective within a class, then diagnosis (assigning an individual to class membership) is an important aid to treatment (Filler et al., 1975). These views have been hotly debated within the behavioral sciences. Behavior therapy in particular has been consistently opposed to the labeling of individuals on the basis of commonalities in the content of behavior without consideration of function. In considering the categories developed within the overall designation of mental retardation, therefore, we need to question whether they serve any of these purposes.

AAMD Classification

In the United States, the prominence and prestige of the American Association on Mental Retardation (formerly AAMD) has meant that the manual of terminology and classification (Grossman, 1977) has set the standard on which other systems are based. The categories of *mild*, *moderate*, *severe*, and *profound* actually reflect extensive clinical experience, with implicit criteria being such "marker" characteristics as ambulatory/nonambulatory, having expressive and receptive verbal language skills, or having concomitant disabilities such as sensory loss, all of which tend to have notable effects on adaptive functioning. So although adaptive behavior was specified as a parallel criterion to IQ score and was a positive move for reducing the more blatant errors of relying on IQ score alone, the emphasis on adaptive functioning has tended to define the categories in terms of what individuals are not able to do. Thus, in the 1963 AAMD classification (Heber, 1961) when adaptive behavior was introduced as a criterion, the result was such statements as "cannot profit from training in self-help" (when describing a school-age child at the profound level) or, when describing preschool-age children at the severely handicapped level, "little or no communicative skills." Thus began a tradition of attempting to describe the various levels in terms of what people could not do or in what setting they should receive services (e.g., in an institution). This represents a very serious error in logic because if you define a category in terms of what will happen to members of that category, you are creating the conditions most supportive of self-fulfilling prophecies—not designing treatment or

planning social and educational services to meet a need. Seltzer (1983) has pointed out that the 1987 revision of the Developmental Disabilities Act (PL 95-602) provided a functionally oriented definition whereby persons living on their own and not needing services would no longer be classified as developmentally disabled, even though they might once have been labeled as mentally retarded. (The *Diagnostic and Statistical Manual of Mental Disorders-III-Revised [DSM III-R]* [APA, 1987] specifically allows for the removal of the mental retardation diagnosis under similar circumstances.)

In the AAMD system, severe mental retardation is defined as having an IQ score between 26 and 40 (for adults, a mental age [MA] of approximately 3–5 years), and profound mental retardation as having an IQ score of 25 and below (an MA of below 3 years for an adult, regardless of chronological age). Adaptive behavior is not, of course, operationally defined. Not surprisingly, in a survey of state definitions of mental retardation, Frankenberger and Harper (1988) found that 73% of the states provided criteria for IQ and its measurement, but only 12% specified criteria for adaptive behavior. (It is interesting that five states did not include measured IQ score in their definition.) Another review of state departments of mental retardation/developmental disabilities (Lowitzer, Utley, & Baumeister, 1987) found that only 22 states were using the AAMD classification system exclusively. Various authors (e.g., Cleland, 1979; Smith & Polloway, 1979) have pointed out that researchers often fail to use accurate AAMD terminology and criteria—for instance, in a review of almost 600 articles, Taylor (1980) found that 20% included subjects who had been incorrectly classified based on the IQ scores obtained, and only 28% of the research articles actually used the AAMD classification system.

APA Classification

It would seem obvious that inconsistency in the use of labels within a classification system further reduces the communication the system is supposed to facilitate. This becomes especially noticeable in the different usages that have evolved in different disciplines. The manual of the American Psychiatric Association, *DSM-*

III-R (APA, 1987), follows the AAMD system very closely, classifying severe mental retardation as having an IQ score between 20 to 25 and 35 to 40, and profound mental retardation as having an IQ score below 20–25, with commensurate impairments in adaptive functioning. (The five–IQ-point flexibility in cut-offs is based on the assumption that "an IQ score is generally thought to involve an error of measurement of approximately five points" [APA, 1987, p. 28], which is an unusual way of dealing with measurement error and the confidence intervals associated with a given score.) *DSM-III-R* has some benefits over previous versions. First, the terminology and implicit assumptions are much more in line with current advances in policy; for example, the phrase "people with mental retardation" is used throughout. Second, mental retardation as a diagnosis should be identified on Axis II (developmental disorders) rather than Axis I (clinical psychiatric syndromes), although this can create a new labeling phenomenon, the "dually diagnosed" client that is critiqued later in this chapter. Third, the descriptive material is freer of biased assumptions than in the past. For example, clients with severe mental retardation are described as follows: "most adapt well to life in the community in group homes or with their families" (APA, 1987, p. 33). Another good example of expressing needs in a positive direction is that for those with profound mental retardation: "Motor development and self-care and communication skills may improve if appropriate training is provided" (APA, 1987, p. 33).

Educational Classifications

Educational classifications have not always been preferable to the psychiatric nosology. Educators are equally likely to express the traditional groupings in terms of what children with severe handicaps will not be able to do (e.g., Sinclair & Forness, 1983). The earlier educational categories of "educable" (IQ scores of 50–75) and "trainable" (IQ scores of 30–50) were particularly regrettable in implying that some children are neither (whatever the differential terminology itself might mean). As Zigler et al. (1984) put it, "how much any individual can learn is an empirical matter and not an assumptive or defi-

nitional one" (p. 222). It was this particularly narrow concept of what was involved in education that was the conceptual parallel of excluding children with severe disabilities from the educational system entirely. As state education systems in more recent years have tried to eliminate these terms and promote less categorical designations, new subclassifications have emerged. In California, for instance, the 1974 state master plan recognized four categories for "data collection and reporting purposes" only: one of these four, "severely handicapped," included all "trainable" mentally retarded children, those with multiple handicaps, and autism. Thus, it is not uncommon in educational settings to consider all those students with measured IQ scores of 50 or below as "severely handicapped."

Validity of Classification Systems

It is interesting that in this quite extensive literature on what is essentially the internal reliability of classification within the construct of mental retardation, there is virtually no consideration given to the validity of the proposed categories. What meaningful differences either in needs or treatments are actually conveyed by the classification of someone as severely mentally retarded? In an interesting study, Bjaanes, Butler, and Kelly (1981) demonstrated that in various residential settings, the more severely handicapped the clients were designated, the fewer habilitation services they actually received. Predictive validity appears to be equally lacking. For a 6-year period, Schalock and Harper (1981) reported a steady decrease in mean IQ scores of clients newly placed in independent living arrangements, indicating that less restrictive placement decisions are a function of changing social policy (and possibly the technical capabilities of the community facilities) rather than of the value of "level of mental retardation" for decision making.

Conclusions

In conclusion, it can be seen that even within the formal classification systems there is some disagreement regarding criteria and definition. Also, there is rather good evidence that within both the official service delivery systems and within the corpus of published research on mental retardation, there is considerable inconsistency in the use of the terminology and criteria of any particular classification system. What does seem extremely clear is that it can be repeatedly discerned that IQ scores provide the critical criteria on which classification is based. Smith and Polloway (1979) found that fewer than 10% of the research publications on mental retardation provided any description of the participants' adaptive behavior. The parallel criterion for mental retardation of deficits in adaptive behavior is ambiguous, mostly because of the limitations of formal measures of adaptive behavior or agreement as to what that construct means. However, there is some evidence that in practice, when an individual is assigned a classificatory level of mental retardation different than would be indicated by IQ score alone, the tendency is for the level to be set *higher* than the IQ score indicated (Roszkowski & Spreat, 1981). Presumably, adaptive behavior estimates can have constructive effects, given that the validity of the classification system is unknown and services are provided on the basis of prior expectancies that rarely have the opportunity to be contradicted (Seltzer & Seltzer, 1983).

Even if there was a formal, widely accepted measure of adaptive functioning—as many psychologists apparently wish to see (Coulter, 1980)—the AAMD definition is problematic since certain "scores" in both IQ and adaptive behavior measures need to be obtained. If some ideal adaptive behavior measure was developed and it correlated fairly highly with IQ scores (for reasons other than the two instruments contain the same item content; Meyers, Nihira, & Zetlin, 1979), then the concepts would prove to be redundant and both scores would not be needed. If the correlation were low, however, indicating that they are tapping orthogonal constructs, then the numbers of individuals actually obtaining low scores on both measures would be much smaller than is currently the case. While this might be desirable, it clearly shows that in order to further understand the problems in the use of IQ score and the development of alternatives, we need to consider the nature of IQ tests and the constructs of intelligence and adaptive behavior. These three topics are discussed next.

SPECIFIC PROBLEMS OF IQ TESTS FOR PEOPLE WITH SEVERE DISABILITIES

Rather than attempting the daunting task of critiquing standardized testing in general, a brief commentary is offered on certain psychometric problems that surround test administration to individuals with severe disabilities, starting with reliability. When children with mental retardation are tested on different occasions not too distant in time, there tends to be adequate (.8–.9) correlation between two administrations of exactly the same IQ test (Sattler, 1988). However, while overall correlations may be significant, disagreements on individual cases may be considerable (Silverstein, 1982). Tests are revised and appear in new editions. For subjects with mental retardation the correlation between old and new versions is acceptable for some tests (e.g., the Stanford-Binet; Lukens, 1988) and not for others. For instance, Goldman (1987) reported that the lower individuals with mental retardation had scored on the Wechsler Adult Intelligence Scale (WAIS; Wechsler, 1955) the relatively higher they scored on the Wechsler Adult Intelligence Scale–Revised (WAIS-R; Wechsler, 1981), with 64% of subjects originally classified as moderately mentally retarded needing to be reclassified as mildly mentally retarded on the basis of WAIS-R IQ scores. Flynn (1985) points out that in general both the Wechsler Intelligence Scale for Children–Revised (WISC-R; Wechsler, 1974) and the WAIS-R produce considerably lower scores than their predecessors, so that the original versions' cut-off score of 70 for mental retardation was far too lenient: "Because of obsolescence and sampling problems, there is at present no coherent criterion of mental retardation" (p. 243).

When considering the intratest reliability of the Wechsler series, people with mental retardation characteristically show considerable scatter in subtest scale scores (Coolidge, Rakoff, Schwellenbach, Bracken, & Walker, 1986), which casts doubt on any neuropsychological inferences about profiles. Intertest variability also tends to be higher for persons with mental retardation than for the general population (e.g., Bloom, Reese, Altshuler, Meckler, & Raskin,

1983; Covin & Sattler, 1985; Spitz, 1986). This is particularly interesting when the comparison test is based on theoretical assumptions regarding the cognitive processing required for academic tasks, such as the Kaufman Assessment Battery for Children (K-ABC: Kaufman & Kaufman, 1983). Naglieri (1985) reported that the best predictor of academic achievement in elementary-age children with mental retardation was the K-ABC Achievement Scale, not the composite "mental processing" score ($r = .29$) or the WISC-R (Wechsler, 1974) full scale score ($r = .44$).

This widespread variability in test scores—which increases with the severity of mental retardation—can be attributed to a number of factors. Some of these are serious technical shortcomings in the tests, such as scoring practices (Spitz, 1988); for instance, a 16-year-old student administered the WAIS-R (Wechsler, 1981) who fails to get a single correct answer throughout the test receives an IQ score of 46. Assigning scores through extrapolation greatly reduces the reliability of the test. There is a tendency, therefore, for school-age students with severe mental retardation to be administered tests designed for very young children, such as the Bayley Scales of Infant Development (Bayley, 1969). These measures are heavily influenced by perceptual and motor abilities and themselves have very low correlations with each other (Simeonsson, Huntington, & Parse, 1980) and with other IQ tests (Dunst & Rheingrover, 1982).

Variability may also be a reality of the performance of people with severe disabilities, since common characteristics such as sensory or motor impairments, medical fragility, and limited verbal comprehension render such individuals particularly vulnerable to seemingly minor variations in the presentation of a task. It cannot be assumed that the conditions under which nonhandicapped individuals take tests are even remotely similar to the conditions under which persons with severe handicaps are examined. For instance, preschool children with disabilities show greater decrements in test performance when tested by an unfamiliar person than do their nondisabled peers (Fuchs, Fuchs, Power & Dailey, 1985). Also, the literature on what happens to performance when one deliberately reinforces test behavior (see Evans & Nelson, 1977) indicates that to the extent external reinforcement improves performance, it does so differentially. The more disadvantaged or disabled the subject, the greater the benefit. This suggests that the motivational and attributional sets for someone with severe disabilities cannot be assumed to be the same as for someone who understands the nature of a test and its personal implications.

There are many factors, of course, that affect test performance—comprehension of the instructions, motivation to excel, anxiety, noncompliance, familiarity with the culture represented by the test, and so on. Some of these factors provide a major source for determining bias and other problems with testing in general. However, all of these factors are mitigated somewhat when one observes a pattern of performance in which the testee performs some of the items correctly—the easier ones—and then begins to fail as the items become progressively more difficult. This pattern is critical evidence for the clinician to establish the validity of the testing procedure. But persons with severe handicaps can usually complete only a very few items in the typical test and thus important data for interpreting performance are lost.

Some commentators (e.g., Spitz, 1986) have suggested that the technical problems for IQ tests within mental retardation arise from the inadequate sampling practices at the lower ranges of intelligence. It is true that the Wechsler Intelligence Scale for Children (WISC; Wechsler; 1967) standardization sample included 2.5% of children with mental retardation living in institutions, whereas the WISC-R (Wechsler, 1974) sample had no such group. However, this would have served only to lower the mean IQ score for the WISC sample (by slightly less than one IQ point). The real problem arises from erroneous assumptions regarding the nature of mental retardation and intelligence, starting with the fundamental assumption that it must be normally distributed. A good example of this bias can be seen in the original WAIS (Wechsler, 1955) in which Wechsler overadjusted the IQs of older people with mental retardation because he believed, incorrectly, that there would be a greater age decline in persons with mental retardation than in nonhandicapped people. Basic assumptions about intelligence—which, after all, is what the tests supposedly measure—therefore need to be considered.

NATURE OF INTELLIGENCE

Thus far, and in keeping with other commentators on this topic, I have refrained from ever referring to IQ tests as intelligence tests, since the currently available IQ tests seem to reflect scholastic aptitude. That is, validity is limited to their being somewhat predictive of school grades. Referring to them as "intelligence tests" implies a validity they do not possess and reifies the concept of intelligence as scores on the test. McClelland (1973) has remarked rather poignantly that:

> psychologists used to say as a kind of "in" joke that intelligence is what the intelligence tests measure. That seems to be uncomfortably near the whole truth and nothing but the truth. But what's funny about it, when the public took us more seriously than we did ourselves and used the tests to screen people out of opportunities for education and high-status jobs? And why call excellence at these test games "intelligence"? (p. 2)

The question then remains as to what *should* be called intelligence, and whether there is any substance to the construct independent of test scores. In considering these matters it might be useful to adopt Sternberg's (1985) distinction between implicit and explicit theories of intelligence. Implicit theories are those conceptions of the nature of intelligence that people already have. It could be claimed (e.g., Neisser, 1979) that intelligence is no more than the discrepancy between an actual person and some ideal or prototype of what society judges as clever. This is a relativistic approach, somewhat akin to the labeling theory of mental retardation, and has numerous weaknesses, the chief being that it is a theory of word meaning, defining one word in terms of other words (e.g., "ability to profit by experience," "ability to think abstractly," "reasons logically and well").

Implicit theories should, however, form the basis for explicit theories, which are formulated around data from people performing tasks thought to be related to the construct. There are basically two types of explicit theory: 1) differential approaches, based on the psychometric strategies of trying to discover the commonalities (factors) that underlie individual differences in test performance; and 2) cognitive approaches that attempt to analyze differences in information processing that would account for superior performance on various basic laboratory tasks. A good example of this latter type of test would be the speed with which an individual can access lexical information stored in long-term memory by comparing judgment (reaction) times to decide whether a pair of letters are the same in name (Aa, bB) or the same physically (AA, bb). Although we might hope that ultimately this information-processing approach will elucidate the basic elements of cognition necessary for everyday functioning in those with severe disabilities, it is clear that they rely heavily on a narrow range of predominantly adult verbal repertoires. Laypersons' views of being smart generally show that our ordinary conceptions of intelligence encompass social competence and practical wisdom as components just as important as verbal reasoning and knowledge. In the differential (psychometric) tradition, neither implicit theories of intelligence nor contemporary research on information processing have had much impact, since test content is selected on largely statistical grounds—which items show large enough individual differences to produce variability and which correlate best with the school performance criterion.

Because tests purport to be aids to prediction, and not to be concerned with the content of the items per se (as would be the case with criterion-based measures), the actual items selected for IQ tests have been quite arbitrary. This has long been a major criticism of tests, one to which the test designers are apparently quite immune: The standard is only whether the item correlates with the predictor. Binet selected the kinds of tasks that teachers of the time were asking children to do in classrooms, and basically similar items have continued in the modern Stanford-Binet (Terman & Merrill, 1973). In the Wechsler (1955, 1967, 1974, 1981) series of tests there was never a major implicit theory of intelligence guiding development of subtests and items. Whenever the implicit theory is articulated, it is easier to evaluate the content of the test in addition to its raw psychometric properties. Thus, for example, the Kaufman and Kaufman (1983) assessment battery for children is based on Luria's (1963) theory of simultaneous versus successive processing, but that theory has not been supported by empirical research in cognitive psychology. The K-ABC also emphasizes associative learning that has been shown not to be the sort of process that differentiates people with mental retardation from nonhandicapped individuals.

Sternberg's (1985) "triarchic" theory of human intelligence has some interest. It contains three subtheories. The first subtheory suggests that the sociocultural context does largely define intelligent behavior, which thus involves adaptation to a present environment, selection of a more optimal environment, and shaping a present environment so that it better fits one's interests and values. The second subtheory, which is experiential, proposes that within a given environment, intelligence is displayed when one is: 1) confronted with a relatively novel task, and 2) actively automatizing performance on a given task in a given situation. The third subtheory is of the components that underlie intelligent behavior—how mental mechanisms work. Three important groups are suggested: 1) metacomponents that control one's information processing, monitor it, and evaluate it; 2) performance components that execute the plans; and 3) knowledge acquisition components that selectively encode new information to allow learning to take place. This kind of theory has considerable potential for the study of mental retardation, since it is so expansive. It does not address how or why a person gets institutionalized, but shows that "intelligence" can be contained in how one can take advantage of a certain situation. Training someone in metamemory might help on some tasks, but it will not assist a person if his or her new environment is so novel that previously learned information cannot be used or accessed.

Existing tests measure only products of intellectual functioning—in Sternberg's (1985) theory they measure only the outcomes of knowledge-acquisition components (e.g., vocabulary

or reading), and to some extent performance components involving encoding and comparison with stored information, such as analogies. Tests of this kind are often called "fluid ability" tests (e.g., Picture Arrangement in the Wechsler [1955, 1967, 1974, 1981] series). Comparisons between groups (such as between cultures, socioeconomic groups, or those with different handicapping conditions) would be particularly unfair if the test's elements are differentially novel across groups.

Another approach to understanding the nature of mental retardation has been to compare directly the learning differences between persons designated as mildly mentally retarded and those not thus labeled. There is an odd bias in such research, in that logically it should make as much sense to study differences between persons showing a spread of more than 30 IQ points at some other location on the distribution (e.g., children having an average IQ score with those having IQ scores between 130 and 145). In fact, this virtually never happens, suggesting that children diagnosed as mildly mentally retarded are perceived as distinctly different in some way. When the psychology of learning was dominated by theories of basic animal learning, interest focused on whether differences could be found in simple associative learning and discrimination tasks. In his major review of this type of experimental research, Estes (1970) concluded that there were no or only minor differences between persons with and without mental retardation on simple classical and operant conditioning paradigms. Thus, depending on how "learning" is to be defined, the simple assumption that people with mental retardation are "slow learners" is false—this has important implications for views that some people cannot learn at all. Differences in discrimination learning (using artificial laboratory tasks), as investigated by Zeaman and House (e.g., 1963), in a well-known program of research, seem to be related to taking longer to attend to the relevant stimulus dimension of the task, not to slower learning once the subjects have attended. This attentional characteristic was shown to be typical of younger children, so that differences are minimized when children are matched for "mental age." Much of this research was fueled by the classic controversy as to whether the learning processes in children with mental retardation were the same (but delayed) or different. This uproductive controversy partially hinged on beliefs regarding fixed deficits. For instance, Ellis (1963) once argued that subjects with low IQ scores have more rapidly fading memory traces, although Belmont and Butterfield (1971), in reviewing the evidence, concluded that observed differences were in the use of memory strategies. Ellis went on to claim that "few processes seem 'normal' in the retarded. Indeed, studies that find normal functions in any task are suspect" (p. 52).

More recent cognitive theories of learning have improved the situation somewhat. Most cognitive theories make some kind of analogy to computers, such as the classic distinction between control processes (the software) and structural components (the hardware). This concept further heightened the notion that persons with retardation tend to have structural deficits (e.g., Fisher & Zeaman, 1973), so that training cannot enhance "intelligence." However, in an important series of studies over a number of years, Campione, Brown, and Ferrara (1982) have made a much more productive distinction between skills that can be instructed easily and those that require greater effort and ingenuity on the part of the teacher. Although a considerable injustice to the richness of their research, two major conclusions have emerged: 1) that children diagnosed as mentally retarded show a relative lack of *spontaneous* strategy use in cognitive tasks; and 2) that after being trained in strategy use, children with intellectual handicaps are less likely to transfer such strategies to new tasks.

ADAPTIVE BEHAVIOR AND COMPETENCE

As already explained, the professional popularity of the concept of adaptive behavior emerged from the obvious truth that IQ-test-score information did not relate sufficiently closely to what people could actually do in a practical, everyday sense. But the concept has quickly become murky and elusive. From its Latin root meaning "to fit," the concept of adaptive behavior has come to imply alteration to an-

other setting. Both meanings remain in the construct of adaptive behavior: the skills that will help an individual *fit* into a social niche, and the ability to *change* one's behavior to suit the demands of a situation. In both cases the situation could be imposed from outside; thus, the behavior that is very adaptive for an institution might not be suited to a natural community setting. Adaptive behavior is not the opposite of maladaptive behavior, since the latter denotes specific acts judged highly undesirable or inappropriate. However, the recent recognition that such excess behavior may be thought of as an individual's attempt to cope with a situation (e.g., Durand, in press) has made it clearer that maladaptive behavior is a form of adaptation judged socially undesirable. It has not yet been determined whether maladaptive behavior is better than no behavior at all, but it seems likely that many types of excess behavior are indicative of responsiveness to environmental conditions (Evans & Scotti, 1989).

As no one has effectively defined or measured adaptability as self-adjustment of behavior, the concept has become virtually synonymous with such constructs as daily competence, life skills, and functional behavior (Evans & Meyer, 1984). Attempts to measure adaptive behavior have thus been no more than static lists of things that a person can do, with the emphasis—to use the definition from the AAMD classification manual (Grossman, 1977)—on "personal independence" and "social responsibility" (Witt & Martens, 1984). The better known first-generation instruments are the Vineland Social Maturity Scale (Doll, 1953), the AAMD Adaptive Behavior Scale (ABS) (Nihira, Foster, Shellhaas, & Leland 1969), the Balthazar Scales of Adaptive Behavior (Balthazar, 1972), and the Cain-Levine Social Competency Scale (Cain, Levine, & Elzey, 1963).

At one level these instruments reflect specific behaviors that seem important and thus should have clinical utility (Evans & Nelson, 1977). Unfortunately, however, they have typically not been used as criterion-referenced measures and were, instead, approached from a psychometric perspective, particularly the widely used and studied Vineland Social Maturity Scale (Doll,

1953) and the AAMD Adaptive Behavior Scale (Nihira et al., 1969). The ABS, for instance, which is divided into parts relating to personal independence or to specific maladaptive behaviors, has been interpreted as a series of items yielding an overall score. But qualifiers such as "occasionally" and "frequently" are hard to judge accurately (MacDonald, 1988), and the ABS has low interrater reliability (Isett & Spreat, 1979; Spreat, 1982) as well as correlating poorly with direct observation of ward behavior (Marks & Rodd-Marks, 1980). Despite (or perhaps because of) these inadequacies, ABS scores correlate very highly with IQ scores (e.g., Christian & Malone, 1973; Futterman & Arndt, 1983), thus raising serious doubts as to the ABS's discriminant validity. In fact, three domains of the ABS (economic activity, language development, and number/time concepts) are sometimes referred to as the "cognitive triad" and can essentially replace standardized IQ test scores for classifying different levels of mental retardation (McLaren & Richards, 1986). Thus, the adaptive behavior concept comes full circle!

There is considerable mention in the literature regarding what the ABS (Nihira et al., 1969) might "predict," as though it were an ability measure, but it seems to correlate with no other parameters of interest. Since program and placement decisions are often based on ABS scores, correlations with these criteria are not indications of predictive validity, as claimed (Futterman & Arndt, 1983). If ABS scores correlated with *success* in community placement, or predicted differential treatment outcomes, then one could imagine some use for the measure and the construct. However, the only consistent finding is that placement success relates to scores on Part Two of the scale (Thiel, 1981), specifically the factor representing aggressive and disruptive behaviors.

Second-generation measures seem to offer somewhat greater promise. Two instruments in this category stand out: the revised Vineland Adaptive Behavior Scales (Sparrow, Balla, & Cicchetti, 1984) and the Scales of Independent Behavior (SIB) (Bruininks, Woodcock, Weatherman, & Hill, 1984). Despite improvement over previous measures, the purpose and utility of these measures have not been well thought out. Neither measure is based on a theory of skilled behavior that includes executive processes in addition to the physical elements of the task. Whether a person can "write a letter" or "prepare a snack" depends on whether they have been taught these skills, whether they have the opportunity to perform them, and the standards of mastery imposed by the environment (Evans, Brown, Weed, Spry, & Owen, 1987). Creating scores by adding up the number of such items provides little usefulness as a criterion outcome measure.

NEUROPSYCHOLOGICAL CONCEPTS OF SEVERE DISABILITY

It seems self-evident that people differ in their abilities and that very general abilities, such as learning from past experiences, would contribute greatly to the skill differences seen between someone who is not handicapped and someone who is judged to be severely mentally retarded. There may be other barriers to general competence, such as a specific brain deficit that interferes with the acquisition, processing, or retrieval of information. Thus, neuropsychological studies of learning and functioning following brain trauma provide some interesting comparison points for mental retardation. Similarly, there are behaviors that might interfere with the opportunity to benefit from standard forms of instruction—such as distractibility when instruction involves inconspicuous cues, disruptive behavior that reduces instructional time, or social deficits that restrict learning through interaction with others.

Clearly, neurological damage is the axis point in the causal pathways of many clinical syndromes that result in severe mental retardation. Fetal alcohol syndrome, for instance, represents a set of dysmorphic characteristics resulting from the toxic effect of alcohol consumption on fetal development; mental retardation arises from the specific insult to neural tissue. Of course it is not known whether the mental retardation of one syndrome is qualitatively similar to that of another. Also, autopsies of people who were mentally retarded reveal specific neuropathological abnormalities only about 50% of the time. But as progress in neuroscience continues, it should be possible, at least, to relate general areas of deficit to the sites, nature, and specificity of the brain dysfunction.

The difficulty arises because much of the relevant evidence comes from studies of people who have sustained brain damage as a result of illness, closed head injury, or cerebral vascular accident. Such individuals generally show a loss in capabilities they once had, sometimes to such a degree that they are functionally equivalent in skill level to someone who is developmentally disabled. But because of the history of prior learning and experience, these people are typically rather different from someone whose brain dysfunction, if any, occurred early in life. Another difference may be in the type of damage. A bullet wound, stroke, or tumor may have far-reaching consequences but still be more specific and localized than a disruption of brain activity or structure early in life that affects all subsequent brain development.

Despite these very major differences, it would seem plausible to think that the assessment of the nature of the organic deficit in someone with severe mental retardation would help ascertain where the cognitive support would be especially needed. Unfortunately, this has not proved to be the case thus far, for an interesting reason. Psychological and related neuropsychological tests have identified a variety of cognitive processes for which people with known brain damage show deficits. However, training programs designed to remedy these directly—known as cognitive retraining—have not yielded very satisfactory results (Benedict, 1989). Increasingly it is being suggested that people with head injury be taught directly the skills that they may lack (Godfrey & Knight, 1988). Essentially this duplicates the dominant perspective in education for persons with severe disabilities. Similarly, the cognitive tasks and the pattern of deficit yielded does not predict at all well the general outcome for the individual, in terms of day-to-day functioning, holding a job, or maintaining social and family relationships. Subtle differences in cognitive processing may make a difference between being a chess master and enjoying a game of checkers, or between being a fighter pilot and

being a reasonably safe driver, but they do not differentiate between people on such dimensions as doing one's laundry, enjoying TV, shopping, or having fun at a park.

Neuropsychological deficits are inferred from relatively poor performance on one type of task compared to performance on some other tasks. This requires that the tasks are all equally comprehensible to people with severe handicaps. Otherwise poor performance is incorrectly attributed to the neuropsychological function supposedly "tapped" by the task. McCaffrey and Isaac (1985) provide an example of this erroneous reasoning: People with moderate mental retardation showed deficits in "planning and regulation of simple behavioral tasks" as evidenced by lack of task persistence and by inflexibility, which the authors took as signs of frontal lobe dysfunction.

"DUAL DIAGNOSIS"

The nature and cause of behavior problems in addition to the intellectual deficits of mental retardation must be of importance in the design of programs that produce maximal learning or sustain the most effective performance. Imagine one were teaching functional skills to an individual judged to be severely intellectually handicapped. After a number of trials of seemingly well-designed instruction, the person was not paying attention, not rehearsing steps taught, and showing minimal acquisition. This lack of involvement clearly represents a barrier to habilitation as well as to functioning. If the person was judged to be depressed, that would have both meaning and implications for continued treatment. The meaning comes from the assumption that the person is exhibiting a syndrome or a collection of characteristics over and above the apathy observed. For example, the person might exhibit other "symptoms" not observed in the educational context, such as disturbed sleep patterns, poor appetite, and sad affect. These signs could reasonably permit the identification of an emergent difficulty—depression.

The depression could be caused by a variety of circumstances—perhaps the loss of a parent or friend, systematic experience of failure, limited reinforcement, or some organic origin. Determining such causes would assist in designing intervention for the depressed behavior, but either way the treatment of depression should be taken into account when proceeding with the instructional program. However, in one survey of psychologists' practices, the modal response to the question of the extent to which a psychiatric diagnosis improved or refined interventions was "makes no difference" for persons with severe or profound disabilities (Jacobson & Ackerman, 1989). Note that treating the depression need not precede the functional skills training, since it may be, depending on how the depression is functionally analyzed, that success with acquiring skills could be the avenue for changing the depressed behavior. This is one reason why the concept of "dual diagnosis" is potentially so damaging: The individual does not have two comparable sets of needs, but rather has interacting, complementary needs.

It may be seen from this example that the recognition of an emotional disorder is particularly important when there is a change in a person's prior status. Warren, Holroyd, and Folstein (1989), for example, described a number of persons with Down syndrome who showed a serious loss of previous adaptive skills. Although under 35 years of age, in most cases the individuals had been given a diagnosis of Alzheimer's disease, which is prevalent in older persons with Down syndrome. However, all responded well to treatment with antidepressant medication. The identification of a change in behavior, the specific identification of symptoms, and a positive response to a carefully designed treatment is much more convincing evidence of specific psychiatric disorder than surveys based on the labels assigned by a psychiatrist after referral (e.g., Eaton & Menolascino, 1982) or a checklist of behaviors and symptoms (e.g., Iverson & Fox, 1989). In fact, such checklists as that developed by Senatore, Matson, and Kazdin (1985) inevitably confound item content with functional competence (e.g., the item "complains of frequent and excessive pain").

Also, psychiatric terminology tends to be subjective and based on implicit standards. Menolascino, Levitas, and Greiner (1986), in explaining why persons with mental retardation are "vulnerable to mental illness," described people with mental retardation as having "primitive thinking, e.g., magical thinking, confusion of reality/fantasy" and thinking that "tends to be concrete and rigid," and as showing "increased utilization of nonadaptive defenses (e.g., denial, . . . regression, projection, etc.)" (p. 1063). Psychiatric symptoms are sometimes so vaguely defined that they lose what little specificity they have when describing people with severe mental retardation whose life experiences have never extended beyond the highly abnormal social environment of a large institution. Reiss (1982), for example, diagnosed "schizophrenia" in almost 50% of persons with severe mental retardation referred to a mental health clinic. However, instead of using accepted objective criteria, the signs of schizophrenia were "thought disorder," "flat affect," and "inappropriate silliness." In a survey of adolescents with developmental disabilities and emotional disturbance, Russell and Tanguay (1981) diagnosed as "psychotic" a 14-year-old boy with brain damage who "was able to communicate only through grunts and gestures and appeared to be hallucinating" (p. 571).

Clinicians unfamiliar with people with severe disabilities and unable to use their alternative forms of communication should be particularly cautious in using highly subjective psychiatric terminology. Especially dangerous is when the usual clinical criteria for a syndrome are changed because the person is severely disabled. Sovner and Hurley (1983), for instance, write: "The mentally retarded often lack the requisite verbal and conceptual skills necessary to communicate their feeling states. Aggressive acting out, withdrawal, and/or somatic complaints may be observed *instead* [italics added] of classic depressive complaints, e.g., feelings of hopelessness" (p. 66). Not surprisingly, Fraser, Leudar, Gray, and Campbell (1986), found no connection at all between specific behavior problems (e.g., self-injury, aggression) identified by a behavioral rating scale and the diagnoses given people with mental retardation by psychiatrists using a structured interview.

Of special interest might be the interaction between the cognitive deficits that characterize mental retardation and the expression of an emotional difficulty, such as a phobia. Phobias are defined as unreasonably intense or irrational fears, implying an element of judgment concerning risks and consequences. A person with severe mental retardation may fear an apparently harmless situation because he or she does not understand it, not because of some prior traumatic experience. The emotional reaction can still usefully be conceptualized as a phobia, but the treatment might focus on increasing understanding—an educative strategy. It is certainly helpful to the design of programs to recognize that a person's refusal to, for instance, go to a shopping mall is a fear rather than simple noncompliance. Reiss and his colleagues have used the phrase "diagnostic overshadowing" to describe findings in which information that a person was mentally retarded reduced the likelihood that clinical judges would consider phobic behavior to be an example of emotional disturbance (Reiss, Levitan, & Szyszko, 1982; Reiss & Szyszko, 1983). But it is not helpful then to label the person as *both* mentally retarded and phobic as two distinctive diagnoses.

Why then has the concept of dual diagnosis gained such rapid popularity? One possibility is that it is a ploy by mental health professionals to obtain third-party insurance reimbursements for services to persons with severe mental retardation and their families. Specifically, an individual whose diagnosis is mental retardation is rarely eligible for psychotherapy services as defined by private insurance providers. However, if the person can also be diagnosed as having a mental illness, to which problems can be attributed, then psychotherapy can be reimbursed. Similarly, in public facilities there is often a major distinction between mental health services and mental retardation services. Thus, the client with mental retardation who also exhibits behavioral characteristics labeled as schizophrenia, conduct disorder, or affective disorder represents an enigma and a source of conflict over responsibility for agencies (Reiss, Levitan, & McNally, 1982). For example, the National Association for the Dually Diagnosed (note the terminology) has called on community mental health centers not to deny services to people with mental retardation. The association's publicity brochure states that there are three primary therapies: psychotherapy, pharmacology, and "training in social skills [that] can alleviate much of the emotional anguish suffered by the dually diagnosed." The creation of this third entity, "the dually diagnosed," absolves both service delivery systems from accepting the need to think functionally about programs: "the introduction of a new label, 'dual diagnosis,' is highly inappropriate, unnecessary, and potentially destructive" (Szymanski & Grossman, 1984, p. 155).

PROFESSIONAL ISSUES IN DIAGNOSTIC TESTING AND CLASSIFICATION

Meehl (1973) wrote a famous essay entitled "Why I do not attend case conferences." Similarly, the present chapter could be called "Why I don't give psychological tests." Of course I do, on occasion, administer tests, just as Meehl probably slipped into one or two case conferences. Psychological tests represent a possible source of information about a client—what one thinks about this information and what one does with it is surely the essence of the debate (Ysseldyke & Marston, 1988). It is the inappropriate inferences and applications that constitute the professional problem. Thus, the topic of testing and diagnosis is not completely reviewed without some brief discussion of major conceptual approaches.

When people who seemed to lack certain basic abilities were isolated from the rest of society by institutionalization, the predictive functions of IQ tests were critical. It would be presumed that the presence of mental retardation caused the low IQ score. However, the low IQ score is known first in time and is used to predict the cause, mental retardation. Based on the test results, the "treatment" of institutionalization followed; however, it was never considered that the placement and the services provided would in any way rectify or mitigate the mental retardation. Therefore, there was little point in thinking of the test scores as predictive. If the test scores predict that after long periods of institutionalization the person would still be considered mentally retarded, the prediction would be accurate but the treatment ineffective. Conversely, if the test score had been erroneous, the deficit environment of the institution might have resulted in developmental delays, so that the test then becomes a self-fulfilling predictor.

We have, however, evolved to the interesting point at which the designation of someone as mentally retarded has no implications for type of living arrangement, school, or community in which that person will function. No particular "treatment"—residential program, special class, or clinical intervention—follows automatically from observation that an individual lacks certain or even many abilities. Thus, the IQ score establishes a category that is irrelevant with respect to programs, since the programs are the same for all individuals, regardless of IQ score. Now, of course, the educational programs would not be identical in variables such as pace, content, independence of discovery, and so on, for every student. Thus, the critical question becomes the nature of individual learner characteristics and how their advantages and disadvantages can be capitalized for the individual's maximum benefit. Thus, we should not be interested in measures with predictive power, but in measures that provide useful information for maximizing growth and development. IQ tests clearly fail in this regard.

CONCLUSIONS AND RECOMMENDATIONS

An interesting dilemma exists. The only formal method for diagnosing someone as severely mentally retarded is a given score on an IQ test. The IQ test and the resultant score have, as seen from this chapter, no other function. Yet the IQ tests are developed outside any set of psychological principles having to do with deficits in cognitive processes. Further, they are designed, psychometrically, on assumptions that seem largely erroneous—such as the normal distribution assumption of a unitary construct of intelligence. More specifically, even within the rules of psychometrics, the tests are constructed with little or no regard for the performance of people with sensory, motor, and cognitive disabilities.

Individuals undoubtedly differ in abilities and have unique educational needs. It is becoming increasingly recognized that the principles and tactics developed to educate children apply equally well to all children, regardless of the diversity of these needs. As these assumptions become accepted on the basis of moral principles or human rights, the classification of children becomes both unattainable and irrelevant. But that will not eliminate mental retardation, since there will continue to be a group of individuals who have very limited abilities and who will show serious skill deficits on the tasks that are required by our present society.

The concept of severe intellectual disability is a meaningful one and it is not a societal construction. Individuals who have the most severe handicaps are those who require extraordinary supports and opportunities in order to allow them to gain a wide range of skills. That many skills are attainable by people fitting this designation is proof of the general value of the approach, compared, for instance, with the traditional testing approach that has served to separate and isolate individuals to no demonstrable benefit. The degree to which such skills have been acquired further supports the value of identifying individuals in terms of their needs rather than in terms of their deficits.

In this reality, the process of psychological assessment is fundamentally different from traditional testing. In rare situations, tests might be part of this process, especially at a time when alternative and better sources of information are unobtainable. The process is to gather and coordinate information that will guide the educational and clinical strategies and decisions. This information has to be in a form that can be used and that is why, for psychological assessment, it is organized around psychological principles. The task of the assessor is to translate those principles. For example, if parents report that a child recognized a relative that he or she had not seen for a number of years, this information is coded psychologically across a variety of dimensions. First comes the question of accuracy and veridicality. Perhaps the parents did not really observe recognition behavior at all, either because they are distorting reality or because the cues they used to make the judgment of recognition were ambiguous. Second is the level of what this information means for psychological processes—for instance, it says something about long-term visual retention (memory). If the child had been assumed to have few abilities, then this particular accomplishment would have to be judged relative to others that the child has, and relative to the skills displayed by others. Finally, the information must be translated into the terms and concepts of others, such as the implications of this visual retention skill for teaching other behaviors.

Rules and procedures may need to be developed to ensure that psychologists are able to make use of information in this fashion. These procedures would then take the place of psychometric principles. Tests need to be evaluated not simply on their properties as measurement devices, but in terms of their application. Two standards must be documented: that the assessment procedure yields a unique intervention design (utility), *and* that the specific design results in a better outcome for the trainee than would have been otherwise observed (treatment validity).

The following list sums up my insights and recommendations regarding the use of tests as diagnostic and prescriptive tools:

1.   IQ tests, as currently constituted, have no place in the assessment of individuals with severe intellectual disabilities. However, they continue to be valuable in documenting the learning, memory, and other cognitive strengths of persons with severe motor and/or sensory impairments only—provided that such tests are adapted for alternative response modes.

2.   Extrapolation of scores or the derivation of IQ scores from scales designed for use with infants or for other special purposes is an especially hazardous practice that provides some continued professional expectation that scores can be meaningfully assigned to people falling within the lower ranges.

3.   The concept of severe intellectual disability is a meaningful one as long as individuals so identified are described in terms of educational and other service needs, as in the TASH definition, rather than in terms of expected functional limitations. Furthermore, it must be remembered that individuals designated within such a category are as different from each other psychologically as are individuals within any other socially identified category.

4.   Alternative perspectives to assessment based on advances in neuropsychology have not yet shown any utility for persons with severe intellectual disabilities. In fact, the reverse seems more true: The educational and rehabilitative techniques that have emerged as best practices for persons with severe developmental disabilities appear to have considerable value for persons with disabilities acquired through head injury and other neurological trauma.

5.   Measures of adaptive behavior, originally hailed as a valuable supplement to IQ testing, have followed in the psychometric tradition and have become "scales" containing lists of poorly defined competencies. They seem ill suited as criterion-referenced measures, as measures of learning style, or as starting points for individualized curricula. The concept and its operational definition needs full reexamination.

6.   Sophisticated theories of intelligence, not tied to psychometric IQ measurement, provide useful insights into the nature of learning and the cognitive structures underlying information processing. Future efforts to better relate assessment to educational strategies and curricular individuation could benefit from research and theory in cognitive processes.

7.   Tests and other measures are only as useful as the way in which they are used. No measure is ipso facto without value unless it provides purely capricious data. The most serious problem with IQ testing and diagnostic procedures has been the way these have been used by professionals in the field. There should be continuing efforts to educate psychologists and professionals in related disciplines on the cessation of classifying and categorizing children in favor of a "radical reconceptualization of the assessment process" (Ysseldyke, Reynolds, & Weinberg, 1984, p. 23).

8.   People with severe disabilities are likely to have an array of related and unrelated emotional difficulties, in roughly the same proportion as do other citizens. The cognitive disabilities may influence this picture, either by exacerbating social adjustment difficulties or by mimicking psychiatric disorders. In either event, the concept of "dual diagnosis" is unnecessary. Instead of enabling an understanding of the personal, social, and community needs of the individual, the concept is likely to perpetuate

undesirable classification and categorization. Continued efforts must be made to resist this additional opportunity for the denigration of persons with severe disabilities.

REFERENCES

Abramowicz, H.K., & Richardson, S.A. (1975). Epidemiology of severe mental retardation in children: Community studies. *American Journal of Mental Deficiency, 80,* 18–39.

Adams, J. (1973). Adaptive behavior and measured intelligence in the classification of mental retardation. *American Journal of Mental Deficiency, 78,* 77–81.

American Psychiatric Association. (1987). *Diagnostic and statistical manual of mental disorders-III-revised.* Washington, DC: Author.

Balthazar, E.E. (1972). *The Balthazar Scales of Adaptive Behavior I: The Scales of Functional Independence.* Palo Alto, CA: Consulting Psychologists Press.

Baumeister, A.A., & Muma, J.R. (1975). On defining mental retardation. *Journal of Special Education, 9,* 293–306.

Bayley, N. (1969). *Manual for the Bayley Scales of Infant Development.* New York: The Psychological Corporation.

Belmont, J.M., & Butterfield, E.C. (1971). Learning strategies as determinants of memory deficiencies. *Cognitive Psychology, 2,* 411–420.

Benedict, R.H.B. (1989). The effectiveness of cognitive remediation strategies for victims of traumatic head injury: A review of the literature. *Clinical Psychology Review, 9,* 605–626.

Binet, A., & Simon, T. (1905). Methodes nouvelles pour le diagnostic du niveau intellectuel des anormaux [New methods for the diagnosis of intellectual abnormalities]. *L'Annee Psychologique, 11,* 191–244.

Bjaanes, A.T., Butler, E.W., & Kelly, B.R. (1981). Placement type and client functional level as factors in provision of services aimed at increasing adjustment. In R.H. Bruininks, C.E. Meyers, B.B. Sigford, & K.C. Lakin (Eds.), *Deinstitutionalization and community adjustment of mentally retarded people* (pp. 87–101). Washington, DC: American Association on Mental Deficiency.

Block, N.J., & Dworkin, G. (Eds.) (1976). *The IQ controversy.* New York: Pantheon.

Bloom, A.S., Reese, A., Altshuler, L., Meckler, C.L., & Raskin, L. (1983). IQ discrepancy between the Binet and WISC-R in children with developmental problems. *Journal of Clinical Psychology, 39,* 600–603.

Bruininks, R., Woodcock, R., Weatherman, R., & Hill, B. (1984). *Scales of Independent Behavior: Woodcock-Johnson Psycho-Educational Battery, Part 4.* Allen, TX: DLM/Teaching Resources.

Cain, L.F., Levine, S., & Elzey, F.F. (1963). *Manual for the Cain-Levine Social Competency Scale.* Palo Alto, CA: Consulting Psychologists Press.

Campione, J.C., Brown, A.L., & Ferrara, R.A. (1982). Mental retardation and intelligence. In R.J. Sternberg (Ed.), *Handbook of human intelligence* (pp. 247–269). Cambridge, England: Cambridge University Press.

Cattell, J.M. (1890). Mental tests and measurements. *Mind, 15,* 373–381.

Christian, W.P., & Malone, D.R. (1973). Relationships among three measures used in screening the mentally retarded for placement in special education. *Psychological Reports, 33,* 415–418.

Cleland, C.C. (1979). Mislabeling and replication: Methodological caveats. *American Journal of Mental Deficiency, 83,* 648–649.

Coolidge, F.L., Rakoff, R.J., Schwellenbach, L.D., Bracken, D.D., & Walker, S.H. (1986). WAIS profiles in mentally retarded adults. *Journal of Mental Deficiency Research, 30,* 15–17.

Coulter, W.A. (1980). Adaptive behavior and professional disfavor: Controversies and trends for school psychologists. *School Psychology Review, 9,* 67–74.

Covin, T.M., & Sattler, J.M. (1985). A longitudinal study of the Stanford-Binet and the WISC-R with special education students. *Psychology in the Schools, 22,* 274–276.

Doll, E.A. (1953). *The measurement of social competence: A manual for the Vineland Social Maturity Scale.* Circle Pines, MN: American Guidance Service.

Dunst, C.J., & Rheingrover, R.M. (1982). Discontinuity and instability in early development: Implications for assessment. In J.T. Neisworth (Ed.), *Assessment in special education* (pp. 54–72). Rockville, MD: Aspen.

Durand, V.M. (in press). *Functional communication training: An intervention program for severe behavior problems.* New York: Guilford Press.

Eaton, L.F., & Menolascino, F.J. (1982). Psychiatric disorders in the mentally retarded: Types, problems, and challenges. *American Journal of Psychiatry, 139,* 1297–1303.

Ellis, N.R. (1963). The stimulus trace and behavioral inadequacy. In N.R. Ellis (Ed.), *Handbook of mental deficiency* (pp. 134–158). New York: McGraw-Hill.

Estes, W.K. (1970). *Learning theory and mental development.* New York: Academic Press.

Evans, I.M., Brown, F.A., Weed, K.A., Spry, K.M., & Owen, V. (1987). The assessment of functional competencies: A behavioral approach to the evaluation of programs for children with disabilities. In R.J. Prinz (Ed.), *Advances in behavioral assessment of children and families* (Vol. 3, pp. 93–121). Greenwich, CT: JAI Press.

Evans, I.M., & Meyer, L.H. (1984). Basic life skills. In J.E. Ysseldyke (Ed.), *School psychology: State of the art* (pp. 37–56). Minneapolis, MN: National School Psychology Inservice Training Network.

Evans, I.M., & Nelson, R.O. (1977). Assessment of child behavior problems. In A.R. Ciminero, K.S. Calhoun, & H.E. Adams (Eds.), *Handbook of behavioral assessment* (pp. 603–682). New York: John Wiley & Sons.

Evans, I.M., & Scotti, J.R. (1989). Defining meaningful outcomes for persons with profound disabilities. In F. Brown & D. Lehr (Eds.), *Persons with profound disabilities: Issues and practices* (pp. 83–107). Baltimore: Paul H. Brookes Publishing Co.

Filler, J.W., Robinson, C., Smith, R.A., Vincent-Smith, L.J., Bricker, D.D., & Bricker, W.A. (1975). Mental retardation. In N. Hobbs (Ed.), *Issues in the classification of children* (Vol. 1, pp. 194–238) San Francisco: Jossey-Bass.

Fisher, M.A., & Zeaman, D. (1973). An attention-retention theory of retardate discrimination learning. In N.R. Ellis (Ed.), *International review of research in mental retardation* (Vol. 6, pp. 171–251). New York: Academic Press.

Flynn, J.R. (1985). Wechsler intelligence tests: Do we really have a criterion of mental retardation? *American Journal of Mental Deficiency, 90,* 236–244.

Frankenberger, W., & Harper, J. (1988). States' definitions and procedures for identifying children with mental retardation: Comparison of 1981–1982 and 1985–1986 guidelines. *Mental Retardation, 26,* 133–136.

Fraser, W.I., Leudar, I., Gray, J., & Campbell, I. (1986). Psychiatric and behaviour disturbance in mental handicap. *Journal of Mental Deficiency Research, 30,* 49–57.

Fuchs, D., Fuchs, L.S., Power, M.H., & Dailey, A.M. (1985). Bias in the assessment of handicapped children. *American Educational Research Journal, 22,* 185–198.

Futterman, A.D., & Arndt, S. (1983). The construct and predictive validity of adaptive behavior. *American Journal of Mental Deficiency, 87,* 546–550.

Godfrey, H.P.D., & Knight, R.G. (1988). Memory training and behavioral rehabilitation of a severely head-injured adult. *Archives of Physical Medicine and Rehabilitation, 69,* 458–460.

Goldman, J.J. (1987). Differential WAIS/WAIS-R IQ discrepancies among institutionalized mentally retarded persons. *American Journal of Mental Deficiency, 91,* 633–635.

Gould, S.J. (1981). *The mismeasure of man.* New York: Norton.

Grossman, H.J. (Ed.). (1977). *Manual on terminology and classification in mental retardation.* Washington, DC: American Association on Mental Deficiency.

Heber, R. (1961). A manual on terminology and classification in mental retardation. *American Journal of Mental Deficiency, 65* (Monograph Supplement [Rev.]).

Herrnstein, R.J. (1973). *IQ in the meritocracy.* Boston: Little, Brown.

Isett, R.D., & Spreat, S. (1979). Test-retest and interrater reliability of the AAMD Adaptive Behavior Scale. *American Journal of Mental Deficiency, 84,* 93–95.

Iverson, J.C., & Fox, R.A. (1989). Prevalence of psychopathology among mentally retarded adults. *Research in Developmental Disabilities, 10,* 77–83.

Jacobson, J.W., & Ackerman, L.J. (1989). Psychological services for persons with mental retardation and psychiatric impairments. *Mental Retardation, 27,* 33–36.

Jencks, C. (1972). *Inequality: A reassessment of family and schooling in America.* New York: Basic Books.

Kamin, L.J. (1974). *The science and politics of IQ.* Hillsdale, NJ: Lawrence Erlbaum Associates.

Kaufman, A.S., & Kaufman, N.L. (1983). *Kaufman Assessment Battery for Children (K-ABC).* Circle Pines, MN: American Guidance Service.

Landesman-Dwyer, S., & Butterfield, E.C. (1983). Mental retardation: Developmental issues in cognitive and social adaptation. In M. Lewis (Ed.), *Origins of intelligence: Infancy and early childhood* (2nd. ed., pp. 479–520). New York: Plenum.

Lowitzer, A.C., Utley, C.A., & Baumeister, A.A. (1987). AAMD's 1983 *Classification in Mental Retardation* as utilized by state mental retardation/developmental disabilities agencies. *Mental Retardation, 25,* 287–291.

Lukens, J. (1988). Comparison of the fourth edition and the L-M edition of the Stanford-Binet used with mentally retarded persons. *Journal of School Psychology, 26,* 87–89.

Luria, A. (1963). *The mentally retarded child.* New York: Pergamon Press.

Lutz, C., & Levine, R.A. (1983). Culture and intelligence in infancy: An ethnopsychological view. In M. Lewis (Ed.), *Origins of intelligence: Infancy and early childhood* (2nd ed., pp. 327–346). New York: Plenum.

MacDonald, L. (1988). Improving the reliability of a maladaptive behavior scale. *American Journal on Mental Retardation, 92,* 381–384.

Marks, H.E., & Rodd-Marks, J. (1980). On an attempt to assess and predict adaptive behavior of institutionalized mentally retarded clients. *American Journal of Mental Deficiency, 85,* 195.

McCaffrey, R.J., & Isaac, W. (1985). Preliminary data on the presence of neuropsychological deficits in adults who are mentally retarded. *Mental Retardation, 25,* 63–66.

McClelland, D.C. (1973). Testing for competence rather than "intelligence." *American Psychologist, 28,* 1–14.

McLaren, K.P., & Richards, H.C. (1986). Adaptive

Behavior Scale cognitive triad: Discrimination and classification of institutionalized mentally retarded adults. *American Journal of Mental Deficiency*, *91*, 304–307.

Meehl, P.E. (1973). Why I do not attend case conferences. In P.E. Meehl, *Psychodiagnosis: Selected papers* (pp. 225–302). New York: Norton.

Menolascino, F.J., Levitas, A., & Greiner, C. (1986). The nature and types of mental illness in the mentally retarded. *Psychopharmacology Bulletin*, *22*, 1060–1071.

Mercer, J. (1973). *Labeling the mentally retarded.* Berkeley: University of California Press.

Meyers, C.E., Nihira, K., & Zetlin, A. (1979). The measurement of adaptive behavior. In N.R. Ellis (Ed.), *Handbook of mental deficiency: Psychological theory and research* (2nd ed., pp. 431–481). Hillsdale, NJ: Lawrence Erlbaum Associates.

Naglieri, J.A. (1985). Assessment of mentally retarded children with the Kaufman Assessment Battery for Children. *American Journal of Mental Deficiency*, *89*, 367–371.

Neisser, U. (1979). The concept of intelligence. *Intelligence*, *3*, 217–227.

Nihira, K., Foster, R., Shellhaas, M., & Leland, H. (1969). *AAMD Adaptive Behavior Scale.* Washington, DC: American Association on Mental Deficiency.

Reiss, S. (1982). Psychopathology and mental retardation: Survey of a development disabilities mental health program. *Mental Retardation*, *20*, 128–132.

Reiss, S., Levitan, G.W., & McNally, R.J. (1982). Emotionally disturbed mentally retarded people: An underserved population. *American Psychologist*, *37*, 361–367.

Reiss, S., Levitan, G.W., & Szyszko, J. (1982). Emotional disturbance and mental retardation: Diagnostic overshadowing. *American Journal of Mental Deficiency*, *86*, 567–574.

Reiss, S., & Szyszko, J. (1983). Diagnostic overshadowing and professional experience with mentally retarded persons. *American Journal of Mental Deficiency*, *87*, 396–402.

Roszkowski, M., & Spreat, S. (1981). A comparison of the psychometric and clinical methods of determining level of mental retardation. *Applied Research in Mental Retardation*, *2*, 359–366.

Russell, A.T., & Tanguay, P.E. (1981). Mental illness and mental retardation: Cause or coincidence? *American Journal of Mental Deficiency*, *85*, 570–574.

Sattler, J.M. (1988). *Assessment of children* (3rd ed.). San Diego: Author.

Scarr, S. (1981). Testing for children: Assessment and the many determinants of intellectual competence. *American Psychologist*, *36*, 1159–1166.

Schalock, R.L., & Harper, R.S. (1981). A systems approach to community living skills training. In R.H. Bruininks, C.E. Meyers, B.B. Sigford, & K.C. Lakin (Eds.), *Deinstitutionalization and community adjustment of mentally retarded people* (pp.

128–141). Washington, DC: American Association on Mental Deficiency.

Seltzer, G.B. (1983). Systems of classification. In J.L. Matson & J.A. Mulick (Eds.), *Handbook of mental retardation* (pp. 143–156) New York: Pergamon Press.

Seltzer, M.M., & Seltzer, G.B. (1983). Classification and social status. In J.L. Matson & J.A. Mulick (Eds.), *Handbook of mental retardation* (pp. 185–200) New York: Pergamon Press.

Silverstein, A.B. (1982). Note on the constancy of the IQ. *American Journal of Mental Deficiency*, *87*, 227–228.

Simeonsson, R.J., Huntington, G.S., & Parse, S.A. (1980). Assessment of children with severe handicaps: Multiple problems—multivariate goals. *Journal of The Association for the Severely Handicapped*, *5*, 55–72.

Sinclair, E., & Forness, S. (1983). Classification: Educational issues. In J.L. Matson & J.A. Mulick (Eds.), *Handbook of mental retardation* (pp. 171–183). New York: Pergamon Press.

Smith, J.D., & Polloway, E.A. (1979). The dimension of adaptive behavior in mental retardation research: An analysis of recent practices. *American Journal of Mental Deficiency*, *84*, 203–206.

Sovner, R., & Hurley, A.D. (1983). Do the mentally retarded suffer from affective illness? *Archives of General Psychiatry*, *40*, 61–67.

Sparrow, S., Balla, D., & Cicchetti, D. (1984). *Manual for the Vineland Adaptive Behavior Scales.* Circle Pines, MN: American Guidance Service.

Spitz, H.H. (1986). Disparities in mentally retarded persons' IQs derived from different intelligence tests. *American Journal of Mental Deficiency*, *90*, 588–591.

Spitz, H.H. (1988). Inverse relationship between the WISC-R/WAIS-R score disparity and IQ level in the lower range of intelligence. *American Journal on Mental Retardation*, *92*, 376–378.

Spreat, S. (1982). The AAMD Adaptive Behavior Scale. *Journal of School Psychology*, *20*, 45–56.

Sternberg, R.J. (1985). *Beyond IQ: A triarchic theory of human intelligence.* Cambridge, England: Cambridge University Press.

Szymanski, L., & Grossman, H. (1984). Dual implications of "dual diagnosis." *Mental Retardation*, *22*, 155–156.

Taylor, R.L. (1980). Use of the AAMD classification system: A review of recent research. *American Journal of Mental Deficiency*, *85*, 116–119.

Terman, L.M., & Merrill, M.A. (1973). *Stanford-Binet intelligence scale.* Boston: Houghton-Mifflin.

Thiel, G.W. (1981). Relationship of IQ, adaptive behavior, age, and environmental demand to community-placement success of mentally retarded adults. *American Journal of Mental Deficiency*, *86*, 208–211.

Turnbull, H.R., & Wheat, M.J. (1983). Legal responses to classification. In J.L. Matson & J.A.

Mulick (Eds.), *Handbook of mental retardation* (pp. 157–170). New York: Pergamon Press.

Warren, A.C., Holroyd, S., & Folstein, M.F. (1989). Major depression in Down's syndrome. *British Journal of Psychiatry, 155,* 202–205.

Wechsler, D. (1955). *Manual for the Wechsler Adult Intelligence Scale.* New York: Psychological Corporation.

Wechsler, D. (1967). *Manual for the Wechsler Intelligence Scale for Children.* New York: Psychological Corporation.

Wechsler, D. (1974). *Wechsler Intelligence Scale for Children–Revised.* New York: Psychological Corporation.

Wechsler, D. (1981). *Manual for the Wechsler Adult Intelligence Scale–Revised.* New York: Psychological Corporation.

Witt, J., & Martens, B. (1984). Adaptive behavior: Tests and assessment issues. *School Psychology Review, 13,* 478–484.

Ysseldyke, J.E., & Marston, D. (1988). Issues in the psychological evaluation of children. In V.B. Van Hasselt, P.S. Strain, & M. Hersen (Eds.), *Handbook of developmental and physical disabilities* (pp. 21–37). New York: Pergamon Press.

Ysseldyke, J.E., Reynolds, M., & Weinberg, R. (1984). *School psychology: A blueprint for training and practice.* Unpublished manuscript, University of Minnesota, Minneapolis.

Zeaman, D., & House, B.J. (1963). The role of attention in retardate discrimination learning. In N.R. Ellis (Ed.), *Handbook of mental deficiency* (pp. 159–223). New York: McGraw-Hill.

Zigler, E., Balla, D., & Hodapp, R. (1984). On the definition and classification of mental retardation. *American Journal of Mental Deficiency, 89,* 215–230.

◇ **CHAPTER 3** ◇

Functional Assessment
Dynamic and Domain Properties

ROBERT GAYLORD-ROSS
San Francisco State University, San Francisco, California

DIANE BROWDER
Lehigh University, Bethlehem, Pennsylvania

We approach the topic of assessment with caution, if not resistance. Assessment has not always served persons with severe handicaps well. Historically, the main "treatment" for such persons involved conducting exhaustive assessments. The assessment findings tended to emphasize the deficits and other negative aspects of the individual. Often clinical and sometimes obscure diagnostic labels resulted from the assessment. Most troubling, the assessment report usually had few guidelines or suggestions for subsequent intervention. Rather, the report was likely to be "shelved," having little impact on later education or therapy. Thus, in some quarters, assessment has become a dirty word. Service providers have often avoided spending much time on assessment, and instead have proceeded directly into teaching activity. More likely, assessments were completed for the purposes of labeling, funding, and planning (individualized education program [IEP]) requirements.

In contrast to this bleak portrayal of traditional assessment, a new approach to assessment is proving its utility and gaining a number of adherents. *Functional assessment* is an approach that attempts to provide information that will be of direct benefit to the individual. Functional assessment has been a broadly defined term, but the following are some of its main characteristics:

1. It focuses on practical, *independent living skills* that enable the person to survive and succeed in the real world.
2. It has an *ecological* emphasis that looks at the individual functioning in his or her surrounding environment.
3. It examines the *process* of learning and performance.
4. It suggests *intervention* techniques that may be successful.
5. It specifies ongoing monitoring procedures that can *evaluate* treatment progress.

Functional assessment thus parallels the curricular changes in the severely handicapped field that have emphasized a "functional" approach. It has avoided past pitfalls that stress the deficits of the individual in clinical isolation, while describing skills the person has attained and how they can be utilized in the environment. Furthermore, it does not usually report scores or labels. It describes the learning process and suggests intervention strategies. Thus, assessment is not episodic; it is formative, as it interacts with ongoing instruction and evaluation. Wherever possible, the individual participates in assessment, with his or her preferences and choices being considered.

The purpose of this chapter is to review the advances of functional assessment. A domain approach organizes the discussion as follows: behavioral, vocational, social, home, school and community, and related skill areas. The review points to advances and limitations. While not proposing a new assessment instrument, certain proven procedures are described and new approaches are advanced. The style of writing is intended to be "functional" so that the reader can take this information and apply it to his or her own circumstances.

BEHAVIOR MANAGEMENT

Historically, problem behaviors were the first class of behaviors to be addressed with systematic instruction. Emerging from this deficit context, problem behaviors such as aggression, self-stimulation, and self-injury were portrayed as the primary defining characteristics of the individual. As the functional curriculum approach emerged, positive skills became the primary characteristics to be addressed. Problem behaviors were then dealt with within the context of simultaneously teaching functional skills. An unresolved debate has questioned whether it is first necessary to suppress disruptive behaviors with behavior modification procedures before substantive skill learning can proceed (cf. Koegel & Covert, 1972). The functional skill view would argue that both skill building and behavior modification can proceed concurrently, with improvements in both domains. A stronger, yet unproven assertion, is that the early introduction of a functional curriculum can actually prevent the appearance of most problem behaviors.

The field of behavioral assessment has developed from within the behavior modification and applied behavior analysis disciplines. In many respects, the notion of behavioral assessment overlaps with the concept of functional assessment. For example, Hawkins (1979) described a five-phase model of behavioral assessment congruent with our description of functional assessment. Hawkins stated:

1. There is an initial screening phase that grossly and briefly determines what kind of program is appropriate for the person.
2. A diagnostic phase assesses the specific characteristics of the problem. Such a detailed functional analysis may be approached with multiple measures including behavioral observations (in vivo or in laboratory), checklist inventories, and standardized normative tests.
3. There is an intervention formulation phase, where pilot trials of the treatment may be assessed.
4. An ongoing monitoring and evaluation system is designed to be used during the implementation of intervention.

5. A follow-up phase collects maintenance information.

Besides noting the similarities between behavioral assessment and functional assessment, it is apparent how assessment and treatment interweave. Both include the formative notions of evaluation and assessment (Irvin, 1988). Rather than having summative or one-shot assessments, the assessment process monitors behavioral development throughout the treatment regimen. Although there is this repeated measure notion, it is still likely that most of the assessment effort will occur in the early phases (the first, second, and third phases of Hawkins's [1979] model).

Decision Models

The formative notion of assessment has been particularly advanced within the behavior reduction framework. During the first 20 years of the behavior modification field, a number of treatment procedures received empirical validation. Some of these procedures included: differential reinforcement of alternative behavior, time out, differential reinforcement of incompatible behavior, and overcorrection. A number of investigators felt the need to take stock of these procedures and set guidelines for their selection.

Both Gaylord-Ross (1980) and Evans and Meyer (1985) advanced decision models to assist the practitioner in the behavior intervention process. These decision models included the following sequence:

1. Determination of the seriousness of the behavior to warrant behavioral intervention
2. Ruling out of alternative etiologies such as biomedical and pharmacological factors
3. Accumulation of quantitative baseline data
4. Conducting of a functional analysis of behavior
5. Possible selection of an ecological intervention (e.g., learning in a larger room)
6. Possible selection of a positive reinforcement intervention
7. Possible selection of an antecedent stimulus arrangement (e.g., modifying task difficulty to easier materials)
8. Possible selection of negative consequence procedures

Extensive information is collected throughout the treatment sequence. Yet, the repeated-measures graph of the target behavior(s) becomes the central data set. The functional analysis of the cause of the behavior (e.g., peer reinforcement) guides a decision for treatment selection. Further, data collection evaluates the effectiveness of the treatment. If it is not completely successful, a subsequent intervention may be selected.

Although visual inspection of the repeated-measures graph (i.e., baseline to treatment A; treatment A to treatment B) has been the primary way to assess treatment effectiveness, the additional criterion of social validity has been added and required before a final determination can be made. Social validity is discussed throughout this chapter as a necessary criterion in functional assessment. Social validity entails that a substantive change in the client has occurred. It asserts that a visual decrease in responding on a graph may not constitute significant treatment success. Social validity is determined in two ways. The first is that a normative (or situationally acceptable) criterion states that the behavior would have decreased within the range of a nonclinical sample of peers. For example, a sample of classmates in the targeted child's class may only be out of their seat during instruction from zero to three times (per pupil) during a school day. The successful treatment of "out-of-seat" behavior would have to reduce the targeted child's frequency to within this range.

The second way of determining social validity involves subjective judgment. A number of significant others (peers, teachers, parents) would indicate whether the client's targeted and related behaviors were not troublesome or had improved substantially. The subjective judgment is made from observing the client in the criterion or other settings, or by viewing videotapes of his or her behavior in these settings. Responses are given on a series of questions, usually in a Likert-scale format. Subjective judgments may be obtained at the end of treatment (and at follow up). For more precise discrimination, they may be given before (pretest) and after (posttest) treatment.

Social validity is important in determining the significance of treatment effectiveness. When used in conjunction with repeated-measures observational data, one can be fairly confident in obtaining treatment success. Also, social validity measures have the advantage of being fairly easy to implement.

Implementation

A central topic of this chapter is the ease and likelihood of implementation of different assessment procedures. We feel that there is a critical crisis between theory and practice in the severely handicapped field. By theory we do not refer to an esoteric model of learning or research on, for example, the conditional probability of a social interaction sequence. Rather, we are referring to the fundamental data collection that may be done in model demonstration classes, in preservice practicum experiences, and in exemplary public school classrooms. There appears to be a real resistance and decline in data collection in typical school programs (W. Rosenberg, personal communication, 1987). In spite of inservice programs and attendance at professional meetings, there appears to be an entropy in the use of simple recording procedures. Peck et al. (1989), for example, found great difficulty in implementing simple systematic instructional procedures with a well-intentioned inservice group.

If repeated measurement is in fact poorly implemented in the field, we may wish to explore alternative models of measurement and evaluation. A functional assessment approach might be a more reasonable way to proceed. Rather than expecting repeated measures of skill acquisition on a daily basis, we might conduct intermittent assessment probes. The simplest approach would be to have a pretest immediately before intervention, a posttest probe immediately after intervention, and a follow-up probe 1–12 months after training.

Repeated measurement in the behavior problem domain has been less of an issue. When a disruptive behavior appears, it tends to draw the attention of many persons. Often it becomes the top priority in a person's educational program. The individual may be in a program with a teacher trained to deal with behavior disorders and/or have consultants with similar skills.

Thus, there is a greater need, as well as attending professionals who may increase the chances of a more careful monitoring of the problem behavior. When a behavior is particularly serious (causing much damage or possible suspension), or when a new or intrusive treatment procedure is used, there is again likely to be much attention drawn to the student, with careful monitoring in place.

Thus, the intensive assessment of behavioral problems and interventions is likely to occur. Such assessment may include repeated measure, behavioral observation across treatment conditions. While this chapter does not discuss measurement techniques (see Gaylord-Ross & Holvoet, 1985; Johnston & Pennypacher 1981), a variety of direct recording procedures that might be used include: event recording, duration measures, time sampling, and response latency. Such direct measurement should be complemented with social validity measurement. These two measures, used in the context of a treatment decision model, should provide a powerful assessment-treatment approach.

Aptitude by Treatment Interaction: Communicative Functioning

Decision models have certainly led to a coordination of assessment and intervention efforts. Yet, the decision model leaves the practitioner to collate information on an individual-by-individual basis. A more powerful social science would first classify individuals along some personality, behavioral, or ability dimension. Then, experimental research would verify that a certain group(s) along the dimension would benefit from a particular intervention and that another group would advance with a different treatment. This notion of "aptitude by treatment interaction" was originally postulated by Cronbach and Snow (1977).

The work of Carr and Durand (1985) has advanced the field of behavior treatment so that a particular aptitude by treatment interaction has been empirically established. Carr (1977) originally postulated that self-injury (and a number of other aberrant behaviors) were motivated either by positive reinforcement (gain), negative reinforcement (escape), or intrinsic reinforcement (the response itself was pleasurable). Carr

and Durand expanded this notion to state that the individual was communicating both his or her state of affairs and his or her desire to move to another condition. More specifically, a person might misbehave to obtain social attention or informational assistance. Conversely, the individual might misbehave to escape or terminate the aversive demands of a teacher or a perplexing instructional task.

Interestingly, Durand (1982) has developed a standardized instrument, the Motivation Assessment Scale, that will classify persons with severe disabilities into "gainers" or "escapers," when the problem behavior is serving either communicative function. The instrument is in a checklist format, and is thus relatively easy to complete. Durand has documented its fine psychometric reliability and validity.

Durand, Crimmins, Caulfield, and Taylor (1989) have impressively taken the final step of offering interventions tailored to whether the person is attempting to escape or avoid something. For example, a student who was demonstrating self-injurious behavior to escape a difficult task was taught the communicative response of seeking instructional assistance from a teacher. The teacher modified the task so the student could succeed. By eliminating the motivation to self-injure in order to escape a difficult task, the behavior decreased. When another difficult task arose, rather than self-injure, the student communicated the need for instructional assistance to the teacher. This impressive melding of assessment and intervention will hopefully serve as a model for other aptitude-by-treatment interaction research in the field (Reichle, 1990). For the practitioner, the Motivation Assessment Scale (Durand, 1982) should serve as a useful classification device to help design interventions.

VOCATIONAL EDUCATION

Traditional vocational assessment did not serve persons with severe disabilities well. Career education models (Brolin, 1978) saw little work potential for persons below the level of moderate mental retardation. Rehabilitation assessment determined that most persons with moderate, severe, or profound mental retardation were incapable of nonsheltered employment. As with other outmoded forms of assessment, progressive intervention models passed it by. That is, as part of the integration movement, teachers started training their students in real work sites. Some of this community-based vocational training led to permanent jobs as the student transitioned to the adult world. Cumulatively, more demonstrations were made with the "supported employment" model (Rusch, 1986; Wehman, 1981), showing that adults with severe disabilities could work in real employment settings. An ecobehavioral analysis (Chadsey-Rusch & Rusch, 1988) showed that, given the presence of a temporary or permanent job coach (instructor) at the work site, an individual with severe disabilities could learn the required job tasks and display an array of general work behaviors.

Given the demonstrated success of an ecobehavioral employment model, there still remain a number of assessment issues to be addressed. It should be remembered that social validity not only determines the behavior criteria of treatment success, but it can also evaluate the appropriateness of treatment goals (Wolf, 1978). In terms of vocational education, the question becomes what should be taught during a training experience. The main tactic is to collect information by asking consumers what they feel is important. In this regard, employers are the potential consumers of employees with severe disabilities. Rusch (1979) and his colleagues have done extensive surveys of what employers feel are key work skills. Job-task performance, general work behaviors (e.g., grooming), related social skills, and the absence of antisocial skills were reported. Some researchers have tried to determine whether general work behaviors or job-task performance is more critical. Both skills appear in the employer surveys, with general work behaviors cited more frequently. Further, Greenspan and Schoultz (1981) and Hanley-Maxwell, Rusch, Chadsey-Rusch, and Renzaglia (1986) found that job-task performance accounts for approximately 40% of terminations, with up to 50% caused by general work behaviors. It appears then that there is not a simple answer to this question, and educators will have to give considerable attention to both skills. Thus, the assessor will have to examine a wide range of skills from both domains. Rusch,

Schutz, Mithaug, Stewart, and Mar (1982) developed a standardized instrument, the Vocational Assessment Curriculum Guide, to assist in this process.

Rather than assess important vocational skills by spanning those voiced by a wide range of employers, it may be possible to identify particular skills that are articulated in one's local community. Thus, F. Brown, Evans, Weed, and Owen (1987) developed an environmental assessment strategy for determining goals by tapping into local needs. The assessment identifies the types of employers who might hire persons with severe disabilities. The skills needed for jobs in these settings are then enumerated. Also, parents provide input regarding their expectations for employment and the skill levels and interests of their child. The assessment then recommends the kind of vocational training needed. The recommendation specifies the types of skills, settings, and materials that must be included in training.

Probably the most valuable vocational assessment information is that obtained from previous training experiences. Gaylord-Ross, Forte, Storey, Gaylord-Ross, and Jameson (1987) and Sailor et al. (1986) have recommended a "rotational assessment" procedure. That is, contemporary secondary vocational training should place a student in a series of work experiences in real employment settings. Professionals should gather information from these experiences that indicates the relative skillfulness of the student in different settings and the preferences of the student for different work settings. To accomplish this, the sequence of placements should reflect different contexts (factory, office, outdoors) and different levels of difficulty (manual and cognitive dexterity). A cumulative data base should emerge related to the abilities and preferences of the individual. This information may ultimately be used in placing the student in a permanent position upon leaving school. This vocational rotational assessment may further continue during the adult years.

At present, a number of school programs pass school leavers on to adult agencies with a permanent job. The adult agency is to provide follow-up support services. Yet, when the individual is terminated from a job, the adult agency returns the client to a segregated program rather than replace them in nonsheltered employment (Moe, personal communication, 1988). For this reason, some schools have developed adult education programs that keep the graduate within the service provision of the school. Whether within-agency or across-agency transition occurs, it is important to assess the projected resources to support job placements. To this end, Gaylord-Ross (1986) developed a model for the situational assessment of students transitioning into supported employment. The model includes environmental assessment and rotational assessment, and also identifies the agencies and resources that will lead to effective transition.

Instructional support is the main type of resource needed for follow-along employment services. Supported employment has developed two types of support models: individual placement and group placement. In the individual placement model a single instructor (job coach) teaches the person the various steps of the position at the work site. When the individual shows mastery, the job coach gradually begins to fade out of the work setting. Ultimately, the person with disabilities works independently and is under the supervision of a co-worker. In the group placement model, a number of workers with disabilities remain under the permanent supervision of a job coach. Thus, persons with more challenging needs may be able to be retained in nonsheltered work. Even in the group model, though, the job coach attempts to fade the degree of his or her supervision at the work site. This may include systematic fading through distancing oneself from the client, or transferring supervisory control to other co-workers.

As just stated, in both individual and group models the job coach attempts to fade his or her supervisory and instructional presence. Thus, it may be useful to explore assessment procedures that predict the nature of this important fading process. The assessment may document particular fading procedures that have worked with a client (e.g., time delay). It may then attempt to determine the "zone of proximal development," a notion developed by Vygotsky (1986), and previously used with students with mild handicaps (Rothman & Semmel, 1990). This theory attempts to predict independent performance by assessing maximal performance under intensive

instructional guidance. That is, the person's maximal performance is assessed when he or she is receiving intensive instructional support (e.g., full physical prompts). The difference between performing under intensive and minimal prompts is the zone of proximal development. This concept may be helpful in assessing the potential performance of persons with severe disabilities.

SOCIAL BEHAVIOR ASSESSMENT

Social behavior development may be the key benefit accruing from integrated programs. The contacts that persons with severe disabilities make with nondisabled people should lead to attitudinal changes, social skills enhancement, and an improved quality of life. It is, therefore, important to assess the social abilities and skills of students with severe disabilities. Such functional assessment may guide instructional programs and maximize integrated social contact and social skills development.

Unfortunately, there has been relatively little work directly assessing the social behavior of persons with severe disabilities. In spite of all of the activity related to social integration, most assessment has been in a research context, with much attention given to measuring the attitudes of nondisabled persons (Voeltz, 1980). The research evaluating social skills interventions, though, appears to hold considerable promise for functional assessment (Brady & McEvoy, 1989).

As in other content domains, the original and main work in social behavior assessment has been with standardized tests. For example, the Vineland Social Maturity Scale has been used with some individuals with severe disabilities. While it provides a gross index of social functioning, it is not reliable for persons with more severe disabilities. Of greater import, it provides little information for designing interventions. Some other, more comprehensive assessments have attempted to follow a developmental model. For example, the CAPE scales use the notion of developmental pinpoints to sequentially assess and suggest goals for intervention (M. Cohen, Gross, & Haring, 1976). Unfortunately, the CAPE has received little field dissemination or validation.

In contrast, the Assessment of Social Competence (ASC) has been developed and validated specifically for use with persons with disabilities in both program planning and evaluation (Meyer et al., 1985). The ASC is organized into 11 functions intended to represent meaningful dimensions of social competence (e.g., Initiate, Self-Regulate, Follow Rules, Indicate Preference). Assessment progresses from the earliest manifestations of these functions to mastery levels of performance by adults, thus reflecting a developmental hierarchy. However, unlike more traditional developmental measures, each level of social skill on the ASC is reflected in functional and immediately useful strategies that an individual might employ to accomplish that function. Thus, value is attached to each level of development, even though the goal would be to increase the complexity of social competence on each of the functions through direct social skills instruction. The ASC has undergone extensive psychometric validation in a series of reliability and validity studies conducted with relatively large samples of children and youth as well as young adults with disabilities (Meyer, Cole, McQuarter, & Reichle, 1990). To date, the ASC is the most comprehensive criterion-referenced assessment alternative to direct observation of individual social skill targets, and should be useful in both descriptive and intervention social skills research and programming.

Environmental Assessment

As in other domains, some useful environmental approaches have emerged in assessing social behaviors. The environmental inventory strategy has been used to identify critical environments and subenvironments in which the student will subsequently have to perform (e.g., residential, work). These settings are then visited, with the most important social behaviors identified as assessment and instructional goals. Williams, Hamre-Nietupski, Pumpian, Marks, and Wheeler (1978) and Falvey, Brown, Lyon, Baumgart and Schroeder (1980) exhaustively applied this environmental inventory strategy for social behaviors.

Ecobehavioral Assessment

The ecobehavioral perspective (Rogers-Warren & Warren 1977) has provided a useful approach to functional assessment. As the phrase implies,

ecobehavioral assessment collects information about the individual and social behaviors in the surrounding social ecology. MacDonald and Horstmeier (1978) applied ecobehavioral assessment to social language development and interventions. Chadsey-Rusch and Gonzalez (1988) have been most instrumental in developing this approach in respect to its application to work settings. Chadsey-Rusch and Rusch (1988) identified three factors in the ecology of the workplace: physical ecology, organizational ecology, and social ecology. A review of assessment and intervention variables was subsequently made. Behaviors were assessed with the social validity notion of what are normative rates of social behaviors in regular contexts. For example, Chadsey-Rusch and Gonzalez (1988) observed nondisabled workers in fast-food settings to emit high rates of joking and teasing behaviors, but near-zero rates of positively reinforcing behaviors. This normative information could then be used to target behaviors for training (e.g., giving and receiving jokes and teasing).

Social Support Networks

The key aspect of the social ecology is the social network of persons in the life of the individual with disabilities. Community-based living has at times been criticized because some individuals with severe disabilities have been isolated, with few significant others in their lives. Loneliness and isolation are, of course, related to a low quality of life. Thus, it may be important to assess the richness of an individual's social network. If the person has few or no acquaintances in school, for example, it may lead to the establishment of a social intervention program (e.g., Special Friends [Campbell, 1989]).

There has been a recent growing interest in the support provided by social networks. Besides offering friendship and supervisory assistance, social support networks may provide a buffer to life stresses (S. Cohen & Wills, 1985). Social support research has distinguished between "perceived availability" and actual support given. Some types of social support include: instructional assistance, material gain, crisis counseling, creative inspiration, and emotional aid. Park, Tappe, Cameto, and Gaylord-Ross (1988) developed a social support network scale for persons with disabilities (cf. Horner, McDonnell, &

Bellamy, 1986). It assesses the different types of social support just mentioned, and also enumerates the number of significant others in community, school, work, and residential contexts. Thus, a lattice of the person's social network may be constructed. The questionnaire may, therefore, be useful as an assessment tool that identifies need areas for social intervention, as well as sectors where the person has an adequate or rich social support system.

Reciprocity is another relevant aspect of social support. Horner et al. (1986) assessed the amount of social support individuals with severe disabilities give to others as well as the amount of support they receive. This giving-to-receiving ratio is referred to as reciprocity. Horner et al. found that nondisabled persons roughly have a one-to-one reciprocity ratio between giving and receiving. In contrast, persons with disabilities receive much more social support than they give. On the one hand, this is understandable given the support systems developed to supervise and assist persons with disabilities. On the other hand, this unequal ratio may reflect the dependent status and personality style of persons with disabilities. Thus, unequal reciprocity may indicate a need for social skills training to provide support to one's friends and associates. Such assessment intervention prescriptions have yet to be developed, but they do offer exciting possibilities for ecobehavioral education.

Social Skills Training

Social skills training has undoubtedly provided the main data base for social behavior development in integrated settings. Social skills training has increased the quantity and quality of interactions between nondisabled persons and persons with severe disabilities. The training tactics have either taught a nondisabled peer to induce interactions (Strain & Odom, 1986), or trained the persons with disabilities to initiate and elaborate interactions (Haring, Roger, Lee, Breen, & Gaylord-Ross, 1986). The research has used a variety of single-case designs that had a baseline phase followed by one or more treatment phases. From an assessment perspective, the repeated measurement of social behavior in part or all of the baseline phase could be considered equivalent to a functional behavioral assessment (Haw-

kins, 1979). That is, educators could replicate the procedures of baseline measurement to obtain functional assessments of social behaviors.

It would be useful to enumerate some of the important features of this research. Many studies have attempted to train initiation and greeting responses (e.g., Haring, 1982). An initiation would entail approaching another person and making some gestural or verbal introduction. A greeting could be an initiation response or a response to an initiation (Odom & Strain, 1984). Nonverbal behaviors such as eye contact or body posture are a second set of social responses that have undergone training. Elaborating or expanding a social exchange is probably the most important and difficult social skill. This behavior may be measured in a number of ways:

1. Duration (in seconds) of a verbal and/or nonverbal exchange (Gaylord-Ross, Haring, Breen, & Pitts-Conway, 1984)
2. Proportion of responses given by the person with disabilities to the nondisabled person (Odom & Strain, 1984)
3. Number of turns taken within an interaction in a verbal or nonverbal exchange (Hunt, Alwell, & Goetz, 1986)
4. Substance or topic of the verbal or nonverbal exchanges (e.g., question, sharing play materials)

More molecular types of analysis (e.g., sequential probability analysis [Strain, 1984]), would probably be too complex for a service delivery context. Termination is the final phase of an interaction after initiation and elaboration (Gaylord-Ross & Pitts-Conway, 1983). Terminations are statements or gestures indicating the end of an exchange.

In many ways, the topics and content of social skills training overlap with areas in applied linguistics and pragmatics. Thus, Gaylord-Ross, Stremel-Campbell, and Storey (1985) outlined important linguistic behaviors that could be addressed in social skills training, including:

1. Protest/rejection
2. Requesting continuation of an object/activity
3. Requesting object/action or choice
4. Repeating

5. Social (greeting; "Thank you")
6. Calling
7. Requesting attention to self
8. Requesting attention to a referent (object, activity, event)
9. Offer
10. Answer ("Yes/No"; "What is the question?")
11. Request permission
12. Comment
13. Request answer
14. Give unknown information

In addition to measuring discrete social behaviors, social skills training has used social validity procedures to evaluate treatment effectiveness. Such procedures could be used as measures during functional assessment. One social validity criterion, normative rate, samples the behavioral rate of a nondisabled group to determine a goal for the performance of participants with severe disabilities. For example, Storey and Gaylord-Ross (1987) observed the rate of positive and negative verbalizations of individuals in a pool hall in order to set criteria for a conversational training program (while playing pool) with persons with disabilities.

A second social validity criterion is subjective judgment. That is, a number of significant others globally rate whether a person is performing well (normally), or has improved in performance over time. For example, Forte, Storey, and Gaylord-Ross (1989) had business and special educators rate the social interactions of students with disabilities in a work setting. The observers filled out brief questionnaires after they observed pretraining and posttraining vignettes on videotape. The ratings showed that the social competence of the students improved as a function of the training. Thus, social validity measures may be used as pretest measures to assess performance and assess goals, and as posttest measures of treatment gains.

ASSESSMENT IN AND FOR THE HOME

In the few available published instruments for assessment of individuals with severe disabilities such as adaptive behavior scales, attention traditionally has been given to assessment of self-care skills such as toileting, hand washing, and dressing. However, making an a priori assumption that self-care is a critical skill area for all individuals with severe disabilities may be a perpetuation of "readiness" models of curriculum planning. While independence in self-care may enhance options for work and community living, the lack of independence need not preclude either obtaining a job or living in one's own home or apartment if other options such as hiring personal assistants are considered.

The alternative to making the assumption that all people with severe disabilities should have objectives in self-care is to use the ecological inventory process to weigh self-care deficits against other skills needed for home and public environments. Earlier in this chapter, consideration was given to identifying skills needed for work placements. Prioritization of skills needed for home environments is now considered.

When applying the "top down" curriculum planning approach delineated by L. Brown, Branston, Hamre-Nietupski, Pumpian, Certo, and Gruenewald (1979) to assessment planning, the first step is to consider an individual's relevant home environments. These might include, for example, a current home placement with parents, a future home placement in a supervised apartment, and respite care. The assessment purpose for an ecological inventory is to identify those skills that are most important to participation in a given environment. This information can then be used for student assessment by noting which of the skills identified by the inventory the student does or does not have. In an ecological inventory of the home environment, the parents are the best qualified to provide this information and thus, a well-done domestic assessment requires developing a parent-professional partnership as well as designing an assessment protocol to collect relevant information.

Parent-Professional Partnership for Assessment

Parental input in the assessment and IEP development process is required by PL 94-142. This input is especially critical in assessing skills for the home. Research on the extent to which professionals have been successful in encouraging this involvement provides mixed reviews. For example, Salisbury and Evans (1988) found parents of students with special needs to be significantly more involved in their students' education than parents of students who were nonhandicapped. However, a series of studies on parental participation in IEP development suggests that the parents' role is often a passive one (Turnbull & Turnbull, 1986). In a study conducted by Lynch and Stein (1982), differences for level of participation were found for the disability type, family life-cycle stage (e.g., student's age), and cultural background. Turnbull and Turnbull suggested ways to increase active parental involvement by addressing barriers to participation such as: 1) providing child care or transportation to conferences, 2) becoming sensitive to cultural and language differences, 3) providing information on the school program, 4) negotiating the meeting to work around both parents' and professionals' time constraints, and 5) avoiding professionals' intimidation of parents (e.g., not outnumbering parents in meetings and avoiding the use of jargon). Since homes are where the myriad of cultural differences in our society may be most apparent, the teacher may be wise to invest time in a home visit to gain further understanding of the student's cultural heritage, as well as specifics of skill priorities.

Besides encouraging parental involvement for identifying IEP objectives and for culturally sensitive curriculum planning, the assessment process also provides the opportunity for role clarification related to domestic skills instruction. Specifically, the teacher needs to identify the extent to which parents want to be involved in teaching/assessment of the student's skills for the home. Having a child with special needs places increased stress on a family, which varies depending on the child's temperament, responsiveness, and caregiving needs (Beckman, 1983). Additionally, other family needs such as economic demands or health problems can temporarily influence the extent to which parents can be involved in ongoing instruction of skills for the home. During the ecological assessment process, the teacher may want to suggest a range of involvement from anecdotal reports of progress to participation in training of skills to clarify the extent of involvement the parents prefer. When caregivers are paid staff (e.g., in a group

home) rather than family members, this role clarification is especially important since home instruction may be a defined part of the staff's responsibility.

Options for Skill Screening

Several options exist for identifying both the skills needed for the home environment and the parents' current priorities. To foster involvement, using an interview format with the parent in a home visit may best meet the dual goals of identifying skills and collaborating with the family. Alternatively, the teacher might use a telephone interview or mail correspondence to gather information. The assessment protocol used to gather information might be a skills checklist, a question-and-answer format, a discrepancy analysis, or the parents' direct observation of the student in the home. Samples of each of these formats are shown in Form 3.1.

From this screening, skills may be identified for housekeeping, personal grooming, meal preparation, family recreation, and so on. Sometimes further assessment is needed to specify the IEP objective. For example, parents may identify the need for the student to have some recreational skills for home. Direct assessment of several recreational options, such as task analytic assessment of using leisure materials and observations of the student's preferences, may be beneficial in selecting a range of activities to target. Wuerch and Voeltz (1982) provided illustrations of this assessment process and specific leisure skill ideas.

ASSESSMENT FOR SCHOOL AND COMMUNITY INTEGRATION

Community-based instruction and public school integration have become important components of educational programs for individuals with severe disabilities. The assessment process needs to reflect the priorities of increasing students' participation in their schools and communities. This chapter cannot fully address the wealth of information now available on community-based instruction and regular class integration. Rather, clues for the assessment process are gleaned from samples of this literature.

FORM 3.1

METHODS TO ASSESS CURRENT HOME SKILLS IN COOPERATION WITH CAREGIVERS

Example: Skills Checklist

Directions: Please check how well Sally performs each of the following activities. If Sally's performance varies, note which is *typical* (most frequently observed). Ratings: 1 = independent, no help needed; 2 = semi-independent, occasional reminders, help needed; 3 = partial participation, performs some components of task without assistance; 4 = no skills yet in this activity. Place an asterisk next to items most important to you.

_____ 1. Bathing
_____ 2. Hair grooming
_____ 3. Meal preparation
_____ 4. (and so on)

Example: Question/Answer Format

1. What does Sally do for herself, or do to help you, with her routine of getting a bath? What would you like for her to learn to do?
2. Tell me about the family's mealtime routine and Sally's typical activities during meal preparation.
   a.
   b.
   c.
   d. (and so on)

Example: Schedule Discrepancy Analysis

Directions: Please note the care you usually provide for Sally at each of the designated times and the skills Sally performs alone. Under "Discrepant Skills," list anything you would like for Sally to learn to do as part of this caregiving routine. Place an asterisk next to your top priorities.

Time/Activity	Caregiver	Sally	Discrepant Skills
7:30 Wake Up	*Wakes up Sally*		*Respond to clock*
8:45 Bathroom	*Toilets Sally*	*Sits alone on toilet*	*Approach toilet* * *Pants up & down*
8:00 Dressing (and so on)	*Dresses Sally*	*Points to choice of shirts*	*Other dressing Choices Dressing skills*

Example: Direct Observation

Directions: Note level of assistance needed for each skill in each routine. Levels of assistance: V = verbal cue to begin/finish; VV = repeated verbal directions to perform task, M = model, PP = partial physical guidance, P = full guidance, X = does not do. Place an asterisk next to each skill that is your priority for Sally's next IEP.

	Monday	Tuesday	Wednesday
Routine: Preparing for school bus			
_____ 1. Put coat on	P	P	P
_____ 2. Put hat on	VV	V	X
_____ 3. Grasp and carry bookbag	X	X	X
_____ 4. Walk to bus	P	P	P
Routine: Afternoon snack			
_____ 1. Get out food for snack	X	X	X
_____ 2. Pour drink			
_____ 3. (and so on)			

School Integration

In 1975, Kaufman, Gottlieb, Agard, and Kukic proposed that mainstreaming for individuals with mild disabilities should focus on three types of integration: temporal (being in proximity with nondisabled students), academic, and social. These three forms of integration are also applicable to individuals with severe disabilities and can help guide the assessment planning. Sometimes the first step in furthering integration is to obtain temporal integration—getting students access to public schools and activities within them such as lunch in the cafeteria, extracurricular activities, and regular classes. Parents can be important allies in making the transition to temporal integration (Hamre-Nietupski, Krajewski, Nietupski, Ostercamp, & Sensor, 1988).

Besides gaining students' access to the mainstream, this temporal integration should be tapped further to meet each student's individualized educational needs. This will require assessment for "academic" or instructional integration and for social integration. Since other sections of this chapter provide information on assessing students' social and instructional priorities, further consideration is now given to how to relate these skills to school integration.

The two components of assessment for integration planning are activity selection and problem solving for meaningful participation within activities. Ford and Davern (1989) described several types of activities that might be targeted for within school integration such as academic classes, community-based instruction with nondisabled students, alternative uses for the self-contained special education classroom space, extracurricular activities, and peer networks. To get started in this activity selection, the teacher might adapt the L. Brown, Branston, et al. (1979) idea of delineating environments, subenvironments, and activities to the school. An example of a school delineation is shown in Form 3.2.

Once possible activities are delineated, the teacher will want to consider meaningful participation through matching IEP objectives to the setting and considering how the setting suggests the need for new objectives. This planning is also shown in Form 3.2 as "Integration Ideas for Sally." If possible, it would be helpful to let Sally try several of these integration ideas to observe the extent of her skill generalization and to discern the feasibility of skill instruction in this setting in a nonintrusive manner, and then to note her preferences for each. From several pos-

---

FORM 3.2

ENVIRONMENTAL DELINEATION TO IDENTIFY SCHOOL ACTIVITIES FOR INTEGRATION

Site: Farmer Elementary School

Environment: "All Purpose" room (Cafetorium)

Subenvironments: Stage, large room, kitchen

Subenvironment Priority: Large room

Activities of Students from Regular Classes
1. Breakfast program
2. Lunch
3. Assemblies
4. Peer instruction in reading by Ms. Brown's class on Wednesday at 2:00 P.M.
5. Help the custodian clean up

Integration Ideas for Sally
1. Social greetings (IEP objective) and listen to peer-instructed story reading
2. Communicate likes/dislikes (IEP objective) while attending assemblies with peer from peer network
3. Open lunch box (IEP objective) and eat with Ms. Jones's fourth-grade lunch
4. Share pictures of rock groups and new fashions to participate in lunch conversation (new IEP objective suggested by observation of fourth graders at lunch)

sibilities, the most meaningful integration for Sally could be selected.

Community Integration

Earlier in this chapter, assessment for integrated home and work environments was described. Community integration also requires being able to use the array of public and business services in one's home community. The focus on using these services is often referred to as "community-based instruction." Although community-based instruction has been a focus in the field of severe disabilities for over a decade, Aveno's (1989) survey of community residential facilities suggested that individuals with disabilities are significantly less involved in community activities than a comparison group of community members without disabilities. Aveno noted that social pressure to avoid public embarrassment by an insensitive public may be one factor in these diminished social excursions. Using the full range of public services in a community requires obtaining specific skills such as purchasing and bus riding, which have often been the focus of community-based instruction research. However, attention also needs to be given to "blending" in public settings by teaching appropriate social protocol and avoiding instructional procedures that stigmatize the student (Aveno, 1989).

Thus, assessment for use of community services might be conceptualized as having three concurrent priorities: 1) identifying skills to increase normalized use of the service (e.g., selecting a purchase), 2) identifying social skills and ways to compensate for unusual behavior for "blending" in public (e.g., keeping hands in coat pockets as an alternative to hand flapping; using greetings in "friendly" environments such as a small town store or avoiding social contact in "cool" environments such as an urban elevator), and 3) assessing the impact of the student's use of the facility and teaching strategies on public reaction.

To identify skills for normalized use of the environment, an ecological inventory of ways the public uses the facility can be useful. Students with severe disabilities may not achieve independent use of the facility and thus, partial participation may be the goal. This partial participa-tion may be most meaningful for the student if it focuses on increasing his or her choice or control in the environment (Sailor, Gee, Goetz, & Graham, 1988). For motivation, it may also be important that the response or response chain end with the "critical effect" of the activity such as consuming a purchased food item (Donnellan & Neel, 1986). Because of the wide range of community facilities, it may also be most efficient to train a generalizable response or response chain. The general case instruction methodology provides a format for this generalization planning (Horner et al., 1986). This format can also be used to assess generalization deficits for IEP planning, as shown in Form 3.3. In the example in the form, the student needs instruction across variations of doors, item displays, cashier counters, and cashier styles (e.g., stating price only, not bagging items). Concurrent instruction across the first three sites would provide this generalization training as the student had no difficulty with the variations that exist at Kate's (e.g., clerk takes items from shelf for customer).

The second priority of identifying social skills for "blending" in public settings can be addressed by targeting in vivo intervention. Hill, Wehman, and Horst (1982) decreased bizarre stereotypes (e.g., jumping up and down, hand flapping) and also taught pinball skills to facilitate normalized use of a recreational facility. Similarly, Gaylord-Ross et al. (1984) taught social interactions as well as leisure material use to facilitate social integration in a high school setting. Determining which behaviors or behavioral deficits will create problems in public cannot always be inferred from school-based observations. In vivo assessment to compare the student's behavior to those typical for his or her age group, as illustrated by Browder (1987), may be the best approach to identify discrepant skills for social blending.

The third priority of assessing public reaction focuses on assessment of the setting to improve blending of the student and/or instructional strategies. To assess public reaction, either the general public or store employees might be informally interviewed or "polled." Phillips, Reid, Korabek, and Hursh (1988) gave a questionnaire to store employees to assess the acceptability of

FORM 3.3

GENERAL CASE ASSESSMENT FOR ONE-ITEM PURCHASE

Instructional Universe: Convenience stores in Lehigh Valley, PA

Generic responses: task analysis (TA)	Assessment Data: Sites to sample stimulus/response (SR) variation (parentheses show S/R variation for that TA step in that site)				Assessment Summary: generalization deficits
	Penn Supreme	Nick's	7-11	Kate's	
1. Enter store	+ (electric door)	− (push)	− (pull)	− (push)	Push/pull door
2. Locate item	− (multiple aisles)	− (display case)	− (aisles)	+ (behind clerk)	Scan aisles and cases
3. Pick out item	+ (bottom shelf)	− (open case)	− (top shelf)	+ (clerk selects)	Shelf location and opening case
4. Take item to counter	+ (large counter)	− (small counter)	− (small counter)	N/A	Size/location of counter
5. Wait in line	+	+	+	N/A	Mastered
6. Pay cashier	− (clerk states price)	+ (clerk extends hand)	− (clerk states price)	− (clerk states price)	Verbal cue
7. Take change/ item	− (change with no bag)	− (no bag)	− (change and bag)	+ (bag)	Unbagged item Change cups
8. Leave store	+ (electric door)	− (pull)	− (push)	− (pull)	Push/pull
Number Correct/ Total Responses:	5/8	2/8	1/8	3/6	
Date of Probe:	Nov. 3	Nov. 10	Nov. 12	Nov. 15	

Above example of general case assessment for one-item purchase is based on Horner, McDonnell, and Bellamy (1986). Prior to this assessment, the teacher defined the range of stimulus and response-variation (not shown). The results of assessing purchasing skills at four convenience stores (Penn Supreme, Nick's, 7-11, Kate's) that sample this variation are shown. (+ = independent correct, − = incorrect or needed prompting, NA = not applicable to that site.)

community-based instruction to teach language skills. An alternative is to have an acquaintance observe the student and teacher from a distance, noting what behavior gets stares or comments from the general public. For example, in an observation of this type, conducted by a supervisor who pretended to be unacquainted with the student and teacher, stares and negative comments occurred when the teacher unzipped the young man's coat. To strangers seated across the restaurant, the scenario appeared to be an intimate exchange of one adult undressing another in pub-

lic. The negative attention was easily avoided by having the student keep his coat on as did many of the customers in the facility.

ASSESSMENT OF RELATED SKILLS: COMMUNICATION, MOTOR SKILLS, AND FUNCTIONAL ACADEMICS

In the developmental model of curriculum development often used in preschool education, content areas for instruction include communication, fine motor skills, gross motor skills, cognitive skills, and preacademics. The influence of this model on the education of individuals with severe disabilities is apparent when these content areas are the instructional focus out of context of daily activities. For individuals whose priorities are skills for increased community integration (i.e., "life skills"), communication, motor skills, and academics may be viewed as "related" to activities of daily living. F. Brown et al. (1987) described routines for assessment according to core skills (i.e., the daily living skill per se) and skills that enhance or enrich the routine. A student with severe disabilities may be able to learn core skills for a routine such as grocery shopping or meal preparation with no change in his or her current communication or motor competence. However, if taught in the context of these activities, related skills such as communicating menu choice and grasping small objects may enhance the student's independence within the activity and may have generalizable benefits to other activities requiring choice or grasp. One such enhancement may be to teach the student to express preference or choice in the context of daily routines (Houghton, Bronicki, & Guess, 1987). Thus, one way to identify related skills that are "functional" to activities of daily living is to select the core skills first and then review these skills to identify related skills that can enhance or extend the activity.

A second approach is to assess the student's competence using a skill sequence for communication, motor skills, or functional academics and then schedule selected skills across activities for generalized use. For example, in the Individualized Curriculum Sequencing (ICS) model (Mulligan, Guess, Holvoet, & Brown, 1980), targeting discrete responses such as reaching and grasping, selecting a choice, and maintaining head control might be taught within several daily routines such as grooming, snack preparation, and leisure activities. The ICS model has been shown to promote generalization of targeted skills to novel activities (Bambara, Warren, & Komisar, 1988). The difference between the ICS model and the developmental curriculum model is that the related skills are: 1) efficient and appropriate for the student's age—not necessarily the next language or motor skill in normal development, and 2) taught in the context of age-

appropriate activities—not as "communication lessons" or "motor lessons."

For language and motor skills it is also important to develop assessment in collaboration with speech/language, occupational, and physical therapists. Sometimes the therapist may have greater expertise in identifying the most efficient "form" to be taught (e.g., picture wallet, use of a walker) and the teacher may have more expertise in the "functions" to be taught (e.g., using the wallet to place an order in a restaurant; use of the walker to get to the cafeteria). However, in multidisciplinary programming both therapists and teacher should discuss both aspects of skills to be taught. Even when related skills instruction is "therapeutic," incorporating it into skills of daily living is feasible and enhances generalization. This integration of therapeutic services for related skills can even be incorporated in community-based instruction (Rainforth & York, 1987). Thus, the assessment of related skills requires identifying target responses and planning ways to incorporate the skills instruction in daily routines.

Form 3.4 illustrates the two methods for assessment of related skills. In the first, skills are selected from a review of daily routines. In the second, skills from a sequence are planned into daily routines for generalized use.

DYNAMIC ASSESSMENT OF PERSONS WITH SEVERE DISABILITIES

The limitations of standardized assessments and inventories have been discussed. Such traditional notions of assessment have been replaced with functional, environmental approaches. While environmental assessment well serves the practical needs of educators, we may ask whether more interesting assessment models may be designed (i.e., earlier notions of assessment that refer to abilities that cut across tasks and circumstances) that pertain to the key issue of generalization. That is, while the community-referenced training movement has been based on the premise that it would induce superior generalization, relatively little data have been accumulated showing generalization across settings (cf. Horner et al., 1986). What might be occurring is Stokes and Baer's (1977) notion of

FORM 3.4

RELATED SKILLS ASSESSMENT

Method: Enhance Domain Activities

Routine	Potential Related Skills to Assess
1. Meal preparation	*Motor* Reach and grasp; operate blender with switch *Verbal* Communicate menu choice; ask for help *Academic* Count measures

Method: Assess Related Skills Sequence and Build Into Functional Activities

Skills Sequence	Ideas for Functional Use
+ 1. Palmar grasp	(mastered)
+ 2. 3-jaw chuck	(mastered)
− 3. Pincer grasp	Coin use for vending machine; buttoning

or

Skills Sequence Assessment Results	ICS Activity Ideas
Communication: Point to choice	1. Cooking—choose food, grasp utensil, head up to view preparation
Motor: Maintain grasp. Hold head up.	2. Gardening—choose plant, grasp plant, grasp watering can, head up to look at plant

ICS = Individualized Curriculum Sequencing (Mulligan, Guess, Holvoet, & Brown, 1980). (+ = independent correct, − = incorrect or needed prompting.)

"sequential programming." That is, the person is merely retrained anew in the subsequent work setting with few transfer effects resulting from previous work experiences. Controlled research will determine whether this null hypothesis may be confirmed or rejected. It may also be useful to apply an assessment approach to examine generalization and other dynamic properties of learning.

A Proposal for Dynamic Assessment

A dynamic assessment centers around the four phases of learning (White & Haring, 1976): acquisition, production, generalization, and maintenance. While it could be used in conjunction with environmental assessment, it does not emphasize the content of performance.

The individual must first demonstrate acquisition learning. To avoid floor or ceiling effects, a task of intermediate difficulty would be selected. On repeated probes the person would perform at the 40%–60% range. Tasks that are viewed as functional in a person's life would be preferred. Next, effective cues and consequences would be identified. They might be selected from previous work, but they should be validated as part of assessment. A procedure such as Striefel's (1974) might be used to identify powerful reinforcers. Next, a systematic instructional program would be implemented. The program would include effective cues and consequences, as well as a task analysis. Repeated trials and sessions would be run until some learning criterion (e.g., 100%) was reached. The graphed data would indicate a "rate of learning" curve. Further validation would be provided as to the effectiveness of particular cues and consequences. Adaptations that were needed to reach criterion would be noted. If criterion could not be reached, implications for partial participation (Baumgart et al., 1980) would be stated.

Production assessment would proceed after acquisition assessment. A task would be identified that could be performed at a faster rate and/or for a longer duration. Preferably, the acquisition task would be used, unless it was felt there was no room for improvement in production dimensions. As in acquisition assessment, effective cues and consequences would be identified. Then, a production instructional program would be written and implemented. Contingent reinforcement and prompting techniques would be used to increase rate or stamina. The acceleration in production across training sessions would be graphed and noted. Effective production procedures would be highlighted.

Next a generalization assessment would be conducted. The task used in the acquisition or production assessment would be presented to the student. The task would be presented in a different setting (or subsetting) and by different people. For example, if the student had to stack lunch trays in the school cafeteria during acquisition and production, he or she could be taken to the faculty cafeteria to do the same task. If perfect generalization did not occur on the probe trial, repeated training trials would be conducted in the generalization setting until criterion had been reached. Generalization performance would be reported in terms of the number of training trials to criterion, or in a similar metric. Again, the degree of generalization and effective techniques to promote generalization would be reported.

Finally, after 3 months had passed since the last training session, a maintenance assessment would be conducted. The acquisition and production task would be presented in the criterion setting. If criterion performance was not displayed, a series of booster training sessions would be conducted until criterion errors reached maintenance performance (trials or sessions to criterion). Again, techniques to facilitate maintenance would be noted.

Content Considerations

Data and information gathered from a single task across the different phases of learning would be synthesized and would thus present a profile of a particular learning style. Useful information related to effective teaching techniques should emerge. Still, it could be pointed out that information from a single task or content domain may not be reliable or may not accurately reflect the total ability repertoire of the individual. Therefore, the functional assessment procedure needs to be replicated on several other task domains. This would ensure the representativeness and ecological validity of the assessment process.

The important task domains may vary according to professional philosophy. A common set of functional domains has been personal management, vocational, social/leisure, and community. Other relevant domains might be academic and residential. Domains articulated from a developmental framework have been communication and motor. Four domains should be selected for the dynamic assessment. The four-phase assessment (i.e., acquisition, production, generalization, and maintenance) should be replicated in each of the four domains. Preferably, tasks from the student's IEP would be selected for assessment. This would integrate the assessment-curriculum intervention process, and would increase the chances of assessment recommendations being followed in teaching practice. Furthermore, since assessments are typically mandated, it would force the teacher to participate in data-based, systematic procedures. This participation might spill over into actual teaching practice throughout the year. Thus, the problem of quality teacher practices might be rectified through dynamic assessment.

Most important, the dynamic assessment presents a profile of the learning characteristics of the individual. When there is a consistency of learning style in performance across task domains, clear information may be provided about: 1) the rate of learning in the different phases; 2) the amount and types of instructional support needed to facilitate learning; and 3) the ability of the student to generalize across settings, persons, and materials. When little or no generalization occurs with a variety of procedures, a sequential programming strategy might be inferred. If substantive generalization appears, the types of transfer strategies that work (e.g., sufficient exemplars, general case) may be noted.

When there is inconsistent replication across task domains, a more complex interpretation will result. For example, a student may show impressive generalization on one task and little generalization on three others. Such an effect would indicate the "potential" for generalization and prompt a further inquiry into what promotes and what deters transfer of learning.

Dynamic assessment is thus an ongoing process that portrays and inquires about learning styles and effective instructional procedures. In addition, when there is little evidence of generalization or independent functioning, there may be an indication for an intensive service delivery system (e.g., group supported employment placement), where continued cues and consequences are provided by an instructor.

The proposed dynamic assessment approach is in a schematic form. There is a need for its further conceptual development and field testing. We feel this effort would be worthwhile, since it would move the current state of functional assessment beyond its content-referenced form. The predominant integration movement assumes a degree of generalization of training results across community-referenced environments. The proposed dynamic assessment would key training efforts to individual learning styles and encourage practical instructional decision making.

Consideration for Practice

The dynamic assessment of students with severe disabilities is intended to improve educational practice in a number of ways. As has been stated, it should gather critical learning style data related to generalization assets and deficits. The assessment might identify generalization strategies that work, thus providing strategies for teachers. It may also identify areas of need where generalization skills ought to be learned. In addition, by conducting such a dynamic assessment, it may force some teachers, for the

first time, to address issues of generalization and maintenance, as well as data-based instruction. Dynamic assessment may thus indirectly improve teaching practice.

It should be noted that our suggestion for dynamic assessment is not a call for the resuscitation of ability constructs that are highly inferential and focus upon the deficits of the individual with disabilities. Rather, the assessment process is quite pragmatic in having educators collate past and current instructional data from functional tasks. Furthermore, we do not expect stereotyped generalizations about the student to emerge that would stigmatize or suggest separate (segregated) placements. Rather, practiced learning and teaching strategies might develop that would have a favorable impact on the pupil's future education.

SUMMARY OF ASSESSMENT FOR SKILL SELECTION

The tradition of assessment in special education has been to identify innate abilities or traits of individuals through the use of instruments such as the IQ test. This approach is losing credibility as the advantages of behavioral assessment for educational planning become apparent. For individuals with mild disabilities, "curriculum-based assessment" to pinpoint academic objectives and document service need is the current assessment trend (Shapiro & Kratochwill, 1988). In developing assessment for individuals with severe disabilities it is also important to focus on the outcome of educational planning. Ability and train assessment has often been an excuse for denial of service to this population. Even current skill level may not be relevant if the outcome objective is supported employment and community living, since these are now viewed by many as "rights" rather than privileges to be earned through skill acquisition.

For individuals with severe disabilities, there is no established curriculum for "curriculum-based assessment" for educational planning. Although some are emerging, such as the IMPACT Curriculum (Donnellan & Neel, 1986; Neel & Billingsley, 1989), that may lend themselves to future curriculum-based assessment, the current "best practice" is to identify an individualized life skills "curriculum" through ecological inventories, and then to use these skill lists for skill screening of the student using teacher-made informal assessments (e.g., see Form 3.1). This can be a time-consuming and arduous process for teachers; resources such as published curricula, activity catalogs, files of ecological inventories for a community, and published skills check-

lists may expedite the process. Our dynamic assessment proposal offers an efficient and curricular-referenced approach to this process. Through dynamic and domain assessment approaches, teachers may be able to accurately assess both their communities and their students to achieve the goal of developing IEPs that enhance community integration.

REFERENCES

Aveno, A. (1989). Community involvement of persons with severe retardation living in community residences. *Exceptional Children, 55,* 309–314.

Bambara, L.M., Warren, S.F., & Komisar, S. (1988). The Individualized Curriculum Sequencing model: Effects on skill acquisition and generalization. *Journal of The Association for Persons with Severe Handicaps, 15,* 8–19.

Baumgart, D., Brown, L., Pumpian, I., Nisbet, J., Ford, A., Sweet, M., Ranieri, L., Hansen, L., & Schroeder, J. (1980). The principle of partial participation and individualized adaptations in educational programs for severely handicapped students. In L. Brown, M. Falvey, I. Pumpian, D. Baumgart, J. Nisbet, A. Ford, J. Schroeder, & R. Loomis (Eds.) *Curricular strategies for teaching severely handicapped students functional skills in school and nonschool environments* (Vol. 10, pp. 155–175). Madison, WI: Madison Metropolitan School District.

Beckman, P. (1983). Influence of selected child characteristics on stress in families of handicapped infants. *American Journal on Mental Deficiency, 88,* 150–156.

Brady, M., & McEvoy, M. (1989). Social skills training as an integration strategy. In R. Gaylord-Ross (Ed.), *Integration strategies for students with handicaps* (pp. 213–231). Baltimore: Paul H. Brookes Publishing Co.

Brolin, D.E. (1978). *Life centered career education: A competency based approach.* Reston, VA: Council for Exceptional Children.

Browder, D.M. (1987). *Assessment of individuals with severe handicaps: An applied behavior approach to life skills assessment.* Baltimore: Paul H. Brookes Publishing Co.

Brown, F., Evans, I.M., Weed, K.A., & Owen, V. (1987). Delineating functional competencies: A component model. *Journal of The Association for Persons with Severe Handicaps, 12,* 117–124.

Brown, L., Branston, M.B., Hamre-Nietupski, S., Pumpian, I., Certo, N. & Gruenewald, L.A. (1979). A strategy for developing chronological age appropriate and functional curriculum content for severely handicapped adolescents and young adults. *Journal of The Association for the Severely Handicapped, 13*(1), 81–90.

Brown, L., Branston-McClean, M., Baumgart, D., Vincent, L., Falvey, M., & Schroeder, J. (1979). Using the characteristics of current and subsequent least restrictive environments as factors in the development of curricular content for severely handicapped students. *TASH Review, 4,* 407–424.

Campbell, P.H. (1989). Students with physical disabilities. In R. Gaylord-Ross (Ed.), *Integration strategies for students with handicaps* (pp. 53–76). Baltimore: Paul H. Brookes Publishing Co.

Carr, E.G. (1977). The motivation of self-injurious behavior: A review of some hypotheses. *Psychological Bulletin, 84,* 800–816.

Carr, E.G., & Durand, V.M. (1985). Reducing behavior problems through functional communication training. *Journal of Applied Behavior Analysis, 18* 111–126.

Chadsey-Rusch, J., & Gonzalez, P. (1988). Social ecology of the workplace: Employers' perceptions vs. direct observation. *Research in Developmental Disabilities, 9,* 229–245.

Chadsey-Rusch, J., & Rusch, F.R. (1988). Ecology of the workplace. In R. Gaylord-Ross (Ed.), *Vocational education for persons with handicaps* (pp. 234–256). Mountain View, CA: Mayfield.

Cohen, M., Gross, P., & Haring, N. (1976). Developmental pinpoints. In N. Haring & L. Brown (Eds.), *Teaching the severely handicapped* (Vol. 1). New York: Grune & Stratton.

Cohen, S., & Wills, T.A. (1985). Stress, social support, and the buffering hypothesis. *Psychological Bulletin, 98*(2) 310–357.

Cronbach, L.J., & Snow, R.E. (1977). *Aptitudes and instructional methods: A handbook for research on interactions.* New York: Irvington.

Donnellan, A., & Neel, R.S. (1986). New directions in educating students with autism. In R.H. Horner, L.H. Meyer, & H.D.B. Fredericks (Eds.), *Education of learners with severe handicaps: Exemplary service strategies* (pp. 99–126). Baltimore: Paul H. Brooks Publishing Co.

Durand, V.M. (1982). Motivation Assessment Scale: In M. Hersen & A. Bellack (Eds.), *Dictionary of behavior assessment techniques* (pp. 309–310). Elmsford, NY: Pergamon Press.

Durand, V.M., Crimmins, D.B., Caulfield, M., & Taylor, J. (1989). Reinforcer assessment I: Using problem behavior to select reinforcers. *Journal of The Association for Persons with Severe Handicaps, 14,* 113–126.

Evans, I.M., & Meyer, L.H. (1985). *An educative approach to behavior problems: A practical decision model for interventions with severely handicapped learners.* Baltimore: Paul H. Brookes Publishing Co.

Falvey, M., Brown, L., Lyon, S., Baumgart, D., & Schroeder, J. (1980). Strategies for using cues and correction procedures. In W. Sailor, B. Wilcox, & L. Brown (Eds.), *Methods of instruction for severely handicapped students* (pp. 109–134). Baltimore: Paul H. Brookes Publishing Co.

Ford, A., & Davern, L. (1989). Moving forward with school integration: Strategies for involving students with severe handicaps in the life of the school. In R. Gaylord-Ross (Ed.), *Integration strategies for students with handicaps* (pp. 11–13). Baltimore: Paul H. Brookes Publishing Co.

Forte, J., Storey, K., & Gaylord-Ross, R. (1989). The social validation of community vocational training in technological work settings. *Education and Training of the Mentally Retarded, 24,* 149–156.

Gaylord-Ross, R.J. (1980). A decision model for the treatment of aberrant behavior in applied settings. In W. Sailor, B. Wilcox, & L. Brown (Eds.), *Methods of instruction for severely handicapped students* (pp. 135–158). Baltimore: Paul H. Brookes Publishing Co.

Gaylord-Ross, R. (1986). The role of assessment in transitional, supported employment. *Career Development for Exceptional Individuals, 9,* 129–134.

Gaylord-Ross, R., Forte, J., Storey, K., Gaylord-Ross, C., & Jameson, D. (1987). Community-referenced instruction in technological work settings. *Exceptional Children, 54,* 112–120.

Gaylord-Ross, R., Haring, T.G., Breen C., & Pitts-Conway, V. (1984). Training and generalization of social interaction skills with autistic youth. *Journal of Applied Behavior Analysis, 17,* 229–247.

Gaylord-Ross, R., & Holvoet, J. (1985). *Strategies for educating students with severe handicaps.* Boston: Little, Brown.

Gaylord-Ross, R., & Pitts-Conway, V. (1983). Social behavior development in integrated secondary autistic programs. In N. Certo, N. Haring, & R. York (Eds.), *Public school integration of the severely handicapped: Rational issues and progressive alternatives* (pp. 197–220). Baltimore: Paul H. Brookes Publishing Co.

Gaylord-Ross, R., Stremel-Campbell, K., & Storey, K. (1985). Social skill training in natural contexts In R.H. Horner, L.H. Meyer, & H.D.B. Fredericks (Eds.), *Education of learners with severe handicaps: Exemplary service strategies* (pp. 58–73). Baltimore: Paul H. Brookes Publishing Co.

Greenspan, S., & Shoultz, B. (1981). Why mentally retarded adults lose their jobs: Social incompetence as a factor in work adjustment. *Applied Research in Mental Retardation, 2,* 23–38.

Hamre-Nietupski, S., Krajewski, L., Nietupski, J., Ostercamp, D., & Sensor, K. (1988). Parent/professional partnership in advocacy: Developing *Association for Persons with Severe Handicaps, 13,* 251–259

Hanley-Maxwell, C., Rusch, F.R., Chadsey-Rusch, J., & Renzaglia, A. (1986). Factors contributing to job terminations. *Journal of The Association for Persons with Severe Handicaps, 11,* 45–52.

Haring, T.G. (1982). Training and generalization of greeting response behaviors to severely emotionally disturbed pupils. In R. Gaylord-Ross, T.G. Haring, C. Breen, & V. Pitts-Conway (Eds.), *Social integration of severely handicapped and autistic students* (pp. 132–165). San Francisco: San Francisco State University.

Haring, T., Roger, B., Lee, M., Breen, C., & Gaylord-Ross, R. (1986). Teaching social language to moderately handicapped students. *Journal of Applied Behavior Analysis, 19,* 159–171.

Hawkins, R.P. (1979). The functions of assessment: Implication for selection and development of devices for assessing repertoires in clinical, educational, and other settings. *Journal of Applied Behavior Analysis, 12,* 501–516.

Hill, J.W., Wehman, P., & Horst, G. (1982). Toward generalization of appropriate leisure and social behavior in severely handicapped youth: Pinball-machine use. *Journal of The Association for the Severely Handicapped, 6(4),* 38–44.

Horner, R.H., McDonnell, J.J., & Bellamy, G.T. (1986). Teaching generalized skills: General case instruction in simulation and community settings. In R.H. Horner, L.H. Meyer, & H.D.B. Fredericks (Eds.), *Education of learners with severe handicaps: Exemplary service strategies* (pp. 289–314). Baltimore: Paul H. Brookes PublishingCo.

Houghton, J., Bronicki, G.J.B., & Guess, D. (1987). Opportunities to express preferences and make choices among students with severe disabilities in classroom settings. *Journal of the Association for Persons with Severe Handicaps, 12,* 18–27.

Hunt, P., Alwell, M., & Goetz, L. (1986). Decreasing problem behaviors through a communication board technique. *Journal of The Association for Persons with Severe Handicaps, 13,* 20–27.

Irvin, L. (1988). Vocational assessment in school and rehabilitation programs. In R. Gaylord-Ross (Ed.), *Vocational education for persons with handicaps* (pp.111–141). Mountain View, CA: Mayfield.

Johnston, J. M., & Pennypacher, H.S. (1981). *Strategies and tactics of human behavioral research.* Hillsdale, NJ: Lawrence Erlbaum Associates.

Kaufman, M.J., Gottlieb, J., Agard, J.A., & Kukic, M.B. (1975). Mainstreaming: Toward an explication of the concept. *Focus on Exceptional Children, 7,* 1–12.

Koegel, R.L., & Covert, A. (1972). The relationship of self-stimulation to learning in autistic children. *Journal of Applied Behavior Analysis, 5,* 381–387.

Lynch, E.W., & Stein, R. (1982). Perspectives on parent participation in special education. *Exceptional Education Quarterly, 3*(2), 56–63.

MacDonald, J., & Horstmeier, D. (1978). *Environmental language intervention program.* Columbus, OH: Charles E. Merrill.

Meyer, L.H., Cole, D.A., McQuarter, R., & Reichle, J. (1990). Validation of the *Assessment of Social Competence (ASC)* in children and young adults with developmental disabilities. *Journal of the Association for Persons with Severe Handicaps, 15,* 57–68.

Meyer, L.H., Reichle, J., McQuarter, R., Cole, D., Vandercook, T., Evans, I., Neel, R., & Kishi, G. (1985). *Assessment of social competence (ASC): A scale of social competence functions.* Minneapolis: University of Minnesota.

Mulligan, M., Guess, D., Holvoet, J., & Brown, F. (1980). The individualized curriculum sequencing model (I): Implications from research on massed, distributed, or spaced trial learning. *Journal of The Association for the Severely Handicapped, 5,* 325–336.

Neel, R.S., & Billingsley, F.F. (1989). *IMPACT: A functional curriculum handbook for students with moderate to severe disabilities.* Baltimore: Paul H. Brookes Publishing Co.

Odom, S.L., & Strain, P.S. (1984). A comparison of peer-initiation and teacher-antecedent interventions for promoting reciprocal social interaction of autistic preschoolers. *Journal of Applied Behavior Analysis, 19,* 59–72.

Park, H.S., Tappe, P., Cameto, R., & Gaylord-Ross, R. (1988). *The social support questionnaire.* Unpublished instrument, San Francisco State University.

Peck, C.A., Richarz, S.A., Peterson, K., Hayden, L., Mineur, L., Wandschneider, M. (1989). An ecological process model for implementing the least restrictive environment mandate in early childhood programs. In R. Gaylord-Ross (Ed.), *Integration strategies for students with handicaps* (pp. 281–298). Baltimore: Paul H. Brookes Publishing Co.

Phillips, J.F., Reid, D.H., Korabek, C.A., & Hursh, D.E. (1988). Community-based instruction with profoundly mentally retarded persons: Client and public responsiveness. *Research in Developmental Disabilities, 9*(1) 3–21.

Rainforth, B., & York, J. (1987). Integrating related services in community instruction. *Journal of the Association for Persons with Severe Handicaps, 12,* 190–198.

Reichle, J. (1990). Communication research. In R. Gaylord-Ross (Ed.), *Issues and research in special education* (Vol. 1). New York: Teachers College Press.

Rogers-Warren, A., & Warren, S. (1977). *Ecological perspectives in behavior analysis* (Proceedings of the Kansas Conference on Ecology and Behavior Analysis, held at the University of Kansas, Lawrence). Baltimore: University Park Press.

Rothman, H., & Semmel, M.J. (1990). Dynamic as-

sessment. In R. Gaylord-Ross (Ed.), *Issues and research in special education* (Vol. 1). New York: Teachers College Press.

Rusch, F.R. (1979). Toward the validation of social/vocational survival skills. *Mental Retardation, 17,* 143–145.

Rusch, F.R. (Ed.). (1986). *Competitive employment issues and strategies.* Baltimore: Paul H. Brookes Publishing Co.

Rusch, F.R., Schutz, R.P., Mithaug, D.E., Stewart, J.E., & Mar, D.W. (1982). *Vocational assessment and curriculum guide.* Seattle: Exceptional Education.

Sailor, W., Gee, K., Goetz, L., & Graham, N. (1988). Progress in educating students with the most severe disabilities: Is there any? *Journal of The Association for Persons with Severe Handicaps, 13,* 87–99.

Sailor, W., Halvorsen, A., Anderson, J., Goetz, L., Gee, K., Doering, K., & Hunt, P. (1986). Community intensive instruction. In R.H. Horner, L.H. Meyer, & H.D.B. Fredericks (Eds.), *Education of learners with severe handicaps: Exemplary service strategies* (pp. 251–288). Baltimore: Paul H. Brookes Publishing Co.

Salisbury, C., & Evans, I.M. (1988). Comparison of parental involvement in regular and special education. *Journal of The Association for Persons with Severe Handicaps, 13,* 268–272.

Shapiro, E.S., & Kratochwill, T.R. (1988). *Behavioral assessment in schools: Conceptual foundations and practical applications.* New York: Guilford Press.

Stokes, J.J., & Baer, D.M. (1977). An implicit technology of generalization. *Journal of Applied Behavior Analysis, 10,* 367–379.

Storey, K., & Gaylord-Ross, R. (1987). Increasing positive social interactions by handicapped individuals during a recreational activity using a multicomponent treatment package. *Research in Developmental Disabilities, 8,* 627–649.

Strain, P.S., & Odom, S.L. (1986). Innovations in the education of preshool children with severe handicaps. In R.H. Horner, L.H. Meyer, & H.D.B. Fredericks (Eds.), *Education of learners with severe handicaps: Exemplary service strategies,* (pp.61–98). Baltimore: Paul H. Brookes Publishing Co.

Striefel, S. (1974). *Measuring behavior 7: Teaching a child to imitate.* Lawrence, KS: H & H Enterprises.

Turnbull, A.P., & Turnbull, H.R., III. (1986). *Families, professionals, and exceptionality: A special partnership.* Columbus, OH: Charles E. Merrill.

Voeltz, L. (1980). Children's attitudes toward handicapped peers. *American Journal of Mental Deficiency, 84,* 455–465.

Vygotsky, L.S. (1986). *Thought and language.* Cambridge, MA: MIT Press.

Wehman, P. (1981). *Competitive employment: New horizons for severely disabled individuals.* Baltimore: Paul H. Brookes Publishing Co.

White, O.R., & Haring, N.G. (1976). *Exceptional*

teaching: A multimedia training package. Columbus, OH: Charles E. Merrill.

Williams, W., Hamre-Nietupski, S., Pumpian, I., Marks, J.M., & Wheeler, J. (1978). Teaching social skills. In M.W. Snell (Ed.), *Systematic instruction of the moderately and severely handicapped* (pp. 182–195). Columbus, OH: Charles E. Merrill.

Wolf, M.M. (1978). Social validity: The case for sub-jective measurement, or how applied behavior analysis is finding its heart. *Journal of Applied Behavior Analysis, 11,* 201–214.

Wuerch, B.B., & Voeltz, L.M. (1982). *Longitudinal leisure skills for severely handicapped learners: The Ho'onanea curriculum component.* Baltimore: Paul H. Brookes Publishing Co.

◇ **CHAPTER 4** ◇

Educating All Students
The Future is Now

FRED P. ORELOVE
Virginia Commonwealth University, Richmond, Virginia

It was 1979 when the most recent version of the "educability" debate began. The current rendition of "Who is educable? Who deserves services?" started with the publication of three articles in *Exceptional Children* (Burton & Hirshoren, 1979a, 1979b; Sontag, Certo, & Button, 1979). The point-counterpoint-rebuttal nature of those articles had emotional overtones, but generally conveyed relatively little of the passion that was to come. The substance of the *Exceptional Children* trilogy lay in the display of proof that individuals with very significant disabilities could in fact acquire skills (i.e., learn).

Two years later, the debate exploded with the publication of the inaugural issue of *Analysis and Intervention in Developmental Disabilities (AIDD)*, devoted entirely to the question "Are all children educable?" The children referred to in the question were those who "were until recently considered 'untrainable' or 'custodial' cases, . . . [most of whom showed] extremely little promise of becoming creative, productive citizens even with the most heroic efforts of today's most skilled behavior therapists" (Kauffman, 1981, p. 2).

The educability debate took on a rather different tone. While concerns about educating children inherently carry political baggage, the educability issue became openly political and passionate. The *educational* questions ("What do we know? What do we need to learn?"), characterized by Stainback and Stainback's (1983) review of the literature, gave way to *policy* questions ("Are all children capable of benefiting from an education? Do all children belong in school?").

Some of the passion undoubtedly had its roots in earlier (but not so much earlier!) days, when identical labels of "ineducable" were applied to

individuals with moderate mental retardation (Goldberg & Cruickshank, 1958) and, more recently, to individuals with severe disabilities (Blatt, 1987). Indeed, virtually every generation discovers a new group of children on whom to hang the "ineducable" tag, a phenomenon Baer (1984, p. 298) refers to as "one of our oldest and most self-destructive social dramas: 'Us vs. Them.' " The educational "Maginot Line" continues to be redrawn. Thus, the issue of educability commands our attention because it is so familiar and, instinctively, it seems so wrong.

Today's version of the educability question evokes passion and concern and merits our respect for other reasons as well. Special education has grown significantly in the past decade. While it certainly has not solved all the problems of helping individuals with severe disabilities, there has accrued a certain confidence borne of the success in creating integrated services, placing people in jobs, and teaching a wide range of skills. This professional confidence, coupled with confidence by many in the seemingly limitless instructional technology, has made it possible to begin looking at people who present the most difficult challenges.

Those very successes, in fact, have made it *necessary* to take a closer look at those learners who traditionally have been excluded. Many states and school districts decided to serve the "most capable" (read "less trouble") first. That left those individuals with profound disabilities back in the institutions or the segregated centers. It is now time to go back and get those people. Relatedly, one keeps hearing the challenge echoing: "Sure, you can do it with *these* folks, but what about *those* folks?" To be sure, many professionals relish the challenge to figure out what to do about "those" folks. Many others have simply recognized that the rights of individuals with the most significant disabilities have been abrogated, that their treatment has been unequal, if not altogether neglected. It simply is *right* to be concerned about them.

Finally, the practical reality is that improved neonatal technology for children with serious physical and medical impairments has created greater numbers of children in school programs who are demanding our attention. These children are visible enough for school districts to begin formulating policy and procedures and for courts to begin issuing decisions forced by schools and parents alike.

A recent court case (*Timothy W. v. Rochester, New Hampshire, School District*, 1989) embodies the central issues involved in the educability debate. Timothy W., who was almost 9 years old when the original action was filed in November, 1984, was born with severe respiratory problems. He shortly thereafter experienced an intracranial hemorrhage, subdural effusions, seizures, hydrocephalus, and meningitis. According to the court summary, Timothy is multiply handicapped and profoundly mentally retarded. He has cerebral palsy (spastic quadriplegia) and a seizure disorder and is cortically blind. Timothy was denied education by the Rochester, New Hampshire, schools because they believed him to be incapable of benefiting from an education. The district court supported the school district, denying Timothy the right to an education. The United States Court of Appeals, however, reversed the lower court, and issued an unambiguous ruling:

> The statutory language of the [Education for All Handicapped Children] Act, its legislative history, and the case law construing it, mandate that all handicapped children, regardless of the severity of their handicap, are entitled to a public education. The district court erred in requiring a benefit/eligibility test as a prerequisite to implicating the Act. School districts cannot avoid the provisions of the Act by returning to the practices that were widespread prior to the Act's passage . . . of unilaterally excluding certain handicapped children from a public education on the ground that they are uneducable. (*Timothy W.*, 1989, pp. 972–973)

Therefore, the question "Shall we educate or not?" is moot legally, as well as philosophically (Baer, 1981). As the appellate court in *Timothy*

W. revealed, the law is unequivocal on this point. (See also Dussault, 1989, for a legal analysis of this issue.) The court, however, also held the following:

> Educational methodologies in [basic functional life skills] are not static, but are constantly evolving and improving. It is the school district's responsibility to avail itself of these new approaches in providing an education program geared to each child's individual needs. The only question for the school district to determine, in conjunction with the child's parents, is what constitutes an appropriate individualized education program (IEP) for the handicapped child. (*Timothy W.*, 1989, p. 973)

Thus, the case is out of the courtroom, but the ball (and Timothy) are back in *our* court. We have come full circle from asking what we know about teaching people with the greatest learning, behavioral, and physical challenges to questioning *whether* to do so, and, finally, wondering *how* to do so. What do we know about how to offer Timothy and his global brothers and sisters the best education possible? What do we still need to learn? That is the focus of this chapter.

The chapter is organized around the following two basic questions: 1) What constitutes an appropriate education for students with profound disabilities? and 2) What strategies are available for teaching students with profound disabilities? For each question, a brief summary is provided of what we know (or think we know), followed by suggestions for what we might examine next as a profession. The empirical questions and data are suffused with—and, it is hoped, driven by—concerns about our values. First, however, the chapter examines the kind of person to whom we are referring.

WHAT GROUP OF INDIVIDUALS ARE WE ADDRESSING?

One of the single biggest indicators of how far we need to go is that professionals still are trying to define and describe exactly whom they are talking about. No disability label is immune to periodic reexamination and recategorization by well-meaning professional organizations. In the case of "profoundly handicapped" (or "the most severely handicapped"), however, the struggle is to pin down the category for the first time. The benefit of doing so for encouraging research is obvious (Holvoet, 1989). But, as Holvoet stated, "if labeling is allowed in order to promote studies and advocacy issues, research persons in these areas have a strong obligation to use the labels in the most judicious and nonharmful manner possible" (p. 64).

Another potential benefit of accurately describing the population is to provide a common basis for professional discussion. Some of the early educability debate was clouded by confusion about exactly which people were being discussed. Part of the confusion, of course, was created by the description of the "extremely debilitated group" that Kauffman (1981) provided in the editor's introduction to the special issue of *AIDD* on educability. (Ultimately, it is recognized, the subtle discriminations between categories of individuals become meaningless in comparison to the substance of the issues at stake.)

It has become increasingly clear that even if the field is unable to arrive at a simple, coherent definition—which is difficult for a complex, heterogeneous group of people—it is at least getting better at describing the characteristics of this group (Ferguson, 1985; Rainforth, 1982; Sailor, Gee, Goetz, & Graham, 1988; Snell & Carney, in press; Thompson & Guess, 1989). In a qualitative study involving 6 teachers of students with the "most profound disabilities," Thompson and Guess listed four major descriptors that characterized that group of children: limited level of awareness, limited response repertoires, no system of communication, and medical complications. Those four descriptors are consistent with the working definition of "the most severely handicapped" offered by Sailor et al.:

> Many of these students have various orthopedic and sensory disabilities and may have little or no voluntary control over their movements. Many are medically at risk, chronically ill, or medically dependent, while others have extremely severe behavior disorders. These students often do not demonstrate any obvious choices or preferences, may show no signs of anticipation, or show very little affect. Their self-injurious or assaultive behavior may be so severe that they are restricted from participation in many environments. (1988, p. 89)

Ultimately, even the term "profound" becomes relative (Thompson & Guess, 1989). Nevertheless, I am speaking here of individuals who, as one of the teachers in the Thompson and Guess study stated, "are really different from the students we typically think of as students in (SMH) programs" (1989, p. 10). The issues and data discussed in the remainder of this chapter are built on this foundation. Because most research studies fail to provide a clear, reliable description of their subjects (Holvoet, 1989), there is necessarily an imperfect match between what we know and for whom that knowledge is relevant or applicable. In considering specific studies for discussion, this chapter errs, it is hoped, on the conservative side. While that shrinks the data base, it also reduces to some degree one's concerns about the validity of the procedures and results.

WHAT CONSTITUTES AN APPROPRIATE EDUCATION FOR STUDENTS WITH PROFOUND DISABILITIES?

Present Knowledge

Consider the following quote from the decision of the U.S. Court of Appeals in the *Timothy W.* case: "The only question for the school district to determine . . . is what constitutes an appropriate individualized education program (IEP) for the handicapped child." On the surface, this statement seems innocuous. Professionals and parents sit around a table and hammer out an IEP. But wait a minute. This IEP is for a child described by the schools as unteachable. This child cannot see. He has seizures. He cannot walk and he can hardly move. What, then, should the IEP contain? Should the goals be aimed at making Timothy independent? Will he be a productive, participating member of society? Should we teach him to be happy? How will we know? What do we think *Timothy* wants to do? How do we find out? What exactly *is* the purpose of school, anyway?

Once professionals commit to teaching learners with profound disabilities, they confront the question of *what* to teach. By extension, they quickly find themselves asking questions about meaningfulness, appropriateness, and quality of life. The question "What is an *appropriate* education for students with the most severe disabilities?" cannot be answered simply by consulting a curriculum guide or conducting an ecological inventory. Kauffman and Krouse (1981) threw down the gauntlet when they challenged: "Formulating consensual definitions of *education, meaningful skill,* and *significant progress* will be difficult, but it is a task we can not avoid" (p. 56, italics in original). This section offers some perspectives on each of these three terms. It does so under the explicit assumption that all children are capable of benefiting from systematic instruction and are entitled, educationally and legally, to a public school education.

What is "Education?"

This question demands a relatively brief answer. Kauffman and Krouse (1981) conceded that "all children probably are educable if education is defined as acceleration of any operant response" (pp. 55–56). It is argued here that an education is the sum total of planned and incidental experiences and activities that occur within the school and community, the main thrust of which has been developed jointly by the child's teacher, parents, and other relevant professionals through the IEP process. If those planned activities for a particular child consist solely of accelerating operant responses, so be it. (One assumes, of course, that the professionals acted with knowledge of the students and conducted careful assessments prior to formulating the objectives.) In other words, someone must have thought those goals were meaningful.

What are "Meaningful Skills"?

This question must first be answered with another question: "Meaningful for whom?" (Orelove, 1984). Some have argued that social validation be used to determine the social significance of goals (Van Houten, 1979; Wolf, 1978). That is, are the specific targeted skills what society wants and values? Miller (1982) carefully refuted this approach on both philosophical and practical grounds. In any event, our society operates its public schools through local school boards, who hire and authorize its officials (superintendents and their staff) to perform their jobs as they are professionally trained.

Thus, it typically falls to the professionals (particularly the teachers) to select instructional goals and, hence, to determine the direction and purpose of their students' education. In choosing goals for the "typical" learner who has a severe disability, the professional has a difficult job, because there usually are hundreds of possible skills the student could be taught, but there is only so much time. Nevertheless, the teacher often approaches the task of choosing goals as equivalent to choosing what specific *skills* the student should acquire. The situation becomes even more complex when deciding what to teach a person with more restricted response repertoires and limited sensory intake. Holvoet (1989) pointedly observed that professionals' focus is not just on behavior change, but also on changing individuals with disabilities to be more like "normal" people. In doing this, Holvoet argued, we are emphasizing what is important to *us*, not necessarily what is important to the learner. A distressing (but, unfortunately, common) example of this occurs each time we eliminate a behavior we consider distasteful without replacing it with an equally or more useful behavior (Evans & Scotti, 1989; Holvoet, 1989).

We are left with examining our motives carefully in selecting instructional targets and, in particular, with asking ourselves: "How could this be meaningful for the student?" Evans and Scotti (1989) offered several provocative ideas. Although they focus on outcome measures, which the next section addresses more specifically, the concepts are useful in making decisions about choosing goals.

It seems clear that choosing goals for most learners with profound disabilities can not be predicated solely, if at all, on the environmental or ecological inventory approach (L. Brown et al., 1979; Helmstetter, 1989). Such an approach assumes a rather straightforward translation from skills required to function in a particular setting to skills to be developed in an individual student. The students addressed here, however, have response repertoires so limited as to render a straight skill development approach impractical. Even with extensive use of partial participation (Baumgart et al., 1982), the behavior often becomes sliced so fine that the resulting individual units of behavior have no clear function for the individual.

An alternative is to focus on teaching a repertoire of *effective* behaviors, those that produce an effect upon the social environment (Evans &

Scotti, 1989). The social environment includes the learners' peers, teachers, parents, and caregivers, among others. (Methods of organizing the environment to facilitate this are described in subsequent sections.) The value of effective behaviors lies in their life beyond the simple response itself. Dunst, Cushing, and Vance (1985) demonstrated how small behaviors (in their study, the response was fixated head turning in infants with profound mental retardation and multiple handicaps) can have higher order effects by exciting and engaging others in the environment to alter their own behaviors and style and frequency of interacting. Thus, the behavior itself, however small in scale, may trigger an avalanche by affecting other individuals, who, in turn, are more likely to occasion other behaviors in the learner.

This interactive model of behavior change (which Dunst et al., 1985, called a "social systems perspective") was clearly characterized by Hawkins (1984), as he discussed the meaningfulness of educational change for his daughter, Karrie, who has a significant disability:

> If anyone were to be the judge of whether a particular behavior change is "meaningful" it should certainly not be the general taxpayer alone, who has no idea how rewarding it is to see your retarded 19 year old acquire the skill of toilet flushing on command or pointing to food when she wants a second helping. . . . It is functional for the taxpayer even though his or her answer to the question, "Is this meaningful?" might well be, "No" or, "Not enough to pay for." And, although we cannot readily say how much Karrie's being able to flush the toilet enhances her personal reinforcement/punishment ratio, I can testify that it enhances mine as a parent. (p. 285)

Evans and Scotti (1989) also offered some "rules" for choosing behavioral targets, as follows:

> One rule might be that if a primary and important caregiver has a particular personal concern, such as self-stimulatory behavior in public, then improving that particular behavior in that context could have some priority as an outcome. . . . A second rule is that if the undesirable behavior would attract a great deal of negative public attention and avoidance, then again it might be a priority. . . . A third consideration is related to the presence of a few other behaviors that make people likeable, despite other specific negative habits. Some persons with profound handicaps are much more likely to attract the

attention, interest, and liking of caregivers than others. (p. 101)

In choosing to reduce or eliminate any excess (i.e., extra, unwanted) behaviors, it is critical that alternative behaviors that serve the same or similar functions for the individual be taught in place of the original behavior (Carr & Durand, 1985; Evans & Meyer, 1985). It is recognized here that we will be unable to teach enough skills, or the "right" skills, to make all children equally appealing and, hence, approachable. Clearly, we should not always place the burden on the child to change to please everyone else. Service providers will also have to change some of their own behaviors and perceptions, which in some ways may be more difficult than teaching children thought to be "ineducable."

Finally, Holvoet (1989) took a wide-angle view that forces us to think carefully in determining "meaningful" skills. Her discussion of research is equally applicable to classroom teaching and other services:

> If professionals believe that to be happy and have a good quality of life, a person must be able to partake in the rituals of job, housework, shopping, keeping oneself neat and clean, and taking care not to offend others, then research efforts must focus on ways to achieve these goals. . . . If, however, researchers and "helping" professionals wish to stand behind the value of these individuals, *as they are,* not as they wish to change them to be, then research might need to focus more on what type of impact these individuals may have on others, how persons with profound handicaps develop the skills they do, and what needs their current behaviors fulfill. (Holvoet, 1989, p. 70)

What is "Significant Progress"?

The discussion in the preceding section about effective behaviors and higher order effects provides some clues to answer this question. The qualifying word "significant" can be operationalized by again asking, "Significant to whom?" As the earlier quote by Hawkins (1984, p. 285) suggests, parents and other caring individuals in the student's life may be in the best position to answer that question.

As for assessing "progress," professionals who work with individuals with profound disabilities are in need of some new outcome measures or new applications of old ones. Evans and Scotti (1989) suggested several. First, changes in the level of a learner's excess behavior may signal problems with the learner's educational program or may be indicative of other negative circumstances. Second, indices that reflect the learner's emotional state (e.g., facial expression, vocalization, physiological measures such as pulse) would be most useful for persons who are unable to say what they are feeling. Third, the amount of time an individual spends continuously involved in an (unforced) activity could indicate the degree to which the person is enjoying the activity. For example, Miller (1982) observed that a "person who repeatedly emits a response to generate a reinforcing consequence is giving testimony that such reinforcers are meaningful or of value to her or him" (p. 7). Fourth, "behavioral complexity" might be employed; this term refers to the proportion of different behaviors observed to occur within a specific time interval. As Evans and Scotti (1989) noted, however, no normative comparisons currently are available to make complete meaning of the data that would result from this measure.

Another way of looking at progress presents itself in the Component Model of Functional Competence (F. Brown, Evans, Weed, & Owen, 1987; Evans, Brown, Weed, Spry, & Owen, 1987; Evans & Scotti, 1989). The model is built on the notion of critical effects and is organized around behavioral routines (activities that achieve critical effects) across three domains: personal management, leisure, and work. Evans and Scotti proposed that a learner with a profound disability who could initiate a routine only, without being able to perform the core of the routine, could be said to participate meaningfully. For example, "an individual [*sic*] providing a signal that he needs to be toileted would generally be preferred over the complete lack of any component of the toileting routine" (p. 92).

Finally, various motor measures might be used to determine significant progress. Landesman-Dwyer and Sackett (1978), for example, measured increases in eye movement, head and facial movement, and trunk and limb movements in persons who were nonambulatory and profoundly mentally retarded. To the degree to which those movements made individuals more comfortable or gave them greater access to people, either directly or indirectly, they could be said to be "significant." Naturally, one would choose movements that were more likely to be shaped into more complex behaviors or that by themselves could be used to initiate actions or engagement. Evans and Scotti (1989) described two other possible motor measures. The first is endurance of simple to complex motor actions to enable individuals to gain physical benefits. The second measure is eye movements, which might be measured electronically.

In short, "meaningful skills" and "significant progress" can be operationalized. Teachers confronting learners with the most severe disabilities might do well to avoid being drawn into established patterns of translating needed skills wholesale into IEP goals and objectives. Rather, they might look at the behaviors, however small and fleeting, and skills those students exhibit and become keen observers of those behaviors, with all their nuances. The teachers in the Thompson and Guess (1989) study talked about placing great value on increasing levels of awareness and looking for indications that students were reacting to environmental input, including eye flutters and subtle changes in expression.

In addition, professionals who work with very challenging students will need to rely more heavily on parents in all phases of the students' educational lives. Tawney (1984) described a project (Next Step) to train parents to evaluate the quality of their children's IEP and educational programs. Tawney's point is well taken: "If I were the parent of a severely handicapped child, and you, as public school administrators, teachers, or behavior analysts, told me that my child was ineducable, despite your best faith efforts to train/educate him or her, I would start asking some questions" (p. 293). Those questions, which span evaluation, program development, and accountability, are well worth examining. No teacher who asked those questions of himself or herself, and honestly responded to them, could fail to be a better teacher.

Future Needs

This section provides several suggestions for future research and development activities to help address the question, "What constitutes an appropriate education?"

Conduct Research on Feelings and Beliefs

To determine an appropriate education for individuals with profound disabilities, it first seems necessary to understand their needs. Knowing someone well leads to greater caring and an appreciation for the necessity of choosing goals and activities wisely. It would be useful to conduct qualitative research on the feelings and beliefs of individuals with the most severe disabilities and their families. The study by Thompson and Guess (1989) could serve as a model, with the methodology altered to secure information from people who are nonverbal.

Teach History, Law, and Policy

As Blatt said, "For a child to change, his teacher has to change" (1981, p. 29). The field needs to do a better job educating prospective and current teachers in educational/social history, law, and policy. Teachers will do a better job if they are committed to the students with whom they work. Greater commitment will result from an understanding of the ways in which individuals with disabilities represent a disenfranchised minority (Biklen & Knoll, 1987). It is important to appreciate the social, as well as the educational, context in which schools and teachers operate. Making teachers more aware of these things will make them better teachers by making them more dedicated, *caring* teachers.

Examine the IEP Process

Much has been written about the ways in which IEPs are developed and the ways in which parents are involved or excluded (e.g., Hawkins & Hawkins, 1981). It has been suggested in previous sections of this chapter that the involvement of parents and other care providers is especially critical in developing instructional content for learners with profound disabilities. It would be worthwhile for educators and researchers to explore the processes by which IEPs are developed for persons with severe disabilities, particularly with respect to parent participation.

Continue Work on Curriculum Models

Noonan and Reese (1984) suggest that research and curriculum development be conducted to de-termine questions of educational benefit. There is an even more basic need to determine the benefits of various curriculum models for selecting content for learners with profound disabilities. Each of the most prominent models (developmental model, environmental model, Individualized Curriculum Sequencing model) has benefits, but also some clear drawbacks (Brinker, 1985a).

Conduct Longitudinal Research on Adult Needs

One of the established strategies for selecting instructional goals is to focus on those skills the learner needs to function in his or her adult life. But we actually know very little about the adult lives of individuals with the most significant disabilities, since relatively few of them have had the opportunity to live in the community. It would be useful to begin obtaining a data base on the social, domestic, and vocational activities and needs of those adults.

Conduct Research on Higher Order Effects

Dunst et al. (1985) recommend that we systematically collect data to determine the second- and third-order effects of operant learning in individuals with profound disabilities. Such data certainly would provide some direction on what behaviors would provide the greatest chance of social pay-offs. This type of research would involve looking not just at children, but also at those people in the environment whom the children influence and by whom they are influenced. In general, research that paid greater attention to the entire social context of learning could pay great dividends.

Conduct Research on Functions of Behaviors

Some recent work on the communicative functions of excess behaviors (e.g., Carr & Durand, 1985) has been extremely beneficial in helping us to formulate more humane and effective strategies for reducing difficult behaviors. This line of research needs to be continued for individuals with profound disabilities, many of whom exhibit multiple, challenging forms of behaviors. In addition, Holvoet (1989) suggests that similar research be conducted on the functions of spontaneous, adaptive behavior. Understanding the *functions* of behavior will help us choose those behaviors that have the greatest potential for being meaningful for a particular individual.

Explore Quality-of-Life Issues

Sailor et al. asserted that "quantifying 'quality of life' in a way that allows for measurement of outcomes of educational programs for persons with the most severe disabilities is one of the greatest challenges we face in the coming decade" (1988, p. 89). This statement relates in part to the need to further develop more sensitive outcome measures. It also concerns a marriage of measurement and values, epitomized by the earlier quote by Holvoet (1989, p. 70). Conducting research on quality of life forces the researcher to ask the question, "What is meaningful?"

WHAT STRATEGIES ARE AVAILABLE FOR TEACHING STUDENTS WITH PROFOUND DISABILITIES?

Perhaps the most divisive issue in the educability debate has centered on the degree to which individuals with the most severe disabilities are viewed as capable of learning. Those who have argued in the negative have followed one of two lines of reasoning. The first cites inherent limitations on the student's impaired organic function. Ellis (1979) has stated this case more fervently than most, claiming that behavior modification is useless against a damaged central nervous system. Moreover, Ellis stated, "Without . . . normally functioning tissue, adaptive behavior does not occur" (1979, p. 29). The second line of reasoning, which is used more commonly, is that the technology itself has limits. As Bailey claimed, "To suggest . . . that we have a technology capable of *habilitating* this type of client is misleading at best and unethical at worst" (1981, p. 48).

Those who have taken the position that all individuals should be considered educable (Baer, 1981; Hawkins & Hawkins, 1981; Marshall & Marks, 1981; Roos, 1979) claim that the training technology is still largely unexplored. Baer summarized this point as follows: "A child cannot be declared unteachable in fact until teaching has been tried and has failed; teaching is too large a set of procedures . . . to have been tried and to have failed in its entirety" (1981, p. 96).

Despite the hopeful prognosis by many in the field, based on enthusiasm for a powerful instructional technology, it is true that the data base is sorely lacking (Tawney, 1984). The situation continues to improve gradually, particularly over the past several years, as the profession continues to renew its commitment to those individuals with the most severe disabilities. This section examines some of the literature with respect to strategies for teaching skills and behaviors to these individuals. The focus is on research designed to influence outcomes, what Sailor et al. (1988) termed "dependent variable" research. As is evident, the research in this field is limited.

Demonstrations of Awareness and Change

The early part of the modern era of research with individuals considered profoundly handicapped (i.e., the 1960s and 1970s) seems to have been concerned with demonstrating that such individuals could do something, or, more accurately, were "conditionable." The nature of the behaviors or tasks themselves were subordinate to the evidence that change occurred as a result of an intervention or stimulus. The famous study by Fuller (1949), in which a young man was taught to raise his arm through continuous reinforcement, gave birth to similar research (e.g., Murphy & Doughty, 1977; Rice, 1968; Rice & McDaniel, 1966; Rice, McDaniel, Stallings, & Gatz, 1967). Later research (Haskett & Hollar, 1978; Utley, Duncan, Strain, & Scanlon, 1983) took the demonstrations of simple conditioning of gross motor behaviors a step further by showing that children with profound disabilities were able to discriminate contingent from noncontingent events. In the Utley et al. study, 4 young children received vision stimulation (Christmas lights) either contingently, by visually fixating at a night light, or noncontingently. All children demonstrated longer duration of visual fixation to the sensory stimulation display during sessions of contingent stimulation. Haskett and Hollar discussed the importance of their own work as follows: "These results are thus at odds with the notion that profoundly retarded persons learn only with the greatest difficulty (if at all) or that they prefer relatively sterile, invariant environments over those affording visual and auditory stimuli" (1978, p. 66). A practical application of this early work on simple operant conditioning can be found in Goetz, Gee, Baldwin, and Sailor (1982), who established a reliable operant response to an auditory cue in students with profound disabilities. This linkage allowed students to participate in formal audiological assessment.

In addition to establishing contingency awareness, Haskett and Hollar (1978) also demonstrated that children with profound disabilities were able to be reinforced by sensory stimulation (see also Bailey & Meyerson, 1969). These studies, among others, gave rise to additional research that showed that some individuals with the most severe disabilities demonstrated consistent preferences for selected reinforcers. The majority of work in this area concentrated on the presentation of sensory reinforcers, primarily tactile, visual, and auditory (e.g., Dewson & Whiteley, 1987; Fehr, Wacker, Trezise, Lennon, & Meyerson, 1979; Gutierrez-Griep, 1984; Wacker, Berg, Wiggins, Muldoon, & Cavanaugh, 1985).

Indeed, several recent studies (Green et al., 1988; Pace, Ivancic, Edwards, Iwata, & Page, 1985; Wacker et al., 1985) examined procedures for identifying reinforcer preferences for students with profound disabilities, a traditional problem for many teachers. None of the studies, unfortunately, evaluated reinforcer selection procedures in an applied, functional manner. Two of them (Green et al., 1988; Pace et al., 1985) were conducted in training centers, and the process for selecting the potential reinforcing stimuli and, in some cases, the target behaviors, was based on convenience, rather than similarity to naturally occurring situations. Nevertheless, the research clearly revealed how individualized and consistent the choice of reinforcers was for participants. Those data, plus the finding by Green et al. (1988) that caregivers' opinions of student preferences were remarkably invalid, suggest that staff take the time to assess carefully the reinforcing value of consequent events.

A recent study by Wacker, Wiggins, Fowler,

and Berg (1988) not only avoided the problem of nonfunctionality of the previous work, but cleverly extended and applied previous findings within functional programs. Students with profound disabilities were taught to use microswitches to activate prerecorded messages that signaled the teacher to attend to them. The students also used the device to make requests of other staff in the school and community. This study's use of social reinforcement extends our knowledge of reinforcing events beyond edibles and sensory reinforcers. Moreover, Wacker et al. (1988) applied microswitch technology in functional activities both at school and in the community.

Teaching Functional Skills

It is clear that the profession and technology have passed the stage where demonstrations of simple change are necessary or useful. The IEPs of students with profound disabilities contain various goals, all of which, it is hoped, are "meaningful" or have "significance." This section reviews research and demonstrations with individuals with profound disabilities within several curricular domains: communication, self-help, motor, and community living.

Communication Skills

As Reichle, York, and Eynon (1989) have observed, few empirically based studies have been conducted with individuals with profound disabilities with respect to establishing skills leading to social interactions. Fortunately, some excellent work in the communication area focused on learners with the most severe disabilities has appeared in the past few years. Most of this literature is devoted to describing models for understanding communication development and to suggesting specific assessment and intervention strategies. Although much empirical research remains to be conducted, practitioners now have a relative wealth of strategies to try with a group of learners, few of whom possess the skills to control their environment (i.e., to communicate their needs and desires). This section very briefly summarizes some of the recent work in this area.

Noonan and Siegel-Causey (in press) describe strategies for establishing initial communication repertoires. These strategies are subsumed under the four areas described below.

1. *Enhancing sensitivity* Caregiver sensitivity to early communication attempts has been shown to be vital to further communication. Enhancing sensitivity is possible through: 1) being familiar with the student's nonsymbolic behavior (e.g., opening mouth, turning head), and 2) assigning meaning or intentionality to the student's nonsymbolic behavior (e.g., smacking his or her lips when he or she has finished a bite of food).

2. *Increasing opportunities* Learning to communicate requires ensuring opportunities to do so. Caregivers can increase opportunities by: 1) perceiving students' communication needs through noting situations that are highly motivating or that might promote communication; 2) creating communication opportunities by delaying anticipation of students' needs and desires; and 3) interrupting students in the middle of a behavioral sequence and requiring a communicative response to continue.

3. *Sequencing experiences* It is helpful to organize daily activities into a regular, sequential format to allow learners to become familiar with the recurrent patterns. Sequencing experiences may be facilitated by: 1) providing natural, recurring events (e.g., daily dressing and meals, leisure activities); and 2) responding contingently to student behaviors immediately and reliably.

4. *Utilizing movement* Noonan and Siegel-Causey (in press) suggest that the movement-based approach of van Dijk (e.g., 1986) could be extended and adapted to include children with significant disabilities. As they observe, the van Dijk model was designed for students with sensory impairments, but no motor or physical impairments. While Writer (1987) has noted that little empirical research exists on the efficacy of the approach, two studies do suggest a direction for further work. In the first study, Sternberg, Pegnatore, and Hill (1983) successfully employed a prelanguage communication procedure to increase communication awareness responses in four children with profound mental retardation. The procedure consisted generally of the experimenter sitting in close physical contact with the student and moving with the student, while simultaneously verbalizing the actions that were taking place. The various awareness responses included reaching toward the experimenter, cooing, and smiling. The second study (Sternberg, McNerney, & Pegnatore, 1985) extended the earlier work by using similar techniques to develop "co-active imitative behaviors" (clapping hands, placing hands on knees, jumping) with 3 students with profound disabilities.

It is well known that many of the students with the most severe disabilities not only are nonverbal, but have significant impairments in movement and vision and hearing. Thus, much of the recent work in communication has concentrated on nonsymbolic communication. Siegel-Causey and Downing (1987) have described numerous instructional techniques for facilitating development of nonsymbolic behaviors for communicative purposes. The strategies are designed for learners with dual sensory impairments, a traditionally underserved group. Most of the techniques Siegel-Causey and Downing described are also applicable to students with profound disabilities who are *not* sensory impaired. The basic thrust of their approach is to promote behaviors that lead from unintentional to intentional communication at a nonsymbolic level. After presenting general guidelines for promoting communicative competence (e.g., teach within natural routines, use functional settings with nondisabled peers, provide activities that promote communication frequently throughout the day), Siegel-Causey and Downing described nine intervention strategies:

1. Sensitivity to individual preferences and dislikes
2. Compensation for lack of distance senses
3. Responsivity to the individual's attempts to communicate
4. Consistency in instructional structure and format
5. Providing contingencies
6. Creating a need to communicate
7. Incorporating time-delay into adult responses
8. Establishing a cooperative social environment
9. Increasing expectations for communicative behavior (1987, pp. 30–31)

For each of the nine strategies, a variety of more specific strategies are provided for the caregiver to attempt. For example, under "establishing a cooperative social environment," Siegel-Causey and Downing suggest the following: "Establish situations for peer interaction that incorporate turn taking *and* physical contact during the individual's play/recreational periods. . . . As much as possible, encourage the individual to participate in reciprocal roles of an activity (pushing/pulling a wagon) . . . " (1987, p. 40). (A complete review of the literature on nonsymbolic processes has been performed by Siegel-Causey, Ernst, & Guess, 1987.)

Reichle et al. (1989) have explored another level of communicative competence for persons with profound disabilities in the form of initiating, maintaining, and terminating interactions. The authors use as a basis the class of skills called "indicating preferences." One of the first steps in teaching students to indicate preference is to help them to obtain desired objects as a way of teaching them that their actions exert control over the environment. Teaching this skill is contingent on discovering objects that are sufficiently motivating to the student. The reinforcer selection studies cited previously (i.e., Wacker et al., 1985, 1988) could be useful toward this end.

After determining reinforcing events, the teacher (therapist, parent, etc.) seeks discrete voluntary behaviors in the student that could be used to approximate self-selecting. These might range from looking and changes in facial expression to reaching and vocalizing. "The target behavior is the one that: 1) is under the most precise voluntary control; 2) is relatively easy to execute, motorically . . . ; and 3) can be physically prompted by the interventionist, if necessary" (Reichle et al., 1989, p. 196).

Finally, a study by Stremel-Campbell and Matthews (1987) is worth noting. The authors reviewed the communication/language IEPs and educational programs for over 200 children with dual sensory impairments and summarized the major weaknesses, as follows:

1. A large number of "stimulation" programs for children without systematic intervention goals or data;
2. Overall, a lack of receptive "input" that includes gesture or tactile cues so the child can learn to construct meanings about his world;
3. A large number of expressive objectives of sign training signs—even though the children may not be demonstrating prelinguistic com-

munication and have had the same objective for 2–5 years without demonstrating progress;
4. A lack of training being conducted in ongoing natural routines without utilizing objects and activities that the child is interested in; and
5. A lack of programmatic communication objectives in which turn-taking, joint attention, joint action sequences are trained. (Stremel-Campbell & Matthews, 1987, p. 162)

We know enough to know what does *not* work, and we also know a fair amount about what probably *does* work, or at least has a reasonable chance of succeeding. Obviously, communication skills in individuals with profound disabilities cannot be taught in isolation. The task of pulling it together lies ahead, but there is good reason to be optimistic.

Self-Help Skills

This area spans such diverse skills as dressing, eating, toileting, and grooming. For this reason, it is impossible to treat the topic comprehensively in this section. Moreover, since many individuals with the most severe disabilities also have significant motor and sensory disabilities, as well as associated health impairments, it is difficult and admittedly artificial to address specific teaching strategies without addressing the students' total physical needs. Given this caveat, this section nevertheless highlights a few notable studies that have discussed some ways to teach individuals with profound handicaps.

In the realm of mealtime skills, Orelove and Sobsey have summarized nine major categories of intervention: "1) modifying position of the student, 2) modifying foods, 3) modifying utensils, 4) modifying feeding schedules, 5) modifying presentation of foods, 6) modifying the mealtime environment, 7) modifying physical assistance, 8) providing sensory stimulation, and 9) providing specific training" (1987, p. 225). A review of these nine categories reveals that some strategies (e.g., providing sensory stimulation, modifying schedules) focus on the environmental antecedents, whereas others (e.g., providing specific training, modifying presentation of foods) rely more on the activities within the eating situation itself.

Several empirical studies are noteworthy for their application of various teaching procedures to individuals with profound disabilities. Thompson, Iwata, and Poynter (1979) taught a 10-year-old boy with multiple disabilities (profound retardation, cerebral palsy, hearing and vision loss) to reduce his tongue thrust and to chew more appropriately through contingent reinforcement and mild punishment (gently pushing his tongue back in his mouth). Sobsey and Orelove (1984) applied a package of oral stimulation procedures to facilitate eating skills, such as lip closure and swallowing, and to decrease interfering behaviors, such as spilling. Ulicny, Thompson, Favell, and Thompson (1985) taught a 16-year-old girl with profound disabilities, who previously had made no progress in eating, to transfer food from her tray to her mouth without assistance. They used a variation of the "mini-meal" technique (Azrin & Armstrong, 1973; Stimbert, Minor, & McCoy, 1977), in which meals are divided into smaller portions and served hourly. Apart from the studies cited, there is little empirical literature on strategies for working with individuals who lack key oral-motor skills, such as lip closure, swallowing, and chewing. This relative lack of research may stem partly from the practical difficulties of observing and measuring such behaviors. This is a prime area of research on which therapists and special educators can collaborate (Sobsey & Orelove, 1983).

Many individuals with multiple disabilities are physically unable to perform key components of toileting sequences. As a result, they are usually schedule trained. Regardless, a few studies with individuals with profound mental retardation offer some strategies for toilet training. The reader is encouraged to consult Lancioni and Ceccarani (1981), Richmond (1983), and Smith, Britton, Johnson, and Thomas (1975). Few data are available, unfortunately, that compare approaches, and most studies were conducted in residential settings. There is also a marked use of aversive consequences within many of the toileting programs, although the efficacy of such procedures has not been assessed. There is good reason to believe, in fact, that such aversive techniques not only are unnecessary, but are detrimental to long-term success and to positive relationships between the student and the caregiver. Once again, a team approach to conducting research on toileting, one that would include educators, therapists, and medical personnel, would greatly bolster a critical, yet understudied, area.

As Snell (1987) has noted, even less attention has been given in the research literature to study of dressing skills training. Snell also has observed that improvement in the dressing skills of institutionalized individuals with profound mental retardation taught by traditional operant methods has been gradual. The typical approach has been to adapt clothing whenever possible and to employ various prompting hierarchies (e.g., graduated guidance), while incorporating partial participation (i.e., requiring parts of a dressing sequence or different forms of the steps in the chain). Perhaps the key piece of research remains the study by Azrin, Schaeffer, and Wesolowski (1976), who taught adults to remove and put on five garments as an entire sequence. Snell summarized the training techniques as follows:

> Long instructional sessions (3 hours); the instruction of all steps simultaneously in a forward progression; extensive use of manual guidance early in learning . . . ; systematic application and fading of prompts; continuous use of praise and stroking contingent upon any effort to follow instruction or guidance; the requirement of visual attention to the task; and the initial involvement of two trainers so that praise, stroking, and manual guidance could be provided. (1987, p. 382)

An attempt to replicate the Azrin et al. study met with only partial success (Diorio & Konarski, 1984). Although the participants made individual gains, 1 person failed to reach criterion on undressing, and all 3 failed to acquire independent dressing skills.

In short, the literature on teaching self-help skills to individuals with profound disabilities is spotty. There are few systematic replications of procedures, and many studies rely on complex packages of techniques that rarely are employed separately to determine the effectiveness of individual components. Many of the procedures used with individuals with severe disabilities certainly could be adapted for persons with profound disabilities.

Motor Skills

This area in some ways is the most critical for individuals with profound disabilities and the most challenging for their caregivers. Students' movement and posture are directly linked not only to their health and comfort, but to their ability to communicate, to take in information, and, generally, to participate in activities at school and in the community.

Indeed, a glance at Jennifer's IEP (Bostrom, 1983), a 3-year-old girl with degenerative brain disease, reveals the following goals: 1) move her left leg when heel cord stretch is being performed by an adult, 2) move her head when given verbal and physical cues in a supine or supported sitting position, and 3) hold her head straight while in a supine position. These sorts of goals often typify the educational planning for children with multiple disabilities, yet our knowledge about how to plan successful interventions remains somewhat rudimentary.

We know a bit more about how to shape whole units of motor behaviors into meaningful skills or how to increase the rate or intensity of existing movements. Various researchers have used prompting and reinforcement, sometimes delivered contingently through microswitches, to improve students' head control (Ball, McCrady, & Hart, 1975; Caro & Renzaglia, 1986; Maloney & Kurtz, 1982), posture (Burch, Clegg, & Bailey, 1987), sitting (Kuharski, Rues, Cook, & Guess, 1985), and reaching and grasping (Correa, Poulson, & Salzberg, 1984).

Despite these successful demonstrations, Campbell reminded us that "disorders in posture and movement abilities are frequently so severe in individuals with profound disabilities that remediation cannot be achieved through currently used treatment and intervention approaches" (1989, p. 164). Campbell (1989) summarized two alternative approaches that have greater promise for persons with profound disabilities. The first is a *prevention-intervention* approach, in which programming is designed to prevent further development of physical disabilities. Campbell (1989) described several strategies under this approach, including positioning to maintain muscle length and using passive deep pressure on muscles. The second is a *compensatory* approach, in which compensation for the severity of the disability is made. The two most common types of compensation are adaptive equipment (e.g., to facilitate an individual's position)

and switch interface devices (see Campbell, 1987a; 1987c; Rainforth & York, 1987; and York & Rainforth, 1987).

Two of the difficulties in developing motor skills are training movements that are functional for the student and integrating therapeutic and instructional methodologies. Campbell (1987a) described a model for doing both and provided examples. Perhaps more than any other single area, the incorporation of motor behaviors within meaningful activities requires the collaboration of a team of individuals (Campbell, 1987b; Orelove & Sobsey, 1987).

Community Living Skills

In an area conspicuous by its lack of a body of research with individuals with profound disabilities, one recent study deserves mention. Gee, Graham, Lee, and Goetz (1988) worked with 3 children who are medically fragile and considered "the most seriously challenged." All 3 were nonambulatory and had no formal communication system; their instructional objectives centered on increasing their ability to receive information and to gain control over their environment. For each child, the dependent measure was acquisition of four to six specific motor and sensory behaviors. A thorough process for selecting target measures was used, involving the use of "natural contexts and ongoing routines" (Gee et al., 1988, p. 6). Individualized operant instructional procedures were written to teach each skill. The independent variable was the use of interspersed trials, and the trainers used only naturally occurring opportunities for instruction. The students increased their levels of competence on 8 of the 15 skills taught; no student completed the final criterion level on every skill. This study, as have many others with individuals with moderate or severe disabilities, suggested that training in the natural environment, despite the initial practical obstacles, yields superior results instructionally.

Reducing Excess Behaviors

Individuals with the most severe disabilities engage in numerous, and often multiple forms, of behaviors that range from being annoying to others to being personally life threatening. A brief discussion of this topic is relevant here for several reasons. First, many of the most challenging of these behaviors interfere with attempts to develop other, more acceptable skills, thereby perpetuating the image of the individual as "ineducable." Second, the exhibition of excess behaviors (especially aggressive or destructive behaviors) sometimes is used by school administrators as the sole reason for trying to exclude individuals with profound disabilities from programs. Third, it is essential to understand that excess behaviors and adaptive behaviors generally are two different sides of the same coin. Reducing one behavior cannot be viewed in the absence of strengthening another behavior.

This final point is a key element of what has been termed an *educative* approach to behavior problems (Evans & Meyer, 1985; Meyer & Evans, 1989). In contrasting this approach to an "eliminative" approach, Meyer and Evans described four major assumptions:

> First, *the major purpose of habilitative services is to encourage adaptive behavior and to promote maximum participation by the individual in meaningful daily experiences. . . .* Second, *not all behavior problems are equal priority targets for behavior change. . . .* Third, *even when a behavior problem is a priority, the most effective strategy to reduce it is to replace it with a skill that accomplishes its function for the individual. . . .* Fourth, *even when a behavior problem is a priority and there will be a decelerative program to change it, interventions to do this must be normalized. . . .* (1989, pp. 14–15)

In a stunning application of an educative approach, Berkman and Meyer (1988) worked with a 45-year-old man who exhibited multiple and severe self-injurious behaviors. The authors instituted a four-component intervention plan, which included: 1) changing the stimulus conditions associated with self-injury, 2) teaching positive alternative behaviors, 3) involving the individual in all phases of decision making regarding his daily schedule of activities, and 4) providing for back-up crisis-management procedures to prevent further self-injury. Outcomes included a dramatic decrease in all forms of self-injurious behavior, as well as maintenance and generalization of those changes to integrated community environments.

Future Needs

Once again, this section highlights some of the needs for research and demonstration in educating those children with the most challenging disabilities.

Conduct Research on Instructional Formats

The language of instructional programming for individuals with severe disabilities is replete with terms such as "forward and backward chaining," "least prompts," "graduated guidance," "time delay," and "interspersed trials." While we know relatively little about which types of prompting, chaining, and trial presentation formats work best for a given student with a severe disability on a given task or activity, we know even less about those same questions for individuals who present the most severe challenges.

Research by Steege, Wacker, and McMahon (1987) and a review by Ault, Wolery, Doyle, and Gast (1989) have suggested some directions for the field. Steege et al. compared two stimulus prompt strategies used to teach students with severe disabilities four community living skills. In the first strategy, termed "traditional," the trainer reinforced correct performance on each task step. If the student failed to initiate a response within 5 seconds, the trainer provided successively more restrictive instructional prompts until the student gave the desired response. The second strategy, termed "prescriptive," was similar to the traditional technique, but data from each trial were used to prescribe the level of prompt to be delivered during the next trial. Both techniques were equally effective, although the prescriptive strategy was more efficient.

Ault et al. (1989) performed a comparative review of studies that used instructional strategies with persons with either moderate or severe disabilities. Procedures were evaluated on their effectiveness and efficiency. The authors made four recommendations for future research and practice, which could apply equally to work with individuals with more significant disabilities: 1) conduct more studies comparing the effectiveness and efficiency of instructional strategies, 2) conduct investigations of the specific variables of single strategies to identify the most efficient use of each procedure, 3) expand the efficiency measures to assess whether students learn information not directly targeted for instruction, and 4) conduct research to determine which strategy is best to use with given types of students and skills.

In conducting studies on instructional strategies with learners with profound disabilities, researchers will need to control and to plan for the wider range of input to and output from these individuals. The presentation of instructional materials and antecedent and consequent events will be dramatically influenced by the degree and type of sensory function/loss, the extent of alertness, the ability to maintain posture and to orient to stimuli, the type and quality of movement, the rate of responding, and so forth. It will be critical for researchers to describe carefully the learners' sensory, physical, and behavioral characteristics to allow a body of research to be generated in a careful fashion.

There are also nonempirical issues to be explored in the area of instructional programming. For example, if prompts can never be faded or reduced, are they still useful? Partial participation suggests that some steps in a sequence may always need to be performed by the instructor. What if an entire sequence consists of such steps (and they cannot be replaced through adaptations, such as microswitches)? A point comes when the teacher, parent, and other professionals ask if the effort is worth including the task or activity on the IEP. It is suggested here that issues of instructional efficiency be weighed against the student's dignity and the parents' desires and perceptions.

Conduct Research on Motivation and Attention

Holvoet (1989) has observed that many individuals with profound disabilities seem unresponsive to the environment, yet it is not clear to what degree this is the result of central nervous system damage, learned helplessness, ill-chosen reinforcers, and so forth. Recent work on biobehavioral states (Guess et al., 1988; Rainforth,

1982) has provided a potentially rich avenue for further research. Guess et al. suggested two primary areas: 1) identifying more sensitive measures for assessing the level of awareness of self and the environment for students who show minimal alertness to the environment, and 2) examining biological/physiological conditions that potentially affect state conditions (e.g., medications, seizures, nutrition).

In addition, Holvoet (1989) suggested that further research be done on students' perception of contingency relationships and on various types of stimulation and reinforcers. She hypothesized that individuals who receive things noncontingently and without asking for them may have greater difficulty perceiving contingency relationships and, hence, may have a more difficult time learning. Holvoet also suggested that individuals with profound disabilities, because of their central nervous system dysfunction, may be more motivated by stimuli that are received by their primitive senses (i.e., olfactory, tactile, and vestibular-proprioceptive).

Examine the Use of Technology

Warren, Horn, and Hill stated that "technological innovation can and should promote actual learning of new skills within the target domain, and increase and optimize teacher-learner contact" (1987, p. 285). Warren et al. further observed that "to date very few technological education innovations have been subjected to any type of empirical analysis of effectiveness along these dimensions" (1987, p. 285) and specifically critiqued the scant research performed to date.

The use of technology thus far has been limited mainly to simple microswitches to activate toys and vocational apparatus. The use of more sophisticated technology, such as microcomputer-mediated instruction of motor skills (see Warren et al., 1987), has been limited to demonstration projects or to an individual child or program that had access to someone particularly resourceful. Even in cases where teachers have been taught to construct microswitches, the educational goals often become subservient to—or unrelated to—the switches themselves. Thus, there is good reason to be extremely cautious about the application of technology to individuals with profound disabilities (indeed, the recent book by F. Brown & Lehr [1989] contained no mention of the subject). Yet interdisciplinary efforts between medicine, education, biomedical engineering, physical and occupational therapy, and other fields are long overdue in designing devices that take students' complex motor, sensory, and behavioral skills and needs into consideration. Particularly needed are adaptations and devices that are simple and affordable, and thus readily available to schools with few resources.

Examine Services for
Individuals who are Medically Fragile

As the number of students with complex health care needs (including those considered medically fragile) has increased, school programs have had to reexamine how to deliver necessary educational and related services. Mulligan-Ault, Guess, Struth, and Thomas (1988) have observed that many such individuals have been treated as patients rather than as students. Moreover, the questions of *who* should be providing health care services, and *how* those services should be integrated into the school day, are being legitimately raised. Since many of these students are absent from school a great deal (Thompson & Guess, 1989), concerns with regression and recoupment of skills need to be explored.

Conduct Research
on Special Needs of Families

The extraordinary needs of children with the most severe disabilities, especially those with multiple health concerns, places extraordinary demands on families. At the same time, it is critical that parents be given opportunities to be involved in educational planning for their children. The problem is that many families simply do not have the time (cf. Featherstone, 1980).

A second issue around parents concerns the role they often are asked to assume as interventionists. Kogan, Tyler, and Turner (1974) studied a group of mothers as they interacted with their young children with cerebral palsy during play and therapy sessions. When mothers were performing therapy, both mother and child dis-

played greater amounts of negative behaviors than when they were playing, which persisted over the 2 years of the study. Moreover, the mothers progressively became less friendly and warm during both play and therapy sessions as the study progressed. Kogan et al. hypothesized that "parents may be concentrating most heavily on deficits and failing to appreciate or respond to areas of competence and uncomplicated development; that is, they are focusing on the area which provides them with the least positive feedback" (1974, p. 525).

It would be worthwhile to examine how professionals interact with parents who have children with the most severe disabilities and the degree to which it is appropriate to expect them to be able to participate in planning and intervention. It would be unwise to expect parents to act as interventionists at the expense of being parents, with the attendant responsibility for nurturing their own emotional growth, as well as that of their child.

Conduct Work on
Peer Interactions/Relationships

There is good documentation of the beneficial effects of integrated services on nonhandicapped students, in terms of their increased acceptance and support (e.g., Biklen, Corrigan, & Quick, 1989; Brinker, 1985b; Brinker & Thorpe, 1986; Haring, Breen, Pitts-Conway, Lee, & Gaylord-Ross, 1987; Voeltz, 1982). There is also empirical support for increases in the interactive behavior of students with severe disabilities as a function of structured intervention in integrated settings (e.g., Breen, Haring, Pitts-Conway, & Gaylord-Ross, 1985; Cole, Meyer, Vandercook, & McQuarter, 1986).

However, little has been done in either of these areas with respect to individuals with the most severe disabilities. Demonstrating clear benefits for both groups would have important implications for social policy and for the delivery of educational services. Research on these topics could combine the methodologies currently being used to study reciprocal horizontal social interactions (cf. Halvorsen & Sailor, in press) and those contained within the communication studies with nonverbal individuals described previously in this chapter.

Continue to Develop Supportive Systems

This final recommendation is different from those preceding, in that it is more of a plea to refine and expand what is already happening to include individuals with the most severe disabilities. Sailor et al. (1988) have described some of what needs to be done: establish policies and programs for full integration, expand community-referenced curricula and programs, increase interdisciplinary involvement, and establish greater opportunities for work and community living. To a large degree, we need to avoid getting trapped in another version of the "readiness" model, wherein we learn everything about people with profound disabilities before we offer them the full range of services to which they are entitled. The only way we can answer the question "What strategies are available for teaching individuals with profound disabilities?" is to do so in the community, in fully integrated settings.

CONCLUSION

This chapter began by underscoring that the educability debate is over 10 years old. In another decade, we reach the beginning of a new millennium. Over the long haul, there is nothing magical about one year over another. The idea of the year "2000," however, is sobering. It gives rise to a sense of a passage of time that is more dramatic than when we move from, say, 1991 to 1992. The idea of the year 2000 seems so remote and, yet, most of us will still be around, still teaching and writing and researching. It would be magnificent, indeed, to write a follow-up chapter in the year 2000 that talks about the advances of the past 10 years and looks ahead to the next century. Those past 10 years begin right now. There is much work to do. Timothy W.'s successors await.

It is fitting to close with the words of Burton Blatt, taken from his final book, published posthumously in 1987:

> The educability hypothesis has suffered both at the hands of those who would not consider it (in spite of any evidence), and by those who insist on propagating it (in spite of a paucity of evidence). Like the ideas of normalization, deinstitutionalization, conservatism, or liberalism, the educability hypothesis is powered (or dismissed) by the conception one has of what human beings ought to be like and what opportunities they ought to have. Whether the educability hypothesis is true or not must await further and better examination. But what may be even more important is the idea that people should be treated—in schools, in developmental facilities, by their families, by society—*as if* they can change, *as if* careful systematic intervention on their behalf will make a difference. (p. 58)

REFERENCES

Ault, M.J., Wolery, M., Doyle, P.M., & Gast, D.L. (1989). Review of comparative studies in the instruction of students with moderate and severe handicaps. *Exceptional Children, 55,* 346–356.

Azrin, N., & Armstrong, P. (1973). The "minimeal"—A method for teaching eating skills to the profoundly retarded. *Mental Retardation, 11,* 9–13.

Azrin, N.H., Schaeffer, R.M., & Wesolowski, M.D. (1976). A rapid method of teaching profoundly retarded persons to dress by a reinforcement-guidance method. *Mental Retardation, 14*(6), 29–33.

Baer, D.M. (1981). A hung jury and a Scottish verdict: "Not proven." *Analysis and Intervention in Developmental Disabilities, 1,* 91–97.

Baer, D.M. (1984). We already have multiple jeopardy: Why try for unending jeopardy? In W.L. Heward, T. Heron, D. Hill, & J. Trap-Porter (Eds.), *Behavior analysis in education* (pp. 296–299). Columbus, OH: Charles E. Merrill.

Bailey, J.S. (1981). Wanted: A rational search for the limiting conditions of habilitation in the retarded. *Analysis and Intervention in Developmental Disabilities, 1,* 45–52.

Bailey, J.S., & Meyerson, L. (1969). Vibration as a reinforcer with a profoundly retarded child. *Journal of Applied Behavior Analysis, 2,* 135–137.

Ball, T.S., McCrady, R.E., & Hart, A.D. (1975). Automated reinforcement of head postures in two cerebral palsied retarded children. *Perceptual and Motor Skills, 40,* 619–622.

Baumgart, D., Brown, L., Pumpian, I., Nisbet, J., Ford, A., Sweet, M., Messina, R., & Schroeder, J. (1982). Principle of partial participation and individualized adaptations in educational programs for severely handicapped students. *Journal of The Association for the Severely Handicapped, 1*(2), 17–27.

Berkman, K.A., & Meyer, L.H. (1988). Alternative strategies and multiple outcomes in the remediation of severe self-injury: Going "all out" nonaversively. *Journal of The Association for Persons with Severe Handicaps, 13,* 76–86.

Biklen, D., Corrigan, C., & Quick, D. (1989). Beyond obligation: Students' relations with each other in integrated classes. In D.K. Lipsky & A. Gartner (Eds.), *Beyond separate education: Quality education for all* (pp. 207–221). Baltimore: Paul H. Brookes Publishing Co.

Biklen, D., & Knoll, J. (1987). The disabled minority. In S. Taylor, D. Biklen, & J. Knoll (Eds.), *Community integration for people with severe disabilities* (pp. 3–24). New York: Teachers College Press.

Blatt, B. (1981). *In and out of mental retardation: Essays on educability, disability, and human policy.* Baltimore: University Park Press.

Blatt, B. (1987). *The conquest of mental retardation.* Austin, TX: PRO-ED.

Bostrom, S. (1983). Jennifer. *Journal of The Association for the Severely Handicapped, 8,* 58–62.

Breen, C., Haring, T., Pitts-Conway, V., & Gaylord-Ross, R. (1985). The training and generalization of social interaction during breaktime at two job sites in the natural environment. *Journal of The Association for Persons with Severe Handicaps, 10,* 41–50.

Brinker, R.P. (1985a). Curricula without recipes: A challenge to teachers and a promise to severely mentally retarded students. In D. Bricker & J. Filler (Eds.), *Severe mental retardation: From theory to practice* (pp. 208–229). Reston, VA: Council for Exceptional Children.

Brinker, R.P. (1985b). Interactions between severely mentally retarded students and other students in integrated and segregated public school settings. *American Journal of Mental Deficiency, 89,* 587–594.

Brinker, R.P., & Thorpe, M. (1986). Features of integrated educational ecologies that predict social behavior among severely mentally retarded and nonretarded students. *American Journal of Mental Deficiency, 91,* 150–159.

Brown, F., Evans, I.M., Weed, K.A., & Owen, V. (1987). Delineating functional competencies: A component model. *Journal of The Association for Persons with Severe Handicaps, 12,* 117–124.

Brown, F., & Lehr, D.H. (Eds.). (1989). *Persons with profound disabilities: Issues and practices.* Baltimore: Paul H. Brookes Publishing Co.

Brown, L., Branston-McClean, M.B., Baumgart, D., Vincent, L., Falvey, M., & Schroeder, J. (1979). Using the characteristics of current and subsequent least restrictive environments in the development of curricular content for severely handicapped students. *AAESPH Review, 4*(4), 407–424.

Burch, M., Clegg, J., & Bailey, J. (1987). Automated contingent reinforcement of correct posture. *Research in Developmental Disabilities, 8,* 15–20.

Burton, T.A., & Hirshoren, A. (1979a). The education of severely and profoundly retarded children: Are we sacrificing the child to the concept? *Exceptional Children, 45,* 598–602.

Burton, T.A., & Hirshoren, A. (1979b). Some further thoughts and clarifications on the education of severely and profoundly retarded children. *Exceptional Children, 45,* 618–625.

Campbell, P.H. (1987a). Integrated programming for students with multiple handicaps. In L. Goetz, D. Guess, & K. Stremel-Campbell (Eds.), *Innovative program design for individuals with dual sensory impairments* (pp. 159–188). Baltimore: Paul H. Brookes Publishing Co.

Campbell, P.H. (1987b). The integrated programming team: An approach for coordinating professionals of various disciplines in programs for students with severe and multiple handicaps. *Journal of The Association for Persons with Severe Handicaps, 12,* 107–116.

Campbell, P.H. (1987c). Physical management and handling procedures with students with movement dysfunction. In M.E. Snell (Ed.), *Systematic instruction of persons with severe handicaps* (3rd ed., pp. 174–187). Columbus, OH: Charles E. Merrill.

Campbell, P.H. (1989). Dysfunction in posture and movement in individuals with profound disabilities: Issues and practices. In F. Brown & D.H. Lehr (Eds.), *Persons with profound disabilities: Issues and practices* (pp. 163–189). Baltimore: Paul H. Brookes Publishing Co.

Caro, P., & Renzaglia, A. (1986). *Teaching contingency awareness and head control to young children with severe handicaps.* Unpublished manuscript, University of Illinois at Urbana-Champaign.

Carr, E.G., & Durand, V.M. (1985). Reducing behavior problems through functional communication training. *Journal of Applied Behavior Analysis, 18,* 111–126.

Cole, D.A., Meyer, L.M., Vandercook, T., & McQuarter, R.J. (1986). Interactions between peers with and without severe handicaps: The dynamics of teacher intervention. *American Journal of Mental Deficiency, 91,* 160–169.

Correa, V.I., Poulson, C.L., & Salzberg, C.L. (1984). Training and generalization of reach-grasp behavior in blind, retarded young children. *Journal of Applied Behavior Analysis, 17,* 57–69.

Dewson, M., & Whiteley, J. (1987). Sensory reinforcement of head turning with nonambulatory, profoundly mentally retarded persons. *Research in Developmental Disabilities, 8,* 413–426.

Diorio, M.S., & Konarski, E.A. (1984). Evaluation of a method for teaching dressing skills to profoundly mentally retarded persons. *American Journal of Mental Deficiency, 89*(3), 307–309.

Dunst, C.J., Cushing, P.J., & Vance, S.D. (1985). Response-contingent learning in profoundly handicapped infants: A social systems perspective. *Analysis and Intervention in Developmental Disabilities, 5,* 33–47.

Dussault, W.L.E. (1989). Is a policy of exclusion based upon severity of disability legally defensible? In F. Brown & D.H. Lehr (Eds.), *Persons with profound disabilities: Issues and practices* (pp. 45–59). Baltimore: Paul H. Brookes Publishing Co.

Ellis, N.R. (1979). The Partlow case: A reply to Dr. Roos. *Law and Psychology Review, 5*, 15–49.

Evans, I.M., Brown, F.A., Weed, K.A., Spry, K.M., & Owen, V. (1987). The assessment of functional competencies: A behavioral approach to the evaluation of programs for children with disabilities. In R.J. Prinz (Ed.), *Advances in behavioral assessment of children and families* (Vol. 3, pp. 93–121). Greenwich, CT: JAI Press.

Evans, I.M., & Meyer, L.H. (1985). *An educative approach to behavior problems: A practical decision model for interventions with severely handicapped learners.* Baltimore: Paul H. Brookes Publishing Co.

Evans, I.M., & Scotti, J.R. (1989). Defining meaningful outcomes for persons with profound disabilities. In F. Brown & D.H. Lehr (Eds.), *Persons with profound disabilities: Issues and practices* (pp. 83–107). Baltimore: Paul H. Brookes Publishing Co.

Featherstone, H. (1980). *A difference in the family.* New York: Basic Books.

Fehr, M., Wacker, D., Trezise, J., Lennon, R., & Meyerson, L. (1979). Visual, auditory, and vibratory stimulation as reinforcers for profoundly retarded children. *Rehabilitation Psychology, 26*, 201–209.

Ferguson, D. (1985). The ideal and the real: The working out of public policy in curricula for severely handicapped students. *Remedial and Special Education, 6*, 52–60.

Fuller, P.R. (1949). Operant conditioning of a vegetative human organism. *American Journal of Psychology, 62*, 587–599.

Gee, K., Graham, N., Lee, M., & Goetz, L. (1988). *The future is now: Acquisition of basic sensory and motor skills within natural, integrated contents with students facing the most serious challenges.* Unpublished manuscript, San Francisco State University.

Goetz, L., Gee, K., Baldwin, M., & Sailor, W. (1982). Classroom-based sensory assessment procedures for severely handicapped students: Case studies of a stimulus transfer paradigm. *Analysis and Intervention in Developmental Disabilities, 2*, 171–185.

Goldberg, I., & Cruickshank, W. (1958). The trainable but noneducable: Whose responsibility? *National Educational Association Journal, 47*, 622–623.

Green, C.W., Reid, D.H., White, L.K., Halford, R.C., Brittain, D.P., & Gardner, S.M. (1988). Identifying reinforcers for persons with profound handicaps: Staff opinion versus systematic assessment of preferences. *Journal of Applied Behavior Analysis, 21*, 31–43.

Guess, D., Mulligan-Ault, M., Roberts, S., Struth, J., Siegel-Causey, E., Thompson, B., Bronicki, G.J.B., & Guy, B. (1988). Implications of biobehavioral states for the education and treatment of students with the most profoundly handicapping conditions. *Journal of The Association for Persons with Severe Handicaps, 13*, 163–174.

Gutierrez-Griep, R. (1984). Student preference of sensory reinforcers. *Education and Training of the Mentally Retarded, 19*, 108–113.

Halvorsen, A., & Sailor, W. (in press). Integration of students with severe and profound disabilities: A review of research. In R. Gaylord-Ross (Ed.), *Issues and research in special education* (Vol. 1). New York: Teachers College Press.

Haring, T.G., Breen, C., Pitts-Conway, V., Lee, M., & Gaylord-Ross, R. (1987). Adolescent peer tutoring and special friend experiences. *Journal of The Association for Persons with Severe Handicaps, 12*, 280–286.

Haskett, J., & Hollar, W.D. (1978). Sensory reinforcement and contingency awareness of profoundly retarded children. *American Journal of Mental Deficiency, 83*, 60–68.

Hawkins, R.P. (1984). What is "meaningful" behavior change in a severely/profoundly retarded learner: The view of a behavior analytic parent. In W.L. Heward, T. Heron, D. Hill, & J. Trap-Porter (Eds.), *Behavior analysis in education* (pp. 282–286). Columbus, OH: Charles E. Merrill.

Hawkins, R.P., & Hawkins, K.K. (1981). Parental observations on the education of severely retarded children: Can it be done in the classroom? *Analysis and Intervention in Developmental Disabilities, 1*, 13–22.

Helmstetter, E. (1989). Curriculum for school-age students: The ecological model. In F. Brown & D.H. Lehr (Eds.), *Persons with profound disabilities: Issues and practices* (pp. 239–263). Baltimore: Paul H. Brookes Publishing Co.

Holvoet, J.F. (1989). Research with persons labeled profoundly retarded: Issues and ideas. In F. Brown & D.H. Lehr (Eds.), *Persons with profound disabilities: Issues and practices* (pp. 61–82). Baltimore: Paul H. Brookes Publishing Co.

Kauffman, J.M. (1981). Editor's introduction. *Analysis and Intervention in Developmental Disabilities, 1*, 1–3.

Kauffman, J.M., & Krouse, J. (1981). The cult of educability: Searching for the substance of things hoped for; the evidence of things not seen. *Analysis and Intervention in Developmental Disabilities, 1*, 53–60.

Kogan, K.L., Tyler, N., & Turner, P. (1974). The process of interpersonal adaptation between mothers and their cerebral palsied children. *Developmental Medicine and Child Neurology, 16*, 518–527.

Kuharski, T., Rues, J., Cook, D., & Guess, D. (1985). Effects of vestibular stimulation on sitting behaviors among preschoolers with severe handicaps. *Journal of The Association for Persons with Severe Handicaps, 10*, 137–145.

Lancioni, G.E., & Ceccarani, P.S. (1981). Teaching independent toileting within the normal daily program: Two studies with profoundly retarded children. *Behavior Research of Severe Developmental Disabilities, 2,* 79–96.

Landesman-Dwyer, S., & Sackett, G.P. (1978). Behavioral changes in nonambulatory, profoundly mentally retarded individuals. In C.E. Myers (Ed.), *Quality of life in severely and profoundly mentally retarded people: Research foundations for improvement* (pp. 55–144). Washington, DC: American Association on Mental Deficiency.

Maloney, F.P., & Kurtz, P.A. (1982). The use of a mercury switch head control device in profoundly retarded, multiply handicapped children. *Physical and Occupational Therapy in Pediatrics, 2*(4), 11–17.

Marshall, A.M., & Marks, H.E. (1981). Implementation of "zero reject" training in an institutional setting. *Analysis and Intervention in Developmental Disabilities, 1,* 23–35.

Meyer, L.H., & Evans, I.M. (1989). *Nonaversive intervention for behavior problems: A manual for home and community.* Baltimore: Paul H. Brookes Publishing Co.

Miller, J.M. (1982). *The educability debate: A question of rights, values, and responsibilities.* Unpublished manuscript, University of Virginia, Charlottesville.

Mulligan-Ault, M., Guess, D., Struth, L., & Thomas, B. (1988). Implementation of health- related procedures in classrooms for students with severe multiple impairments. *Journal of The Association for Persons with Severe Handicaps, 13,* 100–109.

Murphy, R., & Doughty, N. (1977). Establishment of controlled arm movements in profoundly retarded students using response contingent vibratory stimulation. *American Journal of Mental Deficiency, 82,* 212–216.

Noonan, M.J., & Reese, R.M. (1984). Educability: Public policy and the role of research. *Journal of The Association for Persons with Severe Handicaps, 9,* 8–15.

Noonan, M.J., & Siegel-Causey, E. (in press). Special needs of students with severe handicaps. In L. McCormick & R.L. Schiefelbusch (Eds.), *Early language intervention* (2nd ed.). Columbus, OH: Charles E. Merrill.

Orelove, F.P. (1984). The educability debate: A review and a look ahead. In W.L. Heward, T. Heron, D. Hill, & J. Trap-Porter (Eds.), *Behavior analysis in education* (pp. 271–281). Columbus, OH: Charles E. Merrill.

Orelove, F.P., & Sobsey, D. (1987). *Educating children with multiple disabilities: A transdisciplinary approach.* Baltimore: Paul H. Brookes Publishing Co.

Pace, G.M., Ivancic, M.T., Edwards, G.L., Iwata, B.A., & Page, T.J. (1985). Assessment of stimulus preference and reinforcer value with profoundly retarded individuals. *Journal of Applied Behavior Analysis, 18,* 249–255.

Rainforth, B. (1982). Biobehavioral state and orienting: Implications for educating profoundly retarded students. *Journal of The Association for the Severely Handicapped, 6,* 33–37.

Rainforth, B., & York, J. (1987). Handling and positioning. In F.P. Orelove & D. Sobsey, *Educating children with multiple disabilities: A transdisciplinary approach* (pp. 67–101). Baltimore: Paul H. Brookes Publishing Co.

Reichle, J., York, J., & Eynon, D. (1989). Influence of indicating preferences for initiating, maintaining, and terminating interactions. In F. Brown & D.H. Lehr (Eds.), *Persons with profound disabilities: Issues and practices* (pp. 191–211). Baltimore: Paul H. Brookes Publishing Co.

Rice, H.K. (1968). Operant behavior in vegetative patients, III: Methodological considerations. *Psychological Record, 18,* 297–302.

Rice, H.K., & McDaniel, M.W. (1966). Operant behavior in vegetative patients. *Psychological Record, 16,* 279–281.

Rice, H.K., McDaniel, M.W., Stallings, V.D., & Gatz, M.J. (1967). Operant behavior in vegetative patients, II. *Psychological Record, 17,* 449–460.

Richmond, G. (1983). Shaping bladder and bowel continence in developmentally retarded preschool children. *Journal of Autism and Developmental Disorders, 13,* 197–205.

Roos, P. (1979). Custodial care for the "subtrainable"—Revisiting an old myth. *Law and Psychology Review, 5,* 1–14.

Sailor, W., Gee, K., Goetz, L., & Graham, N. (1988). Progress in educating students with the most severe disabilities: Is there any? *Journal of The Association for Persons with Severe Handicaps, 13*(2), 87–99.

Siegel-Causey, E., & Downing, J. (1987). Nonsymbolic communication development. In L. Goetz, D. Guess, & K. Stremel-Campbell (Eds.), *Innovative program design for individuals with dual sensory impairments* (pp. 15–48). Baltimore: Paul H. Brookes Publishing Co.

Siegel-Causey, E., Ernst, B., & Guess, D. (1987). Elements of nonsymbolic communication and early interactional processes. In M. Bullis (Ed.), *Communication development in young children with deaf-blindness: Literature review III* (pp. 57–102). Monmouth: Oregon State University, Communication Skills Center for Young Children with Deaf-Blindness.

Smith, P.S., Britton, P.G., Johnson, M., & Thomas, D.A. (1975). Problems involved in toilet training profoundly mentally handicapped adults. *Behaviour Research and Therapy, 13,* 301–307.

Snell, M.E. (Ed.). (1987). *Systematic instruction of persons with severe handicaps* (3rd ed.). Columbus, OH: Charles E. Merrill.

Snell, M.E., & Carney, I.H. (in press). Persons with profound mental retardation and multiple handicaps. In J. Matson & D. Dietz (Eds.), *Introduc-*

tion to mental retardation. Glenview, IL: Scott, Foresman.

Sobsey, R.J., & Orelove, F.P. (1983). Conducting transdisciplinary research with severely handicapped individuals. *Education and Treatment of Children, 6,* 311–371.

Sobsey, R., & Orelove, F.P. (1984). Neurophysiological facilitation of eating skills in children with severe handicaps. *Journal of The Association for Persons with Severe Handicaps, 9,* 98–110.

Sontag, E., Certo, N., & Button, J.E. (1979). On a distinction between the education of the severely and profoundly handicapped and a doctrine of limitations. *Exeptional Children, 45,* 604–616.

Stainback, W., & Stainback, S. (1983). A review of research on the educability of profoundly retarded persons. *Education and Training of the Mentally Retarded, 18,* 90–100.

Steege, M.W., Wacker, D.P., & McMahon, C.M. (1987). Evaluation of the effectiveness and efficiency of two stimulus prompt strategies with severely handicapped students. *Journal of Applied Behavior Analysis, 20,* 293–299.

Sternberg, L., McNerney, C.D., & Pegnatore, L. (1985). Developing co-active imitative behaviors with profoundly mentally handicapped students. *Education and Training of the Mentally Retarded, 20,* 260–267.

Sternberg, L., Pegnatore, L., & Hill, C. (1983). Establishing interactive communication behaviors with profoundly mentally handicapped students. *Journal of The Association for the Severely Handicapped, 8,* 39–46.

Stimbert, V.E., Minor, J.W., & McCoy, J.R. (1977). Intensive feeding training with retarded children. *Behavior Modification, 1,* 517–529.

Stremel-Campbell, K., & Matthews, J. (1987). Development of emergent language. In M. Bullis (Ed.), *Communication development in young children with deaf-blindness: Literature review III* (pp. 141–183). Monmouth: Oregon State University, Communication Skills Center for Young Children with Deaf-Blindness.

Tawney, J.W. (1984). The pragmatics of the educability issue: Some questions which logically precede the assumption of ineducability. In W.C. Heward, T. Heron, D. Hill, & J. Trap-Porter (Eds.), *Behavior analysis in education* (pp. 287–295). Columbus, OH: Charles E. Merrill.

Thompson, B., & Guess, D. (1989). Students who experience the most profound disabilities: Teacher perspectives. In F. Brown & D.H. Lehr (Eds.), *Persons with profound disabilities: Issues and practices* (pp. 3–41). Baltimore: Paul H. Brookes Publishing Co.

Thompson, G., Iwata, B., & Poynter, H. (1979). Operant control of pathological tongue thrust in spastic cerebral palsy. *Journal of Applied Behavior Analysis, 12,* 325–333.

Timothy W. v. Rochester, New Hampshire, School District, 875 F.2nd 954 (1st Cir. 1989).

Ulicny, G.R., Thompson, S.K., Favell, J.E., & Thompson, M.S. (1985). The active assessment of educability: A case study. *Journal of The Association for Persons with Severe Handicaps, 10,* 111–114.

Utley, B., Duncan, D., Strain, P., & Scanlon, K. (1983). Effects of contingent and noncontingent vision stimulation on visual fixation in multiply handicapped children. *Journal of The Association for the Severely Handicapped, 8,* 29–42.

van Dijk, J. (1986). An educational curriculum for deaf-blind multihandicapped persons. In D. Ellis (Ed.), *Sensory impairments in mentally handicapped people* (pp. 374–382). London: Croom-Helm.

Van Houten, R. (1979). Social validation: The evolution of standards of competency for target behaviors. *Journal of Applied Behavior Analysis, 12,* 581–591.

Voeltz, L.M. (1982). Effects of structured interactions with severely handicapped peers on children's attitudes. *American Journal of Mental Deficiency, 86,* 380–390.

Wacker, D.P., Berg, W.K., Wiggins, B., Muldoon, M., & Cavanaugh, J. (1985). Evaluation of reinforcer preferences for profoundly handicapped students. *Journal of Applied Behavior Analysis, 18,* 173–178.

Wacker, D.P., Wiggins, B., Fowler, M., & Berg, W.K. (1988). Training students with profound or multiple handicaps to make requests via microswitches. *Journal of Applied Behavior Analysis, 21,* 331–343.

Warren, S.F., Horn, E.H., & Hill, E.W. (1987). Some innovative educational applications of advanced technologies. In L. Goetz, D. Guess, & K. Stremel-Campbell (Eds.), *Innovative program design for individuals with dual sensory impairments* (pp. 283–309). Baltimore: Paul H. Brookes Publishing Co.

Wolf, M.W. (1978). Social validity: The case for subjective measurement. *Journal of Applied Behavior Analysis, 11,* 203–314.

Writer, J. (1987). A movement-based approach to the education of students who are sensory impaired/multihandicapped. In L. Goetz, D. Guess, & K. Stremel-Campbell (Eds.), *Innovative program design for individuals with dual sensory impairments* (pp. 191–223). Baltimore: Paul H. Brookes Publishing Co.

York, J., & Rainforth, B. (1987). Developing instructional adaptations. In F.P. Orelove & D. Sobsey, *Educating children with multiple disabilities: A transdisciplinary approach.* (pp. 183–217). Baltimore: Paul H. Brookes Publishing Co.

CHAPTER 5

Telling New Stories

The Search for Capacity Among People with Severe Handicaps

JOHN O'BRIEN
Responsive Systems Associates, Lithonia, Georgia

BETH MOUNT
Graphic Futures, West Hartford, Connecticut

Some stories enhance life;
others degrade it.
So we must be careful
about the stories we tell,
about the ways we define
ourselves and other people.

—Burton Blatt (1987, p. 142)

Consider these two stories:

I

Mr. Davis has a mental age of 3 years, 2 months. IQ = 18. Severe impairment of adaptive behavior, severe range of mental retardation. Becomes agitated and out of control. Takes [medicines] for psychosis.

Severely limited verbal ability; inability to comprehend abstract concepts. Learns through imitation. Has learned to unlock the Coke machine and restock it, and to crank a power mower and operate it.

His family is uncooperative. They break appointments and do not follow through on behavior management plans.

II

Ed lives with his mother and sister in [housing project]. Ten of his relatives live nearby and they visit back and forth frequently. His father spends little time with him, but two of his sisters have been very helpful when there are crises. His family agree that he will live with one or another of them for the rest of his life.

Ed is at home in his neighborhood. He visits extended family members and neighbors daily. He goes to local stores with his sisters and helps with shopping. He goes to church.

Ed dresses neatly, is usually friendly, and shakes hands with people when he meets them. He is a very big man, with limited ability to speak. When he gets frustrated and upset he cusses and "talks" to himself in a loud voice. These characteristics often frighten other people who do not know him well. He has been excluded from the work activity center because he acts "out of control" there. He has broken some furniture and punched holes in the walls there and scares some of the staff people very much.

Ed likes people and enjoys visiting in the neighborhood. He loves music, dancing, and sweeping. He likes loading vending machines and operating mechanical equipment. He likes to go shopping. He likes to cook for himself and for other people and can fix several meals on the stove at home. He likes to hang clothes and bring them in off the line. He likes to stack cord wood and help people move furniture. He prefers tasks that require strength and a lot of large muscle movement.

Both of these stories were told to help the same man. But they differ in the way they were constructed, in their purpose, in their consequences, and in the assumptions they shape about human development and human services organization.

DIFFERENT RULES FOR CONSTRUCTION

A multidisciplinary team told the first story in its required annual review of Mr. Davis's progress. They integrated data from psychological, social work, nursing, speech therapy, and occupational therapy assessments with data about Mr. Davis's performance in the day program. They determined objectives for the next year, recommended additional therapy services, and made a placement recommendation. The team was un-

certain about the extent to which Mr. Davis's behavior problems are an expression of psychotic
illness and agreed to seek a psychiatric evaluation to settle the question. Mr. Davis was not at
the meeting because he had acted out violently
that day and staff had sent him home to his
mother in compliance with the team's behavior
management plan. Though the social worker
sent an invitation, no one from his family attended. The meeting took 20 minutes.

A group of people who know and care about
Mr. Davis and his family told the second story as
part of a collective search for a better response to
his situation. An outside facilitator, conducting
research for her doctoral dissertation (Mount,
1987), met Mr. Davis and his family at the suggestion of the day program director. With his
mother and sister and two direct service workers,
the facilitator organized a personal futures planning meeting (see O'Brien, 1987, for a description of this process). Staff people from the day
program joined Mr. Davis, members of his extended family, neighbors, and church members
at the family's church on a Sunday afternoon.
They told stories about Mr. Davis and his family,
expressed their concerns for his situation and
their ideas about his future, shared information
about opportunities in the neighborhood, and
came up with suggested next steps. Several people, including program staff, took personal responsibility for action steps and agreed to meet
again to review progress, without the facilitator.
The facilitator recorded the meeting on large
posters, using color-coded graphic symbols and
quotations from participants. Mr. Davis sat with
one of his sisters during the meeting. He asked
for, and carried home, the poster that described
the group's ideas about his future. The meeting
took 2 hours.

DIFFERENT PURPOSES

Professionals told the first story in compliance
with state regulations in order to control the routine work of direct service staff. Their story justifies Mr. Davis's eligibility for the program and
the program's responses to his problem behaviors. It takes existing service arrangements as a
given.

People who know Mr. Davis and his family
told the second story voluntarily in order to discover actions that will reveal capacities in him,
in the people who care about him, and in his
neighborhood. Their story justifies action to expand his opportunities and learn better ways to
support him. It calls for changes in existing service arrangements from the time and place of
planning meetings to the mission and activities
of the day program.

DIFFERENT CONSEQUENCES

The people who told the first story selected objectives for Mr. Davis that would increase his
time on task on the assembly contract at the center, increase his accuracy in performing a letter-
folding simulation to improve his fine motor coordination, and ready him to prepare meals by
identifying menu items from pictures of the four
food groups. Noting an increase in his problem
behavior, they recommended his admission to a
psychiatric hospital for evaluation and mental
health treatment. Noting his unmet need for
speech therapy and his mother's difficulty in following through on required programs, they recommended post–psychiatric hospital placement
in the regional mental retardation institution for
intensive training. While the plan arising from
their meeting was being typed, Mr. Davis was
excluded from the program in response to staff
concern for their safety and the safety of other
clients.

The people who told the second story responded to their account of Mr. Davis's preferences and neighborhood resources to deal with
the idleness resulting from his exclusion from
the day program and the threat of institutionalization. They decided that he preferred hard physical work and work with machines to sedentary
tasks requiring fine movements. Within 3 days,
one of his sisters and a direct service staff person
had developed an opportunity for him to load
soft-drink vending machines at three convenience stores in his neighborhood. Within 2
weeks, another sister and a neighbor had begun
to create a schedule of lawn mowing, firewood
stacking, and yard work that he and one of his
cousins could share, with occasional assistance

from a center staff person. They recognized his ability to help out at home and encouraged his mother to increase her expectations of regular and reliable performance. They acknowledged that he was a welcome visitor in many neighborhood homes and shared what they had learned about how to understand his communication and deal with his occasional episodes of talking to himself and "blowing off steam." They agreed that there was no reason for Mr. Davis to go to the psychiatric hospital or the mental retardation institution.

The tellers of the second story did not aim for perfection, and they have not achieved it. Three years after this process began, Mr. Davis still loads machines and does outside work daily, but these activities do not add up to a full-time job and he receives very little cash for his efforts. He remains active and helpful around his house and among his neighbors. He has had no help to improve his ability to communicate, though there have been several unproductive referrals. He continues to talk to himself but has not had a frightening episode in more than a year. A number of the people who gathered at the first meeting still meet regularly to share what they are doing and learning about Mr. Davis and what they might do together next.

DIFFERENT ASSUMPTIONS, DIFFERENT ORGANIZATIONS

Organizations are systems for interpreting their actions and their environments; for telling stories about what has happened, about what events mean, and about what to do next (Daft & Weick, 1984). Assumptions about effective organization and human development shape, and in turn are shaped by, the ways human services organizations make sense of their world.

The first story assumes that professional people who share very little of Mr. Davis's daily life can speak the most important words about him. These words have power because they are objective data, the (often quantitative) results of scientific procedures. Things will be better for Mr. Davis if he, his family, and direct service workers, non-experts all, listen to and obey professional plans. The second story assumes that

Mr. Davis himself, and those who share and shape his daily life, should be the primary speakers. Knowledge and the power to effectively bind action arise primarily from personal commitment, careful listening, and shared action. When available technology is insufficient to cure, the role of experts is to listen and cooperate.

The first story assumes that Mr. Davis remains the same person no matter where and how you meet him. What needs to be known about him is disclosed by viewing him in isolation from his social context (Sarason, 1981). His measured intelligence fixes his potential for development unequivocally and dictates his future (Gould, 1981). The second story assumes that Mr. Davis's life can only be understood in context. He is both unable to meet the prerequisites for cooking and able to fix meals. He is both dangerous and friendly. He is both "that big crazy boy" and a welcome guest in some people's homes. He is both unable to speak and able to dance. His potential for development is the product of his efforts and the efforts of his allies and assistants (Bronfenbrenner, 1977). He can only be revealed when people join with him to create his future. In this sense, his potential is unknown and unknowable apart from what action he and the others he relies upon decide to do together.

The first story assumes that Mr. Davis will be helped if the tellers exhaustively catalogue his deficiencies. Their conversation is dominated by what he can't do, what he won't do, and why he doesn't. The second story assumes that capacity, interest, and preference make the foundation of effective help. What he likes, what he wants to do, and his vocation among us centers the storytelling and action.

The first story assumes that human services exist to change Mr. Davis. Accurate classification leads to appropriate placement and good diagnosis leads to proper prescription. If Mr. Davis complies with the prescribed program, he will progress as far as he is able (Biklen, 1988). Services change by learning to do better what they are currently doing. The second story assumes that human services exist to assist Mr. Davis by supporting him, his family, and friends to develop and pursue community opportunities

(O'Brien & Lyle, 1988). Services develop by learning to do new things in new ways (Argyris & Schon, 1978).

The first story assumes that reliable and effective service results from hierarchical structures controlled by rational argument among experts who find preexisting answers by standard examination (Weick & Browning, 1986). Impersonal statements, standardized scores, quantified objectives, linear logic, and appeals to authority shape the organization. The second story assumes that reliable and effective service results from collaboration across organizational boundaries influenced by shared visions and shaped by negotiation of multiple differences. Answers don't preexist, they are constructed by the way people organize to find them (Maturana & Varela, 1980) and communicated in the narratives people share (Weick, 1987). Personal testimony, graphic images, shared food, music, laughter and tears, and creative action shape the organization.

NEW DIRECTIONS, NEW STORIES

Raymond Kilroy's vision compels attention to new directions for himself, for other people with severe disabilities, and for all of us.

> We are moving away from emphasizing my needs toward building upon my capacities. We are moving away from providing services to me in some facility toward building bridges with me to communities and neighborhood associations. We are moving away from programming me and other people with disabilities toward empowering us and our families to acquire the support we want. We are moving away from focusing on my deficits to focusing on my competence. We are moving away from specialized disability organizations so that we can develop and sustain relationships with people who will depend upon people like me and upon whom people like me can depend. (Kilroy, 1987, p. 4)

To move toward this future we must all learn to listen to, to tell, and to act on new stories, stories whose theme is action to discover capacity.

REFERENCES

Argyris, C., & Schon, D. (1978). *Organizational learning: A theory of action perspective*. Reading, MA: Addison-Wesley.

Biklen, D. (1988). The myth of clinical judgement. *Journal of Social Issues, 44*(1), 127–140.

Blatt, B. (1987). *The conquest of mental retardation*. Austin, TX: PRO-ED.

Bronfenbrenner, U. (1977). Toward an experimental ecology of human development. *American Psychologist, 32*, 513–531.

Daft, R., & Weick, K. (1984). Toward a model of organizations as interpretation systems. *Academy of Management Review, 9*, 284–295.

Gould, S. (1981). *The mismeasure of man*. New York: Norton.

Kilroy, R. (1987). *Testimony to the United States Senate Subcommittee on the Handicapped*, Washington, DC.

Maturana, H., & Varela, F. (1980). *Autopoiesis and cognition*. Boston: Reidel.

Mount, B. (1987). *Personal futures planning: Finding directions for change*. Unpublished doctoral dissertation, University of Georgia, Athens.

O'Brien, J. (1987). A guide to life-style planning: Using *The Activities Catalog* to integrate services and natural support systems. In B. Wilcox & G.T. Bellamy, *A comprehensive guide to* The Activities Catalog: An alternative curriculum for youth and adults with severe disabilities (pp. 175–189). Baltimore: Paul H. Brookes Publishing Co.

O'Brien, J., & Lyle, C. (1988). *Framework for accomplishment*. Atlanta: Responsive Systems Associates.

Sarason, S. (1981). *Psychology misdirected*. New York: Free Press.

Weick, K. (1987). Organizational culture as a source of high reliability. *California Management Review, 29*, 112–127.

Weick, K., & Browning, L. (1986). Argument and narration in organization communication. *Journal of Management, 12*, 243–259.

◇ **CHAPTER 6** ◇

Evaluating Evaluation
A "Fictional" Play

MARY ULRICH
West Chester, Ohio

PROLOGUE

It is 1975. Mom, Dad, and 10-month-old Aaron are sitting in the neurologist's office. After a 30-minute evaluation:

Doctor: You have reasons to be concerned. We will conduct more tests, but my evaluations show your son will always be in *special* school.

Dad: Of course, Doctor, my wife and I are both teachers. We would insist the school be something special.

Doctor: I don't think you understand.

Now it is 1980. In a conference room at the large downtown education center, Mom, Dad, and 13 professionals sit around a large rectangular table. Aaron, Tommy (his 3-year-old brother), and the babysitter are nearby doing puzzles and rolling a large ball.

Psychologist: Aaron is now 5 years old and school age. He is untestable. His IQ is below 50, so he is to go to the segregated special school. Aaron is so lucky, our three new segregated schools and workshops are beautiful. He will be happy and safe . . . . When he gets to the school his new teacher will write some objectives.

Mom/Dad: Here is a copy of our evaluation and goals to meet Aaron's needs (*Table 6.1*). We are with Aaron for 18 hours each day, 365 days a year. We feel we know our son.

It's 1982. Aaron is 7. It is the "Impartial Hearing for Aaron vs. Superintendent." The independent evaluator is beginning her report.

Dr. F.: Regular evaluation tools are not very helpful, so I've submitted a summary of my 35-page educational evaluation (*Table 6.2*).

ACT ONE

It is a spring afternoon in 1985. Aaron, a young man of 10 who has severe learning challenges,

Table 6.1. Parents' goals for Aaron and for Tommy

If you fail to plan, you plan to fail!
Build a dream and the dream will build you!
—Dr. Robert Schuller

1980 Dream Plan for Aaron Ulrich:

Aaron will be educated in a public school with his non-handicapped brother and neighbors. He will have a functional curriculum that looks at the needs in his life spaces (vocational, recreation-leisure, domestic, general community functioning). His out-of-school activities will evolve around his family and his own friends, interests, and talents. He will be in age-appropriate settings: elementary school, 5–10; junior high, 11–13; senior high, 14–21; job in community, 22. He will begin vocational training now at age 5 so he will be able to perform the job. Aaron will use the ongoing supported services model. If he isn't able to be a dish washer, then he can be a dish-washer's helper . . . there is some job he will be able to do with success. At the appropriate time, Aaron will move to a supported apartment to live with one or two friends. He will continue to be interdependent in many ways, and will have self-esteem and confidence in the things he does and be a contributor to his family, his extended family, and his community.

1980 Dream Plan for Tommy Ulrich:

Tommy will be educated in a public school with his handicapped brother and neighbors. He will have a functional curriculum that looks at the needs in his life spaces (academic, vocational, recreation-leisure, domestic, general community functioning). His out-of-school activities will evolve around his family and his own friends, interests, and talents. He will be in age-appropriate settings. He will make a career choice and pursue training (vocational, university, apprentice). At the appropriate time, Tommy will move to his own home, probably marry, and begin his own family. He will have self-esteem and confidence in the things he does, and be a contributor to his family, his extended family, and his community.

his mother, and Dr. Sam Smith, the school psychologist, are sitting in the supply closet of Aaron's local elementary school.

Dr. S.: (*Shaking hands*) It is nice to meet you. I'm sorry, but this is the only empty space in the school.

Mom: We are very excited to begin this re-

93

Table 6.2.   Independent evaluator's report summary

Sample of educational needs (according to testimony and current IEP)	Current placement in regular school	Proposed placement in integrated school
A. Individualized instruction	A. 5 students in the class; the 5 students were grouped according to content needs; some students worked on their printing skills while Aaron worked on manual signing.	A. 12 students in the class; *all 12* worked on pegboards, engaged in a "hat" activity, sang songs, and then listened to a record.
B. Chronological-age expectations	B. Aaron received instruction on how to walk to his classroom independently; Aaron received instruction on how to use the regular bathroom independently— his teacher indicated that she was concerned about how his nonhandicapped peers might perceive him if he were to have a "toileting accident."	B. Hands were held of students as they walked down the halls; diapers of students were changed in the classroom; other students were learning how to use a bathroom that was located in the classroom. Students sat on the toilet with the door wide open; there was no apparent concern for privacy.
C. Emphasis on acquiring independence and functional skills in meaningful contexts	C. During large group activities, Aaron sat at his desk and received praise for sitting and listening.	C. Two students who had difficulty attending were strapped into their chairs.
D. Preparation for adult functioning	D. The teacher indicated that 10 or more trips were made each year for the purposes of community instruction.	D. More than 90% of the 1980 graduates of this school became clients of the sheltered work activity center (located on the same grounds as the school). The teacher indicated that the students do not receive community instruction until they progress to one of the adolescent classes.
E. Maximization of physical development	E. Aaron's classroom was located on the second floor; he was learning to climb the stairs at least three times daily with alternating feet.	E. During the hearing, the administrator mentioned stairs were purchased for the classrooms so that students could practice walking up and down them.
F. Development of social and communicative skills	F. Nonhandicapped students were observed greeting Aaron by name; information was passed along like, "Hey, Aaron, your bus is here." He has participated in field trips with regular education students and the "little brother" program; Aaron was learning how to say "Hi" and gesture in response to the greetings of others; he was learning how to use pictures to communicate messages in the classroom. "Reducing inappropriate vocalizations" was an objective of	F. Of the 240 students at this school, *all* have severe disabilities. Students were observed body rocking, emitting incessant irrelevant vocalizations, and performing other maladaptive actions; yet, in many cases, no teacher intervention was provided.

(continued)

Table 6.2. *(continued)*

Sample of educational needs (according to testimony and current IEP)	Current placement in regular school	Proposed placement in integrated school
	Aaron's educational program.	

- -

Comments: Based on the sample of educational needs expressed during the hearing by school district personnel and those needs currently identified in Aaron's IEP, which of the two placements would provide an enabling environment? the least restrictive environment? Or more to the point, how can we justify the removal of Aaron from a regular educational environment?

---

evaluation. Aaron has been in school since he was 13 months old and now we are halfway through his educational career. Over the last 10 years we have learned that Aaron does best on tasks that make sense to him.

Dr. S. *(Nodding)*: I've observed Aaron in his classroom this week and it's all pretty new to me, but the teacher, Mrs. . . . what's her name?

Mom: Mrs. Jones.

Dr. S.: Mrs. Jones does seem to be energetic. Initially, I had some concerns about the multihandicapped class being in this building, but things seem to be going smoothly. It doesn't seem to be taking anything away from the regular students' schooling.

Aaron: *(Unrolling the large roll of construction paper)* Whee . . . *(When Mom stops him he bites his hand)*

Dr. S.: Aaron certainly has pretty red hair. Now, to begin this evaluation, why don't you tell me about your pregnancy?

Mom: *(Exasperated, looks up at the ceiling).* Aaron is our first child . . . . *(Camera fades)*

Aaron is seated at a horseshoe-shaped table that has one leg shorter than the other. He begins rocking the table. He giggles at the noise.

Dr. S.: *(Pulling wood testing device from Black Kit)* Aaron, let's put this little red block in this first little box. Watch me.

(Aaron gives eye contact)

Dr. S.: *(Psychologist with Ph.D., a grown man, then demonstratively leans over table and puts the little block in the first compartment)* See!

(Aaron claps)

Dr. S.: OK, Aaron, now it's your turn.

(Aaron tries to copy, but after several attempts throws the block across the room)

Dr. S.: *(Pulling out the Bayley Infant Scale)* Aaron, put the raisin in the cup.

Aaron: *(Eats the raisin)* Drink.

Dr. S.: *(Frustrated)* Aaron, let's look at some pictures. You can get a drink when we're finished. If we stop for a drink now, we'll never get *done*.

Aaron: *(Pulling the leftover Christmas decorations off the shelf, gets up from the table)* All done.

(Dr. S., gently assisting Aaron back to his chair, shows Aaron a picture of a one-dimensional, black-and-white line drawing of a man's leather dress shoe.)

Mom: Aaron uses that word all the time. *(Pointing to Aaron's foot)* Could he identify his own? He has never worn that style before.

Dr. S.: No, we must use this picture, or it would invalidate the test!

(Aaron takes picture and starts licking and flipping it)

ACT TWO

Spring, 1988. Aaron, now 13, his mother, and Dr. Carol Brooke, the school psychologist, are sitting in the speech room of the local junior high school.

Psychologist: *(Shaking hands)* It is nice to meet you. The speech therapist is out today so we are fortunate to be able to use this room.

Mom: We are very excited to begin this re-evaluation. Aaron has been in school since he was 13 months old and we only have 8 more years to prepare him for all the skills he will need to live, work, and recreate in his community. The teachers are trying to do a functional, community-based curriculum, but are struggling with questions about Aaron's learning style. We go to the mall one month, the bowling alley another month, the park another, and though the teachers are working very hard, we really have no current level of functioning in the community environments. No useful evaluation material. Each year we must pull IEP [individualized education program] objectives out of the air instead of getting goals that are based on evaluation data.

Psychologist: (*Smiling*) Your teachers really are patient with the children. I went with the class to the vocational site at the Pizza Place. Aaron did a great job cleaning windows and mirrors, rolling the bread sticks, and folding the pizza boxes. The teachers did seem frustrated about not having time to do the functional assessments. They admitted they usually just stick the psychologists' report in the drawer.

Mom: Did you get the functional assessment articles and tools I sent in last month? I know it's a lot of information, but people from TASH are willing to help. If you have any questions about the DeKalb, Syracuse, or REACH materials, I've put the phone numbers on them. I've already completed a "Dream Plan" for Aaron and the "Life Space Analysis."

Psychologist: It looks interesting. But, I've devoted this whole week to evaluating Aaron, and I haven't gotten to the reading material yet.

Several weeks later, 12 people are seated around a table in the back of the multihandicapped classroom. Mr. Long, the principal, opens the IEP meeting. In the background, Aaron is listening to records with a headset.

Principal: (*Smiling at Mom and Dad*) I enjoy seeing Aaron at the afterschool intramural basketball games cheering for his brother.

Dad: Yes, it's great having both the boys at the same school.

Principal: We are here to conduct the annual review, discuss Aaron's reevaluation, and write his IEP for next year. Now we only have an hour, so let's begin. You have all received copies previously. Dr. Brooke, would you summarize your report?

Psychologist: (*Referring to her report:*

Table 6.3) I spent a whole week testing him on several occasions so he wouldn't be tired or feel I was an unfamiliar person.

Principal: Evaluations were also completed by the OT [occupational therapist], PT [physical therapist], teacher, language therapist, and the bus driver; these are in your packets. (*Looks at parents*)

Mom: I'd like to pass around Aaron's "Dream Plan," the "24-hour Life Space Analysis," and the "Current and Future Environments" inventories. This is our best guess of where Aaron is heading.

(*The parents' report goes around the tables from professional to professional. It eventually comes back to the parents. No one knows what to do with it.*)

Principal: Now, everyone has submitted their suggested goals to Mrs. Amend, Aaron's teacher. These have been placed into the domains and were distributed last week. Does ev-

---

Table 6.3.   Report summary

Aaron is 13 years old.

INTELLIGENCE: Six subtests were administered on the Stanford-Binet IV. Raw scores of zero were obtained on all but one subtest. He did not point to required body parts on a picture of a person . . . .

ACHIEVEMENT: Aaron is not working on readiness academic skills; no achievement measures would be appropriate.

SOCIAL-EMOTIONAL: Aaron is isolated in that he does not attempt to interact with his peers, but he does not physically avoid them . . . .

ADAPTIVE-BEHAVIOR: Aaron's Adaptive Behavior Social Quotient score indicates that at this point in his life, Aaron is dependent upon adults for his care and safety. Many skills that are demonstrated at school have not generalized to other settings . . . .

RECOMMENDATIONS:
1. Aaron is going to learn proportionately fewer skills than 99% of the population. He is going to need an increased number of teaching trials. He will forget skills he does not practice. It takes a longer time for him to recoup skills he forgot. He has problems with transfer and generalization.
2. Standardized intelligence testing is not adequate to assess Aaron's cognitive functioning. Therefore, it is very important to continually assess in his natural environment and measure his growth in those goals leading toward optimum independence as an adult.
3. To promote generalization of skills it is necessary for those cues and scripts used by school personnel to be adopted by Aaron's family and practiced frequently.

eryone have their copy of the draft IEP? (*All nod*)

Since Mrs. Amend is the leader of our transdisciplinary team, let's have her put this all together. Dr. Brooke had agreed to be secretary for writing down the goals for the final copy of the IEP. (*Principal looks at clock*)

Teacher: Any questions about Page 1 of the draft?

Mom: Aaron has learned a lot of new skills this year. I love the fact that he can find his own homeroom. Even though it's only 6 minutes long, it's 6 minutes of increased contact with the regular students. Aaron is getting on the bus more quickly. The OT and PT plans for starting on his stronger right foot, and the bus driver's "planned ignoring" are working well. I am excited that this year we are writing *one* IEP instead of five separate ones (one for Speech, OT, PT, Adapted PE [physical education], Teacher).

Dad: I am still concerned that the IEP goals in this year's draft are disjointed. I really think the vocational component of Aaron's program, with the two daily in-school jobs and two times a week community-based jobs, is a model. I know you are all talented and caring people. Aaron is very lucky.

Mom: (*Turning to psychologist*) This evaluation must have been very frustrating. (*Psychologist smiles and nods*) Before we write down any goals I would like to share the standards I've decided to use:

1. Does this goal increase Aaron's opportunity for interactions with others?
2. Does it increase his opportunity to make choices?
3. Does the goal enhance the way others will look at him? (Normalization)
4. Does the goal increase his independence doing functional skills in their natural environments?

Teacher: Let's begin—Domestic Domain

1. Aaron will eat at the proper speed, size, and consistencies of food without a monitor (adult/peer).

Dad/Mom: Great, all the goals on Page 1 are fine.

(*Teacher continues and goals are transcribed*)

Teacher: What about Page 6—Recreation/Leisure Domain?

Dad: I need some information on Goal 4.

Teacher: (*Reads aloud Goal 4*) To improve gross motor skills and physical fitness. 4a) Aaron will throw a ball, stepping with opposition on three of five trials.

Dad: I would like to be able to play toss with Aaron in the yard. That would be a skill Aaron could use his whole life.

Adapted PE Teacher: No, that's a different skill than 4a. In Special Olympics, Aaron has to throw the softball and then we measure it.

Dad: Is anyone catching the ball?

Adapted PE Teacher: No, that's not the activity. (*Smiling*) Aaron stands by a line, throws the ball on the gym floor, and then we measure the distance. In my evaluation, this and the frisbee throw were the only events in which Aaron would have success.

Mom: When you and I throw a ball, do we usually throw it on the ground?

Adapted PE Teacher: But this is an event in Special Olympics. We throw softballs and frisbees on the floor so we can measure the distance. Aaron still throws pretty randomly, but at least he can participate. We've been practicing this for weeks.

Dad: You know, we have this dangerous problem at home. Aaron has been throwing the ball into the street and watching it bounce. Do you think he's practicing his ball throw? (*Referring to the psychologist's report*)

Mom: Maybe he can generalize some things like ball throwing and not generalize other things like safety. Could we make a goal where Aaron learns to toss the ball to a friend? It would be more normal and get Aaron to look at others.

Adapted PE Teacher: But Special Olympics . . . .

Dad: Aaron is NOT to participate in Special Olympics if they can't have functional normal activities that Aaron will use in regular recreation settings. We want activities that will carry over to his adult life. Not waste time on 1-day events Aaron will then have to unlearn.

Teacher: (*Secretly winks at Dad and Mom*) Goal 4c) Aaron will participate in a variety of games using correct motor patterns and following directions 70% of the time.

Mom: Does that mean Aaron is only working on 70% or part of the directions with 100% accuracy? Some days, some directions, other days, different directions? Some days he doesn't have to follow directions?

Dad: We're not trying to be smart, but it's 100% or nothing. Remember last year's goal that "Aaron will independently maneuver the shopping center parking lot 60% of the time." What happens the other part of the percentage could be deadly! If I give Aaron a direction, I expect him to follow it 100% of the time. (*Smiling*) Aaron will be successful if he then follows it as often as his brother does! (*Mom smiles*)

Supervisor: As you know, for the last 3 years we have been working on our own curriculum. We only have one typist and no word processor, so it's taking longer than expected. Our district is unique from every other district in the world. Some of the problems we're encountering here will be solved when OUR curriculum is finished in a couple of months.

Mom: Couldn't we use DeKalb's or Syracuse's curriculum until ours is finished?

Supervisor: As I explained at your IEP last year, our curriculum has to be tailor made to just this district.

Dad: In regular fifth grade, when the district is adopting a new science curriculum, does the district just let the teachers "wing it" for a year or 2 or 3 until the typist gets finished?

Mom: Couldn't we be doing the ecological assessments and some record keeping now so we could actually see what Aaron is learning?

Supervisor: You're going to love it.

Mom: (*Gives a sigh*) Please give me a copy as soon as possible.

Teacher: I would like a copy too.

Principal: We only have a couple of minutes left; we'll finish writing this all up and (*looking at parents*) we'll send it to you.

(*Everyone starts talking and getting up to leave*)

Dad: Aaron has nothing to do in the summer. Here is a list of his behaviors from last year. (*Table 6.4*) We strongly feel Aaron needs the structure and extra learning time of an extended school year. We'd like to add that to the IEP. We're really concerned that Aaron's summer is not nearly as meaningful as the kinds of experiences Tommy has. (*Table 6.5*)

Table 6.4.   Aaron's behavior around home—Summer, 1984

Destroyed Tommy's toys
Broke TV
Broke stereo
Punched out and crawled through screen door and windows
Ran trucks over car hood—requiring paint job on car
Bit and pinched everyone
Slammed doors between rooms
Turned on water faucets
Put pool balls and ? in dryer—now dryer makes loud noises

Principal: (*Shaking hands with Dad*) That's an issue we'll have to discuss with the Director of Special Services. Gosh, it's been great to see you. You have two fine sons. Let's keep in touch about the unresolved issues.

THE END

AN EPILOGUE

In the preceding "fictitious" story, the psychologist was right about "achievement" when she reported that Aaron was not working on academic readiness skills. But in fact, Aaron has "achieved" many new skills this year. He can independently present his wallet when paying at the grocery. He has learned to give his food order at McDonald's using his augmented communication system; he now independently rides the regular school bus with his brother and neighbors; he can sort silverware at home and at his job site . . . .

As a parent, I have my own criteria of evaluation. Does my child have any friends? Does anyone value my child enough to want to be near him without being paid? The highlight of last year was when one of the typical kids asked if Aaron could go to band. "He likes music, and he should be in this class." (This fifth grader and the band director evaluated Aaron and decided he could play in the rhythm section.) How many functional tasks or parts of tasks can my child do this year that he wouldn't do last year? How many choices does he get to make? Is he any more independent? Is my life easier?

For years and years, people were told by the experts that they had to go into the hospital for minor operations, because that was the only way the insurance companies would cover the bills.

Table 6.5. Comparison of Tommy and Aaron's Summer, 1984, activities (and costs)

| Tommy Ulrich (age 9) | | Aaron Ulrich (age 10) | |
Activities	Cost	Activities	Cost
Family vacation	(same)	Family vacation	(same)
Cub Scout camp (7 days) (regular kids only)	$ 40	Camp Happiness (special only)	$385
		Y Camp (4 days) (special unit/regular and special kids)	$120
Summer School (3 hours/day)		Summer School (3 hours/ day)	
Computer class (10 days)	$ 15	MH class (5 weeks or 25 days) (Overlapped with Camp Happiness)	$265
Science in the outdoors (10 days)	$ 15		
Swim camp (7 hours/5 days) (regular kids only)	$ 15		
Cub Scout outings Reds games picnic	$ 5		
PYO baseball league (12 weeks long— two–three practices/games/week, picnic and tournament)	$ 20		
Party with friends	(same)	Party with classmates	(same)
Overnights friends cousins			
Options not chosen Gymnastics camp Church camp Art class Soccer league Foreign language class			
TOTAL	**$110**	**TOTAL**	**$770**
Note: This is a *partial* list.		Note: This is a *complete* list.	

Today, *outpatient* surgery is the general practice. "Whole life" insurance was once the standard; now the industry's bread and butter is "term" insurance. Remember when the experts said it was too dangerous for fathers to be in the delivery room? Or for mothers to be awake during delivery? Now, they have "birthing suites" for the whole family! Ask the experts in one of America's major corporations what happens when you insist on doing things the way you've always done them!

In 1978, Nicholas Hobbs said, "Parents have to be recognized as special educators, the true experts on their children; and professional people—teachers, pediatricians, psychologists, and others—have to learn to be consultants to parents." Parents have important information that must be included in the evaluation. Parent inventories and other tools that include their input will help them feel confident about the information they know and the direction in which they are heading. The problem of evaluation has become asking the "usual" questions: This is not the same as asking "useful" questions. Good IEPs, meaningful long- and short-term goals, effective behavioral intervention, integrated therapy, and increased social interactions all depend on evaluations. If we truly become a transdisciplinary team and all use the "eyes" of expertise (including the expertise of parenting), we can help build the future based on the needs of individuals, not on the needs of the system.

In the past, parents have eagerly gone to evaluations for help; bared their souls; shared their hopes, dreams, and fears; and entrusted their greatest treasure—their child. And, time and again, we have been betrayed by useless tests and wasted years of inappropriate training and meaningless experiences. Right now, when I evaluate evaluations they are conspicuously on the low end of the bell curve.

In 3 years, my son's "Act Three," another re-evaluation, will start again with the same handshake. But will we meet the challenge? Will the evaluation tools and final recommendations be the same???

◇ **CHAPTER 7** ◇

Assessment
Current Concerns and Future Directions

ADRIANA L. SCHULER
LINDA PEREZ

San Francisco State University, San Francisco, California

Given ongoing pressures to upgrade the assessment and education of individuals with severe disabilities, it is time to critically reappraise the theoretical models and concepts that underlie current practices. For instance, with regard to assessment, it could be argued that the proliferation of psychometric testing practices has served to restrict the lives of individuals with disabilities. The implicit focus on what someone cannot do, the preoccupation with norms, and the lack of concern for context is likely to undermine perceived competence, as attention is being diverted from more creative and adaptive behaviors in more relevant settings.

Additional concerns about current practices are raised by the extreme challenges involved in the assessment of individuals with severe disabilities. For example, common assessment formats are useless when someone's sensory, motor, verbal, or conceptual idiosyncrasies interfere with standardized test administration. No pure behavioral measures of isolated skills can ever be obtained, since the domains being sampled are inavoidably "contaminated." Even when traditional measures seem applicable, they may need to be modified to such an extent that scores become meaningless, complicating the interpretation of assessment findings. These practical concerns are closely intertwined with the need to reappraise the theoretical foundation of current assessment practices.

This chapter examines the conceptual underpinnings of prevailing assessment practices, as they have become increasingly challenged by changing perspectives on learning, develop-

ment, and behavior organization. Based on these current reconceptualizations, and the type of expertise that has evolved in attempting to assess individuals with severe disabilities properly, suggestions are made for future practices. The need for a *comprehensive* assessment involving multiple measures and contexts is emphasized.

HISTORICAL CONSIDERATIONS AND CURRENT PRACTICES

The term "assessment" does not necessarily refer to any particular practices, value judgments, or attitudes. It merely refers to a process of close examination and evaluation, and not to any specific content. Nevertheless, most of us equate the term "assessment" with particular tests, protocols, scores, referrals, placement procedures, and the like. While assessment can serve a variety of functions, its most prevalent use has been in diagnosis and identification, in reference to special education placement and/or the provision of other related services. Besides placement issues, prevailing assessment practices have been shaped by psychometric constructs, deficiency models, and behavioral stimulus-response notions of learning. Despite their fundamental differences, these disciplines are highly enmeshed when it comes to assessment practices. Due to their common theoretical orientation, behavioral and psychometric constructs have readily blended with notions of deficiency and segregation that continue to dominate the field of special education. The premise of such an approach is that effective remediation is based on the ac-

The authors want to thank Charles Peck, J.R. Podratz, and Barry Prizant for the inspiration, comments, suggestions, and support provided throughout the preparation of this manuscript.

curate diagnosis of symptomatic deficiencies, which then become the focus of remedial efforts, overlooking the adaptive functions of the behavior of concern.

A major attraction of the disease model and notions of deficiency has been its documented effectiveness in medical domains. Adoption of such a model has allowed practitioners to diagnose the cause of disease or dysfunction, to isolate it, and to treat it accordingly. After all, isolation reduces the dangers of contamination. With regard to assessment, the deficiency model suggests that symptoms of underlying pathologies are identified. When applied to education and human behavior in general, such models divert from the adaptive functions of behavior to a more restrictive examination of its topography. Overt behaviors are taken at face value in a quest for objective symptoms and accurate diagnosis. Since single, context-free measures are typically pursued, contextual variation is being masked. The assessment approach adopted, therefore, serves to validate the deficiency model.

The danger with a deficiency approach to assessment is that the disease model tends to legitimize the isolation and segregation of individuals with disabilities. It provides an avenue for society to channel its discomfort with deviance when common expectations and norms are violated. For instance, a temper tantrum is more comfortably interpreted as resulting from a seizure disorder or sensory deficit than as environmentally induced, or as a personal "statement." Violations of expectations are readily dismissed as a sign of pathology, and, therefore, are easier to manage.

A related concern has to do with the fact that the measures used are not as objective as presumed. Even if the measure is obtained in a seemingly objective fashion, it still reflects the values and beliefs of the test constructors. When major decisions are made about the quality of the lives of individuals with disabilities, this becomes a serious consideration.

Another concern has to do with the highly structured nature of traditional assessments, which is, to some extent, imposed by psychometric considerations. In order to allow for norm-based comparisons, behaviors and performance are examined in response to specific instructions and testing materials. Given the inherent structure, it could even be argued that compliance is being tested more than adaptive and/or creative capacities, since responses to the instructions of others are being examined rather than any self-initiated behavior. The type of motivational mechanisms that underlie behavior in more meaningful contexts is being replaced by the motivation to look good and/or please the examiner and/or relevant others.

The constraints imposed by the psychometric model force us to examine individuals in contexts that do not require any initiation, self-evaluation, or any other form of self-regulatory behavior. To put it differently, highly structured assessments do not take into consideration the type of adaptive problem-solving capabilities that are most critical to everyday coping skills and life satisfaction. This issue deserves the close attention of special educators, since structure seems the hallmark of special education; the students enrolled typically require more structure than is available in less restrictive settings.

It has become increasingly clear that a large proportion of students enrolled in special education programs have trouble in imposing structure upon their own behavior; skills in the areas of planning, self-evaluation, and self-monitoring are typically lacking (Torgesen, 1981). In fact, limitations in these and related metacognitive abilities may be the primary characteristic of students with learning and behavior problems (Brown & Campione, 1986; Torgesen, 1981). These types of problems are not easily substantiated by highly structured traditional assessment devices, or by any type of assessment that fails to examine the underlying thought processes. The high degree of structure inherent in traditional psychometric assessment preempts the need for self-regulation; behavior is observed when external structure is applied. This oversight may serve to explain why it has been so difficult to pinpoint the exact nature of milder disabilities. What fails to be assessed is how a student performs when external structure is either not provided, or is provided only to a limited degree.

Common assumptions and beliefs about what causes disorders or disabilities, how children learn, and what constitutes development have shaped current assessment practices, even if not acknowledged. As is explained in the next section, both preoccupation with quantification of observable behaviors and search for objectivity are commensurate with static notions of learning and development. The time has come to critically examine common beliefs about learning and development, and deficiency.

COMMON BELIEFS ABOUT LEARNING AND DEVELOPMENT

Views of learning as a passive and linear process continue to dominate the field of special education, and perpetuate current assessment practices. It is often assumed that the learning process can be reduced to a series of linear steps, an assumption that invites modular approaches to education. Such an approach lends itself well to task analysis, step-by-step instruction, and related forms of educational "technology." New skills are depicted as "add-ons" rather than as the result of more pervasive restructuring processes. The learner is viewed as the passive consumer of carefully defined instructional stimuli without any a priori notions of the material presented. This conceptualization of learning as linear and orderly is congruent with the idea of predictable sequences and prerequisites, leading to the assessment of supposedly related behaviors out of context. For instance, communicative ability may be equated with automatic responses to pictures, or with manual imitation skills. The need for more naturalistic observation is conveniently preempted on the basis of these presumed relationships between observed and nonobserved behaviors.

The orientation discussed above typically leads to assessment devices that examine the product of learning rather than the underlying thought processes, and they are carried out in a highly structured context-stripped fashion. For instance, developmental status and behavior are evaluated through standardized tests and developmental checklists that: 1) are designed around normally observed skill sequences, 2) emphasize prerequisites, and 3) make generalizations on the basis of the presence or absence of component pieces of more complex skills.

Static views of learning and assessment as described above have been fueled by noninterac-

tive accounts of learning and development. For instance, major theoreticians, such as Skinner, Chomsky, and Piaget, have not emphasized social interaction as a major developmental force or learning mechanism. Skinner portrays others merely as deliverers of contingencies, Chomsky sees them as largely irrelevant to language learning, and Piaget portrays children in their solitary quest for knowledge. Social interaction in the context of assessment is likely viewed as an interfering source of error rather than as a legitimate assessment parameter. Moreover, the search for objective measures has served to deemphasize social interaction, and to approach the individuals involved with suspicion.

Views of development as unidimensional have also had an impact on assessment practices and on the ways the assessment process is conceptualized. It has typically been believed that the accomplishment of major developmental milestones speaks to advances in underlying mental processes, and that those cut across a number of tasks and domains. For instance, the appearance of language is often attributed to gains in powers of symbolic representation, which should, therefore, be paralleled by gains in symbolic domains, such as play, drawing, and so on (for a discussion of this issue, see Wolff & Gardner, 1981). Such beliefs are paralleled by unidimensional views of intelligence that have surfaced in the elusive search for the so-called g-factor. It has often been assumed that there is such a thing as generalized cognitive ability, which is the subtratum of all mental activity, and which can be captured in a single measure or score. Within this framework it is understandable that assessment tends to be equated with the assignment of a single score, which is believed to quantify the basic mental ability.

DEVELOPMENT RECONSIDERED

Prevailing assessment practices are being challenged by reconceptualizations of development and learning, which are at odds with the assumptions just discussed. First, as mentioned above, social interaction is increasingly viewed as a critical mediating force in development (for a recent review of this issue, see Schuler & Perez, 1988). Fueled by a greater appreciation of the role

of caregivers, or rather of the reciprocal transactions between caregivers and infants, transactional accounts of early development have proliferated. The terms "mediation" and "scaffolding"
are increasingly used in reference to the ways
in which caregivers arrange their infants' learning environments to maximize predictability and
foster competence. Transactional accounts of
learning and development have thus become
commonplace (e.g., see Bruner, 1975; Feuerstein, 1980; Snow, 1984), highlighting the mediating effects of caregivers.

Second, learning is becoming viewed as an
active and nonlinear process. Learners are motivated not only by external rewards, but also by
the desire to predict, detect contingencies (Lewis,
1985), and impose order upon otherwise random
stimulus input. As stated by Donaldson (1978),
children are invested in making sense out of the
objects, people, and events that surround them.
From day one children are viewed as active gen-
erators and testers of hypotheses who are engaged in a continuous mental restructuring process. This same notion of restructuring serves
to contradict linear notions of learning: New
knowledge and insights are seen as "rebuilts"
rather than "add-ons." This perspective of learning as an active process directly contradicts past
images of young children as clean slates or
empty buckets (James, 1890; Watson, 1919).

Third, unidimensional notions of development have become increasingly challenged. For
instance, Gould (1981) has argued most eloquently against the notion of generalized and
fixed cognitive skills, uncovering the dangerous
social ramifications of such beliefs. Gardner
(1983) introduced the notion of "multiple intel-
ligences," claiming that human mental activities
are the conglomerate of a number of distinct
modes of mind, which differ in terms of their
neuropsychological make-up and can operate
relatively independently.

FUTURE DIRECTIONS

Given the drawbacks of traditional assessment
practices, which tend to be deficiency oriented,
highly structured, and based upon outdated
static conceptualizations of learning and development, this section presents a number of recommendations for the future.

Concern for Function

The desire to describe and quantify behaviors
precisely and to segment them into component
pieces has diverted attention away from functions and intentions, which elude precise quantification and breakdown. To put it differently,
the *structure* of behavior has often received
much more attention than its *function*. Moreover,
preoccupation with deficiency has led to the dis-
missal of deviant behaviors as pathological without consideration of their possible adaptive function. The behaviors were viewed as confirmation
of particular diagnoses, and not as of functional
relevance to the individual of concern. This may
be best exemplified by the ways speech/language
services to students with severe disabilities have
been conceptualized. Speech/language programming has traditionally been divorced from behavior development, since the communicative
functions of many undesirable behaviors, such as
echolalia, tantrums, headbanging, and so forth
(for a more detailed discussion of these matters,
see Schuler & Prizant, 1987) were typically not
considered.

Behaviors have often been taught because
they were observable and measurable, and/or
were part of an a priori specified instructional
sequence. Consequently, interventionists have
depended heavily on extrinsic sources of reinforcement, thereby decreasing chances of generalization to more natural contexts. A more functional orientation is critical to the selection of
relevant objectives that boost motivation. The
current trend to complete so-called ecological
inventories in an attempt to assess what should
be learned to operate successfully in subsequent
living environments represents a promising example of assessment that is not only instructionally referenced, but also ecologically validated. The intent to assess which skills will be
meaningful in targeted real-life environments
presents yet another dimension of functional
assessment.

Matters of
Context and Competence

Alternative assessments need to be explored that
lend themselves to look at the functions of the
behaviors observed. These types of assessments
cannot take place in context-stripped environ-

ments, since contextual variables need to be identified. Moreover, the identification of those conditions that foster the greatest levels of competence is critical to avoid continued perceptions of deficiency. It is important to realize that the types of assessments that are being proposed are radically different from more traditional ones, which sample behavior within a single and strictly controlled context. In fact, contextual variation needs to be assessed in search for those contexts that are most conducive to the demonstration of competence. In addition, efforts should be made to identify which types of "intelligence" and modes of learning afford the greatest amounts of competence. It has been pointed out by Gardner (1983) and Goldman and Gardner (1989) that schools and assessment practices have traditionally favored linguistic and mathematical types of intelligence over interpersonal, musical, spatial, or physical forms of intelligence.

The types of assessments proposed are in line with more dynamic notions of assessments that focus on the learning process, and more specifically, on the ability to learn when provided with specified environmental support. This notion is congruent with Vygotsky's (1978) construct of the "zone of proximal development," referring to what individuals can do with the facilitation of others as opposed to independently (for an overview, see Campione, Brown, & Bryant, 1985). This help may take many different forms. For instance, a sequence of qualitatively organized prompts could be used (Campione, in press). When serving the needs of students with the most severe disabilities, the notions of assistance and support need to be viewed in their broadest sense. Relevant others can supply additional materials, and provide more supportive environments, motivation, and rapport, as well as adopt highly nurturant interaction styles.

Ultimately, assessments should be developed that compare independent performance with performance under various configurations of environmental support. Rather than being viewed as measurement error, discrepancies in performance across contexts may be indicative of

emerging skills, which are inherently context dependent. A formalized description of contextual variation may help to account for discrepancies between observers, tests, and test scores, and make previously "untestable" individuals more readily assessed in a fashion that is meaningful to instruction. In addition, such forms of assessments as explored by Peck (1989) may help to settle disputes regarding interobserver reliability and generalization, since changes in context are not probed rather than controlled for.

Need for Qualitative Measures

New appreciation of the active role that infants take in imposing order upon otherwise random stimulus input, and of the important mediating role that caregivers play in enabling them to do so, makes it necessary to evaluate active thought processes. Rather than merely examining responses to external stimuli, issues such as self-initiation need to be considered. An individual's ability to structure and regulate his or her own environment needs to be appraised instead of how that individual operates under externally imposed structure. The assessment of play may serve as a case in point, as it examines a person's ability to plan and regulate his or her own behavior guided by active imagery and self-talk (for a more detailed discussion, see Perez, 1987). The challenge here is the identification of proper measurement and evaluation procedures. Since the behaviors involved are not always easily observable or quantifiable, more qualitative descriptions are in place. The type of information sought may not be readily captured in a single score. While precise specification of observational criteria will be of great help, more subjective clinical judgments are required. What is needed is a new appreciation of the assessor as an active constructor and evaluator of hypotheses rather than merely an administrator of prepackaged tests. After all, high reliability ratings are most easily obtained when the most trivial questions are asked. The professional identity of assessors and educators at large may need to be readjusted in the process of change.

REFERENCES

Brown, A.L., & Campione, J.C. (1986). Psychological theory and the study of learning disabilities. *American Psychologist, 41*(10), 1059–1068.

Bruner, J.S. (1975). The ontogenesis of speech acts. *Journal of Child Language, 2,* 1–20.
Campione, J.C. (in press). Assisted assessment: A

taxonomy of approaches and an outline of strengths and weaknesses. *Journal of Learning Disabilities*.

Campione, J.C., Brown, A.L., & Bryant, N.R. (1985). Individual differences in learning and memory. In R.J. Sternberg (Ed.), *Human abilities: An information processing approach* (pp. 103–126). New York: W.H. Freeman & Co.

Donaldson, M. (1978). *Children's minds*. New York: Norton.

Feuerstein, R. (1980). *Instrumental enrichment: An intervention program for cognitive modifiability*. Baltimore: University Park Press.

Gardner, H. (1983). *Frames of mind*. New York: Basic Books.

Goldman, J., & Gardner, H. (1989). Multiple paths to educational effectiveness. In D.K. Lipsky & A. Gartner (Eds.), *Beyond separate education: Quality education for all* (pp. 121–139). Baltimore: Paul H. Brookes Publishing Co.

Gould, S.J. (1981) *The mismeasure of man*. New York: Norton.

James, W. (1890). *The principles of psychology*. New York: Holt.

Lewis, M. (1985). Developmental principles and their implications for at-risk and handicapped infants. In M. Hanson (Ed.), *Atypical infant development* (pp. 3–24). Baltimore: University Park Press.

Peck, C.A. (1989). Assessment of social communicative competence: Evaluating environments. *Seminars in Speech and Language, 10*(1), 1–15.

Perez, L. (1987). *Comparison of play behaviors of preschool premature infants of very low birthweight and their normal peers*. Unpublished doctoral dissertation, University of California, Berkeley.

Schuler, A.L., & Perez, L. (1988). The role of social interaction in the development of thinking skills. In E.L. Meyen, G.A. Vergason, & R.J. Whelan (Eds.), *Effective instructional strategies for exceptional children* (pp. 259–275). Denver, CO: Love Publishing Co.

Schuler, A., & Prizant, B. (1987). Facilitating communication: Pre-language approaches. In D. Cohen & A. Donnellan (Eds.), *Handbook of autism and atypical development* (pp. 301–316). New York: John Wiley & Sons.

Snow, C.E. (1984). Parent-child interaction and the development of communicative ability. In R.L. Schiefelbusch & J. Pickar (Eds.), *The acquisition of communicative competence* (pp. 69–107). Baltimore: University Park Press.

Torgesen, J.K. (1981). The relationship between memory and attention in learning disabilities. *Exceptional Education Quarterly, 3*, 51–59.

Vygotsky, L.S. (1978). *Mind in society: The development of higher psychological processes*. Cambridge, MA: Harvard University Press.

Watson, J.B. (1919). *Behavior from the standpoint of a behaviorist*. Philadelphia: J.B. Lippincott.

Wolff, D., & Gardner, H. (1981). On the structure of early symbolization. In R.L. Schiefelbusch & D.D. Bricker (Eds.), *Early language* (pp. 287–329). Baltimore: University Park Press.

♦ SECTION II ♦

DEINSTITUTIONALIZATION AND COMMUNITY SERVICES

Nearly 25 years ago, Blatt and Kaplan (1966) published their famous exposé of institutional life in their pictorial essay *Christmas in Purgatory* and Senator Robert Kennedy, after visiting several institutions in 1965, announced his negative reactions to millions of Americans through the news media. The myth of the protective environment of congregate living for persons with mental retardation would seem to have been shattered forever, particularly as subsequent investigations continued to document intolerable conditions, depersonalization, and even abuse in these large hospitals in various parts of the world. Before long, a growing consensus emerged that such facilities by their very nature were incapable of being habilitative, and the "deinstitutionalization" movement began. In their place, professionals and advocates called for the development of community services that would support persons with disabilities in a manner that was more reflective of the way that others who did not have disabilities chose to live, work, and spend their leisure time.

However, it has now become clear that the transition from large institutions to the community will be a complex process. As the review chapters in this section make clear, we have demonstrated the potential to enable everyone—no matter how severe his or her disabilities—to participate in family-scale living, work on a meaningful job for pay, recreate in the community, and develop personally satisfying social relationships with others. Yet, the overwhelming majority of our resources are still being expended upon institutions and large-scale "group" homes, segregated sheltered workshops and day activity centers, and handicapped-only recreation programs. The TASH resolutions reprinted in this section recognize that until funding, capital investment, and all other resources shift to support for individuals in their families and community, most persons with disabilities will continue to be deprived of the opportunity to enjoy a meaningful lifestyle. Well-funded institutions cannot be replaced by poorly funded community services. The chapters in this section remind us of our original intentions and the directions needed to develop the kinds of community services that could finally make institutions and segregation no more than unfortunate and embarrassing memories of the past.

REFERENCES

Blatt, B., & Kaplan, F. (1966). *Christmas in Purgatory: A photographic essay on mental retardation*. Boston: Allyn & Bacon.

DOCUMENT II.1

Deinstitutionalization Policy

The Association for Persons with Severe Handicaps believes that a mutual consideration for both quality services and quality of life is necessary, and that this mutual consideration cannot be achieved in environments which segregate persons with disabilities from the community. Thus, TASH calls for the termination of services, activities, and environments which: (a) remove children from their homes and neighborhoods, and citizens from their home communities; (b) require that persons with disabilities live under circumstances that would not be considered acceptable for persons within that same age range were they not disabled, including institutions and large scale group homes and ICF/MRs; (c) rely exclusively upon paid caregiver and other professionalized relationships to the detriment of more normalized social support networks, family systems, peer relationships, and friendships; and (d) stigmatize persons with disabilities by portraying them as individuals in need of help, care, and sympathy rather than dignity, respect, mutual companionship, and enjoyment.

TASH believes that both the commitment and the technology now exist to achieve alternative, truly community-based services. TASH calls upon the professional and advocacy community to work toward community-based options that reflect the full range of choices that are available to persons without disabilities. These choices minimally include:

1. The right to live in normalized, community-based homes, including living with parents, self-selected roommates, and varied groupings and environments considered desirable, appropriate, and chosen by persons without disabilities at particular ages in their lives;
2. The right to attend the same school he or she would attend if s/he did not have a disability and to receive at that school the individualized educational services which are appropriate for his or her needs without compromise to the development of interactions with peers (whether or not those peers themselves have a disability) throughout the school years;
3. The right of access to a variety of vocational training opportunities which allow for daily interactions with co-workers, employers, and (where relevant) consumers who do not have disabilities regardless of level or type of disability;
4. The right to participate in the kinds of extracurricular, recreational, and other leisure experiences enjoyed by typical peers and citizens; and
5. The right to daily and longitudinal social interactions with peers and other citizens (without regard to disability) that are oriented toward developing a variety of relationships, social support networks, friendships, and the ultimate goal of a normalized social status for individuals with disabilities.

FURTHER, TASH supports the expenditure of government funds in support of families pursuing community integration.

ORIGINALLY ADOPTED OCTOBER 1979
REVISED NOVEMBER 1986

*　*　*　*　*

Resolution Opposing Capital Investment in Institutional Settings in the State of New York

WHEREAS, TASH has previously called for a cessation of capital investment in institutional settings and redirection of resources to integrated community services; and

WHEREAS, Certain officials in the New York State Office of Mental Retardation and Developmental Disabilities are engaged in a multi-million dollar project to construct new facilities on the grounds of state institutions, and are planning to build over 1,000 "beds" at institutions throughout New York State;

THEREFORE BE IT RESOLVED, THAT TASH calls upon Governor Mario Cuomo and the New York State Legislature to take the following steps:

1. Stop all new construction and major renovation of buildings on institutional grounds;
2. Close all institutional buildings that do not meet safety standards at the earliest possible time;
3. Develop a long-term plan to phase out institutions and fund alternative uses for institutional facilities;
4. Redirect capital and operating funds for institutions into the community.

BE IT FURTHER RESOLVED, THAT the President of TASH shall notify all responsible New York officials of this resolution.

ORIGINALLY ADOPTED DECEMBER 1985

* * * * *

Gramm Rudman Resolution

WHEREAS, Federal programming in recent years has opened doors to independent, productive, community living for persons with the most severe handicaps, providing opportunities for success never before thought possible in educational, vocational, and social growth, and which would not have been possible without incentives provided by the federal government; and

WHEREAS, The nation is now beginning to celebrate the tenth anniversary of the Education for the Handicapped Act (EHA), which is the foundation for current and future successes for persons with severe and profound handicaps, and which resulted in the declaration by Congress that every child with a handicap, no matter how severe, be guaranteed the right to an education appropriate to his or her individual needs and capabilities; and

WHEREAS, Within the framework of EHA, persons, who in earlier times would have been relegated to a lifetime of institutionalization, are now living at home with their families, attending school like other children in their neighborhoods, and gaining skills that will enable them to live and work with support in their own communities; and

WHEREAS, The framework of EHA will be seriously weakened by the Gramm Rudman budget reduction proposals as passed by the House and Senate and such weakening would result in serious curtailment of EHA programs, hitting hardest those people most in need of EHA protection; and

WHEREAS, Congress has recognized that deinstitutionalization is essential social response to the needs of persons with mental retardation, and has created programs providing services necessary for community living within Medicaid through the Medicaid Waiver and the ICF/MR; and

WHEREAS, A reduction in Medicaid funds would not result in a reduction of total public money for persons who would be forced back into an institution, but would simply reconfigure federal/state responsibility with the money flowing to the institution rather than buying services in the community; and

WHEREAS, In many cases SSI is the only income available to persons with severe mental retardation, and any reductions in this program could be life-threatening to these people who are unable without this assistance to provide for themselves; and

WHEREAS, Section 202 housing for persons with handicaps and who are elderly is a crucial resource for persons in need of publicly provided living space, but is only a limited and preliminary response to the housing needs of persons with severe handicaps, and more money is urgently needed for living facilities; and

WHEREAS, Early intervention is one of the greatest hopes for prevention of severe and profound mental retardation, and initiatives through the federally funded maternal and child health programs have resulted in the good health of babies that otherwise would have been severely handicapped, as well as in children who function with less severe retardation than would have been possible without interventive services; and

WHEREAS, The Gramm Rudman budget reduction proposals currently before you seriously threaten the very core of these programs and would set persons with severe handicaps back twenty years; and

WHEREAS, Protection of each of these programs which touch the lives of millions of Americans has been hard sought since 1981; and

WHEREAS, The threat of reduction has resulted in the past, and will continue to result, in a loud national outcry from educators, health care specialists, service providers, consumers, and their families.

THEREFORE BE IT RESOLVED, THAT the members of The Association for Persons with Severe Handicaps unanimously and adamantly urge members of the U.S. House of Representatives and Senate to protect each of the programs outlined from the Gramm Rudman or any other automatic budget cutting plans.

ORIGINALLY ADOPTED NOVEMBER 1985

*   *   *   *   *

DOCUMENT II.4

Policy Statement for Cessation of Capital Investment in Segregated Settings

WHEREAS, TASH policy supports the right of all people with severe handicaps to receive services in integrated environments; federal and state fiscal policies, including Medicaid, encourage capital investment in segregated institutions, workshops, and other settings; virtually every state in the nation has invested financial resources in construction or renovation of one or more of the following: large residential settings, segregated workshops, day activity centers and separate "disabled-only" schools, and in other segregated services; and such investment perpetuates an inappropriate, restrictive, and outmoded model of services; and

RESOLVED, THAT TASH calls for a cessation of capital investment in renovation and construction in large residential settings, separate work and activity settings, segregated schooling, and other segregated centers, and redirection of resources to integrated community services.

ORIGINALLY ADOPTED OCTOBER 1981
REVISED OCTOBER 1987

*   *   *   *   *

CHAPTER 8

Living it Up!
An Analysis of Research on Community Living

JAN NISBET

MARSHA CLARK

SUSAN COVERT

University of New Hampshire, Durham, New Hampshire

Twenty years ago, during the wave of deinstitutionalization and public realization that residential facilities for persons with severe disabilities were cruel and dehumanizing, small group homes were the solution. In 1979, even after attending a Program Analysis of Service Systems (PASS) workshop, there was little or no question that small group homes of six or eight people could, through decorating and arranging, be like yours and mine. As a field we attempted to validate the success of small-group living arrangements in comparison to the mammoth institutions for persons with severe disabilities through numerous studies (see Brook, 1973; Herz, Endicott, Spitzer, & Mesnikoff, 1971; Krowinski & Fitt, 1978; Levenson et al., 1977; Mosher & Menn, 1978; Pasamanick, Scarpitti, & Dinitz, 1967; Stein, Test, & Marx, 1975; Washburn, Vannicelli, Longabaugh, & Scheff, 1976; Wilder, Levin, & Zwerling, 1966). Variables such as size, resident composition, location, staff training, cost, property values, neighborhood responses, and "client" interactions and progress have also been analyzed. Although not unequivocal, basically the research can be summarized as follows:

1. Persons with disabilities who move out of large residential environments do better in smaller ones when there is sufficient attention paid to their individual characteristics.

2. Differences that are observed across small community living arrangements have more to do with an interaction between numerous factors (e.g., those delineated above and those inherent to communities) than to one single variable.

3. When individuals with disabilities or their families are provided with individualized support, there are greater chances of programmatic success and satisfaction.

RESEARCH AGENDAS

The research that sets a direction for individualized supports in community living is scant. Most of the data serve to validate or evaluate current practices, to prove that something is better or worse. Unlike the field of physics or engineering, research does not typically drive practices in community living. Instead, model demonstrations serve as the foundation for replication, further development, and research. There is not

---

Marc Gold, in his book *Marc Gold: "Did I Say That?"* provided retrospective analyses of articles he had written during his academic and professional career. He admitted both great writing and that that was flawed. We would like to adapt his strategy here and apply it to intent: We will never attempt to conduct a comprehensive literature review on community living again. There are many articles and books that pertain to community living, roughly over 2,000. We chose to examine only those that were published after 1980. Because of the rapid expansion and changes in philosophy, we felt that it was both impossible and uninteresting to examine ancient literature. Some references were made to earlier studies if they provided the clear basis for future work. Studies that were conducted in institutional environments were ignored, for obvious reasons. Studies that claimed to be conducted in community settings, but really were conducted in group homes of over 12, were virtually ignored with a few exceptions. In many research endeavors it was difficult to determine whether the persons involved were severely disabled. We erred on the side of inclusion rather then exclusion.

one parametric or nonparametric study that has proved that developing individualized support options for persons with severe disabilities in their local communities is better than placement in group living arrangements. But, as a field, we have embraced this idea. Because, as a group concerned about the lives of persons with severe disabilities, we know it is the *right* thing to do. The opposition asks, "But where are your data?"; and then we conduct the studies. In this regard, research is used to verify and validate the fundamental rights of persons with disabilities rather than to set new directions.

Strategies for financing individual apartments and homes, arranging personal supports, developing formal and informal networks and friendships, and facilitating learning in the community are presented at national and state conferences, but are not published in recognized journals. There are few books. What we as a field really need to know, we do not. Maybe some do, but most do not. As we move from formal structures, such as group homes, to less formal supports, such as supported apartments, family living arrangements, home ownership and cooperative living, and full community participation, the variables become difficult to describe. Quantitative analysis, in many regards, seems inappropriate. Ethnographic research strategies such as interviews and participant-observation techniques (Bogdan & Biklen, 1982) that attempt to capture community, lifestyles, events, and interactions appear more appropriate given the direction of the field and the needs of persons with disabilities and their families. "A qualitative study can contribute an analysis of how people interact with the community, how staff relate to people in this type of setting, and of issues in individualized planning which can inform any effort to assure that people with severe disabilities are being integrated into the community" (Knoll & Olsen, 1988, p. 14).

Vanier (1979) described two essential elements of life in the community: 1) interpersonal relationships, a sense of belonging; and 2) an orientation of life to a common goal and common witness. Almost 10 years later, these aspects of community and their relationships to persons with severe disabilities had hardly been studied. By 1988, there were at least 14 reviews on community living and adjustment (see Balla,

1976; Baroff, 1980; Craig & McCarver, 1984; Freedman, 1976; Haney, 1988; Haney & Heal, 1987; Heal & Fujiura, 1984; Heal, Sigelman, & Switsky, 1978; Landesman-Dwyer, 1981; McCarver & Craig, 1974; Peck, Blackburn, & White-Blackburn, 1980; Pilewski & Heal, 1980; Sigelman, Novak, Heal, & Switzsky, 1980; Windle, Stewart, & Brown, 1961; Zigler & Balla, 1977).

A criticism of this research is its focus on individual-level factors at the expense of group, organizational, and community variables. This is a serious problem because of the lack of correlation between individual-level variables (e.g., intellectual and physical abilities) and community living success (Haney, 1988). Thus, variables such as staff commitment and training may be stronger contributors to community living success than the level of mental retardation or adaptive behavior.

Butterfield (1982) criticized community living research and discussed the consequences of bias. He suggested that most of the research to date was scientifically uninteresting and provided little guidance for improving living arrangements. Butterfield also suggested that when differences are found among and between those who live in "specialized" living arrangements it is difficult to attribute the differences to the living arrangement, characteristics of the people who were assigned to the living arrangement, or to an interaction of the arrangement with people's characteristics. The lack of random assignment always defeats the scientific purpose of comparing people in different living environments. However, he further noted that studies done for social or clinical reasons are not rendered invalid because of a selection bias.

> For example, if the question is whether people who receive care in a special living arrangement advance to the point of being able to subsist outside the arrangement, then selection bias is irrelevant, because the question is about people who are selected for the arrangement not the interaction between the two. (Butterfield, 1982, p. 248)

CASE STUDIES AND PERSONAL REPORTS

There are few case studies of persons with severe disabilities living in their own homes and well integrated into their communities (Taylor, Racino, Knoll, & Lutfiyya, 1987). Most studies are based on group home experiences (see Bercovici, 1983; Heshusius, 1981; Rothman & Rothman, 1984). Qualitative researchers (Bogdan & Taylor, 1982; Edgerton, 1967; Edgerton & Bercovici, 1976; Edgerton, Bollinger, & Herr, 1984; Rothman & Rothman, 1984) have provided some of this information, but it is sparse and frequently based on individuals in group or boarding homes. Balla, Butterfield, and Zigler (1973) suggested that observing persons in the community and studying their daily routines would provide expansive information for researchers and providers. Bjannes and Butler (1974) used naturalistic observation to describe activities that distinguished facilities that encouraged competent and normalizing behaviors versus those that did not. Other studies that used naturalistic observation procedures across different sizes and types of facilities resulted in conclusions that a community living arrangement could not be considered an "a priori normalizing environment" (Chadsey-Rusch, 1985, p. 398); and that internal and external supports were needed to facilitate normalization.

Edgerton (1967), Edgerton and Bercovici (1976), and Edgerton and Langness (1978) have provided the most expansive base for ethnographic research. These studies of successful integration have primarily involved observations and interviews with persons with mild disabilities. Bogdan and Taylor (1982) in *Inside Out: The Social Meaning of Retardation* provided another example of qualitative research through the use of personal interviews with three previously institutionalized adults. Personal reports of the effects of community living on the lives of persons with disabilities can also be read in books such as *On Our Own: Patient-Controlled Alternatives to the Mental Health System* (Chamberlin, 1978), *Disabled We Stand* (Sutherland, 1981) and *We Can Speak for Ourselves: Self-Advocacy by Mentally Handicapped People* (Williams & Shoultz, 1982).

WHAT IS COMMUNITY LIVING?

As the focus of the research agenda is "community living," it is important to have an understanding of this concept. Although community living appears to be relatively easy to define, it involves more than simply living in a residence. There is a difference between living in a community and being integrated into the community (Kregel, Wehman, Seyfarth, & Marshall, 1986). Programs can easily be community based (i.e., located in the community) without being integrated (Bachrach, 1981). In fact, Landesman and Vietze (1987) noted the following as characteristics of institutionalization in the community: rigid administrative organization, inadequate social interaction, insufficient resource utilization, and limited relationships with others. As used here, community living encompasses the integration of individuals with disabilities into the community and addresses the social, recreational, vocational, and/or educational needs of individuals in that community. The homes should be small, individualized, cooperative living situations where individuals with disabilities have input on living companions, self-care routines, friends, community activities, and others on a daily basis (Janicki, 1981).

Options for community living include the natural family, adoptive families, foster homes, supervised apartments, and supportive living arrangements (S.J. Taylor, 1987a). The key to each of these options is that they are all home environments that encourage social interactions, vocational development, and independence by providing the support necessary to individuals with disabilities and their families. These home environments are homes that persons with disabilities live in with their families, or that they personally rent or own, and that cannot be taken away from them. These homes are in contrast to homes owned or rented by a state or local agency, where persons with disabilities can be removed without consideration of the individuals' desires or the needs of their families (Knoll & Ford, 1987). Additionally, a home can be arranged according to the personal choice of the individual who resides there and not according to the group wishes or the requirements of an anonymous agency.

S.J. Taylor (1987b) summarized six basic assumptions/principles associated with the present interpretation of community integration:

1. All individuals with disabilities can and should live in the community. Community

living can be accessible to *all* persons with disabilities, without exception.

2. In addition to being integrated into regular neighborhoods, individuals with disabilities must also be integrated into work and community settings.

3. People with disabilities and their families need support to live in the community. Support has been given to institutions and group homes to provide assistance to individuals with disabilities, yet the same level of support is not afforded families. Financial, social, and professional support needs to be provided to families.

4. People with disabilities and their neighbors should be encouraged to develop lasting, meaningful social relations.

5. Individuals with disabilities should be given the opportunity to learn. This includes an array of social, educational, and vocational skills that would enable persons to function more independently.

6. Individuals with disabilities and their families should be actively involved in the design, implementation, monitoring, and evaluation of services. This helps to ensure that needs and wishes are attained and maintained.

In sum, community living is an encompassing concept that focuses on integrated, individualized, community residency for individuals with disabilities, that is closely linked to addressing their educational and vocational needs, and social relationships, networks, and support.

MOVEMENT INTO THE COMMUNITY

Shift from Institution to Community Living Options

The total number of persons with mental retardation living in institutions is approximately the same today as 50 years ago. However, as of 1986, facilities of 15 and fewer residents had a somewhat greater total of persons than state institutions (104,189 and 103,049, respectively) (Lakin, Hill, White, & Wright, 1988). This change may be partly attributed to litigation that confronted the efficacy of institutionalization. According to Willer and Intagliata (1984), court

decisions regarding deinstitutionalization have established three precedents: increased restrictions placed on who should be considered for admission (*Welsch v. Likins,* 1977; *Wyatt v. Stickney,* 1972); lack of consideration of institutional placement prior to attempting all community alternatives (*Welsch v. Likins,* 1977; *Wyatt v. Stickney,* 1972); and restrictions on the length of placement in an institution (*Wyatt v. Stickney,* 1972).

The precedent for community living was set by two cases: *Wyatt v. Stickney* (1972), which embraced the concepts of normalization and least restrictive environment; and *Halderman v. Pennhurst State School and Hospital* (1977), which required deinstitutionalization. There has been a rapid increase in the number of community-based living options for individuals with disabilities since the Halderman case, with similar court cases occurring in other states. The number of individuals with disabilities residing in institutions has decreased by 100,000, from a daily average of 194,650 in 1967 to 94,696 in 1987 (White, Lakin, Hill, Wright, & Bruininks, 1988). Reasons other than court-ordered deinstitutionalization have stimulated the movement toward community living options: advocacy by parents and consumers, demonstration by individuals with disabilities of their ability to live independently or semi-independently in the community, documented improvement by individuals with disabilities who have resided in the community, and understanding of the need to teach functional skills in the natural environment.

A study conducted in 1982 by Hauber and colleagues surveyed every state regarding the public and private residential options for individuals with disabilities (Hauber et al., 1984). Community living options were divided into eight categories: small group residence (1–6-bed and 7–15-bed facilities); large private group residence (16–63-, 64–299-, and 300 + -bed facilities); large public group residence; specialized foster care; semi-independent living; supervised living arrangement; personal care; and specialized nursing care. The most noticeable finding was the wide variation in services among the states. When the data were compiled, the findings indicated that although there were more specialized foster homes than any other single type of model, more individuals with disabilities lived in facilities that housed over 300 individuals. There were more 1–6-bed group homes than 7–15-bed group homes. While this study included alternatives to group and foster homes, the number of semi-independent options (306) and supervised living arrangements (185) was comparatively small.

A more recent study by Lakin et al. (1988) reported a decrease in the number of individuals with mental retardation residing at state institutions for more than 16 persons and an increase in the number of those residing in community facilities. They noted that in 1967 the overwhelming majority of individuals with disabilities who were residing outside the family were in large state institutions; by 1986 the majority were living in community facilities.

Data on size and placement during the latter part of the 1970s present conflicting results. While 73% of the community living options served 10 or fewer individuals, over half of individuals with disabilities were served in facilities that housed more than 30 people (Bruininks, Kudla, Hauber, Hill, & Wieck, 1981). Lakin et al. (1988) analyzed the changing trend of large versus small residential facilities for individuals with mental retardation for the years 1977, 1982, and 1986. While the numbers of persons with disabilities living in facilities of 15 or less increased during this period, more people still live in residences housing 16 or more individuals. Thus, while there has been a growth in the number of community facilities, the majority of individuals with disabilities do not live in home-style environments. Finally, Hill, Lakin, and Bruininks (1984) summarized and compared the results of two national surveys of residential facilities for people with mental retardation. The results showed similar trends for children and adults with disabilities. They found a decreasing number of children in out-of-home residential care and an increasing proportion of persons with severe/profound handicaps in community-based residences.

Changes in Skills as the Result of Deinstitutionalization

A longitudinal study (Conroy & Bradley, 1985) of the *Halderman* case was conducted to mea-

sure, among other things: the change in the residents as a result of community versus institutional placement, the impact of institutionalization on the families and the communities, and the costs of deinstitutionalization. Individuals who left Pennhurst were placed in community living arrangements (CLAs) that housed an average of three people and generally no more than six. The CLAs were located in regular residential locations. Adaptive behavioral data were collected on 176 people who resided at Pennhurst from 1978 to 1980 and who then lived in CLAs in 1983 and 1984. While at Pennhurst, the individuals demonstrated no gains in adaptive behavior, whereas there was a significant increase in adaptive behavior after placement in the community. Growth was noted after the initial placement and continued a year after residing in the community. In interviews with selected consumers before and after community placement, satisfaction was reliably assessed. While at Pennhurst, the residents generally expressed satisfaction. However, after movement to community residences, they expressed a significant increase in satisfaction as compared to those who remained at Pennhurst. The community living arrangements also were rated higher on scales of normalization and individualization. Conroy and Bradley noted two other significant findings: 1) the more normalized the setting, the more progress that person was likely to make; and 2) individuals placed with fewer people did significantly better than those placed with greater numbers. In sum, the smaller the number of residents, the greater the increase in adaptive behavior.

Sokol-Kessler, Conroy, Feinstein, Lemanowicz, and McGurrin (1983) collected behavioral data on 713 residents of public institutions in 1978 and 1980. The same data were collected on individuals living in the community. By matching the individuals on adaptive behavior measures, the authors concluded that residents of institutions made no significant developmental progress over a 2-year period of time, whereas those in the community made significant developmental progress in the reduction of maladaptive behavior. Conroy, Efthimiou, and Lemanowicz (1982) reported that deinstitutionalization was associated with significant gains in adaptive behavior. Matched clients who remained at the institution (i.e., Pennhurst) did not show gains.

Aanes and Moen (1976); Bell, Schoenrock, and Bensburg (1981); Soforenko and Macy (1977); and Thompson and Carey (1980) all found improvement in various measures of adaptive functioning as a result of moving from more to less restrictive environments. Eating, cleanliness, appearance, socialization, kitchen duties, clothing care, language and communication development, interpersonal relationships, time skills, knowledge of community services, and ability to use recreation/leisure resources were examined. Minor differences in the length and duration of skill gain over time were reported. The amount, type, and quality of instructional opportunities were not included in these studies, and one should assume that change in environment and provision of opportunity facilitates skill acquisition. This is consistent with the findings of O'Neill, Brown, Gordon, Schonhorn, and Greer (1981) who used "activity pattern indicators" (Brown, Diller, Fordyce, Jacobs, & Gordon, 1980) with 26 persons prior, during, and after a move from an institution to supervised apartments.

Landesman-Dwyer (1981) reported the only large study of the effects of living arrangements to which persons with mental retardation were assigned. She constructed 49 trios of persons with retardation. The trios were matched for sex, adaptive behavior, age, length of institutionalization, and medical and behavioral characteristics. One member of each trio was randomly selected for assignment to a different living arrangement, another member was randomly selected for movement to a new arrangement, and the third remained in the old arrangement. Baseline data were collected, and outcome data were collected a year later. Landesman-Dwyer found small but reliable effects of changed living arrangements. The nature of the effects varied with the behavioral characteristics of the residents prior to their move. Close (1977) did the only other study in which residents with mental retardation were randomly assigned to living arrangements. He found larger effects than did Landesman-Dwyer. That is, smaller "family-style" residences correlated with improved adaptive behavior. However, there were differences in

"programming" between the two sets of living arrangements.

Resident Characteristics Influencing Movement into Community Options

The notion of a continuum of services is based on the idea that persons with various levels of disability require different types of environments and supports. Personal characteristics, therefore, dictated the types of living arrangements. Those with the most severe disabilities were in the most restrictive settings. A body of research exists that is based on the notion that personal characteristics rather than the intensity and types of supports are key to success in the community. For example, Schalock and Harper (1979) trained 79 clients residing in group homes, foster homes, and family situations and placed them in supervised or independent apartments and houses. The 69 who remained in those settings after 2 years had strengths in such areas as symbolic operations, personal maintenance, clothing care and use, socially appropriate behavior, and functional academics. Those who returned to more restrictive environments had adaptive behavior deficits, and problems with money management, cleanliness, social behavior, and meal preparation. The adaptive behavior skills that proved to be significant predictors of community success were: personal maintenance, communication, food preparation, community use and clothing care (Rotegard, Bruininks, Holman, & Lakin, 1985). Intagliata and Willer (1982) compared 49 persons who lived in the community and then were re-institutionalized with 255 who did not return to more restrictive placements. Those who returned had significantly less developed social skills, less regular contact with friends in the community, and less behavioral control. Interestingly, those who returned to the institution were more likely to be independent travelers. Sternlicht (1978) found that self-care skills were the most significant predictor of successful foster care placements. Unacceptable behavior and poor health were the best predictors of unsuccessful placements. Similar research by Nihira, Foster, Shellhaas, and Leland (1974), comparing approximately 25 successful and unsuccessful community placements, found behavior and self-help as best predictors of success. These claims were based on descriptive statistics and personal knowledge of the residents. However, within the research design there was no significant difference.

Crnic and Pym (1979) found by interviewing staff that resident motivation and coping skills, social interaction, and service agency support were required to facilitate a successful transition to semi-independent living. Sutter, Mayeda, Call, Yanagi, and Yee (1980) reported that the 17 of the 60 persons who returned to an institution had significantly better self-help and social skills, but significantly more severe behavior problems. Unfortunately, there are virtually no data on the role that personal contacts, socioeconomic status of the family, service delivery philosophy and organization, and community networks have on return to more restrictive environments. Information regarding these variables would create a better understanding of all the influences that contribute to placement in more restrictive settings.

Are We Saving Money?

Cost is an issue that is generally raised whenever deinstitutionalization and community living are discussed. Numerous studies have been conducted that compare the costs of community residential facilities (see Baker, Seltzer, & Seltzer, 1977; Heal & Daniels, 1978; O'Connor, 1976; O'Connor & Morris, 1978; Templeman, Gage, & Fredericks, 1982) or have compared the cost of public institutions with that of community residential facilities (see Mayeda & Wai, 1975; Minnesota Developmental Disabilities Planning, 1982; Nihira, 1979; Wieck & Bruininks, 1980). In all, the cost of community living arrangements was less than that of institutionalization. Some of the difference in cost could be accounted for by union expenses associated with the institution. In the Pennhurst follow-up study, Conroy and Bradley (1985) indicated that the differences in cost could be related to the fact that those individuals residing in community living arrangements could utilize services such as church, library, and fire safety that were available to others in the community, thus reducing the expenses. Also, community programs tend to use a "generalist" approach, where the staff perform a number of responsibilities instead of only one specific task, as occurred at the institution. Finally, there appears to be little relationship between the individual's needs and the cost of the CLA. Rather than developing placements based on need, people were more likely to be placed in a residence based on availability. Conroy and Bradley noted that this system of placement is contrary to the intent of the court-ordered deinstitutionalization.

Jones, Conroy, Feinstein, and Lemanowicz (1984) matched 70 institutionalized and deinstitutionalized adults. They found that the deinstitutionalized group required less public money than the institutionalized group, although the financial burden shifted substantially from federal sources to state and local funding sources when people moved to the community. Templeman et al. (1982) over a 5-year period of time compared the cost of children in an institution, a group home, and a single-family residence. They estimated a 57% savings when children were living in a group home versus an institution. Also, family support and respite care have assisted families in ways that prevent costly out-of-home placements. However, cost analyses of these programs have not been widely conducted.

The Medicaid Waiver has been the most significant contributor for funds for community services. In 1982, Bruininks, Kudla, Wieck, and Hauber reported that among 2,000 community residential facility directors, 46% cited the lack of an available continuum of comprehensive services as a major problem in community placement. Colombatto et al. (1982) indicated that only 33% of institution directors thought that persons with severe disabilities could be served in the community given the current resources. The number decreased to 10% when persons with labels of profoundly handicapped were considered.

Nerney, Conley, and Nisbet (1989) analyzed the costs of providing community living services in Nebraska, New Hampshire, and Michigan. They analyzed three service regions in their entirety and concluded that the least expensive option was family care. However, when community residences were compared, the authors found that the costs, in general, are higher when persons with severe disabilities are grouped homogeneously. That is, if persons with severe disabilities are placed together, the costs are greater than when they live with persons with less significant disabilities. However, 90% of federal dollars are expended in large mental retardation/developmental disability programs that serve only 5% of all persons with developmental disabilities (Braddock, Howes, & Hemp, 1984).

RESEARCH ON COMMUNITY LIVING ARRANGEMENTS

There is a small body of research on small community-based options and their relationship to personal gain and community integration. Community living research has focused on three major subject populations, the individual with developmental disabilities, the caregiver, and the place in which the individual resides (Heal, 1985). Doucett and Freedman (1981) reviewed many instruments that have been used to assess community integration. The majority of instruments focused on where people received services, the frequency and types of interactions, and the utilization of generic services. Heal and Laidlaw (1980) suggested measures in the six following domains as important to the integration process: approximation to normalization, social and self-care competence, the individual's satisfaction, others' satisfaction, residential climate, and cost. Bersani (1987a) and the staff at the Center on Human Policy at Syracuse University developed a Community Integration Inventory that is organized to collect descriptive data regarding where, with whom, what settings, and types and frequency of interactions. It is more comprehensive than others and attempts to break down the daily, weekly, and monthly routines of persons with severe disabilities.

The most common outcome measure used in the community integration literature has been some index of the individual's success in the community (Bell et al., 1981; Gollay, Freedman, Wyngaarden, & Kurtz, 1978; Heal et al., 1978; Rosen, Kiuitz, Clark, & Floor, 1970; Schalock, Harper, & Genung, 1981; G.B. Seltzer, 1981; Windle et al., 1961). Outcome measures most commonly used are those such as: who remained in the community or returned to the institution; competence in community survival skills; move-

ment through the continuum of human services; affiliation; acceptance; satisfaction with community, jobs, or residence; arrangement of staff-resident interactions; critical incidents; and cost (Heal, 1985).

Since 1979, approximately 11 reviews have addressed residential and community living issues including research on institutionalization (Birenbaum & Seiffer, 1976; Scheerenberger, 1976; Zigler & Balla, 1977) and on deinstitutionalization (Craig & McCarver, 1984; Heal et al., 1978; McCarver & Craig, 1974; Pilewski & Heal, 1980). Balla (1976) and Baroff (1980) examined the relationship between facility size and quality of care. Landesman-Dwyer (1981) studied successful participation in community life according to an extensive set of variables. Haney and Heal (1987) reviewed all relevant comparative studies obtained from *Psychological Abstracts* from January, 1970, to September, 1984, and the subsequent examination, and specifically reviewed 20 articles. Five areas of investigation included: community versus institutional residence; home versus institutional residence; group home and community living arrangement versus institutional residence; foster care versus institutional residence; and various other community alternatives.

What's Happening in Group Homes?

Group homes are no longer considered the housing model of choice for persons with severe disabilities. Alternatives such as supported apartments, home ownership and cooperatives, family support and care, and shared living are increasingly popular practices and concepts, as they are individualized to meet the needs of the person. However, because the majority of research has focused on group homes, the research on group homes is addressed here (however irrelevant to the current community living agenda). Rotegard et al. (1985) suggested that:

> living in the community does not alone have inherently normalizing effects on the behavior or competency of mentally retarded persons in residential facilities. Various authors/researchers have found the essence of normalization of the environment to be the opportunity for control of personal space, the chances for positive social interaction, the personalization of the physical setting, and/or the encouragement of socialization. (p.161)

Characteristics of residents, their caregivers, and facilities have been used to predict resident changes (Novak & Heal, 1980). Changes as a function of time, relocation from one facility to another, and specific interventions have also been included as independent variables.

Adaptive Behavior

Adaptive behavior has been defined as "the effectiveness or degree with which individuals meet the standards of personal independence and social responsibility expected for age and cultural group" (Grossman, 1983, p.1). Using this definition, general adaptive behaviors would include community living skills, social interaction skills, leisure skills, and vocational skills. Willer and Intagliata (1982) found that when the level of mental retardation was controlled, group home residents exhibited significantly lower ratings of improvement in adaptive behavior and significantly higher ratings in improvement in community living skills. In a follow-up study, Willer and Intagliata (1984) investigated the effect of different residential alternatives on adaptive behavior using a posttest-only design. The difficulty in comparing settings is obvious because of the fact that individuals were placed in different settings according to personal and environmental characteristics. However, the researchers concluded that those placed in their natural homes were the most severely disabled and exhibited the greatest degree of behavioral deficit. They improved the least in functioning and demonstrated no improvement in adaptive behavior. Foster care residents improved in self-care skills, as well as some community living skills, and showed a decrease in behavior problems over time. Group home residents exhibited the most improvement in some community living skills, but had high rates of maladaptive behavior. Residents of health care facilities (i.e. nursing homes) exhibited more behavior problems than any other group.

Eyman, Demaine, and Lei (1979) examined the relationship between residential facilities' Program Assessment of Service Systems (PASS 3) (Wolfensberger & Glenn, 1975) scores and adaptive behavior through the use of path analysis in foster care and board-and-care homes. The results indicated that the number of PASS factors with high scores appeared to be significantly related to positive adaptive behavior change. Hull and Thompson (1980) examined the relationship between certain residential variables and adaptive behavior improvement with 369 individuals. Seven variables associated with the residential environment (activities promoting social integration, appearance, transportation, community resources, social protection, resident-staff interaction, and quality of the physical setting) were highly correlated ($r = .75$) with adaptive behavior (IQ, resident satisfaction with the residence, resident independence, and problem behavior). Suedfeld (1980) provided empirical support that the negative aspects of severely restricted environmental stimulation were not uniform across subjects. In fact, the author reported that some individuals appeared to enjoy or prefer conditions perceived by others as very oppressive or intolerable. The interpretation that oppression was enjoyable is subjective and unfortunate.

Larson and Lakin (1989) reviewed 16 studies that conducted follow-up research on individuals with disabilities who had left institutions and were living in community facilities of less than 15 people (see Table 8.1). All of the studies minimally reported movement toward improved adaptive skills as a result of their living in the community. Thirteen of the studies reported significant improvement in adaptive skills or in the self-care/domestic area. Only one of the studies noted a decrease in skills, and that occurred in the vocational domain.

Social Interaction in Group Homes

Landesman-Dwyer, Sackett, and Kleinman (1980a), in their study of 20 group homes, used 10 separate behavioral or environmental categories to collect 16,000 hours of behavioral samples and concluded that: 1) age and level of retardation were correlated with activity levels; 2) small group homes did not maximize social behavior; 3) positive social behavior was associated with homogeneous grouping of residents; 4) parent visitations contributed to inactive behavior; and 5) residents in older buildings showed more community interaction than those living in new, specially designed group homes (cited in Chadsey-Rusch, 1985). The authors

Table 8.1. Behavioral outcomes associated with movement from state institutions to small (15 or fewer persons) community living arrangements

Author, date, & type of study	State	# Subjects	Age	Time (months)	Level of retardation		BEHAVIORAL OUTCOMES		
					Mild/moderate	Severe/profound	Adaptive behavior		Problem behavior
							General/overall	Specific domains	
Bradley, Conroy, Covert, & Feinstein (1986)	NH	160	A & C	72	X	X	+ +	+ d	0
Close (1977)	OR	12	A	12		X			
Colorado Division of Developmental Disabilities (1982)	CO	115	A & C	12	X	X	+	+ + a	
Conroy & Bradley (1985)	PA	383[a]	A & C	72[a]	X	X	+ +		+
Conroy, Efthimiou, & Lemanowicz (1982)	PA	140	A	24	X	X	+ +		+[a]
Conroy, Feinstein, & Lemanowicz (1988)	CT	207	A	24	X	X	+ +	+ + d	- -
D'Amico, Hannah, Milhouse, & Froleich (1978)	WV	13	A & C	6, 12[b]	X	X	+ + [a] + + [d]	+ + a,b,c,f 0,d,e	
Eastwood & Fisher (1988)	N.E. USA	98	A	24–48		X		+ + c + a	
Feinstein, Lemanowicz, Spreat, & Conroy (1986)	LA	103	A & C	9, 18	X	X	+ +		+ +
Horner, Stoner, & Ferguson (1988)	OR	23	A & C	60	X	X		+ + a,c,f	+
Kleinberg & Galligan (1983)	NY	20	A	4, 8, 12	X	X		+ + a[b],b,c 0e,g –d	
O'Neill, Brown, Gordon, & Schonhorn (1985)	NY	27	A	3, 9	X	X		+ + a,b[e]	
D. B. Rosen (1985)	AR	116	A	24	X	X	+ +	+ + a,d,e,f	
Schroeder & Hanes (1978)	NC	38	A	12	X	X	+ +		
State of Wisconsin (1986)	WI	24	A	18	X	X		+ + b,c, d,f + a	
Thompson & Carey (1980)	MN	8	A	24	X	X	+[f]	+ a,b,f	0

From Larson, S.A., & Lakin, K.C. (1989). Deinstitutionalization of persons with mental retardation: Behavioral outcomes. *Journal of The Association for Persons with Severe Handicaps, 14,* 324–332; reprinted by permission.

[a] This study included six groups, all of which showed significant gains; the largest group measured over the longest time is reported here.

[b] Domestic skills increased significantly, but grooming skills showed no overall change.

[c] IQ above 20.

[d] IQ below 20.

[e] Significant increases were found in 4 of 16 subcategories in these skill areas.

[f] Mean differences were not tested for statistical significance.

Age   A = adult; C = children; A & C = adults and children.

Outcomes   + + = statistically significant improvement after move to the community; + = improvement after move but not statistically significant; 0 = no change after move; – – = decline after move but not statistically significant; – = statistically significant decline after move to the community.

Adaptive behavior domains   a = self-care, domestic; b = communication/language; c = social skills; d = vocational; e = academic; f = community living; g = recreation/leisure.

also found that more social interaction among peers was found in smaller group homes. Staff behavior and interactions with residents was not related to facility size. In a study of friendship and affiliation, Landesman-Dwyer, Berkson, and Romer (1979) found that: social interaction generally occurred within dyads rather than larger size groups; and the frequency of social interactions was correlated not with sex or level of mental retardation, but rather with the group home characteristics. With an increase in group home size, the number of interactions increased. However, size did not necessarily affect intensity of relationships. Homogeneity of groupings and sex ratios did. Stephen J. Taylor, Director of the Center for Human Policy (1984), criticized much of this research as reflecting the "cocktail party effect". That is, with larger groups of people, there is an increased likelihood of interactions.

Krauss and Erickson (1988) collected data on informal supports provided by family, friends, and professionals for 49 aging persons with mental retardation who lived either with their family, in a community residence, or in an institution. The results indicated that family members are the predominant social network for older individuals who reside at home. In contrast, individuals who lived in community settings or institutions had an equivalent number of family, friend, and professional social supports. These findings are consistent with those of Willer and Intagliata (1981).

Berkson and Romer (1980) and Romer and Berkson (1980a, 1980b) studied the social ecology of residential and work settings. In general, they found that personal characteristics (i.e., attractiveness, intelligence, communicative abilities) were significant predictors of interactiveness, that opposite-sex relationships were "stronger" than same-sex relationships, and that persons with moderate levels of intelligence interacted extensively with those possessing both higher and lower levels of intelligence. Clearly, similar results might be expected from persons who are not disabled.

Kishi, Teelucksingh, Zollers, Park-Lee, and Meyer (1988) administered a life-choice survey adapted from a measure by Meyer, St. Peter, and Park-Lee (1986) to 42 nonretarded adults and 24 adults with mental retardation. They found that persons living in group homes "generally do not have choices about fundamental matters of living and persons identified as lowest functioning in each home had more limited choices than did those ranked highest functioning" (p. 434). Research designed to evaluate interventions that provide more choice-making opportunities and modify practices of support staff is needed.

Impact of Size of Residential Facilities

The size of residential programs has been the clearest focus of research, policy, and programmatic discussion in the field of community living and severe disabilities. Using the Physical Environment Scale, Rotegard, Hill, and Bruininks (1983) found that characteristics of a homelike environment decreased as size increased. Facilities housing less than 16 persons were found to be the most homelike. Residences with eight or less persons facilitated autonomy and activity among the residents. Bjannes and Butler (1974) controlled for resident ability and other resident and staff characteristics and found that very small facilities fostered overprotectiveness and "clients" were less autonomous than those in larger homes. MacEachron (1983) speculated that more normal social and physical environments would facilitate normal social and interactional behavior.

Size as a variable in itself is not directly related to quality of care (Bercovici, 1981; Hull & Thompson, 1980; King, Raynes, & Tizard, 1971; McCormick, Balla, & Zigler, 1975). Landesman-Dwyer, Sackett, and Kleinman (1980b) reported that social groupings were more important than the actual size of the facility. Landesman-Dwyer (1981) noted:

No single study is without flaws: neither can definitive answers be obtained from a handful of investigations. The findings are provocative in so far as they challenge the notion all retarded people should or would prefer to live in very small homes or apartments. The matter of size should be related to clients' age, past experiences, ability level, and current life situation. Courts and states are deciding prematurely that facilities that serve more than three people or six people, or 10 people, etc., cannot provide habilitating and normalizing experiences. There simply are not enough data available to support these major policy decisions. Theoretically and practically, the advantages of having a range in the size of community-based options are considerable. (p. 225)

Today, with virtually no research on small supported living arrangements, persons concerned about community living for persons with severe disabilities consider the above statements antiquated and regressive.

Role of Staff in Residential Environments

Fiorelli, Margolis, Heverly, Rothchild, and Keating (1982) described the formulation of a curriculum development model for training resident advisors. The competency clusters included: advocacy and legal rights; behavior change, case management, definition and causes; group process, human development, individual program design, implementation, and evaluation; instructional analysis, medically complex and multiply handicapped; normalization; problem solving; program maintenance; severe and profound disabilities; and vocational appraisal. Overall, the authors evaluated the curriculum as successsful in improving staff competencies.

The role that staff play in instructing persons with disabilities has only recently been questioned. Bercovici (1981) found that residential staff discouraged residents from maintaining contact with friends. Janicki (1981) observed that staff members typically interacted with residents in ways to control their behavior. Staff in general were undertrained and did not have a clear sense of their role (Backus, 1983). Elder (1980) found that human services staff had knowledge of only 40%–60% of other agencies, services, and supports in their communities. Baker et al. (1977), in a survey of community residential facilities, found that houseparents remained, on an average, for less than 2 years. In a study that examined the differences in staff behavior as a function of the size of the facility, Felce et al. (1987) examined the density of staff encouragement of appropriate behavior in various residential settings. They found that appropriate contingent attention of positive behavior was three times greater in small homes than in large community units.

Knoll and Ford (1987) outlined residential service providers' roles to include the following: 1) to build relationships and natural supports, 2) to secure community involvement, 3) to facil-

itate active participation, 4) to use nonintrusive interventions, 5) to help access privacy and personal space, 6) to involve in natural routines, 7) to recognize and use age-appropriate activities, 8) to provide real choices, 9) to minimize "dead-time," and 10) to personalize the full experience. Lakin et al. (1988) described strategies for promoting stability of direct care staff. They suggested that services: maximize the use of people who promise stability; maximize the new and potential employees' knowledge of and ability to perform the job role; communicate that direct care is valued and valuable; maximize potentially attractive aspects of the direct care role; ensure that positions are well designed and adequately supplemented; and maximize compensation to employees.

Community Integration

There are numerous other works that discuss group home and other living arrangements. J.A. Sherman, Sheldon, Morris, Strouse, and Reese (1984) described a community-based residential program for mentally retarded adults, called the Teaching-Family Model. The model included: family-style atmosphere; skills-training curriculum; motivational systems; self-government system; and other model components such as consultation, workshops, and evaluations. Jacobs (1986) described a supported apartment program in Madison, Wisconsin, called Community Options. Although not data based, these program descriptions report success and improved living conditions for persons with severe disabilities. Singer, Close, Irvin, Gersten, and Sailor (1984) described an alternative to the institution for young people with severely handicapping conditions in a rural community. Similar to the findings in the Pennhurst-related work and that of Close (1977), they found that youth with severe handicaps who were labeled as multiply handicapped, nonambulatory, aggressive, or resistive can learn new adaptive skills in a training home setting, and that their rate of growth is significantly higher than comparable persons in the institution.

Setting Variables

Variables related to setting include: type of living arrangement, size of living arrangement, unit size, staff-to-resident ratio, administrator-to–direct care ratio, degree of normalization, enriching characteristics of the environment, primary interactors, and social climate (Heal, 1985). Griffin, Landers, and Patterson (1974) examined changes in the social behavior of persons with mental retardation as a function of social density (e.g., number of people in the setting). They concluded that fewer persons and more privacy did not necessarily have a positive effect on social behavior. In light of this finding, Reizenstein and McBride (1978) explained that service programs often describe themselves physically to reflect their idealized images, but that programs' defined life spaces must always be tested against actual experiences within the environment (cited in Rotegard et al., 1985). Similar to other research efforts of this type, the activities in which persons were engaged were not described or controlled. Therefore, findings of this nature must be interpreted with caution.

Geographic Location

Bjannes and Butler (1974) suggested that the geographic location of the facility and the involvement of the caregiver in the daily aspects of behavior appeared to relate to the development of independent functioning and social competence of the residents. This suggestion and findings based on a small study are consistent with common sense. That is, if persons with severe disabilities are living in a location accessible to stores, transportation, recreation/leisure, and vocational opportunities, then their opportunities to learn activities related to community functioning are greater. Those in more isolated and rural settings are likely to have an arduous time accessing generic community services and environments.

Social Behavior

Kendrick (1987) compared the social lives of those living in group homes with those living in supported apartments. His methodology was based on interviews, observations, and examinations of the daily schedules of the residents. He found that persons in supported living arrangements were more isolated and participated less frequently in their communities than did persons living in group homes. Clearly, Kendrick is not suggesting that the field return to the notion of group living arrangements, but rather that care

should be taken not to assume that setting alone, independent of other factors such as friendship, supports, and location, facilitates community integration that will significantly change the lives of individuals with disabilities. This is consistent with Bogdan and Taylor's (1987) warning:

> People can be placed in the community and experience segregation, isolation, and loneliness. This is not to say that moving people out of institutions is an unworthy pursuit. To the contrary, for people to be part of the community, they must be in the community. . . . What we are saying is that community placement is simply a means to an end, and not the ultimate goal. . . . We know far less about how people make friends and how those who are different come to be accepted. In the next wave, we will need a sociology of acceptance. (p. 210)

Saxby, Thomas, Felce, and deKock (1986) examined the use of shops, cafés, and public houses by adults with severe and profound mental disabilities. They found that nonsocial participation while shopping or in bars and cafés occupied 29% and 36% of the time respectively. These figures were somewhat lower than engagement levels within the homes, but the level of social interaction between staff and residents was similar.

Landlords and Neighborhoods

The relationships among persons with severe disabilities and their neighbors has been primarily examined in the context of property values and attitudes. According to the work of M.M. Seltzer (1985), 25%–50% of community living arrangements are contested by landlords and neighbors. The reasons most frequently cited for contesting these arrangements are related to fear of decline in property values, safety, and the possibility of increased traffic congestion. Salend and Giek (1988) interviewed 25 landlords to examine their perspectives about independent living arrangements. A significant number of them indicated they had problems renting to individuals with disabilities. The authors suggested that those "individuals demonstrating the ability to be self-sufficient could be placed in independent living arrangements, and those lacking the skills necessary for independent living could receive training to increase their readiness" (p. 89). The notion of readiness, unfortunately, continues to pervade the literature. Curricula such as that proposed by Bauman and Iwata (1977); Crnic and Pym (1979); Schalock (1975); and Vogelsburg, Williamson, and Friedl (1980) were mentioned to facilitate the necessary training.

Research on neighborhood acceptance of group homes is extensive. M.M. Seltzer (1985) noted that 25%–50% of group homes have experienced neighborhood resistance which diminishes over time. The author provided an analysis of both high-profile and low-profile approaches to developing community residences, emphasizing that the low-profile approach may be equal if not superior to the high-profile. Carefully structured community educational experiences were also suggested. Burchard, Hasazi, Gordon, Yoe, and Simoneau (1986) used G.B. Seltzer's (1981) satisfaction survey to compare residents in group homes, natural homes, and supervised apartments. They found individuals living in apartments to be more satisfied than those in the other two settings.

Although neighborhood resistance has been extensively studied (e.g., Ashmore, 1975; Cornhill Association, 1978; Sigelman, 1976), the involvement of neighbors in the lives of persons with severe disabilities has not. With the exception of Perske's *New Life in the Neighborhood*, (1980) and *Circle of Friends* (1988), the primary findings are that neighbors are not involved with individuals outside of residential settings (Baker et al., 1977; Moreau, Novak, & Sigelman, 1980). Because the primary focus of the majority of these studies is neighborhood acceptance of group living arrangements—unfamiliar entities to many—most of the findings can only be interpreted as resistance to group living arrangements rather than to individuals with disabilities. Future research should focus on neighborhood resistance to adults with severe disabilities who own their own homes.

SUPPORTED LIVING

Supported living is used generally to describe small living arrangements where flexible support is provided as necessary. "Supported living is defined as persons with disabilities living where and with whom they want, for as long as they want, with the ongoing support needed to

sustain that choice" (Bellamy & Horner, 1987, p. 506). Supported living, like supported employment, is viewed as an alternative to intermediate care facilities for the mentally retarded (ICFs/MR) or large group homes, and focuses on the individual needs of the resident rather than on service models. It includes accountability for life-style options; diversity of residential options; individually determined support; and broad technology of residential support (Boles, Horner, & Bellamy, 1988).

Based on an extensive evaluation of Centennial Services in Greely, Colorado, O'Brien and Lyle-O'Brien (1989) described five characteristics that accounted for change in the personal lives of persons receiving residential support services:

1. The successful redesign of the program focused most available resources on supporting individual people in their choice of homes.
2. A vision of communities that included all people in positive ways animated the Residential Support Program (RSP).
3. RSP maintained open organizational boundries.
4. RSP staff had a sense of themselves as a cohesive team pioneering important new approaches in hostile territory.
5. Staff combined personal commitment with practical knowledge. Unencumbered by clinical perspectives and professional procedures, many staff wanted to do "whatever it takes" to support people.

These features contributed to a change from congregated living situations to individualized living arrangements in the community. Other reports, published by the Center on Human Policy at Syracuse University, developed through program visitations that included extensive observations and interviews, recognized the role of leadership and staff behavior and organization on successful change.

Burchard et al. (1986) and Halpern, Close, and Nelson (1985) examined semi-independent living arrangements, using qualitative research methods. The individuals with disabilities presented their own perspectives on daily experiences and future goals, satisfaction with services, and social outlets. Aspects of home and neighborhood, employment and finances, social relations, and community services were also described. Program administrators, program staff, and individual clients were interviewed. Although relevant to the field, the persons described did not have severe disabilities.

Types of Supported Living Options

There are increasing numbers of state-of-the-art community living programs throughout the country. Unfortunately, the research and professional literature does not reflect this change and little or no data are available (Taylor, 1987a). The research is scant compared to studies conducted on families who have children with disabilities, foster care and special needs adoption, integrated education, and supported employment. In the programs that have been described, one common component is the individualized nature of the service option that fits the placement to the individual and not the individual to any available program. Some of these programs include: Options in Community Living in Wisconsin; Supervised Apartments in Region V, Nebraska; Supported Independence in Macomb, Oakland; Seven Counties Services in Louisville, Kentucky; Residential, Inc. in Ohio; Centennial Developmental Services in Evans, Colorado; and Beta Hostels in Attleboro, Massachusetts. These programs or support services share several basic features including: 1) paid support by live-in staff, on-call staff, paid roommates or companions, paid neighbors, or attendants; 2) individualization and flexibility; 3) a focus on the individual rather than the facility; 4) a belief that people live in homes, not "slots" or "facilities"; and 5) consumer and family involvement in planning and quality assurance.

Various supported living models exist. These include apartments, shared housing, home ownership with agency supersivion, collectives, and cooperatives. L'Arche, a well-known community support program for adults, is located in 16 different countries. The program is based on: 1) the value of the person with mental handicaps, 2) the importance of mutual relationships, 3) the importance of a sense of community, and 4) spiritual dimensions. Wehbring and Ogren (1975) compared seven residential programs for persons

with mental handicaps. They reported that L'Arche had the strongest sense of community. The term "community" was undefined and measured subjectively by the researchers. Katz and Bender (1976) described groups such as L'Arche as "vehicles through which these outcast persons can claim and grow towards new identities, redefining themselves and society; can overcome solitariness through identification with a reference group; and sometimes can work towards social ends or social change which they see as important" (p.6).

Research on Needed Skills

The types of skills that persons with severe disabilities need to live in the community were studied by Lovett and Harris (1987) who interviewed 48 adults with mild and moderate disabilities. Vocational and social skillls were rated as most important, followed by personal, academic, and leisure skills. Gollay et al. (1978) studied the experiences of deinstitutionalized adults in the community who listed the following associated necessary skills and problems: 1) finding a job, 2) loneliness, and 3) managing money. The authors also reported, in descending order, that the adults worried most about: 1) being taken advantage of, 2) loss of housing, 3) being sent back to the institution, and 4) being sick or having seizures.

Virtually all of the research conducted to date has focused on persons with disabilities living in rented apartments or homes owned and/or operated by agencies. Very few persons with disabilities own their homes and choose with whom they live. Laux (1988) described financing for home ownership through innovative tax options and investment opportunities. However, few program model descriptions have been published. Future research should focus on the relationship of home ownership to personal choice and satisfaction, empowerment, and community perceptions and attitudes.

CHILDREN AND FAMILIES IN THE COMMUNITY

In many states there has been a virtual end to the institutionalization of children. Children with severe disabilities remain with their own families, are adopted, or are placed in foster care or in pediatric community living situations of various sizes. C.E. Meyers, Bothwick, and Eyman (1985) studied the demographic characteristics and level of mental retardation of approximately 59,000 residents in the California disability service system. Approximately 50% of recipients of services lived in the natural home; 14% lived in family care settings. In two follow-up studies of residents who moved from the institution to the community, the strongest predictor of success was the involvement of families and their understanding of community integration (Schalock et al., 1981; Schalock & Lilly, 1986).

Reasons for Out-of-Home Placement

Covert (1988) conducted 20 interviews: 10 with families who had been forced to place their child out of the home and 10 with families who were able to care for their child in their home. The results of these interviews point to the various needs that different families have and the lack of flexibility in the service system to meet these needs. Numerous factors related to family composition, severity of disability, health needs, and socioeconomic status contributed to the decision to place the child outside of the home. B.R. Sherman (1988) surveyed 377 families who provided care at home and 154 who placed their family member with disabilities outside of the home. Predictors of out-of-home placement included an older family member with disabilities, more severe disabilities, more severe behavior disorders, large-family composition, a perception that caring for the member is disruptive to family life, and a single-parent household. Salisbury (1987), using retrospective research methodology, examined selected characteristics of an intact sample of 56 young children with severe handicaps who resided in community residential facilities. Children with atypical birth histories were placed in community residential facilities earlier than were children in the no-risk group. Records indicated that medical/caregiver demands (41%), behavior (23%), court-ordered placement for abuse/neglect (20%), and family crisis (16%) accounted for reasons for placement.

Cole and Meyer (1989) reported that the decision to seek an out-of-home placement was af-fected by numerous child-related stressors, pre-existent family resources, and new sources of support. Using multiple regressional analyses, they found that child-related stressors were negatively related to parents' plans for placing the child outside the home before age 21 and positively related to plans for placing the child outside the home after age 21. Both internal resources and degree of external resource use was related to maintaining the child at home until age 21. Even after child-related stressors and family characteristics were accounted for, familes who made greater use of external resources were more apt to report plans to keep their child at home until age 21 than were families who did not access these new resources. These findings are consistent with those of Tausig (1985), who found, using retrospective analysis, that individual child variables, family characteristics, and stress-related variables were the best predictors of out-of-home placement requests.

State Support to Families

The provision of services and support designed to meet the needs of the entire family and not only those of the individual with disabilities is a relatively new development in services. In 1972, Pennsylvania became the first state to initiate a family support project. At least 29 states currently provide extensive services and resources to families who care for a disabled family member in the home. Ten states have a cash subsidy program, 10 fund family support services, and 9 offer families a combination of financial assistance and support services. For more than two thirds of these states, the creation of family support services has occured since 1980 (Bates, 1987). Temporary child care as a respite service, however developed and delivered, is considered one part of family support.

Researchers studying families with members with disabilities consistently find that they experience both normative and unusual stress (Singer, Irvin, & Hawkins, 1988). Depending on the family and its own attributes, parents may need assistance dealing with their children with disabilities. To accomplish this, support programs have evolved, most of them designed to assist families to keep their children with severe disabilities at home. Parents who care for a child with severe disabilities may require such supports as: architectural modification to the home, child care, counseling and therapeutic resources, dental and medical care not otherwise covered, specialized diagnosis and evaluation, specialized nutrition and clothing, specialized equipment and supplies, homemaker services, in-home nursing and attendant care, home training and parent courses, recreation and alternative activities, respite care, transportation, specialized utility costs, and vehicle modification (S.J. Taylor et al., 1987, p. 43). While support to families may take a variety of forms; the major goals of any family support program are to: 1) deter unnecessary out-of-home placements, 2) return persons living in institutions back to a family setting, and 3) enhance the care-giving capacity of families (Agosta & Bradley, 1985). The Wisconsin Department of Health and Social Services (1985) explained their Family Support Program as follows: "The program is intended to ensure that ordinary families faced with the extraordinary circumstances that come with having a child with severe disabilities will get the help that they need without having to give up parental responsibility and control" (p. 1).

Families need to be recognized as the primary decision makers in determining what specific services and resources they receive. The acknowledgment that families are in the best position to know their own needs is an underlying tenet in successful family support programs. However, there has been little research to date on this topic. Another important characteristic of exemplary family support programs is built-in flexibility in service options and delivery. Families have unique and differing needs that cannot always be met by a single agency or a standard program model (S.J. Taylor et al., 1987). Families should be offered a range of service options that include the use of existing generic community resources. The identification and coordination of resources and services is an important function of family support programs; too often families are unaware of what assistance is available or are unable to tap into their own natural support systems.

Effective family support programs must not only tolerate a high degree of individualization in service delivery, but also encourage open, creative approaches to problem solving. Neither of these is a characteristic usually associated with the large state and federal bureaucracies that fund social services. It is to the credit of grassroots lobbying efforts by families that the concept of family support is beginning to be accepted at both state and national levels (Covert, 1988). The following model programs offer examples of how three states have chosen to improve their services to families.

Michigan Family Subsidy Act Michigan offers families both an array of support services and financial assistance. The Michigan Family Subsidy Act provides eligible families with $225 a month to be used at the parents' discretion. To qualify for this financial assistance, families must have an annual income of less than $60,000 and have a child (under the age of 18) with severe mental impairments who is living at home. Currently, 2,500 families are enrolled in the program at a cost of $6.7 million to the state. In an evaluation of the Michigan program, a "pre" and "post" survey of families demonstrated that the receipt of the monthly cash subsidy: 1) significantly reduced family stress, particularly financial stress; 2) improved life satisfaction for the mothers; 3) resulted in a decrease in plans to seek out-of-home placements; and 4) meant an increase in family purchases. Lower income families used the subsidy to help pay for basic needs: clothing, special food, transportation, and general household expenses. Families with higher incomes used the subsidy to provide specialized services or equipment for their child and respite for the family (J. Meyers & Marcenco, 1986).

Wisconsin Family Support Program Wisconsin's Family Support Program provides an individualized approach to assisting families. A needs assessment is conducted for eligible families (those who have children with severe disabilities), and an annual family plan is drawn up based on identified needs. The family plan includes: 1) a description of family needs, 2) services to be provided with public or private funding other than the Family Support Program, 3) the availability of community services and an existing family network, 4) a description and estimated cost of services and goods to be funded by the Family Support Program, and 5) an agreement of participation signed by the family and the administering agency. Service coordination is a primary function of the Wisconsin Family Support Program. This includes helping families negotiate the numerous federal and state bureaucracies, as well as assisting families in using generic community services. Up to $3,000 can be allocated per family to fund any needed equipment or service that is documented in the family plan. Services may be paid for directly by the administering agency or in a grant to the family. Families are accountable for dollars spent and must keep receipts (Wisconsin Department of Health and Social Services, 1985).

Family Support Services, Calvert County, Maryland   The Association for Retarded citizens in Calvert County, Maryland, operates the Family Support Services program. Governed by the philosophy "whatever it takes," program staff assist in obtaining those services or resources the family sees as needed in order to care for its family member with disabilities at home. In addition, the program offers a variety of respite options, integrated day care, parent support through a parent group and individual parent counselors, financial support, information referral, and service coordination (Bersani, 1987b). Flexibility, the use of community resources, and the involvement of families are all factors in the success of this program. As Maryland expands its involvement in family support, staff worry that state regulations, paperwork, and stringent accountability measures will affect their ability to continue meeting family needs with the straightforward, individualized approach that has proven so effective (Roundtable discussion, American Association on Mental Retardation, Northeast regional conference, September, 1987, personal communication).

Federal Support to Families

Following the states' initiatives in the development of family support services, federal programs are making needed changes in favor of families and home care. An example of change at the national level is the passage of the 1986 Early Education Amendments to PL 94-142, which called for increased early intervention services for infants and toddlers with disabilities and their families. The amendments included provisions for case management services and the

development of individualized family service plans to ensure that families receive comprehensive and coordinated services from state and community agencies (Campbell, 1987).

At the national policy level, the importance of the family's role is beginning to be recognized. The 1987 U.S. Surgeon General's Report on Children with Special Health Care Needs called for a family-centered, community-based approach to health care. The report recommended, among other things, the facilitation of parent-professional collaboration; the implementation of programs that provide emotional and financial support to families; and the assurance that health care delivery systems are designed to be flexible, accessible, and responsive to families.

A final example of a change at the federal level that would significantly affect families is the proposed Medicaid Home and Community Quality Services Act now before Congress. If enacted, this legislation could reverse the current institutional bias of the Medicaid program, expanding the availability of Medicaid dollars for use in community and home settings. As part of the criteria for participation in the Medicaid program, the bill mandates that states provide case management and individual and family support services (Bergman, 1987).

Informal Supports and Networks

The use of informal supports and networks has only recently been investigated. Social networks have been defined as a group of individuals "who provide information leading the subject to believe (s)he is cared for and loved, esteemed, and a member of a network of mutual obligations" (Cobb, 1976, p.300). Informal supports and networks may be individuals or groups, including relatives, friends, co-workers, neighbors, social clubs or organizations, day-care organizations, babysitters, and religious associations (Dunst, Trivette, & Deal, 1988). Networks have direct and indirect influences on both the parents and the child and may change over time (Cochran & Brassard, 1979). Although networks are important to all families, those families who have a member with disabilities tend to have fewer supports (Friedrich & Friedrich, 1981; Stagg & Catron, 1986). The results of a study conducted in New Hampshire (Covert, 1988) on family support indicates that only 51% of individuals who have a child with disabilities feel that their family is very helpful, while 16% received no assistance. Families reported that there was even less support from neighbors, resulting in a feeling of isolation at times.

Networks have been associated with a range of positive outcomes, such as decreased possibility of institutionalization, increased sense of emotional and psychological well-being, reduction in the dependence on formal service delivery systems, and promotion of social interaction (Branch & Jette, 1982; M.M. Seltzer, Ivry, & Litchfield, 1987). Dunst et al. (1988) concluded that social supports designed specifically to meet the needs of the family can also assist individual members of the family by promoting child-parent well-being, reducing caregiving time demands, increasing positive parent-child interaction, and increasing the parents' perception of the child's level of functioning. Additionally, Dunst et al. stated that, to the extent possible, families should be provided with informal rather than formal networks.

Special Needs Adoption/Foster Care

There have been numerous studies involving families who have children with disabilities. This research has focused on stress reduction, impact on brothers and sisters, the relationship between degree of disability and family integrity, and systems responses to family members. Children with severe disabilities often are at risk for an out-of-home placement because of the impact on the family and the lack of responsiveness on the part of the service system. As a result, some families are forced to place their children outside of the home. These children, particularly if they have severe disabilities, are frequently placed in pediatric nursing homes, intermediate care facilities, or foster homes; with few exceptions, they are not typically considered for adoption. This negative attitude, that children with intense needs are "unadoptable," has resulted from: 1) lack of experience with special needs adoption, 2) reliance on group residential models, and 3) negative stereotypes regarding persons with severe disabilities. The McComb-Oakland Regional Service Delivery System in Michigan has demonstrated, however, that chil-

dren with the most severe disabilities can be adopted. Permanency planning has evolved as a philosophy that embraces each "child's right to a stable home and lasting relationships" (Taylor et al., 1987).

Special Needs Adoption Research

Research on the adoption of children with disabilities has not been expansive (Crnic, Friedrich, & Greenburg, 1983). Krisheff (1977) stated that there was virtually no information for agencies on adoption practices for children with special needs. Although this has changed with the establishment of the National Resource Center for Special Needs Adoption, information on the type of person who is most likely to adopt a child with disabilities is scant, at best. In general, research conducted by DeLeon and Westerberg (1980), Franklin and Massarik (1969a, 1969b, 1969c), Gath (1973, 1983), and Wolkind and Kozaruk (1983) indicated that parents who adopt children with disabilities usually: 1) have strong personalities, 2) have stable relationships, 3) have an outward-looking attitude, 4) have a high degree of determination, 5) are older, 6) are less likely to be in a professional class, 7) have prior familiarity with disabilities, and 8) are motivated to specifically adopt a child with disabilities. Finally, the "large majority of parents view the adoption as successful and the relationship between the parent and child as positive" (Glidden, 1986, p. 10).

Glidden, Valliere, and Herbert (1988) studied 42 families who adopted children with disabilities in an attempt to determine the effect on family functioning. Self-report questionnaires and semistructured interviews revealed positive results. In fact, families who choose to adopt children with disabilities may have more positive experiences than birth families for the following reasons: the adoptive family chose the child, whereas the birth family did not; personal characteristics associated with the wish to adopt; and previous investigators may have overestimated the negative effect that children with mental retardation have on the birth family (Byrne & Cunningham, 1985; Turnbull & Behr, 1986).

Many projects currently funded by state and national agencies have research components. Typically, these include analyses of the rate of adoption disruptions and dissolution, family and child satisfaction measures, pre/posttests after specific training, and overall changes in placement in relation to age, disability, region, and case worker.

Special needs adoption has received increased attention since 1984. However, the Consortium of States (1984) identified adoption as a low priority among child welfare services. As a result, adoption professionals fear that the gains made in the permanency planning movement and in the field of special needs adoption are being lost. After a period of decreasing numbers of children in substitute care, there are an increasing number of protective service reports and investigations, and more children are entering substitute care, particularly older children.

The absence of a central body with up-to-date and state-of-the-art information resulted in the creation of the National Resource Center for Special Needs Adoption in Chelsea, Michigan. This center has an extensive publication list that includes information on: adopting older children and children with handicaps, helping children when they move, adoption resources for mental health professionals, permanency planning, and a manual for professionals working with adoptive families. Hence, there is already an expansive array of information that could be immediately used by persons concerned with special needs adoption. What is absent, however, is information on the utility and effectiveness of these materials on statewide services.

Exemplary Programs

In Massachusetts, Project IMPACT, a placement agency for children with special needs, has coordinated an interagency effort to promote permanency planning for children with developmental disabilities since 1984. The focus of this project is on developing strong relationships for persons currently living in residential facilities. The Rocky Mountain Adoption Exchange involves skill-level training in permanency planning for interdisciplinary teams from social services, including: developmental disabilities, foster care, and adoption; community-centered boards; legal services; and advocacy and parent groups. The University of Kansas–Children's Rehabilitation Unit has a project that focuses on minimizing the

risk of adoption disruption. The successful adoption of children with special needs has resulted in a need for additional information after the placement has been made. A key concept of the project is to link families with resources. In Western Pennsylvania, Project S.T.A.R. has a Specialized Parent Preparation program that offers a time for families to explore their own attitudes, and to learn more about disabilities, parenting, and adoption. A recruitment video "Straight from the Heart" has been made and various other resources are made available for professionals and parents interested in special needs adoption. Michigan's Specialized Adoption Program has also received national attention. Because permanency planning was so successful with children with developmental disabilities, Michigan expanded its commitment to special needs adoption to children with mental health needs. Services provided by the program include: counseling of the birth family toward making a decision about release, the preparation of child assessments, recruitment and adoption work for each child, and postrelease and postadoption services. North Carolina has an adoption project that encourages collaboration between mental health and child welfare systems. In addition to administrative collaboration and participation, services offered include: pre/post placement services, family and the placement of child assessment, and introduction of a mental health worker into the adoption process prior to placement to encourage familiarity and facilitate family therapy if needed (Staff, 1989).

In sum, these projects emphasize parent and professional training and support; pre/postplacement support; the inclusion of a variety of children with special needs into the adoption system; the necessity for emphasizing the building of relationships; adequate intake and assessment procedures; and overall community awareness of the needs of children who have special needs or are labeled as disabled.

Respite Services

Respite services may be categorized according to where the services are provided (i.e., in home or out of home). In-home respite may include services by a trained and licensed homemaker, a sitter/companion who provides services on an as-needed basis, and/or a relative the family contacts. There are many more out-of-home respite services available. These include special families licensed to provide respite to one or two individuals with disabilities, parent cooperative services where parents agree to provide care to one another's children, day-care centers, community recreational options, and respite residences that provide only respite services (Levy & Levy, 1986).

Studies such as that conducted by Cohen (1980) found that when individuals who use respite care were contrasted with those who do not, the users of respite were more likely to report enhanced family functioning, yet were also more likely to be considering out-of-home placement for their child with disabilities (Intagliata, 1986). Intagliata, Gibson, and Rinck (1984) reported that 25 families using respite care programs showed no significant improvements in stress and mental well-being when considered as a single group; however, if the sample was stratified by level of utilization of respite services, the results indicated that those making greatest use of the program had shown improvement, while those who used low or moderate levels of respite did not demonstrate significantly reduced stress levels or improvement in their mental well-being. The availability of respite services may enable family members to become more socially active and in turn reduce their feelings of social isolation (Intagliata, 1986). In a study by Joyce, Singer, and Isralowitz (1983), parents reported that they were able to engage in more social and leisure activities as the result of their participation in a respite program.

Respite services can have a direct and an indirect impact on an individual with disabilities. Parents indicate improve relations with and more positive attitude toward their child with disabilities (Cohen, 1980; Joyce et al., 1983). A study by Wikler, Hanusa, and Stoysheff (1986) demonstrated that when respite services are provided to children who display behavior problems, the behaviors remain at the same level or improve.

The importance of respite services cannot be overemphasized in the picture of community living. Joyce et al. (1983) reported that in a 32-family sample, 30% stated that they would not be able to care for their children without respite services. The California Department of Developmental Services (1986) reported that 47% of a 98-parent sample said that they would consider an out-of-home placement if respite services were unavailable. Cohen (1980) reported that of 107 persons using respite services, a large majority said that they would not be able to cope without it. And when compared with 35 nonuser families, a significantly higher proportion of families indicated that there remained a possibility of out-of-home placement. Edgar, Reid, and Pious (1988) described a Special Sitters program in Seattle that has been replicated in five communities across the nation. A training package was developed, and families with children with disabilities used the service extensively.

FUTURE RESEARCH NEEDS AND AGENDAS

The field of study concerned with persons with severe disabilities will continue to need intervention-related research to examine effective community teaching methodologies, policy-related research that sets a social agenda, analyses of how we are spending money, and attitude-and-perception surveys to assess overall changes. In 1981, Bruininks, Meyers, Sigford, and Lakin provided some general recommendations about research questions and issues. Many of their recommendations continue to be relevant and most have not been thoroughly implemented. They include:

1. *Social interactions involving a community of interested persons and relationships are crucial in community adjustment and should be researched in more detail with the goal of strengthening social opportunities where they are weak.* There is not a substantial research base that describes the process of establishing relationships and involving and building community. Interactions have been categorized and counted but a richer understanding is required. McKnight (1987) described the process of "bridge-building" but its application in local communities has not been analyzed. We need to examine the lives of persons with severe disabilities who are well-connected participating members of their communities and anaylze how they

came to be. A series of case studies that detail the process of inclusion is badly needed.

2. *Avoid equating recidivism with failure to adjust as outcome variables in conducting future studies, and develop more individualized indices of adaptation to the community.* It is clear from the studies presented that individualized indices of adaptation to community hardly exist. For example, although currently there is a large emphasis on persons with severe behavior disorders, there are no studies that describe the reduction of behaviors in the context of integrated settings and community participation. Single-subject research combined with a more thorough understanding of what constitutes success and adaptation in the community would assist community facilitators to plan and implement more appropriate supports. Group data are helpful in analyzing the overall effectiveness of a system but do not provide the close examination of specific strategies targeted toward an individual. Persons involved in the design of community living options for individuals with severe disabilities typically advocate the "one at a time" approach because of their understanding that no one strategy will work for a group. This has been our failure in the past. By first establishing models (e.g., group homes) we fail to truly acknowledge the individual and individual indices of adaptation.

3. *More longitudinal and prospective studies are needed.* There are a number of longitudinal studies that have been conducted (see Table 8.1) that describe group changes as the result of deinstitutionalization or community living. There are few studies that describe the life of a person with severe disabilities in the community over a 1-, 2-, 3-, or 4-year period of time. The field of severe disabilities constantly questions and engages in discussion around issues of friendship and personal relationships. However, there is little information on how relationships grow, change, or deteriorate over time. Additionally, as communities include all of its members with severe disabilities, neighborhoods, schools, and organizations should be examined. Do their roles change? Do attitudes change? Is inclusion easier with time and practice?

4. *Intensive and ethnographic approaches should be utilized to complement the more wide-spread use of large-scale surveys.* Researchers at the Center on Human Policy at Syracuse University and at the University of Oregon have most actively engaged in ethnographic analyses of circumstances related to persons with severe disabilities. They have contributed to a larger understanding of group homes, supervised apartments, supported work settings, and family involvement in community living. Continued support for such efforts is essential to develop a broader understanding of community, social supports, and the evolving role of the service system. The constant critical analysis of our work and involvement from an observer's perspective will force us to recognize the realities of working with people who have complex needs. Ethnographic research will also help to identify the benefits and problems associated with developing and providing community living supports.

5. *Research should more often include persons with disabilities as respondents. We Can Speak for Ourselves* (Williams & Shoultz, 1982), *Disabled We Stand* (Sutherland, 1981), and other books and chapters written by persons with disabilities should continue to be supported and promoted. Additional research should be conducted that asks specific questions of consumers about their perceptions of support and their desires for intervention by the human services system. Satisfaction and empowerment as an outcome of opportunity for choice and community participation should be analyzed.

With the current focus on school and community integration for young people with disabilities and on family support, a new era is evolving. We will not need to ask questions about whether persons with disabilities do better in the community after they have been incarcerated for most of their lives. We will not need to ask whether a group home for 12 persons is good compared to a small supported living situation where individuals have friends and relationships. We will not need to examine the cost-benefit ratio of having people in the community because, it is hoped, they will have always been there. Our research efforts should shift from "Is bigger better than smaller?" to "What is best for persons with severe disabilities and their families?" Our research agendas should move from being comparative to ones that are life enhancing and descriptive, focusing on new directions in supports and services. Finally, our research agenda should shift from a sole focus on children and adults with severe disabilities to communities, friendships, networks, empowerment, and interdependent relationships. Asking questions regarding the impact of persons with severe disabilities on the lives of others and vice versa is a new direction. These studies should be conducted in small supported living arrangements (otherwise known as people's homes) rather than large residential programs or other service settings. Too much of the research to date can be considered irrelevant because of where it was conducted. Frankly, how "clients" interact with one another in board-and-care homes of 30 persons or more is uninteresting. How persons with severe disabilities become involved as homeowners, neighbors, friends, co-workers, and leaders in their communities is more intriguing.

REFERENCES

Aanes, D., & Moen, M. (1976). Adaptive behavior changes of group home residents. *Mental Retardation, 14,* 36–40.

Agosta, J., & Bradley, V. (1985). *Designing programs to support family care for persons with developmental disabilities: Concepts to practice.* Cambridge, MA: Human Services Research Institute.

Ashmore, R.D. (1975). Background considerations in developing strategies for changing attitudes and behavior toward the mentally retarded. In M.J. Begab & S.A. Richardson (Eds.), *The mentally retarded and society: A social science perspective* (pp.159–174). Baltimore: University Park Press.

Bachrach, L.L. (1981). A conceptual approach to deinstitutionalization of the mentally retarded: A perspective from the experience of the mentally ill. In R.H. Bruininks, C.E. Meyers, B.B. Sigford, & K.C. Lakin (Eds.), *Deinstitutionalization and community adjustment of mentally retarded people* (pp. 51–67). Washington, DC: American Association on Mental Deficiency.

Backus, L.H. (1983). *Assessment of training needs of personnel employed in facilities serving developmentally disabled adults in the state of Kansas.* Lawrence: Kansas University Affiliated Facility.

Baker, B.L., Seltzer, G.G., & Selzer, M.M. (1977). *As close as possible: Community residences for retarded adults.* Boston: Little, Brown.

Balla, D.A. (1976). Relationships of institutional size to quality of care: A review of the literature. *American Journal of Mental Deficiency, 81,* 117–124.

Balla, D., Butterfield, E.C., & Zigler, E. (1973). Effects of institutionalization on retarded children: A longitudinal cross-institutional investigation. *American Journal of Mental Deficiency, 78,* 530–549.

Baroff, G.S. (1980) On "size" and quality of residential care: A second look. *Mental Retardation, 18,* 113–117.

Bates, M. (1987). *Family support cash subsidy report provision* (Working paper). Madison: Wisconsin Council on Developmental Disabilities.

Bauman, K.E., & Iwata, B.A. (1977). Maintenance of individual housekeeping skills using scheduling plus self-recording procedures. *Behavior Therapy, 8,* 544–560.

Bell, N.J., Schoenrock, C., & Bensberg, G. (1981). Change over time in the community: Findings of a longitudinal study. In R.H. Bruininks, C.E. Meyers, B.B. Sigford, & K.C. Lakin (Eds.), *Deinstitutionalization and community adjustment of mentally retarded people* (pp. 195–202). Washington, DC: American Association on Mental Deficiency.

Bellamy, G.T., & Horner, R.H. (1987). Beyond high school: Residential and employment options after graduation. In M. Snell (Ed.), *Systematic instruction of persons with severe handicaps* (pp. 491–510). (3rd ed.). Columbus, OH: Charles E. Merrill.

Bercovici, S.M. (1981). Qualitative methods in cultural perspectives in the study of deinstitutionalization. In R.H. Bruininks, C.E. Meyers, B.B. Sigford, & K.C. Lakin (Eds.), *Deinstitutionalization and community adjustment of mentally retarded people* (pp. 133–144). Washington, DC: American Association on Mental Deficiency.

Bercovici, S.M (1983). *Barriers to normalization: The restrictive management of mentally retarded persons.* Baltimore: University Park Press.

Bergman, A. (1987, June). *Family Support Newsletter.* (Available from United Cerebral Palsy, Inc., Government Action Building, 1522 K St., N.W., Washington, DC)

Berkson, G., & Romer, D. (1980). Social ecology of supervised communal facilities for mentally disabled adults: I. Introduction. *American Journal of Mental Deficiency, 85,* 219–228.

Bersani, H.A. (1987a). *Perceived training needs of direct care staff in community residences for adults.* Syracuse, NY: Syracuse University, Center on Human Policy, Research and Training Center on Community Integration.

Bersani, H.A. (1987b). *Site visit to Calvert County Maryland Association for Retarded Citizens family support services.* Syracuse; NY: Syracuse University, Center on Human Policy, Research and Training Center on Community Integration.

Birenbaum, A., & Seiffer, S. (1976). *Resettling retarded adults in a managed community.* New York: Praeger.

Bjannes, A.T., & Butler, E.W. (1974). Environmental variation in community care facilities for mentally retarded persons. *American Journal of Mental Deficiency, 78,* 429–439.

Bogdan, R., & Biklen, S. (1982). *Qualitative research methods for education: An introduction to theory and methods.* Boston: Allyn & Bacon.

Bogdan, R., & Taylor, S.J. (1982). *Inside out: The social meaning of mental retardation.* Toronto: University of Toronto Press.

Bogdan, R., & Taylor, S.J. (1987). Conclusion: The next wave. In S.J. Taylor, D. Biklen, & J. Knoll (Eds.), *Community integration for people with severe disabilities* (pp. 209–213). New York: Teachers College Press.

Boles, S., Horner, R.H., & Bellamy, G.T. (1988). Implementing lasting programs for supported living. In B.L. Ludlow, A.P. Turnbull, & R. Luckasson (Eds.), *Transitions to adult life for people with mental retardation: Principles and practices* (pp. 101–117). Baltimore: Paul H. Brookes Publishing Co.

Braddock, D., Howes, R., & Hemp, R. (1984). *A summary of mental retardation and developmental disabilities expenditures in the United States: F.Y. 1977–1984* (Public Policy Monograph #3). Chicago: University of Illinois at Chicago, Institute for the Study of Developmental Disabilities.

Bradley, V.J., Conroy, J.W., Covert, S.B., & Feinstein, C.S. (1986). *Community options: The New Hampshire Choice.* Cambridge, MA: Human Services Research Institute.

Branch, L.G., & Jette, A.M. (1982). A prospective study of long-term care institutionalization among the aged. *American Journal of Public Health, 72,* 1373–1379.

Brook, B. (1973). An alternative to psychiatric hospitalization for emergency patients. *Hospital and Community Psychiatry, 24,* 621–624.

Brown, M., Diller, L., Fordyce, W., Jacobs, D., & Gordon, W. (1980). Rehabilitation indicators: Their nature and uses for assessment. In B. Bolton & D.W. Cook (Eds.), *Rehabilitation client assessment* (pp. 97–121). Baltimore: University Park Press.

Bruininks, R.H., Kudla, M.J., Hauber, F.A., Hill, B.K, & Wieck, C.A. (1981). Recent growth and status of community residential alternatives. In R.H. Bruininks, C.E. Meyers, B.B. Sigford, & L.C. Lakins, (Eds.) *Deinstitutionalization and community adjustment of mentally retarded people* (pp. 14–27). Washington, DC: American Association on Mental Deficiency.

Bruininks, R.H., Kudla, M.J., Wieck, C.A., & Hauber, F.A. (1982). Management problems in community residential facilities. *Mental Retardation, 18,* 125–130.

Bruininks, R.H., Meyers, C.E., Sigford, B.B., & Lakin, R.C. (Eds.). (1981). *Deinstitutionalization and community adjustment of mentally retarded people.* Washington, DC: American Association on Mental Deficiency.

Burchard, S.N., Hasazi, J.E., Gordon, K.R., Yoe, J., & Simoneau, D. (1986). *Community living project: Progress report.* Burlington: University of Vermont, Department of Psychology.

Butterfield, E. (1982). Some basic changes in research facilities. In R. Kugel & A. Shearer (Eds.), *Changing patterns in residential services for the mentally retarded* (pp. 42–46). Washington, DC: President's Committee on Mental Retardation.

Byrne, E.A., & Cunningham, C.C. (1985). The effects of mentally handicapped children on families—A conceptual review. *Journal of Child Psychiatry and Psychology, 26,* 847–867.

California Department of Developmental Services. (1986). *Client development evaluation report.* (Available from author, 1600 9th St., P.O. Box 944202, Sacramento, CA 94244-2020)

Campbell, P.H. (1987). Physical management and handling procedures with movement dysfunction. In M. Snell (Ed.), *Systematic instruction of students with moderate and severe handicaps* (pp. 174–188). Columbus, OH: Charles E. Merrill.

Chadsey-Rusch, J.C. (1985). Community integration and mental retardation: The eco-behavioral approach to service provision and assessment. In R.H. Bruininks & K.C. Lakin (Eds.), *Living and learning in the least restrictive environment* (pp. 245–260). Baltimore: Paul H. Brookes Publishing Co.

Chamberlin, J. (1978). *On our own: Patient-controlled alternatives to the mental health system.* New York: McGraw-Hill.

Close, D.W. (1977). Community living for severely and profoundly retarded adults: A group home study. *Education and Training of the Mentally Retarded, 12,* 256–262.

Cobb, S. (1976). Social support as a moderator of life stress. *Psychosomatic Medicine, 38,* 300–314.

Cochran, M.M., & Brassard, J.A. (1979). Child development and personal social networks. *Child Development, 50,* 601–616.

Cohen, S. (1980). *Final report: Demonstrating model continua of respite care and parent training services for families of persons with developmental disabilities.* New York: City University of New York, Graduate School, Center for Advanced Study in Education, Education Department.

Cole, D.A., & Meyer, L.H. (1989). Impact of needs and resources on family plans to seek out-of-home placement. *American Journal on Mental Retardation, 93,* 380–387.

Colombatto, J.G., Isett, R.D., Roszkansk, M., Spreak, S., D'Onofrio, A., & Alderfer, R. (1982). *Perspectives on deinstitutionalization: A survey of the national superintendents of public residential facilities for the mentally retarded.* Philadelphia: Temple University, Woodhaven Center.

Colorado Division of Developmental Disabilities. (1982). *Colorado's regional center satellite group homes: An evaluation report.* Denver: Author.

Conroy, J.W., & Bradley, V.J. (1985). *The Pennhurst longitudinal study: A report of five years of research and analysis.* Philadelphia: Temple University Developmental Disabilities Center.

Conroy, J., Efthimiou, J., & Lemanowicz, J. (1982). A matched comparison of the developmental growth of institutionalized and deinstitutionalized mentally retarded clients. *American Journal of Mental Deficiency, 86,* 581–587.

Conroy, J.W., Feinstein, C.S., & Lemanowicz, J.A. (1988). *Results of the longitudinal study of CARC v. Thorne Class members* (Report No. 7). Philadelphia: Temple University, Developmental Disabilities Center.

Consortium of States. (1984). *National report on adoption.* City, MI: Author.

Cornhill Association. (1978, April). *Elements of a community acceptance strategy for community programs for the mentally disabled.* Boston: Massachusetts Department of Mental Health.

Covert, S. (1988). *A study of family support needs in New Hampshire.* Durham, NH: Institute on Disability.

Craig, E.M., & McCarver, R.B. (1984). Community placement and adjustment of deinstitutionalized clients: Issues and findings. In N.W. Gray & N.R. Ellis (Eds.), *International review of research in mental retardation* (Vol. 12, pp. 95–122). New York: Academic Press.

Crnic, K.A., & Pym, H.A. (1979). Training mentally retarded adults independent living skills. *Mental Retardation, 17,* 13–16.

Crnic, K.A., Friedrich, W.N., & Greenburg, M.T. (1983). Adaptation of families with mentally retarded children: A model of stress, coping, and family ecology. *American Journal of Mental Deficiency, 89,* 125–138.

D'Amico, M.L., Hannah, M.A., Milhouse, J.A., & Froleich, A.K. (1978). *Evaluation of adaptive behavior: Institutional vs. community placements and treatment for the mentally retarded.* Stillwater: Oklahoma State University, National Clearinghouse of Rehabilitation Materials.

DeLeon, J., & Westerberg, J. (1980). *Who adopts retarded children?* Unpublished manuscript.

Doucett, J., & Freedman, R. (1981). *Progress test for the developmentally disabled: An evaluation.* Cambridge, MA: Ware Press.

Dunst, C., Trivette, C., & Deal, A. (1988). *Enabling and empowering families: Principles and guidelines for practice.* Cambridge, MA: Brookline Books.

Eastwood, E.A., & Fisher, G.A. (1988). Skill acquisition among matched samples of institutionalized and community-based persons with mental retardation. *American Journal on Mental Retardation, 93,* 75–83.

Edgar, E.B., Reid, P.C., & Pious, C.C. (1988). Special sitters: Youth as respite care providers. *Mental Retardation, 26,* 33.

Edgerton, R.B. (1967). *The cloak of competence: Stigma in the lives of the mentally retarded.* Berkeley: University of California Press.

Edgerton, R.B., & Bercovici, S. (1976). The cloak of competence: Years later. *American Journal of Mental Deficiency, 80,* 485–497.

Edgerton, R.B., Bollinger, M., & Herr, B. (1984). The cloak of competence: After two decades. *American Journal of Mental Deficiency, 88,* 345–351.

Edgerton, R.B., & Langness, L.L. (1978). Observing mentally retarded persons in community settings: An anthropological perspective. In G.P. Sackett (Ed.), *Observing behavior: Volume I. Theory and applications in mental retardation* (pp. 335–348). Baltimore: University Park Press.

Elder, J.O. (1980). Essential components in development of interagency collaboration. In J.O. Elder & P.R. Magrab (Eds.), *Coordinating services to handicapped children: A handbook for interagency collaboration* (pp. 181–201). Baltimore: Paul H. Brookes Publishing Co.

Eyman, R.K., Demaine, G.C., & Lei, T. (1979). Relationship between community environments and resident changes in adaptive behavior: A path model. *American Journal of Mental Deficiency, 83,* 330–338.

Feinstein, C.S. Lemanowicz, J.A., Spreat, S., & Conroy, J.W. (1986). *Report to the special master in the case of Gary W. v. the State of Louisiana.* Philadelphia: Temple University, Developmental Disabilities Center.

Felce, D., Saxby H., deKock, U., Repp, A., Ager, A., & Blunder, R. (1987). To what behaviors do attending adults respond? A replication. *American Journal of Mental Deficiency, 91,* 496–504.

Fiorelli, J.S., Margolis, H., Heverly, M.A., Rothchild, E., & Keating, D.J. (1982). Training resident advisors to provide community residential services: A university based program. *Journal of The Association for the Severely Handicapped, 7*(1), 13–20.

Franklin, D.S., & Massarik, F. (1969a). The adoption of children with medical conditions: Part I. Process and outcomes [Special issue]. *Child Welfare, 46.*

Franklin, D.S., & Massarik, F. (1969b). The adoption of children with medical conditions: Part II. The families today [Special issue]. *Child Welfare, 47.*

Franklin, D.S., & Massarik, F. (1969c). The adoption of children with medical conditions: Part III. Discussion and conclusions [Special issue]. *Child Welfare, 48.*

Freedman, R. (1976). Approaches to defining and measuring the community adjustment of mentally retarded persons: A review of the literature (Vol. 1) (Project report). Cambridge, MA: Abt Associates.

Friedrich, W.N., & Friedrich, W.L. (1981). Psychosocial assets of parents of handicapped and nonhandicapped children. *American Journal of Mental Deficiency, 85,* 551–553.

Gath, A. (1973). The impact of an abnormal child upon the parents. *British Journal of Psychiatry, 130,* 405–410.

Gath, A. (1983). Mentally retarded children in substitute and natural families. *Adoption & Fostering, 7*(1), 35–40.

Glidden, L.M. (1986). Families who adopt mentally retarded children: Who, why, and what happens. In J.J. Gallagher & P.M. Vietze (Eds.), *Families of handicapped persons: Research, programs and policy issues* (pp. 129–142). Baltimore: Paul H. Brookes Publishing Co.

Glidden, L.M., Valliere, V., & Herbert, S. (1988). Adopted children with mental retardation: Positive family impact. *Mental Retardation, 26,* 119.

Gold, M. (1980). *Marc Gold: "Did I say that?"* Champaign, Il: Research Press.

Gollay, Freedman, Wyngaarden, & Kurtz (1978). *Coming back: The community experience of deinstitutionalization of mentally retarded people.* Cambridge, MA: A.B.T. Books.

Griffin, J.C., Landers, W.F., & Patterson, E.T. (1974). *Behavior architecture: Effects of the physical environment on the behavior of the retarded.* Lubbock: Texas Technical University Research and Training Center in Mental Retardation.

Grossman, H.J. (Ed.). (1983). *Classification in mental retardation.* Washington, DC: American Association on Mental Deficiency.

Halderman v. Pennhurst State School and Hospital, 446 F. Supp. 1295, 1314–1320 (E.D. Pa., 1977).

Halpern, A.S., Close, D.W., & Nelson, D.J. (1985). *On my own.* Baltimore: Paul H. Brookes Publishing Co.

Haney, J.I. (1988). Empirical support for deinstitutionalization. In L.W. Heal, J.I. Haney, & A.R.N. Amado (Eds.), *Integration of developmentally disabled individuals into the community* (pp. 37–58). Baltimore: Paul H. Brookes Publishing Co.

Haney, J.I., & Heal, L.W. (1987). The relationship of residential environment differences to adaptive behavior of mentally retarded individuals: A review and critique of research. In J.A. Mulick & R.F. Antonak, *Transitions in mental retardation: Advocacy, technology and science* (pp. 89–102). Norwood, NJ: Ablex.

Hauber, F.A., Bruininks, R.H., Hill, B.K., Lakin, K.C., Scheerenberger, R.C., & White, C.C. (1984). National census of residential facilities: A profile of facilities and residents. *American Journal of Mental Deficiency, 89,* 236–245.

Heal, L.W. (1985). Methodology for community institutional research. In R.H. Bruininks & K.C. Lakin (Eds.), *Living and learning in the least restrictive environment* (pp.199–224). Baltimore: Paul H. Brookes Publishing Co.

Heal, L.W., & Daniels, B.S. (1978). A cost effectiveness analysis of residential alternatives. *Mental Retardation, 3,* 35–49.

Heal, L.W., & Fujiura, G. (1984). Methodological considerations in research on residential alternatives for developmentally disabled persons. In N.R. Ellis & N.W. Bray (Eds.), *International review of research in mental retardation* (Vol. 12, pp. 205–244). New York: Academic Press.

Heal, L.W., & Laidlaw, T.J. (1980). Evolution of residential alternatives. In A.R. Novak & L.W. Heal (Eds.), *Integration of developmentally disabled individuals into the community* (pp. 141–162). Baltimore: Paul H. Brookes Publishing Co.

Heal, L.W., Sigelman, C.K., & Switzky, H.N. (1978). Research on community residential alternatives for the mentally retarded. In N.R. Ellis (Eds.), *International review of research in mental retardation* (Vol. 9, pp. 209–249). New York: Academic Press.

Herz, M., Endicott, J., Spitzer, R., & Mensnikoff, A. (1971). Day vs. inpatient hospitalization: A controlled study. *American Journal of Psychiatry, 127,* 107–117.

Heshusis, L. (1981). *Meaning in life as experienced by persons labelled retarded in a group home.* Springfield, IL: Charles C Thomas.

Hill, B.K., Lakin, K.C., & Bruininks, R.H. (1984). Trends in residential services for people who are mentally retarded. *Journal of The Association for persons with severe handicaps, 9,* 243–250.

Horner, R.H., Stoner, S.K., & Ferguson, D.L. (1988). *An activity-based analysis of deinstitutionalization: The effects of community re-entry on the lives of residents leaving Oregon's Fairview Training Center.* Salem: University of Oregon, Specialized Training Program of the Center on Human Development.

Hull, S.T., & Thompson, S.C. (1980). Predicting adoptive functioning of mentally retarded persons in community settings. *American Journal of Mental Deficiency, 85,* 253–261.

Intagliata, J. (1986). Reassessing the impact of respite care services. A review of outcome evaluation studies. In C.L. Salisbury & J. Intagliata (Eds)., *Respite care: Support for persons with developmental disabilities and their families* (pp. 263–288). Baltimore: Paul H. Brookes Publishing Co.

Intagliata, J., Gibson, B., & Rinck, R. (1984, May). *Evaluating the impact of respite care on respite utilization and family well-being.* Paper presented at the Annual Conference of the Association on Mental Deficiency, Minneapolis, MN.

Intagliata, J., & Willer, B. (1982). Reinstitutionalization of mentally retarded persons into family-care and group homes. *American Journal of Mental Deficiency, 87,* 34–39.

Jacobs, P.A. (1986). Studies of the fragile (x) syndrome in populations of mentally retarded individuals in Hawaii. *American Journal of Medical Genetics, 23,* 567–572.

Janicki, M.P. (1981). Personal growth and community residence environments. In H.C. Hywood & J.R. Newbrough (Eds.), *Living environments for devel-*

opmentally retarded persons (pp. 59–101). Baltimore: University Park Press.

Jones, P.A., Conroy, S.W., Feinstein, C.S., & Lemanowicz, J.A. (1984). A matched comparison study of cost effectiveness: Institutionalization and deinstitutionalized people. *Journal of The Association for Persons with Severe Handicaps, 9,* 304–313.

Joyce, K., Singer, M., & Isralowitz, R. (1983). Impact of respite care on parents' perception of quality of life. *Mental Retardation, 21,* 153–156.

Katz, A.H., & Bender, E.I. (1976). *The strength in us.* New York: New Viewpoints.

Kendrick, M. (1987). *Study of individuals in group homes and supported apartments.* Unpublished manuscript.

King, R.D., Raynes, N.V., & Tizard, S. (1971). *Patterns of residential care: Sociological studies in institutions for handicapped children.* London: Routledge and Kegan Paul.

Kishi, G., Teelucksingh, B., Zollers., N., Park-Lee, S., & Meyer, L. (1988). Daily decision-making in community residences: A social comparison of adults with and without mental retardation. *American Journal on Mental Retardation, 92,* 430–435.

Kleinberg, J., & Galligan, B. (1983). Effects of deinstitutionalization on adaptive behavior of mentally retarded adults. *American Journal of Mental Deficiency, 88,* 21–27.

Knoll, A., & Ford, A. (1987). Beyond caregiving: A reconceptualization of the role of the residential service provider. In S.J. Taylor, D. Biklen, & J. Knoll (Eds.), *Community integration for people with severe disabilities* (pp. 129–146). New York: Teachers College Press.

Knoll, A., & Olsen, C. (1988). *The use of qualitative research methodology to examine community integration.* Unpublished manuscript.

Krauss, M.W., & Erickson, M. (1988). Informal support networks among aging persons with mental retardation: A pilot study. *Mental Retardation, 26,* 197–201.

Kregel, J., Wehman, P., Seyfarth, J., & Marshall, K. (1986). Community integration of young adults with mental retardation: Transition from school to adulthood. *Education and Training of the Mentally Retarded, 21,* 35–42.

Krisheff, C.H. (1977). Adoption agency services for the retarded. *Mental Retardation, 15*(1), 38–39.

Krowinski, W., & Fitt, D. (1978). *On the clinical efficiency and cost effectiveness of psychiatric partial hospitalization versus traditional inpatient care with six month follow up data.* Unpublished report to Capital Blue Cross Reading Hospital and Medical Center, Day Treatment Center, Reading, PA.

Lakin, K.C., Hill, B.K., White, C.C., & Wright, E.A. (1988). *Longitudinal change and interstate variability in the size of residential facilities for persons with mental retardation.* Minneapolis: University of Minnesota, Center for Residential and Community Services.

Landesman, S., & Vietze, P. (1987). *Living environments and mental retardation* (N.I.C.H.D. Mental Retardation Research Centers Series). Washington, DC: American Association on Mental Retardation.

Landesman-Dwyer, S. (1981). Living in the community. *American Journal of Mental Deficiency, 86,* 223–234.

Landesman-Dwyer, S., Berkson, G., & Romer, D. (1979). Affiliation and friendship of mentally retarded residents in group homes. *American Journal of Mental Deficiency, 83,* 571–580.

Landesman-Dwyer, S., Sackett, G.P., & Kleinman, J.S. (1980a). Relationship of size of resident and staff behavior in small community residences. *American Journal of Mental Deficiency, 85,* 6–17.

Landesman-Dwyer, S., Sackett, G.P., & Kleinman, J.S. (1980b). *Small community residences: Does size really matter?* Unpublished manuscript, University of Washington, Seattle.

Larson, S., & Lakin, C. (1989). Deinstitutionalization of persons with mental retardation: Behavioral outcomes. *Journal of The Association for Persons with Severe Handicaps, 14,* 324–332.

Laux, R. (1988). *Creative financing of consumer-owned housing.* Portsmouth, NH: Creative Management Associates.

Levenson, A., Lord, C., Sermas, C., Thornby, J., Sullender, W., & Comstock, B. (1977). Acute schizophrenia: An effective out patient treatment approach as an alternative to full time hospitalization. *Diseases of the Nervous System, 23,* 242–245.

Levy, J.M., & Levy, P.H. (1986). Issues and models in the delivery of respite services. In C.L. Salisbury & J. Intagliata (Eds.), *Respite care: Support for persons with developmental disabilities and their families.* (pp. 99–116). Baltimore: Paul H. Brookes Publishing Co.

Lovett, D.L., & Harris, M.B. (1987). Identification of important living skills for adults with mental retardation. *Mental Retardation, 25,* 351–356.

MacEachron, A.E. (1983). Institutional reform and adaptive functioning of mentally retarded persons: A field experiment. *American Journal of Mental Deficiency, 88* 2–12.

Mayeda, T., & Wai, F. (1975). *The cost of long term developmental disabilities care.* Pomona: University of California: Los Angeles, Neuropsychiatric Institute.

McCarver, R.B., & Craig, E.M. (1974). Placement of the retarded in the community: Prognosis and outcome. In N.R. Ellis (Ed.), *International review of research in mental retardation* (Vol. 7, pp. 143–207). New York: Academic Press.

McCormick, M., Balla, D., & Zigler, E. (1975). Resident care practices in institutions for retarded persons: A cross-institutional, cross-cultural study. *American Journal of Mental Deficiency, 80,* 1–17.

McKnight, J.L. (1987). Regenerating community. *Social Policy, 18,* 54–58.

Meyer, L.H., St. Peter, S., & Park-Lee, S. (1986,

November). *The validation of social skills for successful performance in community environments by young adults with moderate to severe/profound disabilities.* Paper presented at the 20th annual meeting of the Association for the Advancement of Behavior Therapy, Chicago.

Meyers, C.E., Bothwick, S.A., & Eyman, R.K. (1985). Place of residence by age, ethnicity and level of retardation of the mentally retarded/developmentally disabled population of California. *American Journal of Mental Retardation, 90,* 266–270.

Meyers, J., & Marcenco, M. (1986). *An evaluation of Michigan's family support subsidy program: Coping with the cost.* Detroit: Wayne State University, Developmental Disabilities Institute.

Minnesota Developmental Disabilities Planning. (1982). *The financial status of Minnesota developmental achievement centers:* 1980–1982. Minneapolis: John H. Nubra.

Moreau, F.A., Novak, A.R., & Sigelman, C.K. (1980). Physical and social integration of developmentally disabled individuals into the community. In A.R. Novak & L.W. Heal (Eds.), *Integration of developmentally disabled individuals into the community* (pp. 91–106). Baltimore: Paul H. Brookes Publishing Co.

Mosher, L., & Menn, A. (1978) Community residential treatment for schizophrenia: Two year follow up. *Hospital and Community Psychiatry, 29,* 715–723.

Nerney, T., Conley, R., & Nisbet, J. (1989). *A residential cost analysis of three regional service delivery systems for persons with developmental disabilities.* Unpublished manuscript.

Nihira, L. (1979). *Costs for care of matched developmentally disabled clients in three settings.* Pomona: University of California, Los Angeles, Neuropsychiatric Institute, Research Group at Lanteron State Hospital.

Nihira, K., Foster, R., Shellhaas, M., & Leland, A. (1974). *Adaptive Behavior Scale: Manual.* Washington, DC: American Association on Mental Deficiency.

Novak, A., & Heal, L.W. (1980). *Integration of developmentally disabled persons into the community.* Baltimore: Paul H. Brookes Publishing Co.

O'Brien, J., & Lyle-O'Brien, C. (1989). *Settling down: Creating personal supports for people who rely on the residential supports of centennial services.* Lithonia, GA: Responsive Systems Associates.

O'Connor, G. (1976). *Home is a good place* (Monograph No. 2). Washington, DC: American Association on Mental Deficiency.

O'Connor, G., & Morris, L. (1978). *A research approach to cost analysis and program budgeting of community research facilities.* Eugene: University of Oregon, Rehabilitation, Research, and Training Center in Mental Retardation.

O'Neill, J., Brown, M., Gordon, W., & Schonhorn, R. (1985). The impact of deinstitutionalization on activities and skills of severely/profoundly mentally retarded multiply-handicapped adults. *Applied Research in Mental Retardation, 6,* 361–371.

O'Neill, J., Brown, M., Gordon, W., Schonhorn, R., & Greer, E. (1981). Activity patterns of mentally retarded adults in institutions and communities: A longitudinal study. *Applied Research in Mental Retardation, 2,* 367–379.

Pasamanick, B., Scarpitti, F., & Dinitz, S. (1967). *Schizophrenics and the community.* New York: Appleton-Century-Crofts.

Peck, C.A., Blackburn, T.C., & White-Blackburn, G. (1980). Making it work: A review of the empirical literature on community living arrangements. In T. Apolloni, J. Cappuccilli, & T.P. Cooke (Eds.), *Achievements in residential services for persons with disabilities: Toward excellence* (pp. 147–167). Baltimore: University Park Press.

Pilewski, M.E., & Heal, L.W. (1980). Empirical support for deinstitutionalization. In A.R. Novak & L.W. Heal (Eds.), *Integration of developmentally disabled individuals into the community* (pp. 21–34). Baltimore: Paul H. Brookes Publishing Co.

Perske, R. (1988). *New life in the neighborhood.* Nashville, TN: Abingdon Press.

Perske, R. (1988). *A circle of friends.* Nashville, TN: Abingdon Press.

Reizenstein, J., & McBride, W. (1978). Designing for mentally retarded people: A socioenvironmental evaluation of New England Villages, Inc. In A. Friedman, C. Zimring, & E. Zube (Eds.), *Environmental design evaluation* (pp. 53–72). New York: Plenum.

Romer, D., & Berkson, G. (1980a). Social ecology of supervised communal facilities for mentally disabled adults: II. Predictors. *American Journal of Mental Deficiency, 85,* 229–242.

Romer, D., & Berkson, G. (1980b). Social ecology of supervised communal facilities for mentally disabled adults: III. Predictors of social choice. *American Journal of Mental Deficiency, 85,* 243–252.

Rosen, D.B. (1985). *Differences in adaptive behavior of institutionalized and deinstitutionalized mentally retarded adults.* Ann Arbor, MI: University Microfilms International (DA8508127).

Rosen, M., Kiuitz, M.S., Clark, G.R., & Floor, L. (1970). Prediction of post-institutional adjustment of mentally retarded adults. *American Journal of Mental Deficiency, 74,* 726–734.

Rotegard, L.L., Bruininks, R.H., Holman, J.G., & Lakin, K.C. (1985). Environmental aspects of deinstitutionalization. In R.H. Bruininks & K.C. Lakin (Eds.), *Living and learning in the least restrictive environment* (pp. 155–184). Baltimore: Paul H. Brookes Publishing Co.

Rotegard, L.L., Hill, B.K., & Bruininks, R.H. (1983). Environmental characteristics of residential facilities for mentally retarded people in the United

States. *American Journal of Mental Deficiency, 83,* 49–56.

Rothman, D.J., & Rothman, S.M. (1984). *The Willowbrook wars.* New York: Harper & Row.

Salend, S.J., & Giek, K.A., (1988). Independent living arrangements with the mentally retarded: The landlords' perspective. *Mental Retardation, 26,* 89–92.

Salisbury, C. (1987). Stressors of parents with young handicapped and nonhandicapped children. *Journal of the Division for Early Childhood, 11,* 154–160.

Saxby, H., Thomas, M., Felce, D., & deKock, U. (1986). The use of shops, cafes and public houses by severely and profoundly mentally handicapped adults. *British Journal of Mental Subnormality, 32,* 69–81.

Schalock, R.L. (1975). *Independent Living Screening Test and remediation manual.* Hastings: Mid-Nebraska Mental Retardation Services.

Schalock, R.L., & Harper, R.S. (1979). Training in independent living can be done. *Journal of the Rehabilitation Administration, 3,* 129–132.

Schalock, R.L., Harper, R.S., & Genung, T. (1981). Community integration of mentally retarded adults: Community placement and program success. *American Journal of Mental Deficiency, 85,* 478–488.

Schalock, R.L., & Lilly, M.A. (1986). Placement from community based mental retardation programs: How well do clients do after 8 to 10 years? *American Journal of Mental Deficiency, 90,* 669–676.

Scheerenberger, R.C. (1976). *Deinstitutionalization and institutional reform.* Springfield, IL: Charles C Thomas.

Schroeder, S.R., & Hanes, C. (1978). Assessment of progress of institutionalized and deinstitutionalized retarded adults: A matched-control comparison. *Mental retardation, 16,* 147–148.

Seltzer, G.B. (1981). Community residential adjustment: The relationship among environment, performance and satisfaction. *American Journal of Mental Deficiency, 85,* 624–630.

Seltzer, M.M. (1985). Informal supports of elderly mentally retarded persons. *American Journal of Mental Deficiency, 90,* 259–265.

Seltzer, M.M., Ivry, J., & Litchfield, L.C. (1987). Family members as case managers: Partnership between the formal and informal support networks. *The Gerontologist, 27,* 722–728.

Sherman, B.R. (1988). Predictors of the decision to place developmentally disabled members in residential care. *American Journal on Mental Retardation, 92,* 344–351.

Sherman, J.A., Sheldon, J.B., Morris, K., Strouse, M., & Reese, R.M. (1984). A community based residential program for mentally retarded adults: An adoption of the teaching-family model. In S.C Paine, G.T. Bellamy, & B. Wilcox (Eds.), *Human*

services that work (pp. 167–179). Baltimore: Paul H. Brookes Publishing Co.

Sigelman, C.K. (1976). A Machiavelli for planners. Community attitudes and selection of a group home site. *Mental Retardation, 14*(1), 26–29.

Sigelman, C.K, Novak, A.R., Heal, L.W., & Switzky, H.N. (1980). Factors that affect the success of community placement. In A.R. Novak & L.W. Heal (Eds.), *Integration of developmentally disabled individuals into the community* (pp. 57–74). Baltimore: Paul H. Brookes Publishing Co.

Singer, G.H., Close, D.W., Irvin, L.K., Gersten, R., & Sailor, W. (1984). An alternative to the institution for young people with severely handicapping conditions in a rural community. *Journal of The Association for Persons with Severe Handicaps, 9,* 251.

Singer, G.H.S., Irvin, L.K., & Hawkins, N.E. (1988). Stress management training for parents of severely handicapped children. *Mental Retardation, 26,* 269–277.

Soforenko, A.Z., & Macy, T.W. (1977). A study of the characteristics and life status of persons discharged from a large state institution for the mentally retarded from the years 1969–1977 (Monograph 1). Columbus: Ohio State University.

Sokol-Kessler, L., Conroy, J., Feinstein, C., Lemanowicz, J., & McGurrin, M. (1983). *Developmental progress in institutional and community settings* (Pennhurst study report pc-83-2). Philadelphia: Temple University Developmental Disability Center.

Staff. (1989). *The Roundtable, 4*(1).

Stagg, V., & Catron, T. (1986). Networks of social supports for parents of handicapped children. In R.R. Fewell & P.F. Vadasy, *Families of handicapped children* (pp. 279–296). Austin, TX: PRO-ED.

State of Wisconsin, Bureau of Evaluation, Division of Policy and Budget. (1986). *Evaluation of the community integration program.* Madison: Authors.

Stein, L., Test, M., & Marx, A. (1975). Alternative to the hospital: A controlled study. *American Journal of Psychiatry, 132,* 517–521.

Sternlicht, M. (1978). Variables affecting foster care placement of institutionalized retarded residents. *Mental Retardation, 16,* 25–28.

Suedfeld, P. (1980). *Restricted environmental stimulation.* New York: John Wiley & Sons.

Sutherland, A.T. (1981). *Disabled we stand.* Bloomington: Indiana University Press.

Sutter, P., Mayeda, T., Call, T., Yanagi, G., & Yee, S. (1980). Comparison of successful and unsuccessful community placed mentally retarded persons. *American Journal of Mental Deficiency, 85,* 262–267.

Tausig, M. (1985). Factors in family decision-making about placement for developmentally disabled individuals. *American Journal of Mental Deficiency, 89,* 352–361.

Taylor, J.D. (1980). A comparison of the adaptive behavior of retarded individuals successfully and unsuccessfully placed in group homes. *Education and Training of the Mentally Retarded, 2,* 56–64.

Taylor, S.J. (1984). Public policy and deinstitutionalization. *Mental Retardation Systems, 1*(1).

Taylor, S.J. (1987a). Continuum traps. In S.J. Taylor, D. Biklen, & J. Knoll (Eds.), *Community integration for people with severe disabilities* (pp. 25–35.). New York: Teachers College Press.

Taylor, S.J. (1987b). Introduction. In S.J. Taylor, D. Biklen, & J. Knoll (Eds.), *Community integration for people with severe disabilities* (pp. xv–xx). New York: Teachers College Press.

Taylor, S.J., Racino, J., Knoll, J., & Lutfiyya, Z. (1987). *The nonrestrictive environment; Community integration for people with the most severe disabilities.* Syracuse, NY: Human Policy Press.

Templeman, D., Gage, M.A., & Fredericks, H.D. (1982). Cost effectiveness of the group home. *Journal of The Association for the Severely Handicapped, 6*(4), 11–16.

Thompson, T., & Carey, A. (1980). Structured normalization: Intellectual and adaptive behavior changes in a residential setting. *Mental Retardation, 18,* 193–197.

Turnbull, H.R., III, & Behr, R. (1986). Presidential address, 1986. Public policy and professional behavior. *Mental Retardation, 24,* 265–275.

United States Surgeon General (1987). *Children with special health care needs campaign '87: Commitment to family centered care for children with special health care needs.* Washington, DC: United States Department of Health and Human Services.

Vanier, J. (1979). *Community and growth.* New York: Paulist Press.

Vogelsburg, R.T., Williams, W.W., & Freidl, M. (1980). Facilitating systems change for the severely handicapped: Secondary and adult services. *Journal of The Association for the Severely Handicapped, 5*(1), 73–85.

Washburn, S., Vannicelli, M., Longabaugh, R., & Scheff, B. (1976). A controlled comparison of psychiatric day treatment and inpatient hospitalization. *Journal of Consulting and Clinical Psychiatry, 44,* 665–675.

Wehbring, K., & Ogren, C. (1975). *Community residences of mentally retarded people.* Arlington, TX: National Association for Retarded Citizens.

Welsch v. Likins, 373 R. Supp. 487, 502 (D.Minn. 1974), aff'd in part and vacated and remanded in part, 550 F.2d 1122 (8th Cir. 1977).

White, C.C., Lakin, K.C., Hill, B.K., Wright, E.A., & Bruininks, R.H. (1988). *Persons with mental retardation in state operated residential facilities: Year ending June 30, 1987 with longitudinal trends from 1950 to 1987.* Minneapolis: University of Minnesota, Center for Residential and Community Services.

Wieck, C.A., & Bruininks, R.H. (1980) *The cost of public and community residential care for mentally retarded people in the United States* (Project Report #9). Minneapolis: University of Minnesota, Developmental Disabilities Project on Residential Services and Community Adjustment.

Wikler, L.M., Hanusa, D., & Stoysheff, J. (1986). Home-based respite care, the child with developmental disabilities, and family stress: Some theoretical and pragmatic aspects of process evaluation. In C.L. Salisbury & J. Intagliata (Eds.), *Respite care: Support for persons with developmental disabilities and their families* (pp. 243–261). Baltimore: Paul H. Brookes Publishing Co.

Wilder, J., Levin, G., & Zwerling, I. (1966). A two year follow up evaluation of acute psychotic patients treated in a day hospital. *American Journal of Psychiatry, 122,* 1095–1111.

Willer, B., & Intagliata, J. (1981). Social environment as predictors of adjustment of deinstitutionalized mentally retarded adults. *American Journal of Mental Deficiency, 86,* 252–259.

Willer, B., & Intagliata, J. (1982). Comparison of family care and group homes as alternatives to institutions. *American Journal of Mental Deficiency, 86,* 588–595.

Willer, B., & Intagliata, J. (1984). *The promises and realities of deinstitutionalization: Life in the community for mentally retarded persons.* Baltimore: University Park Press.

Williams, P., & Shoultz, B. (1982). *We can speak for ourselves: Self-advocacy by mentally handicapped people.* Bloomington: Indiana University Press.

Windle, C., Stewart, E., & Brown, E. (1961). Reasons for community failure of released patients. *American Journal of Mental Deficiency, 66,* 213–217.

Wisconsin Department of Health and Social Services. (1985). *Family support program: Guidelines and procedures.* Madison: Author.

Wolfensberger, W., & Glenn, A. (1975). *Program analysis of service systems.* Toronto: National Institute on Mental Retardation.

Wolkind, S., & Kozaruk, A. (1983). *Children with special needs: A review of children with medical problems placed by the Adoption Resource Exchange form 1974–77* (Report to the Department of Health and Social Services). London: London Hospital Medical College Family Research Unit.

Wyatt v. Stickney, 344 F. Supp. 373, 387 (M.D. Ala. 1972), aff'd sub nom, Wyatt v. Aderholt, 503 F.2d 1305 (5th Cir. 1974).

Zigler, E., & Balla, D.A. (1977). Impact of institutional experience on the behavior and development of retarded persons. *American Journal of Mental Deficiency, 82,* 1–11.

CHAPTER 9

Supported Employment
Emerging Opportunities
for Employment Integration

Frank R. Rusch

Janis Chadsey-Rusch

John R. Johnson

University of Illinois at Urbana-Champaign, Champaign, Illinois

Traditional views of persons with severe handicaps continue to pose enormous challenges to contemporary educational and rehabilitation practices. Although Congress enacted the Rehabilitation Act of 1973 (PL 93-112) and the Education for All Handicapped Children Act of 1975 (PL 94-142), persons with severe handicaps have not fully enjoyed the goals envisioned by legislation. Education legislation was designed to remove restrictions that had denied persons with handicaps equal access to educational opportunities. PL 94-142 sought to encourage educational integration. PL 93-112 sought to encourage more individuals with a handicap to enter the work force by removing unnecessary obstacles to hiring and in their working conditions (Rusch & Phelps, 1987). The results of legislative action, however, have been slow to form for persons with severe handicaps.

Contemporary educational and rehabilitation practices also are posing enormous challenges to traditional educational and rehabilitation efforts. Today, contemporary approaches to employment have rendered traditional practices obsolete in many parts of the United States. The ideological and technological advances in education and rehabilitation are beginning to have an impact in human services.

The purpose of this chapter is to review research related to supported employment and the impact it has had for persons with severe handicaps. First, this chapter introduces supported employment, including a description of placement approaches and model program characteristics. Second, research related to benefit-cost analysis and consumer wages, social integration, and ongoing support is overviewed. In an effort to clarify supported employment–related outcomes in relation to persons with severe handicaps, we compare and contrast wages, level of integration, and amount of support reported for persons with severe handicaps as well as for persons with other handicaps. Finally, unresolved issues and suggestions for future research are discussed.

In general, when we reference persons with severe handicaps we typically refer to individuals with severe mental retardation. This should not suggest, however, that supported employment is inappropriate for individuals with other disabilities (e.g., multiple handicaps, mental illness). However, the majority of the research conducted to date has focused upon individuals with mental retardation.

INTRODUCTION TO SUPPORTED EMPLOYMENT

A fairly recent employment option that has demonstrated enormous success across a wide range of persons with diverse disabilities has been a model of employment services called "supported employment" (Bellamy, Rhodes, Mank, & Albin, 1988; Kiernan & Stark, 1986; Rusch, 1986a; Wehman, 1981). Numerous federal initiatives and emerging legislation have resulted in a significant allocation of federal and state resources for supported employment (Rusch & Hughes, in press; Rusch & Phelps, 1987; Wehman, Moon, Everson, Wood, & Barcus, 1988; Will, 1986). One of the most significant pieces of legislation to date in the area of supported employment has been the Rehabilitation Act Amendments of 1986 (PL 99-506), which authorized a new formula grant for the State Supported Employment Services Program in addition to allowing state rehabilitation agencies to purchase supported employment–related services (e.g., situational assessment, job placement, training). The *Federal Register* (1987) published rules and regulations governing the implementation of this act; according to the rules and regulations, the purpose of the amendments was to "assist States in developing and implementing collaborative programs with appropriate public agencies and private nonprofit organizations for training and traditionally time-limited post-employment services leading to supported employment for individuals with severe handicaps" (p. 30546). The rules and regulations also stipulated that the supported employment program is intended "to provide services to individuals who because of the severity of their handicaps would not traditionally be eligible for vocational services. Individuals who are eligible for services under the program must not be able to function independently in employment without intensive on-going support services for the duration of their employment" (*Federal Register*, 1987, p. 30546). Finally, the rules and regulations defined supported employment as "competitive work in an integrated work setting for individuals who, because of their handicaps, need ongoing support services to perform that work" (*Federal Register*, 1987, p. 30546). The rules and regulations also defined the three critical elements of supported employment: *competitive work* in an *integrated work setting* with *ongoing support services*. The Rehabilitation Act Amendments of 1986 are thus an acknowledgment of the failure of traditional adult services programs to provide bonafide employment services to persons with severe disabilities, including those with severe handicaps, and a recognition that most if not all persons with handicaps have the right to community-based and remunerative employment.

The data generated by supported employment programs around the country have indicated that: 1) persons with disabilities of any type and severity can earn significantly greater wages in supported employment than in sheltered programs (Hill, Wehman, Kregel, Banks, & Metzler, 1987; Noble & Conley, 1987; Tines, Rusch, McCaughrin, & Conley, in press); 2) employers have shown a strong commitment to the employment of persons with handicaps, indicating that persons who do not have handicaps do not have to be isolated from persons with handicaps (Mithaug, 1979); and 3) supported employment programs are more cost-effective in the long run than day activity, work activity, and regular workshop programs (Noble & Conley, 1987; Tines et al., in press).

There are several major differences between supported employment and traditional adult services programs. First, supported employment emphasizes integrated employment, whereas adult day programs emphasize vocational and nonvocational services in segregated settings. Second, supported employment emphasizes competitive work for wages that start at or above the minimum wage. Most adult services programs consider wages as an ancillary outcome of sheltered employment, where the sheltered employment is a greater priority than wages. Finally, supported employment was not initially designed as a continuum of services but as a zero-reject service delivery option (Wehman & Moon, 1988).

An individual may be employed through one of several different types of supported employment program models, such as the individual placement model, the clustered placement model, or the mobile work crew model. However, the objective is competitive employment, regardless of the model—not movement through a continuum of services. The criteria used to determine which placement model is best for certain employees is still being studied; however, individual placement models appear to be more favorable than clustered placement or mobile work crew models.

Most persons with severe handicaps will require ongoing training and assistance in a variety of areas to be successful on the job. Traditionally, regardless of disability type or severity, employment services have not included ongoing support. Job placement, job match, and job maintenance services now available through supported employment programs were traditionally considered solely the responsibility of the individual or the employing agencies. Once he or she was employed, it was up to the individual to learn how to do the job and to keep the job. However, proponents of supported employment have designed service models that assist individuals in acquiring, learning, and keeping their jobs. Ongoing support has rendered the concept that a person must be "ready" for employment obsolete and indefensible. If effective ongoing support is provided, then such support does away with the need for "readiness training."

Placement Approaches

As stated, there are three primary placement approaches to supported employment. These approaches include: 1) individual placement model, 2) clustered placement model, and 3) mobile work crew model. Table 9.1 displays some of the distinguishing characteristics of the three approaches.

Typically, when implementing the *individual placement* model, an employment specialist locates a job in a conventional, private-sector company, and then places the individual with a disability into the job (Bellamy et al., 1988). Continuous on-site training is provided until the supported employee performs the job within acceptable standards. Over time, the type and level of assistance provided are decreased, although at least two contacts per month are provided for the duration of the employment (Wehman & Moon, 1988).

The *clustered placement* model (also referred to as the *enclave* model) differs from the individual placement model in that a group of individuals, typically less than eight, work in close proximity, often performing the same work. Typically, follow-up staff provide continuous training and support for the duration of the employment period, not just during the initial training period (Bellamy et al., 1988). Clustered placements are located within a community-based business referred to as the "host company," and on-site support is provided through the ongoing presence of an employment specialist who serves as a work supervisor.

Mobile work crews typically consist of less than eight supported employees who provide specialized contract services throughout a community (Wehman & Moon, 1988). Services often are provided from a van (thus the reference to "mobile") and include janitorial or groundskeeping work. Training and continuous supervision are provided by an on-site work supervisor.

Program Components

Supported employment should be viewed as an intervention package containing several components that contribute to its effectiveness (Lagomarcino, 1986; Vogelsberg, 1986; Wehman, 1986). The following components of supported employment have been identified by Trach (in press), Trach and Rusch (in press), and others (e.g., McDonnell, Nofs, Hardman, & Chambless, in press; Wacker, Fromm-Steege, Berg, & Flynn, in press): 1) community survey and job analysis, 2) job match and placement, 3) job training, 4) follow-up services, and 5) interagency coordination.

Table 9.1. Supported employment approaches

Approach	Description	Degree of support
Individual placement model	A single individual is hired by an employer to perform a job	Job coach trains and assists the employee and gradually decreases the amount of support
Clustered placement model	A group of six to eight persons who work at a specific location in a community business or industry	Continuous training and supervision provided by the job coach who may be employed by the company
Mobile work crew	A small group of three to five persons work out of a van at several locations in the community with the supervision of a job coach	Continuous training and supervision provided by the job coach

Typically, employment specialists conduct *community surveys and job analyses* by surveying the community for potential job placement sites through phone calls, mail correspondence, and personal contacts with prospective employers. Direct observation of potential job sites then is conducted to identify vocational and social skills that are requisite for placement in those sites.

Job match and placement involve assessing employee characteristics in relation to job requisites. The employment specialist matches information obtained from the community survey and specific job analysis to an employee's vocational and social skills assessment information to determine an appropriate job match. Usually, employment options are made available to the potential employee, with the supported employee encouraged to participate in his or her own placement selection. Additionally, no individual is excluded from employment (a zero-reject feature) and the opportunity for increased wages and job advancement for each employee is considered.

Following placement, the employment specialist assists the supported employee to perform required job tasks through *job training*. Procedures the employment specialist typically uses include systematic training techniques (e.g., applied behavior analysis), job modifications to adapt the job to an employee's particular disability, and planning for the maintenance of work behavior acquired during training. Specifically, the employment specialist conducts a task analysis of the vocational and social aspects of a job, develops training strategies, determines criteria for acceptable performance, teaches the supported employee to perform the desired work behaviors, and plans for the continuance of the performance.

Finally, the employment specialist provides *follow-up services* to assist individuals in maintaining their employment after job skills have been acquired. Typically, the amount of support required lessens over time, and employment specialists should be able to identify and enlist natural support available in the workplace, utilizing both setting variables (e.g., clocks, whistles, pictures) and interpersonal variables (e.g., co-workers). Additionally, employment specialists promote the social acceptance of the supported

employee by using social validation methodology (Hughes, Rusch, & Curl, in press).

Interagency coordination refers to the ongoing coordination of all services provided by agencies that influence the job placement and retention of the supported employee. These services include, for example, social skills training and travel training provided by an employee's guardian, residence supervisor, or case coordinator (Schalock & Kiernan, in press).

Summary

Wages and integration are major outcomes of recent rehabilitation legislation. Wages earned typically are at or above minimum wage. The primary intent of the Rehabilitation Act Amendments of 1986 is also that supported employees be provided with equal opportunities for physical and social contact with co-workers and the general public.

A characteristic that distinguishes supported employment from other services is the provision of ongoing support for the duration of the employment. This support usually includes direct training at the work site as well as assistance in job-related activities away from the work site. The amount and intensity of support provided is determined individually according to the needs of the supported employee. Programs that provide on-site assessment and training services, but that do not provide ongoing support, would be considered time-limited services rather than supported employment.

Supported employment is specifically designed to overcome impediments to employment for persons with severe handicaps. These individuals usually are unable to gain access to, or derive lasting benefit from, traditional vocational training and employment programs. Supported employment combines features that make employment possible and meaningful for these individuals and for society.

OVERVIEW OF RESEARCH

Although supported employment has emerged as a viable alternative to sheltered employment, several problems have emerged. Our review of outcome data from published and unpublished articles reveals that on the average individuals with severe handicaps constitute less than 10% of the total number of individuals served by supported employment—and this may be a conservative estimate. Table 9.2 compiles data indicating the severity of disabilities experienced by persons benefiting from supported employment programs throughout the United States. The average percentage of persons with severe handicaps reported by studies in this table is approximately 7% of the total number of persons benefiting from supported employment.

Kiernan, McGaughey, and Schalock (1986), for example, reported data in a national employment survey of adults with developmental disabilities. Of the total number of adults included in their sample ($N = 112,996$), nearly 58% were reported as being placed or served in sheltered employment and only 20% ($n = 22,513$) were: placed in a transitional training/employment program (5.6%), placed in a supported employment program (3.7%), or competitively employed (10.6%). Kiernan et al. also reported that of the 1,662 persons included in the sample for the "detailed survey" whose current employment environment was transitional, supported, or competitive, persons with severe handicaps represented only 3.3% ($n = 55$) of the sample. Of the total number of persons whose current environment was only categorized as supported employment ($n = 259$), only about 8% of the sample comprised individuals with severe handicaps.

Interestingly, the language of the rules and regulations for the Rehabilitation Act of Amendments of 1986 makes it very clear that supported employment was "intended to provide services to individuals who because of the severity of their handicaps would not traditionally be eligible for vocational services" (*Federal Register,* 1987, p. 30546). Our research, as well as research reported by Kiernan et al. (1986) and Kregel and Wehman (1989), suggests that persons with severe handicaps are still not meaningfully employed or benefiting from contemporary employment services.

In this section, we overview research that has emerged in relation to wages and benefit-cost analyses, integration, and ongoing support; each of these features represent the distinguishing characteristics of supported employment. Although the intent of this chapter is to review re-

search conducted with persons with severe handicaps, data bases including persons with other handicapping conditions are presented for comparison because existing literature focusing upon persons with severe handicaps is limited.

Wages and Benefit-Cost Analyses

Earning a wage is a measure of one's worth in our society. Indeed, youth in this country aspire to obtain a job that will help them and/or their families achieve some degree of self-sufficiency. Supported employment results in increased wages to consumers regardless of their disabilities and their prior work histories (Conley & Noble, 1990). Considerable evidence also suggests that supported employment is a cost-effective alternative to traditional adult services programs serving persons with handicaps. Typically, a program's effectiveness is evaluated by comparing one program's outcomes with those of the available alternatives. Economic assessment of supported employment has become an important aspect of the evaluation procedures applied to federal and state programs that emerged in the 1980s (Noble & Conley, 1987). The economic efficiency of supported employment has been evaluated primarily through benefit-cost analysis.

Findings reported by several studies conducting benefit-cost analyses over 1- to 3-year periods in the late 1970s and early 1980s suggest that although supported employment programs' costs were greater than their benefits to society and taxpayers, costs gradually decreased and benefits increased. For example, Noble and Conley (1987) found that all forms of supported employment (i.e., individual placements, clustered placements, and mobile work crews) were more productive in terms of earnings and less costly than adult day care, work activity centers, and sheltered workshop alternatives. Hill et al. (1987) provided one of the most detailed analyses of the financial impact that supported employment has had on consumers with moderate and severe mental retardation. Although costs initially were greater than benefits during the first 3 years of operation, benefits began to exceed costs by the fourth year, and benefits continued to increase while costs decreased over an 8-year period. Hill et al. found that the net bene-

Table 9.2. Measure of disability by selected supported employment programs (SEPs)

Reference	Name and location of SEP	Placement models	Period of study	Disability descriptors	Sample descriptors
Hill, Wehman, Kregel, Banks, & Metzler, 1987	Virginia Commonwealth University, Richmond Rehabilitation and Training Center (VCU, RRTC); Richmond, VA	Individual	9/78–6/86	Percentage of total clients placed: Mild = 33% Moderate = 15% Severe = 6% Other = 10% Median IQ = 48	Number of clients placed = 214 Mild and other = 97 Moderate and severe = 117
Kiernan, McGaughey, & Schalock, 1986	National Employment Survey	Not specified	1984–1986	Above 70 IQ = 53 Mild = 127 Moderate = 59 Severe/profound = 20	Number of persons whose current employment environment is supported employment: n = 259
Lagomarcino, 1986	Community Services Program; Champaign, IL	Individual, enclave, mobile crew	1975–1985	Percentage of total persons employed: Mild = 46% Moderate = 26% Severe = 2% Mentally ill = 16% Other = 10%	Number of persons employed = 134
Lam, 1986	WI	Individual, enclave	Unknown	Mean IQ = 64 Range = 30–102	Number of clients = 50
Major & Baffuto, 1989	Project HIRE; NJ	Individual	7/85–11/87	IQ 70+ = 12% Mild = 59% Moderate = 23% Severe = 6% Mean IQ = 57 MDN IQ = 55 Range = 25–89	Number of consumers who obtained jobs: n = 395
Moss, Dineen, & Ford, 1986	Employment Training Program; Seattle, WA	Individual	1975–1985	Mean IQ = 56 Range = 30–65	Number of active clients = 70

Citation	Program; Location	Model	Dates	Client characteristics	Number
Noble & Conley, 1987	Specialized Training Program (STP); Eugene, OR	Benchwork	Unknown	Mean IQ = 30 Untestable = 45	Number of clients = 213
Noble & Conley, 1987	Physio-Control; OR	Enclave	Unknown	Mean IQ = 40 Range = 22–45	Number of clients = 14
Noble & Conley, 1987	VCU, RRTC; Cerebral Palsy Center; Richmond, VA	Individual	Unknown	Mean IQ = 97 Range = 75–120	Number of clients = 10
Rusch, Hughes, & Johnson, 1988	Illinois Supported Employment Project; IL	Individual, enclave, mobile crew	2/86–12/87	Mean Percent: 1986 / 1987 — Borderline IQ 70-84: 22.98 / 16.77; Mild: 42.19 / 43.39; Moderate: 23.49 / 26.55; Severe: 6.37 / 9.10; Profound: 1.65 / 2.08; Other (85+): 2.98 / 2.19	Average number of persons employed for 23 months: n = 164 (1986), n = 253
Schalock & Lilley, 1986	Mid-Nebraska Mental Retardation Services; NE	Unknown	1976–1986	Mean IQ = 67 SD = 12 Range = 40–91	Number of clients placed = 85
Vogelsberg, 1986	Transition I; VT	Individual, enclave	4/80–11/84	Mean IQ = 61 MDN IQ = 62 Range = 45–79	Number of workers = 36
Vogelsberg, 1986	Transition II; VT	Individual, enclave	11/81–11/84	Mean IQ = 55 MDN IQ = 59 Range = 10–73	Number of workers = 25
Vogelsberg, 1986	Transition III; VT	Individual, enclave	3/84–11/84	Mean IQ = 66 MDN IQ = 67 Range = 56–73	Number of workers = 12

fit to each worker was $6,815 and the net benefit to the taxpayer was $7,111 per supported employee. Similarly, McCaughrin (1988) found that for every dollar invested in supported employment, the taxpayer received $2.21 in return over an 8-year period. In Illinois (McCaughrin, Rusch, Conley, & Tines, 1989), 500 supported employees increased society's net benefit by 9% and the taxpayers' net benefit by 18% in the second year.

Schneider, Rusch, Henderson, and Geske (1981) compared the net cost to society of sheltered employment to the costs associated with supported employment. Based upon 2 years of available data, projected net costs to society were made for 5-, 10-, and 20-year periods. Schneider et al. concluded that by the fifth year the supported employment program would begin to provide a benefit to society. This finding was contrasted with the net cost to society of sheltered employment, which remained constant over time. Interestingly, Tines et al. (in press) found Schneider et al's. projections of the net benefit to society were grossly underestimated when compared to actual benefits. In fact, Schneider et al's. projected program costs were much greater than actual program costs, projected employee earnings were less than actual individual earnings, and the projected net benefit to society was less than the actual net benefit to society. In retrospect, Schneider et al. assumed that follow-up service patterns evident after 2 years of employment would continue well into the future. Consequently, they projected a fixed cost over time that was too high. In effect, the supported employees required less and less support over time as they adapted to their employment. Also, Schneider et al. calculated future earnings based upon the assumption that these supported employees would not earn significantly more wages in the future. In fact, these employees' earnings increased several fold after the third year of employment, reflecting increased benefits and employment stability (i.e., tenure).

In Illinois, in March, 1989, there were 568 supported employees participating in the statewide initiative in supported employment. Table 9.3 displays the number of persons employed and their average monthly salaries. Persons with severe mental retardation represented only 6% of

Table 9.3. Number and average monthly income by category of disability employed in Illinois Supported Employment Program (N = 568; March, 1989)[a]

Disability category	Number	Monthly income
Learning disability	20	$319
Mild mental retardation	230	$324
Moderate mental retardation	120	$386
Severe mental retardation	32	$192
Profound mental retardation	4	$ 40
Mental illness	82	$310
Sensory impairments	8	$397
Traumatic brain injury	5	$185
Physical disability	29	$529
Health impaired	8	$456
Substance abuse	1	$151
Autism	8	$176
Not reported	21	—

[a]21 incomplete files.

the total employed; however, these individuals earned approximately $2,300 annually.

In contrast, individuals with severe handicaps who were previously enrolled in adult activity programs in Illinois earned less than $40 per month or approximately $480 annually. In addition, data reported by model supported employment programs in March of 1989 indicated that one supported employee with profound mental retardation earned $360 per month. Also, no supported employee earned less than $1.48 per hour. Data in Illinois suggest that persons with severe handicaps who are supported in employment benefit greatly from integrated employment when considering wages; however, these same persons appear to be significantly underrepresented compared to other disability groups.

Summary

Supported employment has resulted in new opportunities, never before available, for persons with severe handicaps. These opportunities include earning wages. Available data suggest that all supported employees earn wages above those they would have earned had they remained in their alternate programs (e.g., extended sheltered employment, work activity, adult day care). However, it is clear that these wages are low in comparison to the earnings of the general public.

Supported employment is also a program alternative that is financially attractive to the taxpayer. Clearly, the cost of supported employment is less than those costs reported by alternate sheltered programs.

Although wages are important, there are a number of other benefits to supported employment that are not cost related (cf. Martin, Schneider, Rusch, & Geske, 1982). In the next section of this chapter, we overview available research related to the benefits of working in integrated environments.

Integration

Most work settings are very social settings. Typically, employees interact with their supervisors and co-workers about job-related matters, such as the job tasks that need to be done and the best way to accomplish these tasks (Chadsey-Rusch & Gonzalez, 1988). In addition, co-workers interact frequently about non-job-related matters, such as the weather, current events, and leisure pursuits (Chadsey-Rusch & Gonzalez, 1988). More importantly, employment settings provide opportunities for the formation of friendships (Pogrebin, 1987), social support (House, 1981), and social experiences outside of work; consequently, the workplace helps to create a sense of community (Klein & D'Aunno, 1986).

Federal regulations stipulate that supported employment must occur in integrated settings. Integrated work settings are defined as settings where: 1) most co-workers are not handicapped, and 2) individuals with handicaps are not part of a work group consisting only of others with handicaps, or are part of a small work group of not more than eight individuals with handicaps (*Federal Register*, 1987). Clearly, this definition of integration is narrow, focusing only on the physical proximity of integration.

Unfortunately, there is a scarcity of research related to integration in supported employment. The small amount of research that has been conducted generally has focused only on social interactions and has not included persons with severe handicaps. Instead, persons with mild and moderate mental retardation typically have formed the primary subject pool. Even though few studies have involved individuals with severe handicaps, we review related research in order to draw implications for persons with severe handicaps.

For illustrative purposes, integration can be characterized by two general types of interactions that occur in work settings: task and nontask. As discussed earlier, task-related interactions are those involving job-related matters and nontask interactions are those involving topics unrelated to work (e.g., greetings or conversations about family or leisure pursuits). Research related to these two general classes of interactions are reviewed below.

Task-Related Interactions

An important skill involved in being able to acquire and maintain a job is the ability to initiate and respond to interactions from others regarding job tasks. Gabarro (1987) has referred to working relationships as interpersonal relationships that are task based. Task-related interactions have been suggested by employers as being important (Rusch, Schutz, & Agran, 1982; Salzberg, Agran, & Lignugaris/Kraft, 1986) and have begun to be validated by studies involving direct observations in integrated employment settings (e.g., Chadsey-Rusch & Gonzalez, 1988; Chadsey-Rusch, Gonzalez, Tines, & Johnson, 1989; Lignugaris/Kraft, Rule, Salzberg, & Stowitschek, 1986; Lignugaris/Kraft, Salzberg, Rule, & Stowitschek, 1988).

In Lignugaris/Kraft et al. (1986), for example, direct observation methods were used to study the pattern and content of social interactions of employees with handicaps and those who were not handicapped. In this study, the individuals with handicaps were described as being mildly and moderately mentally retarded; however, no IQ scores were reported so it is not possible to determine how many employees were mildly mentally retarded. Also, from the available setting description, it is difficult to determine if the observations took place in a supported employment setting; however, because the study involved employees without handicaps, there appeared to be opportunities for interactions to occur between employees with and without disabilities. Lignugaris/Kraft et al. (1986) reported that conversations regarding work-related topics occurred two thirds of the time, and that there were no differences between workers with and without handicaps regarding these work-related interactions.

In their most recent study, Lignugaris/Kraft et

al. (1988) again compared the interaction patterns between a group of workers with mild and moderate disabilities and a group of workers without disabilities who were working in the same setting as in the study just described (i.e., nonprofit business). In this investigation, however, Lignugaris/Kraft et al. (1988) used a different research methodology (i.e., anecdotal recordings) to collect information. The findings from this study indicated that interactions were frequent, that the target workers interacted more with co-workers than with supervisors, and that commands and asking for information were the most frequently observed topic areas. Additionally, differences were found in the interaction patterns between the workers with and without disabilities. Employees with disabilities were more likely to interact with other employees with disabilities, and nondisabled employees interacted more frequently with their same counterparts. Workers with disabilities received more commands and were less involved in teasing and joking interactions. Workers without disabilities were involved in fewer greetings and were asked for information more often during work than employees with disabilities.

Similar results were reported by Chadsey-Rusch et al. (1989). In this study, which involved employees with mild and moderate mental retardation (M IQ $= 63.6$, $SD = 15.1$), task-related interactions occurred more often than nontask-related interactions during work periods; there also was no statistically significant difference between the employees in relation to frequency of task-related interactions. The observations in this study occurred in individual placement supported employment sites in food service and light industry; however, the subjects observed had been successfully placed (on the same job after approximately 3 years) and received follow-up only on a very intermittent basis (typically two contacts per month).

Two recent studies have been conducted with students with moderate and severe handicaps receiving training in integrated employment settings (Chadsey-Rusch, 1988; Storey & Knutson, in press). Storey and Knutson directly observed the social interactions of 6 nonhandicapped workers, and 5 students with moderate and severe handicaps (no IQ score was given) and 1 individual who was served by an employment agency for adults with disabilities. Although Storey and Knutson did not find any significant differences between the two groups in the frequency of interactions, exploratory data analysis of individual categories revealed that the students with handicaps were less likely to be engaged in interactions with their co-workers or involved in work or personal conversations. However, the students were more likely to be involved in interactions with their school supervisor, and received more compliments and instruction than nonhandicapped workers.

Similar results were found by Chadsey-Rusch (1988). In this study, a group of 10 students with severe/profound handicaps were directly observed upon arrival at school, during lunch, and in community-based job training sites. Chadsey-Rusch (1988) reported that in the employment sites, 87% of all interactions were task related, initiated primarily by school supervisors, and consisted of directions, questions, praise, information, and criticism. Across all observational conditions, interactions with peers (both handicapped and nonhandicapped) constituted only 1% of all the interactions.

Although it is difficult to draw conclusions from these studies for persons with severe handicaps, some tentative implications can be suggested. These results do confirm that job-related interactions occur and that it may be important for supported employees to be able to initiate and respond to such interactions, particularly with respect to job acquisition and maintenance. In the Chadsey-Rusch et al. (1989) study, for example, the workers with handicaps participated just as frequently as their nonhandicapped counterparts in task-related interactions, and they had been successfully employed for several years. Although it is difficult to state that there is a functional relationship between being successfully employed and being able to initiate and respond to task-related interactions, we believe that integration might be enhanced by being able to participate in interactions about job-related topics.

Students with severe handicaps who are being trained in community-based job sites are quite likely to be involved in task-related interactions; however, most of these interactions are with school supervisors rather than with nonhandicapped co-workers. As students with severe handicaps enter the work force, it remains to be seen if task-related interactions predominate, and if co-workers play more of a role by taking part in these types of interactions. Future research is needed to determine the types of interactions in which persons with severe handicaps engage and what the implications of these interactions are for integration.

Non-Task-Related Interactions

Task-related interactions are important and may relate to overall job maintenance. However, non-task interactions may be just as important, particularly with regard to the implications they might have for the formation of friendships. Frequently, friendships develop on the job. For example, Verbrugge (1979) reported that adults often name work colleagues among their closest friends. Even adolescents report that many of their friendships were established at work settings (Zetlin & Murtaugh, 1988). In a recent review, Nisbet and Hagner (1988) also described the importance of interpersonal relationships within work settings.

Friendships are likely to develop in the workplace for at least three reasons: 1) workers are in close proximity to one another, 2) they share common interests and experiences, and 3) they have the opportunity to provide help and support to one another (Verbrugge, 1979). Close proximity is important for developing friendships because it provides the opportunity for interactions. As a relationship develops, it is not always necessary for two people to be in constant close physical proximity (e.g., such as sharing an apartment or working side by side), but at some point in the relationship, physical proximity will provide the opportunity for interactions to occur and for friendships to form. For example, opportunities to interact may occur during lunch and breaks, or at company-sponsored events, such as parties or bowling or baseball leagues. In addition, the physical layout of a setting may promote interactions if people work in close proximity to one another and few physical barriers exist.

In addition to proximity, similar interests, backgrounds, attitudes, and personality appear to contribute to friendship formation (Festinger, 1950; Izard, 1960; Veitch & Griffitt, 1973). Pogrebin (1987) suggested that we prefer people who are similar to us and that our friends typically live, work, and recreate where we do. At work, co-workers definitely have one thing in common—their jobs. Thus, co-workers are involved in similar types of experiences for a good portion of their day. As has been suggested, social interactions center frequently around job-related topics and events that occur in the workplace (Chadsey-Rusch & Gonzalez, 1988; Lignugaris/Kraft et al., 1986).

Two prominent theories in friendship formation suggest that relationships are regarded more positively if the individuals involved in the relationship perceive it to be more rewarding than costly (Altman & Taylor, 1973; Levinger & Snoek, 1972). Although difficult to define, the rewards of friendship have included emotional support and help, trust, acceptance, companionship, ego enhancement, and stimulation (Ginsburg, Gottman, & Parker, 1986). It is very possible that these kinds of rewards can be provided by co-workers. For example, many of us have probably been involved in an unpleasant situation at work that was improved because of the help and support provided by a co-worker. In addition, co-workers may provide support about non-work-related matters. The workplace provides the opportunity for interactions of this type to occur, and these interactions can contribute to the formation of friendships.

Supported employment has increased the opportunity for close physical proximity between persons with and without handicaps. Because there are more adults with handicaps working in integrated employment settings, we do know that we have made strides in creating the opportunities for friendships to develop. Where these opportunities exist, however, it would be helpful to know the kind of relationships that individuals with handicaps have with their co-workers, the kind of interactions in which they engage, and how they feel about their relationships. Little information exists to address any of these issues.

After directly observing interactions in individual supported employment sites, Chadsey-Rusch et al. (1989) found that workers with mental retardation were just as likely to be involved in job-related interactions as nonhandicapped workers, but were less likely to be involved in non-work-related interactions during lunch and break and work periods. Thus, even though these workers were in close proximity to their co-workers, they were not involved in the type of interactions that might contribute to friendship formations with nonhandicapped co-workers.

Rusch, Hughes, and Johnson (1988) have been exploring the issue of integration and co-worker involvement by looking at the types of support provided by co-workers to target employees (or persons with handicaps). Essentially, Rusch, Hughes, and Johnson (1988) have identified a number of relationships that exist in supported employment settings: training, associating, befriending, advocating, collecting data, and evaluating. In the training relationship, the co-worker provides on-the-job training to the target employee. An associating relationship indicates that a co-worker merely interacts with the target employee at some time, whereas befriending means that the co-worker interacts with the target employee outside the work setting. When co-workers advocate, they protect, optimize, and support the target employee's employment status. If co-workers assume an evaluating relationship, they provide feedback regarding a target employee's social and work performance.

Rusch, Hughes, and Johnson (1988) studied the frequency of the different types of co-worker involvement with supported employees throughout the state of Illinois. Of interest was how many supported employees had experienced some type of involvement with nonhandicapped co-workers over a 5-month period. They found that, on the average, more supported employees (n = 309) tended to experience co-worker associating (79%) followed by evaluating (62%), training (52%), advocating (37%), befriending (23%), and data collection (17%). A total of 31 persons with severe handicaps were included in the sample. This group, as a whole, consistently demonstrated significantly less involvement with nonhandicapped co-workers than any other single group. For example, on the average, approximately 45% of all supported employees with borderline, mild, and moderate mental retardation had experienced some type of co-worker involvement. In comparison, on the average, only 22% of the individuals with severe handicaps had experienced some type of co-worker involvement. Even more disappointing is the fact that almost all of the individuals with severe handicaps had not experienced some type of befriending (98%), advocating (92%), or training (72%) from their co-workers.

This type of information is helpful in suggesting that interactions do occur between workers with and without handicaps in supported employment programs. However, the types of interactions or relationships that do occur may not be the kind that indicate that friendships are developing. In particular, the befriending category was very low for all individuals with handicaps and especially low for those persons with severe mental retardation. Since the associating category is quite broad by definition, it is possible that those individuals involved in an associating relationship may find their relationship with their co-workers change over time to more of a befriending relationship. However, Rusch, Hughes, and Johnson (1988) did not find a change in co-worker involvement over time. It may have been that the period of time under investigation in the study was too short; future research is clearly warranted in this area.

Subsequent to the Rusch, Hughes, and Johnson (1988) investigation, Rusch, Johnson, and Hughes (in press) analyzed patterns of co-worker involvement among 264 supported employees in relation to level of disability versus placement approach (i.e., individual, clustered, crew). Results indicated that supported employees extensively associate with their nonhandicapped co-workers. However, Rusch et al. (in press) found that supported employees who were employed in mobile work crews were much less involved with co-workers. Supported employees who were individually placed or who worked in clustered placements were more involved with co-workers. These findings are not surprising. Typically, mobile work crews consist of eight or fewer supported employees performing subcontract work. These employees are often transported by a company van to different settings to perform janitorial or maintenance jobs and these jobs are usually performed when the contracting agency is no longer open to the public. For example, a mobile work crew may clean a bank after the nonhandicapped co-workers have worked their shifts. In fact, in the Rusch et al. (in press) study, only one out of six supported employees with moderate or severe mental retardation employed in a crew engaged in an interaction over a 6-month period.

Summary and Conclusions

Because of the paucity of research, few conclusions can be drawn about the status of integration between persons with and without severe handicaps in supported employment settings. It appears that nonhandicapped workers are likely to interact with workers with handicaps about job-related matters, and their involvement has typically been one of associating, evaluating, and training. However, there have been fewer interactions about non-job-related matters, and not many nonhandicapped workers have befriended workers with handicaps. If friendships are not developing, we do not know whether these workers with handicaps are lonely. It is possible that some supported employees may have developed friends outside the workplace. However, if this is not the case, and if individuals are lonely and would like more friends, it would seem to be important to develop strategies to facilitate friendships. As we continue to make strides by enabling persons with severe handicaps to work in integrated employment settings, we must not be content with mere physical integration and job maintenance. We must determine if workers have friends and support and if they are lonely. The work setting is one place where friendships and support can be facilitated, and we should develop strategies to do so.

Additionally, research also points to the possibility that nondisabled co-workers do associate with supported employees, unless these supported employees are members of mobile work crews. Findings suggest that the type of supported employment placement is an important measure of the number of persons for whom co-worker involvement had occurred.

Ongoing Support

A unique characteristic of supported employment is the provision of ongoing support. Federal regulations have mandated that sup-

ported employees receive a minimum of two contacts per month for the duration of their employment. This provision differentiates supported employment from transitional or time-limited follow-up contacts where follow-up may be even less frequent and the expectation is that support eventually will be terminated (Rusch, 1986b).

Although ongoing support has not been clearly defined by legislators and policymakers, support services typically are provided by employment training specialists. As discussed, this support includes surveying communities for job possibilities, matching potential employees to identified jobs, placing target employees into these jobs, and providing postplacement support that results in the target employee remaining employed. Additionally, employment training specialists provide cooperating agencies (e.g., residential programs, case management services) with information and assistance to coordinate their ongoing support of the target employee.

Ongoing support can be thought to comprise three primary functions. The first is the provision of those services necessary for a target employee to acquire, perform, and keep a job successfully. The second function of ongoing support is to improve the quality of one's employment status. This may involve creating conditions that allow greater interaction among supported employees and their co-workers. It may also involve helping supported employees acquire benefits, promotions, raises, and/or new responsibilities. These outcomes usually are the result of an employment training specialist providing information to co-workers. The third function of ongoing support is the provision of services to individuals who, following a term of employment, experience a change in their job status. These changes may be desirable, such as when an employees changes jobs to obtain better wages; conversely, these changes may be the result of a layoff or firing.

An implicit assumption in the provision of ongoing support is that all persons with handicaps should have the opportunity for integrated employment. A second assumption is that the provision of ongoing support should vary with respect to individual need. With these assumptions in mind, the remainder of this section is devoted to a review of research related to the provision of ongoing support provided by employment training specialists and co-workers, but organized around job maintenance and job enhancement. Additionally, we discuss the reasons why target employees separate from their jobs. This final discussion is important because an analysis of job separations may reveal why so few persons with severe handicaps are actually entering supported employment.

Employment-Related Services

The first function of ongoing support was described as providing services to assist individuals in acquiring, performing, and keeping a job. The literature is replete with reviews of maintenance and generalization strategies that have addressed learning in work settings (cf. Baer, Wolf, & Risley, 1968; Berg, Wacker, & Flynn, in press; Gifford, Rusch, Martin, & White, 1984; Stokes & Baer, 1977; Wacker & Berg, 1986). The number of studies, however, that have focused on the amount of training and intervention provided to supported employees is limited. Wehman et al. (1985) suggested that follow-up provided to 3 employees decreased significantly over time, with the majority of the decrease occurring after a 2-month period. Kregel, Hill, and Banks (1988) analyzed employment

training specialists' time provided to supported employees during their first 52 weeks of employment. Kregel et al. reported a substantial decrease in the average hours of intervention provided within the first 10 weeks of employment to 51 persons.

Postplacement follow-up support is also fairly narrowly focused. Typically, follow-up assumes fairly intense and constant levels of support provided to supported employees throughout the term of their employment. Recently, Johnson and Rusch (in press) analyzed hours of direct training per month provided by employment training specialists. They found that the hours of direct training provided to supported employees did not change over time, except when supported employees were placed individually. Johnson and Rusch speculated that training hours did not decline for clustered and mobile crew placement approaches because these placement approaches typically were marketed and developed in a fashion where the expectation existed for the employment specialist to be continually present at the work site. Table 9.4 displays the mean hours of direct training per month provided by employment specialists over a 12-month period. These data show that supported employees placed individually receive less support over time, with an average of 18 hours of training provided per

Table 9.4.   Mean hours of direct training per month provided by employment specialists to all supported employees employed for 12 consecutive months, by type of disability and supported employment

Month	All persons $N = 78$	Type of disability			Type of supported employment		
		Mild $n = 40$	Moderate $n = 31$	Severe $n = 7$	Individual $n = 36$	Clustered $n = 40$	Mobile crew $n = 2$
1	23.4	15.3	26.2	57.3	21.9	25.8	4.0
2	25.0	17.6	24.3	69.5	17.5	32.9	0.5
3	22.9	13.9	24.6	67.6	13.5	32.5	0.5
4	22.18	13.0	19.8	85.3	8.7	35.4	1.0
5	21.8	12.6	22.6	70.4	9.6	33.7	2.0
6	25.4	17.9	21.0	87.0	11.8	38.8	0.5
7	23.4	15.3	20.8	80.8	9.7	36.8	0.5
8	19.4	14.0	16.2	64.7	6.6	31.9	0.5
9	20.1	12.7	17.1	75.1	7.6	32.0	5.0
10	20.2	13.5	15.9	77.4	7.0	33.0	0.5
11	20.0	13.7	15.3	76.5	6.7	32.8	2.5
12	19.8	11.2	15.8	86.7	5.1	33.7	6.0

From Johnson, J.R., & Rusch, F.R. (in press). Analysis of direct training hours received by supported employment consumers. *American Journal on Mental Retardation*; reprinted with permission.

month during the first 3 months of employment versus an average of 6 hours of training during the 10th, 11th, and 12th months. In stark contrast, 40 supported employees who were placed with a group of peers received more than 33 hours of training on the average during the 10th, 11th, and 12th months versus 31 hours of training during the first 3 months of employment. Table 9.4 also states that supported employees with severe handicaps receive between 57 and 87 hours of training each month of their employment; supported employees with mild handicaps between 11 and 18 hours; and supported employees with moderate handicaps between 15 and 26 hours of training.

Extending Employee Competence

Few studies have focused upon extending employee competence. Extending employee competence requires that we focus upon teaching individuals strategies that they can use to adapt to their roles as employees and to the expectations that exist in most human performance situations.

Research over the past 10 years has shown that employees encounter new expectations for performance and often new responsibilities throughout their employment. These new expectations require that employees adapt their performance in ways that will result in acceptable judgments by work supervisors and co-workers—the significant others in the workplace. Therefore, individual competence must be recognized as an important focus of our training support (Berg et al., in press). Two strategies have been proposed by Hughes et al. (in press) whereby the employment specialist helps the supported employee to: 1) identify independence objectives in relation to the demands of the workplace, and 2) learn independence.

Employment specialists typically conduct situational assessments to determine job-related requirements and supported employees' abilities in relation to meeting these requirements. Methods that the employment specialist often use include interviews and observation of actual performance of job tasks. For example, Crouch, Rusch, and Karlan (1984) asked supervisors in a food service setting to specify the times that work tasks were to be started and completed. Supervisor evaluations indicated that 3 employees

failed to get their work done on time. Next, these supported employees were observed to identify the time they started and completed their required job tasks. Direct observation indicated that the supported employees rarely met the supervisors' criteria.

When problem areas are identified in which the supported employee is not performing independently, strategies are implemented by the employment specialist that result in improved employee performance independent of ongoing specialist assistance. Procedures have emerged as a result of recent research that shows that supported employees may be active participants in promoting their own independent performance (Mithaug, Martin, Husch, Agran, & Rusch, 1988). These procedures consist of the supported employee: 1) making a decision, 2) performing independently, 3) evaluating performance, and 4) adjusting future performance as a result of self-evaluation (Mithaug et al., 1988).

During *decision making,* employees are taught to identify the tasks they are assigned; during *independent performance,* employees complete the work assignment by performing the work as scheduled. Typically, supported employees are assisted initially in the acquisition of planning, scheduling, and managing their own behavior (cf. Rusch, Martin, & White, 1985). During *self-evaluation,* employees monitor their own performance by self-recording work outcomes, such as the time they begin and end work, the amount of work completed, and the accuracy of the work (Connis, 1979). By comparing these outcomes with their own expectations, employees learn to conclude whether they met their own goals, which allows them an opportunity to evaluate and plan for future work performance.

During *adjustment,* employees decide if changes need to be made the next time they perform the task(s). Adjustments may consist of changes in starting or ending times, task selection or set-up, or accuracy of task completion. If an employee's performance meets the goals established during decision making, little or no adjustment will be required. Performance that does not meet these goals will require a change in task or method of task completion.

By extending employee competence, employment specialists help supported employees adapt to changing expectations for performance and increasing responsibilities and opportunities on the job. We recommend that employment specialists who are extending individual competence by promoting independence allow supported employees to adjust their performance in relation to the varying demands and expanding opportunities of their jobs.

Sometimes assistance provided by the employment specialist cannot be extended solely to the supported employee. Consequently, behavior management must be transferred to stimuli or significant others in the work environment (Rusch & Kazdin, 1981). We contend that natural support, including both setting variables and significant others such as co-workers, exists in abundance in the workplace. Thus, employment specialists should be able to identify and enlist necessary support from either the work environment or co-workers. The following section introduces recent efforts to identify co-workers to support an employee's job status.

Co-worker Involvement

Because of their consistent presence in the work environment and the possibility that they may be performing the same or similar tasks as the target employee, co-workers are a potentially powerful resource of ongoing support for target employees in adapting to new work environments independent of employment training specialists (Nisbet & Hagner, 1988; Rusch, 1986b; Rusch & Minch, 1988; Shafer, 1986; Wehman & Kregel, 1985). For example, Crouch et al. (1984) taught co-workers to prompt employees with moderate mental retardation to use their wrist watches to facilitate initiation and completion of job tasks at appropriate times. Other co-workers present in the setting also reminded the employees to look at their watches, using cues in the form of "Don't forget to get your job done on time; use your watch." The target employees demonstrated that they could start and complete their jobs on time with the support of their co-workers.

Responsibility for evaluating and providing assistance to target employees may be transferred systemically to work supervisors and co-workers who are naturally present in the environ-

ment, when target employees cannot assume full responsibility for their own performance. For example, Wehman, Hill, and Koehler (1979) transferred verbal prompting provided by an employment specialist to that provided by the work supervisor of a kitchen employee with moderate mental retardation. The employment specialist gradually removed himself from the vicinity of the employee.

Rusch and Menchetti (1981) taught co-workers to deliver a warning to a food service employee with moderate mental retardation for noncompliance to requests by supervisors, co-workers, and cooks. Co-workers also were taught to report the results of the intervention to follow-up staff. Wilson, Schepis, and Mason-Main (1987) withdrew the employment specialist from the kitchen (the actual work area) to the dining area of a restaurant, after which only periodic site visits were made to evaluate the work behavior of an employee with moderate mental retardation. Additionally, prompts and feedback were provided by the restaurant owners and the co-workers.

Job-Status Change

One function of ongoing support involves the provision of services to individuals who have experienced a change in their employment status. Lagomarcino (1990) indicated that of the 613 individuals with severe disabilities who have been employed in Illinois since November, 1985, 184 (30%) have been separated from at least one job. *Separation* refers to a change in the job status of an employee that takes one of three forms: 1) the employee is terminated by the employer for poor production skills, for not being able to keep up with the demands of the position, or for social reasons; 2) the employee is laid off by the employer for economic reasons or as a result of the seasonal nature of the work; or 3) the employee takes a better job.

Job separation studies typically report case studies of individual programs that focus upon individual placements of persons with mental retardation. For example, Greenspan and Shoultz (1981) reported on the primary reason for involuntary termination from competitive employment for 30 individuals with mild to moderate mental retardation and found that social incompetence played at least as important a role in explaining job failure as did poor production. Hanley-Maxwell, Rusch, Chadsey-Rusch, and Renzaglia (1986) reported similar findings among 51 individuals.

Lagomarcino (1990) identified 184 individuals who had separated from a total of 204 jobs between November 1, 1985 and November 1, 1987. Twenty-one percent of the job separation group consisted of individuals with moderate/severe/profound handicaps. Individual adjustment on the job, which included social-related and production-related reasons, was most often cited as the reason for persons' losing their jobs (35%). Social-related reasons (e.g., poor social skills, poor work attitude, poor attendance) accounted for 65% of the job separations in this category. Production-related reasons (e.g., work rate too slow, low-quality work) accounted for the remaining 35% in this category. Examination of all 204 separations indicate that social-related reasons constituted 23% of *all* job separations, whereas production-related reasons constituted only 12% of all job separations. Job separation as a result of the economy (e.g., temporary layoff, business closed, seasonal layoff) constituted 33% of all separations. It should be noted that 16.5% of these separations came from two agencies in an area of Illinois where the unemployment rate ranges from 12% to 15% and the models that were implemented were predominantly mobile work crews and clustered enclaves in industrial settings.

Lagomarcino (1990) noted that approximately 10% of the individuals who were separated from their jobs took better jobs or it was determined that they no longer needed the ongoing support provided through supported employment. Forty-four job separations were categorized as "other." The majority of the separations in this category were due to individuals moving out of the area (*n* = 16). Thirteen individuals were separated from supported employment because of medical and health problems.

In relation to disability category, Lagomarcino (1990) found that 33% of all job separations for the borderline/mild mental retardation disability group were due to poor individual adjust-

ment on the job. Interestingly, all of these reasons were social related rather than production related. In contrast, although poor individual adjustment on the job accounted for 39% of job separations in the moderate/severe/profound mental retardation disability group, the job separations were fairly evenly distributed across social- and production-related reasons. Approximately 50% of all job separations in the moderate/severe/profound mental retardation disability group occurred due to the economic situation of the employer or because of seasonal layoffs. As would probably be expected, most of the individuals who took a better job or no longer needed ongoing support were in the borderline/mild mental retardation disability category.

In relation to placement approach, Lagomarcino (1990) stated that poor individual adjustment on the job accounted for approximately 40% of all job separations among individual and clustered placements. In contrast, poor individual adjustment to the job accounted for only 11% of job separations among the mobile work crew placements. The characteristics of the employment settings may partially explain this difference. As noted earlier, individual and clustered placements typically provide more opportunities for interactions with nonhandicapped co-workers than do mobile work crews. Therefore, social skills play a major role in the success of an individual employed in the community. Finally, economic reasons accounted for over 60% of all job separations from the mobile work crew placement model. Individual and clustered placements were significantly lower in this area (21% and 31%, respectively), which also would be expected. Typically, crews are formed as a result of subcontracts that are bid and won by local rehabilitation agencies. It is not uncommon for these agencies to undermine their own business success by underbidding available contracts. Essentially, the profit margin is too low to assume the continued success of the new business.

Summary and Conclusions

The intent of supported employment is to provide assistance to individuals with handicaps who are not able to function in competitive employment without ongoing support. These persons require extensive ongoing support to participate in integrated community services and to enjoy a quality of life that may be realized by people with few or no disabilities. Historically, legislative intent has not paralleled implementation, and the history of supported employment may prove to be no different. Supported employment has been conceptualized and implemented by state vocational rehabilitation agencies to varying degrees and to a wide range of persons with and without handicaps. Employment results in at least two possibilities. The first is that support is provided to persons who do not need it; the second is that we fail to provide support to target employees who need "ongoing support" in order to remain employed.

Existing supported employment rules and regulations pose problems to the field because, as a profession, we are not technically capable of predetermining likely support. We know that individuals adapt to their work environments. As they become more skilled, they should in turn require less support. Of interest, however, is research that suggests that ongoing support does not decrease or increase over time (Johnson & Rusch, in press). It seems that we do not systematically withdraw our support regardless of whether we are serving persons with severe mental retardation or mild mental retardation, placed individually or placed in groups.

We also know that integration, which is mandated by the Rehabilitation Act, results in new opportunities for persons with and without disabilities to interact. For example, nonhandicapped co-workers are assuming nonprescribed roles, including associating with target employees during breaks, training target employees to perform new tasks, and providing feedback to target employees about their work performance (Rusch et al., in press).

There is a long-standing historical precedent for too little support; only recently has legislation allowed us to consider too much support to be an issue. Existing job separation data force us to take a closer look at several issues related to supported employment for persons with handicaps. First, given the population currently being served, one must wonder if persons with borderline to mild mental retardation are in their "least restrictive" work environment. In fact, we

may be providing too much support for some employees through supported employment.

Second, we must emphasize more effective vocational training opportunities for supported employees in advance of their employment. It is not surprising that a large percentage of the persons in the job separation group had difficulty adjusting to their jobs given the fact that most of these individuals were previously employed in sheltered workshops or work activity centers. Community employment settings contrast sharply with these sheltered settings, requiring individuals with handicaps to interact daily with nonhandicapped co-workers, to adapt and adjusts to changing work demands, and to meet production demands that are usually much more difficult than those encountered during their sheltered employment.

UNRESOLVED ISSUES AND SUGGESTIONS FOR FUTURE RESEARCH

We conclude this chapter with a discussion of issues we believe may be the most critical to the future development and implementation of supported employment. We organize these issues and suggested areas of research along the same three characteristics of supported employment just discussed: wages and benefit-cost analyses, integration, and ongoing support.

Wages and Benefit-Cost Analyses

A sizable amount of research has been conducted on the costs versus the benefits of supported employment. This literature has attempted to address the benefits of supported employment to society, taxpayers, and consumers. At the present time, however, persons with borderline and mild handicaps are clearly outnumbering employees with moderate, severe, and profound handicaps. It may be that service providers are enrolling persons with less severe disabilities in their initial efforts to build a capacity to deliver supported employment. Consequently, costs of supported employment for persons with severe versus mild handicaps may differ from those that have been reported to date. We believe that it may be entirely possible that the costs of supported employment are high due to high levels of job turnover associated with employees with mild handicaps. The costs of supported employment have been shown to decrease substantially over time when employees stabilize on the job (McCaughrin, 1988). Benefit-cost analyses that consider the costs of supported employment services related to job placement and training versus long-term support seem warranted.

Future research that begins to identify the costs associated with placement approaches also seems warranted. Currently, we do not have information related to the costs of utilizing group placement approaches versus the individual placement approach. Hill et al. (1987) reported data that relates to their efforts to place persons individually; Tines et al. (1990) aggregated costs associated with individual placements, clustered placements, and mobile work crews. We believe that the costs of mobile work crews may be exorbitant when considering the costs associated with failed business practices. Lagomarcino (1990) found that 33% of all job separations associated with crews were a result of either temporary layoffs, failed businesses, or seasonal layoffs.

Integration

To date, researchers primarily have considered the financial benefits of supported employment. And, indeed, these benefits have been impressive; in particular, employees with severe handicaps earn more money and their earnings appear to increase over time as a result of their employment. "Quality of life" has only recently been recognized as an important dimension of competitive employment (Matson & Rusch, 1986). However, exactly what constitutes quality of life is complex and so far a consensus on its definition does not exist (Landesman, 1986). Some dimensions of quality of life mentioned in the literature are derived from rights-to-equal-treatment legislation (Rusch, Rose, & Greenwood, 1988). By placing individuals in an integrated setting where the opportunity for increased earnings and interactions with nondisabled co-workers exists, it is believed that supported employees will ultimately participate more fully in generic services often available to everyone in the local community (Hill et al., 1987).

We believe that integration does improve one's quality of life; however, very little data exist in relation to employee satisfaction with changes in one's place of employment, type of tasks performed, and the environment in which one resides. Because we are uncertain of how to define integration we have stressed close physical proximity to nonhandicapped workers as a critical factor. We have not focused upon the texture and quality of interactions with co-workers. We believe that integration can only occur when supported employees interact with their co-workers about job-related and non-job-related matters on the job and during lunch and breaks as well as after working hours. Because there have been so few investigations involving supported employees with severe handicaps, the need to describe the nature and type of interactions that occur between these employees and workers without handicaps continues to exist.

Placement approach may be the single most important factor influencing co-worker involvement. Based upon the study conducted by Rusch et al. (in press), the mobile work crew approach to placement should be avoided. The individual placement approach should be the first approach considered, followed by placing a small number of supported employees in the same business. When this latter approach is utilized, however, the individuals should be dispersed throughout the work environment with opportunities to take breaks and eat lunch with co-workers who are not handicapped.

If a person is determined not to be "integrated," then research needs to be done that assesses this impact on both workers with and without handicaps. For example, it would seem to be important to know, from a co-worker's perspective, what the effects are of working alongside a worker with severe handicaps. It would also be important to assess the feelings of the person with severe handicaps. For example, if little integration was apparent, it would be important to know if the person with severe handicaps was lonely. It is possible for people to have friends and support outside of work, such that this level of integration might not be needed at work. However, if it was determined that an individual was not integrated and was lonely, then procedures should be developed to promote integration. Few intervention studies have been conducted to promote integration between persons with severe handicaps and persons without handicaps in supported employment settings; the research done with less handicapped populations in the area of social skills training (Chadsey-Rusch, 1986), though, might prove useful as a beginning point.

It may also be possible that the types of jobs that supported employees acquire result in different levels of integration. Table 9.5 overviews the job categories of supported employees with moderate and severe/profound mental retardation. Most of these jobs are entry level. Traditionally, entry-level occupations are held by persons entering the job force for the first time. Over time they gain work experiences and move on to better paying and more desirable occupations. Characteristically, we can conclude that this changing work force diminishes supported employees' opportunities to enter into long-term relationships with persons who are not handicapped. Research is needed to address the social

impact of traditional entry-level employment versus nontraditional employment on, for example, friendship formation.

Ongoing Support

Ongoing support has typically involved a diverse conglomeration of services that may or may not be well orchestrated (cf. Trach & Rusch, in press). As a result, the effectiveness of ongoing support has been difficult, if not altogether impossible, to evaluate. Questions related to how much ongoing support is enough, and what kinds of employment outcomes are derived from specific types of ongoing support services remain unanswered.

A second problem is that we have not been very innovative in the development of ongoing support. Typically, the individual's behavior is the focus of ongoing support. Research also must focus on the extent to which the development of co-worker/employer support is a major contributor to job retention and success. An-

Table 9.5. Job categories of supported employees in Illinois ($N = 700$)

Job category	All placements	Moderate retardation	Severe/profound retardation
Assembly	47	6	5
Janitorial	128	30	5
Food service	50	14	4
Packer	27	5	1
Dish washer	31	12	3
Kitchen worker	16	4	0
Material handler/porter	36	7	12
Painter/helper	4	1	0
Maintenance	65	8	3
Machine operator/semiskilled	37	9	0
Housekeeper	43	11	2
Clerk/clerical	59	12	0
Hospital worker	3	0	0
Factory worker	20	2	0
Launderer	20	3	5
Unskilled sorter	43	6	1
Other	1	0	0
Child care	9	0	0
Unknown/unreported	60	4	2
Unemployed (terminated)	0	0	0
Work area supervisor	1	0	0
TOTAL	700	134	43

other major area of untapped potential for the development of support services is the technological progress in the development of computer software, hardware, and microswitches. This technology has tremendous potential in the area of providing support to individuals with severe sensory/physical disabilities.

Another area that requires serious long-term study is the configuration of costs of ongoing support required for individuals with severe handicaps. Current research indicates that critical costs associated with ongoing support may remain stable over time (cf. Johnson & Rusch, in press). This research may be interpreted as a disincentive for rehabilitation agencies considering implementing supported employment services. The question is: What kinds of services need to be developed so that persons with severe handicaps are no more and no less difficult to serve than individuals with less severe handicaps?

Another major area for continued study is related to the experience and training of employment specialists. As was previously stated, the withdrawal of supervision and training and the development of co-worker/employer support may require a level of expertise not shared by most employment specialists at this time (Winking, Trach, Rusch, & Tines, 1989). Additionally, the effects of staff turnover on the job performance and tenure of supported employees have yet to be examined (Winking et al., 1989).

Finally, new and innovative means of getting employers to assume more responsibility for the employment and training of supported employees need to be developed (Nisbet & Hagner, 1988). If employers are going to benefit from the employment of persons with handicaps from a business and financial standpoint it seems reasonable to expect a greater investment of employer resources.

IN THE FINAL ANALYSIS

Recent changes in rehabilitation legislation (PL 99-506) have reflected a major shift from a cost-containment, cost-effective approach to a zero-reject, equal opportunity focus (DeStefano & Snauwaert, 1989; Wehman, 1988). This new focus poses enormous conflicts in services provi-

sion, particularly when legislation is not accompanied by increases in federal funds to support the new focus. Supported employment has been a disappointing development in relation to the expectation multiple consumers have formed as a result of model program research and development (cf. Rusch, 1990). For example, our focus upon costs is overshadowed by the belief that supported employment should be cost-effective. The costs of supported employment should only be considered from the perspective of human costs associated with our failure to stimulate employment opportunities for persons who wish to work.

Public Law 99-506 defined supported employment as "competitive work in an integrated work setting for individuals who, because of their handicaps, need ongoing support services to perform that work" (*Federal Register*, 1987, p. 30546). We should be concerned over the interpretation of integration. Integration is the defining characteristic of supported employment. Integrated employment is achieved when persons with severe handicaps are afforded an equal opportunity to participate in the workplace. An integrated workplace is formed only when individual differences are accepted and individual competence is maximized.

Rusch (1990) pointed out that "we are not very advanced in our understanding of what defines integration, its goals and its standards. Many of our goals for integration focus upon how *we* define quality of life" (p. xvi). These goals have followed fairly narrow conceptual paradigms. Typically, we merely focus upon physical integration without regard to the texture of participation and the richness of opportunity to become an equal participant in the workplace. We, for example, focus upon the ratio of persons with and without severe disabilities who are working in one setting as opposed to what the supported employee personally gains as a result of participation (e.g., new friends, job satisfaction, increased competence) (Rusch, 1990).

We enter the last decade of this century with many expectations—and these expectations will continue to grow and to challenge the status quo. We should expect a period of litigation to precede entitled adult services; we should continue to urge a massive increase in research funds to study emerging issues and strategies for implementing supported employment services; and we should focus our material efforts in a cooperative fashion that advances employment opportunities for persons with severe handicaps. "While significant gains have been made, there is much more ground to cover, and many, many promises to keep" (Prehm, 1986, p. xii).

REFERENCES

Altman, I., & Taylor, D.A. (1973). *Social penetration: The development of interpersonal relationships*. New York: Holt.

Baer, D.M., Wolf, M.M., & Risley, T.R. (1968). Some current dimensions of applied behavior analysis. *Journal of Applied Behavior Analysis, 1*, 91–97.

Bellamy, G.T., Rhodes, L.E., Mank, D.M., & Albin, J.M. (1988). *Supported employment: A community implementation guide*. Baltimore: Paul H. Brookes Publishing Co.

Berg, W.K., Wacker, D.P., & Flynn, T.H. (in press). Teaching generalization and maintenance of work behavior. In F.R. Rusch (Ed.), *Supported employment models, methods, and issues*. DeKalb, IL: Sycamore Publishing Co.

Chadsey-Rusch, J. (1986). Identifying and teaching valued social behaviors in competitive employment settings. In F.R. Rusch (Ed.), *Competitive employment issues and strategies* (pp. 273–287). Baltimore: Paul H. Brookes Publishing Co.

Chadsey-Rusch, J. (1988). *Social ecology of the workplace: Implications for graduating high school students with severe handicaps*. Champaign: University of Illinois, Transition Institute at Illinois.

Chadsey-Rusch, J., & Gonzalez, P. (1988). Social ecology of the workplace: Employers' perceptions versus direct observation. *Research in Developmental Disabilities, 9*, 229–245.

Chadsey-Rusch, J., Gonzalez, P., Tines, J., & Johnson, J.R. (1989). Social ecology of the workplace: An examination of contextual variables affecting the social interactions of employees with and without mental retardation. *American Journal on Mental Retardation, 94*, 141–150.

Conley, R.W., & Noble, J.H. (1990). Benefit-cost analysis of supported employment. In F.R. Rusch (Ed.), *Supported employment models, methods, and issues* (pp. 271–287). DeKalb, IL: Sycamore Publishing Co.

Connis, R. (1979). The effects of sequential pictorial cues, self-recording, and praise on the job task sequencing of retarded adults. *Journal of Applied Behavior Analysis, 12*, 355–361.

Crouch, K.P., Rusch, F.R., & Karlan, G.P. (1984). Competitive employment: Utilizing the correspondence training paradigm to enhance productivity. *Education and Training in Mental Retardation, 19*, 268–275.

DeStefano, L., & Snauwaert, D. (1989). *A value-critical approach to transition policy analysis*. Champaign: University of Illinois, Transition Institute at Illinois.

Federal Register. (1987, August 14). The State Supported Employment Services Program, *52*(157), 30546–30552.

Festinger, L. (1950). Laboratory experiments: The role of group belongingness. In J.G. Miller (Ed.), *Experiments in social process* (pp. 31–46). New York: McGraw-Hill.

Gabarro, J.J. (1987). The development of working relationships. In J.W. Lorsch (Ed.), *Handbook of organizational behavior* (pp. 172–314). Englewood Cliffs, NJ: Prentice-Hall.

Gifford, J.L., Rusch, F.R., Martin, J.E., & White, D.M. (1984). Autonomy and adaptability in work behavior of retarded clients. In N.R. Ellis & N.W. Bray (Eds.), *International review of research in mental retardation* (Vol. 12, pp. 285–318). New York: Academic Press.

Ginsberg, D., Gottman, J., & Parker, J. (1986). The importance of friendship. In J. Gottman & J. Parker (Eds.), *Conversations of friends* (pp. 3–48). New York: Cambridge University Press.

Greenspan, S., & Shoultz, B. (1981). Why mentally retarded adults lose their jobs. Social competence as a factor in work adjustment. *Applied Research in Mental Retardation, 2*(1), 23–38.

Hanley-Maxwell, C., Rusch, F.R., Chadsey-Rusch, J., & Renzaglia, A. (1986). Factors contributing to job terminations. *Journal of The Association for Persons with Severe Handicaps, 11*, 45–52.

Hill, M., & Wehman, P. (1983). Cost benefit analysis of placing moderately and severely handicapped individuals into competitive employment. *Journal of The Association for the Severely Handicapped, 8*, 30–38.

Hill, M., Wehman, P., Kregel, J., Banks, P.D., & Metzler, H.M.D. (1987). Employment outcomes for people with moderate and severe disabilities: An eight-year longitudinal analysis of supported competitive employment. *Journal of The Association for Persons with Severe Handicaps, 12*, 182–189.

House, J.S. (1981). *Work stress and social support*. Reading, MA: Addison-Wesley.

Hughes, C., Rusch, F.R., & Curl, R.M. (in press). Extending individual competence, developing natural support, and promoting social acceptance. In F.R. Rusch (Ed.), *Supported employment models, methods, and issues*. DeKalb, IL: Sycamore Publishing Co.

Izard, C.E. (1960). Personality, similarity, and friendship. *Journal of Abnormal and Social Psychology, 61*, 47–51.

Johnson, J.R., & Rusch, F.R. (in press). Analysis of direct training hours received by supported employment consumers. *American Journal on Mental Retardation.*

Kiernan, W.E., McGaughey, M.J., & Schalock, R.L. (1986). *National employment survey for adults with developmental disabilities* (Technical Report). Boston: The Children's Hospital, The Developmental Evaluation Clinic.

Kiernan, W.E., & Stark, J.A. (Eds.). (1986). *Pathways to employment for adults with developmental disabilities.* Baltimore: Paul H. Brookes Publishing Co.

Klein, K.J., & D'Aunno, T.A. (1986). Psychological sense of community in the workplace. *Journal of Community Psychology, 16*, 175–187.

Kregel, J., Hill, M., & Banks, P.D. (1988). Analysis of employment specialist intervention time in supported competitive employment. *American Journal on Mental Retardation, 93*, 200–208.

Kregel, J., & Wehman, P. (in press). Supported employment: Promises deferred for persons with severe handicaps. *Journal of The Association for Persons with Severe Handicaps, 14*, 293–303.

Lagomarcino, T.R. (1986). Community services: Using the supported work model within an adult service agency. In F.R. Rusch (Ed.), *Competitive employment issues and strategies* (pp. 65–75). Baltimore: Paul H. Brookes Publishing Co.

Lagomarcino, T.R. (1990). Job separation issues in supported employment. In F.R. Rusch (Ed.), *Supported employment models, methods, and issues* (pp. 301–316). DeKalb, IL: Sycamore Publishing Co.

Lagomarcino, T.R., Hughes, C., & Rusch, F.R. (1988). *Utilizing self-management to teach independence on the job.* Manuscript submitted for publication.

Lam, C.S. (1986). Comparison of sheltered and supported work programs: A pilot study. *Rehabilitation Counseling Bulletin, 30*(2), 66–82.

Landesman, S. (1986). Quality of life and personal life satisfaction: Definition and measurement issues. *Mental Retardation, 24*, 141–143.

Levinger, G., & Snoek, J.D. (1972). *Attractions in relationships: A new look at interpersonal attraction.* Cambridge, MA: General Learning Press.

Lignugaris/Kraft, B., Rule, S., Salzberg, C.L., & Stowitschek, J.J. (1986). Social interpersonal skills of handicapped and nonhandicapped adults at work. *Journal of Employment Counseling, 23*, 20–30.

Lignugaris/Kraft, B., Salzberg, C.L., Rule, S., & Stowitschek, J.J (1988). Social-vocational skills of workers with and without mental retardation in two community employment sites. *Mental Retardation, 26*, 297–305.

Major, T., & Baffuto, T. (1989). Supported competitive employment in New Jersey. In P. Wehman & J. Kregel (Eds.), *Supported employment for persons with disabilities: Focus on excellence* (pp. 207–223). New York: Human Sciences Press.

Martin, J., Schneider, K., Rusch, F., & Geske, T.

(1982). Training mentally retarded individuals for competitive employment: Benefits of transitional employment. *Exceptional Education Quarterly, 3*, 58–66.

Matson, J.L., & Rusch, F.R. (1986). Quality of life: Does competitive employment make a difference? In F.R. Rusch (Ed.), *Competitive employment issues and strategies* (pp. 331–337). Baltimore: Paul H. Brookes Publishing Co.

McCaughrin, W.B. (1988). *Longitudinal trends of competitive employment for developmentally disabled adults: A benefit-cost analysis.* Unpublished doctoral dissertation, University of Illinois at Urbana-Champaign.

McCaughrin, W.B., Rusch, F.R., Conley, R.W., & Tines, J. (1989). *Benefit-cost analysis of supported employment in Illinois: The first two years.* Unpublished manuscript.

McDonnell, J., Nofs, D., Hardman, M., & Chambless, C. (in press). An analysis of the procedural components of supported employment programs associated with worker outcomes. *Journal of Applied Behavior Analysis.*

Mithaug, D. (1979). Negative employer attitudes toward hiring the handicapped: Fact or fiction? *Journal of Contemporary Business, 8*, 19–26.

Mithaug, D., Martin, J.E., Husch, J.V., Agran, M., & Rusch, F.R. (1988). *When will persons in supported employment need less support?* Colorado Springs, CO: Ascent Publications.

Moss, J.W., Dineen, J.P., & Ford, L.H. (1986). University of Washington employment training program. In F.R. Rusch (Ed.), *Competitive employment issues and strategies* (pp. 77–85). Baltimore: Paul H. Brookes Publishing Co.

Nisbet, J., & Hagner, D. (1988). Natural supports in the workplace: A reexamination of supported employment. *Journal of The Association for Persons with Severe Handicaps, 13*, 260–267.

Noble, J.H., & Conley, R.W. (1987). Accumulating evidence on the benefits and costs of supported and transitional employment for persons with severe disabilities. *Journal of The Association for Persons with Severe Handicaps, 12*, 163–174.

Pogrebin, L.C. (1987). *Among friends.* New York: McGraw-Hill.

Prehm, H. (1986). Foreword. In F.R. Rusch (Ed.), *Competitive employment issues and strategies* (pp. xi–xii). Baltimore: Paul H. Brookes Publishing Co.

Rusch, F.R. (Ed.). (1986a). *Competitive employment issues and strategies.* Baltimore: Paul H. Brookes Publishing Co.

Rusch, F.R. (1986b). Developing a long-term follow-up program. In F.R. Rusch (Ed.), *Competitive employment issues and strategies* (pp. 225–232). Baltimore: Paul H. Brookes Publishing Co.

Rusch, F.R. (1990). Preface. In F.R. Rusch (Ed.), *Supported employment models, methods, and issues* (pp. xv–xvi). DeKalb, IL: Sycamore Publishing Co.

Rusch, F.R., & Hughes, C. (in press). Overview of supported employment and the influence of applied behavior analysis. *Journal of Applied Behavior Analysis*.

Rusch, F.R., Hughes, C., & Johnson, J. (1988). *An analysis of the type and level of co-worker involvement with supported employees*. Champaign: University of Illinois, Transition Institute at Illinois.

Rusch, F.R., Johnson, J.R., & Hughes, C. (in press). Analysis of co-worker involvement in relation to level of disability versus placement approach among supported employees. *Journal of The Association for Persons with Severe Handicaps*.

Rusch, F.R., & Kazdin, A.E. (1981). Toward a methodology of withdrawal designs for assessment of response maintenance. *Journal of Applied Behavior Analysis*, *14*, 131–140.

Rusch, F.R., Martin, J.E., & White, D.M. (1985). Competitive employment: Teaching mentally retarded employers to maintain their work behavior. *Education and Training of the Mentally Retarded*, *20*, 182–189.

Rusch, F.R., & Menchetti, B.M. (1981). Increasing compliant work behaviors in a non-sheltered setting. *Mental Retardation*, *19*, 107–112.

Rusch, F.R., & Minch, K.E. (1988). Identification of co-worker involvement in supported employment: A review and analysis. *Research in Development Disabilities*, *9*, 247–254.

Rusch, F.R., & Phelps, L.A. (1987). Secondary special education and transition from school to work: A national priority. *Exceptional Children*, *53*, 487–492.

Rusch, F.R., Rose, T., & Greenwood, C.R. (1988). *Introduction to behavior analysis in special education*. Englewood Cliffs, NJ: Prentice-Hall.

Rusch, F.R., Schutz, R.P., & Agran, M. (1982). Validating entry-level survival skills for service occupations: Implications for curriculum development. *Journal of The Association for the Severely Handicapped*, *7*(3), 32–41.

Salzberg, C.L., Agran, M., & Lignugaris/Kraft, B. (1986). Behaviors that contribute to entry-level employment: A profile of five jobs. *Applied Research in Mental Retardation*, *1*, 299–314.

Schalock, R.L., & Kiernan, W.E. (in press). Interagency service delivery coordination. In F.R. Rusch (Ed.), *Supported employment models, methods, and issues*. DeKalb, IL: Sycamore Publishing Co.

Schalock, R.L., & Lilley, M.A. (1986). Placement from community-based mental retardation programs: How well do clients do after 8 to 10 years? *American Journal of Mental Deficiency*, *90*, 669–676.

Schneider, K., Rusch, F.R., Henderson, R.A., & Geske, T.G. (1981). Competitive employment for mentally retarded persons: Costs versus benefits. In W. Halloran (Ed.), *Funding and cost analysis* (Policy paper series: Document 8). Champaign: Uni-

versity of Illinois, Leadership Training Institute–Vocational and Special Education. (Reprinted in *Interchange*, [1982, March], pp. 1–6).

Shafer, M.S. (1986). Utilizing co-workers as change agents. In F.R. Rusch (Ed.), *Competitive employment issues and strategies* (pp. 215–224). Baltimore: Paul H. Brookes Publishing Co.

Stokes, T., & Baer, D. (1977). An implicit technology of generalization. *Journal of Applied Behavior Analysis*, *10*, 349–367.

Storey, K., & Knutson, N. (in press). A comparative analysis of social interactions of workers with and without disabilities in integrated work sites: A pilot study. *Education and Training in Mental Retardation*.

Tines, J., Rusch, F.R., McCaughrin, W.B., & Conley, R.W. (in press). Benefit-cost analysis of supported employment in Illinois: A statewide evaluation. *American Journal on Mental Retardation*.

Trach, J.S. (in press). Supported employment program characteristics. In F.R. Rusch (Ed.), *Supported employment models, methods, and issues*. DeKalb, IL: Sycamore Publishing Co.

Trach, J.S., & Rusch, F.R. (in press). Supported employment program evaluation: Evaluating degree of implementation and selected outcomes. *American Journal on Mental Retardation*.

Veitch, R., & Griffitt, W. (1973). Attitude commitment: Its impact on the similarity-attraction relationship. *Bulletin of the Psychonomic Society*, *1*, 295–297.

Verbrugge, L.M. (1979). Multiplexity in adult friendships. *Social Forces*, *57*(4), 1286–1304.

Vogelsberg, R.T. (1986). Competitive employment in Vermont. In F.R. Rusch (Ed.), *Competitive employment issues and strategies* (pp. 35–49). Baltimore: Paul H. Brookes Publishing Co.

Wacker, D.P., & Berg, W.K. (1986). Generalizing and maintaining work behavior. In F.R. Rusch (Ed.), *Competitive employment issues and strategies* (pp. 129–140). Baltimore: Paul H. Brookes Publishing Co.

Wacker, D.P., Fromm-Steege, L., Berg, W.K., & Flynn, T.H. (in press). Supported employment as an intervention package: A preliminary analysis of internal validity. *Journal of Applied Behavior Analysis*.

Wehman, P. (1981). *Competitive employment: New horizons for severely disabled individuals*. Baltimore: Paul H. Brookes Publishing Co.

Wehman, P. (1986). Competitive employment in Virginia. In F.R. Rusch (Ed.), *Competitive employment issues and strategies* (pp. 23–33). Baltimore: Paul H. Brookes Publishing Co.

Wehman, P. (1988). Supported employment: Toward equal employment opportunity for persons with severe disabilities. *Mental Retardation*, *26*, 357–361.

Wehman, P., Hill, M., Hill, J.W., Brooke, V., Pendleton, P., Britt, C., & Cattey, T.J. (1985). Competitive employment for persons with mental retardation: A follow-up six years later. *Mental Retardation, 6,* 274–281.

Wehman, P., Hill, J.W., & Koehler, F. (1979). Placement of developmentally disabled individuals into competitive employment: Three case studies. *Education and Training of the Mentally Retarded, 14,* 269–276.

Wehman, P., & Kregel, J. (1985). A supported work approach to competitive employment of individuals with moderate and severe handicaps. *Journal of The Association for Persons with Severe Handicaps, 10,* 3–11.

Wehman, P., & Moon, M.S. (1988). *Vocational rehabilitation and supported employment.* Baltimore: Paul H. Brookes Publishing Co.

Wehman, P., Moon, M.S., Everson, J.M., Wood, W., & Barcus, J.M. (1988). *Transition from school to work: New challenges for youth with severe disabil-*

ities. Baltimore: Paul H. Brookes Publishing Co.

Will, M. (1986). Let us pause and reflect—but not too long. *Exceptional Children, 51,* 11–16.

Wilson, P.G., Schepis, M.M., & Mason-Main, M. (1987). In vivo use of picture prompt training to increase independent work at a restaurant. *Journal of The Association for Persons with Severe Handicaps, 12,* 145–150.

Winking, D.L., Trach, J.S., Rusch, F.R., & Tines, J. (1989). Profile of Illinois supported employment specialists: An analysis of educational background, experience, and related employment variables. *Journal of The Association for Persons with Severe Handicaps, 14,* 278–282.

Zetlin, A.G., & Murtaugh, M. (1988). Friendship patterns of mildly learning handicapped and nonhandicapped high school students. *American Journal on Mental Retardation, 92,* 447–454.

◇ **CHAPTER 10** ◇

Recreation and Leisure
A Review of the Literature and Recommendations for Future Directions

JOHN DATTILO

The Pennsylvania State University, University Park, Pennsylvania

Contained in this chapter is a review of the literature devoted to leisure for persons with severe disabilities that is relevant to the TASH *Deinstitutionalization Policy* resolution (Document II.1, this volume) the *Gramm Rudman Resolution (Document II.2, this volume)*, and the *Policy Statement for Cessation of Capital Investment in Segregated Settings* (Document II.3, this volume). The chapter is organized into five major sections: 1) implications of TASH resolutions on leisure services delivery, 2) current status of leisure services for persons with severe disabilities, 3) research supporting the principles espoused by the TASH resolutions: rationale for leisure education, 4) suggested protocols for developing leisure assessments and services embracing those principles, and 5) recommendations for research priorities.

IMPLICATIONS OF TASH RESOLUTIONS ON LEISURE SERVICES DELIVERY

The TASH *Deinstitutionalization Policy* (Document II.1, this volume) encourages efforts promoting community-based options for individuals with severe disabilities reflecting the full range of choices available to persons without disabilities. Practitioners and researchers alike have long recognized the intimate relationship between freedom of choice and leisure (Witt, Ellis, & Niles, 1984). According to Bregha (1985), leisure is the most precious expression of our freedom. Therefore, "leisure" is frequently defined as an individual's perception of freedom to choose to participate in meaningful, enjoyable, or satisfying experiences (Iso-Ahola, 1980; Neu-

linger, 1982). As individuals encounter positive emotions associated with the leisure experience, they will be motivated intrinsically to participate (Dattilo, 1986). That is, people will desire to participate simply to be involved in the experience, not for some external reward. The goal in providing leisure services for persons with severe disabilities should be to provide these individuals with the skills and opportunities required for them to perceive that they are free to participate in such chosen experiences.

Rago and Cleland (1978) stated that the focus of education for persons with severe disabilities should be on fostering skills that encourage individuals to maximize their happiness. Therefore, all persons with disabilities should receive assistance and encouragement related to leisure involvement (Reiter & Levi, 1981). Professionals must prepare persons with severe disabilities for leisure in a way that brings personal rewards and enables them to contribute to the life of their community. Therefore, federal and state support is needed for professionals and families to assist persons with severe disabilities in experiencing happiness and satisfaction through leisure involvement in the community.

The TASH *Policy Statement for Cessation of Capital Investment in Segregated Settings* (Document II.3, this volume) supports the right of individuals with severe disabilities to receive services in their communities. As individuals move from institutional and restrictive environments, services intended to facilitate the leisure experience must move with them. Therefore, community-based leisure instruction must occur in a systematic and deliberate manner to provide the support necessary for individuals with severe disabilities to achieve a standard of living commensurate with their same-age peers who do not possess disabilities.

Scheerenberger (1987) described the philosophy of deinstitutionalization as seeking greater emphasis on freedom, independence, individuality, mobility, personalized life experiences, and a high degree of interaction in a free society. Although for at least a decade our rhetoric has called for deinstitutionalizing persons with disabilities and the creation of community-based services, the development of these services has lagged behind this rhetoric (Baroff, 1986). One particular service that has not been addressed adequately is leisure. It is clear that every attempt should be made to provide leisure services for persons with severe disabilities in an integrated fashion within the community.

The TASH *Gramm Rudman Resolution* (Document II.2, this volume) recognizes the value of previous incentives provided by the federal government guaranteeing the right of all individuals to an education that affords them the opportunity to gain skills. These skills should enable people to live with support in their community. A major component of the educational services provided to persons with severe disabilities is the leisure domain. The TASH resolution was passed to urge members of the House of Representatives and the Senate to protect each of the programs designed to improve the quality of life of people with severe disabilities that were threatened by the enactment of the Gramm Rudman budget reduction proposal. This includes ensuring the existence of programs dedicated to facilitating independent leisure functioning for persons with severe disabilities.

According to Dattilo (in press), when people are grouped together and then separated from others, for whatever reason, the differences rather than the similarities between the groups appear to become the focus of attention. In effect, when people are separated from other people in a society, they do not experience equal opportunities to receive services. Although integration has been described as consisting of those practices that maximize a person's participation in the mainstream of society, integration is only meaningful if it involves social integration and acceptance, and not merely physical presence

(Wolfensburger, 1972). Hutchison and Lord (1979) described integration of persons with disabilities into recreation activities as: 1) experiencing participation and enjoyment similar to peers who do not possess disabilities, 2) upgrading skills and confidence, 3) participating in community activities of their choice, and 4) encouraging self-confidence and the perception of dignity. Schleien and Ray (1988) encouraged the development of integrated recreation opportunities by establishing communication linkages between persons and agencies concerned about community leisure services, conducting accessibility surveys, and providing comprehensive staff training. To prevent the termination of leisure services threatened by budget reduction proposals such as Gramm Rudman, concerted efforts convincing policymakers of the importance of such services must occur.

CURRENT STATUS OF LEISURE SERVICES FOR PERSONS WITH SEVERE DISABILITIES

To examine the current status of leisure services for individuals with severe disabilities, this section reviews the literature describing existing needs and leisure patterns of people with severe disabilities. More specifically, the absence of systematic efforts to facilitate integrated community-based leisure participation is addressed.

Leisure Lifestyles of Persons with Severe Disabilities

Individuals with severe disabilities have an excess of free time (Burke & Cohen, 1977; Katz & Yekutiel, 1974; Stanfield, 1973; Wehman & Moon, 1985), and typically may not use their free time in constructive ways (Sternberg & Adams, 1982; Wehman & Schleien, 1981). Based on the premise that effective use of free time is critical in the adjustment of persons with severe disabilities, Katz and Yekutiel surveyed 128 parents concerning the leisure and social problems of their children with disabilities. The investigators observed significant problems in the leisure domain that resulted in a greatly restricted range of available recreation activities. Ball, Chasey, Hawkins, and Verhoven (1976) observed that persons with severe disabilities typically have more unoccupied free time than other people because they frequently lack skills to participate in recreation activities. Wehman and Schleien (1980) also highlighted this issue: They reported that leisure skills selection for individuals with severe disabilities, especially those individuals who are older, is often not consistent with the chronological age of the individual, and instead involves the use of age-inappropriate materials and activities.

Absence of Integration into Community Recreation

Researchers have examined the leisure patterns of individuals with severe disabilities and have reported a clear absence of integration into community recreation opportunities. Luckey and Shapiro (1974) observed that individuals with severe disabilities often lack a knowledge of available leisure resources, which frequently results in adjustment problems in the community. Gollay, Freedman, Wyngaarden, and Kurtz (1978) conducted an investigation of 440 persons who had been deinstitutionalized, many of whom possessed severe disabilities; they found that these individuals most often participated in passive and solitary recreation activities. Based on these results, Gollay (1981) concluded that persons with severe disabilities were less integrated in recreation activities than were other individuals with disabilities. Other researchers have reported that many individuals with mental retardation, including those with severe disabilities, spend their free time inside their homes rather than participating in community recreation activities (Salzberg & Langford, 1981; Wehman, Schleien, & Kiernan, 1980). Cheseldine and Jeffree (1981) surveyed 214 families having at least one member with a mental disability; some of the families included an adolescent with severe disabilities. Based on their findings, Cheseldine and Jeffree concluded that the adolescents were experiencing problems developing a satisfying leisure lifestyle because of their: 1) lack of information regarding existing leisure resources, 2) lack of skills necessary for participation, 3) lack of friends with whom to participate in recreation activities, and 4) parent-imposed restrictions. They argued that these barriers were responsible for adolescents' primarily participating in solitary, passive, and family-oriented activities that restricted their choice of leisure experiences. Based upon that study of a small group of persons with developmental disabilities, Crapps, Langone, and Swaim (1985) observed that all participants, regardless of degree of disability, spent an extremely limited amount of free time participating in community recreation environments. These conclusions were supported by Kregel, Wehman, Seyfarth, and Marshall (1986), who surveyed 300 young adults with mild, moderate, and severe mental retardation and found that the majority of their recreation pursuits were passive, home-based activities.

Inadequate Community-Based Leisure Services for Persons with Severe Disabilities

Clearly, there is a strong need to develop effective leisure services delivery systems in the community. Quilitch and Gray (1974) evaluated a teaching program to normalize and reintegrate persons with severe disabilities into society, and found that participants no longer took part in recreation activities after the instructional program was terminated. They maintained that such findings underscore the need to provide leisure instruction within the community while systematically programming for generalization and maintenance. Schleien, Porter, and Wehman (1979) administered an assessment of leisure skill needs of persons with developmental disabilities, including those with severe disabilities. Of 128 agencies providing services to individuals with mental retardation, 68% of those agencies indicated they offered less than adequate or no leisure skills training for their clients. The majority of the agencies surveyed reported they could improve programs if appropriate instructional materials and professional expertise were made available to them. Orelove, Wehman, and Wood (1982) observed that the majority of those recreation programs that do exist for people with disabilities are still segregated, especially those programs serving persons with severe disabilities. In an attempt to determine the quantity and quality of recreation services offered in the state of Minnesota, Schleien and Werder (1985) administered a needs assessment to 405 agencies providing recreation for persons with disabilities, many of which provided services for persons with severe disabilities. They also found that a commitment to the least restrictive environment is not reflected in existing leisure programs; agencies reported that segregated programs (e.g., Special Olympics, special camps) were the prevalent organizational format for leisure instruction and programming opportunities.

Baker and Geiger (1988) compiled a comprehensive list of competencies from the 13 programs that were funded under the Pennsylvania Division of Personnel Preparation's Transition in 1987. Of the 38 content areas that were reportedly addressed by those programs providing services for individuals with all degrees of disability, the competency area that was addressed by the least number of programs and received the least amount of emphasis within programs was "instruction in recreation and leisure skills." This absence of recreation and leisure content in programs designed to facilitate each child's effective transition into adulthood demonstrates a clear need for expanding leisure services for persons with severe disabilities, and parallels the absence of integrated options at other ages.

RESEARCH SUPPORTING TASH RESOLUTIONS: RATIONALE FOR LEISURE EDUCATION

Wade and Hoover (1985) identified a lack of education and training for persons with disabilities as a major constraint to their developing a sense of control during leisure participation. To overcome the lack of knowledge many people with disabilities possess about leisure-time options, the efforts of professionals in this domain must include the exploration of participants' leisure attitudes, the increasing of participants' understanding of leisure, and the enhancing of participants' awareness of available opportunities (Lanagan & Dattilo, 1989). Bregha (1985) suggested that leisure understanding, awareness, and control can be accomplished through leisure education. The goal of leisure education is to encourage people to make effective leisure choices

(Ross, 1983). A comprehensive leisure education program can help participants develop leisure behaviors and skills (Peterson & Gunn, 1984), and allow them to realize that their behaviors can have an effect on the environment. Iso-Ahola and Weissinger (1987) determined that feelings of boredom can be decreased by a knowledge of leisure attitudes, an awareness of the psychological value of leisure self-motivation, and a diverse leisure repertoire. Leisure education provides a vehicle for developing an awareness of recreation activities and leisure resources and for acquiring skills necessary for participation throughout the life span (Howe-Murphy & Charboneau, 1987). As a result of leisure education, individuals should be able to enhance the quality of their lives, understand the opportunities and challenges of leisure, determine the impact of leisure on their lives, and acquire knowledge and skills facilitating leisure participation (Mundy & Odum, 1979).

Wilcox and Bellamy (1982) stated that a rationale for leisure education for persons with severe disabilities can be provided by examining: 1) effects of leisure education on collateral curriculum areas, 2) effects of leisure education on maladaptive response repertoires, 3) acquisition of leisure skills preparing individuals for community adjustment in least restrictive environments, and 4) leisure education as a component of appropriate preparation for quality of life consistent with normalization. According to the authors, it is important to involve parents, treatment team members, professionals working in the community, and the individual with severe disabilities when developing a leisure education plan.

Beck-Ford and Brown (1984) developed a systematic leisure education model designed for young adults with severe disabilities that provided a sequence of learning experiences, incorporated opportunities available in the community, addressed aspects of the "leisure education" process, and provided guidelines for the development of individual step-by-step programs. Based on the early work of Mundy (1976), the authors explained that the "leisure education" process includes: 1) leisure awareness, 2) self-awareness, 3) decision making, 4) social interaction, and 5) leisure and related skills.

In an attempt to stimulate development and support of leisure services that embody the intent of the TASH *Deinstitutionalization Policy* (Document II.1, this volume) encouraging community-based options, the TASH *Policy Statement for Cessation of Capital Investment in Segregated Settings* (Document II.4, this volume) supporting the right to receive services in least restrictive environments, and the TASH *Gramm Rudman Resolution* (Document II.3, this volume) recognizing the right to education that enables people to live in their community, the following sections contain a description of relevant literature, including empirical investigations, supporting the need, value, and relevance of leisure instruction. Collectively, the reported research promotes the development of a comprehensive approach to leisure education for individuals with severe disabilities. Leisure education programs should include the following goals for persons with severe disabilities: 1) demonstrate competence through choice/decision making, 2) be aware of age-appropriate community-based leisure behaviors, 3) demonstrate social interaction skills, 4) understand the availability of leisure resources, and 5) learn leisure participation skills. Each of the five goals of leisure education are briefly introduced and findings of empirical investigations supporting the establishment and achievement of these goals are reported.

Goal 1: Demonstrate Competence through Choice/Decision Making

Introduction

Crapps et al. (1985) proposed that successful community integration should include not only quantitative aspects (how much a person actually participates in the community) but qualitative aspects as well. The authors made the distinction between "passive integration," involving a person in an environment or recreation activity planned and implemented by a supervising practitioner, and "active integration," including choices and decision making relative to environments, activities, and so forth by participants. Therefore, a critical component of the provision of leisure services for individuals with severe disabilities is incorporation of choice (Dattilo &

Barnett, 1985; Ford et al., 1984; Nietupski & Svoboda, 1982; Utley, Duncan, Strain, & Scanlon, 1983).

Unfortunately, choice making among individuals with severe disabilities continues to be an area that receives little attention from practitioners and researchers (Shevin & Klein, 1984; Wuerch & Voeltz, 1982). As a result, activities are frequently offered as passive stimulation with no thought given to determine individual's preferences (Reid, 1975). These preferences should be of major concern when developing leisure programs (Certo, Schleien, & Hunter, 1983; Falvey, 1986; Graham, 1981; Gutierrez-Griep, 1984; Wehman & Schleien, 1980). If practitioners are to provide opportunities for participants with severe disabilities to demonstrate leisure preferences, it is critical that they develop strategies to recognize the exhibition of preferences by people unable to indicate choices through conventional means (Guess & Siegel-Causey, 1985; Houghton, Bronicki, & Guess, 1987; Martin, Burke, & Findlay, 1985).

In an attempt to address the unmet leisure education needs of adolescents with severe disabilities, Wuerch and Voeltz (1982) developed a leisure activities curriculum that provided adolescents with opportunities to learn and select leisure activities during their free time. The three major goals of the project were to: 1) develop leisure skills that are both developmentally and age appropriate, and generalizable to integrated community settings; 2) encourage development of self-initiated leisure skills that are enjoyable, and 3) facilitate cooperative leisure planning by all people concerned about the development of individuals with severe disabilities. Their curriculum component includes explicit instruction in choice making for all students, and they reported that every youth in their field tests was able to learn to make a meaningful choice.

Dattilo (1985) utilized recommendations by Wehman, Renzaglia, Berry, Schultz, and Karan (1978) to facilitate the development of self-initiated leisure as an aspect of a comprehensive leisure curriculum for persons with severe disabilities, and suggestions by Nietupski and Svoboda (1982) to teach these individuals to self-initiate and terminate their leisure experiences. Specifically, Dattilo (1985) presented systematic techniques to encourage choosing behaviors. Designed in an attempt to stimulate practitioners to provide opportunities for choice and encourage the exhibition of choosing behaviors by participants with severe disabilities, these procedures include: 1) teaching functional skills, 2) increasing leisure understanding, 3) reinforcing choosing behaviors, 4) modifying and adapting elements of the experience, 5) determining choices, 6) determining pleasure and displeasure, and 7) measuring participation. Schleien, Tuckner, and Heyne (1985) identified self-initiated, independent leisure functioning in natural environments as the ultimate goal of leisure instruction for persons with severe disabilities. To facilitate acquisition of this goal, the authors recommended that instructional programs address generalization of acquired skills to natural environments.

Research

In response to the observation that little research had been conducted with the expressed purpose of systematically assessing preferences of individuals with severe disabilities (Rynders & Friedlander, 1972), investigators have demonstrated that, given the opportunity, individuals with severe disabilities can make differential selections (Favell & Cannon, 1976; Fehr, Wacker, Trezise, Lennon, & Meyerson, 1979; Hill, 1980). Caro and Renzaglia (1985), Gutierrez-Griep (1984), and Wacker, Berg, Wiggins, Muldoon, and Cavanaugh (1985) demonstrated that individuals with severe disabilities offered a choice among recreation activities by activating adaptive switches displayed consistent individual preferences, often maintained over time. Rietveld (1983) systematically trained children with severe disabilities to exhibit choice behaviors. The successful training procedure developed by Rietveld concentrated on instruction to accelerate the following behaviors: 1) scanning available alternatives prior to selecting an activity, 2) selecting new activities following the conclusion of an activity, and 3) completing activities following distractions from adults or peers.

Dattilo and Rusch (1985), Goodall and Corbett (1982), and Utley et al. (1983) emphasized

the importance of providing contingent responses to choices made by individuals with severe disabilities and empirically demonstrated that these individuals preferred activities that were administered contingently. To assess their individual leisure preferences systematically, Dattilo (1986) incorporated the use of adaptive switches connected to a computer that provided immediate and contingent recreation activities to three children with severe disabilities. This procedure was replicated (Dattilo, 1987a) and then further refined and tested across different recreation activities and participants (Dattilo, 1988; Dattilo & Mirenda, 1987).

Pace, Ivancic, Edwards, Iwata, and Page (1985) applied a procedure measuring approach behaviors to various materials, allowing the investigators to determine the preferences of 6 individuals with severe disabilities. In response to a successful replication of the procedure across 5 different participants with severe disabilities, Green et al. (1988) concluded that the preferences of persons with severe disabilities can be identified with a reasonable degree of reliability. The aforementioned investigations illustrate that the leisure preferences of persons with severe disabilities can be assessed accurately while providing participants with enjoyable opportunities to demonstrate control over their environments.

Based on Williams, Hamre-Nietupski, Pumpian, McDaniel-Marks, and Wheeler's (1978) recommendations to teach persons with severe disabilities to initiate, sustain, and terminate leisure involvement, Nietupski and Svoboda (1982) successfully taught 6 adults with severe disabilities to self-initiate, sustain, and terminate a cooperative recreation activity. The investigators reported that participants continued to self-initiate, sustain, and terminate the recreation activity weeks after instruction was completed. Results of the investigation were replicated using a different recreation activity by Duffy and Nietupski (1985). The effectiveness of these investigations supports contentions that persons with severe disabilities can learn functional leisure skills by increasing their ability to initiate, sustain, and terminate activity involvement.

Nietupski et al. (1986) successfully administered choice-training procedures developed by

Wuerch and Voeltz (1982) to 3 participants with moderate/severe disabilities in an attempt to facilitate self-initiated and sustained leisure skills. The authors observed that once participants were given a concrete method of self-initiating (e.g., selecting activities from a pictorial "choice chart") on a consistent basis, they demonstrated choice-making skills. Therefore, Nietupski and his colleagues (1986) recommended that practitioners provide frequent opportunities for choice making in a structured fashion, rather than assuming individuals with severe disabilities lack self-initiation skills.

Schleien and Larson (1986) implemented and evaluated a leisure education program designed to teach the complete and functional use of a community recreation center by 2 adults with severe disabilities. The leisure education program included strategies designed to enhance chronologically age-appropriate, functional, recreational activity participation (Wehman & Schleien, 1981) and choice training (Wuerch & Voeltz, 1982). Results indicated that individuals with severe disabilities could acquire age-appropriate leisure skills to use a recreation center independently, access a neighborhood center in the absence of a care provider, and communicate personal preferences of recreation activities to community recreation professionals.

Goal 2: Be Aware of Age-Appropriate Community-Based Leisure Behaviors

Introduction

It is extremely important for individuals with severe disabilities to develop age-appropriate, community-based leisure skill repertoires to facilitate successful integration into the community (Falvey, 1986; Martin et al. 1985; Schleien et al., 1985). Ford et al. (1984) suggested that leisure skills be developed on the basis of those activities performed by individuals who are not disabled in a wide variety of integrated community environments. Therefore, practitioners should encourage persons with severe disabilities to acquire leisure skills that are age appropriate and comparable to those of their peers (Wehman & Moon, 1985). Practitioners should teach only those leisure skills that have the potential of

being performed in the presence of, or in interaction with, peers without disabilities (Schleien & Ray, 1988; Silberman, 1987).

Research

Wehman et al. (1978) recognized the need for persons with severe disabilities to develop a repertoire of leisure skills and conducted a study employing a task analysis leisure instruction program for 2 people with severe disabilities. Results of the investigation demonstrated the importance of teaching age-appropriate leisure skills to persons with severe disabilities to expand their leisure repertoire and thus provide them with increased choice for leisure involvement.

To avoid the use of infant and preschool recreation materials for adults with severe disabilities, Horst, Wehman, Hill, and Bailey (1981) recommended expanding the range of chronologically age-appropriate leisure skill options. Therefore, the authors conducted an investigation using a task analytic approach that taught individuals to use a variety of recreation materials (i.e., frisbee, cassette player, electronic bowling). Hill, Wehman, and Horst (1982) conducted an investigation demonstrating the ability of 3 individuals with severe disabilities to acquire and generalize skills facilitating participation in chronologically age-appropriate recreation activities. The results of the investigation underscore the value of leisure instruction occurring in the community.

Voeltz, Wuerch, and Bockhaut (1982) noted that practitioners must assist persons with severe disabilities in developing age-appropriate leisure-time activity repertoires if those persons are to adjust to integrated community environments (Ball et al., 1976; Birenbaum & Re, 1979; Brown, Branston, et al. 1979; Wehman & Schleien, 1981; Wilcox & Bellamy, 1982). However, Voeltz et al. reported that documentation of accurate performance of a recreation activity skill during training sessions is a limited evaluation of the effectiveness of leisure education programs; they recommended inclusion of documentation providing evidence that community residents value skills displayed by persons with severe disabilities. Therefore, they conducted an investigation demonstrating the feasibility of employing social validation procedures to evaluate the applied significance of a leisure intervention program designed for youth with severe disabilities.

Dyer, Schwartz, and Luce (1984) conducted an investigation examining the functional value of materials and tasks as well as the age appropriateness of tasks. Following completion of the intervention strategy that was based on the description of age-appropriate functional skills presented by Brown, Branston, et al. (1979), the investigators observed that participants with severe disabilities engaged in functional and age-appropriate activities for increased durations.

Jeffree and Cheseldine (1984) demonstrated that 10 adolescents with severe disabilities could acquire the skills needed to play table games. Their participation in the table games permitted them to interact with other people while engaged in an age-appropriate recreation activity. Jeffree and Cheseldine concluded that once a repertoire of leisure skills has been acquired by persons with severe disabilities, decisions can be made regarding better use of free time.

Hamre-Nietupski, Nietupski, Sandvig, Sandvig, and Ayres (1984) recommended the following considerations when selecting age-appropriate recreation activities for persons with severe disabilities who are deaf/blind: 1) sensory input provided by the activity, 2) motoric movements required for participation, and 3) reaction speed needed to use materials. In an attempt to illustrate these considerations, the authors conducted an investigation involving attachment of permanent tactile prompts on materials, stabilization of materials, enhancement of visual and auditory feedback by materials, and simplification of the task. Hamre-Nietupski et al. concluded that use of a task adaptation strategy in conjunction with systematic instruction can result in the acquisition of age-appropriate leisure skills for persons with severe disabilities who are deaf/blind.

Based on the observation that the majority of investigations demonstrating the acquisition of leisure skills by persons with severe disabilities have focused only on the acquisition of specific skills, Schleien, Certo, and Muccino (1984) conducted an investigation to demonstrate the ability of an adolescent with severe disabilities to acquire and maintain skills required in a community-based recreation activity (bowling). The investigators employed a task-analyzed instructional sequence based on skill and setting

information generated from an ecological inventory in conjunction with systematic behavioral teaching techniques. The adolescent effectively learned the recreation activity and generalized this learning across both setting and materials.

Goal 3: Demonstrate Social Interaction Skills

Introduction

It appears that inadequate social behavior is a major need area for individuals with severe disabilities (Mayhew, Enyart, & Anderson, 1978; Wacker, Berg, & Moore, 1984; Wehman, 1977a; Wehman & Bates, 1978). The absence of important social skills is particularly noticeable during leisure participation and game situations (Marlowe, 1979). However, systematic leisure instruction can stimulate social interaction (Dattilo, 1987b). Specifically, Falvey (1986) suggested that opportunities to interact with all peers should be a dimension of every leisure program for persons with severe disabilities.

Research

Morris and Dolker (1974) increased cooperative play behavior of persons with severe disabilities by applying two specific intervention techniques. One intervention involved pairing children with limited interaction skills with children demonstrating frequent cooperative play behaviors; the other intervention required the use of an instructor directed to shape the individuals' cooperative recreation skills. Similarly, Strain (1975) conducted an investigation examining the effect of a specific cooperative activity (dramatics) on the social play behaviors of children with severe disabilities. The investigator observed a positive functional relationship between social play and dramatic activities. However, generalization and maintenance of these behaviors did not occur.

Based on the assumption that constructive interaction between persons with and without severe disabilities is important in the development of social skills used in recreation activities, Rynders, Johnson, Johnson, and Schmidt (1980) compared the effects of cooperative, competitive, and individualistic goal structures on interpersonal interaction and attraction of 30 junior high school students, 12 of whom possessed severe disabilities. Results of the investigation indicated that a cooperative goal structure employed in a recreation activity promoted significantly more praise, encouragement, and support from teenagers without disabilities toward those with severe disabilities than did either a competitive or an individualistic goal structure.

Hill et al. (1982) observed that instruction of age-appropriate leisure skills may prepare persons with severe disabilities for their least restrictive environments and increase their opportunity to interact with their peers in a social setting. Unfortunately, the majority of research directed toward teaching leisure skills to persons with severe disabilities has simply focused on increasing people's independent use of age-appropriate recreation materials rather than concentrating on teaching them to play with others while participating in age-appropriate activities (Wacker et al., 1984). Therefore, Wacker et al. (1984) paired 4 adolescents with severe disabilities on age-appropriate games and observed an acceleration of on-task behavior during participation in cooperative recreation activities.

Keogh, Faw, Whitman, and Reid (1984) implemented a self-instructional procedure consisting of modeling, verbal prompts, manual guidance, and feedback to teach 2 adolescents with severe disabilities to play table games and successfully interact with other participants. Results of the study indicated that adolescents with severe disabilities can acquire complex skills permitting them to interact with other participants while playing a table game. In a similar investigation, Realon, Favell, Stirewalt, and Phillips (1986) demonstrated that persons with severe disabilities can be taught to provide interactions and recreation materials to others during periods of free time.

Unfortunately, many investigators examining the development of social skills for individuals with severe disabilities have provided incomplete descriptions of programs and lacked methodological control (Dattilo, 1987b; Marchetti and Matson, 1981). Singh and Millichamp (1987) observed that, with few exceptions (i.e., Cone, Anderson, Harris, Goff, & Fox, 1978; Keogh et al., 1984; Spangler & Marshall, 1983), documented training strategies developing independent and social play skills for persons with severe disabilities have not provided sufficient

generalization training and descriptions concerning changes in collateral behaviors. Therefore, the investigators incorporated prompting procedures and a maintenance program to teach 8 adults with severe disabilities to learn, maintain, and generalize independent and social play skills. Singh and Millichamp concluded that the intervention procedures were effective in facilitating acquisition and maintenance of independent and social play and decelerating inappropriate play.

In response to the goal of providing learning environments facilitating cooperative leisure and social integration, Schleien, Krotee, Mustonen, Kelterborn, and Schermer (1987) conducted an investigation examining the effects of a recreational program on social, recreation, and adaptive behaviors of 2 children with severe disabilities who demonstrated autistic behaviors. Following implementation of a systematic training program including: 1) concern for personal activity preferences, 2) employment of cooperative group structures, and 3) application of "Special Friends" training techniques, the investigators observed that participants' appropriate play behavior and orientation to play objects and peers positively increased across a variety of recreation activities and settings while inappropriate play behavior decreased substantially. These findings were replicated in a pilot study conducted by Schleien, Heyne, and Berken (1988) across 6 participants with severe disabilities who also demonstrated autistic behaviors. In addition to positive increases in appropriate play behavior and orientation to play objects, Schleien et al. (1988) observed that acceptance by participants without disabilities toward their peers with severe disabilities changed in a positive direction. The investigators concluded that integration of persons with severe disabilities into recreation activities and programs is both feasible and beneficial for all people involved in the process.

Goal 4: Understand Availability of Leisure Resources

Introduction

It is extremely important for persons with severe disabilities to acquire leisure skills and knowledge of leisure resources. However, the critical issue is not simply to gain an awareness of community resources, but rather to become an active participant in community life (Richler, 1984). Therefore, a comprehensive approach to leisure education encouraging community involvement must be developed to integrate persons with severe disabilities successfully into leisure opportunities available in the community.

Research

More empirical evidence demonstrating effectiveness of comprehensive leisure education programs for people with severe disabilities is needed. One such investigation involved Anderson and Allen (1985) testing the utility of a leisure education program, originally developed by Joswiak (1979), on persons with severe disabilities. The leisure education program emphasizing the development of an awareness of leisure resources within the home and community was administered to 40 individuals with mental retardation, the majority of whom possessed severe disabilities. Upon completion of their study, Anderson and Allen concluded that participation in the leisure education program emphasizing knowledge of leisure resources appeared to enhance the frequency of activity involvement.

The responsibility of all professionals is to provide programs with the best potential for helping participants benefit from leisure (Fain, 1986). Lanagan and Dattilo (1989) demonstrated that a leisure education program emphasizing awareness of leisure resources can produce a higher incidence of involvement than a recreation participation program and shows the potential for knowledge retention. The favorable and sustained results for leisure education may mean a little leisure education goes a long way. Therefore, professionals should consider the inclusion of leisure education programs teaching participants about available community resources when attempting to provide comprehensive leisure services to individuals with severe disabilities.

Goal 5: Learn
Leisure Participation Skills

Introduction

One challenge for practitioners attempting to facilitate leisure involvement for persons with se-

vere disabilities is teaching participants to select materials that facilitate leisure involvement (Davis, 1987). Although material selection is only one type of leisure participation skill, examples of instruction in this area are prevalent. Based on the observations that persons with severe disabilities lack spontaneity and inappropriately use play materials, Wehman (1977a) recommended the use of task analysis, skill sequencing, shaping, chaining, prompting, fading, modeling, and reinforcer sampling when developing play behavior in persons with severe disabilities. In addition, Wehman (1979a, 1979b) delineated several parameters to assess the play skills of individuals with severe disabilities: 1) conditions of the play session, 2) action on play materials, 3) range of play materials, 4) toy preference, 5) duration of play, and 6) cooperative interaction. Once this analysis has occurred, Wehman (1979a, 1979b) recommended arranging recreation environments by working with antecedents (i.e., proximity of toys, selection of play materials, provision of instructions, implementation of prompting and fading) and consequences (i.e., positive tangible, social, and intrinsic reinforcement).

Since many children with severe disabilities may lack sustained, independent toy play, Bambara, Spiegel-McGill, Shores, and Fox (1984) noted that the naturally reinforcing qualities of reactive toys may serve to enhance the maintenance of newly developed play skills once a play training program has been terminated. Therefore, Bambara et al. suggested the following considerations when choosing toys for persons with severe disabilities: 1) requirement of frequent manipulations to produce and sustain sensory feedback, 2) age appropriateness, and 3) preference of sensory feedback by the individual participant.

Although there are methodological problems associated with many of the investigations examining leisure materials for persons with disabilities, valuable instructional strategies have been developed from these efforts. For example, task analysis has become one of the primary tools in teaching skills to individuals with severe disabilities (Wade & Gold, 1978; Wehman, 1978b). Leisure instruction employing task analysis has demonstrated the importance of using reinforcers that are naturally occurring in the environment (i.e., verbal praise, participation in enjoyable activities), rather than "artificial" reinforcers that eventually require systematic fading (i.e., food, tokens).

Research

Data-based investigations have been conducted to examine conditions influencing engagement with leisure materials by persons with severe disabilities (Bambara et al., 1984; Favell & Cannon, 1976; Greer, Becker, Saxe, & Mirabella, 1985; Jones, Favell, Lattimore, & Risley, 1984; Reid, Willis, Jarmon, & Brown, 1978; Switzky, Ludwign, & Haywood, 1979). Based on the premise that systematic instructional programming should occur in conjunction with the provision of leisure materials, investigations have been examining this issue (Flavell, 1973; Hopper & Wambold, 1978; Kazdin & Erickson, 1975; Kissell & Whitman, 1977; Paloutzian, Hasazi, Streifel, & Edgar, 1971; Wambold & Baily, 1979; Wehman, 1976, 1977c; 1978a; Wehman, Karan, and Rettie, 1976; Wehman & Marchant, 1978; Whitman, Mercurio, & Caponigri, 1970). These studies have provided evidence to support the use of various leisure instructional procedures for individuals with severe disabilities. However, the focus of many of these investigations has been either to decrease inappropriate behaviors by increasing frequency and duration of toy manipulation or to determine the reinforcing properties of various toys rather than developing comprehensive leisure programs.

Following an extensive and comprehensive review of the literature on leisure services for persons with severe disabilities, Nietupski, Ayres, and Hamre-Nietupski (1983) observed that most of the aforementioned investigations examining material selection were conducted in an institutionalized setting and often used relatively imprecise terminology. Therefore, in an attempt to develop more effective and precise instructional procedures, many investigators have employed the use of task analysis instruction to teach leisure skills (Day & Day, 1977; Haring, 1985; Reid et al., 1978; Wambold & Baily, 1979; Wehman &

Marchant, 1978; Wehman & Rettie, 1975). More specifically, research has focused on teaching strategies designed to systematically develop more chronologically age appropriate lifelong leisure skills for individuals with severe disabilities. The following activities have been successfully taught: table games (Bates & Renzaglia, 1982; Jeffree & Cheseldine, 1984; Johnson & Bailey, 1977; Marchant & Wehman, 1979; Mithaug & Wolfe, 1976; Nietupski & Svoboda, 1982; Spitz & Winters, 1977; Wehman et al., 1978); use of a stereo or cassette player (Hamre-Nietupski et al., 1984; Horst, Wehman, Hill, & Bailey, 1981; Matson & Marchetti, 1980); pinball, electronic, and video games (Hill et al., 1982; Horst et al., 1980; Powers & Ball, 1983; Sedlak, Doyle, & Schloss, 1982); camera use and photography (Giangreco, 1983; Wehman et al., 1980); drawing (Dixon, 1984); phone skills for recreation (Nietupski & Williams, 1976); darts (Schleien, Wehman, & Kiernan, 1981); dancing (Lagomarcino, Reid, Ivancic, & Faw, 1984); miniature golf (Banks & Aveno, 1986); weaving (Johnson & Bailey, 1977); games and hobbies (Dixon, 1984; Marchant, 1979); and cooking (Schleien, Ash, Kiernan, & Wehman, 1981).

As demonstrated by the investigations listed above, there appears to be an intentional and systematic movement away from isolated activity instruction conducted within an institutional setting toward development of age-appropriate lifelong leisure skills performed within an individual's home community. This movement, supported by the TASH resolutions, must continue to receive support in order for individuals with severe disabilities to experience satisfying leisure lifestyles contributing to the enhancement of their quality of life.

SUGGESTED PROTOCOLS FOR DEVELOPING LEISURE ASSESSMENTS AND SERVICES

A review of the literature reveals development of protocols, models, and guidelines intended to meet some of the previously mentioned leisure education goals. In this section, several of the more noteworthy attempts to develop leisure assessments and service delivery systems to meet the needs of persons with severe disabilities are presented.

Leisure Assessments

An important component of the application of an effective leisure curriculum is the development of systematic assessment procedures (Dattilo, in press). Because of the complexity and breadth of leisure and the implications of severe disabilities on leisure participation, development of effective assessment procedures is critical (Wehman & Schleien, 1980).

Wehman (1977b) developed a multiple-level assessment strategy for play of persons with severe disabilities based on the belief that persons with severe disabilities are capable of learning complex leisure skills when individualized instruction and materials are employed. The assessment strategy addressed the following types of play: 1) exploratory, 2) toy, 3) social, and 4) game.

Wehman and Schleien (1980) identified the following leisure skill areas to be addressed when developing a functional assessment for persons with severe disabilities: 1) proficiency of leisure skills, 2) duration of activity, 3) discrimination between appropriate and inappropriate object manipulation, 4) leisure preference, 5) frequency of interactions, and 6) direction of interactions. The authors stated that while the leisure skill variables are important in developing effective leisure programs, it is equally important to review the following systematic criteria for skill selection: 1) leisure skill preference, 2) functional level and specific educational needs, 3) physical characteristics, 4) age-appropriate level of skill, 5) access to materials and events, and 6) home environment.

Joswiak (1980) constructed a leisure assessment procedure for persons with developmental disabilities, including those with severe disabilities, that incorporated both the concern for the person's leisure skills, interests, and awareness and the underlying components of recreation activities. The author recommended inclusion of the following components in a leisure assessment report: 1) relevant background data, 2) leisure skills demonstration (i.e., expressive, mental, physical), and 3) the actual independent demonstration of leisure and social skills.

Wuerch and Voeltz (1982) developed a leisure activity selection checklist to evaluate the appropriateness of new leisure activities and materials as potential content for a leisure education program for persons with severe disabilities. The checklist allows practitioners to rate activities relative to normalization (i.e., age appropriateness, attraction, flexibility, degree of supervision, longitudinal application), individualization (i.e., skill-level flexibility, prosthetic capabilities, reinforcement power), and environment (i.e., availability, durability, safety, noxiousness, expense).

Patterson (1983) described an individualized leisure assessment instrument for children and adolescents with severe disabilities that focused on individuals' responses to the environment and their initiation of interaction with the environment. The leisure assessment instrument contained the following components: 1) reaction to others, 2) reaction to objects, 3) attention seeking, 4) interaction with objects, 5) self-concept, and 6) interaction with others.

Certo et al. (1983) presented a systematic ecological assessment inventory designed to facilitate age-appropriate community recreation participation by persons with severe disabilities. The inventory is divided into three interrelated areas including: 1) skill selection and skill/facility description (i.e., appropriateness and description of skill, facility, and social environment), 2) component skills and adaptations for partial participation (i.e., physical, perceptual, interpersonal, academic, decision making), and 3) supportive skills (i.e., leisure preparation, transportation, legal issues, orientation).

Dattilo (1984) recommended the use of criterion-referenced instruments when attempting to assess the leisure skills of persons with severe disabilities. The author identified the following possible ways that may facilitate the assessment of leisure skills for persons with severe disabilities: 1) application of task analysis, 2) incorporation of activity analysis, 3) utilization of behavioral observations, 4) implementation of adaptations and modifications, and 5) consideration of logistical requirements.

It is useful for practitioners to examine the total environment in which the person with severe disabilities will attempt to participate in a recreation activity (Dattilo, in press). Environmental analysis inventories provide practitioners with a systematic approach to analyze the leisure context and facilitate the leisure involvement of persons with severe disabilities (Certo et al., 1983). Use of the inventory helps heighten public awareness and increases the sensitivity of all persons involved in integrating community leisure services (Schleien & Ray, 1988). According to Schleien and Ray, an environmental analysis inventory provides a step-by-step procedure for integration into community leisure services, an individualized approach to community recreation participation, helpful information for the planning and delivery of leisure services, and an identification of skills compared to peers who do not have disabilities.

Leisure Services

Wehman and Schleien (1980) recommended the inclusion of the following characteristics when designing and implementing leisure programs for individuals with severe disabilities: 1) fun and enjoyment, 2) constructive or purposeful behavior, 3) participation (even if it is only partial participation), and 4) self-initiated behavior and choice. More specifically, the authors identified several factors that should be considered when selecting leisure skills for instruction: 1) chronological age appropriateness, 2) attitudes of family members, 3) availability of leisure materials in the home, 4) types of available community resources, and 5) attitude, aptitude, and skills of the participant. Based on the philosophy of partial participation (Baumgart et al., 1982), Wehman et al. (1980) provided guidelines for adapting leisure programs relative to materials, devices, rules, procedures, environment, skill sequence, and lead-up activities.

Ford et al. (1984) expanded the curriculum developed by Brown, Branston, et al. (1979) and proposed the following components for leisure instruction: 1) administer a leisure activities inventory, 2) summarize leisure program information, 3) establish leisure program priorities, 4) conduct a discrepancy analysis, 5) use partial participation and propose individual adaptation, 6) determine individualized instructional objec-

tives, and 7) design an instructional program. The authors expressed the opinion that an individualized leisure program must be viewed as a continuous process of asking and answering questions, selecting and analyzing objectives and measurement strategies, and implementing teaching strategies that are designed to meet the constantly changing leisure needs of an evolving and unique person.

Wehman, Renzaglia, and Bates (1985) identified the following characteristics of an appropriate leisure skills instruction program for persons with severe disabilities: 1) incorporation of normalization and age appropriateness, 2) promotion of integration with peers, 3) presentation of participation opportunities, 4) implementation of behavioral instruction, 5) completion of task analysis and instruction by objectives, 6) collection of evaluation and objective data, 7) provision of instruction in natural settings, and 8) support for accessing community-based recreation facilities. Similarly, Schnorr and Bender (1982) described a project intended to enhance the leisure lifestyle for persons with severe disabilities. A useful product of the project was the development of a curriculum guide containing 85 leisure learning units.

Fine, Welch-Burke, and Fondario (1985) proposed a model as a framework for the development of a leisure skills curriculum for persons with severe disabilities that contained the following steps: 1) observation and assessment of the individual, 2) formulation of goals designed to develop appropriate leisure behaviors, 3) implementation of instructional methods to facilitate acquisition of goals, 4) encouragement of appropriate utilization and generalization of the leisure skills, and 5) facilitation of an awareness of leisure resources that encourages self-initiated leisure involvement. Compton and Touchstone (1977) proposed a similar model that emphasized individualized therapeutic recreation services for persons with severe disabilities.

Gaylord-Ross and Holvoet (1985) suggested that practitioners should develop a systematic leisure curriculum for persons with severe disabilities that incorporates task analysis, branching, use of prosthetic devices, and partial participation. In addition, Martin et al. (1985) described a systematic strategy for devising a functional curriculum, including a leisure component, for adolescents with severe disabilities. Martin et al. suggested that practitioners provide activities to participants based on: 1) chronological age appropriateness, 2) observed preferential behavior, 3) perceived participant needs, and 4) relevance and availability of materials.

Putnam, Werder, and Schleien (1985) made suggestions for developing leisure services for persons with disabilities, including those individuals with severe disabilities, based on the following concerns: 1) qualitative aspects of leisure involvement, 2) participants' individual preferences, 3) implications of participation on people's quality of life, 4) normalization, and 5) each individual's least restrictive environment. The authors identified the following recent trends that should be addressed when developing a leisure curriculum: 1) community-referenced instruction incorporating environmental inventories (Bellamy & Wilcox, 1982; Brown, Branston-McClean, et al., 1979; Certo et al., 1983), 2) age-appropriate programs (Wehman & Schleien, 1981; Wuerch & Voeltz, 1982), and 3) individualized programs responding to individual preferences (Granzin & Williams, 1978; Witt & Groom, 1979). In addition, Putnam et al. strongly advocated leisure participation in community settings and provided useful guidelines to facilitate this participation that included conducting a needs assessment of community leisure services, identifying inhibitors and facilitators of leisure participation, developing and supporting leisure programs fostering community involvement, and accessing guidelines developed to establish community leisure services for all persons with disabilities (i.e., Bates & Renzaglia, 1979; Certo et al., 1983; Reynolds, 1981; Vaughn & Winslow, 1979).

Falvey (1986) identified the following activity dimensions to consider when designing, developing, and implementing leisure programs for persons with severe disabilities: 1) chronological age appropriateness, 2) opportunity for interaction with all peers, 3) variety, 4) accessibility, 5) preference by participants and families, 6) relevance to other environments, 7) potential for adaptation, and 8) reasonable time requirements. To facilitate implementation of an effective leisure curriculum, Falvey recommended

inclusion of components originally identified by Williams, Brown, and Certo (1975). Components for instructional programs involved answering the following questions:

1.   What activity should be taught?
2.   Why should an activity be taught?
3.   Where should an activity be taught?
4.   How should an activity be taught?
5.   What performance criteria should be sought?
6.   What materials should be used?
7.   What measurement strategies should be used?

Pollingue and Cobb (1986) developed a model designed to provide continuous age-appropriate participation of persons with all levels of mental retardation in existing community recreation resources. The model was based on the principle of normalization emphasizing community integration, community-based training utilizing an ecological inventory strategy, and interagency collaboration combining existing resources. The authors identified three primary phases of a leisure education model: 1) assessment (i.e., leisure patterns, community resources, leisure choices and planning), 2) implementation (i.e., leisure skills acquisition, community skills training, supervised and unsupervised aspects), and 3) evaluation (i.e., adaptation, maintenance, follow-up). The leisure education model developed by Pollingue and Cobb was an attempt to develop a structure facilitating systematic presentation of alternatives for using free time in natural settings by persons with moderate and severe mental retardation.

Although Davis (1987) identified reduction of inappropriate behaviors during free time, preparation for integrated settings, improvement of communication skills, enhanced fitness, and acceleration of socialization skills as important goals for leisure programs established to provide services to persons with severe disabilities, the author identified the primary goal for these programs as provision of an environment that promotes healthy and enjoyable use of free time. Considering the unique need of individuals with severe disabilities who are autistic, Davis identified the following special considerations in administering leisure services: 1) appropriateness of materials, 2) person's motor proficiency, 3) person's cognitive level, 4) ability to reduce practitioner control, 5) activity complexity and task analysis, 6) amount of structure in activity, 7) ability to increase complexity of steps, 8) opportunities for physical contact, 9) encouragement of mutual dependence, 10) ability to reduce physical contact, 11) person's positioning, 12) structuring of language, and 13) ability to increase number of participants.

Silberman (1987) presented a report developed by the recreation and leisure working group of the National Conference on the Transition of Profoundly/Multiply Handicapped Deaf-Blind Youth identifying the following leisure goals for persons with severe disabilities: 1) provide leisure opportunities on a daily basis, 2) develop skills facilitating optimal performance, 3) acquire isolated skills, 4) develop interaction and group recreation skills, 5) participate in chronologically age-appropriate recreation activities and materials, 6) communicate choices and preferences, and 7) interact with others. In addition, Silberman reported that leisure programs for persons with severe disabilities who are deaf/blind should do the following: 1) coordinate with all aspects of a person's life, 2) include individual and group participation options, 3) occur in variable locations, 4) provide opportunities for integration with peers, 5) provide appropriate transportation, 6) consider family preferences, 7) provide a range of skills facilitating development of a leisure repertoire, 8) encourage communication of choices, 9) provide skill building to facilitate decision making, and 10) conduct assessment of individual capabilities and analysis of activities determining level of participation.

RECOMMENDATIONS
FOR FUTURE RESEARCH
SUPPORTING TASH RESOLUTIONS

The following recommendations for research priorities to meet the leisure needs of persons with severe disabilities are intended to encourage future services and research dedicated to enhancing the leisure lifestyles of individuals with severe disabilities. There are some useful demonstration projects reported in the literature that highlight community-based recreation programs as well as some empirical evidence demonstrating the effectiveness of innovative procedures intended to enhance leisure participation of persons with severe disabilities. However, there appears to be a discrepancy between these innovative programs reported in the literature and typical leisure services experienced by persons with severe disabilities residing in this country. Recommendations for research intended to enhance leisure services delivery for persons with severe disabilities are also presented. Although a review of the literature provided evidence of programs and research designed to increase the independence of individuals with severe disabilities relative to their leisure participation, there continues to exist a need for additional efforts that increase knowledge and awareness of the value of leisure instruction for persons with severe disabilities. Recommendations for research to further the development and validation of meaningful leisure activities are:

1. Examine the impact of *administrative structures* that provide support for persons with severe disabilities attempting to access existing community recreation opportunities

2. Determine effective *leisure services delivery systems* promoting successful integration of persons with severe disabilities into community life

3. Analyze *procedures intended to examine and eliminate barriers* to active leisure participation for persons with severe disabilities

4. Evaluate services designed to assist community professionals in providing *accessible leisure programs* meeting the needs of all citizens

5. Ascertain what *federal and state initiatives* are required to stimulate integrated community leisure services facilitating participation by persons with severe disabilities

6. Identify *age-appropriate leisure skills* that appear to be most valuable for lifelong community leisure participation for persons with severe disabilities

7. Examine *leisure services providers' per-*

ceptions about characteristics needed for successful integration of persons with severe disabilities into their programs

8. Determine degree and quality of *social interaction* that occurs when individuals with severe disabilities participate in community-based recreation activities

9. Assess effectiveness of procedures designed to stimulate *social interaction* between persons with disabilities and other individuals attending community recreation events

10. Analyze *comprehensive leisure education programs* promoting independence by persons with severe disabilities and encourage community involvement

11. Examine available *opportunities for choice and decisions* that persons with severe disabilities have relative to their free time

12. Evaluate interventions promoting *self-determined leisure participation* for persons with severe disabilities

13. Examine amount of *satisfaction and enjoyment* persons with severe disabilities express regarding their community leisure involvement

14. Ascertain *degree of assistance* required for individuals with severe disabilities to successfully participate in community recreation programs

15. Examine *perceptions of family members and guardians* about leisure needs of persons with severe disabilities and possible solutions for removal of barriers to leisure involvement

16. Assess effectiveness of instructional procedures designed to teach persons with se-

vere disabilities to understand and utilize available *leisure resources*

17. Develop *leisure profiles* of persons with severe disabilities to help identify areas for improvement and development

18. Initiate *longitudinal investigations* to measure long-range effectiveness of interventions intended to facilitate independent leisure participation for persons with severe disabilities

19. Demonstrate feasibility of employing *social validation procedures* to evaluate applied significance of leisure interventions designed for persons with severe disabilities

20. Determine *validity and reliability of leisure assessment and evaluation instruments* examining leisure patterns and needs of persons with severe disabilities

21. Determine effectiveness of leisure education programs on individuals with severe disabilities who possess *multiple disabling conditions* (e.g., deaf/blind)

Recommendations for future research efforts devoted to enhancing leisure involvement for persons with severe disabilities have been made to encourage the generation of knowledge and practice embracing the philosophies communicated in the TASH resolutions. The recommendations are intended to generate empirical evidence to encourage community-based leisure options for persons with severe disabilities, promote leisure service delivery occurring in typical community environments, and stimulate leisure education designed to enable persons with severe disabilities to live and actively participate in their community.

REFERENCES

Anderson, S.C., & Allen, L.R. (1985). Effects of a leisure education program on activity involvement and social interaction of mentally retarded persons. *Adapted Physical Activity Quarterly, 2*(2), 107–116.

Baker, B.C., & Geiger, W.L. (1988). *Preparing transition specialists: Competencies of thirteen programs.* Vienna, VA: Dissemin/Action Program.

Ball, W.L., Chasey, W.C., Hawkins, D.E., & Verhoven, P.J. (1976). The need for leisure education for handicapped children and youth. *Journal of Physical Education and Recreation, 47,* 53–55.

Bambara, L.M., Spiegel-McGill, P., Shores, R.E., & Fox J.J. (1984). A comparison of reactive and nonreactive toys on severely handicapped children's manipulative play. *Journal of The Association for Persons with Severe Handicaps, 9,* 142–149.

Banks, R., & Aveno, A. (1986). Adapted miniature golf: A community leisure program for students with severe disabilities. *Journal of The Association for Persons with Severe Hanicaps, 11,* 209–215.

Baroff, G.S. (1986). *Mental retardation: Nature, cause, and management* (2nd ed.). Washington, DC: Hemisphere.

Bates, P., & Renzaglia, A. (1979). Community-based recreation programs. In P. Wehman (Ed.), *Recreation programming for developmentally disabled persons* (pp. 97–126). Baltimore: University Park Press.

Bates, P., & Renzaglia, A. (1982). Language instruction with a profoundly retarded adolescent: The use of a table game in the acquisition of verbal labeling skills. *Education and Treatment of Children, 5,* 13–22.

Baumgart, D., Brown, L., Pumpian, I., Nisbet, J., Ford, A., Sweet, M., Messina, R., & Schroeder, J. (1982). The principle of partial participation and individualized adaptations in educational programs for severely handicapped students. *Journal of The Association for the Severely Handicapped, 7*(2), 17–27.

Beck-Ford, V., & Brown, R. (1984). *Leisure training and rehabilitation.* Springfield, IL: Charles C Thomas.

Bellamy, G.T., & Wilcox, B. (1982). *Secondary education for severely handicapped students; Guidelines for quality services.* Eugene: University of Oregon, Center of Human Development.

Birenbaum, A., & Re, M.A. (1979). Resettling mentally retarded adults in the community—almost 4 years later. *American Journal of Mental Deficiency, 83,* 323–329.

Bregha, F.J. (1985). Leisure and freedom re-examined. In T.A. Goodale & P.A. Witt (Eds.), *Recreation and leisure: Issues in an era of change* (2nd ed., pp. 35–43). State College, PA: Venture.

Brown, L., Branston, M.B., Hamre-Nietupski, S., Pumpian, I., Certo, N., & Gruenwald, L. (1979). A strategy for developing chronoligical age-appropriate and functional curricular content for severely handicapped adolescents and young adults. *Journal of Special Education, 13,* 81–90.

Brown, L., Branston-McClean, M.B., Baumgart, D., Vincent, L., Falvey, M., & Schroeder, J. (1979). Using the characteristics of current and subsequent least restrictive environments in the development of curricular content for severely handicapped students. *AAESPH Review, 4,* 407–424.

Burke, D., & Cohen, M. (1977). The quest for competence in serving the severely/profoundly handicapped: A critical analysis of personnel preparation programs. In E. Sontag, J. Smith, & N. Certo (Eds.), *Educational programming for the severely and profoundly handicapped* (pp. 445–465). Reston, VA: Council for Exceptional Children.

Caro, P., & Renzaglia, A. (1985, December). *Teaching contingency awareness and head control to young children with severe handicaps.* Paper presented at the 12th Annual TASH Conference, Boston, MA.

Certo, N.J., Schleien, S.J., & Hunter, D. (1983). An ecological assessment inventory to facilitate community recreation participation by severely disabled individuals. *Therapeutic Recreation Journal, 17*(3), 29–38.

Cheseldine, S.E., & Jeffree, D.M. (1981). Mentally handicapped adolescents: Their use of leisure. *Journal of Mental Deficiency Research, 25,* 49–59.

Compton, D.M., & Touchstone, W.A. (1977). Individualizing therapeutic recreation services for severely and profoundly handicapped. In G. Hitzhusen, G. O'Morrow, J. Oliver, & K. Hamilton (Eds.), *Expanding horizons in therapeutic recreation* (Vol. IV, pp. 17–28). Columbia, MO: Department of Recreation and Park Administration.

Cone, J.D., Anderson, J.A., Harris, F.C., Goff, D.K., & Fox, S.R. (1978). Developing and maintaining social interaction in profoundly retarded young males. *Journal of Abnormal Child Psychology, 6,* 351–360.

Crapps, J.M., Langone, J., & Swaim, S. (1985). Quantity and quality of participation in community environments by mentally retarded adults. *Education and Training of the Mentally Retarded, 20,* 123–129.

Dattilo, J. (1984). Therapeutic recreation assessment for individuals with severe handicaps. In G. Hitzhusen (Ed.), *Expanding horizons in therapeutic recreation* (Vol. X, pp. 146–157). Columbia: Curators, University of Missouri.

Dattilo, J. (1985). Incorporating choice into therapeutic recreation programming for individuals with severe handicaps. In G. Hitzhusen (Ed.), *Expanding horizons in therapeutic recreation* (Vol. XI, pp. 63–83). Columbia: Curators, University of Missouri.

Dattilo, J. (1986). Computerized assessment of preferences for persons with severe handicaps. *Journal of Applied Behavior Analysis, 19,* 445–448.

Dattilo, J. (1987a). Computerized assessment of leisure preferences: A replication. *Education and Training in Mental Retardation, 22,* 128–133.

Dattilo, J. (1987b). Recreation and leisure literature for individuals with mental retardation: Implications for outdoor recreation. *Therapeutic Recreation Journal, 21*(1), 9–17.

Dattilo, J. (1988). Assessing music preferences of persons with severe disabilities. *Therapeutic Recreation Journal, 21*(2), 12–23.

Dattilo, J. (in press). Mental retardation. In D.R. Austin & M.E. Crawford (Eds.), *Therapeutic recreation service: An introduction.* Englewood Cliffs, NJ: Prentice-Hall.

Dattilo, J., & Barnett, L.A. (1985). Therapeutic recreation for individuals with severe handicaps: An analysis of the relationship between choice and pleasure. *Therapeutic Recreation Journal, 19*(3), 79–91.

Dattilo, J., & Mirenda, P. (1987). An application of a leisure preference assessment protocol for persons with severe handicaps. *Journal of The Association for Persons with Severe Handicaps, 12,* 306–311.

Dattilo, J., & Rusch, F. (1985). Effects of choice on behavior: Leisure participation for persons with severe handicaps. *Journal of The Association for Persons with Severe Handicaps, 11,* 194–199.

Davis, D.H. (1987). Issues in development of a recreational program for autistic individuals with severe cognitive and behavioral disorders. In D.J. Cohen & A.M. Donnellan (Eds.), *Handbook of autism and pervasive developmental disorders* (pp. 371–383). Silver Spring, MD: V.H. Winston & Sons.

Day, R.M., & Day, H.M. (1977). Leisure skills instruction for the moderately and severely retarded: A demonstration program. *Education and Training of the Mentally Retarded, 12,* 128–131.

Dixon, J.R. (1984). Teaching and evaluating activity content with individuals labeled as mentally retarded. In G. Hitzhusen (Ed.), *Expanding horizons in therapeutic recreation* (Vol. X, pp. 230–244). Columbia: Curators, University of Missouri.

Duffy, A.T., & Nietupski, J. (1985). Acquisition and maintenance of video game initiation, sustaining and termination skills. *Education and Training of the Mentally Retarded, 20,* 157–162.

Dyer, K., Schwartz, I.S., & Luce, S.C. (1984). A supervision program for increasing functional activities for severely handicapped students in a residential setting. *Journal of Applied Behavior Analysis, 17,* 249–259.

Fain, G.S. (1986). Leisure: A moral imperative. *Mental Retardation, 24*(5), 261–263.

Falvey, M.A. (1986). *Community based curriculum: Instructional strategies for students with severe handicaps* (2nd ed.). Baltimore: Paul H. Brookes Publishing Co.

Favell, J., & Cannon, P. (1976). Evaluation of entertainment materials for severely retarded persons. *American Journal of Mental Deficiency, 81,* 357–362.

Fehr, M., Wacker, D., Trezise, J., Lennon, R., & Meyerson, L. (1979). Visual, auditory, and vibratory stimulation as reinforcers for profoundly retarded children. *Rehabilitation Psychology, 26,* 201–209.

Fine, A.H., Welch-Burke, C.S., & Fondario, L.J. (1985). A developmental model for integration of leisure programming in the education of individuals with mental retardation. *Mental Retardation, 23,* 289–296.

Flavell, J. (1973). Reduction of stereotypes by reinforcement of toy play. *Mental Retardation, 11,* 21–23.

Ford, A., Brown, L., Pumpian, I., Baumgart, D., Nisbet, J., Schroeder, J., & Loomis, R. (1984). Strategies for developing individual recreation/leisure plans for adolescent and young adult severely handicapped students. In N. Certo, N. Haring, & R. York (Eds.), *Public school integration of severely handicapped students: Rational issues and progressive alternatives* (pp. 245–275). Baltimore: Paul H. Brookes Publishing Co.

Gaylord-Ross, R.J., & Holvoet, J.F. (1985). *Strategies for educating students with severe handicaps.* Boston: Little, Brown.

Giangreco, M. (1983). Teaching basic photography

skills to a severely handicapped young adult using simulated materials. *Journal of The Association for the Severely Handicapped, 8,* 43–49.

Gollay, E. (1981). Some conceptual and methodological issues in studying the community adjustment of deinstitutionalized mentally retarded people. In R.H. Bruininks, C.E. Meyers, B.B. Sigford, & K.C. Lakin (Eds.). *Deinstitutionalization and community adjustment of mentally retarded people* (pp. 86–106). Washington, DC: American Association on Mental Deficiency.

Gollay, E., Freedman, R., Wyngaarden, M., & Kurtz, N. (1978). *Coming back: The community experience of deinstitutionalized mentally retarded people.* Cambridge, MA: Abt Books.

Goodall, E., & Corbett, J. (1982). Relationships between sensory stimulation and stereotyped behavior in severely mentally retarded and autistic children. *Journal of Mental Deficiency Research, 26,* 163–175.

Graham, B. (1981). Analysis of the effectiveness of two alternative choice training procedures on the free time behavior of two severely handicapped youth. In L.A. Voeltz, J.A. Apffel, & B.B. Wuerch (Eds.), *Leisure activities training for severely handicapped students: Instructional and evaluation strategies* (pp. 137–210). Honolulu: Department of Special Education at University of Hawaii.

Granzin, K.L., & Williams, R.H. (1978). Patterns of behavioral characteristics as indicants of recreation preferences: A canonical analysis. *Research Quarterly, 49*(2), 135–145.

Green, C.W., Reid, D.H., White, L.K., Halford, R.C., Brittain, D.P., & Gardner, S.M. (1988). Identifying reinforcers for persons with profound handicaps: Staff opinion versus systematic assessment of preferences. *Journal of Applied Behavior Analysis, 21,* 31–44.

Greer, R.D., Becker, B.J., Saxe, C.D., & Mirabella, R.F. (1985). Conditioning histories and setting stimuli controlling engagement in stereotype or toy play. *Analysis and Intervention in Developmental Disabilities, 5,* 269–284.

Guess, D., & Siegel-Causey, E. (1985). Behavioral control and education of severely handicapped students: Who's doing what to whom? and why? In D. Bricker & J. Filler (Eds.), *Severe mental retardation: From theory to practice* (pp. 230–244). Lancaster, PA: Division of Mental Retardation of the Council for Exceptional Children.

Gutierrez-Griep, R. (1984). Student preference of sensory reinforcers. *Education and Training of the Mentally Retarded, 19,* 108–113.

Hamre-Nietupski, S., Nietupski, J., Sandvig, R., Sandvig, M.B., & Ayres, B. (1984). Leisure skills instruction in a community residential setting with young adults who are deaf/blind severely handicapped. *Journal of The Association for Persons with Severe Handicaps, 9,* 49–53.

Haring, T.G. (1985). Teaching between-class generalization to toy play behavior to handicapped children. *Journal of Applied Behavior Analysis, 18,* 127–139.

Hill, J. (1980). Use of an automated recreational device to facilitate independent leisure and motor behavior in a profoundly retarded male. In P. Wehman & J.W. Hill (Eds.), *Instructional programming for severely handicapped youth: A community integration approach* (pp. 101–113). Richmond: Virginia Commonwealth University, School of Education.

Hill, J., Wehman, P., & Horst, G. (1982). Toward generalization of appropriate leisure and social behavior in severely handicapped youth: Pinball machine use. *Journal of The Association for the Severely Handicapped, 6*(4), 38–44.

Hopper, C., & Wambold, C. (1978). Improving the independent play of severely, mentally retarded children. *Education and Training of the Mentally Retarded, 13,* 42–46.

Horst, G., Wehman, P., Hill, J.W., & Bailey, C. (1980). Developing chronologically age-appropriate leisure skills in severely multihandicapped adolescents: Three case studies. In P. Wehman & J.W. Hill (Eds.), *Instructional programming for severely handicapped youth: A community integration approach.* Richmond: Virginia Commonwealth University, School of Educaiton.

Horst, G., Wehman, P., Hill, J., & Bailey, C. (1981). Developing age-appropriate leisure skills in severely handicapped adolescents. *Teaching Exceptional Children, 4,* 11–15.

Houghton, J., Bronicki, G.J., & Guess, D. (1987). Opportunities to express preferences and make choices among students with severe disabilities in classroom settings. *Journal of The Association for Persons with Severe Handicaps, 12,* 18–27.

Howe-Murphy, R., & Charboneau, B.G. (1987). *Therapeutic recreation intervention: An ecological perspective.* Englewood Cliffs, NJ: Prentice-Hall.

Hutchison, P., & Lord, J. (1979). *Recreation integration: Issues and alternatives in leisure services and community involvement.* Ottawa, Ontario: Leisurability.

Iso-Ahola, S. (1980). *The social psychology of leisure and recreation.* Dubuque, IA: William C. Brown.

Iso-Ahola, S.E., & Weissinger, E. (1987). Leisure and boredom. *Journal of Social and Clinical Psychology, 5*(3), 356–364.

Jeffree, D.M., & Cheseldine, S.E. (1984). Leisure intervention and the interaction patterns of severely mentally retarded adolescents: A pilot study. *American Journal of Mental Deficiency, 88,* 619–624.

Johnson, M.S., & Bailey, J.S. (1977). Leisure training in a half-way house. *Journal of Applied Behavior Analysis, 10,* 273–282.

Jones, J.L., Favell, J.E., Lattimore, J., & Risley, T.R. (1984). Improving independent engagement of nonambulatory multihandicapped persons through the systematic analysis of leisure materials. *Analysis and Intervention in Developmental Disabilities, 4,* 313–332.

Joswiak, K.F. (1979). *Leisure counseling program materials for the developmentally disabled.* Washington, DC: Hawkins & Associates.

Joswiak, K.F. (1980). Recreation therapy assessment with developmentally disabled persons. *Therapeutic Recreation Journal, 14*(4), 29–38.

Katz, S., & Yekutiel, E. (1974). Leisure time problems of mentally retarded graduates of training programs. *Mental Retardation, 12,* 54–57.

Kazdin, A.E., & Erickson, L. (1975). Developing responsiveness to instructions in severely and profoundly retarded residents. *Journal of Behavior Therapy and Experimental Psychiatry, 6,* 17–21.

Keogh, D.A., Faw, G.D., Whitman, T.L., & Reid, D.H. (1984). Enhancing leisure skills in severely retarded adolescents through a self-instructional treatment package. *Analysis and Intervention in Developmental Disabilities, 4,* 333–351.

Kissell, R.C., & Whitman, T.L. (1977). An examination of the direct and generalized effects of a play-training and over-correction procedure upon the self-stimulatory behavior of a profoundly retarded boy. *AAESPH Review, 2,* 131–146.

Kregel, J., Wehman, P., Seyfarth, J., & Marshall, K. (1986). Community integration of young adults with mental retardation: Transition from school to adulthood. *Education and Training of the Mentally Retarded, 21,* 35–42.

Lagomarcino, A., Reid, D.H., Ivancic, M.T., & Faw, G.D. (1984). Leisure-dance instruction for severely and profoundly retarded persons: Teaching an intermediate community-living skill. *Journal of Applied Behavior Analysis, 17,* 71–84.

Lanagan, D., & Dattilo, J. (1989). The effects of a leisure education program on individuals with mental retardation. *Therapeutic Recreation Journal, 23*(4).

Luckey, R., & Shapiro, I.G. (1974). Recreation: An essential aspect of habilitative programming. *Mental Retardation, 12,* 33–36.

Marchant, J. (1979). Teaching games and hobbies. In P. Wehman (Ed.), *Recreation programming for disabled persons* (pp. 79–86). Baltimore: University Park Press.

Marchant, J., & Wehman, P. (1979). Teaching table games to severely retarded children. *Mental Retardation, 6,* 150–151.

Marchetti, A., & Matson, J.L. (1981). Skills for community adjustment. In J.L. Matson & J.R. McCartney (Eds.), *Handbook of behavior modification with the mentally retarded* (pp. 228–244). New York: Plenum.

Marlowe, M. (1979). The games analysis intervention: A procedure to increase the peer acceptance and social adjustment of a retarded child. *Education and Training of the Mentally Retarded, 14,* 262–268.

Martin, M., Burke, M.E., & Findlay, S. (1985). A systematic strategy for devising functional curricula for severely handicapped adolescents. *Australia & New Zealand Journal of Developmental Disabilities, 11*, 169–178.

Matson, J.L., & Marchetti, A. (1980). A comparison of leisure skills training procedures for the mentally retarded. *Applied Research in Mental Retardation, 1*, 113–122.

Mayhew, G., Enyart, P., & Anderson, J. (1978). Social reinforcement and the naturally occurring responses of severely and profoundly retarded adolescents. *American Journal of Mental Deficiency, 83*, 164–170.

Mithaug, D.E., & Wolfe, M.S. (1976). Employing task arrangements and verbal contingencies to promote verbalizations between retarded children. *Journal of Applied Behavior Analysis, 9*, 301–314.

Morris, R.J., & Dolker, M. (1974). Developing cooperative play in socially withdrawn retarded children. *Mental Retardation, 12*, 24–27.

Mundy, J. (1976). Conceptualization and program design. *Journal of Physical Education and Recreation*, 41–43.

Mundy, J., & Odum, L. (1979). *Leisure education: Theory and practice*. New York: John Wiley & Sons.

Neulinger, J. (1982). *The psychology of leisure: Research approaches to study of leisure* (2nd ed.). Springfield, IL: Charles C Thomas.

Nietupski, J., Ayres, B., & Hamre-Nietupski, S. (1983). A review of recreation/leisure skills research with moderately, severely, and profoundly mentally handicapped individuals. *Australia & New Zealand Journal of Developmental Disabilities, 9*, 161–176.

Nietupski, J., Hamre-Nietupski, S., Green, K., Varnum-Teeter, K., Twedt, B., LePera, D., Scebold, K., & Hanrahan, M. (1986). Self-initiated and sustained leisure activity participation by students with moderate/severe handicaps. *Education and Training of the Mentally Retarded, 21*, 259–264.

Nietupski, J., & Svoboda, R. (1982). Teaching a cooperative leisure skill to severely handicapped adults. *Education and Training of the Mentally Retarded, 17*, 38–43.

Nietupski, J., & Williams, W. (1976). Teaching selected telephone-related social skills to severely handicapped students. *Child Study Journal, 6*(3), 139–153.

Orelove, F.P., Wehman, P., & Wood, J. (1982). An evaluative review of Special Olympics: Implications for community integration. *Education and Training of the Mentally Retarded, 17*, 325–329.

Pace, G., Ivancic, M., Edwards, G., Iwata, B., & Page, T. (1985). Assessment of stimulus preferences and reinforcers values with profoundly retarded individuals. *Journal of Applied Behavior Analysis, 18*, 249–255.

Paloutzian, R., Hasazi, J., Streifel, J., & Edgar, D.

(1971). Promotion of positive social interaction in severely retarded young children. *American Journal of Mental Deficiency, 75*, 519–524.

Patterson, R.A. (1983). Development and utilization of an individualized assessment instrument for children and adolescents with severe and profound disabilities. In G. Hitzhusen (Ed.), *Expanding horizons in therapeutic recreation* (Vol. X, pp. 85–102). Columbia: Curators, University of Missouri.

Peterson, C.A., & Gunn, S.L. (1984). *Therapeutic recreation program design: Principles and procedures* (2nd ed.). Englewood Cliffs, NJ: Prentice-Hall.

Pollingue, A.B., & Cobb, H.B. (1986). Leisure education: A model facilitating community integration for moderately/severely mentally retarded adults. *Therapeutic Recreation Journal, 20*(3), 54–62.

Powers, J., & Ball, T.S. (1983). Video games to augment leisure programming in a state hospital residence for developmentally disabled clients. *Journal of Special Education Technology, 6*, 48–57.

Putnam, J.W., Werder, J.K., & Schleien, S.J. (1985). Leisure and recreation services for handicapped persons. In K.C. Lakin & R.H. Bruininks (Eds.), *Strategies for achieving community integration of developmentally disabled citizens* (pp. 253–274). Baltimore: Paul H. Brookes Publishing Co.

Quilitch, H.R., & Gray, J.D. (1974). Purposeful activity for the PMR: A demonstration project. *Mental Retardation, 12*, 28–29.

Rago, W.V., & Cleland, C.C. (1978). Future direction of the profoundly retarded. *Education and Training of the Mentally Retarded, 13*, 184–186.

Realon, R., Favell, J.E., Stirewalt, S.C., & Phillips, J.F. (1986). Teaching severely handicapped persons to provide leisure activities to peers. *Analysis and Intervention in Developmental Disabilities, 6*, 203–219.

Reid, D.H. (1975). *An analysis of variables affecting leisure activity behavior of multihandicapped retarded persons*. Unpublished doctoral dissertation, Florida State University, Tallahassee.

Reid, D.H., Willis, B., Jarmon, P., & Brown, K. (1978). Increasing leisure activity of physically disabled retarded persons through modifying resource availability. *AAESPH Review, 3*, 78–93.

Reiter, S., & Levi, A.M. (1981). Leisure activities of mentally retarded adults. *American Journal of Mental Deficiency, 86*, 301–302.

Reynolds, R. (1981). A guideline to leisure skills programming for handicapped individuals. In P. Wehman & S. Schleien (Eds.), *Leisure programs for handicapped persons: Adaptations, techniques, and curriculum* (pp. 1–13). Baltimore: University Park Press.

Richler, D. (1984). Access to community resources: The invisible barriers to integration. *Journal of Leisurability, 11*(2), 4–11.

Rietveld, C.M. (1983). The training of choice behaviors in Down's syndrome and nonretarded preschool children. *Australia & New Zealand Journal of Developmental Disabilities, 9,* 75–83.

Ross, C.D. (1983). Leisure in the deinstitutionalization process: A vehicle for change. *Journal of Leisurability, 10*(1), 13–19.

Rynders, J., & Friedlander, B. (1972). Preferences in institutionalized severely retarded children for selected visual stimulus material presented as operant reinforcement. *American Journal of Mental Deficiency, 76,* 568–573.

Rynders, J.E., Johnson, R., Johnson, D., & Schmidt, B. (1980). Producing positive interaction among Down syndrome and nonhandicapped teenagers through cooperative goal structuring. *American Journal of Mental Deficiency, 85,* 268–273.

Salzberg, C.L., & Langford, C.A. (1981). Community integration of mentally retarded adults through leisure activity. *Mental Retardation, 19,* 127–131.

Scheerenberger, R.C. (1987). *A history of mental retardation: A quarter century of promise.* Baltimore: Paul H. Brookes Publishing Co.

Schleien, S.J., Ash, T., Kiernan, J., & Wehman, P. (1981). Developing independent cooking skills in a profoundly retarded woman. *Journal of The Association for the Severely Handicapped, 6*(2), 23–29.

Schleien, S.J., Certo, N.J., & Muccino, A. (1984). Acquisition of leisure skills by a severely handicapped adolescent: A data based instructional program. *Education and Training of the Mentally Retarded, 19,* 297–305.

Schleien, S.J., Heyne, L.A., & Berken, S.B. (1988). Integrating physical education to teach appropriate play skills to learners with autism: A pilot study. *Adapted Physical Activity Quarterly, 5,* 182–192.

Schleien, S.J., Krotee, M.L., Mustonen, T., Kelterborn, B., & Schermer, A.D. (1987). The effect of integrating children with autism into a physical activity and recreation setting. *Therapeutic Recreation Journal, 21*(4), 52–62.

Schleien, S.J., & Larson, A. (1986). Adult leisure education for the independent use of a community recreation center. *Journal of The Association for Persons with Severe Handicaps, 11,* 39–44.

Schleien, S.J., Porter, R., & Wehman, P. (1979). An assessment of the leisure skill needs of developmentally disabled individuals. *Therapeutic Recreation Journal, 12*(3), 16–21.

Schleien, S.J., & Ray, M.T. (1988). *Community recreation and persons with disabilities: Strategies for integration.* Balitmore: Paul H. Brookes Publishing Co.

Schleien, S.J., Tuckner, B., & Heyne, L. (1985). Leisure education programs for the severely disabled student. *Parks and Recreation, 20*(1), 74–78.

Schleien, S.J., Wehman, P., & Kiernan, J. (1981). Teaching leisure skills to severely handicapped adults: An age-appropriate darts game. *Journal of Applied Behavior Analysis, 14,* 513–519.

Schleien, S.J., & Werder, J. (1985). Perceived responsibilities of special recreation services in Minnesota. *Therapeutic Recreation Journal, 19*(3), 51–62.

Schnorr, J., & Bender, M. (1982). Project SELF: Special education for leisure fulfillment. *Therapeutic Recreation Journal, 14*(3), 9–16.

Sedlak, R., Doyle, M., & Schloss, P. (1982). Video games: A training and generalization demonstration with severely retarded adolescents. *Education and Training of the Mentally Retarded, 17,* 332–336.

Shevin, M., & Klein, N. (1984). The importance of choice-making skills for students with severe disabilities. *Journal of The Association for Persons with Severe Handicaps, 9,* 159–166.

Silberman, R. (1987). Report of the working group on recreation and leisure. In A.M. Covert & H.D. Fredericks (Eds.), *Transition for persons with deaf blindness and other profound handicaps: State of the art* (pp. 141–146). Monmouth, OR: Teaching Research Publications.

Singh, N.N., & Millichamp, C.J. (1987). Independent and social play among profoundly mentally retarded adults: Training, maintenance, generalization, and long-term follow-up. *Journal of Applied Behavior Analysis, 20,* 23–34.

Spangler, P.F., & Marshall, A.M. (1983). The unit play manager as facilitator of purposeful activities among institutionalized profoundly and severely retarded boys. *Journal of Applied Behavior Analysis, 16,* 345–349.

Spitz, H.H., & Winters, G. (1977). The tic tac toe performance of trainable and educable retarded junior high school students. *Intelligence, 4,* 31–40.

Stanfield, J.S. (1973). Graduation: What happens to the retarded child when he grows up? *Exceptional Children, 39,* 548–553.

Sternberg, L., & Adams, G. (1982). *Educating severely and profoundly handicapped students.* Rockville, MD: Aspen.

Strain, P. (1975). Increasing social play of severely retarded preschoolers with socio-dramatic activities. *Mental Retardation, 13,* 7–9.

Switzky, H.N., Ludwign, L., & Haywood, C. (1979). Exploration and play in retarded and nonretarded children: Effects of object complexity and age. *American Journal of Mental Deficiency, 83,* 637–644.

Utley, B., Duncan, D., Strain, P., & Scanlon, K. (1983). Effects of contingent and noncontingent vision stimulation on visual fixation in multiply handicapped children. *Journal of The Association for the Severely Handicapped, 8*(3), 29–42.

Vaughn, J., & Winslow, R. (1979). *Guidelines for community based recreation programs for special populations.* Alexandria, VA: National Therapeutic Recreation Society.

Voeltz, L., Wuerch, B., & Bockhaut, C. (1982). Social validation of leisure activities training with severely handicapped youth. *Journal of The Association for the Severely Handicapped, 7*(4), 3–13.

Wacker, D.P., Berg, W.K., & Moore, S.J. (1984). Increasing on-task performance of students with severe handicaps on cooperative games. *Education and Training for the Mentally Retarded, 19,* 183–190.

Wacker, D.P., Berg, W., Wiggins, B., Muldoon, M., & Cavanaugh, J. (1985). Evaluation of reinforcer preferences for profoundly handicapped students. *Journal of Applied Behavior Analysis, 18,* 173–178.

Wade, M.G., & Gold, M.W. (1978). Removing some of the limitations of mentally retarded workers by improving job design. *Human Factors, 20,* 339–348.

Wade, M.G., & Hoover, J.H. (1985). Mental retardation as a constraint on leisure. In M.G. Wade (Ed.), *Constraints on leisure* (pp. 83–110). Springfield, IL: Charles C Thomas.

Wambold, C., & Baily, R. (1979). Improving the leisure-time behaviors of severely/profoundly mentally retarded children through toy play. *AAESPH Review, 4,* 237–250.

Wehman, P. (1976). Selection of play materials for the severely handicapped: A continuing dilemma. *Education and Training of the Mentally Retarded, 11,* 46–50.

Wehman, P. (1977a). Applications of behavior modification techniques to play problems of the severely and profoundly retarded. *Therapeutic Recreation Journal, 11,* 16–22.

Wehman, P. (1977b). Developing play behaviors in the severely and profoundly retarded. In P. Wehman, *Helping the mentally retarded acquire play skills: A behavioral approach* (pp. 73–123). Springfield, IL: Charles C Thomas.

Wehman, P. (1977c). Research on leisure time and the severely developmentally disabled. *Rehabilitation Literature, 38,* 98–105.

Wehman, P. (1978a). Effects of different environmental conditions on leisure time activity of the severely and profoundly handicapped. *Journal of Special Education, 12*(2), 183–193.

Wehman, P. (1978b). Task analysis in recreation programs for mentally retarded persons. *Leisurability, 5,* 13–20.

Wehman, P. (1979a). *Curriculum design for the severely and profoundly handicapped.* New York: Human Services.

Wehman, P. (1979b). Teaching recreation skills to severely and profoundly handicapped persons. In R. York & E. Edgar (Eds.), *Teaching the severely handicapped* (Vol. 4, pp. 64–86). Columbus, OH: Special Press.

Wehman, P., & Bates, P. (1978). Education for severely and profoundly handicapped persons: A review. *Rehabilitation Literature, 39,* 2–14.

Wehman, P., Karan, O., & Rettie, C. (1976). Developing independent play in three severely retarded women. *Psychological Reports, 39,* 995–998.

Wehman, P., & Marchant, J.A. (1978). Improving free play skills of severely retarded children. *American Journal of Occupational Therapy, 32,* 100–104.

Wehman, P., & Moon, M.S. (1985). Designing and implementing leisure programs for individuals with severe handicaps. In M.P. Brady & P.L. Gunter (Eds.), *Integrating moderately and severely handicapped learners: Strategies that work* (pp. 214–237). Springfield, IL: Charles C Thomas.

Wehman, P., Renzaglia, A., & Bates, P. (1985). *Functional living skills for moderately and severely handicapped individuals.* Austin, TX: PRO-ED.

Wehman, P., Renzaglia, A., Berry, G., Schultz, R., & Karan, O. (1978). Developing a leisure skill repertoire in severely and profoundly handicapped persons. *AAESPH Review, 3,* 162–172.

Wehman, P., & Rettie, C. (1975). Increasing actions on play materials by severely retarded women through social reinforcement. *Therapeutic Recreation Journal, 9*(4), 173–178.

Wehman, P., & Schleien, S. (1980). Assessment and selection of leisure skills for severely handicapped individuals. *Education and Training of the Mentally Retarded, 15,* 50–57.

Wehman, P., & Schleien, S. (1981). *Leisure programs for handicapped persons: Adaptations, techniques, and curriculum.* Baltimore: University Park Press.

Wehman, P., Schleien, S., & Kiernan, J. (1980). Age appropriate recreation programs for severely handicapped youth and adults. *Journal of The Association for the Severely Handicapped, 5,* 394–407.

Whitman, T.L., Mercurio, J., & Caponigri, V. (1970). Development of social response in two severely retarded children. *Journal of Applied Behavior Analysis, 3,* 133–138.

Wilcox, B., & Bellamy, G.T. (1982). *Design of high school programs for severely handicapped students.* Baltimore: Paul H. Brookes Publishing Co.

Williams, W., Brown, L., & Certo, N. (1975). Basic components of instructional programs. In L. Brown, T. Crowner, W. Williams, & R. York (Eds.), *Madison's alternative for zero exclusion: A book of readings* (Vol. 5). Madison, WI: Madison Public Schools.

Williams, W., Hamre-Nietupski, S., Pumpian, L., McDaniel-Marks, J., & Wheeler, J. (1978). Teaching social skills. In M.E. Snell (Ed.), *Systematic instruction of the moderately and severely handicapped* (pp. 281–300). Columbus, OH: Charles E. Merrill.

Witt, P.A., Ellis, G., & Niles, S.H. (1984). Leisure counseling with special populations. In T.E. Dowd (Ed.), *Leisure counseling: Concepts and applica-*

tions (pp. 198–213). Springfield, IL: Charles C Thomas.

Witt, P.A., & Groom, R. (1979). Dangers and problems associated with current approaches to developing leisure interest finders. *Therapeutic Recreation Journal, 13*(1), 19–31.

Wolfensburger, W. (1972). *The principle of normalization in human services.* Toronto: National Institute on Mental Retardation.

Wuerch, B.B., & Voeltz, L.M. (1982). *Longitudinal leisure skills for severely handicapped learners: The Ho'onanea curriculum component.* Baltimore: Paul H. Brookes Publishing Co.

CHAPTER 11

Social Relationships

Thomas G. Haring

University of California, Santa Barbara, California

People with severe disabilities have a right to live normalized lives in community-based homes, attend schools with chronologically age-matched peers, participate in work, and enjoy a full range of life-enhancing experiences. The technology is emerging to achieve the community-based services needed to realize these rights for all persons with severe disabilities. Given a commitment to these rights, as well as an emerging technology, it is critical to ask at this point in time toward what path our technology should be directed in order to create a full range of options for integrated life-span development. In order to answer this question, it is important to define integration and then specify how our existing technologies of behavior change can assist individuals with severe disabilities in achieving a socially integrated lifestyle. This chapter develops the argument that a careful linkage between commitment to goals and the currently existing behavioral technology must occur if integrated lifestyles for people with severe handicaps are to be realized.

FUNCTIONAL INTEGRATION VERSUS SOCIAL INTEGRATION

As the field's model of service delivery moves from a logic of segregation to a model of community integration it is important to recognize that integration is not a unitary concept. As integrated services are begun, the first level of integration can be termed *functional integration.* Functional integration is defined as the specification of natural settings and the programming of functions within those settings. Thus, there are four basic types of natural settings: vocational, home and neighborhood, community, and school. Within each of these settings there is a primary function for which the setting was designed. The primary purpose of a home is as a space to provide shelter for sleeping, meal preparation, and

recreation. The primary function of the school is to teach the skills necessary for productive adult living and an appreciation and understanding of our culture. When functional integration is achieved, a goal that many integrated programs are currently meeting, there is little functional necessity for social interaction or social relationships. Thus, from a purely functional perspective, it is entirely possible to live a fully integrated lifestyle, and yet be maximally socially segregated. Many people who are elderly in our society experience just such a lifestyle.

An integrated though socially segregated lifestyle, while within our current legal mandates for services, does not achieve the end that is intended by the current emphasis on deinstitutionalization and community-based services. That end needs to include the development and maintenance of a network of friends and acquaintances. If all of a person's friends and acquaintances are from the same social group, and if that social group is routinely devalued by the majority, then that person is functionally segregated regardless of the amount of time spent in the proximity of others or the normalized quality of the environment in which that person functions. Although people with severe disabilities living in community settings typically have relatively rich social networks, frequently these networks comprise only other people with disabilities (Romer & Heller, 1983).

Social integration is defined as the full participation in social interactions within natural environments to the ultimate extent that the people encountered within that environment are part of a stable social network. The achievement of such a social network means that a person can participate within relationships that vary along a continuum from stable, yet casual acquaintances, to more intimate friendships and relationships. A major indicator of integrated programming is an active effort to promote and facilitate the development of social interaction skills so that people with severe handicaps have the necessary behavioral repertoire to enter social networks. The ultimate product of integration is participation in social relationships across the entire range of human intimacy and support dimensions from casual relationships with clerks in stores to the maintenance of long-term friendships.

This position, that social interaction within a stable social network is the ultimate indicator of integrated, community-based services, while entirely consistent with current best-practices models (e.g., Horner, Meyer, & Fredericks, 1986), is not necessarily an outgrowth of our current construct of integration. This has been shown in a study conducted by Meyer, Eichinger, and Park-Lee (1987). Within this research, experts rated 123 program quality indicators. A factor analysis was conducted to identify clusters of items that relate to program quality. From that factor analysis, the first factor was labeled by the authors "Integration." This factor included items that emphasized participation in integrated environments, teaching skills in the natural environment, integration within normal school-based activities, and participation by special education staff in professional and extracurricular activities with regular education staff. It also included administrative arrangements, such as classroom location and riding regular school buses. This finding implies that experts within the field view social interaction and physical proximity with nonhandicapped people as a central construct to a definition of integrated services. However, an interesting and potentially powerful conceptual separation is evident by analyzing the components of another factor from this analysis that included social interaction items. This factor was labeled "Criterion of Ultimate Functioning." Within this factor, items stressed preparation for living in least restrictive environments, including preparation for competitive employment or supported work, and the development of domestic skills.

If items within the Criterion of Ultimate Functioning factor are examined closely, the three social items associated with this factor stress teaching social skills directly and the attainment of social acceptance. Similarly, the other (nonsocial) items loading on this factor also stressed training and preparation to live in the community and hold a normalized job. As defined before, these items are indicative of social integration. In contrast, the Integration factor is largely functional integration. That is, this factor stresses administrative variables, spatial arrangements, and scheduling that create a context for social interaction, but do not involve the direct teaching of skills needed to enhance participation in the social milieu of the school.

Social integration and functional integration represent two separable (though correlated and interrelated) conceptual components of a larger construct of integration. The major focus on integration to date has been in the area of functional integration. Clearly, functional integration is a necessary prerequisite for social integration. The central thesis of this chapter is that social integration, and the attainment of social relationships within normal environments, is an integral component of a construct of integration. An assumption is that social interaction skills and social relationships will not usually develop as a passive consequence of functional integration. Instead, *active* programming efforts (i.e., direct instruction of social interaction skills, planned modifications of social interaction contexts, and the initiation of supported social relationships) are required to achieve the goals of integrated lifestyles for people with severe handicaps. The major purpose of this chapter is to review procedures that have been described and validated to directly teach social interactions and to develop the skills necessary to participate in social relationships that are central to the attainment of integrated, community-based services.

Before reviewing the current research concerning the teaching of social skills necessary for the establishment of social networks, a brief rationale for considering social relationships as a primary outcome of integrated programming is offered.

RATIONALE FOR THE CENTRALITY OF SOCIAL NETWORKS TO THE CONSTRUCT OF INTEGRATION

Social relationships should be viewed as a key indicator and defining characteristic of integrated services for at least the following reasons:

1. *Social relationships contribute substantially to quality of life.* Few nonhandicapped people would choose to live a life of social isolation, yet many people with mental retardation living in community settings report feelings of loneliness and isolation. This problem was illustrated in a study by Bercovici (1981). She found that in 6 out of the 10 group homes that were studied, staff members tended to discourage or prohibit residents from maintaining contacts or friendships with others outside of the program. It is clear that feelings of self-fulfillment and satisfaction with one's life are highly associated with the attainment of a stable social network (e.g., McKinney, Fitzgerald, & Strommen, 1982). The development of intimacy (not necessarily physical intimacy) versus isolation is a central theme in adolescent and adult development and is clearly a theme that is not solely an issue for people with disabilities (cf. Erikson, 1959).

2. *Social interaction skills, ideally produced within the context of an ongoing relationship with another person, are necessary for functional participation in many critical activities.* For example, it is frequently necessary to ask for help when making purchases. It is necessary to interact socially with cashiers to attend movies and other life-enhancing recreational events. Indeed, the nonverbal exchange behaviors that are characteristic of completing a purchase are identical in pattern to the exchange behaviors of playing a game or holding a conversation and are equally social in that they involve a reciprocal exchange of responses between two people.

3. *Many critical skills are maintained over time by complex, remote schedules of reinforcement but are maintained on an immediate basis by the socially reinforcing aspects of interacting with people with whom you have a relationship.* For example, the typical high school student does not attend school to learn subject matter and is not reinforced on a daily basis by grades. Instead, a major motivation for attending school is to gain contact with a personal network of social relationships. Similarly, in many vocational settings, the key daily reinforcers are not monetary, but the social contacts available at the job site. Certainly, the longer term complex contingencies of school and work are powerful determinants of behavior (see Michael, 1986, for a theoretical analysis), but in the absence of daily social contingencies these are often insufficient to maintain behavior. Thus, social networks provide a major source of reinforcement for engaging in behavioral repertoires that are sometimes aversive, but absolutely necessary for living within modern communities.

4. *There is a relationship between social skills use and the lessening of a need for programming based on behavioral control.* For example, the research by Carr and Durand (1985) has had a powerful impact on viewing the instruction of social communicative skills as a primary treatment for seriously disruptive and potentially life-threatening self-injurious behaviors. From this perspective, all behaviors, including aberrant responses, are viewed as potentially communicative attempts to control the behavior of others (e.g., to escape unwanted tasks). Thus, the building of social competence is a significant means toward reducing challenging behaviors that serve to stigmatize some people with severe handicaps and that *seemingly* justify increased social isolation of the individual by service providers.

5. *There is an increasing awareness that* disability *is more an attitude held by professionals and nonhandicapped people than it is a property or defining characteristic of the person with disabilities* (Gartner & Lipsky, 1987; Lane, 1988). The greatest obstacles created for people with disabilities are social barriers that the nondisabled world has created and maintained. Sociological analyses have indicated that such social barriers may reflect an underlying ideology that people with disabilities are not fully human (Goffman, 1963; Wolfensberger, 1972). At the broadest level, it is only when social integration has been achieved that it can be assumed that people with severe disabilities are fully accredited members of communities and that the ultimate goal of integration is met.

Thus, there are many reasons to view the development of social relationships as central to the construct of integration. At the level of the individual, social relationships are seen as an important source of happiness and self-perceptions of quality of life. At the pragmatic level, social interaction, preferably within the context of a stable social network, is an important means for engaging in functional skills, maintaining complex repertoires in the absence of direct tangible reinforcement, and reducing aberrant responding. At the broadest societal level, social integration is an important indicator that people with severe disabilities are accepted as fully human members of a common, pluralistic culture.

EXISTING DATA BASE OF TECHNOLOGIES FOR BUILDING SOCIAL RELATIONSHIPS

There has been a 20-year history of research that relates to the establishment of social skills for persons with severe disabilities. An examination of this literature indicates that the majority of the work done to date has focused on using specific behaviorally based instructional procedures in order to train new social skills, predominantly in the area of play skills with preschool children. Although recent experimental work continues to investigate new instructional techniques as well as new critical skills to teach, there has been an expansion of the social skills and relationship literature in several new directions. The major organizing topics for this review of the existing data base to support the feasibility of directly teaching social interaction skills are: enhancement of contextual variables, direct skills training, and supported relationships.

It is a central assumption of this chapter that the achievement of social networks for people with severe disabilities is dependent on two factors: 1) direct instruction of social skills and 2) direct and indirect facilitation of social relationships. Facilitation of social relationships can be based on either directly facilitating a relationship by structuring the context of the interactions (e.g., establishing a school-based friendship program), or indirectly by changing the social environment via increasing acceptance and accommodation of human differences.

Contextual Enhancement

Contextual enhancement refers to intervention efforts aimed at optimizing the environmental support for the development and maintenance of a social interaction repertoire. Methods to enhance the environmental support for social interactions involve a variety of different means. One important aspect of environmental enhancement concerns an analysis of the physical parameters of a setting to arrange the environment and the objects within the environment to facilitate interaction. Other major approaches have sought to modify the social characteristics of the environment so that a student's initial attempts at social interaction are maximally reinforced and shaped.

Gaylord-Ross and Haring (1987) proposed a conceptual model to guide social interaction research that views dyadic interaction as a reciprocal exchange between two people within an environmental context. The environmental context influences social behavior in several salient ways: 1) it provides stimuli that can supply the raw material for interactions (i.e., the environment contains stimuli such as games or interesting occurrences that can structure interactions), 2) it partially determines the range and variation of behaviors that are acceptable, and 3) it determines the social roles of participants and their responses to social inputs. Baer, Wolf, and Risley (1987) have also introduced the idea of contextualism as a major construct in evaluating the effectiveness of interventions.

To date, social skills research with students with severe handicaps has been concerned with the training of social exchange responses at the dyadic level. That is, the primary focus of prior research has been to train social interaction skills with little reference to the application of these skills to related contexts, the impact that contextual variation *should* exert on modifying appropriate social repertoires, or the reactions of interactants within an extant context to changes in the social repertoire. It should be recognized that there are powerful determinants of social responding (hence, potential foci of intervention) located beyond the level of the dyad. Thus, interventions designed solely to affect responding within the dyad ignore the impact of other variables on reciprocal social behavior—the ability of learners with severe handicaps to respond in natural social contexts may be artificially limited by a technology that focuses solely on responding within the dyad. The importance of contextual factors in research and training of social behavior has been indicated by researchers from diverse backgrounds and theoretical perspectives (cf. Baer, Wolf, & Risley, 1987; Bronfenbrenner, 1979; Endler & Magnusson, 1976; Kantor, 1981; Wolfensberger, 1983).

Behavioral Conceptualizations

A powerful determinant of social behavior is the context in which the behavior occurs. Many behavior analysts have described these contextual variables as *setting events* (W.H. Brown, Bryson-Brockman, & Fox, 1986; Wahler & Fox, 1981). Kantor (1959) defined setting events as those immediate circumstances that influence the occurrence or nonoccurrence of behavior beyond the immediate antecedent social cues and consequences.

A dramatic demonstration of the potential power of manipulating contextual variables is Horner's (1980) research on the effects of environmental enrichment on the behavior of children with profound handicaps. By simply adding a large number of toys into an institutional environment, the study demonstrated a doubling of appropriate adaptive behaviors while substantially reducing the occurrence of several classes of maladaptive behaviors.

Ethnographic Research

The power of social context variables in determining behavior has been described by researchers using naturalistic, field-observation methodologies. The work of Barker and colleagues (e.g., Barker, 1968; Barker, Wright, Barker, & Schoggen, 1961) is regarded as prototypic research in this area (cf. Brandt, 1972). Barker's research involved detailed observations of naturally occurring behavior in a small town in Kansas. Setting events were described as being the most powerful determiners of people's behavior. For example, children were found to change their pattern of behavior drastically from one setting to another. Within any one setting, the social behavior of children who otherwise differed greatly, was consistent. The impact of using field-observation methodology to guide theory development with students with severe

handicaps is showing a promising beginning in the design of residential, transition, and vocational programs (e.g., Zetlin & Turner, 1985).

Chadsey-Rusch and Rusch (1988) developed a line of research with students with severe handicaps within vocational settings that describes the types of social interactions occurring between co-workers. Chadsey-Rusch and Gonzales (1988) found that many social interactions within the workplace were based on either the exchange of information, or teasing and joking. Collecting data on the social contextual characteristics of settings provides an important mechanism for the identification of skills needed to be maximally integrated into natural social environments.

Classroom, Grouping, and Instructional Design Factors

From a special education perspective, Peck and Cooke (1983) referred to a number of important contextual variables that merit investigation in the design of instructional environments for learners with severe handicaps. These include educational activity, group size, peer familiarity, ratio of children with handicaps to nonhandicapped children, availability of play materials, and group structure. Still other important variables include the amount of space available (Black, Freeman, & Montgomery, 1975), classroom organization and structural use of space, and academic versus free-play interactions (Gaylord-Ross & Pitts-Conway, 1984; McHale & Simeonsson, 1980). Organizational variables specific to special education classrooms can affect the subsequent social interaction of peers. These variables, broadly conceived, are characteristic of the environments to which students are exposed. As such, these variables shape the characteristics of social contexts.

Social Climate

In addition to physical and organizational aspects of the environment, other social contextual variables have been identified as having a potentially powerful influence on responding. One important class of variables has been described as *social climate* (Moos, 1973, 1974). Social climate is determined by the affective atmosphere of a classroom. Clearly, some classroom environments are more supportive of social initiations than others and a delineation of those social-affective characteristics that support interactions are an important addition to our understanding of teaching social responding.

Peck (1986) conducted research on classroom social climate variables by systematically investigating the impact of contextual variables, such as student opportunities for making choices, and the responsivity of teachers to the social initiation attempts by students with severe handicaps. He found that by increasing adult attentiveness to child initiations, the level of social initiations produced by students with severe handicaps increased and was associated with increases in the affective climate of the classroom.

Social Responsiveness

From the perspective of the child, the social responsiveness of an environment is as critical as the physical aspects of the environment in terms of the facilitation of social responding. Intervention efforts to change the social environment within which students function have been referred to as *milieu teaching* (Kaiser, Alpert, & Warren, 1987). Increased environmental responsiveness is especially important in reinforcing students' initial attempts at social interactions (Koegel, O'Dell, & Dunlap, 1988; Peck, Tomlinson, Schuler, Theimer, & Haring, 1984). For example, it is important to reinforce precursors to verbal language, such as eye-gaze behavior and hand gestures, in order to teach students that their behaviors have functional effects within environments. Once a student can reliably produce certain *functions* (e.g., requesting by pointing), it is much easier to insert other responses into the extant response class. In fact, nonverbal communication skills may often be more generalizable to other contexts than rotely learned verbal responses. The social responsiveness of adults and peers within a setting can have a substantial impact on the level of social and communicative responding within a given context and has consequences for the longitudinal social development of the student.

A major variable affecting the social responsiveness of an environment is the degree of child directedness as opposed to adult directedness of interactions (Guess & Siegel-Causey, 1985). For example, Koegel, Dyer, and Bell (1987) demonstrated substantial increases in autistic children's social behavior as a function of child-preferred activities. The programming of choices (e.g., Dattilo & Rusch, 1985) is an important means to extend control of leisure as well as instructional interactions to students.

The most extensively developed instructional methodology in the area of adult responsiveness to the communicative initiations of children within naturally motivating contexts was introduced by Hart and Risley (1968, 1975, 1980) in their investigations of incidental teaching and has been subsequently modified by several researchers (e.g., Halle, 1987; Rogers-Warren & Warren, 1980). In general, incidental and other milieu teaching procedures are based on a service provider being aware of a student's motivational state at a given point in time to achieve an event or obtain a desired object. The service provider reinforces a student's initial attempts to communicate, even if this initial form does not correspond to normalized modes of communication. Following this, the service provider generally models a more normalized social form and provides access to the desired event or object. These procedures share a reliance on adult-arranged control of social episodes, but also stress the importance of being aware of a child's communicative intent and reinforcing attempts at social interaction regardless of the accuracy of the response. Incidental teaching procedures have been used to teach children to self-initiate communicative behavior and enhance generalization of social responses within an extant repertoire (e.g., McGee, Krantz, & McClannahan, 1985).

The delay procedure (Halle, Marshall, & Spradlin, 1979) is a modification of the incidental teaching procedure. With this technique, the adult focuses attention on a child after a child indicates interest in an environmental event or object. Using this procedure, teachers wait up to 15 seconds prior to providing a prompt for the child to communicate. This procedure has been shown to increase students' initiation of responses. Modified incidental teaching procedures have proven to be successful in teaching receptive language skills (McGee, Krantz, Mason, & Mc-Clannahan, 1983) and requesting (Carr & Kologinsky, 1983), as well as in increasing the overall level of social initiations within natural contexts (Haring, Neetz, Lovinger, Peck, & Semmel, 1987).

Summary

A diverse research literature from several theoretical orientations points to the potential power of contextual variables in shaping competent social interactions. Contextual models of social behavior indicate that the quality and quantity of social responding can be influenced by the contextual control of social responding. This is an innovative approach to research in social skills training as, to date, the predominant focus of research efforts has been based on evaluating the effectiveness of interventions designed to facilitate the rate of social exchanges within the conceptual unit of the dyad. Social context variables are important determiners of the social responding of nonhandicapped people. Only recently has this perspective been extended to normalizing the responding of students with severe handicaps. The continued development of research within this area could conceivably provide an important source of methods to increase the quality and validity of social interaction interventions.

Direct Instruction of Social Skills

A pragmatic approach to social skills instruction was first suggested by Strain, Cooke, and Apolloni (1976) and follows closely the social interaction analysis format introduced by Cairns (1979). From this perspective, key events within dyadic social interaction are identified in generic terms. For example, interactions are begun with an *initiation* that represents a broad class of verbal and nonverbal behavior. After an initiation, the interactant might acknowledge the initiation in some way, or might offer an elaboration or an extension of the initiation. Interactions can be maintained by such elaboration and extension responses, or new initiations (i.e., topic shifts) can

be introduced to maintain interactions. In addition, people employ repair strategies to "fix" interactions that have broken down in some way (e.g., restate an idea). Interactions are closed by a class of responses called *terminations*. Once such classes are identified, students can be taught generative response classes to serve those functions within a social interaction.

Pragmatic analyses are consistent with Skinner's (1957) descriptions of verbal behavior that stress a functional as opposed to a structural analysis of language use. In conducting a pragmatic assessment, judgments concerning the effectiveness of a given social event are made by analyzing the effect that the response produced on the subsequent responses of others. The focus of social skills training is to identify pivotal social response classes and teach exemplars of each class until broader generative responding emerges.

Social responding within natural integrated contexts is often based on multioperant responding. Multioperant responding means that a response is under the control of several operant relationships. A response might belong to more than one operant class (e.g., saying "water" as a request for water or as a description of the content of a glass), or the reinforcement of a generalization operant might control the stimulus generalization of a class of responses (e.g., reinforcement for attempting to respond to one class of verbal cues might increase the frequency of attempts to use other classes). An early training study that examined a pragmatic operant that could participate in the multioperant control of social responding involved turn taking within a game-playing context (Baldwin, 1983). There is an emerging technology of teaching pivotal social interaction skills to students with severe handicaps that has included initiations, extensions, conversational responsiveness, peer initiation interventions, and teaching social skills within task analyses.

Initiation, Extension, and Conversational Responsiveness Training

A powerful technique to build social interaction skills is to teach students with disabilities to initiate interactions. Gaylord-Ross and Haring

(1987) discussed the advantages of teaching initiations:

1. *Increased probability of successful interactions.* Students with severe handicaps have more control over interactions. This is important because students can initiate interactions around activities within which they are competent rather than passively waiting for peer initiations that may or may not match their current interests and level of competence.

2. *Increased independence.* Students are less dependent on nonhandicapped peers to engage in interactions. The social image of the persons with disabilities may be enhanced because of greater control over interactions.

3. *Increased frequency of interaction.* Teaching social initiation skills to students with severe handicaps results in increased levels of social behavior compared to baseline levels within natural contexts (e.g., Haring & Lovinger, 1989; Odom & Strain, 1986).

The earliest training efforts to teach individuals with severe handicaps initiation responses involved attempts to program generative greeting responses. An early study concerning teaching generalized greeting responses conducted by Stokes, Baer, and Jackson (1974) has had an impact on our current instructional models. Within this study, a multiple exemplar training format was used with institutionalized adults. This study was not only among the first social skills training studies, it also pioneered one of the most powerful generalization strategies now in use. Within this study, participants were prompted to initiate interactions to one staff member and after the training criterion was met, probes were conducted with people who had not participated in instruction. If the learner had not generalized to all staff members targeted for the study, the learner was instructed to greet another staff member. Teaching with additional staff members continued until generalization to all staff was observed.

While training an initial greeting response is an important first step in teaching social interaction skills, it is clear that initiation responses such as saying "Hi" and gestural waves result in interactions that last only a few seconds. Additional training procedures are needed to teach more elaborate interactions of extended duration. Unfortunately, many such interactions among nonhandicapped people involve ongoing, complex conversations.

An initial study that taught initiation skills that resulted in more extended interactions and that was not dependent on conversational skills was conducted by Gaylord-Ross, Haring, Breen, and Pitts-Conway (1984). Within this study, three nonverbal activities were selected around which students with autism could initiate interactions. The three activities, playing a hand-held video game, listening to a Sony Walkman, and sharing gum, were age-appropriate activities that nonhandicapped students as well as the students with autism enjoyed. The students were trained to approach and offer to share the objects as a means to initiate interactions. Training was conducted with peer "confederates" while the data reported were with untrained nonhandicapped peers naturally encountered within a school courtyard setting as part of the normally scheduled midmorning break. The results indicated that, prior to training, the students with autism never initiated interactions. During the initiation training phase, two of the students initiated interactions at least once during each break, while the third student initiated an average of two interactions per break. Importantly, the mean duration of interactions indicated that the students and the peers interacted for extended periods of time.

Breen, Haring, Pitts-Conway, and Gaylord-Ross (1985) extended the findings of the earlier study by applying the same underlying model of teaching object-centered initiations. Within this research, students were trained to make coffee within a break-time context in actual job sites. After making coffee, the students were taught to offer coffee to nonhandicapped co-workers and participate in break-time conversations. A multiple exemplar format was used to promote generalization across co-workers. As training progressed, generalization probes in the actual break-room were conducted with the observer being as unobtrusive as possible. Training with multiple exemplars of co-workers (actually, confederates of the instructor) continued until generalized initiations were observed. The importance of teaching appropriate break-time behaviors as components of integrated vocational training programs has been well documented (e.g., Storey, Bates, & Hanson, 1984; Sulzbacher, Haines, Peterson, & Swatman, 1984).

Initiation training strategies are fundamental to social interaction training approaches. As these procedures have been developed and extended, it is clear that all initiations are not equal. That is, some initiations (e.g., offering a toy as a bid to start playing) can result in interactions of extended durations. An important current trend in social skills research is to teach responses to students with severe handicaps that can be used to extend and elaborate interactions (e.g., Lalli, 1988). In an example of this approach, Haring, Roger, Lee, Breen, and Gaylord-Ross (1986) trained students to initiate verbal interactions within a cafeteria setting in an elementary school. Of the 3 students trained, only 1 student showed response-response interrelationships between learning initiation responses and the spontaneous generation of elaboration or conversational extension responses. In order to normalize these interactions, all 3 students required instruction in extending conversations.

Wildman, Wildman, and Kelly (1986) reported a similar study that targeted several classes of conversation extension responses such as asking questions of one's partner, and giving information about oneself. The training was shown to be effective in increasing conversational competence, which was independently confirmed with social validity ratings. Downing (1987) was also successful in teaching a generic ability to extend conversational interactions by modeling and reinforcing responses from conversational partners that were relevant and meaningful to the topic under discussion. Finally, Hunt, Alwell, and Goetz (1988) demonstrated that not only could elaboration responses be taught (in this case defined as conversational "turns"), but that the teaching of such responses resulted in decreases in socially inappropriate behaviors.

In summary, social initiation and interaction extension and elaboration skills are an important means to increase the level of social interactions within natural settings. Within these interventions, it is critical to assess not only the increases

in frequencies of social behaviors but also the increases in the normalized quality of social interactions that result from training. Without ongoing monitoring of effectiveness, direct social skills training might produce not only limited generalization, but initiation skills that have non-normalized or ineffective characteristics (e.g., Berler, Gross, & Drabman, 1982).

It is important to survey carefully the social characteristics of the natural environment to select skills for training that are desirable within specific social contexts. This factor, more than any other, explains the success of some studies versus the limited effects reported in other research efforts. An a priori assessment of social interaction behaviors of peers within natural settings should be conducted prior to planning interventions (e.g., Haring et al,, 1986). As discussed earlier, ethnographic techniques are a particularly powerful way to identify subtle social interaction skills that are needed in natural contexts. In addition, the social validity of such interventions should be monitored periodically throughout interventions (rather than in a pretest/posttest manner as is more typical) to ensure that skills being taught are maximally effective in criterion contexts.

A major weakness of this literature is the lack of demonstrated relationships between the acquisition of specific skills and the attainment of the larger objectives for the training of these skills—that is, increased social acceptance. One important way to assess the effects of initiation training interventions is to assess the immediate effects of the initiation of the response on the peer (e.g., Fox, Shores, Lindeman, & Strain, 1986). Those initiation strategies that result in more generally positive responses from peers can then be identified. In addition, it is critical to assess the duration as well as the frequencies of interactions to identify optimal contexts and initiation strategies.

Peer Initiation Interventions

Peer initiation interventions have an extensive history of effectiveness in promoting increased social interaction of children with disabilities (e.g., Hendrickson, Strain, Trembly, & Shores, 1982). Within these strategies, nonhandicapped peers are trained to initiate interactions with students with disabilities. This research has documented that these strategies result in increases in social interactions between students with disabilities and their peers. These effects have been shown to be applicable across students with autism (Odom & Strain, 1986; Strain, Kerr, & Ragland, 1979), children with behavior disorders (Strain & Fox, 1981), children with mental retardation (Lancioni, 1982), and students with severe handicaps (Young & Kerr, 1979). Peer initiation procedures can be applied within school settings, or within home settings by siblings (James & Egel, 1986).

It is important to differentiate between peer initiation interventions, peer tutor interventions (e.g., Gaylord-Ross & Pitts-Conway, 1984; Greenwood et al., 1987), and the use of peer confederates within teacher-directed interventions (e.g., Brady et al., 1984; Gaylord-Ross et al., (1984). With peer initiation strategies, peers are taught to organize play episodes, share toys, respond positively to social responses, and engage in play. Within a peer initiation role, the peer serves as a "social facilitator" for the student with disabilities to enter and participate in play or social interactions. In contrast, peer tutoring indicates a more directly instructional role. For example, peers can be taught to directly train skills needed for social leisure interactions and can be taught to model and directly teach social interaction behavior. Within a peer tutor role, peers function as teachers to directly instruct social skills. Although a common approach (e.g., Donder & Nietupski, 1981; Kohl, Moses, & Stettner-Eaton, 1984), the effects of such procedures in improving more purely social interactions and peer acceptance is still an unresolved issue, although in at least one study (Haring, Breen, Lee, Pitts-Conway, & Gaylord-Ross, 1987), negative effects were not observed.

With peer confederate strategies, a small group of nonhandicapped children are selected as confederates to assist in training that is managed by a teacher. For example, to train students with severe handicaps to greet peers, it is helpful to have a group of confederates to use during training. The student with severe handicaps can be prompted by the teachers to approach the confederate and produce an appropriate greeting.

Multiple confederates are used in a sufficient exemplar format to promote generalization to untrained peers. Each of these procedures can be used alone or in combination to teach social skills and increase the level of social interactions within integrated settings.

Several applications of peer initiation interventions have indicated that the procedures not only resulted in increases for targeted students, but also produced "spillover" effects to nontargeted students (Strain, Shores, & Kerr, 1976). Sasso and Rude (1987) showed that the status of the peers used within the intervention influenced other peers to interact with the student with disabilities. This is a potentially powerful finding because it indicates that Wolfensberger's (1983) concept of social role valorization may operate to increase social acceptance. That is, the social desirability of high-status peers may, in essence, "rub off" on the student with disabilities, thus facilitating broader peer acceptance. Sasso, Hughes, Swanson, and Novak (1987) investigated a technique in which nonhandicapped peers were trained to reinforce untrained nonhandicapped peers for initiating interactions with students with disabilities. The results indicated that the procedure was effective in increasing the level of interaction and that teacher prompting of interaction was largely unnecessary.

This is an unusual finding. Frequently, peer initiation interventions involve direct teacher prompting and reinforcement to maintain socially interactive responses. Recent work by Odom, Hoyson, Jamieson, and Strain (1985) illustrated some potential problems with the application of a peer initiation intervention within an integrated preschool program. Within that study, peers were trained using teacher models to initiate social interactions. The peers were taught to organize play situations, share toys, request toys, assist in activities, and compliment the social behavior of the students with disabilities. Following training the students' social initiations and interactions with peers with disabilities were observed within three contexts. Within these otherwise natural interaction contexts, the nonhandicapped peers received prompts to initiate interactions and token reinforcement for each successful initiation. The results indicated that the peer intervention package (including training in a stimulation setting and prompts and reinforcement in the criterion settings) produced rapid increases in the frequency of positive initiations across all three contexts. Generalization probes were conducted within other social contexts and prompts and reinforcers were not given. Importantly, under unprompted conditions, the nonhandicapped peers did not interact appreciably with the peers with disabilities. In addition, a component analysis was conducted by systematically adding and withdrawing the prompting and the reinforcement procedures within the three criterion contexts. Results indicated that the positive interactions were almost entirely dependent on the use of prompts and rewards by the teacher within those settings.

Given the lack of maintenance of social initiation and the lack of generalization in the absence of direct teacher prompts and reinforcement, the utility of peer initiation interventions as a means to structure ongoing social relationships and social networks should be examined. That is, it appears from these data that the nonhandicapped peers who participate may not develop an increased intrinsic motivation to interact with peers with disabilities. Studies have not yet been conducted to demonstrate that the peers value the interactions with the students with disabilities, view them as more normalized, or have increased their likelihood of interacting with them in the absence of being directed to do so by the teacher. In fairness, these procedures are not designed to build positive relationships, only to increase interactions and teach social interaction skills. It is possible that the use of such procedures over longer durations would result in friendships or indications of more naturally motivated interactive behavior. It is also possible that the major effects of such intervention are to be found not as procedures to shape acceptance, but as procedures to train social skills that will facilitate future interactions. However, at present, it is unclear what the benefits are of applications of these procedures beyond increasing the levels of interactions under teacher-directed conditions. This being the case, it is essential to validate that the procedures result in increased social skills for students with disabilities (not just increases in the frequency of interactions as a function of adult interaction).

Social Skills within Task Analyses of Functional Skills

The final direct social skills instructional strategy to be reviewed involves inserting the instruction of social skills into the task analyses being used to teach the acquisition of functional and critical skills. F. Brown, Evans, Weed, and Owen (1987) argue persuasively that many community-oriented skills cannot be considered learned to a functional level if the social skills that are associated with the functional skills are not taught concurrently. In other words, task analytic instruction needs to include a plan for teaching all of the skills needed under the conditions of the varying demands of natural environments, including social interaction skills.

Shopping is an example of a functional skill often targeted for instruction. However, it is typical to find that task analyses of shopping skills do not include social responses (e.g., McDonnell, 1987). This is a lost opportunity to train social skills as well as to provide a basis for the development of casual relationships between clerks and the student. If the instruction is being carried out in the student's home neighborhood (as it should be), this represents a high opportunity cost.

There are several examples of studies that involved the successful teaching of social skills directly within task analytic instruction of critical skills. For example, Haring, Kennedy, Adams, and Pitts-Conway (1987) taught students with disabilities to generalize shopping skills across multiple community environments. Within the task analysis, skills were separately designated as social responses and functional responses. Functional responses constituted the minimal response repertoire needed to complete purchases across the multiple settings. Social skills extended the repertoire to include interactions with clerks and social politeness responses. Interestingly, within baselines of the skills, the students averaged baseline performance of 40%–80% correct on the functional skills needed to shop while social skills performance in the settings was consistently absent. Given that these students had been in a nationally recognized, "state-of-the-art" community-oriented instructional program, this probably represented the program's emphasis on functional skills and a relative lack of emphasis on the integration of social skills within community training.

Teaching social skills within a task analytic format involves the use of "branching" task analyses. For example, within the shopping study discussed above (Haring, Kennedy, et al., 1987), after the step "Approach the counter" there was a branching step consisting of "If greeted by the cashier, answer 'Hi' or 'Fine' as appropriate" and "If not greeted by the cashier, say 'Hi.'" Within this study, the generalization of social and functional skills was promoted by training within the natural environment and training with videotaped examples of same-age peers making purchases. The social responses of the peers on the videotapes was purposely varied so that students with disabilities would learn a more generic set of social responses rather than specific responses in specific circumstances. Although the functional skills were acquired more easily by the students than the social skills, all 3 students with disabilities performed social skills at criterion level by the end of the study.

An important purpose of functional skills training within the community is not only to promote more independence, but to create the foundation for social relationships within those settings. It is therefore important to survey each setting targeted for instruction to identify people who are routinely in those settings and social interaction skills that are appropriate to those contexts. As an anecdotal example, after teaching the 3 students from the initial study (Haring, Kennedy, et al., 1987) cited above to shop, Haring, Breen, Weiner, Bednersh, and Kennedy (1988) subsequently replicated and extended these procedures with 7 more students. Within the course of training 10 students to shop independently (generally requiring a year of instruction conducted daily) the authors noted many instances of cashiers recognizing the students as repeat customers and showing high degrees of responsivity to their attempts at social interactions. The development of such relationships needs to be viewed not as a side effect of functional skills training, but as a directly programmed main effect, equally as important as the functional skills. In addition, as the recognition that the development of social relationships

is a main effect of training rather than a side effect, the strength of such relationships needs to be assessed directly (e.g., through interviews or questionnaires) to document and monitor the creation of a stable social network.

Supported Relationships

Procedures and validated models to directly promote social relationships within integrated settings have not been developed nearly to the extent of instructional packages designed to teach social skills (Odom & McEvoy, 1988). Although this literature is sparse, there have been some important initial efforts to create programs and procedures to support relationships in a fashion analogous to supported work options in vocational programming. In supported work, service providers engage in a range of functions including recruiting potential employers, developing job sites, training job skills, soliciting feedback from employers as to their satisfaction, and providing longitudinal training and problem solving as needed. Service providers can perform similar functions to create supported relationships, including: 1) recruiting potential peers for participation in friendship interactions, 2) surveying potential social interaction contexts for skills and contexts that would be most beneficial to students, 3) developing specific activities or materials for each identified context, 4) training necessary social interaction skills, 5) surveying peers to assess their satisfaction and increases in the sociometric status of the student with disabilities, and 6) engaging in ongoing support and problem solving to maintain the relationship. There are currently few published examples of programs or studies that have attempted to implement comprehensive programs for supported relationships.

Most of the published material concerning friendship formation between students with severe disabilities and typical students have been anecdotal or descriptive reports of specific friendships. For example, Strully and Strully (1985) described the development of a friendship between their 12-year-old daughter and a classmate. The authors reported that the friendship that was developed was made possible to a great extent by creating a service delivery model whereby their daughter would receive the major portion of her instructional program directly within regular junior high school classes rather than in a segregated, handicapped-only class located on the regular school site. The Strullys believe that the development of such friendships was critical to their daughter's quality of life and that longitudinally, such friendships will be even more important than the acquisition of critical skills to her becoming an integral member of her community.

Although of an anecdotal nature, such reports have had a powerful impact on causing many professionals to rethink the purpose of instruction for students with severe handicaps. It is apparent that there are many innovative efforts to promote friendships within integrated programs. Unfortunately, these efforts are rarely presented in professional journals as program descriptions, or empirically validated. Instead, methods to structure supported friendships are frequently reported by word of mouth within professional conferences or from teacher to teacher. For example, at the 1988 Annual TASH Conference in Washington, D.C., a major strand of the conference was devoted to the development of mainstreamed programs for students with severe handicaps. Several presentations (e.g., Falvey, 1988) gave specific recommendations for assessing the formation of friendships.

Forest (1987) reported the use of "circles" of friends to support integration and relationships. In creating circles, a network of friends is used as a resource for the person with disabilities to increase opportunities for participation in regular education and regular school activities. For example, in planning the integration of one high school–age student, the initial step in this process was to hire a person to facilitate this student's integration into community activities. Within the school setting, the facilitator assisted in getting students without disabilities to know and support this student. As a result of this advocacy and support, within 6 months the student was integrated into a full school day. Within each class, the student received support from one or more nonhandicapped students who made up her circle. Thus, the concept of the circle offers a viable approach to creating and supporting relationships within regular schools. Importantly, this concept stresses the idea of inter-dependence between people as well as independence.

An innovative friendship program has been developed by Breen and Lovinger (1989). At La Colina Junior High School in Santa Barbara, California, students with severe handicaps are assigned to a special education classroom, but attend regular education classes such as art and physical education and all noncurricular activities (e.g., lunch and breaks between classes). In addition to these administrative efforts to include the students with severe handicaps in the mainstream of the school, there is also a program designed to create supported friendships. Within this program, typical students are recruited for participation every school year through a variety of means including awareness training concerning disabilities. In addition, signs are posted inviting students to organizational meetings (where pizza is served) to introduce them to the supported friendship program.

After trying several different approaches, the program is currently structured with several unique characteristics. First, the typical students make a minimum commitment of time that is purposely kept low. For example, a student may commit to a minimum of one, two, or three lunch periods per week. Students may exceed the minimum commitment at any time. This procedure was instituted because many students initially *overcommitted* to the program and became dissatisfied after a month or so of participation. By keeping the initial commitment lower, the majority of the students have successfully maintained a friendship for at least a year.

A second unique aspect of the program is that entire peer groups are recruited for participation, not just individuals. Thus, as the program typically functions, the student with severe disabilities spends the lunch period with a peer group, and follows that peer group throughout its normal social interaction patterns.

A third unique feature is that peer groups meet with the students and the teacher during one lunch period each week for social/leisure interactions. The teacher typically brings in an age-appropriate feature-length film or taped segments of music videos, and provides refreshments. During this time, the teacher informally interviews the peer groups to determine how the nonmonitored lunch-time interactions are proceeding. This provides the teacher with the opportunity to identify potential problems and to provide specific suggestions for how to handle the problems in the future. In addition, it provides the opportunity to identify training objectives for social skills or critical skills that are perceived by the peers as requiring intervention.

There are several examples of supported friendship programs that have been empirically documented. The most thoroughly documented program to provide supported relationships was developed by Meyer (1985). Her approach, referred to as "Special Friends," was implemented on a wide-scale basis and has been experimentally validated (Voeltz, 1980, 1982). Within such friendship-based programs, students with severe disabilities are matched with a nondisabled peer and times for social/leisure interactions are scheduled. An important element in the development of friendship-based programs is the identification of a set of recreational activities that both participants enjoy, that involve age-appropriate materials, and result in normalized participation. To implement friendship-based programs, a validated recreational training curriculum (e.g., Wuerch & Voeltz, 1982) is useful. Activities such as sports, hobbies, and games, as well as activities such as eating lunch and attending school events together, can be included.

One area that has not received sufficient attention is the development of integrated after-school friendship opportunities. To date, the best examples involve integrating students into clubs such as 4-H, Boy Scouts, and other social leisure organizations (Moon & Bunker, 1987). While these contacts provide many opportunities for friendship development, there is a great deal of unused after-school time that is available for social interaction. In fact, it is far more typical to engage in friendship interactions at home after school rather than in school-oriented activities or after-school clubs.

Roger, Haring, Lee, and Gaylord-Ross (in preparation) reported the results of an empirical validation of an after-school program. To set up the program, the classroom teacher surveyed the addresses of her students in special education and the addresses of same-age peers who attended the same school in order to identify students who lived in close proximity to each other. Within this school, the teacher already operated a popular "special friend" program during leisure time in her classroom. Her first recruitment efforts consisted of approaching students who were currently involved in the classroom-based program to see if they would be interested in an after-school program. In addition, during regularly scheduled integrated activities (e.g., art or lunch) the teacher approached highly interactive peers to determine if they were interested in the after-school program. Based on this initial recruitment, 3 nonhandicapped peers were tentatively matched with 3 students with disabilities. Both sets of parents were contacted to determine if they would provide transportation and time to play—all six sets of parents were agreed. After the parents' support was obtained, the teacher conducted environmental inventories in each home to identify social/leisure activities that were age appropriate and enjoyed by both participants. The teacher then began instruction of needed social interaction skills within the special education classroom. Specific game-playing skills, and skills in initiating and maintaining conversations were taught. The results indicated that the training was successfully generalized to the home setting and that the participants enjoyed and continued the interactions after the initial efforts to set up the relationships.

Methods to support the development of friendship interactions are the most direct means to shape social networks for persons with severe handicaps. These efforts represent complex interventions that involve both direct instruction of skills needed to support the relationship and an effort to arrange the environment to allow closer and more regular contact between students. Interventions such as these can operate both from the context of mainstreamed programs, where students with severe handicaps attend regular classes, and also integrated school models, where students attend normal classes, but remain primarily assigned to self-contained special education classrooms. As the review of literature from this section indicated, there are currently many applications of supported friendship programs within school programs. Unfortunately, few of these efforts are being documented and disseminated in print and even fewer have been empirically validated. Those efforts that have been thoroughly developed and tested provide support for this approach and point to future programmatic and research needs that will constitute a new area of investigation.

ARTICULATION BETWEEN INSTRUCTION AND INTEGRATION OUTCOMES

As this review of the literature has indicated, there are a variety of means to create social interaction skills and increase the probability of the formation of meaningful social relationships between students with severe handicaps and nonhandicapped students. The most important conclusion from this review is that although many of the technologies needed to promote social relationships are relatively new, there are a great number of models, including: environmental reengineering, initiation training, peer intervention strategies, direct instruction of social skills within task analyses of functional skills, and importantly, the recent emergence of strategies to create supported friendships. While this review has indicated that each approach continues to require additional validation, a sufficient body of data exists to support the argument that we have a promising technological base for the creation of more meaningful social interaction networks for people with severe handicaps.

In this chapter I have argued that there is an unfortunate conceptual separation within the construct of integration, a separation between efforts to systematically rearrange the school environment to promote maximal contact and efforts to directly train needed social interaction skills. The results of this separation can have serious impact on the creation of meaningful social networks for all citizens. A reliance on environmental rearrangement could quite possibly result in open environments, with little meaningful interaction (Gaylord-Ross & Haring, 1987). Similarly, a concentration on social skills training that is not referenced to the build-up of social relationships could result in individuals who are taught skills that are essentially irrelevant to social interactions under natural conditions or who will remain essentially isolated if efforts to promote opportunities for contact and friendship are

not undertaken. In the remainder of this chapter, I present methods that can create a better articulation between creating opportunities for interaction through integration, and direct training of social skills by keying activities in both areas to the development of relationships. These suggestions constitute a possible plan for the generation of future research.

Template Matching

Hoier and Cone (1987) proposed a model referred to as "template matching" to guide the application of social skills training. This model has several features that provide a data-based linkage between social skills training and the development of stronger social relationships. Students were asked to sort descriptions of social attributes and behavior into two categories: "like my friend" and "not like my friend." The sorting process continued until a list of 10 descriptors was produced. From this list, the three highest rated items were selected for instruction. Within this study, the highest rated items were "sharing," "complimenting," and "praising." After these items were identified, the target student was taught to increase the frequencies of these responses. Ongoing measures to assess the likability of the student performing the template behaviors were conducted. These consisted of three 8-point Likert-type scales that each peer filled out after each scheduled play period (e.g., "How friendly was your peer?"). In adapting this model for use within integrated school programs, it may be useful to change the questions based on the needs at each site and the ages of the students. In addition to yielding quantifiable data, this model would provide teachers with a useful structure for regularly receiving feedback from peers and allow the teacher to qualitatively assess the strength of the relationship, give suggestions for different activities, and watch for signs of peer "burnout."

In summary, the template matching procedure allows the generation of social skills training objectives and content that is generated directly from the peers with whom the subject regularly interacts. In addition, it provides a method to assess the instructional validity of the training not by reference to some arbitrary standard, but by reference to the reactions of the peers to the interactions. Thus, the adoption of this procedure would represent a substantial move toward a better articulation between social skills instruction and achievement of stable social interaction networks. To date, this procedure has not been directly applied to instructional programs for students with severe handicaps; however, it appears to be a feasible procedure that warrants further testing.

The template matching procedure for programming social skills instruction differs substantially from traditional assessments of social validity that are frequently used to increase the relevance of socials skills training. Indeed, it is becoming almost traditional to end chapters on social skills training with a plea for increased concern with assessing the validity of such interventions. However, many of the methods used traditionally to assess the social validity of interventions are not keyed to the increased development of a richer social network. Instead, these procedures frequently employ expert judges or other adults who subjectively evaluate whether social skills increased after intervention and whether the behaviors were qualitatively improved over baseline conditions. For example, Haring et al. (1986) used undergraduate teachers in an education course to subjectively rate increased social competence. This method anchors the qualitative judgment of social validity to adult perceptions of the resultant behavior change rather than peer perception of the validity of the behavior change. Thus, data are not provided to judge whether the training would facilitate better integration into peer groups.

In another commonly used social validity procedure, the students' posttraining data are compared to normative data from nonhandicapped children in similar circumstances (cf. Greenwood, Walker, Todd, & Hops, 1981). Although this procedure does provide an objective standard for judging the social validity of behavior change, there is little reason to believe that a normative standard is sufficient or valid for persons with disabilities. For example, it is possible that a normative standard may underestimate the degree of behavior change required by a person with severe handicaps. On the one hand, if Marc Gold's (1980) "competency/deviancy hypoth-

esis" is correct—that is, the less competence an individual has, the less deviance is tolerated in that person by others—then it would be clear that a normative standard is not valid. On the other hand, it is also possible that a normative standard may overestimate the degree of competence required by a learner with severe disabilities. In a study of peer-tutor and special friend interactions within a high school setting (Haring, Breen, et al., 1987), the peers assessed had overwhelmingly positive levels of social acceptance, yet this group of adolescents with autism, severe mental retardation, and multiple sensory impairments displayed social behavior that was significantly non-normative in nearly all natural contexts. Thus, the critical questions concerning the validity of social skills interventions might not be answered by traditional social validity assessments that are based on expert ratings or normative standards. The preferable approach is to base the judgment of social validity on the reactions of the peers with whom the student interacts or the people whom the student encounters as part of a stable social network.

A Priori Assessment of Peer Response Patterns

Future demonstrations designed to shape social relationships should include more fine-grained analyses of peer social interaction patterns prior to the design of interventions. As discussed earlier, the use of ethnographic and interview methodologies have been demonstrated to be particularly suited to this task. An example of this approach was modeled within the study conducted by Haring et al. (1986). Within that study, peers were extensively interviewed prior to intervention to identify the topics of conversation that typically occurred within given contexts in the school as well as specific ways of introducing topics or greeting friends within those contexts. In another example of collecting data to build validity into training in an a priori way, Haring, Breen, and Laitinen (1989) taught age-appropriate clothing selection skills to 3 adolescent girls attending integrated schools. Clothing selection skills were targeted for instruction because previous research had demonstrated that social acceptance was determined in part by physical appearance (Strain, 1985). Within the study by Haring et al. (1989), a group of 20 peers from the students' school was asked to rate items from a catalog to determine age and situational appropriateness prior to intervention. Items that were rated as appropriate by at least 80% of the peers were selected as training examples. Clearly, such standards change from school to school and from school year to school year. These procedures can be considered as directly analogous to environmental inventories of functional skills. That is, skills—including social skills—cannot be considered functional until the characteristics of the environment are assessed to determine whether that specific setting will support those skills, whether the specific responses identified for training have a use in the setting, and whether the resultant behaviors will enhance the social image of that person in the perception of typical interactants within that setting.

Assessment of Sociometric Status

Another important addition for future research in this area is to develop new procedures to assess, in a dynamic fashion, changes in the sociometric status of students. For example, in the template matching procedure, each of the peers filled out brief questionnaires concerning their perceptions of each of the interactions. While less frequent assessment than this might be more desirable in school-based programs, this type of assessment allows periodic feedback as to the changing strength of the relationships between students as an ongoing process.

Another method that deserves further development is to assess the degree of peer responsiveness to the social initiations of target students. This strategy can be used to identify interventions that result in more positive responses and extend the duration of interactions. For example, Haring and Lovinger (1989) assessed the responsiveness of peers to the initiations of students with severe disabilities within integrated preschool and kindergarten programs. The typical students' affective responses (e.g., enthusiastic inclusion into play or rejection of the social bid) were recorded. Following baseline, two interventions—a peer initiation intervention and a

play training intervention—were introduced. The results indicated that while both procedures increased the overall level of social interaction, the play training procedure resulted in the most favorable peer responses to the initiations by the students with disabilities. Thus, the study represents a preliminary effort to link social skills interventions to the more affective elements of social acceptance.

Methods to Assess Social Networks

A critically needed element in the development of social relationships for persons with severe handicaps is the development of methods to assess the formation of friendship patterns. Peer nomination scales are the most commonly used method of sociometric assessment (Cartledge & Milburn, 1986). When conducting peer nominations in the traditional manner, students are asked, for example, to identify the three students they like best and the three they like least. From these data, it is possible to diagram patterns of friendships, identify cliques, identify popular and unpopular students, and determine how well integrated a student is into the social networks of the school. Unfortunately, there has been little work to date in identifying peer nomination procedures that could be used in integrated programs for persons with severe handicaps, although Strain (1984) has conducted some important preliminary work in this area within integrated preschools.

In conducting peer nomination measures (Asher & Taylor, 1981), students are asked to nominate those within their class with whom they would participate in various activities or those who, in their perception, fit various criteria. For example, Hiroshige (1989) interviewed elementary-age children with questions such as: 1) "Whom would you like to play with?" 2) "Who are your friends?" and 3) "Who would you invite to your birthday party?" In conducting the survey, students are asked to list at least three children for each question.

An advantage of using peer nomination scales is that it is possible to "map" the interrelationships between students in order to determine structural relationships between and within peer groups or cliques. For example, some students can be described as "stars" in that they have the highest rates of nominations by others and tend to form nodal points within such peer nomination networks. Some students are nominated occasionally and are located on the periphery of a group; other students are rarely nominated, and when they are, it is not clear that they fit into any one peer group or clique.

As stated, peer nomination scales have not received substantial validation in use with students with severe handicaps. This is unfortunate in that the use of these scales requires some degree of field testing to determine questions and response forms that are appropriate for different age levels. In addition, as peer nomination items are developed to assess the degree of friendship and participation of persons with severe handicaps within supported education settings, it may be important to validate items that assess not only "best friend" relationships, as is typical when responses are limited to three nominations per item, but also various degrees of acquaintanceships.

In addition to assessing the formation of a stable friendship network within the school, it would also be important to assess the formation of more casual relationships with other nonhandicapped people within the student's neighborhood and community. As with other assessments of social relationships, once a method to assess peer social networks is developed, the next step will be to link such assessments with the identification, instruction, and validation of social skills interventions.

SUMMARY AND CONCLUSION

The creation of social relationships is emerging as one of the most critical outcomes of integrated programming. This chapter has indicated that a sufficient technology of intervention and assessment exists to promote these outcomes more actively. However, although a variety of instructional procedures and models to support relationships exist, there continues to be a paucity of empirical demonstrations that show that the application of these models and procedures will cause increases in the number and strength of social relationships. The use of these technologies to create social networks has not been evaluated.

To create expanded opportunities for social relationships it is important to evaluate not only school-based friendships, but the entire range of social interactions within the context of stable social networks within the home and community.

The following are some specific implications relevant to the concerns of practitioners and parents:

1. *Physically integrated placements are necessary, but not sufficient, for achieving social integration.* Fortunately, a variety of models such as friendship programs and the use of integration facilitators such as circles of friends can be used to increase the probability of social integration. One of the greatest needs for future research is to provide more thorough evaluations and demonstrations of social support mechanisms.

2. *The objectives and results of social skills training programs must be evaluated in terms of their meanings to peers, not adults.* This means that social skills interventions need to be planned in consultation with peers to identify skills that in their view would most enhance participation and likability. In addition, the results of social interaction training programs need to be evaluated in terms of increased participation in stable social relationships. We can no longer be satisfied with the acquisition of skills that are not demonstrated within the context of participation in activities with friends.

3. *Social performance may be enhanced by changing aspects of the social environment as well as by providing increased opportunities for interaction and skill instruction.* Variables such as increasing peer responsiveness, and increasing the climate of acceptance in a school are important considerations "beyond the level of the dyad."

4. *There is a great need for the development of evaluation models that can assess changes in social networks and document the degree of social participation in integrated environments and in supported education.* Although increased use of such methods is needed by researchers, a more important need is to develop simple, database systems that can be used by teachers to develop and monitor social interaction networks.

5. *The creation of social relationships needs to be viewed as a main effect of instruction, not*

as a side effect. That is, as instruction is planned in community settings, integrated classrooms, and school settings, the support and creation of relationships needs to be considered as important as the acquisition of functional skills. Students with severe handicaps should have the right both to instruction of relevant skills needed for more independent living and to support in developing and maintaining social relationships.

A critical issue for the future is to consider more closely the impact of instructional programming on quality of life. Models to create and support relationships as well as more socially valid efforts at social interaction instruction offer considerable potential to shape wider social networks and higher quality interactions. The formation of stable social networks is as important to the achievement of integrated lifestyles as any other major endeavor in the field. While a sufficient organizational and instructional foundation currently exists to develop social relationships and integrated lifestyles more fully, many individuals with severe handicaps continue to lead lives that are functionally segregated. As the concept of integration is expanded to include social as well as functional integration, as social skills training begins to be better referenced to increases in social acceptance, and as we develop better methods to assess the formation of social networks, broader opportunities for establishing friendships will be created and the quality of life experienced by people with severe handicaps will be concomitantly improved and normalized.

REFERENCES

Asher, S.R., & Taylor, A.R. (1981). Social outcomes of mainstreaming: Sociometric assessment and beyond. *Exceptional Education Quarterly, 1,* 13–40.

Baer, D.M., Wolf, M.M., & Risley, T.R. (1987). Some still-current dimensions of applied behavior analysis. *Journal of Applied Behavior Analysis, 20,* 313–328.

Baldwin, M.L. (1983). *Establishing reciprocity in play within dyads of severely handicapped students.* Unpublished doctoral dissertation, University of California–Berkeley.

Barker, R.G. (1968). *Ecological psychology: Concepts and methods for studying the environment of human behavior.* Stanford, CA: Stanford University Press.

Barker, R.G., Wright, H.F., Barker, L.S., & Schoggen, M. (1961). *Specimen records of American and English children.* Lawrence: University of Kansas Press.

Bercovici, S. (1981). Qualitative methods and cultural perspectives in the study of deinstitutionalization. In R.H. Bruininks, C.E. Meyer, B.B. Sigford, & K.C. Lakin (Eds.). *Deinstitutionalization and community adjustment of mentally retarded people* (pp. 133–144). Washington, D.C.: American Association on Mental Deficiency.

Berler, E.S., Gross, A.N., & Drabman, R.S. (1982). Social skills training with children: Proceed with caution. *Journal of Applied Behavior Analysis, 15*(1), 41–53.

Black, N., Freeman, B.J., & Montgomery, J. (1975). Systematic observation of play behavior in autistic children. *Journal of Autism and Developmental Disorders, 5,* 363–371.

Brady, M.P., Shores, R.E., Gunter, P., McElvoy, M.A., Fox, J.J., & White, C. (1984). Generalization of an adolescent's social interaction behavior via multiple peers in a classroom setting. *Journal of The Association for Persons with Severe Handicaps, 9,* 278–286.

Brandt, R.N. (1972). *Studying behavior in natural settings.* Lanham, MD: University Press of America.

Breen, C., Haring, T.G., Pitts-Conway, V, & Gaylord-Ross, R. (1985). The training and genralization of social interaction during breaktime at two job sites in the natural environment. *Journal of The Association for Persons with Severe Handicaps, 10,* 41–50.

Breen, C., & Lovinger, L. (1989, December). *PAL (Partners At Lunch) Club: Evaluation of a program to support social relationships in a junior high school.* Paper presented at the 16th Annual TASH Conference, San Francisco.

Bronfenbrenner, U. (1979). *The ecology of human development.* Harvard University Press.

Brown, F., Evans, I.M., Weed, K.A., & Owen, V. (1987). Delineating functional competencies: A component model. *Journal of The Association for Persons with Severe Handicaps, 12,* 117–124.

Brown, W.H., Bryson-Brockman, W., & Fox, J.J. (1986). The usefulness of J.R. Kantor's setting event concept for research on children's social behavior. *Child and Family Behavior Therapy, 8,* 15–25.

Cairns, R.B. (1979). *Social development: The origins and plasticity of interchanges.* San Francisco: W.H. Freeman.

Carr, E.G., & Durand, V.M. (1985). Reducing behavior problems through functional communication training. *Journal of Applied Behavior Analysis, 18,* 111–126.

Carr, E.G., & Kologinsky, E. (1983). Acquisition of sign language by autistic children II: Spontaneity and generalization effects. *Journal of Applied Behavior Analysis, 16,* 297–314.

Cartledge, G., & Milburn, J.F. (1986). *Teaching social skills to children: Innovational approaches.* Elmsford, NY: Pergamon Press.

Chadsey-Rusch, J., & Gonzales, C. (1988). Social ecology of the workplace: Employer perceptions versus direct observations. *Research in Developmental Disablities, 9,* 229–245.

Chadsey-Rusch, J., & Rusch, F.R. (1988). Ecology of the workplace. In R. Gaylord-Ross (Ed.), *Vocational education for persons with handicaps* (pp. 234–256). Palo Alto, CA: Mayfield.

Dattilo, J., & Rusch, F.R. (1985). Effects of choice on behavior: Leisure participation for persons with severe handicaps. *Journal of The Association for Persons with Severe Handicaps, 10,* 194–199.

Donder, D., & Nietupski, J. (1981). Nonhandicapped adolescents teaching playground skills to their mentally retarded peers: Toward a less restrictive middle school environment. *Education and Training of the Mentally Retarded, 16,* 270–276.

Downing, J. (1987). Conversational skills training: Teaching adolescents with mental retardation to be verbally assertive. *Mental Retardation, 25,* 147–155.

Endler, N.S., & Magnusson, D. (1976). Toward an interactional psychology of personality. *Psychological Bulletin, 83,* 956–974.

Erikson, E.H. (1959). *Identity, youth, and crisis.* New York: Norton.

Falvey, M. (1988, December). *Research on quality characteristics of friendship between students with severe handicaps and their peers without handicaps.* Symposium conducted at the 15th Annual TASH Conference, Washington, DC.

Forest, M. (1987). *More education/integration: A further collection of readings on the integration of children with mental handicaps into the regular school system.* Downsview, Ontario: The G. Allan Roeher Institute, York University.

Fox, J., Shores, R., Lindeman, D., & Strain, P. (1986). Maintaining social initiations of withdrawn handicapped and nonhandicapped preschoolers through a response-dependent fading tactic. *Journal of Abnormal Child Psychology, 14,* 387–396.

Gartner, A., & Lipsky, D.K. (1987). Beyond special education: Toward a quality system for all students. *Harvard Educational Review, 57,* 367–395.

Gaylord-Ross, R., & Haring, T. (1987). Social interaction research for adolescents with severe handicaps. *Behavioral Disorders, 12,* 264–275.

Gaylord-Ross, R.J., Haring, T.G., Breen, C., & Pitts-Conway, V. (1984). The training and generalization of social interaction skills with autistic youth. *Journal of Applied Behavior Analysis, 17,* 229–247.

Gaylord-Ross, R.J., & Pitts-Conway, V. (1984). Social behavior development in integrated secondary autistic programs. In N. Certo, N. Haring, & R. York (Eds.), *Public school integration of severely handicapped students: Rational issues and progressive alternatives* (pp. 197–219). Baltimore: Paul H. Brookes Publishing Co.

Goffman, E. (1963). *Stigma: Notes on the management of spoiled identities.* Englewood Cliffs, NJ: Prentice-Hall.

Gold, M.W. (1980). *Try Another Way training manual.* Champaign, IL: Research Press.

Greenwood, C.R., Dinwiddie, G, Bailey, V., Carta, J., Dorsey, D., Kohler, F.W., Nelson, C., Rotholz, D., & Schulte, D. (1987). Field replication of classwide peer tutoring. *Journal of Applied Behavior Analysis, 20,* 151–160.

Greenwood, C.R., Walker, H.M., Todd, N.M., & Hops, H. (1981). Normative and descriptive analysis of preschool freeplay social initiation rates. *Journal of Pediatric Psychology, 4,* 343–367.

Guess, D., & Siegel-Causey, E. (1985). Behavioral control and education of severely handicapped students: Who's doing what to whom? and why? In D. Bricker & J. Filler (Eds.), *Severe mental retardation: From theory to practice* (pp. 230–244). Washington, DC: Council for Exceptional Children.

Halle, J.W. (1987). Teaching language in the natural environment: An analysis of spontaneity. *Journal of The Association for Persons with Severe Handicaps, 12,* 28–37.

Halle, J., Marshall, A., & Spradlin, J. (1979). Time delay: A technique to increase language use and facilitate generalization in retarded children. *Journal of Applied Behavior Analysis, 12,* 431–439.

Haring, T.G., Breen, C.G., & Laitinen, R. (1989). Stimulus class formation and concept learning: Establishment of within- and between-set generalization and transitive relationships via conditional discrimination procedures. *Journal of the Experimental Analysis of Behavior, 52,* 13–25.

Haring, T.G., Breen, C., Lee, N., Pitts-Conway, V., & Gaylord-Ross, R.J. (1987). Adolescent peer tutoring and special friend experiences. *Journal of The Association for Persons with Severe Handicaps, 12,* 280–286.

Haring, T.G., Breen, C.G., Weiner, J., Bednersh, F., & Kennedy, C.H. (1988). *The effects of concurrent vs. serial teaching application of videotape modeling on generalized pruchasing skills.* Manuscript submitted for publication.

Haring, T.G., Kennedy, C.H., Adams, M.J., & Pitts-Conway, V. (1987). Teaching generalization of purchasing skills across community settings to autistic youth using videotape modeling. *Journal of Applied Behavior Analysis, 20,* 89–96.

Haring, T.G., & Lovinger, L. (1989). Social interaction through teaching generalized play initiation responses to children with autism. *Journal of The Association for Persons with Severe Handicaps, 14,* 58–67.

Haring, T.G., Neetz, J.A., Lovinger, L., Peck, C., &

Semmel, M.I. (1987). Effects of four modified incidental teaching procedures to create opportunities for communication. *Journal of The Association for Persons with Severe Handicaps, 12,* 218–226.

Haring, T.G., Roger, B., Lee, M., Breen, C., & Gaylord-Ross, R.J. (1986). Teaching social language to moderately handicapped students. *Journal of Applied Behavior Analysis, 19,* 159–171.

Hart, B.M., & Risley, T.R. (1968). Establishing use of descriptive adjectives in the spontaneous speech of disadvantaged preschool children. *Journal of Applied Behavior Analysis, 1,* 109–120.

Hart, B.M., & Risley, T.R. (1975). Incidental teaching of language in the preschool. *Journal of Applied Behavior Analysis, 3,* 411–420.

Hart, B.M., & Risley, T.R. (1980). In vivo language interventions: Unanticipated general effects. *Journal of Applied Behavior Analysis, 13,* 407–432.

Hendrickson, J.M., Strain, P.S., Trembly, A., & Shores, R.E. (1982). Interactions of behaviorally handicapped children: Functional effects of peer social initiations. *Behavior Modification, 6,* 323–353.

Hiroshige, J.A. (1989). *Effects of direct instruction of social skills and peer facilitation on free play at recess of students with physical disabilities.* Unpublished doctoral dissertation, University of California–Santa Barbara.

Hoier, T., & Cone, J.D. (1987). Target selection of social skills for children. *Behavior Modification, 11,* 137–163.

Horner, R.D. (1980). The effects of an environmental "enrichment" program on the behavior of institutionalized profoundly retarded children. *Journal of Applied Behavior Analysis, 13,* 473–493.

Horner, R.H., Meyer, L.H., & Fredericks, H.D.B. (Eds.). (1986). *Education of learners with severe handicaps: Exemplary service strategies.* Baltimore: Paul H. Brookes Publishing Co.

Hunt, P., Alwell, N., & Goetz, L. (1988). Acquisition of conversation skills and the reduction of inappropriate social interaction behaviors. *Journal of The Association for Persons with Severe Handicaps, 13,* 20–27.

James, S.D., & Egel, A.L. (1986). A direct prompting strategy for increasing reciprocal interactions between handicapped and nonhandicapped siblings. *Journal of Applied Behavior Analysis, 19,* 173–187.

Kaiser, A.P., Alpert, C.C., & Warren, S.F. (1987). Teaching functional language: Strategies for language intervention. In M.E. Snell (Ed.), *Systematic instruction of persons with severe handicaps* (pp. 247–272). Columbus, OH: Charles E. Merrill.

Kantor, J.R. (1959). *Interbehavioral psychology.* Granville, OH: Principia Press.

Kantor, J.R. (1981). *Interbehavioral philosophy.* Chicago: Principia Press.

Koegel, R.L., Dyer, K., & Bell, C.K. (1987). The influence of child-preferred activities on autistic children's social behavior. *Journal of Applied Behavior Analysis, 20,* 243–252.

Koegel, R.L., O'Dell, M., & Dunlap, G. (1988). Producing speech use in nonverbal autistic children by reinforcing attempts. *Journal of Autism and Developmental Disorders, 18,* 525–538.

Kohl, F.L., Moses, L.C., & Stettner-Eaton, B.A. (1984). A systematic training program for teaching nonhandicapped students to be instructional trainers of severely handicapped schoolmates. In N. Certo, N. Haring, & R. York (Eds.) *Public school integration of severely handicapped students: Rational issues and progressive alternatives* (pp. 185–195). Baltimore: Paul H. Brookes Publishing Co.

Lalli, J.S. (1988, May). *Teaching social language skills to decrease inappropriate verbalizations.* Paper presented at the annual meeting of the Association for Behavior Analysis, Philadelphia.

Lancioni, G.E. (1982). Normal children as tutors to teach social responses to withdrawn mentally retarded schoolmates: Training, maintenance, and generalization. *Journal of Applied Behavior Analysis, 15,* 17–40.

Lane, H. (1988). Is there a psychology of the deaf? *Exceptional Children, 55,* 7–21.

McDonnell, J. (1987). The effects of time delay and increasing prompt hierarchy strategies on the acquisition of purchasing skills by students with severe handicaps. *Journal of The Association for Persons with Severe Handicaps, 12,* 227–236.

McGee, G.G., Krantz, P.J., Mason, D., & McClannahan, L.E. (1983). A modified incidental-teaching procedure for autistic youth: Acquisition and generalization of receptive object labels. *Journal of Applied Behavior Analysis, 16,* 329–338.

McGee, G.G., Krantz, P.J., & McClannahan, L.E. (1985). The facilitative effects of incidental teaching on preposition use by autistic children. *Journal of Applied Behavior Analysis, 18,* 17–31.

McHale, S., & Simeonsson, R.J. (1980). Effects of interaction on nonhandicapped children's attitudes about autistic children. *American Journal of Mental Deficiency, 85,* 18–24.

McKinney, J.P., Fitzgerald, H.E., & Strommen, E.A. (1982). *Developmental psychology: The adolescent and young adult.* Homewood, IL: Dorsey Press.

Meyer, L. (1985, December). *Friendships, or why nonhandicapped children should be friends rather than peer tutors.* Paper presented at the 12th Annual TASH Conference, Boston.

Meyer, L.H., Eichinger, J., & Park-Lee, S. (1987). A validation of program quality indicators in educational services for students with severe disabilities. *Journal of The Association for Persons with Severe Handicaps, 12,* 251–263.

Michael, J. (1986). Repertoire-altering effects of remote contingencies. *Analysis of Verbal Behavior, 4,* 10–18.

Moon, S.M., & Bunker, L. (1987). Recreation and motor skills programming. In M.E. Snell (Ed.),

Systematic instruction of persons with severe handicaps (pp. 214–244). Columbus, OH: Charles E. Merrill.

Moos, R.H. (1973). Conceptualizations of human environments. *American Psychologist, 28,* 652–665.

Moos, R.H. (1974). *Evaluating treatment environments: A social ecological approach.* New York: John Wiley & Sons.

Odom, S.L., Hoyson, M., Jamieson, B., & Strain, P.S. (1985). Increasing handicapped preschoolers' peer interaction: Cross-setting and component analysis. *Journal of Applied Behavior Analysis, 18,* 3–17.

Odom, S.L., & McEvoy, M.A. (1988). Integration of young children with handicaps and normally developing children. In S.L. Odom & M.B. Karnes (Eds.), *Early intervention for infants and children with handicaps: An empirical base* (pp. 241–267). Baltimore: Paul H. Brookes Publishing Co.

Odom, S.L., & Strain, P.S. (1986). A comparison of peer-initiation and teacher antecedent interventions for promoting reciprocal social interaction of autistic preschoolers. *Journal of Applied Behavior Analysis, 19,* 59–72.

Peck, C.A. (1986). Increasing opportunities for social control by children with autism and severe handicaps: Effects on student behavior and perceived classroom climate. *Journal of The Association for Persons with Severe Handicaps, 10,* 183–193.

Peck, C.A., & Cooke, T.P. (1983). Benefits of mainstreaming at the early childhood level: How much can we expect? *Analysis and Intervention in Developmental Disabilities, 3,* 9–22.

Peck, C.A., Tomlinson, C., Schuler, A.C., Theimer, R.K., & Haring, T. (1984). *The social competence curriculum project: A guide to instructional programming for social interactions* (Contract No. 300-83-0353). Washington, DC: U.S. Office of Special Education.

Roger, B., Haring, T.G., Lee, M., & Gaylord-Ross, R. (in preparation). *Promoting integration and social interaction through the development of a nonhandicapped friendship program.*

Rogers-Warren, A., & Warren, S.F. (1980). Mands for verbalization: Facilitating the display of newly taught language. *Behavior Modification, 4,* 361–382.

Romer, D., & Heller, T. (1983). Social adaptation of mentally retarded adults in community settings: A social-ecological approach. *Applied Research in Mental Retardation, 4,* 303–314.

Sasso, G.M., Hughes, G.G., Swanson, H.L., & Novak, C.G. (1987). A comparison of peer initiation interactions in promoting multiple peer initiators. *Education and Training in Mental Retardation, 22,* 150–155.

Sasso, G.M., & Rude, H.A. (1987). Unprogrammed effects of training high-status peers to interact with severely handicapped children. *Journal of Applied Behavior Analysis, 20,* 35–44.

Skinner, B.F. (1957). *Verbal behavior.* New York: Appleton-Century-Crofts.

Stokes, T.F., Baer, D.M., & Jackson, R.L. (1974). Programming the generalization of a greeting response in four retarded children. *Journal of Applied Behavior Analysis, 7,* 599–610.

Storey, K., Bates, P., & Hanson, H.B. (1984). Acquisition and generalization of coffee purchase skills by adults with severe disabilities. *Journal of The Association for Persons with Severe Handicaps, 9,* 178–185.

Strain, P.S. (1984). Social behavior patterns of nonhandicapped and handicapped-developmentally disabled friend pairs in preschools. *Analysis and Intervention in Developmental Disabilities, 4,* 15–28.

Strain, P.S. (1985). Social and nonsocial determinants of acceptability in handicapped preschool children. *Topics in Early Childhood Special Education, 4,* 47–58.

Strain, P.S., Cooke, T.P., Apolloni, T. (1976). *Teaching exceptional children: Assessing and modifying social behavior.* New York: Academic Press.

Strain, P.S., & Fox, J.J. (1981). Peer social interactions and the modification of social withdrawal: A review and future perspective. *Journal of Pediatric Psychology, 6,* 417–433.

Strain, P.S., Kerr, M.M., & Ragland, E.V. (1979). Effects of peer-mediated social initiations and prompt reinforcement procedures on the social behavior of autistic children. *Journal of Autism and Developmental Disorders, 9,* 41–54.

Strain, P., Shores, R.E., & Kerr, M.M. (1976). An experimental analysis of "spillover" effects on the social interaction of behaviorally handicapped preschool children. *Journal of Applied Behavior Analysis, 9,* 31–40.

Strully, J., & Strully, C. (1985). Friendship and our children. *Journal of The Association for Persons with Severe Handicaps, 10,* 224–227.

Sulzbacher, S., Haines, R., Peterson, S.L., & Swatman, F.M. (1984). How to encourage appropriate coffee break behavior. *Teaching Exceptional Children, 19,* 8–12.

Voeltz, L.M. (1980). Children's attitudes toward handicapped peers. *American Journal of Mental Deficiency, 84,* 455–464.

Voeltz, L.M. (1982). Effects of structured interaction with severely handicapped peers on children's attitudes. *American Journal of Mental Deficiency, 86,* 180–190.

Wahler, R.G., & Fox, J.J. (1981). Setting events in applied behavior analysis: Toward a conceptual and methodological expansion. *Journal of Applied Behavior Analysis, 14,* 327–339.

Wildman, B.G., Wildman, H.E., & Kelly, W.J. (1986). Group conversational skills training and social validation with mentally retarded adults. *Applied Research in Mental Retardation, 7,* 443–458.

Wolfensberger, W. (1972). *The principle of normaliza-*

tion in human services. Toronto: National Institute on Mental Retardation.

Wolfensberger, W. (1983). Social role valorization: A proposed new term for the principle of normalization. *Mental Retardation, 21,* 254–259.

Wuerch, B.B., & Voeltz, L.M. (1982). *Longitudinal leisure skills for severely handicapped learners: The Ho'onanea curriculum component.* Baltimore: Paul H. Brookes Publishing Co.

Young, C.C., & Kerr, M.M. (1979). The effect of a retarded child's initiations on the behavior of severely retarded school-aged peers. *Education and Treatment of the Mentally Retarded, 14,* 185–190.

Zetlin, A.G., & Turner, J.L. (1985). Transition from adolescence to adulthood: Perspectives of mentally retarded individuals and their families. *American Journal of Mental Deficiency, 89,* 570–579.

◇ **CHAPTER 12** ◇

Integrated Work
A Rejection of Segregated Enclaves and Mobile Work Crews

Lou Brown
Alice Udvari-Solner
Elise Frattura-Kampschroer
Louanne Davis
Charlotte Ahlgren
Patricia Van Deventer
Jack Jorgensen

University of Wisconsin–Madison and Madison Metropolitan School District, Madison, Wisconsin

When people who are not intellectually disabled are of concern, the a priori cultural assumption is that they should be integrated into all aspects of community life. In fact, complex legal and political safeguards have been established to ensure that citizens without intellectual disabilities function in integrated environments to the greatest extent possible. When people with severe intellectual disabilities are of concern, the a priori cultural assumption is that they must start segregated and then earn or otherwise justify their way into integrated community life. The issue here is the need for the resources and safeguards necessary for all citizens to participate fully in one extremely important part of integrated living—the workplace.

Since World War II, the life expectancies of almost all people in North America have increased dramatically (Siwolop & Mohs, 1985). The cultural solution to the problem of what to do with increasing numbers of adults with severe intellectual disabilities was to confine them to segregated day programs. In 1950, only 6 shel-

tered workshops were operative in the United States; in 1984 there were almost 5,000 (Buckley & Bellamy, 1985; Nelson, 1971). Davis (1987) reported growing waiting lists and many efforts to increase the capacity of existing facilities and to build new ones. Obviously, the majority of adults with severe intellectual disabilities who enter segregated facilities do not move to integrated environments. In fact, studies of the movement of workers from segregated to integrated settings reveal that only 1%–3% actually do so (California Department of Finance, 1979; Minnesota Developmental Disabilities Council, 1982; Zivolich, 1984). In effect, the placement of an adult who is severely intellectually disabled in a segregated day facility has been a sentence to confinement for life. Furthermore, the vast majority of those so confined have regressed and underachieved, and have been denied opportunities to experience interactions with non-disabled people in a healthy variety of integrated environments.

In the early 1970s, the treatment of people

This paper was supported by Grants #G008630388 and #H029D80019 to the University of Wisconsin and the Madison Metropolitan School District from the U.S. Department of Education, Office of Special Education and Rehabilitative Services, Divisions for Educational Services and Personnel Preparation. An expanded version is contained in Brown, L., Udvari-Solner, A., Frattura-Kampschroer, E., Davis, L., & Jorgensen, J. (Eds.). (1987). *Educational programs for students with severe intellectual disabilities, Vol. XVII.* Madison, WI: Madison Metropolitan School District.

with intellectual disabilities was analyzed, and insightful and valid observations that they were unnecessarily excluded, devalued, denied, over-protected, and harmed were made. In response, it was concluded that if such individuals were to be allowed a decent chance in life, many of the attitudes, values, expectations, laws, and regulations associated with their rights, abilities, and opportunities had to change. One way to guide the needed changes was to attempt to live by what became known as the "principle of normalization," which requires that an individual with disabilities be treated and respected as a typical person and integrated into the normal rhythms of everyday life (Nirje, 1969; Wolfensberger, 1972).

The ideology of integration is now being applied to the world of work. In fact, each year more parents/guardians, advocates, and others realize: 1) that the people they represent must be given the chance to do real work next to non-disabled co-workers, 2) that segregation is becoming tremendously expensive and taxpayers are clamoring for more cost-efficient options, and 3) that governmental units are changing laws and regulations and making opportunities and resources available so people with severe intellectual disabilities can be given access to integrated work (Will, 1984a, 1984b).

DAYTIME OPTIONS
CURRENTLY UTILIZED

The nine major daytime options experienced by adults with severe intellectual disabilities are:

1. Home
2. Institution
3. Nursing home
4. Activity center
5. Sheltered workshop
6. Retarded business
7. Mobile work crew
8. Enclave
9. Individually appropriate integrated work environment

Since the goal here is to enhance quality of life through integration, absorption, and support, options 1 through 8 are judged inherently unacceptable. Arguments against the use of the ubi-

quitous sheltered workshop and activity center options have been articulated elsewhere (Brown, Shiraga, Ford, et al., 1986; Brown, Shiraga, York, et al., 1984; The Association for Persons with Severe Handicaps, 1983). Soon segregated workshops and activity centers will be historical footnotes. Unfortunately, some of them are being replaced by segregated enclaves and mobile work crews.

Any benefit that can be realized in segregated enclaves or crews can also be realized in individually appropriate integrated work environments (option 9). However, there are many benefits that can be realized in individually appropriate integrated work environments that can never be realized in enclaves or crews. Thus, enclaves and crews are unnecessarily restrictive.

Trach and Rusch (1987) defined an enclave as "a group of six to eight persons who work as a team at a specific location in a community business or industry" (p. 5); a mobile work crew is referred to as "a small group of three to five persons who work out of a van at several locations in the community with the supervision of a job coach" (p. 5). While variations in size and other characteristics exist across professionals (Bellamy, Rhodes, Mank, & Albin, 1987), these two definitions seem reasonable for purposes here.

Brown, Udvari-Solner, et al. (1987) offered three basic characteristics of an integrated work environment. *First,* if mathematically possible, the general work environment must be naturally proportioned. That is, since approximately 1% of the general population is considered severely intellectually disabled, no more than approximately 1% of all workers who function in a general work environment can be severely intellectually disabled. *Second,* no more than two people with disabilities can function in any immediate work environment. *Third,* a worker with disabilities must function within sight, sound, and reasonable distance of nondisabled co-workers.

Rigid adherence to the natural proportion criterion may be difficult and actually inappropriate under some circumstances. Nevertheless, it is better to err on the side of a natural proportion than it is to accept, tolerate, or attempt to justify violations. A factory, which is considered a general work environment, may employ 500 nondisabled people and 5 with severe intellectual disabilities. A superficial analysis might result in the judgment that the environment is naturally proportioned and therefore integrated. However, a more careful analysis might reveal that the five people with disabilities are: confined to a separate area, supervised 100% of the time by paid professionals, allowed only segregated lunches and breaks, and restricted to social situations in which individualized interactions with non-disabled people are improbable. Thus, while the factory may be naturally proportioned, the immediate work and related environments are segregated and must be redesigned so that no more than two people with disabilities function in sight, sound, and reasonable distance of nondisabled co-workers.

COMPARING THE INTEGRATED WORK ENVIRONMENT AND ENCLAVE OPTIONS

As enclaves and mobile work crews are considered ideologically interchangeable, so the term *enclave* is used here to represent both. A three-step strategy is used to contrast the enclave and the individually appropriate integrated work environment options:

First, five important dimensions that can be used to evaluate aspects of the life space of a worker with severe intellectual disabilities are considered: 1) nature and cost of supervision, 2) nature and cost of transportation, 3) opportunities for work enhancement, 4) opportunities for social relationships, and 5) personalized matching of a worker to a work environment. *Second,* ideological values associated with each dimension are presented. *Third,* the dimensions and the associated values are discussed to contrast the enclave and the individually appropriate integrated work environment options.

Nature and Cost of Supervision

Supervision refers to the time, instruction, assistance, and other personal supports for a worker with severe intellectual disabilities to function effectively in integrated work and related environments. *Artificial supervision* refers to the supports provided that are not available to nondisabled co-workers. In addition, artificial

supervision is paid for with tax and other dollars to which nondisabled co-workers do not have access. *Natural supervision* refers to a worker functioning acceptably with supervision provided primarily by nondisabled co-workers and employers as unobtrusive parts of their typical work routines.

Values

1. Prior to entrance, a prospective environment must offer reasonable opportunities for co-workers without disabilities to assume natural supervisory responsibilities as unobtrusive parts of their typical work routines.

2. When a worker first enters an integrated environment, paid professionals must provide artificial supervision. In addition, the worker should have access to the same training opportunities available to co-workers, if appropriate.

3. The nature of the artificial supervision initially provided must be systematically faded, but can rarely, if ever, be terminated.

4. The goal must be to provide the highest quality of natural supervision and the least artificial supervision at the most reasonable costs over long periods of time.

Discussion

Supervision in enclaves is typically provided by a paid job coach, which is artificial supervision. Bellamy et al. (1987) described supervision in an enclave as "a group of persons with disabilities work[ing] in sufficient proximity to make coordinated training and support services available at all times, not just during the initial training period" (p. 22).

In any work environment that contains more than two people with disabilities the probability of developing natural supervision is limited and the need for long-term and cost-inefficient artificial supervision is maximized for four major reasons. *First,* continuous supervision by paid job coaches prohibits co-workers without disabilities from learning and assuming natural supervisory responsibilities (Hagner, 1988). In fact, the mere presence of a special someone who is paid to supervise often signals to others that it is not their role to be involved. *Second,* a nondisabled co-worker would in all likelihood be unwilling and/or unable to assume natural supervision for more than two workers with disabilities. Even if a nondisabled worker did agree to supervise a group of workers with disabilities, it would almost always disrupt and detract from his or her own productivity. *Third,* when workers with disabilities receive artificial supervision "at all times," many receive it regardless of whether it is needed. *Fourth,* since the nature of an enclave impedes the involvement of nondisabled co-workers in natural supervisory activities and since a job coach is always present, supervision costs rarely decrease over time (Thompson & Wolf, 1989).

Individually appropriate integrated work environments allow reasonable opportunities to develop high-quality, cost-efficient supervision because the process of arranging for a worker with disabilities to function in an integrated environment requires the job developer to evaluate the possibilities of unobtrusive natural supervision. If the development of unobtrusive natural supervision is not feasible, an alternative environment is sought. In addition, the job coach and the employer agree that the artificial supervision provided at the outset will be faded and replaced with individually appropriate amounts and kinds of natural supervision. However, even though supervision by nondisabled co-workers develops and the need for a paid job coach is reduced, the job coach is rarely, if ever, completely removed. The time and money once used for continuous paid supervision can then support other job coach functions, such as providing opportunities for work enhancement and building social relationships in the workplace. Further, as natural supervision increases, more workers can be served by one job coach, which can reduce the average cost of supervision over time.

Nature and Cost of Transportation

Complementary and efficient relationships between where one lives and where one works are important for success in the workplace. Thus, any discussion of transportation to and from work must include information about the nature of the associated domestic environment. Supported family-style homes and apartments that contain no more than two unrelated people with disabilities are the clearly preferred domestic options (Johnson, 1985; Taylor, Racino, Knoll, &

Lutfiyya, 1987). Conversely, group homes and other domestic environments that contain more than two unrelated people with disabilities are rejected. In addition to containing only one or two people with disabilities, supported apartments and homes must be distributed naturally within a community. A neighborhood or area of approximately 1,000 people should contain no more than two geographically dispersed supported homes or apartments.

Values

1.   Work environments should be as close as possible to a worker's home.
2.   Working is so important to personal dignity and cultural respect, anything reasonable must be done to ensure that an individual can get to and from a decent job.
3.   Every community has a finite amount of financial and other resources that can be devoted to the vocational functioning of adults with severe intellectual disabilities. Thus, the less money spent on transportation to and from work, the more money available for other important services or to serve others.
4.   If a worker truly needs a personal attendant, a specialized vehicle, and/or other extraordinary and relatively costly services to get to and from work, so be it.
5.   Whenever reasonable, a worker should use the transportation systems and services used by others who are not disabled.
6.   The supervision and social relationships experienced going to and from work should be the same as those available to nondisabled people, whenever appropriate.

Discussion

When adults with severe intellectual disabilities live in supported homes and apartments that are naturally dispersed geographically, but work in enclaves, it is rare that more than one or two will live close to their place of work. This causes travel to become complicated, lengthy, and costly, and almost always requires artificial supervision. Unfortunately, a common reaction to such travel problems is to extend segregated thought and practice. That is, instead of using public buses, integrated car pools, walking, or other typical modes of transportation, a "special" van or bus is arranged. The image of a cluster of adults with disabilities riding in a cost-inefficient "retarded van" to and from their "retarded enclave" is ideologically unbearable.

Using special buses and vans allows workers with disabilities to be gathered from a wide variety of locations and delivered to an enclave. However, travel time is almost always unnecessarily excessive. Expending the least amount of time in transit is extremely important because many adults with severe intellectual disabilities also experience muscle contractions, spasticity, skin sensitivities, and other physiological difficulties. Functioning in mobility-limiting situations for long periods of time is often unhealthy and in some cases harmful. In addition, when given long periods of time with nothing meaningful to do, some engage in maladaptive actions.

One way to reduce the problems associated with excessive travel time is to create unnatural living environments close to the enclave (e.g., a group home). This close geographic proximity reduces travel time, but again there is the unnecessary, demeaning, and unwanted reality of six to eight adults with disabilities living in a group home and riding to and from an enclave in a "retarded van."

When adults with severe disabilities live in supported homes and apartments that are naturally dispersed geographically and work in individually appropriate integrated environments close to their homes, the least costly and the most typical transportation modes can be utilized. While a few will always need relatively costly specialized transportation options, such as adapted vans, most can learn to walk, wheel, share cabs, ride public buses, or ride in car pools with nondisabled people under natural supervisory conditions.

Certainly it could be argued that adults with disabilities can walk, ride public buses, and travel in integrated car pools to and from their segregated enclaves. They can. In fact, Rhodes and Valenta (1985) reported that all 8 members of an enclave at a biomedical equipment company learned to travel to their enclave in city buses. However, if they can learn to travel in the community with nondisabled people, they can learn to work next to nondisabled co-workers in integrated environments.

Opportunities for Work Enhancement

Work enhancement refers to opportunities to grow vocationally over time. *Horizontal enhancement* refers to opportunities to learn and perform increasing numbers of tasks within a particular difficulty range. *Vertical enhancement* refers to opportunities to learn and perform more complex and possibly higher paying tasks in a slightly more demanding difficulty range.

Values

1. Every worker should be given the opportunities and supports necessary to participate in at least two different activities per half-day of work.

2. Every worker should be given the opportunities and supports necessary to learn increasing numbers of tasks within a particular difficulty range (horizontal enhancement).

3. Every worker should be given the opportunities and supports necessary to learn to participate in work activities within a more demanding difficulty range (vertical enhancement). If a worker cannot function efficiently in a more demanding range, so be it; but opportunities for vertical career advancement must be accessible.

4. If a particular work environment does not allow for reasonable horizontal and vertical enhancement, it can rarely, if ever, be considered acceptable as a permanent placement.

Discussion

Some enclaves offer neither horizontal nor vertical enhancement. For example, there are enclaves in which workers with disabilities are required to put jackets on books or to construct one part of a wooden pallet during their entire work days and careers. In these situations, the range of tasks within a particular level of difficulty is extremely circumscribed and opportunities to learn more complex tasks at the next level of difficulty are essentially nonexistent.

Some enclaves offer horizontal, but not vertical, enhancement. A group of eight adults with intellectual disabilities cleaning the fifth floor of an office building or removing litter from a rest area along a road are examples. In these instances, a worker often has an opportunity to perform an array of tasks within the same level of difficulty such as sweeping, washing windows, picking up trash, and emptying waste baskets. However, he or she must engage in the same activities over extended periods of time, regardless of whether he or she wants, needs, or is capable of a vertical career move. In fact, in some enclaves a contractual arrangement is made for workers with disabilities to perform specific rudimentary tasks. Learning to perform tasks within a higher difficulty range is not allowed because a contract has not been negotiated to do so or because those tasks are being performed by nondisabled workers.

Integrated work environments offer better opportunities to learn new and more complex tasks over time than enclaves for three major reasons. *First,* as part of the initial job development process, the tasks available in a business are considered in relation to the short- and long-term enhancement needs of an individual. An environment that offers reasonable opportunities for horizontal and vertical enhancement is selected over one that does not. *Second,* an individualized enhancement plan can be agreed upon by all parties before work begins. During initial job development, the employer and job coach can select a cluster of tasks considered within the worker's current difficulty range. The worker then begins by learning to perform one task and adds to his or her repertoire until at least two can be performed per half-day of work. Subsequently, an individualized vertical enhancement plan can be designed and implemented. *Third,* one of the best ways to realize horizontal and vertical enhancement is to have an individual with disabilities work within sight, sound, and reasonable distance of a large number of nondisabled co-workers who are engaging in a wide variety of tasks. In such settings, nondisabled co-workers, job coaches, and others are likely to identify new job opportunities.

Opportunities for Social Relationships

Five positive personal interactions between a worker with severe intellectual disabilities and nondisabled co-workers are of concern.

1. *A work companion* is a nondisabled co-worker who teaches, monitors, or helps a worker who is disabled as he or she performs real work in an integrated environment. This assistance includes, but is not limited to, creating adaptations that enhance work performance, dispensing corrective feedback, checking the quality of completed work, and providing needed physical assistance.

2. *A lunch/dinner/break companion* is a nondisabled co-worker who functions with a worker who is disabled during lunch, dinner, or break times. While the nature of the relationship is primarily that of companionship, assistance may be provided.

3. *A before-work companion* is a nondisabled co-worker who socializes with a worker who is disabled before work begins.

4. *A friend* refers to a nondisabled co-worker who develops and maintains a personal relationship with a worker who is disabled. The relationship is reciprocal, shared, mutually satisfying, and extends to nonwork hours and days. The relationship is primarily social in nature and must be nurtured by frequent contacts over extended periods of time.

5. *A travel companion* is a nondisabled person, who may or may not be a co-worker, who travels in a car pool or on a public bus or train, or otherwise functions with a worker who is disabled as they go to and from work.

Values

1. The more disabled a worker, the more important it is that a wide variety of social relationships with nondisabled co-workers be developed.

2. Prior to the selection of a work environment, reasonable opportunities to develop at least the five kinds of social relationships previously delineated must be verified. If an environment disallows or impedes the development of these social relationships, an alternative must be secured.

3. Once a worker enters an environment, individualized, systematic, and long-term strategies that result in the development and maintenance of at least the five kinds of social relationships previously delineated must be designed, implemented, and evaluated.

4. Systematic interventions by paid supervisors will be necessary to arrange and verify

some social relationships. However, the role and presence of paid supervisors should be faded so that relationships are maintained and enhanced by nondisabled co-workers and the worker with disabilities.

5. Social relationships should not be confined to the days, hours, and places of work. They should also be expressed at office parties, office softball and bowling games, picnics, outings, banquets, and other functions that are parts of the camaraderie and spirit of the workplace.

Discussion

When a worker with severe intellectual disabilities functions in an enclave, the development of social relationships with nondisabled co-workers and others is unacceptably restricted for three major reasons. *First,* as the number of people with disabilities in an environment increases, the probability of nondisabled co-workers becoming personally involved with an individual decreases. Since enclaves contain more people with disabilities than almost any social environment can absorb, acceptable ranges of social relationships between enclave members and co-workers without disabilities rarely develop. *Second,* social relationships often emanate from sharing similar experiences gained in common environments and activities. As members of an enclave are set apart from nondisabled workers, many of the typical ways social relationships develop simply cannot be actualized. *Third,* social relationships develop best from individual knowledge, frequent personal contacts, unique combinations of interpersonal styles, privacy, sharing, and trust. Enclaves with their "special boss" are perceived as unnatural in that they are dramatically different from conditions under which nondisabled workers function. These different conditions engender feelings of separateness and groupness, a sense of "us versus them," and social barriers few can overcome.

When a worker functions in an individually appropriate integrated work environment, developing the five kinds of desired social relationships is more probable because the social milieu of a work environment is examined carefully prior to selection. If the development of a reasonable range of social relationships is improbable, the environment is not considered for use. In addition, no more than two workers who are dis-

abled function in the immediate work environment. Under such conditions, nondisabled co-workers who are able and willing to interact are identified, and calculated actions that facilitate the development of social relationships are made. Then, a plan for fading specialized interventions in order to allow the maintenance, monitoring, and enhancement of the relationships is designed, implemented, and evaluated.

Personalized Matching of a Worker to an Environment

The process of determining the unique characteristics of a worker with disabilities and then arranging for effective functioning in an integrated environment that is complementary, enhancing, and supportive is referred to as *personalized matching.* Three personalized matching strategies are of concern.

1. In the *natural match strategy,* comprehensive and valid information about a particular worker is gathered. Then, with the specific worker in mind, comprehensive and valid information about a large number of potential work environments and activities is gathered. If the information clearly indicates the characteristics of the work environment are compatible with the characteristics of the worker, the environment is selected for use. That is, as substantial changes either in the environment or in the worker do not seem necessary, a "natural" match is considered to exist.

2. In the *change the environment strategy,* comprehensive and valid information about a particular worker is gathered. Then, with the specific worker in mind, comprehensive and valid information about a large number of potential work environments and activities is gathered. In some cases, a particular environment is not quite acceptable for use. However, specific changes that will make it more compatible with the unique characteristics of the worker can be made efficiently and expeditiously. The changes are made, an acceptable match is engineered, and the environment is then considered usable.

3. In the *change the worker strategy,* comprehensive and valid information about a particular worker is gathered. Then, with the specific worker in mind, comprehensive and valid information about a large number of potential work

environments and activities is gathered. After considering both clusters of information, it is determined that the demands of a particular environment are inflexible. However, if specific changes in the worker can be made, a compatible match can be generated and so the environment is selected for use. Teaching a worker to use a specialized device that allows the completion of a task within required rate and quality standards and assisting a worker to choose clothing in accordance with company dress codes are examples of this strategy.

Values

1. Comprehensive and valid information about the personal preferences and other unique physical, intellectual, social, and behavioral characteristics of a worker must be gathered.

2. Then, with a particular worker in mind, comprehensive and valid information about a large number of potential vocational environments and activities must be gathered.

3. Finally, after considering all information gathered, a personalized match between a worker and a work environment must be arranged.

Discussion

When personalized matching is considered, enclaves are particularly unacceptable for two major reasons. *First,* only a very restricted range of work environments can tolerate enclaves. Thus, thousands of businesses and even entire communities are overlooked as viable work options because they simply cannot absorb a group of individuals with disabilities. *Second,* when the procedures used to arrange most enclaves are examined, personal and family preferences and other unique characteristics of a worker rarely guide the selection of the work environment and activities. In most instances, the work environment and tasks are preselected and then an individual is forced to fit in. In fact, a strategy typically used to develop enclaves has been outlined by Rhodes and Valenta (1985) and Trach, Rusch, and DeStafano (1987). Specifically, a job developer conducts a community survey to identify potential work environments. Then, specific businesses are contacted and the possibility of employing a group of people with disabilities is discussed. When an employer expresses a willingness to employ a group of workers with disabilities, a contract is negotiated. The work environment is then examined to determine the work performance criteria and social skills necessary to function therein. Workers are then secured to perform the agreed-upon tasks. This strategy almost always lacks the individualization so necessary for personalized job matching. In fact, it is the inverse of the strategy recommended here.

Meaningful personalized matching is more likely in integrated work environments because businesses that can absorb one or two individuals with disabilities are more numerous than those that can absorb a group. If a job coach has access to large numbers of potential work environments, the chances of arranging an acceptable personalized match increase. In addition, personalized matching is inherent to the procedures used to find and develop integrated work environments. That is, comprehensive and valid information about the worker and a variety of vocational environments and activities is gathered. Then, the personal preferences and other unique characteristics of the worker drive the selection of the environment and activities. When a job is developed with an individual worker in mind, the chance of a successful match is greater than when an environment is secured and then a worker is required to meet the associated demands.

SUMMARY AND CONCLUSIONS

On the one hand, consider the young woman with severe intellectual disabilities who rides to and from her job at a local bank in a car pool with nondisabled neighbors. When she arrives at the bank, she "hangs out" with her friends until it is time to punch in. She engages in work activities that were selected based upon her preferences and abilities next to her nondisabled co-workers. She is the only worker with disabilities there and almost all of the supervision she receives comes from nondisabled co-workers. However, occasional assistance is provided by a job coach. Initially, she learned a small set of tasks, but over time she took advantage of opportunities to learn several tasks that were more complex and difficult. She has developed a wide range of social relationships with her co-workers that are actualized before, during, and after work. In sum, she enjoys her job, performs it acceptably, cherishes her interactions with the nondisabled people with whom she works, is safe and comfortable in the surroundings, and is looking forward to the future.

To some, the fact that she has severe intellectual disabilities and works in a bank is remarkable because the cultural stereotype requires that we view her as nonproductive, in need of shelter and someone who is paid to watch her at all times. Fortunately, we now know that individuals with severe intellectual disabilities can and should function in the integrated world of work and that to deny them the opportunity is unfair. Finally, one of the most important purposes of a 21-year public school career is to prepare a student with severe intellectual disabilities to live, work, and play in integrated environments throughout adulthood.

On the other hand, consider the ideological and curricular absurdities of a longitudinal special education program designed to prepare a young woman with severe intellectual disabilities for functioning in an enclave. We could teach her to ride a public bus, to function in an integrated car pool, or to traverse busy streets in her wheelchair. But why bother? When she graduates, a special van with six other people with disabilities will pick her up and take her to and from her enclave. We could teach her to function in a socially acceptable manner with nondisabled students prior to the start of school. This might help her function with nondisabled co-workers prior to the start of work. But why bother? In her enclave she will interact only with six other people with disabilities. We could teach her to work next to nondisabled co-workers. But why bother? In her enclave she is going to be in a special area of the workplace and only six other people with intellectual disabilities will be near her. We could teach her to function in response to the guidance and assistance offered by nondisabled people who are not specifically paid to monitor her. But why bother? A job coach will be in her enclave watching her all the time. We could teach her to take breaks, eat lunch, and go to parties and other social functions with nondisabled people. But why bother? The disabled members of her enclave will eat, take breaks, and socialize together, and they will be unable to establish meaningful social relationships with nondisabled co-workers. In sum, we could teach her to be a citizen in an integrated world, but if she is going to be segregated for life in an enclave, why bother?

REFERENCES

Bellamy, G.T., Rhodes, L.E., Mank, D.M., & Albin, J.M. (1987). *Supported employment: A community implementation guide*. Baltimore: Paul H. Brookes Publishing Co.

Brown, L., Shiraga, B., Ford, A., Nisbet, J., Van Deventer, P., Sweet, M., York, J., & Loomis, R. (1986). Teaching severely handicapped students to perform meaningful work in nonsheltered vocational environments. In R. Morris & B. Blatt (Eds.), *Special education: Research and trends* (pp. 131–189). New York: Pergamon Press.

Brown, L., Shiraga, B., York, J., Kessler, K., Strohm, B., Rogan, P., Sweet, M., Zanella, K., Van Deventer, P., & Loomis, R. (1984). Integrated work opportunities for adults with severe handicaps: The extended training option. *Journal of The Association for Persons With Severe Handicaps, 9*(4), 262–269.

Brown, L., Udvari-Solner, A., Shiraga, B., Long, E., Davis, L., Verban, D., Van Deventer, P., & Jorgensen, J. (1987). The Madison strategy for evaluating the vocational milieu of a worker with severe intellectual disabilities: Version II 1988. In L. Brown, A. Udvari-Solner, E. Frattura-Kampschroer, L. Davis, & J. Jorgensen (Eds.), *Educational programs for students with severe intellectual disabilities* (Vol. XVII, pp. 1–372). Madison, WI: Madison Metropolitan School District.

Buckley, J., & Bellamy, G.T. (1985). National survey of day and vocational programs for adults with severe disabilities: A 1984 profile. In P. Ferguson (Ed.), *Issues in transition research: Economic and social outcomes* (pp. 1–12). Eugene: University of Oregon, Specialized Training Program.

California Department of Finance. (1979). *A review of sheltered workshops and related programs (Phase II): To Assembly Concurrent Resolution No. 2067* (Vol. II, Final Report). Sacramento: State of California.

Davis, S. (1987). *A national status report on waiting lists of people with mental retardation for community services*. Arlington, TX: Association for Retarded Citizens of the United States, National Headquarters.

Hagner, D. (1988). *The social interactions and job supports of employees with severe disabilities within supported employment settings.* Unpublished doctoral dissertation, Syracuse University, Syracuse, NY.

Johnson, T.Z. (1985). *Belonging to the community.* Madison: Wisconsin Council on Developmental Disabilities.

Minnesota Developmental Disabilities Council. (1982). *Policy analysis series: Issues related to Walsch v. Noot* (Paper No. 9). St. Paul, MN: Author.

Nelson, N. (1971). *Workshops for the handicapped in the United States.* Springfield, IL: Charles C Thomas.

Nirje, B. (1969). The normalization principle and its human management implications. In R. Kugel & W. Wolfensberger (Eds.), *Changing patterns in residential services for the mentally retarded* (pp. 179–195). Washington, DC: President's Committee on Mental Retardation.

Rhodes, L.E., & Valenta, L. (1985). Industry-based supported employment: An enclave approach. *Journal of The Association for Persons With Severe Handicaps, 10*(1), 12–20.

Siwolop, S., & Mohs, M. (1985, February). The war on Down syndrome. *Discover,* pp. 67–69.

Taylor, S., Racino, J., Knoll, J., & Lutfiyya, Z. (1987). *The nonrestrictive employment: On community integration for people with the most severe disabilities.* Syracuse, NY: Human Policy Press.

The Association for Persons with Severe Handicaps. (1983). *Position statement on employment for per-*

sons with severe handicaps. Seattle, WA: Author.

Thompson, L., & Wolf, S. (1989). *Supported employment in Michigan: Impact upon persons with severe disabilities—interim report.* Kalamazoo: Western Michigan University, College of Arts and Sciences, The Supported Employment Evaluation Project.

Trach, J.S., & Rusch, F.R. (1987). *Supported employment in Illinois: Program implementation and evaluation* (Vol. I). Urbana-Champaign: University of Illinois, Secondary Transition Intervention Effectiveness Institute.

Trach, J.S., Rusch, F.R., & DeStafano, L. (1987). Supported employment program development: Degree of implementation manual. In J.S. Trach & F.R. Rusch (Eds.), *Supported employment in Illinois: Program implementation and evaluation* (Vol. I, pp. 17–50). Urbana-Champaign: University of Illinois, Secondary Transition Intervention Effectiveness Institute.

Will, M. (1984a). *OSERS programming for the transition of youth with disabilities: Bridges from school to working life.* Washington, DC: U.S. Office of Special Education and Rehabilitative Services.

Will, M. (1984b). *Supported employment services: An OSERS position paper.* Washington, DC: U.S. Department of Education.

Wolfensberger, W. (1972). *The principle of normalization in human services.* Toronto: National Institute on Mental Retardation.

Zivolich, S. (1984). *Regional Center of Orange County survey of day activity programs and developmental centers.* Unpublished manuscript, Regional Center of Orange County, Anaheim, CA.

CHAPTER 13

What's Wrong with the Continuum?
A Metaphorical Analysis

COLLEEN WIECK
Governor's Planning Council on Developmental Disabilities, St. Paul, Minnesota

JEFFREY L. STRULLY
Association for Retarded Citizens in Colorado, Denver, Colorado

An essay describing the problems of the traditional continuum allows us to avoid lengthy reviews of literature on the topic, appropriate citations, and American Psychological Association (APA) style. We have chosen two metaphors to illustrate our concerns with the continuum. The first metaphor should appeal to all air travelers, mostly professionals who fly in and out of states to discuss their latest book. The second metaphor should have a universal appeal because it focuses on "Dr. Ruth–type" sexual guidelines to describe continuum dysfunctions.

CONTINUUM AS AN AIRLINE

Background

The continuum is really a misnomer since it really never meant a continuous series of services. The continuum contained a certain set of fixed points in the areas of education, residences, and adult day programs. For example, in public schools, there were 24-hour state-operated residential schools, special segregated schools, special wings within school buildings, special classrooms within buildings, and special itinerant services. In the residential continuum, there were special 24-hour state-operated institutions, nursing homes, congregate care, community intermediate care facility for the mentally retarded (ICF/MR) services, group homes, supervised apartments, foster care, and living on your own. In day program services, there were day-care settings, day activity programs, day treatment, therapeutic treatment, work components, work activity, sheltered work, enclaves, work stations, and competitive placements.

During the 1970s, several national leaders had a set of overheads depicting the ideal continuum. The diagrams contained a set of boxes drawn along a line from margin to margin. Big boxes represented large-size programs, often reserved for people with the most severe disabilities, while small boxes were less restrictive and served people with mild handicaps. The key to understanding the continuum is that people had to move through the series of buildings or boxes in order to become independent or more independent. Movement depended on earning through learning developmental tasks, achievement of tasks, and graduation to the next level.

Expectations were fixed in the continuum approach. People with the least handicaps and mild disabilities had the best services, best personnel in terms of ratios and training, best surroundings, best materials, and best potential for success. People with the most severe disabilities experienced the opposite. These individuals had the worst services, least services, newest personnel with the poorest ratios and poorest training, worst surroundings, worst materials, and worst potential to succeed.

If progress was not made by individuals in the continuum approach, there would be five consequences. All of these consequences would make conditions worse for people with disabilities:

1. More goals and objectives were added to the individual plan.
2. People stayed in the same placement or were moved backward.
3. Emphasis was placed on personal failure, not environmental failure.
4. New training programs were added.

5. New "kits" from special education catalogues were purchased.

Flying the Unfriendly Skies

As airline travel has become more "user un-
friendly," it is fitting to compare the continuum
with air travel. The continuum has as many
problems as the airlines. Beginning at the federal
level, there are two similar bureaucracies created
to oversee operations. Both the Federal Aviation
Administration (FAA) for airlines and the Health
Care Financing Administration (HCFA) for the
residential continuum have great powers, but
they often approach problems with a certain rigidity and ineffectiveness. The inspections are
not frequent, timely, or thorough. Both agencies
are designed to meet the needs of people; however, both are engrossed in paper shuffling, both
are criticized for not assuring safety, and both
are bogged down in rules and regulations.

If we were to assign labels to the boxes on the
residential continuum using airline jargon, a
Boeing 747 jumbo jet would be considered the
institution. Airline personnel commonly refer to
these craft as "cattle cars." When any service is
that large, then personalized, individualized services are least likely to occur. A McDonnell
Douglas DC-10 is smaller than a 747 but is still
large. There are lots of people who were sent
from a large public institution to a large community facility. People were transferred from one
size to the next, just one size smaller. The Boeing 727 and 737 are smaller than the others but
are still large. Smaller planes are not as homogeneous; some have two seats on one side and three
seats on the other. Again, with the continuum
model, the transfer is always to the next smaller
size. If people finally graduate or can afford a
change, then services can become smaller and
smaller until you fly solo.

The management structure is similar in both
settings. There is a chief executive officer (CEO)
or pilot, a program director or navigator, and
flight attendants or direct care staff. The most
highly trained, best-paid individuals are CEOs.
There is no career ladder in either option. If you
begin in direct care or as a flight attendant, there
is low probability of becoming a pilot or CEO.
Administrators stay behind closed doors during
working hours just as the flight crew stays away

from passengers on the airline. Occasionally
people chat with the pilot or CEO, but usually
those people are either very important or very
rich.

In order to determine where you would fit on
the plane or in the residential continuum, an assessment is necessary. People who travel first
class tend to be those with the least handicaps.
These are the individuals with the most options,
flexibility, and choices (especially food and bev-
erages); who have the most opportunity to get
up, stretch, and move around; and who receive
personalized services. If you are seated in the
middle or the coach, you are probably a person
with moderate disabilities. If you are at the back
of the plane, you are someone with the most severe disabilities. Movement to the front or off
the plane occurs if you learn lots of new skills or
get better. It is hard to learn new skills or get better when you are sitting in a group of nine people, 45 rows away from the front of the line. The
back of the plane has very poor flight attendant-
to-passenger ratios, is often served leftover magazines, or has no services. There is only one exit
from this model, which is very slow but very orderly. Some services on the plane or in the residential continuum come at additional cost, such
as supports and personal services (music, movie,
drinks).

If you do earn your way off the plane, you
would be immediately boarded onto the next
plane to start over. This time there may be six
people in the row and a few less rows, but you
still have to earn your way through. If you travel
often enough, you may be eligible for frequent
flyer coupons or token economies. This means
that you have succeeded at being miserable and
that entitles you to more of the same.

Some individuals can receive more individualized services if they can afford private, exclusive services offered in a Lear Jet or private residential setting on the East Coast. Flying on the
Lear Jet may cost $5,000, while residential rates
are comparable for the month. If the family or
individual wants to be less extravagant, there are
always Piper Cubs or residential services in the
Midwest. Privacy curtains might separate the
passengers rather than more elaborate means.

For those who cannot get any residential care,
respite care would be comparable to a kite, avail-

able locally or borrowed from friends. The Home and Community-Based Waiver is slightly more adventuresome, and comparable to skydiving or hot air balloon rides.

In order to enter the plane or the continuum, there are certain procedures that must be followed. First, you must begin with a ticketing agent or eligibility technician. You can tell them your destination, but they are more interested in forms and numbers. Their idea of quality is processing as many people as possible without eye contact. If your plans do not fit, too bad. The rules are set by someone else. There are lines, and the waiting is unbearable. Sometimes people wait in one line when they should be in another line.

You can leave your luggage or worldly possessions with a skycap or case manager, but you will again lose your identity. You will be just another case number or ticket stub. You are never assured that you will ever get your possessions back. You can carry your possessions with you but you are limited to one bag that meets size specifications. Once on board you are allowed to touch your possessions only during certain periods.

There are times when you are given a standby status, which means you are on a waiting list. Waiting lists occur because planes fill up and there is little movement off. People do not get better, they do not graduate; nor are they interested in a later flight, or coupons for even later flights. In other words, once on board, people do not leave.

Everyone must wait in the terminal. The continuum approach ends here for many people. It is ominous but accurate to say that the continuum is terminal; for many people, it is a dead end with no place to go and no movement.

Departure time can be admission dates and arrival times can be discharge dates. How many times have you heard the following phrases, which describe the status of both flyers and people with disabilities:

Eventually
Not now
Whenever
Most likely
Ultimately
Sometime soon
Sometime
Not yet
By and by
Before long
Anytime
Imminent
Later
About now

The dates and periods must be extended because of air-traffic-controller problems. In this case, the controllers are the three levels of government—local, state, and federal officials. Each level of government gives different directions to the pilots or providers. Traffic delays can be due to funding inadequacies, regulatory contradictions, work slowdowns, strikes, and walkouts. When planes are stacked up and circling, there is stagnation and no one is moving through the continuum. People may spend an eternity on some planes. An equal number may be on standby for years to get onto planes or into services that are out of date and inappropriate. Canceled flights probably mean there is a problem with the provider, instability of services due to low per diems, or labor unrest. The extent of active treatment is limited to the wrong tasks, self-stimulation, and cards.

If major problems do develop, there are limited oxygen masks and seat cushions that convert to life preservers, which are temporary remedies only.

For your own safety, you are forced to sit in an uncomfortable seat, strapped in, discouraged from moving around, exploring, or socializing. You are forced to live with others based on no particular criteria except random assignment. Some get outside views or windows, some get leg room, while others get stuck in the middle. Remember—choices are limited in the continuum. You are forced to fit into slots or preexisting services offered by a provider. Take it or leave it.

Not much happens during a flight or stay. There may be some turbulence. It is a boring time with little stimulation. The environment is totally controlled, including temperature, lighting, interior colors, standard-issue blankets, and pillows. The rattling of food trays and the beverage cart causes a break in the monotony. Meals cause some people to get excited, but only temporarily. High-calorie food keeps people lethargic. There is no family-style dining. People simply sit and wait and sit and wait.

Privacy is nonexistent. There is crowding. Bathrooms are very functional with little privacy, limited toilet paper, and stainless steel fixtures for easy cleaning. If you want to sleep, you are usually in an uncomfortable position. There are never enough pillows and blankets for everyone. Seatbelts become restraints.

The staff often talk as if you are not there. If you have a special request, you are told to wait. When fulfilling the request, you are referred to by an identification code: " '6C' wants tea," " '12D' needs change." The staff are mechanical in their conversations. Natural voice inflections are missing. Repetition and perseveration occur throughout the shift. "Coffee? Coffee? Coffee? Coffee? Coffee?"

New staff or flight attendants try harder. At the beginning, you receive training. Unfortunately, you are taught skills you already know. There are no competency-based tests. Everyone is subjected to seatbelt-buckling lessons whether needed or not.

What is needed is a shift from the continuum to supporting individuals in settings that match need, capacity, interests, and preferences. Airline service is only expected to get worse. We must change our way of thinking about the continuum and move toward a different approach.

CONTINUUM AS PERPETUAL FOREPLAY

The continuum is a lot like perpetual foreplay. People with disabilities try and try, but they never really get to the good stuff. People are forced to stay in certain situations, are allowed to practice with simulated objects, are allowed to watch movies, and can self-actualize until they reach a certain level of performance before they take the next step to nirvana or the big "0" outcomes. The continuum may have made sense 10 or 20 years ago; but as we head into the next century, it is time to stop fooling around and get down to the good stuff. It is time for the "forgotten generation" to become the "me generation"

and have a home, have a career, learn together in regular education classes in their own neighborhoods, have friends, play, and have intimate relationships. The time has come to do away with the continuum.

Edifice Complex

Our human services system and the continuum is based on one major tenet—buildings. Owning a building is wonderful. Owning a series of buildings that people can move in and out of is great. Our system has bought, sold, and leased more buildings than Donald Trump and Harry Helmsley. Our system has been based not on individual needs but on the real estate market. Special buildings for special people. Administrators yearn to be real estate brokers, owners of chains, and land barons. Whenever you go on a tour of a special building, the administrator points out all the rooms, improvements, and planned remodeling. Rarely will a tour focus on people, friendships, and continuity of supports. There is an obsession with bricks and mortar, the continuum aphrodisiac. Our system is deeply mired in funding methodologies, rate structures, financing, mortgages, fair market values, and property allowances. The continuum perpetuates buildings. We need to stop thinking about real estate and start thinking about a moratorium on special construction so that we can focus on *people*.

Based on our collective experience, we have yet to meet any individual who needs a group home because of their 21st chromosome. We know people who need a home of their own, a place to live, a house with some special accommodations or adaptations. Playboy mansions are similar to large community ICF/MR services—people rarely call them home.

The time has come to stop thinking about real estate, fixed assets, buildings, and land prices. It is time to think about people and regular housing stock.

Test Your Erogenous Quotient

When you enter the continuum model of services, you must be assessed. This is similar to going to a newsstand and buying Playboy or Cosmopolitan and taking the latest quiz. "Are you a sensitive spouse?" "What do men (or women) really want?" It is our belief that assessment tools help the authors of the tests but rarely help the individuals tested. The current assessment tools in our field perpetuate the continuum. This is especially true for computerized assessments that can generate a profile on a person with multiple disabilities in 30 nanoseconds and prepare a computerized program plan in 10 microseconds. Assessment tools have become a come-on requiring high expenditures for cheap thrills. Buy a $500 package; spend $2,000 to receive training in Atlanta, Chicago, Las Vegas, or Los Angeles; use 50 hours of direct care time filling out checklists so that you can pinpoint deficiencies rather than strengths, capacities, and choices or preferences.

Assessments always come with manuals. These manuals can be illustrated or use photographs. The more explicit the manual, the more expensive. Color photos cost more than black and white or postcards. The manuals need to be rated like movies: PG = pretty good, R = restrictive settings, and X = Xeroxed from somewhere else. Assessment instruments always make people go through developmental sequences. In a similar fashion, people can progress through beginning stages of sexual expression to more advanced techniques. Unfortunately, stacking blocks, stringing beads, and assembling puzzles is not as stimulating.

Ménage à Trois

This is obviously the beginning number of a team meeting held at least once a year—unless people like harassment, then there may be two group sessions. This group experience occurs when several bodies are brought together—some may know each other, while others may be strangers—and people get to play around with other people's lives. These can be chance get-togethers such as going to a singles' bar. In some instances, there can be high-tech action with videotape equipment, one-way mirrors, and observers. Team meetings or group grope can bring people together to discuss someone they do not know, check each other out, do some talking, and then do drinks for relaxation.

Foreplay

The correct term for foreplay in human services for people with disabilities is *pre*. People must work on getting ready to live, learn, work, and play by going to *pre*living, *pre*academic, *pre*work, and *pre*recreation classes. Most human services programs have worked on preparing people for things that they usually do not need or want or could do without. A common theme song for performance anxiety is, "I Can't Get No Satisfaction."

Myth of Bigger is Better

For male readers only. The continuum concept is based on the assumption that intensive intervention services are provided to the most challenging individuals in the most segregated settings. People with less intensive needs can receive less service in integrated programs. The other assumption is that people who are the most challenging need to be grouped in large numbers in order to hire the right staff in massive quantities and types needed. In addition, there is the belief that the bigger the program, the more peers people with severe disabilities can have. Of course, the peers are people with equally severe disabilities. It is inconceivable that peers could be individuals without disabilities. All of these assumptions are false—after all, "Small is beautiful."

Sadomasochism

In the continuum, people who present significant behavior problems are grouped together, usually in some type of locked unit where there are at least one dozen psychologists who worship B.F. Skinner twice a day or bow to six-cycle logarithmic graph paper altars. It is all right to use intrusive interventions as long as we go through proper procedures. For example, documentation of the problem must occur followed by 12 forms explaining why lower level intervention will not work, then come the signatures from people who really do not care and family members who have been coerced into signing.

If people cannot get their behavior under control, then there are all kinds of bondage or assorted restraints available. Leaving restrictive settings is contingent on working out these problems first, even though the environment is the primary source of the behavior difficulties. It is a rare event when people envision someone with a severe behavior problem living in a less restrictive setting such as an apartment. Instead, peo-

ple visualize new units for special dually diagnosed individuals funded by both mental health
and mental retardation. Possibilities are endless
for new uses of old buildings.

Taboos

The continuum produces many problems that
can be briefly highlighted as deviations. Here are
some examples:

1. Exhibitionism refers to private providers
   who display their wealth ostentatiously from
   the continuum industry.
2. Inhibitions refer to people who do not express their true feelings about limited and
   inappropriate services.
3. Devices/gadgets/aids are offered in catalogues published by an "educational" publisher rather than Frederick's of Hollywood.
4. Voyeurs are those people who travel to other
   states to see best practices or those who watch
   university videos on integration.
5. Dysfunctions are waiting lists including
   people trying to enter the continuum, people trying to move to the next level, and
   people trying to get out of the continuum.
6. Infidelity means living in an ICF/MR but

flirting with the idea of owning your own
home.
7. Cohabilitation refers to living with at least
   two (individual) plans under the same roof.
8. Perversions are plentiful. Building bigger
   and bigger chains of ICF/MR services or developing state-operated community services
   are two prominent perversions.
9. Peep shows occur when licensing agents
   come once a year to determine "quality" by
   checking the water, square footage, and number of people to a bedroom.

FANTASIES: PICTURE A
WORLD WITHOUT A CONTINUUM

The continuum never made any sense—nor will
any other intellectual approach that does not put
the person at the center of the services. The continuum is important to those comfortable with
the status quo and for those who do not want to
see any changes. Picture a world where people
with all types of labels are truly connected with
people who do not have labels. Visualize and
dream about a world that is not overregulated,
overprofessionalized, overserviced, and overbuilt.

CHAPTER 14

Community Living
Lessons for Today

STEVEN J. TAYLOR

JULIE ANN RACINO

Syracuse University, Syracuse, New York

Over the past 5 years, we have studied community living programs for people with the most severe disabilities—the organizations, the practitioners, the lives of people with disabilities, the services and supports, and the governmental and community context. We have also had many opportunities to observe the participation of people with disabilities in the community—their relationships, their associations and activities, and the way in which informal networks and formal systems interact.

The most important lesson we have learned is that we continue to learn. As we traveled the country looking at innovative programs and services and working with states and agencies, we found ourselves constantly refining our thinking about community living, revising our assumptions about how communities and states work, and recalling lessons we previously learned. Let us tell you about some of the lessons as we know them today.

ON DEINSTITUTIONALIZATION

The issue of "institutions versus the community," which has dominated the attention of the field of developmental disabilities for nearly 20 years, is yesterday's issue. That people with severe disabilities can be served in the community is no longer an unproven proposition. An increasing number of places across the country have found ways to support people with the most challenging needs in the community. The primary issue today has to do with how to foster full participation in community life.

Deinstitutionalization is yesterday's issue in the sense that people are now being supported to live in the community. Yet, this is not to ignore the fact that over 90,000 people with mental retardation continue to be confined in public institutions and many more are living in private institutions, residential schools, and nursing homes. Formidable political and administrative obstacles stand in the way of fulfilling the spirit of TASH's resolutions on integration (see Documents II.1, II.2, II.3, and II.4, this volume). Many states continue to invest significant resources in segregated institutions, such as the building of small residential units on the grounds of state institutions in New York State.

ON THE LIMITATIONS
OF SERVICE SYSTEMS

Service systems cannot and should not attempt to provide everything that people need. When people with developmental disabilities rely exclusively on service systems, they cannot become part of their communities. The more service systems provide, the less other people, including family members and friends, may be involved in the person's life. No matter how caring or well intentioned, staff cannot fulfill all of people's needs for friendship and personal relationships.

If people with developmental disabilities are to form relationships with other people, if they are to become part of their community, agencies and staff must be prepared to play new roles. They must learn to support informal social net-

Partial support for this chapter was provided through Cooperative Agreement #G0085CO 3503 with the National Institute on Disability and Rehabilitation Research. The opinions expressed herein are solely those of the authors.

works and to build these networks where they do not exist. In order to do these things, agencies and staff will need to develop a clearer understanding of how relationships are formed and how communities work.

ON RELATIONSHIPS

To be part of the community is to have relationships and roles as a family member, neighbor, schoolmate, friend, casual acquaintance, co-worker, church member, club participant, and/or shopper. It also means experiencing the joys and downfalls of love, the fears and expectations of a new or developing relationship, and the security or discomfort of being known.

Relationships imply reciprocity, a mutuality of giving and receiving. People with developmental disabilities are often denied opportunities to give and contribute. Yet, people with developmental disabilities can and do contribute to communities and they initiate, develop, and maintain relationships with family, friends, and acquaintances. Often this occurs despite daily efforts to define people with developmental disabilities in terms of their deficits and their clienthood.

ON COMMUNITY

Community has many different meanings for people—from a spirit and feeling to a neighborhood or place. Being part of a community means being a part of something larger than yourself, something that touches the lives of other people. Whether it is health care or housing or education or jobs, a commitment to community includes, but does not highlight, people with disabilities. The challenge is to find what can bring us together—not what separates or pulls us apart.

This is not meant to imply that community members will always step forward and include people with disabilities. There will be setbacks and frustrations and times when community will be used as an excuse for denying services and supports to people with disabilities and their families. However, to move from a segregated society requires a new look at the acceptance and strengths that are already present in people and communities, but are often unrecognized and untapped.

ON SUPPORTS, NOT FACILITIES

The field of developmental disabilities has defined its mission in terms of creating specially designed *facilities*—first large ones and now smaller ones—and *programs* into which people must fit. When people with developmental disabilities grow and learn, they often must move from their home, no matter how much they care about the people with whom they live or their neighborhood. Often they must choose between a home in the community or the supports and services they need and desire.

It is time now to shift our attention to creating the supports, both formal and informal, that people with developmental disabilities need to live in a home and participate in the community. Agencies and staff will need to assume new roles in supporting families and people with disabilities to meet the challenges and share the joys of everyday life. Families and individuals with disabilities must move to the foreground, out of the shadow of facilities and programs.

ON FAMILIES AND THEIR CHILDREN

All children, regardless of the severity of their disability, belong in families. With advances in technology, practical experience, and a growing commitment, we can support children to live in birth, adoptive, or foster families, and to develop enduring relationships with adults.

Families know best what are the supports and services they need. These services should be a matter of entitlement, not charity. Families come in different sizes, shapes, and forms. Services should support the entire family as defined by the family, promoting quality lives for all family members. Agencies and staff need to understand better what it means to support families and how schools and other institutions have an impact on family life.

It is important to recognize the unique contributions, perspectives, strengths, and needs of families. At the same time, there must be an awareness that parents and their children may differ in their perspectives on many issues. Agencies and staff must support lifelong relationships between parents and their children, when mutually desired, and also support each child's increased autonomy in moving from adolescence to adulthood.

ON HOMES AND SUPPORTS

People with developmental disabilities, whether married or single, have a right to live in a home in the community. As with other people, they should live in regular housing, in neighborhoods of their choice, and with people of their own choosing. Although often excluded from these opportunities, they should have the option to lease or buy their own homes, to live in a place where their service provider is not their landlord, and to have control over their home environment.

People should be entitled to whatever supports and services are necessary to live in a regular home and participate in community life. People with disabilities and the people close to them are in the best position to define what they need and desire. All people can and do express choices and these should be respected and acted upon. Whenever possible, staff and agencies should work directly for people and be accountable to them. The main challenge today is to become better at understanding people's preferences.

ON LIVING A MEANINGFUL LIFE

The most important thing to know about people with developmental disabilities is that they are ordinary people. They have hopes and dreams, disappointments and sadness, and a way of understanding and relating to the world. This is not to ignore that disability is a difference, only that in addressing people's particular needs, we often lose sight of each individual's human complexity.

All people, whether with or without a disability, should be able to decide how they will live their lives. People with disabilities face the same decisions and complexities that all of us do: the definition of self; the meaning of life; relationships with parents, friends, and those who cross our paths; the daily routines and experiences; and the opportunities we seize, create, postpone, reject, or simply let pass by. The burden of proof must be placed on the government officials or outside parties who wish to curtail or limit the choices in the lifestyles of adults with disabilities.

Just as philosophers throughout the ages have not agreed on the meaning of life, so it is not possible to create a flow chart for life or to catalogue its important aspects. While efforts for pursuing the "good life" for people with disabilities are critical, the endeavor is no less complex than the one all people have faced throughout time.

ON PROFESSIONALS AND CHANGE

The field of developmental disabilities is preoccupied with changing people with developmental disabilities to "fit into" society, making communities more accepting, and educating parents. While these efforts are often full of caring and done with the best intentions, the underlying message seems to be that the world would be a better place if only parents, people with disabilities, and other ordinary people acted and thought more like professionals.

It is time to acknowledge in our day-to-day work that the full integration of people with disabilities will require all of us to change the way we think about schools, homes, work, health care, transportation, and recreation. We will need to see the capacities and strengths in communities and ordinary people as they exist in day-to-day life, drawing on those strengths for the betterment of all of us. To support these changes, agencies, staff, and professionals will need to take on new roles and work as equals with parents, people with disabilities, and ordinary citizens.

ON CHANGING SERVICE SYSTEMS

Change is slow and serendipitous. When it comes to complex human services systems, especially on the state and federal levels, it is impossible to predict with precision the outcomes of any new initiative. Every advance reveals new challenges. Every solution creates its own set of problems. Every plan encounters unanticipated problems in implementation. This is not to question attempts to change service systems. It is to suggest that there are no simple solutions to complex problems and that change can be an agonizingly slow and frustrating process. Change occurs in small steps, with many setbacks along the way.

TASH's work toward Medicaid reform is an important effort to increase the availability of flexible individual- and family-responsive services. While a critical step forward, Medicaid reform will also result in new issues, such as the problems encountered when family supports are funded through Medicaid, and other as yet unanticipated dilemmas.

ON GOVERNMENT

Since change is unpredictable, states, regions, and communities, for that matter, cannot control everything that happens within their borders. Entrenched bureaucracies, political controversies, and reluctant constituencies can thwart the most carefully thought out plans. Governments can create incentives and disincentives. They can encourage some things and discourage other things from happening. But they cannot mandate meaningful lives for people with developmental disabilities.

Many government programs stifle creativity. They create an atmosphere in which bureaucratic compliance is rewarded and innovation and risk taking are punished. Just as governments can inhibit innovation and creativity, they can also foster these things.

ON DIVERSITY

Diversity is a great strength, whether based upon ethnic, cultural, class, individual, or gender differences. Yet, supports, services, and even basic concepts may exclude or limit some people with disabilities from full participation in the community. More often than not, the people will be those who are already disenfranchised— the poor, people of color, and the oppressed of the society. To achieve a society that fully includes people with disabilities, diversity must not only be accepted, but actively fostered.

Without vigilant efforts, concepts that provide guidance on disability issues may undermine the efforts of other oppressed groups in this society.

To support families at the expense of the liberation of women, or people with developmental disabilities at the expense of reform movements for prisons, is to diminish all of us. Concepts that provide guidance for bettering the lives of all people will on a long-term basis benefit people with developmental disabilities.

ON CONCEPTS

Concepts, ideas, and principles can help us get from one place to another. Yet, they must be viewed in historical context. The ideas that guide us today can mislead us tomorrow. Concepts that should be able to move us beyond where we are today include:

Community integration
Informal supports
Friendships
Self-determination
Nonaversives
Own homes
Personal assistance
Circle of friends
Bridge building
Supported jobs
Building community
Choices
Community participation
Permanency planning
Housing and supports
Individualized and flexible supports
Life sharing

Concepts such as normalization, integration, and mainstreaming make sense only in a society where people with disabilities cannot move freely in and out of relationships and participate fully in the community. Having these concepts does not mean we have arrived; it only means that we recognize that people with developmental disabilities have been denied.

As times change, there arises a need to find new concepts and ideas suited to those times. We must be prepared to abandon old concepts and find new ones to guide us through the challenges and dilemmas we will undoubtedly face.

A REDEFINITION OF THE CONTINUUM OF SERVICES— ZERO EXCLUSION MODELS AND SUPPORTS

At the time that compulsory attendance laws were passed in the United States in the latter part of the 19th century, the schools were also compelled to expand the educational system to accommodate the many children and youth who had never before attended school. The majority of these youngsters did not have disabilities, though some might today be diagnosed as having mild disabilities. But it was perhaps inevitable that a class-graded instructional system charged with the responsibility to educate all students quickly moved to various forms of tracking and separating according to ability levels. Students with severe disabilities, for the most part, did not even enter this public school picture until much later, when PL 94-142 (1975) made it clear that everyone had a right to an education. By this time, separate schools and separate classes were the norm in special education, and even the mainstreaming of students with mild disabilities was not a simple matter.

Times have changed, and as the chapters in this section clearly show, there is now considerable evidence regarding the efficacy of integrated educational programs for students with severe disabilities in regular schools and classes. Yet, the "continuum of services" requirement of PL 94-142 is still most likely to be a continuum of increasingly restrictive placements rather than increasingly intensive resources provided to the student who needs them. How can we best enable all students—including those with the most severe disabilities—to attend the same school they would attend if they did not have disabilities *and* receive an individually appropriate education in the regular classroom with their age peers? How must related services be delivered to meet individualized needs in regular schools and classes? What kinds of supports are needed by families in order to keep their school-age child at home with his or her brothers and sisters? And how must the training of the various professionals involved in our educational system be changed to prepare them for the dramatic change from isolated schools and classes to working in the mainstream? The chapters in this section detail both the evidence and promising new ideas about the various components of supported education and the associated services needed during the school years by children and their families.

A REDEFINITION OF THE CONTINUUM OF SERVICES— Zero Exclusion Models and Supports

Resolution on the Redefinition of the Continuum of Services

Children and adults with severe disabilities require specialized and individualized services that traditionally have not been made available in typical school and other community environments. Instead, access to such services has been tied to categorical placements which increasingly isolate persons with disabilities from relationships with their family, peers, and other citizens. In the past, the concept of a continuum of services has been used to foster the notion that persons with severe disabilities must earn the right to lead integrated lives in the community. TASH believes therefore that a redefinition of the continuum is vitally needed.

The Association for Persons with Severe Handicaps believes that specialized and individualized services can be readily and effectively provided in integrated settings, and need not preclude opportunities to develop peer and other social relationships which are so critical to the achievement of full participation in society.

TASH further believes that effective methodologies and models which can be applied in integrated settings now exist, and that the focus of new significant and systematic research and development efforts should now be upon the development, implementation, validation, and dissemination of such alternatives to outdated practices which segregate persons with disabilities from their families, peers, and the community by requiring placement in handicapped-only and categorically-grouped services and settings.

THEREFORE, TASH calls for a redefinition of the continuum of services which emphasizes the attainment of the following characteristics and components:

1. The provision of specialized staff, resources, and services to meet individual needs in the regular classroom, neighborhood school, home and family, and community program and setting;

2. The substantive training and retraining of personnel, both special and generic service professionals—to prepare them for providing instruction to a variety of heterogeneous groups of learners;

3. The systematic shifting of service delivery design and services away from a categorical, homogeneously grouped, and separate model to one which requires integration and thrives on a variety of grouping arrangements;

4. The philosophical and administrative merger of special and regular education and specialized and generic services into one service delivery system, evidenced by the integration of both professional staff and students; and

5. An unambiguous model of the Least Restrictive Environment which is marked without exception by integration into normalized community environments and proximity to family and peers and other citizens who do not have disabilities.

FURTHERMORE, The Association for Persons with Severe Handicaps commits its resources and energies to support and promote such components of an integrated continuum of services, through advocacy, dissemination, research, training, and program development in collaboration with consumers, colleagues, families, professional training programs, research centers, and community services.

ORIGINAL RESOLUTION "I.Q. TESTS" ADOPTED OCTOBER 1979
REVISED NOVEMBER 1986

* * * * *

Position Statement of the Related Services Subcommittee of the TASH Critical Issues Committee

The Association for Persons with Severe Handicaps (TASH) is an international organization whose primary purpose is to advocate and support exemplary models of service delivery for persons with severe handicaps.

Many persons with severe handicaps have complex and challenging needs. The expertise of related services professionals, such as physical therapists, occupational therapists, and speech and language pathologists is frequently required.

TASH believes that related services personnel have expertise and can contribute in the process of integrating persons with severe handicaps into typical home and community life. A high degree of collaboration and sharing of information and skills must occur among families, direct service providers, and related services personnel.

The provision of integrated services requires that related services personnel:

1. Establish priorities with parents/advocates and other team members;
2. Observe and assess persons with handicaps in natural settings;
3. Collaborate with family and team members to provide intervention strategies and adaptations that optimize participation in natural settings;
4. Teach specific and individualized procedures to enhance functional positioning, movement, and communication abilities in natural settings;
5. Evaluate the effectiveness of intervention procedures based on performance outcomes in natural settings.

ORIGINALLY ADOPTED NOVEMBER 1986

*   *   *   *   *

Supported Education Resolution

WHEREAS, TASH policy states that people with disabilities must have the opportunity to achieve full integration into society.

WHEREAS, the Education for the Handicapped Act presumes that students with disabilities attend regular classes and schools, with appropriate supports.

WHEREAS, a number of schools, classes, and programs have effectively integrated students with severe disabilities and students with no disabilities, through supported education.

WHEREAS, many students with disabilities are prohibited from attending regular schools and classrooms or programs with peers who are not disabled.

WHEREAS, in some instances courts have failed to decide in favor of certain students with severe disabilities being integrated and have therefore allowed segregation of students with disabilities to continue.

BE IT RESOLVED THAT TASH affirms its support for students with severe disabilities by:

Working with parents to plan strategies to advocate for integrated education.

Calling upon the court systems to enforce the statutory obligation that students with severe disabilities be educated with students who have no disabilities.

Encouraging the U.S. Department of Education, the U.S. Justice Department, and state departments of education to enforce the presumption of integrated schooling for all students through supported education. Encouraging the U.S. Department of Education and state departments of education to foster the development of program models, research, and training on school, classroom, and program integration.

Encouraging schools and education departments to develop supportive education approaches to ensure that students with severe disabilities are educated with students who do not have disabilities.

Participating as amicus in litigation to achieve integration for students with disabilities.

ORIGINALLY ADOPTED DECEMBER 1988

* * * * *

◇   **CHAPTER 15**   ◇

Supporting the Education of Students with Severe Disabilities in Regular Education Environments

MICHAEL F. GIANGRECO
University of Vermont, Burlington, Vermont

JoANNE W. PUTNAM
University of Montana, Missoula, Montana

Over the past decade and a half, when the term "integration" has been applied to the education of students with severe disabilities, often it has meant placement in self-contained classes in general attendance elementary and secondary schools. Such placement may have included minimal interactions with nondisabled peers that typically took place in nonacademic settings and activities, such as the lunchroom, bus, playground, assemblies, and homeroom. Any participation in regular classes was generally restricted to the "specials" such as physical education, art, music, or the technical arts (e.g., shop). While the movement toward at least this level of integration signaled a vast improvement over placement in separate schools attended only by children with disabilities, the observed limitations and inequities of self-contained special classes have resulted in the challenge to develop a more inclusive model of school integration (McDonnell & Hardman, 1989; Taylor, 1988).

Beginning in the late 1980s and now into the 1990s, the term "integration" is increasingly being replaced by the phrase "full inclusion." Full inclusion refers to the provision of appropriate educational services to all students in regular classes attended by nondisabled students of the same chronological age in their neighborhood school, including students with severe disabilities. Like many other promising practices, the placement of students with severe disabilities in regular classes has been evolving. To date, congruence of regular class placement with the values inherent in PL 94-142 (Lipsky & Gartner, 1989, p. 4) and the logic embedded in the various curricular and programmatic components of a quality educational program (Fox et al., 1987; Meyer, Eichinger, & Park-Lee, 1987) have resulted in successful demonstrations of regular class integration (Ayres, 1988; Berres & Knoblock, 1987; Biklen, 1985, 1988; Brost & Johnson, 1986; Flynn & Kowalczck-McPhee, 1988; Ford & Davern, 1989; Ford, Foster, Searl, & Taylor, 1984; Forest, 1984, 1987; Giangreco & Meyer, 1988; G. Porter, 1988; Schattman, 1989; Thousand & Villa, 1989; Villa & Thousand, 1990; Williams et al., 1986). This evolution has reached the point where program descriptions are more widely available and empirical support has begun to emerge.

The main purpose of this chapter is to review existing literature on students with severe dis-

Partial support for preparation of this chapter was provided through the U.S. Department of Education, Office of Special Education and Rehabilitative Services, Demonstration Projects for Deaf-Blind Children and Youth (HO86H80017) awarded to the Center for Developmental Disabilities at the University of Vermont. The opinions expressed herein do not necessarily reflect the position or policy of the U.S. Department of Education, and no official endorsement should be inferred.

The authors wish to acknowledge Wes Williams, Lu Christie, Rich Villa, Jacque Thousand, and Gloria Kishi for their helpful feedback and suggestions during the preparation of this chapter.

abilities regarding the provision of appropriate special education services in regular education environments. Both the TASH Resolution on the Redefinition of the Continuum of Services (Document III.1, this volume) and the Supported Education Resolution (Document III.3, this volume) challenged the field to move beyond the earlier concept of separate classes in regular schools to the design, implementation, and validation of effective models of full inclusion into regular classrooms and the life of the school. Readers wishing a more detailed history and rationale for this shift in emphasis or a summary of the substantial data base documenting the benefits of integration for students with and without severe disabilities are referred to Bogdan (1983); Forest (1987, 1989); Gartner and Lipsky (1987); Lipsky and Gartner (1989); Meyer and Putnam (1988); Reid (1987); Snell (1988); Snell and Eichner (1989); W. Stainback, Stainback, and Forest (1989); and Thousand et al. (1986).

PARAMETERS OF INCLUSIVE EDUCATION

Peck and Semmel (1982) noted that "the LRE concept defines optimal placement for children with special educational needs as that in which an appropriate instructional program can be delivered with the least abrogation of the child's right to be educated with nonhandicapped peers" (p. 56). Thus, the essence of regular class integration for students with severe disabilities is *providing specially designed instruction in regular education environments.* This interpretation of the law was upheld by the Sixth Circuit Court of Appeals in the case of *Roncker v. Walter* (1983). The court ruled that if a desirable service currently provided in a segregated setting can feasibly be delivered in an integrated setting, it would be inappropriate under PL 94-142 to provide the service in a segregated environment. This was referred to as the "principle of portability" and advanced the legal and logical grounds for providing specially designed instruction in regular education environments.

Within regular classes, the education of students can be broadly characterized along two dimensions: 1) the student's educational and curricular needs, and 2) the supports provided to the

student in order to meet those needs successfully (Giangreco & Meyer, 1988). The student's educational needs would be addressed by particular goals and objectives reflecting prioritized curricular content, delivered to the student in both school and nonschool (community-based) instructional contexts. Any given individual student might be pursuing curricular content that is substantively the same as that for nondisabled age-peers, or he or she might be pursuing a course of study that is extended, modified, or otherwise individualized and might vary greatly from that designed to accommodate the majority of typical students. Supports refer to resources such as school personnel, peer groupings, equipment and prosthetic devices, materials, and various instructional adaptations designed to facilitate inclusion and learning for the student. And, finally, a student might work toward attaining his or her educational goals given the same supports typically available in regular education, or might require extended, modified, or otherwise individualized supports.

Figure 15.1 illustrates four basic options for education within regular education classrooms that reflect these basic parameters of program and support. These options may occur in combinations throughout the course of a week, a day, or even within an individual lesson. In the first option (A), a student's program would be similar to the typical curricular content for a particular grade, and the supports provided would be those generally available in regular education environments: A student eligible for special education services would obviously have needs and require supports beyond this level. Option B might represent a program for a student with a sensory or motor impairment only, but whose curricular goals are virtually identical to those established for age-peers; this student would require certain specialized supports such as the services of an orientation and mobility specialist and/or adaptations such as translation of material into sign language or Braille. Students with severe disabilities are most likely to require the kinds of accommodations represented by the two remaining options (C and D). In some instances (perhaps for a portion of the school day), the student's highly individualized goals might be achievable within the regular classroom with the

SUPPORTS

Supports similar to those
typically
available in regular education

Supports that are extended,
modified, or individualized

	Supports similar to those typically available in regular education	Supports that are extended, modified, or individualized
Educational program similar to regular education	**A** No accommodations required	**B** Support accommodations required
Educational program that is extended, modified, or individualized	**C** Program accommodations required	**D** Program and support accommodations required

P R O G R A M S

Figure 15.1.   Integration options within regular education classroom environments across the dimensions of support and program. (Adapted from Giangreco & Meyer, 1988, p. 256.)

kinds of supports typically available in that setting (option C). In most instances, however, students with severe disabilities will have educational program and support needs that are more extensive and require formal accommodations within the regular classroom (option D). Later in this chapter, we describe both the supports and curricular adaptations that have been proposed to accomplish this.

Local Schooling

Educating students with disabilities in the same schools they would attend if not handicapped is supported by law (Code of Federal Regulations, 1987, §300.552 a, c) and logic (L. Brown, Long, Udvari-Solner, Davis, et al., 1989; Hardman, McDonnell, & McDonnell, 1989; Sailor, 1989). Access and opportunities to participate in the variety of activities valued by a community occurs in the local school, so that social networks can be established and maintained (Froland, Pancost, Chapman, & Kimboko, 1981). Interdependent relationships among people established through these networks have both direct and indirect implications for the quality of a person's life (Meyer & Eichinger, 1987). The kinds of supports offered by such relationships across the life span are personally beneficial by assisting persons to cope with stress; achieve a positive psychosocial adjustment; and establish close, meaningful re-

lationships such as friendships, partnerships, and an adult family unit (Hardman et al. 1989; Snow & Forest, 1987; Strully & Strully, 1985).

Being a member of one's community also creates opportunities for personal growth and achievement that might otherwise be unavailable. For example, Hasazi, Gordon, and Roe (1985) found that a significant percentage of people with disabilities obtained their jobs through social networks of family and friends. Conversely, when the network of family and friends either is not established or is disrupted by placement beyond the boundaries of the neighborhood community: 1) family involvement is compromised, 2) school programs are less likely to reflect curricular content relevant to the community where the student lives and spends his or her nonschool time, 3) access to extracurricular activities may be limited, and 4) other members of the community do not experience the necessary opportunities to develop both the social commitment and skills needed to include individuals who require varying levels of support (Hardman et al., 1989).

Regular education service delivery patterns vary widely depending upon factors such as population density, geography, tradition, and resources (Thousand et al., 1986). Therefore, the ways students move through the schools in different communities will vary accordingly. While the patterns for school-age students may already be established, integrated patterns of service delivery for preschoolers and older students (18–21 years old) require creative and individualized planning. For example, postsecondary-age students might attend programs on college campuses (Frank & Uditsky, 1988; Giangreco & Meyer, 1988; Panitch, 1988; Uditsky & Kappel, 1988). Given the age of the students, this regionalization would be normalized since most 18–21-year-olds who are continuing their education typically attend colleges or technical schools rather than high schools. Further, in rural areas, colleges often are located in regional centers for recreation, social gathering, purchasing, cultural events, and employment. Thus, the regionalization matches students' needs for access to meaningful instructional environments (L. Brown, Long, Udvari-Solner, Davis, et al., 1989).

If students with severe disabilities are to be included in their local schools and follow the patterns of service delivery offered to their nondisabled siblings and neighbors, school personnel must cease confusing intensity of services with location of service delivery (Taylor, 1988). Further, schools must be restructured, both physically and programmatically, to provide better access to all students and to provide educational experiences that reflect the demands of an inclusive life in the community.

Individualized Educational Goals

In recent years, major curricular reform has occurred in educational programs for students with severe disabilities. Past practices of organizing a sequence of educational goals for individual students based upon normative developmental continua in traditional domains such as motor, language, cognitive, socioemotional, and so on were soundly criticized by L. Brown, Nietupski, and Hamre-Nietupski (1976). L. Brown and his colleagues argued that such curricula were fundamentally inappropriate for students with severe handicaps, and by definition, could only result in the acquisition of relatively meaningless, nonfunctional splinter skills across the school career. Alternatively, curricula that were referenced to the demands of current and future domestic, vocational, leisure, and community environments—such that each goal selected for

instruction represented a functional skill that would be of use to students now and as adults—were both feasible and more likely to result in meaningful outcomes for students with severe intellectual handicaps (L. Brown et al., 1976; L. Brown et al., 1979).

These claims were supported in a longitudinal follow-up of the ultimate achievements of two groups of graduates from the Madison, Wisconsin, public schools, one of which had experienced a predominantly developmentally based curriculum and the other a community-referenced, functional curriculum (L. Brown et al., 1987). Further empirical evidence for the effectiveness of an environmentally referenced approach to the education of students with severe disabilities was summarized in Horner, Meyer, and Fredericks (1986) and in Goetz, Guess, and Stremel-Campbell (1987). Finally, widespread consensus regarding the components of functional curricula was documented in a large-scale, national survey conducted by Meyer et al. (1987). Their social validation of "most promising practices" for students with severe disabilities involved a comprehensive survey of the professional literature to identify such practices (including those supported by empirical data) and formal ratings by relevant respondent groups—state directors of special education; prominent parent advocates; and national experts in mental retardation, severe disabilities, behavioral research, and deaf-blindness.

Integration into the community was a prominent feature of the L. Brown et al. (1976) call for action, and this concern led directly to the recommendation that curricula must be referenced to the demands of actual environments. In addition to the L. Brown et al. (1987) follow-up report on the outcomes of graduates, there is preliminary evidence that instruction in an age-appropriate functional activity will be associated with increased skill in social interactions with peers (Vandercook, 1989). Various other reports have documented the successful acquisition and generalization of functional skills that relate to increased social competence and community adjustment (e.g., Snell & Browder, 1986). Clearly, developmentally sequenced curricula for students with severe intellectual handicaps entailed increasingly greater discrepancies between their educational activities and those of same-age, nondisabled peers. Furthermore, such curricula were even associated with practices such as placement of secondary-age students with severe disabilities on elementary school campuses in the early days of integration. Now, however, as the context of educational services has shifted from self-contained classes to regular classes, there is a need to expand existing environmentally referenced curricular approaches to address the demands and opportunities available in those environments (York & Vandercook, in press).

For each student, the individualized education program (IEP) is intended to reflect his or her educational priorities. As regular class placements have increased and received professional support, so have resources for assisting in IEP development, which are based upon the premise of regular class integration. Recent examples include the *Syracuse Community-Referenced Curriculum Guide* (Ford et al., 1989), *The McGill Action Planning System—MAPS* (Vandercook, York, & Forest, 1989), the *Cayuga-Onondaga Assessment for Children with Handicaps, Version 6.0* (Giangreco, Cloninger, & Iverson, 1990), and the *Individual Program Design Procedures Manual* (Williams, Fox, & Fox, 1988). Each of these shares certain features, including: 1) an emphasis upon team decision making, 2) a home-school collaboration component, 3) planning based upon a process that incorporates both ecological analysis and problem-solving techniques, 4) strategies for the selection of prioritized goals for individual students, and 5) an approach for matching individual student goals with regular class schedules and activities. While each of these guides describes program components that have been in use for a period of at least several years in various public school programs (and thus have been "field tested" to some extent), none is accompanied by formal data regarding student outcomes.

Longitudinal Planning and Meaningful Outcomes

Annual goals that signify educational priorities for an individual student have been the hallmark of the IEP, yet exclusive emphasis upon yearly goals could result in an education that is too narrowly focused. The same generic outcomes of schooling that are relevant for nondisabled students may be appropriate for students with disabilities. These include such factors as citizenship, community membership, development of a positive self-image, expansion of meaningful personal relationships, productive use of leisure time, vocational productivity, self-control and competence in personal management, and developing a personal style for ongoing learning (i.e., "learning how to learn"). Thus, just as an exclusive emphasis upon acquiring basic academic skills might be regarded as far too restrictive for nondisabled students, an emphasis upon the mastery of a set of functional skills for students with severe disabilities could unnecessarily limit individuals' abilities to achieve social competence and full citizenship as adults.

Williams et al. (1988) noted that IEP goals have typically not addressed these broader outcomes of schooling that might well require more than a single year to achieve. Earlier, Voeltz and Evans (1983) and Evans and Meyer (1987) expressed a similar concern that expectations and, eventually, evidence regarding meaningful student outcomes should serve as the basis for the selection of prioritized annual goals on the IEP. Similar concerns regarding the value of more generic skills such as decision making as a supplement to more typical functional skills have also appeared (e.g., Guess, Benson, & Siegel-Causey, 1985; Shevin & Klein, 1984). Logically, students in self-contained environments would be most vulnerable to narrow educational experiences, while those who are mainstreamed would be exposed to a wider breadth of opportunity and daily validation of the extent to which prioritized educational goals actually relate to increased social competence.

The regular education curriculum could prove to be a starting point for the identification of the needed breadth of curricular experiences (Giangreco et al., 1990). It may be appropriate to require substantive justification for any significant deviations from the curriculum content and typical educational activities experienced by typical age-peers (Giangreco et al., 1990). While educational models that seek to place individualized student priorities within a more expansive educational context are not new, their availability and reports of their efficacy with students who have severe disabilities have yet to appear in the professional literature.

Instruction in Nonschool Environments

Community-based instruction has become widely accepted as an essential component of educational programming for students with severe disabilities (L. Brown et al., 1976; L. Brown et al., 1983; Falvey, 1989; Sailor et al., 1986; Sailor et al., 1989; Snell & Browder, 1986). The need for direct instruction in the community has been based upon certain assumptions:

1. Students need to learn skills in the environments in which they will ultimately be used.
2. Because students with severe handicaps have difficulty generalizing what they learn across settings, learning those skills directly in the community becomes critical.
3. Because students with severe disabilities require more time to master skills, instruction in the community must also commence at an earlier age than might otherwise be necessary to ensure sufficient learning time.
4. Community-based instruction would also ensure that the essential interaction skills needed for use of skills in the presence of relevant nondisabled persons in the community would be evident.
5. Community-based instruction would by definition entail the simultaneous preparation of the nondisabled population for interactions with those with severe handicaps.

Various recommendations have appeared in the literature regarding the relative proportion of time students should spend in nonschool, community-based instruction versus school-based activities. At one end of the spectrum, the Community Intensive Instructional Model recommends explicit guidelines for increasing amounts of time beginning with once a week for 3–8-year-olds, twice a week for 9–11-year-olds, four times weekly for 12–18-year olds, and 80%–100% of the day off campus by age 19–22 (Sailor et al., 1989). Interestingly, earlier descriptions of this model emphasized fairly high percentages of time off campus for even younger children (e.g., 75% of available instructional time by ages 12 to 16; see Sailor & Guess, 1983, and Sailor et al., 1986). The Sailor et al. (1989) and other recent works have emphasized the importance of the regular education classroom and school setting as the context for essential learning experiences (e.g., Ford et al., 1989). Yet, there continues to be considerable emphasis upon the importance of leaving the regular education setting for community-based instruction, particularly as the student becomes older.

Suggested percentages of time to be spent in various settings may be useful as a rule of thumb to secure currently unavailable learning experiences, but these guidelines can also become problematic if they overshadow individualization based upon unique student needs. Furthermore, there are virtually no empirical data to support such percentages. In fact, there currently exists no research evidence to evaluate the relative importance of school versus nonschool learning environments and experiences in general. (The literature on general case instruction does investigate one aspect of this issue—the extent to which criterion skills can be mastered in various learning situations as a function of the extent to which critical components are replicated. See Horner, McDonnell, & Bellamy, 1986, for a review of this literature). Logically, it is reasonable to propose that because of various learner characteristics, students with severe disabilities may require direct instruction in criterion environments. But it is an empirical question whether the regular classroom environment is or is not the criterion environment for various critical life skills. For example, if one justification for nonschool instruction is that it prepares persons with and those without disabilities for task-related interactions with one another, shared school environments could be similarly justified as the essential context for children to experience those and other more informal social interactions across the life span. How much community-based instruction is essential for the acquisition of critical criterion skills, and how much nonschool instruction can students experience without cost to the potential benefits of learning and social experiences in the mainstream school setting? These are important questions that must be addressed in future work.

MANAGEMENT NEEDS
RELATED TO INSTRUCTION

One of the most important areas of support, and often the simplest to accommodate, are management needs related to instruction. Management needs refer to *aspects of the educational program that are done to or for the student* that must be attended to if the student is to have adequate access to educational opportunities. Unlike student participation in instruction required by IEP goals or general curricula, management needs do not necessarily require any active student response. For example, the courts have established that many health-related procedures such as management of tracheostomy (*Hymes v. Harnett County Board of Education,* 1981), intermittent catheterization (*Irving Independent School District v. Tatro,* 1984; *Tokarcik v. Forest Hills School District,* 1981), and dispensing medication (*Department of Education, State of Hawaii v. Katherine D.,* 1983) are school responsibilities.

In the *Irving* (1984) case, the Supreme Court stated:

> A service that enables a handicapped child to remain at school during the day is an important means of providing the child with meaningful access to education that Congress envisioned. The Act (P. L. 94-142) makes specific provision for services, like transportation, for example, that do no more than enable a child to be physically present in class.

Therefore, services such as tube feeding to provide nutrition and hydration, repositioning to allow for physical comfort and avoid debilitating conditions (e.g., joint contractures, decubitis ulcers), or providing adaptive devices/materials (Bigge, 1988, p. 64; York & Rainforth, 1987) are appropriate management needs, since they are needed by some students merely in order to be in school for a full day. The Supreme Court qualified its support for management services by indicating that, " . . . if a particular medication or treatment may appropriately be administered to a handicapped child other than during the school day, a school is not required to provide nursing services to administer it" (*Irving Independent School District v. Tatro,* 1984).

Three major issues present themselves when management needs are delivered to students who are placed in regular education classes: 1) the relationship between management needs and educational inclusion, 2) the relationship between management needs and student dignity, and 3) the extension of management needs to encompass services that will be increasingly prominent in integrated settings.

The courts have held that students with intensive management needs do not relinquish their right to be educated in the least restrictive environment. The case of *Espino v. Besteiro* (1981) involved the need for an air-conditioned environment for a 7-year-old child who was unable to regulate his own body temperature. The school originally agreed to provide an air-conditioned cubicle to be placed in the classroom. The court interceded and required the school to air condition the entire classroom because the cubicle restricted the student's interactions with peers. Various advances in medical and engineering technology imply that students with increasingly complex management needs will be able to gain access to regular schools and classrooms. Precautions will be required to ensure that attention to management needs does not restrict regular class placement opportunities.

As management needs are attended to, student dignity and privacy must not be violated. Practices that have been associated with self-contained special classes or special schools, such as changing a student's soiled diaper behind a screen in the corner of the classroom or administering postural drainage and suctioning in the presence of other students, are inappropriate in separate classes and become even more aberrant and stigmatizing in regular classes. Such practices may interfere with a learner's self-concept, perpetuate double standards, and do nothing to enhance the perceptions of classmates toward the learner. Regular class placement does not necessarily mean that every service provided to the student occurs in the regular class. Students placed in regular classes could have access in the same school subenvironments used by nonhandicapped students for procedures requiring privacy, for example. Thus, students should change clothes for physical education class in the locker room, have their bowel and bladder needs attended to in a bathroom, and receive medication in the health office. Since adapted materials and devices range from simple and unobtrusive to complex and very obtrusive, care must also be taken to ensure that any potential benefits of using an adaptation are not overshadowed by stigmatizing effects that may draw undue negative attention toward a person with disabilities (Stieler et al., 1977). If students with severe disabilities use the same facilities as their nondisabled counterparts and use the most normalized adaptations available, the likelihood of compromising student dignity can be greatly reduced.

Finally, management can be extended beyond passive therapeutic techniques, adaptations, specialized health procedures, and transportation to include removal of barriers to participation and supports to professionals and families (*Code of Federal Regulations*, 1987, §300.13). For example, regular education students might be taught the augmentative communication system used by a student who is nonverbal. This would be considered a management need because it is done for the student (not necessarily requiring his or her participation) and would be necessary for access to the educational program. Another management need might be consulting with school staff who operate after-school programs. In the case of *Rettig v. Kent City* (1983), the court required the school to provide at least 1 hour per week of extra-curricular activities as a related service for a 10-year-old student with severe disabilities. The court's decision was based, in part, on the *Code of Federal Regulations* (1987, §300.16, Nonacademic Services) which stated, "Each public agency shall take steps to provide nonacademic and extracurricular activities in such a manner as is necessary to afford handicapped children an equal opportunity for participation in those services and activities . . . [and that] they be exposed on an equal basis as nonhandicapped children." Further, in *Stacy G. v. Pasadena Independent School District* (1982), the court directed the school to offer training in behavioral techniques and counseling to the parents of a child with severe retardation and challenging behaviors to help relieve emotional stress, and therefore have an indirect benefit for the child.

Management needs typically are a small but important aspect of the educational program. Strategies to address management needs that support mainstreaming, preserve student dignity, and are expansive in their vision of what is necessary to do for a student can provide clear paths to inclusive opportunities.

CURRICULAR AND INSTRUCTIONAL PRACTICES

As regular and special education professionals work together to deliver appropriate educational programs to students with severe disabilities in the regular classroom, curricular and instructional practices must be identified to facilitate this process. Furthermore, these efforts should be coordinated with parallel reform movements to restructure America's schools and classrooms to better meet the needs of today's diverse student population. For example, educators concerned about the large percentage of students at risk for dropping out of school acknowledge that these statistics may indeed reflect failures to learn, but may also be evidence of schools that fail to teach (Natriello, 1987; Wehlage & Rutter, 1987). In fact, the variety of pressures for reform upon our educational system creates a window of opportunity for collaborative research efforts to validate classroom and instructional organization patterns that promote both achievement and social adjustment for all students in the regular classroom. Various authors concerned about the absence of appropriate mainstream educational opportunities for students with disabilities have advocated for fundamental change in the traditional means of delivering instruction in regular education to solve this dilemma (D. W. Johnson, Johnson, & Maruyama, 1983; Madden & Slavin, 1983; Nevin & Thousand, 1987; Wang & Birch, 1984).

In this section, existing evidence is reviewed regarding those curricular and instructional practices that have been related to: 1) the successful mastery of relevant skills, including evidence on acquisition, generalization, and maintenance of those skills; 2) progress in attainment of meaningful outcomes, such as evidence of social competence in school and nonschool environments; 3) efficient delivery of services to students with severe disabilities within the regular classroom at various age levels; and 4) coordination of services between regular and special education professional staff and resources. As noted earlier in this chapter, the majority of this research has been carried out for two scenarios: 1) effects of relatively limited integration experiences for students with severe disabilities have occurred in situations where these students attend self-contained classes for the majority of the school day, but are exposed to time-limited mainstreaming and/or peer interaction experiences; and 2) the effects of more fundamental alterations to instructional and curricular practices upon students has occurred in mainstream educational arrangements for students with mild to severe disabilities. Thus, the data base is disappointingly limited for evidence regarding full inclusion in mainstream classes for students with severe disabilities. Nevertheless, this section reviews the subset of promising instructional support approaches for which data exist that might be applicable for students with severe learning needs.

Structured Social Contact

Research carried out over a period of many years regarding the social integration of students with mild to moderate disabilities has long documented that mere physical proximity will not result in positive outcomes (Gresham, 1982; Semmel, Gottlieb, & Robinson, 1979). According to some researchers, when students with disabilities are subjected to unstructured integration experiences, they may: 1) be more socially isolated from their peers than are nondisabled students, 2) be less socially accepted than their nondisabled peers (Asher & Taylor, 1981; Bryan, 1974; Gresham, 1982; MacMillan, Jones, & Aloia, 1974), and/or 3) interact more frequently among themselves than with nondisabled students in integrated schools (Peterson & Haralick, 1977; Porter, Ramsey, Tremblay, Iaccobo, & Crawley, 1978). Alternatively, almost any structured effort to have an impact upon the academic and social integration of students with mild to moderate disabilities has had a positive outcome. Programs ranging from teaching social skills to students with disabilities to structuring teacher behavior to model positive inter-

actions with those students in the regular classroom have been associated with increases in peer acceptance and academic performance (for a comprehensive review of this research, see Meyer & Putnam, 1988). (The evidence of the effects of instructional modifications has been even more dramatic, but these data are discussed in the next section.)

On the one hand, research carried out in integrated schools has also documented the positive effects of structured contact upon students over and above the effects of physical proximity alone. On the other hand, Voeltz (1980) found that even without a structured interaction program, the mere presence of students with severe disabilities on campus—even though they attended completely separate self-contained classes—was associated with significantly more positive student attitudes toward persons with disabilities in comparison to the attitudes held by students in schools that were not integrated. But in both her 1980 report and her 1982 follow-up, the most positive acceptance scores occurred in those schools where students with severe disabilities were enrolled in self-contained classes but also participated in a structured recess "special friends" peer interaction program; these results were highly significant in this large-scale investigation involving several schools and a large sample of children (Voeltz, 1980, 1982). In her follow-up study in which nondisabled peers (interviewed several years later as older teenagers) who had or had not participated in the earlier peer interaction program in elementary school, Kishi (1988) found that those students who had experienced either contact or interactions with peers with severe disabilities retained more positive attitudes than those who had had no contact. This follow-up study further suggested that students' positive attitudes increased with age (Kishi, 1988).

Kishi (1988) also reported that several students described negative feelings about situations during the earlier elementary school interaction program when they were asked to "help" or supervise a student with severe disabilities. Apparently, at least some staff members had involved nondisabled students in activities such as feeding despite explicit guidelines for the program prohibiting such interaction experiences

(Voeltz, 1984). Reports of such negative memories years later by nondisabled peers are consistent with various caveats offered by D.W. Johnson and Johnson (1989) in their review. These authors maintained that some of the reasons why physical proximity alone is not sufficient to produce positive relationships include: 1) both peers with and without disabilities will experience an "interaction strain" in initial encounters, 2) normative cultural admonitions to "be kind to someone" with a disability may result in overfriendliness or paternalism in initial encounters that may be likely to decrease over time; and 3) the presence of ambivalent feelings that involve more favorable overt or public attitudes may be experienced along with less favorable nonverbalized feelings toward persons with disabilities. If such issues are valid, it would be particularly important that the interactions between individuals with severe disabilities and their nondisabled peers be carefully structured to offset these phenomena of interaction strain, paternalism, and ambivalent feelings that could become increasingly and openly negative over time. Either physical proximity alone or demanding interactions that place unreasonable responsibilities upon the child without disabilities could ultimately result in decreased social acceptance of persons with disabilities.

Instructional Modifications

It is not surprising that planned integration efforts have posed challenges to schools, given the strong tradition of teacher-directed, whole-class, age-graded instruction with little instructional variability across relatively homogeneous groups of children (Goodlad, 1983). Elementary and secondary teachers typically are unaccustomed to teaching groups of students that would be as diverse as those suggested by full inclusion of students with severe disabilities. Students may also be unaccustomed to learning and working with peers with disabilities; they too may lack the breadth of interpersonal skills needed for meaningful and positive cooperation with peers who seem quite different from other classmates. D.W. Johnson, Johnson, and Holubec (1986) stressed that students are not born collaborators, but must learn the skills required to work effectively with one another. Strain and

Shores (1983) also noted that the absence of interpersonal skills needed by students of varying ability levels to learn together would continue to be a critical barrier to effective integration unless instruction in those skills was provided. Various other educators have also maintained that successful integration will be dependent upon appropriately structured classroom activities and accompanied by teacher guidance and encouragement to maximize learning and interpersonal outcomes (Ballard, Corman, Gottlieb, & Kaufman, 1977; Bricker, 1978; Stainback & Stainback, 1985).

Thus, a major challenge for those involved in integrating students with severe disabilities is to provide specialized instruction to meet individual student needs while also providing opportunities for meaningful peer relationships and participation in classroom activities. Students receiving special services may not always work at the same pace or be guided by the same educational objectives and curricula as their age-peers in the regular classroom. Past practices that involve structuring individualistic learning activities—tutorials—within the regular class have been refered to as "islands in the mainstream" and associated with continuing isolation of those students from their peers and the life of the classroom (Biklen, 1985, p. 18). As Madden and Slavin (1983) noted, "All too often mainstreaming involves putting academically handicapped students in regular classrooms where their learning problems cause them to be resegregated" (p. 552).

One promising approach that involves students of varying ability levels in shared instructional and learning experiences is *cooperative learning* (D.W. Johnson et al., 1986). In cooperative groups, individuals work together to reach common goals (Deutsch, 1949). Cooperative learning situations can be contrasted with learning situations in which an individual's goal attainment is not correlated with group goal attainment (individualistic) or is negatively correlated with others' goal attainments (competitive).

As conceptualized by D.W. Johnson and Johnson (1989), cooperative learning is a teaching strategy that consists of five basic elements. "Positive interdependence" is the first requirement. This means that accomplishment of a group goal is dependent upon members working together—otherwise the goal cannot be achieved. Methods for promoting positive interdependence are: 1) having mutual goals (goal interdependence); 2) utilizing divisions of labor (task interdependence); 3) dividing and/or sharing materials, resources, or information among group members (resource interdependence); 4) assigning students differing roles (role interdependence); and 5) giving joint rewards (reward interdependence). Second, face-to-face verbal (or other communication forms) interactions must occur. Third, students are held individually accountable for mastering the assigned material and contributing to the group's efforts. Insisting upon individual accountability averts the "hitchhiking" phenomenon, where one student does most of the work and the others are viewed as getting a "free ride." Fourth, students are expected to utilize positive interpersonal and small-group skills. Teachers provide specific instructions on how to collaborate in groups (e.g., by providing instruction in social skills such as encouraging others to participate or taking turns). Teachers also spend time monitoring student behaviors, discussing group functioning, and providing students with feedback on their performance. The final essential component of good cooperative learning is group processing, which involves self-evaluation within the group regarding how well the group is functioning and whether group goals are being achieved.

Extensive research on cooperative learning (approximately 600 studies to date) has indicated that in addition to contributing significantly to student achievement, cooperative learning activities result in students who tend to be friendlier, have more of a group orientation, and learn more from one another (D.W. Johnson et al., 1983; D.W. Johnson, Maruyama, Johnson, Nelson, & Skon, 1981). In cooperative learning situations, more helping, encouraging, tutoring, and assisting among students occurs than in competitive or individualistic situations (D.W. Johnson & Johnson, 1986). Cooperative learning experiences also have been found to "promote more differentiated, dynamic, and realistic views (and therefore less stereotypes and static views) of other students (including handicapped peers and students from different ethnic

groups) than do competitive and individualistic learning experiences" (D.W. Johnson & Johnson, 1984, p. 115).

Over 50 studies have been conducted on mainstreaming and cooperative learning. D.W. Johnson et al. (1981) and D.W. Johnson and Johnson (1989) reviewed 41 studies comparing the relative effects of two or more goal structures on interpersonal attraction between students with and without disabilities. Cooperative learning experiences produced greater interpersonal attraction between the two groups of students than did competitive (effect size = 0.70) and individualistic (effect size = 0.16) experiences.

Although most studies on the use of cooperative learning have involved students with mild disabilities, the application of such procedures to students with moderate and severe handicaps is increasing. Studies have been conducted in elementary and secondary school and recreation settings, involving activities as varied as science projects, art, cooking, music, academic and preacademic tasks, and group recreation activities (Eichinger, 1990; Jellison, Brooks, & Huck, 1984; R. Johnson, Johnson, DeWeerdt, Lyons, & Zaidman, 1983; R. Johnson, Rynders, Johnson, Schmidt, & Haiden, 1979; Putnam & Rynders, 1985; Rynders, Johnson, Johnson, & Schmidt, 1980; Wilcox, Sbardellati, & Nevin, 1987). The general findings from this research are that cooperative learning situations are associated with significantly higher levels of certain positive social and verbal interaction behaviors, greater interpersonal attraction on sociometric outcome measures, and academic gains comparable to those in competitive and individualistic situations.

A study by Putnam, Rynders, Johnson, and Johnson (1989) involved students with moderate and severe disabilities in fifth-grade science classes. Social interaction behaviors of students in cooperative groups either receiving or not receiving instruction in cooperative skills were compared. The students receiving cooperative skills instruction interacted more positively with one another than did those who did not receive this instruction. Although the students with disabilities in this study were not expected to attain the same achievements in science as the other students, there was anecdotal evidence that students contributed to their groups' goal attainments in various ways while also working on their own individual instructional objectives. Individual objectives focused on the development of skills such as following instructions, identifying objects, measuring liquids, taking turns, obtaining materials at the back of the room, and communicating effectively.

The Putnam et al. (1989) cooperative learning investigation combined aspects of curriculum overlapping (described later in more detail) as well as partial and extended participation in science activities. These included: 1) having a student with moderate disabilities print the answers to the questions as the other group members spelled the words, and 2) having a student with severe disabilities obtain the equipment from a table and pour water into a container during an experiment on displacement. These examples and others described in Ford and Davern (1989) demonstrate creative teacher planning to include students with severe disabilities in regular class activities. Further research is needed to determine which educational situations are most suited for cooperative learning activities involving heterogeneous groups that include students with severe disabilities.

Curricular Adaptations

A key strategy for incorporating students with severe disabilities into regular classes is through *curricular adaptations,* or modifying curriculum assignments to meet the needs of individual learners. Typically, students with severe disabilities learn at a significantly slower rate than do nondisabled classmates. Therefore, the lesson content expectations placed upon these students must be adjusted to: 1) prevent mismatch between each student's skill level and the lesson content, and 2) promote student success in learning relevant skills. There is evidence to suggest that appropriate curricular choices for students result in success on daily tasks, which are the antecedents to long-term achievement (Gickling & Armstrong, 1978). While curricular adaptations for a student might involve a combination of learning alone and learning in small and large groups, this section focuses on curricular adaptations that provide for learning within heterogeneous groups. This is not meant to imply that

there is never a need to deliver intensive individualized instruction outside of group contexts—an issue not unlike that of deciding how much community-based instruction is needed and justified outside the regular school for each student. However, only the Meyer et al., (1987) social validity study of general guidelines for relative proportions of such learning opportunities provided "empirical" support for promising practices in this area. Clearly, future research is needed to address this issue.

Adapting curricula to meet individual student needs is a task that is familiar to many regular education teachers. Individualization involves establishing personalized goals and objectives for a student and determining effective ways to accomplish them. Two broad options exist for individualized curricular adaptations: 1) multilevel curriculum selection, and 2) curriculum overlapping.

Multilevel Curriculum Selection

Multilevel curriculum selection refers to identifying different goals and objectives for individual students within the same curricular domain and teaching them within the same lesson or activity (C. Campbell, Campbell, Collicott, Perner, & Stone, 1988). For example, a student with severe disabilities integrated into a reading group with his or her second-grade classmates who are learning to read words and simple sentences may be learning to read two to three functional vocabulary items and to match those words to sample objects. Multilevel curriculum selection has occurred in regular education as an adaptation of Bloom's *Taxonomy of Educational Objectives* (1956), including knowledge, comprehension, application, analysis, synthesis, and evaluation goals for different students. For example, in a lesson on money, one student might be learning at knowledge level (e.g., identifying money), another at comprehension level (e.g., understanding the uses of money), and others might be applying their knowledge and comprehension by making purchases and budgeting.

Multilevel curricular selection can involve "partial participation," a concept whereby persons with severe disabilities "can acquire many skills that will allow them to function, at least in part, in a wide variety of least restrictive school and nonschool environments" (Baumgart et al., 1982, p. 19). The assumptions underlying partial participation are that: 1) it is educationally more advantageous than exclusion from age-appropriate environments and activities, 2) it is applicable regardless of the student's degree of dependence or level of functioning, 3) it should be increased through direct systematic instruction, 4) it should result in more positive perceptions of the student by others, and 5) it should commence at an early age to facilitate current and future inclusion in integrated settings (Baumgart et al., 1982).

Multilevel curricular selection can also be consistent with expanded models of participation such as Project SPAN (F. Brown, Evans, Weed, & Owen, 1987). When confronted with teaching behaviors that appear too difficult or seem inappropriate for students with severe disabilities, educators have sometimes limited their participation because they have focused on the "core" skills associated with activities. Exclusive focus on core skills limits the scope of behavioral routines to often have arbitrary beginning and ending points (F. Brown et al., 1987). To address this concern, the Project SPAN model elaborates routines to include extension and enrichment components. Extension components examine the learner's ability to perform the following skills with regard to a particular activity: initiating, preparing, monitoring of quality, monitoring of tempo, problem solving, and terminating. Enrichment components explore the learner's ability to communicate, engage in appropriate social behavior associated with the routine, and indicate choices and preferences. (For a summary of data on student attainment of different components of routines, see Evans, Brown, Weed, Spry, & Owen, 1987).

Curriculum Overlapping

Curriculum overlapping is a variation on multilevel curriculum selection wherein the individually selected goals and objectives to be acquired within the context of a shared group activity are generated from different curricular areas (Giangreco & Meyer, 1988, p. 257). This concept essentially addresses the commonly expressed concern that many academic classes enrolling typical students are simply not relevant to the ed-

ucational needs of students with severe disabilities. For example, the inclusion of these students in classes such as algebra, biology, or mathematics may be regarded as inappropriate because: 1) the curricular content is viewed as nonessential for the lifestyle needs of persons with severe disabilities (as it may be for many typical students as well); 2) the curricular content is regarded as beyond the cognitive capabilities of students with severe disabilities; and 3) even if the information were judged to be important and could be mastered, the modifications necessary for meaningful participation would be so extreme that the academic development of nondisabled students might be jeopardized (Brown, Long, Udvari-Solner, Schwartz, et al., 1989). In the Putnam et al. (1989) cooperative learning study described earlier, the student with severe disabilities was included in a science class in order to master individually appropriate educational goals in other curricular domains, such as social competence, communication, and mobility. To date, there have been virtually no other examples in the published literature of learner outcomes accomplished through the application of the principles of curricular overlapping in the regular classroom, though examples can be found in practice (e.g., Biklen, 1988).

Adaptive Instruction

Adaptive instruction is a comprehensive approach designed to accommodate diversity among students within regular classes that combines or is compatible with many practical and effective components from the aforementioned strategies of multilevel curriculum selection and curriculum overlapping (Wang, Reynolds, & Schwartz, 1988). According to Walberg and Wang (1987), adaptive instruction is based on the premise that "individual students learn in different ways and at varying rates, and a major task for schools is to provide educational experiences that accommodate these differences in order to optimize each student's education" (p. 113). Distinguishing features of the model include:

1. Instruction is based on the assessed capabilities of each student.
2. Materials and procedures permit each stu-

dent to make progress in the mastery of instructional content at a pace suited to his or her abilities and interests.

3. Periodic evaluations of student progress emphasize feedback to individual students regarding mastery.

4. Each student assumes some responsibility for diagnosing his or her needs and abilities, for planning individual learning activities, and for evaluating his or her mastery.

5. Alternative activities and materials are available to aid students in the acquisition of essential academic skills and content.

6. Students have a choice in determining their individual educational goals, outcomes, and activities.

7. Students assist each other in pursuing individual goals, and they cooperate in achieving group goals.

Research involving students with mild disabilities has indicated that exemplary implementations of adaptive instruction programs are associated with achievement levels and classroom processes that are superior to those attained under exemplary traditional instruction (i.e., teacher-directed and group-paced instruction). Various programs are available—each of which has empirical support documenting positive outcomes for students with mild learning handicaps—that incorporate aspects of adaptive instruction, including the Adaptive Learning Environments Model (ALEM) (Wang & Birch, 1984), the Bank Street Model (Gilkeson, Smithberg, Bowman, & Rhine, 1981), and Team Assisted Individualization (Slavin, Madden, & Leavey, 1984). As ALEM has been widely implemented and evaluated in situations involving students with disabilities and is often discussed with reference to the regular education initiative in particular, it is described here in more detail.

ALEM has been field tested for more than a decade at the University of Pittsburgh and elsewhere in a large number of public and private schools (Wang & Birch, 1984). ALEM involves curricular and instructional modifications to support students with mild handicapping conditions and other students with learning difficulties in the regular classroom. Components of the model include: 1) a diagnostic-prescriptive

monitoring system, 2) delabeling of mainstreamed special students, 3) provision of individualized assistance to all students experiencing learning problems based upon periodic performance data, and 4) teaching students self-management skills. The ALEM curriculum combines "direct" or prescriptive instruction with aspects of informal, or open, education thought to be conducive to the attitudes and processes of inquiry, social cooperation, and self-management for learning (Wang, Gennari, & Waxman, 1985). Although ALEM is a promising adaptive learning program model, critics have challenged the evaluation methodology utilized in early reports (Hallahan, Keller, McKinney, Lloyd, & Bryan, 1988). In addition, ALEM has not to date been systematically extended to address the ability of the model to include students with severe disabilities as well. In principle, of course, ALEM involves an alternative to group-paced instructional models, and might thus have considerable potential for providing the kinds of intensive, individualized learning activities needed to complement group experiences such as cooperative learning in the regular classroom.

Other Regular
Education Curricular Modifications

Various other instructional arrangements have been described as having particular promise for instructing students with special needs in regular classrooms. In their review of research and practices, Nevin and Thousand (1987) identified several curricular and instructional approaches that would appear to be supportive of mainstreaming in principle: 1) "mastery learning" (Anderson, 1985; Bloom, 1977, 2) increasing academic learning time (Wilson, 1987), and 3) applied behavior analysis (Berkson & Landesman-Dwyer, 1977; Deno & Mirkin, 1977; Haring, Lovitt, Eaton, & Hansen, 1978).

PEOPLE RESOURCES

Education is first and foremost a labor-intensive undertaking, and the quality of a program is most certainly dependent upon the characteristics of the people involved. Human resources are possibly the most crucial component for the delivery of quality programs to children—interestingly enough, they are also the least studied. At this point in time, while it appears that knowledge and skills regarding exemplary practices are important, even more important may be the ability of the adult personnel to operationalize collaborative teamwork principles in their interactions with one another and with their students.

Perhaps because the inclusion of students with severe disabilities in the regular classroom is so new, we could identify virtually no research regarding the organization of staff and other human resources to facilitate this process. There are, however, working papers, program descriptions, and informal reports of observations of schools and classrooms that have achieved full inclusion. For example, Fenwick (1987) described the advantages and disadvantages of various staffing strategies implemented at the Edward Smith School in Syracuse, New York, where students with autism and other severe disabilities have received special services in the regular classroom for many years. But no data have been provided to support the generalizations drawn regarding preferable practices to facilitate mainstreaming. There is, however, a growing professional literature empirically documenting the effects of various staffing patterns in mainstream services for students with mild disabilities. For example, considerable information is now available regarding components of effective consultation to the regular classroom teacher to meet individual needs (see Fuchs & Fuchs, 1989, for one such report, and Huefner, 1988, for a review of this research). Such evidence should be utilized as a starting point for the organization of staffing resources to support mainstream services for students with severe disabilities (see also Chapter 17, this volume, for a review of personnel preparation needs). In the interim, this final section of this chapter presents an overview of the issues and possible research directions for more formal investigation.

Teachers

At the heart of any regular classroom is the teacher. Managing and providing meaningful instruction to a group of 20–30 children or adolescents is a challenge regardless of the characteristics of individual students. When a student enters the regular classroom with curricular needs that differ from those of his or her classmates and may require intensive instruction, regular education teachers are confronted with a task for which they may be unprepared and that typically requires collaboration and support.

Within the framework of multiple supports, a crucial element of successful integration is for regular class teachers to assume ownership for education of the student with disabilities, just as they would for any other student on their class list. This ownership is vital to the development of an inclusionary climate in the classroom. From a practical standpoint, in order for the input of other school personnel to be truly supportive, the regular class teacher must play a significant role in guiding the process. Logically, whenever a student with disabilities is viewed by the teacher as someone else's primary responsibility, he or she is more likely to be socially and academically isolated within the regular class. Conversely, in classes where teacher behavior and verbalizations indicate ownership as the student's primary teacher, isolated or parallel education would be minimized and inclusion in class activities should be greater. However, we were unable to locate any research investigating the specific effects of teacher behavior within the regular classroom upon students with severe disabilities or their nondisabled peers.

As integration efforts have expanded, new roles have emerged for teachers as collaborators and consultants within the regular classroom. Collaborative team-teaching arrangements have emerged as one type of service delivery configuration designed to utilize the skills of both classroom teachers and teachers prepared to serve as resource consultants in particular specialized need areas (Fenwick, 1987). Thousand and Villa's (1989) recent review suggested that the critical elements for effective team teaching parallel those for cooperative group learning, including: direct interactions, interdependence, use of prosocial skills such as conflict management, communication, trust building, and individual accountability. Whether they are referred to as support facilitators (S. Stainback, Stainback, & Harris, 1989), methods and resource teachers (Campbell et al., 1988), teacher consultants (Huefner, 1988), or education specialists (Thousand et al., 1986), alternative positions have been created and both special education teachers and master teachers with specialized skills are being retrained to fill such roles. For example, the University of Vermont initiated a post–master's degree–level (certificate of advanced study) training program in 1986 to prepare educational specialists (ES) to support students with intensive educational needs in regular classes. By the 1988–1989 school year, 20 educational specialists were serving students in 14 Vermont Supervisory Unions. During the 1989–1990 school year 35 educational specialists served more than half of Vermont's Supervisory Unions.

There are a growing number of districts and schools that utilize consultation and team-teaching staffing models to support mainstream placements for students with severe disabilities. The documentary *Regular Lives,* aired on public television in the United States in 1988, provided several examples of such programs (Biklen, 1988); and entire school districts in certain states in the United States and provinces in Canada now serve virtually all students with severe disabilities by providing consultation to regular class services. Nevertheless, systematic evaluation reports of the components of these efforts and outcomes associated with those components for students have not yet been published.

Related Services Personnel

In addition to consultant teachers serving as integration specialists, a wide array of related services providers are mandated to support the education of students with severe disabilities, including: occupational therapists; physical therapists; speech/language pathologists; and other professionals such as social workers, school psychologists, orientation-and-mobility instructors, nurses, and recreation specialists (as individually appropriate). Much of the service currently provided to students with severe disabilities by these related professionals has been characterized as direct and "pull out," isolated from typical instructional environments (P.H. Campbell, 1987; Giangreco, 1986). As these students access regular classes, related services personnel will be called upon to support those educational programs with services that are compatible with regular education routines. Giangreco, York,

and Rainforth (1989) argued that the first consideration for related services delivery should be carefully designed, indirect/consultative services if those services are to support integration (see also Giangreco, 1989b).

Paraprofessionals

Teacher aides or educational assistants have been used extensively to support students with disabilities placed in regular classes. Service delivery patterns for the use of teacher aides has followed three basic patterns: 1) one aide is assigned to one student full time, 2) one aide is assigned to a small group of students within the same class or school (typically, two to four students), or 3) two or more aides rotate responsibilities for both direct student support and other school duties (e.g., library support, cafeteria work, bus supervision).

Some parents and professionals have expressed concern that the assignment of aides may result in a situation where the least trained of the adults involved with the student has the most responsibility and may often be left to make many day-to-day decisions. Others are concerned that the overreliance on teacher aides interferes with the development of a sense of ownership by the regular classroom teacher for a student with severe disabilities who has a one-to-one aide assigned. While the use of paraprofessionals can be a valuable instructional resource, we could identify no systematic investigations that examined the impact of various paraprofessional service delivery configurations designed to support students with severe disabilities in regular classes. Thus, while documentation is unavailable, reports from school districts suggest that use of a full-time aide for a single student has serious limitations for both school systems and students. First, districts typically have difficulty justifying a full-time aide for every student with special needs placed in a regular class. Second, burnout among aides is said to increase and productivity suffer when their assignments are restricted to the same student exclusively. Third, the presence of a full-time aide for a student may be detrimental by creating unnecessary dependency or because the physical presence of the adult may interfere with the development of peer relationships (York, Vandercook,

Caughey, & Helse-Neff, 1988). The changing role of teacher assistants and the level of dependence upon their services will require modification and individualization in order to keep pace with the call for full inclusion into regular education.

Peers and Classmates

Traditionally, regular education peers have been engaged in both social interactions and peer tutoring relationships with students with severe disabilities (see Chapter 11, this volume, for a comprehensive review of the effects of these patterns upon children's social relationships). Peer tutoring programs have been reported as effective approaches for teaching students with disabilities in regular classes (Maheady, Sacca, & Harper, 1988), and research on this model has documented short-term benefits such as observable academic gains, the modification of undesirable behaviors, and increasing the amounts of individual attention a student receives (Krouse, Gerber, & Kaufman, 1981; Leyser & Gottlieb, 1981). However, as Krouse et al. cautioned, the long-term social effects of this practice have yet to be examined carefully, especially in terms of the ultimate impact of peer tutorial relationships upon peer cooperation and mutual concern.

A more recent development has involved including peers as members of planning teams for students with disabilities so that they become collaborators in educational decision making (Schattman, 1989; Vandercook et al., 1989). In schools in Minnesota, Vermont, and in various locations in Canada, some local planning teams have invited classmates to participate in the design of educational programs based upon the presumption that they have student-centered perspectives that would be relevant to meaningful educational planning. On a less formalized level than planning teams, students often are creative problem solvers who can assist teachers in designing ways for students to become meaningfully involved in regular class activities. Little is known about the effects of peers on planning teams and few procedures or guidelines are available to ensure that student confidentiality is maintained; furthermore, it would seem important that nondisabled students are not called upon to assume a level of responsibility that

makes them uncomfortable. The inclusion of peers on planning teams and as classroom-based problem solvers has potential, but the process must ensure that the intended benefits are forthcoming and safeguards are in place; at least one systematic research effort involving peers in such roles is now ongoing and data will be available regarding various outcomes after a 2-year time period (I.M. Evans & C.L. Salisbury, personal communication, January 8, 1990).

Administrators

School administrators are a vital link in the development and maintenance of integrated education. At some point in the process, changes must be reflected in board of education policies and practices in the form of budgetary accommodations, the redefinition of job roles and functions, and hiring practices (Canadian Education Association, 1985; Giangreco, 1989a; Villa & Thousand, 1990). At a more immediate level, Villa and Thousand suggested that administrators must engage in a variety of supportive measures to facilitate integration, such as creating mechanisms for teamwork and consensus building to occur (e.g., through provision of release time), encouraging and rewarding creativity and collaboration, and developing peer-teacher support networks. Clearly, schoolwide or systemwide integration efforts will require the active support of district-level administrators, with school principals and special education counterparts serving as key people in school-level changes.

RESEARCH RECOMMENDATIONS

1. *We need to examine the effects of various components of full-inclusion models upon academic achievement, social-behavioral skills, social attitudes, and interpersonal relationships between children.* A great deal of research has been carried out in regular education settings where children with and without severe disabilities generally attended separate classes but were exposed to different interaction experiences, such as peer tutoring versus special friendship play relationships. Based upon these data, we can confidently state that virtually any form of structured contact has resulted in more positive

attitudes and experiences than physical exposure alone. There is also some evidence to suggest that less hierarchical friendship interactions will be associated with more positive outcomes than hierarchical tutoring relationships alone, where the nonhandicapped child's only experience with the child with severe disabilities is to serve as a peer tutor. In addition, social contact with non-disabled children has been related to increased mastery of IEP goals by students with severe disabilities, and the research on cooperative learning shows no ill effects associated with integration upon the achievement of nondisabled children participating in isolated learning experiences with children with moderate to severe disabilities (see Meyer & Putnam, 1988, for a comprehensive review of these data).

However, virtually all these data were collected for children who spent the vast majority of their school day in separate environments—that is, in different classrooms. To date, no evidence exists regarding the effects of different components of a full-inclusion model upon student achievement, attitudes, social competence, and friendships. For example, what kind of impact would involvement of typical peers in instructional planning (as in MAPS, Vandercook et al., 1989) have upon children's achievement, friendships, and so on? Would team teaching be more or less facilitative of student mastery of IEP goals in comparison to other staffing models, such as consultant teacher services? Which types of full-inclusion models would ultimately be associated with the development of informal social support networks in the community through the attainment of social competence, positive attitudes, and feelings of friendship by nondisabled children toward their peers with severe disabilities? Many other specific research questions might be and should be formulated once the actual components of various full-inclusion models have been articulated more clearly and field tested in schools and classrooms. But above all, as "integration" has always carried many different meanings ranging from mere physical proximity to actual structured contact between children, "inclusion" must be specified and the important variables relating to outcomes for children must be evaluated systematically.

2. *We need some basis for achieving a bal-*

ance between the needs of students with severe disabilities for intensive skill instruction and community-based instruction on the one hand and regular classroom integration and social interaction experiences on the other. Recommendations continue to abound regarding the percentages of time students with severe disabilities should spend receiving instruction in the community during the school day at various ages— that is, outside the school and thus away from nondisabled peers. These recommendations are based upon the more general evidence that students with severe disabilities do not easily generalize what they have learned in one environment (e.g., the classroom) to another (e.g., the criterion community settings), thus leading to the logical conclusion that new skills should be taught directly to students in those criterion settings—in the community. But while this might seem a logical conclusion, there are no data whatsoever to suggest how much community instruction at what ages is needed. Nor do data exist regarding any possible "costs" that such community-based instruction might incur to the extent that it involves more segregation from peers and the school community. It may simply be impossible to empirically validate the relative effects of spending varying percentages of time in school versus nonschool/community environments across the school years. Historically, this has been the sort of longitudinal research question that we have never been able to answer with any confidence because of both logistical complications and the multiple sources of (intended and unintended) influences upon learner outcomes.

Yet, while we may never acquire the experimental sophistication to answer such a question empirically, we clearly need to temper our eagerness to make enthusiastic and detailed prescriptions based solely upon the biases of the individual writer. Perhaps some combination of a more thorough theoretical exploration of the various implications would help, and researchers might collect some evidence regarding the potential of the school as a source of learning criterion skills at different ages. For example, does the elementary school include potentially valuable learning experiences such as social competence routines (e.g., turn taking, getting ready, finishing, and putting away) and essential early social interaction opportunities (i.e., being part of one's peer group) that do relate to skill mastery and valued social outcomes? How does this compare to the opportunities available to secondary-age students in school versus nonschool settings? In the interim as we await the results of such systematic study, social validation research might be conducted to support the kinds of practices we do implement for students. At the very least, we should have more information about the importance that parents and professionals place on different experiences for children. We might even try to find creative and valid ways to ask the children themselves. . . . And at some level, the question might not be unlike that personal balance that each of us strives to attain between "work" and "play" in our lives: How can we strike a similar balance for a child with severe disabilities?

3. *Much more research and development is needed to validate those aspects of various curricular adaptation models that will result in positive educational outcomes for students.* Within the past 5 years, we have witnessed the emergence of significant support for full inclusion—education for all children in the regular classroom—as a philosophical principle. Entire books have appeared discussing both the principle and the practice of full inclusion. And, we can point to examples of regular classroom instruction, with the needed instructional supports, for individual students with severe disabilities as well as for all students with severe disabilities in some schools and even entire school districts. Nevertheless, there is little that we can tell others about how best to modify and adapt curricula for these students based upon actual data regarding student accomplishments using those approaches. Good ideas such as overlapping curricular objectives to enable us to meet the needs of a student whose educational goals are greatly discrepant from his or her typical peers must be translated into guidelines that have been developed, field tested, and validated on behalf of real children in typical schools.

4. *Research is similarly needed on the effects of varied instructional practices and teacher behaviors upon the academic and social integration of students.* Again, only the research on cooperative learning and any generalizations

we might draw from regular education initiatives such as ALEM (Wang & Birch, 1984) give us any help here. Cooperative learning as an instructional grouping strategy can be related to various positive social and academic outcomes for students in comparison to either individualistic or competitive structures. And ALEM provides one model of individualizing instruction for classrooms that reflect a considerable level of diversity. Areas that beg investigation, however, include the application of various technologies such as computer-assisted instruction (CAI) and even combinations of technology and different grouping and goal structures. A variation of the early aptitude-treatment-interaction (ATI) research might be useful to explore the effects of different teaching styles upon the attainment of different educational goals for students. And finally, can we identify teacher behaviors and variations in teaching styles that are associated with positive learner outcomes and can be taught to teacher trainees and inservice teachers?

5. *If community integration and participation is the ultimate objective of our educational system, we may need to reevaluate the individualized educational objectives traditionally posed both for students with disabilities and those without disabilities.* We know very little about the actual impact of having learned a particular skill upon the individual's success in criterion community environments. For example, we have long focused upon teaching persons with disabilities specific job skills that related to task performance, only to learn that employees most often lost their jobs for reasons that had more to do with social competence than the quality of their work. Vandercook's (1989) study is a rare example of a demonstration that learning a particular skill (e.g., how to play appropriately with an age-appropriate toy) was related to a desirable positive learner outcome (e.g., increased cooperative participation with nondisabled peers). Once again, our decisions about what to teach students—with disabilities and nondisabled—have been based more upon our individual biases and traditions than upon evidence that what students are learning really makes a difference in their lives. This situation is also unlikely to change unless we begin to specify the kinds of long-term, positive outcomes we expect for per-

sons with severe disabilities. In the absence of data, the "criterion of ultimate functioning" posed by L. Brown and his colleagues (1976) was a good start. By now, however, we could begin to track the effects of different emphases in students' IEPs upon their development and social adjustment. Documentation of long-term planning and systematic evaluation of various IEP outcomes should be the focus of longitudinal research efforts and a requirement of daily practice at the state level.

6. *Validated systems-change strategies are needed to assist schools, districts, and regions in their changeover from segregated models to integrated, full-inclusion educational models.* Special education research is historically rooted in educational psychology, a tradition that emphasizes the controlled experiment and intervention at the individual unit of analysis level. Ethnographic research paradigms and multivariate research technologies that allow for the documentation of multiple and unintended influences and effects must be expanded to evaluate systems-change efforts judged to show varying degrees of success. New paradigms or strategies for knowledge production might need to be developed to investigate complex systems-change issues that go far beyond the individual child, teacher-child dyad, or even classroom level. Our rigid adherence to certain paradigms in research and evaluation—reflected most clearly in publication and funding—must give way to increased willingness to utilize alternative evaluative methods that might be equally or better suited to answer the kinds of questions that continue to elude us.

7. *We need to better understand the ways in which professionals who have traditionally functioned as special and regular educators can work together to meet the needs of the diverse student population of today's schools.* Our school districts are staffed by teachers and other professionals who have a history of working with children in isolation from one another. The teacher education programs that train those professionals are similarly separate. How can we best prepare professionals who can both teach children well and work together and support one another in order to do even better? How do we gen-

erate both teacher attitudes and skills that support learning across the full range of students' abilities and needs? Closely related to this staffing issue is more intense scrutiny of the fundamental structure of classrooms: What would be the effects of alternatives to age-graded classes (such as family and other cross-age groupings more common in a country such as New Zealand) upon student learning, behavior, and social relationships? As we come to accept and value the diversity of today's student population, perhaps we can begin to evaluate more fundamental reforms and even major restructuring efforts that could better assist our school system to meet the needs of the children of today who will become the society of tomorrow.

SUMMARY AND CONCLUSIONS

As the field moves toward full-inclusion models in America's schools, we shall continue to confront the challenge of individualizing instruction to meet unique educational needs on behalf of students with severe disabilities. The status of regular class instruction—with special service supports and resources—is at a formative and crucial stage of development. Many educators have pointed to the values that support full inclusion, the clear and compelling failures of exclusionary and segregated models, and the logic of providing services to students in their neighborhood schools and classrooms as perhaps the most promising practice for the coming years. If regular class integration is to move beyond its current status as primarily an exemplary model available only in some regions to a very few children to one that is generally available, both systems-change research and systematic evaluations of the effects of our practices upon outcomes for children will be critical. Such research would not be focused upon whether we should integrate children with disabilities into the regular classroom with their peers—this is a value judgment regarding what we want our society to look like. Instead, research must be designed to gather the necessary information to help in the design of increasingly effective and creative ways to expand the educational and social opportunities to students with all levels of ability and diverse needs. In combination with an inclusionary values base and sound logic and theory to guide us where data continue to be absent, research will continue to serve as an important impetus to shape educational and social policy and practice.

REFERENCES

Anderson, L.W. (1985). A retrospective and prospective view of Bloom's "Learning for Mastery." In M.C. Wang & H.J. Walberg (Eds.), *Adapting instruction to individual differences* (pp. 254–268). Berkeley, CA: McCutchan.

Asher, S.R., & Taylor, A.R. (1981). The social outcomes of mainstreaming: Sociometric assessment and beyond. *Exceptional Education Quarterly, 1,* 13–30.

Ayres, B. (1988, September). Integration: A parent's perspective. *Exceptional Parent,* pp. 22–25.

Ballard, M., Corman, L., Gottlieb, J., & Kaufman, M.J. (1977). Improving the social status of mainstreamed retarded children. *Journal of Educational Psychology, 69,* 605–611.

Baumgart, D., Brown, L., Pumpian, I., Nisbet, J., Ford, A., Sweet, M., Messina, R., & Schroeder, J. (1982). Principle of partial participation and individualized adaptations in educational programs for severely handicapped students. *Journal of The Association for the Severely Handicapped, 7*(2), 17–27.

Berkson, G., & Landesman-Dwyer, S. (1977). Behavioral research on severe and profound mental retardation. *American Journal of Mental Deficiency, 81,* 428–455.

Berres, M., & Knoblock, P. (Eds.). (1987). *Program models for mainstreaming: Integrating students with moderate to severe disabilities.* Rockville, MD: Aspen.

Bigge, J. (1988). *Curriculum based instruction for special education students.* Mountain View, CA: Mayfield.

Biklen, D. (1985). *Achieving the complete school: Strategies for effective mainstreaming.* New York: Teachers College Press.

Biklen, D. (Producer). (1988). *Regular lives* [Video]. Washington, DC: State of the Art.

Bloom, B.S. (1956). *Taxonomy of educational objectives: Handbook I. Cognitive domain.* New York: David McCay Co.

Bogdan, R. (1983). "Does mainstreaming work?" is a silly question. *Phi Delta Kappan, 64,* 427–428.

Bricker, D. (1978). A rationale for the integration of handicapped and nonhandicapped school children. In M.J. Guralnick (Ed.), *Early intervention and the integration of handicapped and nonhandicapped children* (pp. 3–26). Baltimore: University Park Press.

Brost, M., & Johnson, T. (1986, October). *Special education does not mean special classes: Two parents' observations about Louisville, Kentucky's experiences in integrating special and regular education systems and students.* Madison: Wisconsin Coalition for Advocacy.

Brown, F., Evans, I., Weed, K., & Owen, V. (1987). Delineating functional competencies: A component model. *Journal of The Association for Persons with Severe Handicaps, 12,* 117–124.

Brown, L., Branston, M.B., Hamre-Nietupski, S., Pumpian, I., Certo, N., & Gruenewald, L. (1979). A strategy for developing chronological-age-appropriate and functional curricular content for severely handicapped adolescents and young adults. *Journal of Special Education, 13,* 81–90.

Brown, L., Long, E., Udvari-Solner, A., Davis, L. Van Deventer, P., Ahlgren, C., Johnson, F., Gruenewald, L., & Jorgensen, J. (1989). The home school: Why students with severe intellectual disabilities must attend the schools of their brothers, sisters, friends, and neighbors. *Journal of The Association for Persons with Severe Handicaps, 14,* 1–7.

Brown, L., Long, E., Udvari-Solner, A., Schwartz, P., Van Deventer, P., Ahlgren, C., Johnson, F., Gruenewald, L., & Jorgensen, J. (1989). Should students with severe intellectual disabilities be based in regular or special education classrooms in home schools? *Journal of The Association for Persons with Severe Handicaps, 14,* 8–12.

Brown, L., Nietupski, J., & Hamre-Nietupski, S. (1976). The criterion of ultimate functioning and public school services for severely handicapped students. In M.A. Thomas (Ed.), *Hey don't forget about me: Education's investment in the severely, profoundly, and multiply handicapped* (pp. 2–15). Reston, VA: Council for Exceptional Children.

Brown, L., Nisbet, J., Ford, A., Sweet, M., Shiraga, B., York, J., & Loomis, R. (1983). The critical need for nonschool instruction in education programs for severely handicapped students. *Journal of The Association for the Severely Handicapped, 8*(3), 71–77.

Brown, L., Rogan, P., Shiraga, B., Zanella, K., Albright, K., Kessler, K., Bryson, F., Van Deventer, P., & Loomis, R. (1987). *A vocational followup evaluation of the 1984 to 1986 Madison Metropolitan School District graduates with severe intellectual disabilities* (Monograph). Seattle, WA: The Association for Persons with Severe Handicaps.

Bryan, T. (1974). Peer popularity of learning disabled children. *Journal of Learning Disabilities, 7,* 621–625.

Campbell, C., Campbell, S., Collicott, J., Perner, D., & Stone, J. (1988, June). Individualized instruction. *Education New Brunswick—Journal Education, 3,* 17–20.

Campbell, P.H. (1987). The integrated programming team: An approach for coordinating professionals of various disciplines in programs for students with severe and multiple handicaps. *Journal of The Association for Persons with Severe Handicaps, 12,* 107–116.

Canadian Education Association. (1985). *Mainstreaming: Some issues for school boards.* Toronto: Author.

Code of Federal Regulations. (1987, July). *34,* §300–399.

Deno, S., & Mirkin, P. (1977). *Data-based program modification: A manual.* Reston, VA: Council for Exceptional Children.

Department of Education, State of Hawaii v. Katherine D., 727 F.2d 809 (1983).

Deutsch, M. (1949). A theory of cooperation and competition. *Human Relations, 2,* 129–152.

Education for All Handicapped Children Act of 1975, §612, 20 U.S.C. §§1401–1485.

Eichinger, J. (1990). Effects of goal structures on social interaction between elementary level nondisabled students and students with severe disabilities. *Exceptional Children, 56,* 408–417.

Espino v. Besteiro, 520 F.Supp. 905 (1981).

Evans, I.M., Brown, F.A., Weed, K.A., Spry, K.M., & Owen, V. (1987). The assessment of functional competencies: A behavioral approach to the evaluation of programs for children with disabilities. In R.J. Prinz (Ed.), *Advances in behavioral assessment of children and families* (Vol. 3, pp. 93–121). Greenwich, CT: JAI Press.

Evans, I.M., & Meyer, L.M. (1987). Moving to educational validity: A reply to Test, Spooner, and Cooke. *Journal of The Association for Persons with Severe Handicaps, 12,* 103–106.

Falvey, M.A. (1989). *Community-based curriculum: Instructional strategies for students with severe handicaps* (2nd ed.). Baltimore: Paul H. Brookes Publishing Co.

Fenwick, V. (1987). The Edward Smith School program: An integrated public school continuum for autistic children. In M. Berres & P. Knoblock (Eds.), *Program models for mainstreaming: Integrating students with moderate to severe disabilities* (pp. 261–286). Rockville, MD: Aspen.

Flynn, G., & Kowalczck-McPhee, B. (1988). *A school system in transition.* Kitchener, Ontario: Waterloo Region Roman Catholic Separate School Board.

Ford, A., & Davern, L. (1989). Moving forward with school integration: Strategies for involving students with severe handicaps in the life of the school. In R. Gaylord-Ross (Ed.), *Integration strategies for students with handicaps* (pp. 11–33). Baltimore: Paul H. Brookes Publishing Co.

Ford, A., Foster, S.B., Searl, S.J., & Taylor, S.J. (1984). *The Brown School Model Project: A description.* Syracuse, NY: Syracuse University, The Center on Human Policy.

Ford, A., Schnorr, R., Meyer, L., Davern, L., Black, J., & Dempsey, P. (1989). *Syracuse community-referenced curriculum guide for students with moderate and severe disabilities.* Baltimore: Paul H. Brookes Publishing Co.

Forest, M. (1984). *Education/integration: A collection of readings on the integration of children with mental handicaps into regular school systems.* Downsview, Ontario: G. Allan Roeher Institute.

Forest, M. (1987). *More education/integration: A further collection of readings on the integration of children with mental handicaps into regular school systems.* Downsview, Ontario: G. Allan Roeher Institute.

Forest, M. (1989). *It's about relationships.* Toronto: Frontier College Press.

Fox, W., Thousand, J., Williams, W., Fox, T., Towne, P., Reid, R., Conn-Powers, C., & Calcagni, L. (1987). *Best educational practices '87: Educating learners with severe handicaps.* Burlington: University of Vermont, Center for Developmental Disabilities.

Frank, S., & Uditsky, B. (1988). On campus: Integration at university. *Entourage, 3*(3), 33–40.

Froland, C., Pancost, D., Chapman, N., & Kimboko, P. (1981). *Helping networks and human services.* Beverly Hills: Sage Publishing.

Fuchs, D., & Fuchs, L. (1989). Exploring effective and efficient prereferral interventions: A component analysis of behavioral consultation. *School Psychology Review, 18,* 260–279.

Gartner, A., & Lipsky, D. (1987). Beyond special education: Toward a quality system for all students. *Harvard Educational Review, 57,* 367–395.

Giangreco, M.F. (1986). Effects of integrated therapy: A pilot study. *Journal of The Association for Persons with Severe Handicaps, 11,* 205–208.

Giangreco, M.F. (1989a). Facilitating integration of students with severe disabilities. Implications of "planned change" for teacher preparation programs. *Teacher Education and Special Education, 12,* 139–147.

Giangreco, M.F. (1989b). Making related service decisions for students with severe handicaps in public schools: Roles, criteria, and authority. *Dissertation Abstracts International, 50*(6), 1624-A. (University Microfilms No. 8919516)

Giangreco, M.F., Cloninger, C., & Iverson, V. (1990). *Cayuga-Onondaga Assessment for Children with Handicaps—Version 6.0.* Stillwater: National Clearing House of Rehabilitation Training Materials at Oklahoma State University.

Giangreco, M.F., & Meyer, L.H. (1988). Expanding service delivery options in regular schools and classrooms for students with severe disabilities. In J. Graden, J. Zins, & M. Curtis (Eds.), *Alternative educational delivery systems: Enhancing instructional options for all students* (pp. 241–267).

Washington, DC: National Association of School Psychologists.

Giangreco, M.F., York, J., & Rainforth, B. (1989). Providing related services to learners with severe handicaps in educational settings: Pursuing the least restrictive option. *Pediatric Physical Therapy, 1,* 55–63.

Gickling, E., & Armstrong, D.L. (1978). Levels of instructional difficulty as related to on-task behavior, task completion and comprehension. *Journal of Learning Disabilities, 11,* 559–566.

Gilkeson, E.C., Smithberg, L.M., Bowman, G.W., & Rhine, W.R. (1981). Bank Street Model: A developmental-interaction approach. In W.R. Rhine (Ed.) *Making schools more effective: New directions from follow through* (pp. 249–288). New York: Academic Press.

Goetz, L., Guess, D., & Stremel-Campbell, K. (Eds.). (1987). *Innovative program design for individuals with dual sensory impairments.* Baltimore: Paul H. Brookes Publishing Co.

Goodlad, J.I. (1983). A study of schooling: Some findings and hypotheses. *Phi Delta Kappan, 64,* 462–470.

Gresham, F.M. (1982). Misguided mainstreaming: The case for social skills training with handicapped children. *Exceptional Children, 48,* 422–433.

Guess, D., Benson, H.A., & Siegel-Causey, E. (1985). Concepts and issues related to choice-making and autonomy among persons with severe handicaps. *Journal of The Association for Persons With Severe Handicaps, 10,* 79–86.

Hallahan, D.P., Keller, C.E., McKinney, J.D., Lloyd, J.W., & Bryan, T. (1988). Examining the research base of the regular education initiative: Efficacy studies and the Adaptive Learning Environments Model. *Journal of Learning Disabilities, 21*(1), 29–35.

Hardman, M.L., McDonnell, J., & McDonnell, A. (1989). *The inclusive neighborhood school: Educating students with severe disabilities in the least restrictive environment.* Manuscript submitted for publication.

Haring, N., Lovitt, J., Eaton, M., & Hansen, C. (1978). *The fourth R: Research in the classroom.* Columbus, OH: Charles E. Merrill.

Hasazi, S., Gordon, L., & Roe, C. (1985). Factors associated with the employment status of handicapped youth exiting high school from 1979–1983. *Exceptional Children, 51,* 455–469.

Horner, R., McDonnell, J., & Bellamy, G.T. (1986). Teaching generalized skills: General case instruction in simulation and community settings. In R.H. Horner, L.H. Meyer, & H.D.B. Fredericks (Eds.), *Education of learners with severe handicaps: Exemplary service strategies* (pp. 289–314). Baltimore: Paul H. Brookes Publishing Co.

Horner, R.H., Meyer, L.H., & Fredericks, H.D.B. (Eds.). (1986). *Education of learners with severe handicaps: Exemplary service strategies.* Balti-more: Paul H. Brookes Publishing Co.

Huefner, D.S. (1988). The consulting teacher model: Risks and opportunities. *Exceptional Children, 54,* 403–414.

Hymes v. Harnett County Board of Education, 664 F.2d 410 (4th Cir. 1981).

Irving Independent School District v. Tatro, 104 S.Ct. 3371 (1984).

Jellison, J.A., Brooks, B.H., & Huck, A.M. (1984). Structuring small groups and music reinforcement to facilitate positive interactions and acceptance of severely handicapped students in the regular music classroom. *Journal of Research in Music Education, 32,* 243–264.

Johnson, D.W., & Johnson, R.T. (1984). *Cooperation in the classroom.* Edina, MN: Interaction Books.

Johnson, D.W., & Johnson, R.T. (1986). *Cooperation and competition.* New York: Lawrence Erlbaum Associates.

Johnson, D.W., & Johnson, R.T. (1989). Cooperative learning and mainstreaming. In R. Gaylord-Ross (Ed.), *Integration strategies for students with handicaps* (pp. 233–248). Baltimore: Paul H. Brookes Publishing Co.

Johnson, D.W., Johnson, R.T., & Holubec, E.J. (1986). *Circles of learning: Cooperation in the classroom* (rev. ed.). Edina, MN: Interaction Books.

Johnson, D.W., Johnson, R.T., & Maruyama, G. (1983). Interdependence and interpersonal attraction among heterogeneous and homogeneous individuals: A theoretical formulation and a meta-analysis of the research. *Review of Educational Research, 3*(1), 5–54.

Johnson, D., Maruyama, G., Johnson, R., Nelson, D., & Skon, L. (1981). The effects of cooperative, competitive, and individualistic goal structures on achievement: A meta-analysis. *Psychological Bulletin, 89,* 47–62.

Johnson, R., Johnson, D.W., DeWeerdt, N., Lyons, V., & Zaidman, B. (1983). Integrating severely adaptively handicapped seventh-grade students into constructive relationships with nonhandicapped peers in science class. *American Journal of Mental Deficiency, 87*(6), 611–619.

Johnson, R., Rynders, J., Johnson, D.W., Schmidt, B., & Haiden, S. (1979). Producing positive interaction between handicapped and nonhandicapped teenagers through cooperative goal structuring: Implications for mainstreaming. *American Educational Research Journal, 16,* 161–168.

Kishi, G. (1988). Long-term effects of different types of contact between peers with and without severe disabilities: Outcomes of integration efforts in Hawaii. *Dissertation Abstracts International, 50* (2), 412-A. (University Microfilms No. 8901837)

Krouse, J., Gerber, M., & Kaufman, J. (1981). Peer tutoring: Procedures, promises, and unresolved issues. *Exceptional Education Quarterly, 1*(4), 107–115.

Leyser, Y., & Gottlieb, J. (1981). Social status im-

provement of unpopular handicapped and nonhandicapped pupils: A review. *Elementary School Journal, 81*(4), 228–236.

Lipsky, D.K., & Gartner, A. (Eds.). (1989). *Beyond
separate education: Quality education for all*. Baltimore: Paul H. Brookes Publishing Co.

MacMillan, D.L., Jones, R.L., & Aloia, T.F. (1974).
The mentally retarded label: A theoretical analysis
and review of research. *American Journal of Mental Deficiency, 79*, 241–261.

Madden, N.A., & Slavin, R.E. (1983). Mainstreaming students with mild handicaps: Academic and
social outcomes. *Review of Educational Research,
53*, 519–569.

Maheady, L., Sacca, M.K., & Harper, G.F. (1988).
Classwide peer tutoring with mildly handicapped
high school students. *Exceptional Children, 55*(1),
52–59.

McDonnell, A.P., & Hardman, M.H. (1989). The desegregation of America's schools: Strategies for
change. *Journal of The Association for Persons
with Severe Handicaps, 14*, 68–74.

Meyer, L.H., & Eichinger, J. (1987). Program evaluation in support of program development: Needs,
strategies, and future directions. In L. Goetz, D.
Guess, & K. Stremel-Campbell (Eds.), *Innovative
program design for individuals with dual sensory
impairments* (pp. 313–353). Baltimore: Paul H.
Brookes Publishing Co.

Meyer, L.H., Eichinger, J., & Park-Lee, S. (1987). A
validation of program quality indicators in educational services for students with severe disabilities.
*Journal of The Association for Persons with Severe
Handicaps, 12*, 251–263.

Meyer, L.H., & Putnam, J. (1988). Social integration.
In V.B. Van Hasselt, P.S. Strain, & M. Hersen
(Eds.), *Handbook of developmental and physical
disabilities* (pp. 107–133). New York: Pergamon
Press.

Natriello, G. (1987). Introduction. In G. Natriello
(Ed.), *School dropouts: Patterns and policies* (pp.
1–19). New York: Teachers College Press.

Nevin, A., & Thousand, J. (1987). Avoiding or limit-
ing special education referrals: Changes and chal-
lenges. In M.C. Wang, M.C. Reynolds, & H.J.
Walberg (Eds.), *Handbook of special education:
Research and practice* (pp. 273–286). New York:
Pergamon Press.

Panitch, M. (1988). Community college integration:
More than just an education. *Entourage, 3*(3), 26–
32.

Peck, C., & Semmel, M. (1982). Identifying the least
restrictive environment (LRE) for children with severe handicaps: Toward an empirical analysis. *Journal of The Association for the Severely Handicapped, 7*(1), 56–63.

Peterson, N.L., & Haralick, J.G. (1977). Integration
of handicapped and nonhandicapped preschoolers:
An analysis of play behavior and social interaction.

*Education and Training of the Mentally Retarded,
12*, 235–245.

Porter, G. (1988, June). *School integration: Fact, fantasy, or the future?* Paper presented at the International Conference on Special Education, Beijing,
China.

Porter, R.H., Ramsey, B., Tremblay, A., Iaccobo,
M., & Crawley, I. (1978). Social interactions in heterogeneous groups of retarded and normally developing children: An observational study. In G.
Sacket (Ed.), *Observing behavior: Theory and applications in mental retardation* (Vol. 1). Baltimore:
University Park Press.

Putnam, J.W., & Rynders, J.E. (1985). *Effects of
teacher instruction on promoting cooperative interactions between moderately-severely mentally handicapped and nonhandicapped children*. Minneapolis:
University of Minnesota Consortium Institute.

Putnam, J., Rynders, J., Johnson, R., & Johnson, D.
(1989). Collaborative skill instruction for promoting positive interactions between mentally handicapped and nonhandicapped children. *Exceptional
Children, 55*(6), 550–558.

Reid, R. (1987, Fall). Homecoming: The benefits of
educating learning impaired students in their local
schools with their non-disabled peers. *The Deci-
sion-Maker*, pp. 5–6. (Available from Center for
Developmental Disabilities, University of Vermont, Burlington, VT 05405)

Rettig v. Kent City, 539 F. Supp. 769 (1981); 720 F.2d
463 (1983).

Roncker v. Walter, 700 F.2d 1058, cert. denied, 104
S.Ct. 196 (1983).

Rynders, J., Johnson, R., Johnson, D., & Schmidt,
B. (1980). Producing positive interaction among
Down syndrome and nonhandicapped teenagers
through cooperative goal structure. *American Journal of Mental Deficiency, 85*, 268–283.

Sailor, W. (1989). The educational, social, and vocational integration of students with the most severe
disabilities. In D.K. Lipsky & A. Gartner (Eds.),
*Beyond separate education: Quality education for
all* (pp. 53–74). Baltimore: Paul H. Brookes Publishing Co.

Sailor, W., Anderson, J.L., Halvorsen, A.T., Doering, K., Filler, J., & Goetz, L. (1989). *The comprehensive local school: Regular education for all
students with disabilities*. Baltimore: Paul H.
Brookes Publishing Co.

Sailor, W., & Guess, D. (1983). *Severely handicapped
students: An instructional design*. Boston: Houghton Mifflin.

Sailor, W., Halvorsen, A., Anderson, J., Goetz, L.,
Gee, K., Doering, K., & Hunt, P. (1986). Community intensive instruction. In R.H. Horner, L.H.
Meyer, & H.D.B. Fredericks (Eds.), *Education of
learners with severe handicaps: Exemplary service
strategies* (pp. 251–288). Baltimore: Paul H.
Brookes Publishing Co.

Schattman, R. (1989). *Franklin Northwest Supervisory Union: A model for full integration.* Swanton, VT: Franklin NW Supervisory Union.

Semmel, M.I., Gottlieb, J., & Robinson, N.M. (1979). Mainstreaming: Perspectives on educating handicapped children in public schools. In D.C. Berliner (Ed.), *Review of research in education* (pp. 223–278). Washington, DC: American Educational Research Association.

Shevin, M., & Klein, N.K. (1984). The importance of choice-making for students with severe disabilities. *Journal of The Association for Persons with Severe Handicaps, 9,* 159–166.

Slavin, R., Madden, N., & Leavey, M. (1984). Effects of team assisted individualization on mathematics achievement of academically handicapped and nonhandicapped students. *Journal of Educational Psychology, 76,* 813–819.

Snell, M.E. (Ed.). (1986). *Systematic instruction of persons with moderate and severe handicaps* (3rd ed.). Columbus, OH: Charles E. Merrill.

Snell, M.E. (1988). Gartner and Lipsky's *Beyond separate education: Quality education for all—* Messages for TASH. *Journal of The Association for Persons with Severe Handicaps, 13,* 137–140.

Snell, M.E., & Browder, D.M. (1986). Community referenced instruction: Research and issues. *Journal of The Association for Persons with Severe Handicaps, 11,* 1–11.

Snell, M.E., & Eichner, S. (1989). Integration of students with profound disabilities. In F. Brown & D.H. Lehr (Eds.), *Persons with profound disabilities: Issues and practices* (pp. 109–138). Baltimore: Paul H. Brookes Publishing Co.

Snow, J., & Forest, M. (1987). Circles. In M. Forest (Ed.), *More education/integration: A further collection of readings on the integration of children with mental handicaps into regular school systems* (pp. 169–176). Downsview, Ontario: G. Allan Roeher Institute.

Stacy G. v. Pasadena Independent School District, 547 F. Supp. 61 (1982).

Stainback, S., & Stainback, W. (1985). *Integration of students with severe handicaps into regular schools.* Reston, VA: Council for Exceptional Children.

Stainback, S., Stainback, W., & Harris, K. (1989). Support facilitation: An emerging role for special educators. *Teacher Education and Special Education.*

Stieler, S., Agostinelli, Sr., Leditschke, F., McDonnell, E., Stilman, Sr., & Urbacher, U. (1977). Prosthesis in educational intervention. In K. Cochran & R. Andrews (Eds.), *Health and welfare of children: Proceedings of an interdisciplinary seminar* (pp. 175–80). Brisbane, Australia: Queensland University. (ERIC Document Reproduction No. ED 165-439)

Strain, P.S., & Shores, R.E. (1983). A reply to "Misguided Mainstreaming." *Exceptional Children, 50,* 271–273.

Strully, J., & Strully, C. (1985). Friendship and our children. *Journal of The Association for Persons with Severe Handicaps, 10,* 224–227.

Taylor, S.J. (1988). Caught in the continuum: A critical analysis of the principles of the least restrictive environment. *Journal of The Association for Persons with Severe Handicaps, 13,* 41–53.

Thousand, J., Fox, T., Reid, R., Godek, J., Williams, W., & Fox, W. (1986). *The Homecoming Model: Educating students who present intensive educational challenges within regular education environments.* Burlington: University of Vermont, Center for Developmental Disabilities.

Thousand, J.S., & Villa, R.A. (1989). Enhancing success in heterogeneous schools. In S. Stainback, W. Stainback, & M. Forest (Eds.), *Educating all students in the mainstream of regular education* (pp. 89–103). Baltimore: Paul H. Brookes Publishing Co.

Tokarcik v. Forest Hills School District, 665 F.2d 443 (3 cir. 1981).

Uditsky, B., & Kappel, B. (1988). Integrated postsecondary education. *Entourage, 3*(3), 23–26.

Vandercook, T. (1989). *Performance in the criterion situation for students with severe disabilities.* Paper submitted for publication.

Vandercook, T., York, J., & Forest, M. (1989). The McGill Action Planning System (MAPS): A strategy for building the vision. *Journal of The Association for Persons with Severe Handicaps, 14,* 205–215.

Villa, R.A., & Thousand, J.S. (1990). Administrative supports to promote inclusive schooling. In W. Stainback & S. Stainback (Eds.), *Support networks for inclusive schooling: Interdependent integrated education* (pp. 201–218). Baltimore: Paul H. Brookes Publishing Co.

Voeltz, L.M. (1980). Children's attitudes toward handicapped peers. *American Journal of Mental Deficiency, 84,* 455–464.

Voeltz, L.M. (1982). Effects of structured interactions with severely handicapped peers on children's attitudes. *American Journal of Mental Deficiency, 86,* 380–390.

Voeltz, L.M. (1984). Program and curricular adaptations to prepare children for integration. In N. Certo, N. Haring, & R. York (Eds.), *Public school integration of severely handicapped students: Rational issues and progressive alternatives* (pp. 155–183). Baltimore: Paul H. Brookes Publishing Co.

Voeltz, L.M., & Evans, I.M. (1983). Educational validity: Procedures to evaluate outcomes in programs for severely handicapped learners. *Journal of The Association for the Severely Handicapped, 8*(1), 3–15.

Walberg, H.J., & Wang, M.C. (1987). Effective educational practices and provisions for individual differences. In M.C. Wang, M.C. Reynolds, & H.J. Walberg (Eds.), *Handbook of special education: Research and practice* (pp. 113–128). New York: Pergamon Press.

Wang, M.C., & Birch, J.W. (1984). Effective special education in regular classes. *Exceptional Children, 50,* 391–398.

Wang, M., Gennari, P., & Waxman, H. (1985). The Adaptive Learning Environments Model: Design, implementation, and effects. In M. Wang & H. Walberg (Eds.), *Adapting instruction to individual differences* (pp. 191–235). Berkeley, CA: McCutchan.

Wang, M., Reynolds, M., & Schwartz, L. (1988). Adaptive instruction: An alternative educational approach for students with special needs. In J. Graden, J. Zins, & M. Curtis (Eds.), *Alternative educational delivery systems: Enhancing instructional options for all students* (pp. 199–220). Washington, DC: National Association of School Psychologists.

Wehlage, G.G., & Rutter, R.A. (1987). Dropping out: How much do schools contribute to the problem? In G. Natriello (Ed.), *School dropouts: Patterns and policies* (pp. 70–88). New York: Teachers College Press.

Wilcox, J., Sbardellati, E., & Nevin, A. (1987). Integrating a severely handicapped girl in a first grade classroom with cooperative learning groups. *Teaching Exceptional Children, 20*(1), 61–63.

Williams, W., Fox, T., & Fox, W. (1988). *Integrating the instruction of students with intensive educational needs into regular education classrooms: Individual program design procedures manual.* Burlington: University of Vermont, Center for Developmental Disabilities.

Williams, W., Fox, W., Christie, L., Thousand, J., Conn-Powers, M., Carmichael, L., Vogelsburg, R.T., & Hull, M. (1986). Community integration in Vermont. *Journal of The Association for Persons with Severe Handicaps, 11,* 294–299.

Wilson, R. (1987). Direct observation of academic learning time. *Teaching Exceptional Children, 19*(2), 13–17.

York, J., & Rainforth, B. (1987). Developing instructional adaptations. In F.P. Orelove & D. Sobsey (Eds.), *Educating children with multiple disabilities: A transdisciplinary approach* (pp. 183–217). Baltimore: Paul H. Brookes Publishing Co.

York, J., & Vandercook, T. (in press). Strategies for achieving an integrated education for middle school aged learners with severe disabilities. *Remedial and Special Education.*

York, J., Vandercook, T., Caughey, E., & Helse-Neff, C. (1988, December). *Does an "Integration Facilitator" facilitate integration?* Minneapolis: University of Minnesota, Institute on Community Integration.

CHAPTER 16

Supporting Families of Persons with Severe Disabilities
Emerging Findings, Practices, and Questions

GEORGE H.S. SINGER

LARRY K. IRVIN

Oregon Research Institute, Eugene, Oregon

C. Wright Mills (1959) distinguished between "issues" and "troubles": The former are public matters, the latter are personal. Troubles and their resolution are matters of the heart that are commonly described in the many versions of intrapsychic analysis such as cognitive psychology. Issues and their resolution are collective matters as in sociological, historical, and policy analyses. Some problems are best dealt with as troubles whereas others can only be effectively addressed as issues. Successful resolution of troubles yields personal benefits such as knowledge, enrichment, and enablement. Success in resolution of societal issues yields societal benefits such as an improved quality of life, a more humane society, and a society that reifies its values in the institutions that serve its citizens.

In this chapter we expand upon Mills's (1959) ideas by examining evidence for the benefits of resolution of troubles and issues related to family adaptation. We highlight research issues that we believe hold special promise for improving services to families. We believe that we can contribute to resolving troubles by recognizing their origin in collective issues.

There are four major conceptual foundations for the discussion we present in this chapter; some are values assertions, others are empirical issues: 1) the problems and benefits of family home caregiving for families of children with developmental disabilities are part of a much larger social issue concerning the role of families and vulnerable citizens in Western industrial nations; 2) the traditional rationale for public services to families is insufficient and should be replaced with one that emphasizes prevention, promotion, and amelioration; 3) traditional service design for families requires new thinking concerning public and private partnerships and the role of formal and informal support systems; and 4) the focus of psychological services for these families requires expansion and revision to reflect the larger context in which helping professions address both troubles and issues.

VIEW FROM HIGH GROUND

Demographic and Policy Trends

Throughout Western industrialized democracies, several demographic trends are apparent. These include urbanization, declining birth rates, increasing diversity in family structure, and historically novel numbers of dependent elderly persons and individuals with disabilities who require new forms of interdependence. One common factor is a revolution in medical care that enables larger numbers of low-birthweight infants, trauma victims, and extremely elderly persons to survive (Gabel & Kotsch, 1981; Kitchen et al., 1986; Kitchen et al., 1982; Lubchenco et al., 1989).

The writing of this chapter was supported in part by Grants #G008730149-88 and #H023T80013 to the Oregon Research Institute from the United States Department of Education. The views expressed do not reflect those of the funding agency.

At the same time that the numbers of vulnerable citizens (young children, persons with chronic illness, extremely elderly persons, and persons with developmental disabilities) are increasing, the traditional human resources for caregiving have been dramatically diverted. That is, a majority of family members who have traditionally been caregivers in homes have joined the labor force. Concomitantly, the traditional social supports for these primary caregivers—marriage, extended family, and settled community—have eroded.

In response, many European countries, under the influence of democratic socialist movements, have enacted national policies aimed at assisting families to care for their vulnerable family members (Baldwin, 1985; Kahn & Kamerman, 1983). These include generous financial assistance as well as neighborhood-level services for assisting families with public health and social needs (Cohen & Warren, 1987; Garbarino et al., 1980).

Social and demographic conditions in the United States are both similar to and markedly different from those in western Europe, depending upon which variable is of interest. On both continents, the prevalence rates of certain diagnostic groups are increasing due to improved chances of survival associated with new medical technology. For example, the age of survival of children with cystic fibrosis has increased sevenfold since 1960, and has increased twofold or greater for children with spina bifida, leukemia, and congenital heart disease (Werner, 1989). Similarly, improved trauma care has given rise to a cumulative and growing population of persons with traumatic brain injury (Wikler, 1986b). It is estimated that 60,000–70,000 persons annually in the United States suffer from moderate to severe brain injuries; as recently as a decade ago many of these individuals would have died (Bush, 1988). Now many survive with long-lasting disabilities (Bush, 1988). This population is cumulative. Similarly, an estimated 250,000 persons with chronic mental illness are discharged to family care each year (Goldman, 1982). And approximately 5.1 million elderly persons require assistance with some aspect of personal care or home management in order to live in the community; this assistance is primarily offered by family members (American Association of Retired Persons, 1986). And, increasing numbers of very low–birthweight children are surviving with an increased incidence in some handicapping conditions, particularly cerebral palsy.

While the number of persons who need assistance to live normal lives in their own homes and communities is increasing, the number of people available to provide this assistance is declining. In the United States, as in Europe, birth rates and size of families are declining. For example, the percentage of family households with three or fewer members rose from 37% in 1900 to 60% in 1980 (Moroney, 1986). Divorce rates are higher and single parenthood is increasingly common. Further, a majority of men and women work outside of the home during the day.

When viewed from a socioeconomic perspective, home caregiving for vulnerable citizens is a vital national resource (Moroney, 1986). If all of the work that is performed by caregiving families had to be paid for in cash, the costs would consume a notable portion of the gross national product (GNP) (Waring, 1988). Since the late 1800s, in western Europe and the United States, married women have done most of this work as part of the homemaker role. Despite dramatic changes in women's societal roles and gradual shifts in societal values over the past 20 years, mothers continue to do the bulk of the daily work of caring for children with disabilities and chronic illness in the United States as well as in other advanced industrialized nations (Kazak & Marvin, 1984; Wilkin, 1979).

Although the traditional assignment of caregiving tasks to mothers has not changed, other basic elements of women's life careers have changed dramatically. Two trends are most apparent: women's participation in the labor force and an increase in the numbers of single mothers during childrearing years. We focus on women as caregivers not because we believe that fathers, siblings, and extended family should not be primary caregivers, but because the literature and our own extensive experience with caregiving families indicate that mothers still do the bulk of this work.

Since the end of World War II, women have entered the labor force in accelerating numbers.

The rise in the percentage of married women and women with dependent children in the labor force has paralleled this general trend. In 1960, 30% of mothers with children from birth to 17 living at home worked outside of the home, compared with 51.2% in 1980 (Moroney, 1986). At the same time, the numbers of single mothers and impoverished women has increased. These social and demographic trends operate to jeopardize home caregiving. They not only place vulnerable citizens in jeopardy but they place caregiving women at risk as well.

When the labor of caregiving can no longer be performed at home because family members must work outside of the home, someone or some societal institution must "take up the slack." The evidence suggests that one major unplanned, and often undesirable, "solution" to the problem of allocating caregiving labor has arisen. That is, many women have simply taken up a double workload: They work outside of the home, and when they return home each day, they do the additional tasks of caregiving (Wilkin, 1979). When caregivers must remain home because a relative requires constant care, it is at a cost of a lower standard of living or welfare dependence. The pressures of inflation in basic goods such as housing often give family members no choice but to seek outside employment and divert caregiving to either poorly paid daycare providers or unemployed elderly family members and/or siblings. Thus, there are increasing numbers of vulnerable persons who require unusual levels of interdependence and caregiving and there are fewer hours and less intrafamily support available for this role.

Unlike most of western Europe, the differences between upper and lower income families in the United States have widened, and the percentage of children living in poverty has been increasing over the past decade (Kagan, 1989). Poverty and its accompanying higher rates of disability cluster among racial and ethnic minorities. Children from economically poor families are 40% more likely to have a severe functional disability than are children in families with higher incomes (Brady, 1987). The implications of this fact are harsh, given that one in five children now lives in poverty in the United States. The extra financial costs of caring for a child

with a chronic disability hit hardest at the poor and lower middle classes. For example, Sultz, Schlesinger, Mosher, and Feldman (1972), in their study of families of children with chronic illness, found that families in the lowest quartile for gross income were required to expend 16% of their income on extra medical expenses compared to 7.9% and 4.1% in the upper two quartiles.

Also, unlike many western European countries, basic services for all families—such as health care and high-quality public school programs—are not universally available in the United States. Currently some 37 million Americans lack any form of health insurance including coverage for care of children with severe disabilities (Anthony-Bergstone, Zarit, & Gatz, 1988). Rates of homelessness, drug addiction, and reported family violence have all increased in the past decade. Thus, a growing population of persons with severe handicaps must be served by a nation that in many ways has not yet established a basic infrastructure for supporting *all* families (Rodgers, 1982).

The United States has been slower than European countries to adopt a national policy of family support for caregiving families. In the recent, more conservative political climate in the United States, policy innovations have emerged only incrementally. At a national level, there has been a recognition only in principle that we should commit federal resources for families of children with handicaps. PL 99-457 requires that public school service providers develop for the first time a plan of family intervention as a way to assist infants and toddlers with handicaps. However, currently less than 2% of all public funds for persons with developmental disabilities goes to families (Braddock, Hemp, Fujiura, Bachelder, & Mitchell, 1989). Over a decade ago, Wilkin (1979) summarized the situation of caregiving families in England in terms that accurately describe the condition in much of the United States in 1990:

> The term community care for children with mental handicaps refers to care *in* the community and not care *by* the community. The nuclear family is the framework in which the child is cared for. Within the family it is mothers who carry the major burden of care usually with relatively little support from

other family members. The contribution of people outside the family to the practical burden of care is almost negligible. (p. 146)

As we discuss later, those families that are most successful at caregiving often are the ones in which the mother is strongly supported by other family members and that draw upon a variety of community services (e.g., Cole & Meyer, 1989).

Family Caregiver Stress

A sociological view of issues as causes of personal troubles would lead to a prediction that caregivers who are caught between these opposing socioeconomic forces would experience psychosocial difficulties. In fact, there is evidence that home caregiving for vulnerable persons does exact a toll on many people in the absence of adequate formal and informal societal assistance.

Salutogenesis/Bonadaptation versus Pathogenesis/Maladaptation

Before we sketch the case that there is a generic societal problem called *caregiver stress* that has resulted from economic and demographic trends, a few words are needed about the literature on caregiving stress. Just as the problems of caregivers reflect larger societal trends, so the research literature on family home caregiving reflects larger trends in the social sciences. Until recently, the study of family caregiving has reflected a general emphasis in the social sciences on troubles rather than issues, and on pathological effects of difficult circumstances rather than personal benefits and historic achievements in response to stressful circumstances. A.P. Turnbull, Blue-Banning, Behr, and Kerns (1986) noted this bias in the extensive literature on the personal troubles and family strains that arise in some families of children with disabilities. They pointed out that this corpus of knowledge flies in the face of the experience of many families who come to view home caregiving as a natural and beneficial responsibility that brings with it challenges that promote personal benefits. We would add that this literature fails to acknowledge the way in which Western societies gradually are moving toward goals of mutual aid that have been central tenets of Western civil and religious thought for centuries. On an individual level,

home caregiving offers an opportunity for personal enrichment. On a societal level, the creation of adequate supports for families offers the opportunity to achieve the ideals that underpin our culture.

In recent years, health and developmental psychologists have begun to try to account for the ways that people respond to severe life stressors in such a way that they not only survive but also grow and benefit. Social science has been so fixed upon pathology that most of these authors have had to invent words to describe gains that can arise in individuals and families as a result of adversity. Antonovsky (1987) described the process as "salutogenesis," the opposite of pathogenesis. Similarly, McCubbin and Patterson (1983) labeled the opposite of maladaptive family response to crisis as "bonadaptation." Most of the literature on salutogenesis has framed the discussion in terms of personality traits. For example, Antonovsky identified a sense of coherence as the distinguishing trait of persons who benefit from adversity. People with a sense of coherence view the environment as orderly, find a meaning in adversity that accompanies motivated action, and have a sense that they can control environmental or intrapsychic aspects of the situation. Similarly, S.J. Taylor, Knoll, Lehr, and Walker (1989) studied cancer patients who coped well, and characterized them as having a sense of mastery, high self-esteem, and meaning. Summers, Behr, and Turnbull (1989) followed S.J. Taylor et al.'s model in exploring positive adaptation to the presence of a family member with disabilities. And Cole (1986) adapted the notion of bonadaptation from McCubbin and Patterson in order to account for positive outcomes in families of children with severe handicaps.

A problem with Antonovsky's (1987) trait approach is that it assumes that relatively fixed personal characteristics are key determinants. Consequently, it holds few implications for amelioration of distress among those who do not already have these traits. Presumably, personality traits evolve over long periods of time and cannot be induced or learned in the short term.

We proceed on the more optimistic assumption that critical features of personal, familial, and societal coping can in fact be identified and disseminated. On a personal level, we believe that coping skills can be learned through ordinary social learning processes. On the level of the family unit, we believe that group sharing of tasks, effective communication, conflict resolution, and shared meanings can be learned and promoted through the right kinds of social supports. At a societal level, we believe that formal and informal institutions can be strengthened or created in order to promote these positive outcomes.

In this chapter, we try to identify teachable components of skills and malleable social circumstances that may foster acquisition and generalization of these skills. We try to demonstrate the way that some aspects of salutatory personality traits have been taught to some people in difficulty. Similarly, we try to identify characteristics of families that adapt well to caregiving and some of the social circumstances that enable these families to succeed. At a societal level, we describe some of the emerging policies in other democratic industrialized societies that appear to be building a historical achievement of enabling citizens to care for one another in adversity. This approach to family caregiving is concerned not only with the problems and troubles that families suffer but also with the benefits and achievements associated with successful caregiving and its social context. Thus, when we review some of the evidence for personal troubles and family strains it is for the purpose of diagnosis in order to prescribe effective supportive circumstances. We do not believe that the extensive literature on caregiver stress should be interpreted as simply reflecting the biases of family researchers. Nor should it be viewed as an accurate representation of the whole picture. Evidence concerning what personal, familial, and societal variables are associated with positive adaptation to caregiving is equal in importance to evidence that many caregiving families have serious troubles. Taken together, such evidence provides some useful information about ways to alleviate suffering, prevent the conditions that induce distress, and promote the conditions that enable families to arrive at benefits and society to accomplish historical achievements. In this context, the literature on pathogenesis—the negative processes and outcomes in some care-

giving families—is viewed as one useful tool in helping design effective interventions.

Caregiver Stress as a Generic Problem with Generic Solutions

Home caregiving can place considerable pressure upon family members who assist their vulnerable relatives. A growing body of evidence (e.g., Joyce, Singer, & Isralowitz, 1983; Orford, 1987) suggests that, without proper societal support, caregiving exacts a common toll on some primary caregivers. We have recently conducted a meta-analysis of studies of caregivers that compare caregivers with matched controls on measures of psychosocial adjustment (Singer, Irvin, & Yovanoff, in preparation). We searched the literature for studies of caregivers of elderly family members with disabilities, children with handicaps, and family members with traumatic brain injury. In order to qualify for our sample, a study must have used standardized instruments and noncaregiving control groups, and means and standard deviations had to be reported. We believe that the aggregate picture presented by this study does reflect a reality that some (a sizable minority of) caregivers experience. In Table 16.1 we present a "box score" comparison of studies that have examined caregivers of children with severe handicaps and family caregivers of elderly persons with Alzheimer's disease or other severe cognitive impairments. Table 16.1 shows the number of studies reviewed that reported significant differences on selected variables related to well-being between caregivers and noncaregivers. We interpret our meta-analysis results as showing that caregivers commonly are at greater risk for psychological distress than are persons who are not caring for vulnerable relatives. Interestingly, the two studies of parents of children with severe handicaps that did not find a difference in rates of maternal risk for depression compared parents of infants and young children with and without handicaps (Bristol, Gallagher, & Schopler, 1988; Erickson & Upsher, 1989). The nonsignificant differences may be due to elevated levels of distress in mothers of infants, regardless of whether or not the infants have handicaps, and to the fact that the parents who were studied were participants in early intervention programs that provided ex-

Table 16.1. Numbers of studies[a] reporting significant relationships[b] between selected variables related to caregiver stress (number of significant findings/number of relevant studies)

	Stress	Burden	Depression	Support		Social life	Marital satisfaction	Quality of relationship to recipient	Caregiver gender	Finance	Health
				Formal	Informal						
Stress		3/3	2/5	1/2	4/5	3/3	5/5	3/3	2/2	3/3	3/3
Burden					2/2	2/2		2/2	0/2	1/1	
Depression						1/1					
Level of impairment	9/10	8/10	3/4								
Recipient behavior	4/4	4/4									

[a] A total of 31 outcome studies were reviewed and referenced. Of the 31 publications, 13 reported research on families of elderly dementia patients, and 18 reported research on families of children with handicaps. The studies included in this review are: Anthony-Bergstone, Zarit, and Gatz (1988); Beckman, Pokorni, Maza, and Balzer-Martin (1986); Breslau and Davis (1986); Breslau, Staruch, and Mortimer (1982); Bristol, Gallagher, and Schopler (1988); Burdz, Eaton, and Bond (1988); Cantor (1983); Chetwynd (1985); Cummings (1976); Davies (1985); Drinka, Smith, and Drinka (1987); Dyson and Fewell (1986); Ericksohn and Upshur (1989); Fitting, Rabins, Lucas, and Eastham (1986); Friedrich and Friedrich (1981); Gath (1977); Haley, Levine, Brown, and Bartolucci (1987); Holroyd and Guthrie (1979); Holroyd and McArthur (1976); Kazak and Marvin (1984); Montgomery, Gonyea, and Hooyman (1985); Pahl and Quine (1987); Pearson, Verma, and Nellet (1988); Poulshock and Deimling (1984); Pratt, Schmall, Wright, and Cleland (1985); Roach (1984); Salisbury (1987); Wikler (1986b); Winogrond, Fisk, Kirsling, and Keye (1987); Zarit, Reever, and Bach-Peterson (1980); and Zarit, Todd, and Zarit (1986).

[b] Significant relationships are based on correlations and group differences are significant at the .05 level.

tensive social support. The evidence suggests that there is a common phenomenon, caregiver stress, when family members provide home care for children or elderly relatives with severe handicaps. It is important to note that our analysis examined caregiving of persons with some of the most severe handicaps—both severe cognitive impairment and need for assistance with many of the activities of daily living.

Family caregiving is not inevitably a negative experience. A majority (two thirds in most studies) of caregivers are not distressed at any given time. And distress in the present may lead to positive outcomes in the future. Of course, caregiving creates the opportunities for personal growth and a deepening of interpersonal ties. It would be absurd simply to label caregiving, a most human of activities, as a source of pathology. Caregiver stress should be viewed not only on a personal level as a source of troubles, but also as a source of potential benefit to caregivers, families, and society. On a societal level, it should be considered not only as a set of issues, but also as an opportunity for historic achievements. Table 16.1 does not contain evidence of caregiver benefit because such benefit has not yet been systematically assessed—although there has been much testimonial evidence that many people benefit from the caregiver role (Ferguson & Asch, 1989; McCubbin et al., 1983; H.R. Turnbull, Guess, & Turnbull, 1988).

It is important also to note the extent and severity of caregiver stress. First, the measures used in these studies are self-reports of psychological moods and symptoms. The best two instruments are the Center for Epidemiological Studies Depression (CES-D) Scale (Radloff, 1977) and the Beck Depression Inventory (BDI) Beck, Ward, Mendelson, Moch, & Erbaugh, 1961). Both are used as indicators of depressive symptomology. Both have cut-off scores that have been empirically validated. We believe that these measures are best understood as indicators of low morale because clinical depression has to be determined through psychological interviews with trained raters. Low morale is not the same as mental illness. In fact, in the one study in which rates of clinical depression (i.e., mental illness) were examined in caregiving mothers,

no differences were found in the prevalence of clinical depression between caregiving and non-caregiving mothers, although twice as many caregiving mothers reported low morale (i.e., depressive symptomology) (Breslau & Davis, 1986). In studies by Breslau and Davis, Pahl and Quine (1987), and Bristol et al. (1988), approximately 30%–40% of caregiving mothers were demoralized, compared with 15% in the general population.

The research on comparative rates of low morale in parents of children with or without handicaps is equivocal. Those studies that employed large sample sizes and included school-age children have reported significantly higher rates of low morale (Breslau & Davis, 1986; Pahl & Quine, 1987; Singer, Irvin, Irvine, Hawkins, & Cooley, 1989) than have studies that used smaller sample sizes and focused on infants and young children (Bristol et al., 1988). These findings of nonsignificant differences, in addition to small sample size, may be explained by the findings that rates of low morale are elevated in mothers of very young children with handicaps (Radloff & Cox, 1981) and that many parents cope well with the birth of a child with handicaps (Summers et al., 1989).

When family variables are measured, evidence for caregiver stress again emerges. There is evidence for economic stress, social isolation, and sibling distress, as well as some equivocal evidence for higher rates of divorce and lower rates of remarriage. The literature regarding impacts on families of children with severe disabilities has been reviewed in more detail elsewhere (Cole, 1986; Singer & Irvin, 1989b, A.P. Turnbull & Turnbull, 1986). Similar findings of negative family impacts have appeared in studies of families of persons with traumatic brain injury (Livingston & Brooks, 1988), families of persons with chronic mental illness (Abramowitz & Coursey, 1989), and families caring for frail elderly family members (Toseland & Rossiter, 1989). The literature as we have reviewed it suggests that the strains involved in the caregiving role are partly responsible for distress in many families.

The thrust of Mill's (1959) argument about the relationship between personal troubles and societal issues is that when large numbers of people under similar circumstances experience similar personal difficulties, it is likely that the problem is best viewed as a societal issue in which communal solutions to public issues may play a substantial role in ameliorating the personal troubles. In the discussion that follows we describe some of the current public efforts to assist caregiving families with children with developmental disabilities.

When reviewing the current service system for caregiving families, one is immediately struck by the miniscule percentage of public resources put into this area compared with the billions of dollars spent on long-term out-of-home care arrangements for vulnerable persons. For example, only about 2% of all public funds for persons with developmental disabilities goes to various family support services (Braddock et al., 1989). A similarly minute percentage of Medicare funds supports home caregiving for elderly persons (Moroney, 1986). In order to understand this emphasis it is necessary to take a look at the historical assumptions behind public assistance for vulnerable citizens.

Historical Foundations: Tradition of Residualism

It is important to consider the first premises upon which family support services have been founded. Otherwise, the inertia of historical forces is likely to restrict our vision and effectiveness unnecessarily. Moroney (1986) examined the history of family assistance programs in the United States. He asserted that our services have been based upon a residual model in which it is assumed that the great majority of families will fend for themselves, and that only a small *residual* population that fails to fulfill expected societal roles will receive public assistance. The residualist approach provides assistance only after crisis and collapse of normal functioning have occurred. Using the metaphor of a social safety net, assistance is offered from the state only after a family has fallen off the high wire. The starkest demonstration of this fact can be seen in the budgetary figures regarding residential options for persons with handicaps. Again, Braddock et al. (1989) documented that less than 2% of the billions of dollars spent on persons with developmental disabilities

is allocated for family support. The lion's share of the budget goes to supporting persons in institutions. In many cases, public funds are not available for children with handicaps until after parents have given up custody. In effect, society stands ready to help once it is too late.

This residualist tradition has deep historical roots. In ancient Europe, children with handicaps were often abandoned in public to become slaves. In Medieval times, they were frequently abandoned to be raised by the Church. Beginning in the eighteenth century, children with handicaps were expelled from families into disease-ridden public hospitals and foundlings homes (Boswell, 1988). Communities delivered assistance only after children were ejected from natural families. In the contemporary United States, most public resources are not available to caregiving families until they elect to place their children with handicaps out of the home. Until very recently, social insitutions outside of the family have contributed to caregiving only after the family has elected to abrogate normal familial responsibilities by expelling a member with disabilities.

Two other corollaries follow from the residualist perspective: 1) an emphasis on crisis management, and 2) an emphasis on social control. In this historical tradition, public assistance is solely for the purpose of preventing the worst of outcomes and only after informal social systems have failed: Most support services have been established to intervene once a family has begun the process of breakdown. For example, in several states public assistance can only be made available once custody of a child with handicaps is remanded to the state. That is, public help can only be mobilized when conditions have become so adverse that parents are willing to give up legal custody of their children. In this framework, services rarely are designed to promote family well-being or to prevent family breakdown. Promotion and prevention have had little place in a residualist system.

The tradition also carries with it considerable historical baggage from efforts to regulate and control unsuccessful members of society. Social welfare efforts have often been marked by elaborate bureaucracy and extensive efforts to prevent fraud and abuse. According to the residualist logic, a person who needs aid is, de facto, deviant. The recipient of aid is treated as inherently untrustworthy, and decision making about the allocation of support resources is placed in the hands of "experts" who are governed by highly specified procedures. Any use of funds that might be interpreted as contributing to personal gain must be censored in this approach. For example, Agosta (1989b) described a family that needed a washing machine to clean clothes for their daughter, a child with severe disabilities including incontinence. The state family services agency could legally allocate funds so that the parents could take laundry to the laundromat in town (at the added expense of transportation and time), but could not find a way to let the family use money to purchase a used machine. When a creative manager finally came up with a solution, the family was required to display the state seal on the machine to make it evident to all that the state was the ultimate lien holder.

In summary, the residualist tradition not only leads us to ignore family needs until the onset of crises, but it also leads to giving aid in a way that is often impractical, diminishes the self-esteem and sense of empowerment of the recipient, and enmeshes giver and receiver in highly formalized relationships constrained by bureaucracy. Residualism not only limits how much society devotes to its caregiving families but also constrains the *way* in which help is given.

Only recently has public policy been focused to look beyond the residualist perspective. Pressures on caregiving families have mounted steadily during the past decade, and parent advocates have responded with policy initiatives in several states. The limitations of the residualist tradition were clearly expressed by Judge Ellison in the case of *Homeward Bound, Inc., et al. v. Hissom Memorial Center et al.* (1987). He ruled that children have a *constitutional right* to grow up in their own homes and ordered the state of Oklahoma to provide free family support services to parents of children with severe handicaps. His ruling, which highlighted a shift in values away from the residualist tradition, is likely to be a harbinger of future national reforms:

Historically the public policy of Oklahoma has been that persons with mental retardation will only receive support in living environments if the individual leaves home and moves to a state operated institution. The state has provided little or no resources to assist a person to stay home, but has consistently provided immense financial resource to house people away from their own homes. . . . The evidence before this Court is clear that the home, with appropriate supports, is the most likely setting in which to achieve individual growth and development. (*Homeward Bound*, 1987, p. 62)

As we set a new nonresidualist course for the conduct of social policy regarding caregiving families, a new vision of what kind of social contract should exist between caregiving families and society must be developed. First, though, it will be necessary to determine just what it is that families need.

What Families Need

Parents and siblings seem to have a fairly consistent notion of what they need. Several western European nations have established nationwide support systems for families, and a majority of states in the United States now provide some form of family support services (Knoll, Covert, Osuch, O'Connor, & Blaney, 1990), usually as a result of parental advocacy efforts. There is a commonality in the purposes of these new efforts. In a report on the Dutch experience with family support services, Versluys (1986) noted:

Dutch parents articulated the following as important: that parents need time to be alone together, time for their other children, special time with their disabled child, and a chance for family interactions and mutual activities. They also articulated the need to discuss their concerns with someone who understands and appreciates their efforts, but who also can provide practical relief and assistance within the home community. (p. 52)

Not only are there similarities across *societies* in what kinds of supports that family members desire, but there are also similarities in the kinds of supports that are emerging for caregiving families, regardless of the cause of the vulnerable person's disability. There are numerous similarities in effective family support services that have been reported for caregiving families of persons with developmental disabilities (Singer, Irvin, et al., 1989), persons with chronic mental illness (Abramowitz & Coursey, 1989), persons with traumatic brain injury (Rosenthal & Young,

1988), and frail elderly persons (Toseland & Rossiter, 1989). These structural and functional similarities include respite care, financial assistance, in-home assistance with behavioral as well as caregiving tasks, social support from mutual aid organizations, and counseling plus skills training of various coping skills.

The way that help is delivered is also enormously important. Researchers have only recently begun to study the conditions that assist families of persons with severe handicaps to succeed (Cole & Meyer, 1989; Dunst, Trivette, & Deal, 1988; Singer & Irvin, 1989a; Summers et al., 1989). These authors have taken a nonpathological view of families. They have begun to explore what kinds of interventions and community resources can allow families to succeed as home caregivers.

FAMILY SUPPORTS AND FAMILY ADAPTATION THEORY

In this section, we review evidence for a model of stress and coping in families. Stress and coping theory (Billings & Moos, 1985; Lazarus and Folkman, 1984) as applied to families (McCubbin & Patterson, 1983) has been used to organize and synthesize the extensive literature on families of children with severe handicaps (Bristol et al., 1988; Cole, 1986; Friedrich, Wilturner, & Cohen, 1985; Singer & Irvin, 1989b). It provides a useful framework for drawing together information from several fields regarding intervention approaches.

Because the literature has dwelt so exclusively on negative impacts of caregiving, a summary of

this body of knowledge inevitably paints a rather grim picture. Thus we begin this review with a caveat to the reader: Be aware that the medical tradition of emphasizing pathology over wellness and adjustment has dominated this line of work. Evidence of negative impacts of caregiving can be useful in prescribing social remedies. However, such evidence presents only a part of a much more complicated and hopeful picture.

Figure 16.1 presents a model of family stress adapted from the work of Olson et. al. (1983). It shows that positive and negative family adaptations are the product of the interaction of several variables: intrafamily resources, resources from outside of the family, stressors, and the family's way of appraising these events and resources as well as its repertoire of coping skills. Researchers have endeavored to verify this and similar models (Bristol, 1987; Bristol et al., 1988; Cole & Meyer, 1989; Singer, Irvin, & Irvine, in preparation). For example, Bristol used this theoretical framework to determine what variables predict family distress in families of young children with autism. The dependent variables in her study were the quality of parenting, marital satisfaction, and maternal depression. To measure stressors, Bristol assessed stressful life events, characteristics of the children with handicaps, and restrictions on family opportunities due to caregiving demands. To account for intrafamily and external resources, she measured formal and informal sources of social support as well as the family's coping strategies. Maternal appraisals of the stressors were also entered into the regres-

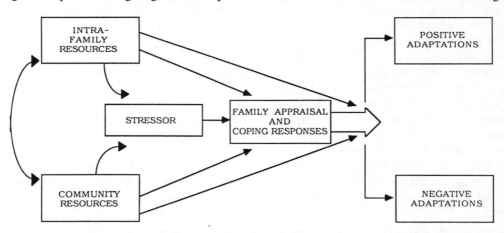

Figure 16.1.   Model of family stress. (Adapted from Olson, McCubbin, Barnes, Larsen, Muxen, & Wilson, 1983.)

sion formula. By combining stressors, resources, coping skills, and appraisals, the model was able to account for 61% of the variance in marital adjustment.

Stressors

In the center of the Olson et al. (1983) model of family stress and adaptation is a set of challenging circumstances, or stressors. It is important to understand the specific sources of challenge and demands for adaptation in caregiving families in order to devise practical ways to promote positive adaptation and to ameliorate maladaptation. In examining stressors, a question immediately arises concerning the unit of analysis. In the extensive literature on stress and its effects on health and morale, the units of analysis have been defined variously as large life-changing events, as minor daily hassles, and as repeated patterns of chronic strain in everyday life.

Major Life Events

Stressors in this line of work are characterized as large, often traumatic events such as a death in the family, a divorce, loss of a job, onset of a serious illness, and so forth (e.g., Ilfeld, 1977). Consistent but modest correlations have been found between major unwanted life events and both physical illness and psychosocial distress (Rahe & Arthur, 1978). The findings would lead us to suspect that desirable interactions between parents and their children with handicaps will be disrupted at times of major unwanted stressors. In some analyses the presence of a family member with disabilities is viewed as a large unit of stress. For example, in his synthesis of the family stress literature, Cole (1986) defined the birth of a child with handicaps as the seminal event that initiates a process of family adaptation. In this case the stressor is viewed as one large traumatic event, the child's birth. Stress can also be analyzed in smaller, more temporally limited units.

Economic Stress and Daily Hassles

Stress also can be defined in terms of common everyday events that disrupt desirable routines. In turn, everyday stressors can be divided into two types: daily hassles and chronic stressors directly related to caregiving. Daily hassles are common, usually relatively small, problems that can be irritating and demoralizing for some people. Kanner, Coyne, Schaefer, and Lazarus (1981) found that daily hassles such as money worries, car troubles, and work pressures are better predictors of depression than are major life events. This line of work suggests that caregiving families that have to cope with many minor problems in daily living would be more vulnerable to demoralization. In a recent study of 229 parents of school-age children with moderate and severe mental retardation we found that a measure of daily hassles correlated significantly with parental depression ($r = .38, p = .000$) (Singer, Irvin, & Irvine, in preparation). Of the top 20 items, the first 6 were financial problems, including not having enough money for emergencies, for necessities, or for extras and problems with car maintenance. Other top-ranked hassles included home repairs, smoking, lack of free time, lack of recreation and entertainment, too much work, too much paperwork, and too much housework. The origin of these hassles cannot be determined from this study; some are likely to be direct or indirect effects of caregiving demands whereas others are best viewed as background conditions that would be present regardless of the caregiving role.

Our research suggests that day-to-day financial hassles create a background of strain in some families. It is no accident that when parent advocates have played a significant role in designing state-level family support services, they have established programs that combine cash grants with social services. Poverty exacerbates caregiver stress by raising the level of background discomfort and danger that sets the context for family life. In turn, family home caregiving can drain family resources or prevent desired participation in the work force. Thus, family support services must take into account the exigencies of economic pressure on caregiving families. The economic costs of home caregiving also can give rise to alterations in expected living patterns. In a majority of both single and two-parent families of children who are nonhandicapped, the parent(s) works outside of the home for money. However, the extra demands of caring for a child with handicaps often make employment difficult for parents in caregiving families. Not only is it more difficult to seek employment, but parents often also must pay for additional expenses incurred in caregiving (Moroney, 1986). In his recent study of 722 families in Illinois, Agosta (1989a) found that 17% of the respondents reported that someone in the household had to give up a paying job to provide home care, 24% reported that someone in the household had to not pursue employment, and 13% reported that someone had to refuse a job promotion.

Chronic Stressors Associated with Caregiving

Stressful events can also be analyzed in terms of frequently repeated patterns of events that overtax family resources. These repeated demands entail both active responding as well as disruption of expected normal routines. For example, family home caregiving may require adjusted daily schedules and activities. These alterations in activity patterns are usually imposed by circumstance rather than willfully chosen. Normal patterns of work, sleep, and recreation can be disrupted. Normal daily routines such as preparing and eating meals may be prolonged and complicated by the vulnerable relative's needs for special food and feeding. Nighttime caregiving may disrupt normal sleep patterns (Pahl & Quine, 1987). And opportunities for culturally normative times of rest and recreation can be reduced. These chronic stressors have a negative impact because they deprive caregivers of other sources of reinforcement that would otherwise be available.

Chronic stressors also may include repeated demands for the caregivers' time and energy (Beckman, 1983; Breslau & Davis, 1986; Gallagher, Beckman, & Cross, 1983; Singer & Irvin, 1989b). In their study of parents of children with handicaps, Breslau, Staruch, and Mortimer (1982) found that the best predictor of maternal depression was the amount of assistance the child required for normal activities of daily life. Chronic caregiving demands can include lifting and transferring, changing and feeding, transporting and supervising, and managing the reactions of outsiders. These stressors appear to have a cumulative effect so that managing a multiplicity of caregiving demands takes a toll (Pahl & Quine, 1987). Another set of demands that can overtax parents arises from problematic child behavior. Severe aberrant behavior is one of the strongest predictors of early out-of-home placement for children (Tausig, 1985). Pahl and Quine found that among parents of children with multiple and severe handicapping conditions, parents who were required to cope repeatedly with serious behavior problems experienced the greatest psychological distress.

Studies of out-of-home placement have suggested that children who repeatedly overtax their caregivers because of serious problem behaviors and/or multiple caregiving demands are at greatest risk of expulsion from the home (e.g., Cole & Meyer, 1989). Further, out-of-home placement or family breakdown is often precipitated by a pile-up of stressors and the sudden onset of major life events (Wikler, 1986b).

Pile-Up of Stressors

Pahl and Quine (1987) conducted a thorough analysis of chronic caregiver stressors in families of children with multiple handicapping conditions in England. They found that the following family stressors were associated with greatest psychological distress in caregiving mothers: child's behavior problems, nighttime disturbance, child's ill health, multiplicity of child's problems, and problems with the child's appearance. They also found that other background factors appeared to exacerbate psychosocial distress: adversity in the family, money worries, and social isolation. In our study of school-age children and their families (Singer, Irvin, & Irvine, in preparation), mothers reported that the most severe chronic stressors associated directly with caregiving fell into three major categories: medical problems, behavioral problems, and difficulties in understanding the child's efforts to communicate.

Caregiver psychosocial distress appears to result often from the pile-up of different kinds of stressors; major life events, daily hassles, and chronic caregiving demands. These, in turn, interact with resources available to the family, including financial status, social support, and coping skills (Bristol et al., 1988; Friedrich et al., 1985; Singer & Irvin, 1989b).

Studies of crises in families of children with handicaps have suggested that some families become dysfunctional when a pile-up of common daily stressors collides with a major unwanted life event (e.g., Wikler, 1986a). The everyday stressors create conditions that place the family at risk by lowering individual morale and straining intrafamily social ties (in some families). They may place the family in a vulnerable position so that when a sudden unwanted life event such as loss of a job, divorce, or serious illness occurs the family is pushed into a crisis in which it becomes temporarily dysfunctional. In the most severe of crises, a family member may become seriously ill or mentally disturbed, a parent may become abusive or neglectful, or social ties may be broken. This last outcome may include ejection of the child from the home (Cole, 1986).

Appraisals and Coping

In order to understand how the sources of stress just discussed affect family support interventions, it is first necessary to discuss the interaction of resources, appraisals, and coping with events. Few events are, by definition, stressors; that is, a severe stressor in one caregiving home may be taken as a matter of course in another. For example, Todis and Singer (in press) conducted a qualitative study of parents who have adopted several children with multiple handicaps. They found that events that conventionally would be viewed as times of great difficulty in many homes (e.g., a child's surgery) were interpreted by these parents as challenges and opportunities for demonstrating mastery. The adoptive parents appeared to take a stance toward conventionally stressful events so that they were not perceived as overtaxing. These appraisals appeared to be facilitated by the fact that the adoptive families had strong sources of intrafamilial and community support. Lazarus and Folkman (1984) presented a theoretical model of the stress appraisal process in which events and resources are inseparable. They posited appraisal as a two-stage process. In the first stage of appraisal, a person perceives an event as potentially harmful or as having already caused harm. In the second stage, the individual surveys the coping resources available in order to adapt to the event. Thus, perceptions of the event and perceptions of resources for responding to it are interwoven.

Cognitive Coping

The notion that cognitive variables play a role in family adaptation has prompted a search for the cognitive strategies that make a difference for coping outcomes. Human cognition is an enormous topic in itself and it should come as no surprise that researchers have attacked the problem of the role of cognition in caregiving adaptation from a wide variety of theoretical approaches. We believe that the most promising approaches to the study of appraisal in family caregiver adaptation can be drawn from research on persons who have effectively coped with life crises (Antonovsky, 1987; Frey, Greenberg, & Fewell, 1989; Summers et al., 1989; Taylor, 1983). Effective cognitive strategies for coping with stressors may be roughly grouped into attributions concerning causality, meaning, and social comparison (e.g., Nixon, 1989).

A characteristic of persons who adapt well to life challenges is that they develop a sense of mastery in regard to their circumstances. The aspects of this trait have been variously described as an internal locus of control, self-efficacy, and mastery (Antonovsky, 1987; Friedrich et al., 1985; Summers et al., 1989). People who are said to have this characteristic describe themselves as able to manage key parts of their external and intrapsychic world. Parents and siblings of children with handicaps may gain a sense of mastery through learning and using a variety of skills including behavioral parent training, advocacy, and stress management skills. Mastery does not necessarily mean that people feel they are able to change or operate upon the external environment in every case. Instrumental action may be balanced with more passive acceptance or faith in others' ability to cope with the situation. Simultaneously, mastery may include skills at altering affective reactions to trying circumstances. For example, forms of relaxation or meditation have been useful to parents in learning to manage stress (Hawkins & Singer, 1989).

Too much emphasis on instrumental control may lead to a sense of failure in the face of intractable circumstances; efforts to improve the situation have to be balanced with ways of accepting it. Passive appraisal strategies such as living one day at a time may contribute to acceptance (Olson et al., 1983). In our work we have attempted to balance control and acceptance by establishing mutual assistance groups in which parents empathetically share common experiences as well as learn behavioral parenting skills and stress management skills.

Friedrich et al. (1985) emphasized the construct of locus of control in their multivariate study of caregiver psychological adaptation. The locus of control construct examines the typical way in which an individual attributes causality to events in life. A person with an internal locus of control is said to believe that he or she can control important events through the use of skill, knowledge, will, or effort; a person with an external locus of control believes more in the influence of less tractable causes such as fate, luck, or divine intervention. In their study of 140 mothers of children with mental retardation, Friedrich et al. found that a measure of locus of control accounted for a small but significant proportion of the variance in marital satisfaction.

One contributor to an internal locus of control is likely to be a person's skill at pinpointing the causes of his or her reactions to events. People who cope well with challenging circumstances are able to see the environment as more orderly than chaotic (Antonovsky, 1987). One behavioral skill that makes up this apparent trait is the ability to pinpoint specific causal events rather than to attribute causality to a relatively undifferentiated fog of phenomena. Wahler (1988) described the way that socially isolated mothers who are caught in negative social networks have difficulty in segmenting the flow of behavior into discrete, observable events (Lazarus & Folkman, 1984). By learning to segment broad attributional statements into more molecular units of thought, mothers were able to disconnect aversive social interactions between adults from their reactions to their child. Similarly, behavior therapists have repeatedly found that self-monitoring skills often have a therapeutic effect (Karoly & Kanfer, 1982). In her study of adaptation to bereavement, Powers (1989) found that widows who were able to pinpoint the cause of their grief and differentiate it from other events had the strongest sense of well-being in the face of recent loss.

People who adapt well to difficult circumstances are able to assign a meaning to the difficulty. This meaning provides them with a linkage to a reference group and provides a kind of cognitive map for reducing uncertainty. Venters (1981) found that the parents of children with cystic fibrosis who adapted best were able to assign a meaning to the disease that was congruent with a belief they held prior to the onset of the illness. Powers (1989) also found that bereaved widows who were coping most successfully attributed a meaning to their loss.

Summers et al. (1989) have embarked upon a line of research that promises to make important contributions to an understanding of the role of cognitive adaptation in caregiving families. They have broken with the pervasive emphasis on pathology and maladaptation in the study of families and stress by looking at predictors of positive perceptions of mastery, meaning, and self-esteem. H.R. Turnbull et al. (1988) pointed out the way that family members of children with severe handicaps, in many cases, come to perceive meaning and benefit from the relationship. They quoted parents who report that their child has brought joy and pride to the family, a richer sense of values, and a greater meaning of love, and has strengthened the family. These meanings usually are stated in broad abstract terms. An understanding of the contextual variables associated with these positive meanings holds promise for assisting families.

Positive social comparison is thought to be one important contextual process in helping people adapt cognitively to threats to health or self-esteem (S.E. Taylor, 1983). Frey et al. (1989) studied parents' self-appraisals compared to other parents in similar circumstances, and they constructed an interesting scale derived from interviews with parents. It measures parental reactions to a set of self-enhancing and self-depreciating statements such as "Others manage to rise to the occasion better than I." In their multiple regression study of 96 mothers and fathers of young children with handicaps, Frey et al. found that parental beliefs were the most powerful correlate of family adjustment variables in a model of stress and coping that included measures of child-related stress, social support, and coping styles. In a later section of this chapter we discuss the implications of the family stress and coping model for family support interventions. The addition of cognition to the model has important ramifications.

A methodological issue arises in adding cognitive processes into the model of family stress and coping. All of the research reviewed so far examines cognition at the individual level. That is, data are collected by asking one family member at a time to respond to questions. However, the theory of family stress and coping posits the family as a collective as the primary unit of analysis. Conceptual problems immediately arise when we try to examine the way that any *group* of people thinks about something. In the field of family sociology and social psychology, researchers have approached the problem in different ways. For example, Moos and Moos (1981) and Olson et al. (1983) administered individual questionnaires to mothers and fathers and then utilized the discrepancies between their scores as a variable in and of itself. Reiss and Olivieri (1983) examined the theory that families develop paradigms—shared ways of interpreting events —and that these shared group perceptions are an important contributor to the way that the family unit adapts to stressful circumstances. Reiss and Olivieri's work is interesting because the notion of a family paradigm derives from laboratory tasks in which family members are required to respond to various analogue challenges. To our knowledge, no one has yet applied this approach to caregiving families. Cole and Meyer (1989) have recently proposed to examine the extent to which family members share beliefs concerning normalization and whether these group cognitions evolve over time. The measurement and study of the concept of shared meanings in different family units require clarification and application before it can be fully integrated into family stress and coping theory.

Coping Skills

Coping with stressful circumstances is partly a matter of appraisal of the stressor and of the resources available for responding to it (Lazarus & Folkman, 1984). Coping is also a matter of the skills that family members utilize in order to solve day-to-day problems as they arise. Several different taxonomies of coping have been developed (e.g., Lazarus & Folkman, 1984; Math-

eny, Aycock, Pugh, Curlette, & Cannella 1986; Olson et al., 1983; Pearlin & Schooler, 1978). We emphasize important distinctions between active problem solving, avoidance of problems, and efforts to manage emotional reactions to problems. Research strongly suggests that people are most likely to have a normal psychiatric profile when they rely primarily on an active problem-solving approach to difficulties rather than self-blame, avoidance, or wishful thinking (Vitaliano, Maiuro, Russo, & Becker, 1987). Behavior therapists have long made communication skills around active problem solving a centerpiece of their interventions for marital and family discord (e.g., Jacobson & Gurman, 1986). Recently, special educators have asserted the value of teaching group problem-solving skills to families of children and young adults with disabilities (Goldfarb, Brotherson, Summers, & Turnbull, 1986). This approach holds promise as a way to enhance family coping skills while further empowering families to make their own choices and evaluate decisions by their own standards. So far, there have been no published studies showing the benefits of family problem solving in these families and thus the approach awaits empirical validation. This is not to say that family problem solving does not have merit; our clinical experience suggests to us that it is one useful set of coping skills that can be taught to some families.

Avoidance coping styles such as trying not to think about a problem, daydreaming, watching TV to get away from a difficulty, and so forth have been associated with poor adjustment in some families (Vitaliano et al., 1987). This finding, however, needs to be qualified by the work of Pearlin and Schooler (1978) who found that people who were faced with intractable problems adapted better when they used more passive coping styles.

There is a third kind of coping that involves neither active attempts to change a stressor nor passive attempts to avoid it. "Secondary coping" involves efforts to manage emotional reactions to stress. One such secondary strategy is "living one day at a time"—focusing on the present and not worrying about future dilemmas. Turnbull, Turnbull, Bronicki, Summers, and Roeder-Gordon (1989) pointed out that this coping style can conflict with active problem-solving efforts and that professionals working with families need to be sensitive to the adaptive power of some secondary coping strategies as well as to the utility of more active problem solving.

Frey et al. (1989) used the family stress and coping model (see Figure 16.1) to predict family adjustment in 48 mothers and 48 fathers of young children with moderate and severe handicaps. They used the framework of family stress and coping that assumes that adjustment is the result of interactions of stressors, resources, appraisals, and coping strategies. Their study introduced some important innovations into the literature because of the careful way in which they studied the role of parental beliefs and coping styles. They measured parental beliefs with a locus of control measure and with a comparative appraisal scale that measured the extent to which parents made self-enhancing or self-derogatory statements when comparing themselves to other parents of children with handicaps. The overall model of child-related stressors, parental beliefs and coping style, and social support (as well as conflict in the social network) accounted for 43% and 50% of the variance respectively in mothers' and fathers' family adjustment.

Intrafamily Resources

Intrafamily resources is the next major component of the family stress and coping model (see Figure 16.1). The evidence is clear that supportive intrafamilial social networks help people to adapt well to caregiving. Friedrich and Friedrich (1981) documented that mothers of children with handicaps who had the lowest stress ratings reported having positive spousal support. In England, Pahl and Quine (1987) found similarly that mothers of children with severe handicaps reported the most positive morale if they had the understanding of a partner and/or if their partner was helpful in sharing the work involved in caregiving. Families that do well with caregiving often function as a mutual support group. McCubbin et al. (1983) found that among families of children with cystic fibrosis, children's health status was best predicted by the extent to which family members cooperated as a team (as perceived by mothers). Similarly, Dunst, Trivette, and Cross (1986) found that social support ac-

counted for unique variance in both the amount of time that mothers interacted with their children with handicaps and in the children's progress.

Instrumental Support

Intrafamily support takes the form of instrumental help as well as expressive/emotional support. In part, intrafamily support consists of the practical ways in which people allocate their time and energy around caregiving tasks or to relieve the caregiver of other competing demands. Thus, the way that work is distributed in the family and family members' satisfaction with it are among key determinants of general satisfaction with caregiving (Dunst, Trivette, & Cross, 1986) and are strong predictors of the quality of observed parenting interactions (Bristol et al. 1988).

Perceived satisfaction with work assignments is more important than the objective distribution of tasks. Kazak and Marvin (1984) found that in families of children with spina bifida, work tasks were allocated along very traditional lines in which the mother provided most of the in-home caregiving and the father worked outside of the home. A majority of the parents were satisfied with this division of labor, and spouses rated their marriages as satisfactory. Other studies, however, have suggested that traditional allocation of household work plus caregiving to mothers and older daughters can be associated with demoralization. Mothers who are assigned disproportionate amounts of caregiving experience increased time demands and decreased well-being (Trivette, 1982). Also, older daughters who are assigned large shares of caregiving roles may be at risk of isolation and depression (Lobato, Faust, & Spirito, 1988).

The traditional gender-based division of labor in the home is likely to be increasingly problematic for caregiving families. A majority of mothers of young children now work outside of the home so that they are required to fill multiple roles as breadwinners, homemakers, and caregivers.

Expressive/Emotional Support

Instrumental social support—who gets up in the middle of the right, who changes the bed linen, who gives out medication, and so on—is only a small part of the picture. The quality of the expressive support exchanged within the family contributes directly and indirectly to parental well-being and to the quality of parenting. In studies of families of children who are not handicapped, the quality of the spousal relationship is predictive of the mother's and the father's adaptation to pregnancy and childbirth, maternal feeding competence, adjustment to mothering, adjustment to fathering, extent of negative affect displayed toward infants, and the extent of active parenting (Goldberg & Easterbrooks, 1984). Similarly, in studies of parents of children with handicaps, expressive spousal support is strongly predictive of the quality of observed maternal and paternal parenting (Bristol et al., 1988).

Studies of marital adjustment indicate that successful couples are characterized by their abilities to solve problems and to communicate without becoming embroiled in anger or depression (Notarius, Benson, & Sloane, 1989). Negative affect during problem-solving interactions clearly discriminates distressed and nondistressed couples. Furthermore, partners in distressed couples are more likely to reciprocate negative interactions. For example, Markman (1979, 1981) found that couples' communication skills and affect predicted their marital satisfaction 3 years after initial assessment.

It would be a mistake to assume that having a child with handicaps, per se, leads to marital distress. Many marriages in families with children with severe handicaps are healthy. In their study of 45 parents of young children with handicaps, Bristol et al. (1988) found that 80% of the mothers reported having satisfactory marriages. And there is some evidence for salutogenesis— that is, some marriages are strengthened by family home caregiving (Kazak & Marvin, 1984). There is reason to be concerned, though, about the impact of family home caregiving on some marriages and also about its impact on remarriage. Some evidence suggests that divorce rates are higher in this population (Tew, Payne, & Lawrence, 1974). According to recent Census Bureau data, twice as many children with severe disabilities live in single-parent families rather than in two-parent families (U.S. Department of Commerce, 1987). Tew et al. studied 59 families of children with handicaps over nearly a decade.

Compared with a control group, they experienced twice the rate of divorce. Because general divorce rates are high, caregiving likely contributes to other destructive processes rather than being the sole cause of divorce.

Although divorce rates are very high and single-parent families are now common during some phases of the life cycle, marriage is still the most popular option for parents. Most individuals who divorce choose to remarry. Little is known about patterns of remarriage in divorced parents of children with handicaps. In her study of single mothers of children with mental retardation, Wikler (1979) found that 80% of the mothers did not expect to remarry, whereas over 70% of divorced mothers in the general population actually do remarry within 5 years of a divorce.

Other evidence suggests that parents are at risk of social isolation due to difficulties in obtaining respite care, fatigue, and perceived negative attitudes from extended family and community members (A.P. Turnbull & Turnbull, 1986). Isolation appears to increase with the age of the child with handicaps. It is likely that higher levels of social isolation make remarriage more difficult by reducing opportunities for social contacts.

Single parents of children with severe handicaps have to face unusual levels of stressors, often with diminished resources. Single parenthood is increasingly common in the general population—67% of children born in the late 1980s will be raised for part of their lives by a single parent (Vincent & Salisbury, 1988). The economic impacts of family home caregiving are augmented by single-parent status. In 1980, the median family income for single-parent households led by mothers was $7,652 compared with $23,930 for families with married couples (Vadasy, 1986). With greatly reduced income, single mothers still must meet the extra medical, child-care, and therapeutic costs of home caregiving.

Other intrafamily subsystems can be affected by the presence of a child with disabilities, including relations with grandparents and between siblings and other family members (Fewell & Vadasy, 1986). Once again there is evidence for considerable variability in the way that other relatives are affected by a child with disabilities.

On the one hand, retrospective studies have indicated that many brothers and sisters believe that they have benefited from life with their sibling with handicaps. Grossman (1972) found that a notable number of siblings were altruistic and socially concerned. On the other hand, there is evidence that some siblings are at risk of social isolation and increased symptoms of depression (Breslau & Prabucki, 1987). Dyson, Edgar, and Crnic (1989) identified intrafamily variables that predicted the self-esteem and behavior problems in siblings of children with handicaps. They conducted a multivariate study of 110 older siblings of children with handicaps under the age of 7 years. They found that parental stress associated with caregiving tasks was the best predictor of sibling self-esteem; the greater the parental stress, the lower the siblings' self-esteem. Sibling behavior problems were predicted by the aspects of the family's functioning as a social unit —that is, siblings were less likely to have behavior problems in families in which members supported one another and in which they encouraged self-expression.

In summary, the way that family members cooperate with one another and the social climate that prevails in a family has important effects on the way that families adapt to living with a child with severe handicaps. It is clear from the emerging evidence that the well-being of all family members is enhanced by intrafamily cooperation. Any systematic attempt to assist families must take into account intrafamily relationships with their potentional for positive as well as negative adaptation.

Community Resources: Social Support from Outside the Family

Community resources, social support from outside of the family, is the final major component of the family stress and coping model (see Figure 16.1). When all of the elements of this model are combined, they provide a framework for organizing and evaluating family support interventions.

Isolation and Perceived Support

A person's perception that adequate social support is available for a variety of needs appears to be an important indicator of general life satisfaction as well as of coping with major life events. By contrast, subjective loneliness and/or the perception of being entangled in nonsupportive social relationships is predictive of ill health as well as poor adaptation to stress (Cutrona & Russell, 1987). Consequently, in looking for causes of caregiver stress/distress, a sensible place to turn is to an examination of the effects of family home caregiving on the caregiver's social relationships both within the family and outside of it.

At the simplest level, the findings regarding the general importance of social support (Dunst, Trivette, & Cross, 1986) would prompt us to ask if there is a relationship between caregiving and troubled social relationships within the family and/or reduced social contact outside of the family. However, simple counts of social ties and satisfaction with them would not be sufficient. Recent research on social support has suggested a much more complex set of issues (e.g. Morgan, 1989; Weiss, 1973).

Not just any social connection will do. A match must exist between the perceived need for support, the kind of support desired, and the source of support in order for a person to feel satisfied with a social tie. And social linkages can be sources of both inadvertent and more deliberately inflicted distress. We briefly review here the evidence regarding social support and caregiving for children with handicaps by first asking generally if support is reduced or strained by caregiving, and then if the match of perceived needs, kinds of support, and sources of support is affected.

People also require social ties from a number of sources outside the family and for a number of different functions. Though not all families of children with severe handicaps experience social isolation, there is reason to believe that they are at unusual risk of separation from a wider community (Stagg & Catron, 1986). Breslau and Prabucki (1987) found that brothers and sisters of children with severe handicaps reported being more isolated than control group peers. Social isolation has been linked to a number of negative mental and physical health outcomes, and is cause for concern (Weiss, 1973).

Why are some families well integrated into informal communities of support while others become isolated? This problem is poorly understood and is an important topic for research. Based on the literature and our clinical experience, family members become isolated because: 1) they are fatigued from caregiving; 2) they have limited opportunities for leisure time because of the difficulty in obtaining child care; 3) they encounter misunderstandings and, sometimes, negative reactions from others regarding their relative with severe handicaps; and 4) their children with handicaps are excluded from the normal social institutions that allow social networks to form. A sense of stigma can be communicated to family members in many ways, ranging from surreptitious stares by strangers in the grocery store to outright rejection by formal organizations. Goode (1980) documented the way that parents of a child with deaf-blindness managed the social presentation of themselves in public settings such as restaurants. These parents developed markedly different styles of introducing their daughter to visitors and strangers in order to mediate others' reactions to her. In our work with mutual aid groups for parents, we have found that parents are frequently interested in exchanging stories and ideas on how to cope with the reactions of strangers to their children with severe handicaps.

Problems of social isolation again point to the linkage of individual troubles with larger social issues. Research and demonstration efforts are needed to explore the impact of a thoroughgoing social integration movement on family isolation. For example, Brown et al. (1989) argued for the need to locate educational placements for students with severe handicaps in their neighborhood schools. They pointed out that the costs of transporting children to special segregated centers or cluster schooling arrangements include the disruption of potential social linkages between neighborhood children. Research is needed to investigate whether neighborhood schooling might also help families to form local social ties with neighbor families and organizations. One initial investigation (Bailey & Winton, 1989) of integrated day-care arrangements for preschoolers with handicaps suggested that families of children who are handicapped and nonhandicapped may not intermingle simply because of physical proximity. Bailey and Winton conducted a sociometric analysis of parents of children who are handicapped and nonhandicapped enrolled in a day-care center over a 9-month period. They mapped the friendship patterns that developed between families and found that, generally, parents of children with and without handicaps did not develop friendships with one another. They concluded that the physical mainstreaming of children may not be sufficient to bring about mainstreaming of family members. Research is needed to investigate those families that do form strong neighborhood ties as well as social arrangements that facilitate family social integration along with the mainstreaming of children in neighborhood schools and child-care arrangements.

Parent-Professional Relationships

Another important area of social support is parent-professional relationships. Life with a family member with disabilities entails much more frequent contact with human services professionals than most people experience. Relationships with professionals, ranging from physicians and nurses to speech/language therapists and special education teachers, are a prominent part of the normal routine for families that include a member with disabilities. There is evidence that professionals can be positive sources of strength and practical assistance as well as sources of stress (e.g., Huang & Heifetz, 1984; Moeller, 1986). Unfortunately, some parents and siblings experience some negative social interactions with helping professionals. Parents report that these interactions can be sources of distress (Doernberg, 1982). One of the most frequently repeated complaints concerns the quality of interactions with medical professionals. Lynch and Stalock (1988) found that 30% of their sample of parents ($N = 50$) reported dissatisfaction with the manner in which a physician informed them of their child's handicapping condition.

Once again, not all parent-professional relationships are conflicted. In fact, there are many parental reports that a variety of professionals can be helpful in terms of their particular expertise as well as in face-to-face exchanges of concern and caring. It is certainly disconcerting for professionals who have dedicated their careers to becoming knowledgeable helpers to find themselves generating discomfort and outright pain in the people whom they intend to serve. The unwanted negative effects of professional intervention require close examination, particularly in the context of efforts to advocate for new services to assist families.

In many ways, the relationships of professional helpers and family members involve the encounter of different cultures. The daily tasks, social contingencies, and roles of the parties differ greatly, even though they all focus upon the same child. Researchers using ethnographic procedures have described the ensuing conflicts as basic clashes in views of the world (Darling, 1983; Singer, Hawkins, Walker, Irvine, & Peters, in preparation). Much of the problem resides in the conditions in which many professionals must work, including stifling levels of bureaucracy, very limited resources, and the residualist role of being asked to provide help once a crisis has already occurred.

Studies of help giving suggest that the way in which the help-giving interaction is structured as well as the interpersonal skills of the professional helper are crucial (Dunst et al., 1988; Huang & Heifetz, 1984). Huang and Heifetz interviewed 28 mothers of young children with mental retardation about professionals who were most and least helpful. They also administered adjective checklists to supplement the interview findings. Parents indicated that four general factors were most important in differentiating helpful and unhelpful professionals. The first concerned personal relatedness. Under this category, adjectives that described helpful professionals were terms such as supportive, warm, enthusiastic, likable, and open-minded. By contrast, unhelpful professionals were described as too busy to spend time with parents, insensitive to worries, and as making the parent feel nervous. A second dimension that parents described centered on the perceived competence of the professionals. The most helpful professionals were perceived by parents as being generally well informed and specifically well informed about their child's problems. By contrast, the least helpful were described as inexperienced and as not knowledgeable. A third dimension in the way that parents differentiated most helpful and least helpful professionals concerned the balance of power in the relationship. The most effective

helpers were able to create a collaborative set in which parents perceived that they were treated as equals, their suggestions were taken seriously, and they were involved in decision making. By contrast, the least helpful professionals were described as dominating, speaking in technical language, demanding, and poor listeners. According to parents, a final dimension that differentiated the most and least helpful professionals concerned efficiency. The most helpful professionals were described as talking to the point and discussing practical goals and management issues versus talking in circles and being inefficient or disorganized. This study (Huang & Heifetz, 1984) suggests that family support professionals not only require training in their area of technical expertise but that they also need to become very proficient in establishing collaborative relationships; listening and communicating effectively; and sharing warmth, enthusiasm, and optimism.

These social and affective skills are not commonly taught in the curricula for many professions. Learning an egalitarian style, listening, and supporting are not skills that are easily acquired from traditional lecture courses. One profession in which much attention has been given to training these skills is the field of counseling psychology. Counselors often learn to interact with their clients through repeated practica as well as lecture classes. Videotaped demonstrations and feedback and individual coaching are common tools of the trade for trainers of counselors. Although these training methods are labor intensive and thus expensive, the literature has suggested that efforts to prepare professionals to support families will fail if trainees do not acquire these essential skills. For example, Dunst et al. (1988) emphasized that the family help giver must establish a relationship of trust with family members in which he or she becomes a trusted confidant. As new family support services are created it will be necessary for universities to create training programs for the workers who will staff these agencies. These programs will require interdisciplinary training across areas of special education, social work, and counseling.

Effective helping is not simply a matter of having direct service staff who are well trained.

The ways in which the service agency structures the relationships between help giver and receiver also matter greatly. For example, studies of help giving have suggested that help is most effectively given when it is offered proactively (Dunst et al., 1988), when the costs in effort and money are reasonable, when the recipient perceives that help is needed, when there is no implication of deviance or stigma in receiving aid, and when it emphasizes family strengths. The administrative and managerial practices of family support agencies can greatly influence the degree to which these approaches to helping are realized in family homes.

Family support helpers in a variety of professions are also most likely to be effective if they have an understanding of family systems, family life cycles, and family stress and coping. Training programs for support personnel will need to transmit theory and information drawn from several fields that have examined the family. The technical knowledge of a specific profession is likely to be necessary but not sufficient for working effectively to assist families.

Summary of Family Stress and Coping

We have compiled some of the evidence concerning a multivariate model of stress and coping in families of children with handicaps. This model suggests that the way that any given family will react to challenging circumstances will result from the interaction of social dynamics within the family unit, cognitive appraisal and coping strategies, practical resources, and social support from outside of the family.

A study by Cole and Meyer (1989) illustrated the utility of this model for explaining family adjustment to children with severe handicaps. This study also serves as a useful bridge to the next section of our chapter because it provides evidence that community supports to families can enhance adaptation. Cole and Meyer surveyed parents of 166 students with severe handicaps in a large metropolitan school district; the study makes an important contribution because it measured the community resources that families utilized. They selected parental intentions concerning placement of their children with severe handicaps prior to age 21 as the dependent variable. Using Olson et al.'s (1983) model of family

stress and coping, they organized several kinds of resources and social supports to determine the best predictors of plans to keep families intact. Once child-related stressors and preexistent family resources were taken into account, families that used more external resources were more apt to plan in-home placement until age 21 for their children. Resources that were most strongly correlated with intentions of keeping a child at home were various forms of in-home and out-of-home respite care; fiscal resources for medical expenses; and availability of professional expertise from physicians, dentists, and special education consultants who could help with family-related and educational concerns. Parents were also asked to evaluate a "wish" list of services that they thought would enhance their ability to maintain a child at home. Parents indicated that several kinds of support would be helpful: increased intrafamilial support from spouse and siblings, fiscal assistance for medical and other household costs, in-home respite care, and access to generic community resources such as recreational programs and public transportation.

In summary, when designing support services for families, we must take into account a number of variables that come into play in the complex process of family home caregiving. In the next section of this chapter we consider the implications of this model for a variety of societal and personal interventions. We draw together intervention research from a variety of disciplines in order to describe promising ways to assist families.

IMPLICATIONS OF FAMILY STRESS AND COPING FOR FAMILY SUPPORT INTERVENTIONS

So far we have described the demographic and socioeconomic trends that are placing families under pressure. We have pointed out that, under these conditions, the role of the family as a resource for citizens who require unusual levels of assistance is threatened regardless of the cause of the disability. Further, we have described the limitations of two frameworks that have governed our thinking about services and about families—residualism and the emphasis on pathology. Finally, we have presented a widely accepted view of family stress and coping (i.e., Figure 16.1) and used it as a framework to review some of the descriptive evidence regarding the various components of the model: stressors, intrafamily resources, appraisal and coping strategies, and community resources. In this section we describe family support interventions that address some portion of the stress and coping model. Whenever it is relevant, we continue to point out our themes of personal troubles rooted in societal issues, common needs among caregiving families, the limits of residualism, and the need to consider multiple variables in assisting families and conducting research.

Reducing Stressors

Family home caregiving for some families at some times entails personal and familial stress. One way to cope with stress is to work actively to reduce its causes. There are four major ways that people have worked actively to reduce or eliminate sources of caregiving stress: 1) respite care, 2) child-focused education, 3) parent training, and 4) fiscal assistance.

Respite Care

Respite care is one of the most consistently requested and yet least available service for families of children with severe disabilities (Salisbury, 1986; Salisbury & Intagliata, 1986; Wikler, 1979). In families with children who are nonhandicapped, parents and siblings normally obtain relief from the care of young children through the use of babysitters, day-care providers, community recreational activities, and visits to the homes of the children's friends. Each of these normal avenues can be impeded when a child experiences severe handicaps. Parents complain that babysitters can be extremely difficult to find because their child requires someone who is more knowledgeable and skilled than the average high school student. Similarly, complex caregiving needs may render grandparents and other extended family members less able to care temporarily for a child with severe disabilities (Slater & Wikler, 1984). When surveyed, parents often rank various forms of respite care among their most preferred of service options (e.g., Agosta, 1989b; Cole & Meyer,

1989; Joyce et al., 1983). For example, in a study of respite care needs in California, Apolloni and Triest (1983) found that 80% of the respondents to their survey viewed respite care as extremely important to their quality of life and 47% stated that they would seriously consider out-of-home placement if respite care were not available.

As Intagliata reviewed the research on respite care at length in 1986, we confine our discussion of it here to studies published since 1986 and to some recent developments in the expansion of generic child-care services. To begin with, Intagliata concluded that there was little evidence to support the claim that respite care reduces family stress. Methodological and service design flaws impeded evaluative research. For example, few studies have been able to utilize randomly assigned control groups and few have measured the effects of regular respite provision over an extended period of time. Further, few have examined respite in the context of other family support services.

There are some important recent exceptions that offer more encouragement regarding the value of respite care. Rimmerman (1989) followed two groups of mothers in Israel for an 18-month period. One group received at least 6 hours of respite care a week compared with a second group that received none. The experimental group reported significantly reduced stress scores on the four factors of the Questionnaire on Resources and Stress (QRS) (Friedrich et al., 1985): parent and family problems, parental pessimism, parental perception of child's characteristics, and parental perception of the child's physical incapacities. There are design issues with this study including the lack of random assignment and the fact that the two comparison groups were each from two different communities. Furthermore, the changes on the QRS, while statistically significant, were so small as to raise questions about their clinical validity. (That is, does a change from a score of 6.07 to 5.67 have any real meaning outside of statistical significance?) However, the study is commendable because it does approach the issue from a longitudinal perspective and measures family stress with an instrument with known psychometric properties. It offers some limited support to the notion that respite care reduces family stress.

It is likely that respite care by itself is necessary but not sufficient to reduce family stress. In a study that we describe in more detail later, Singer, Irvin, et al. (1989) compared randomly assigned groups of parents of children with severe handicaps. One group received 4 hours of respite care a week plus case management services while a second group received a combination of supports including a support group, stress management and behavioral parent training, and extra community-based respite from volunteers. The group receiving the combination of treatments experienced significant reductions in anxiety and depression. The authors provided evidence that these reductions were clinically as well as statistically significant. A follow-up probe showed that the treatment effects maintained 1 year later. This study suggests that respite care is most likely to help families when it is one part of a comprehensive package of supports. From our experience in this and related studies, it is likely that parents of children with intensive caregiving needs require many hours of respite care a week for it to reduce family stress effectively.

The way that respite services are offered plays an important role in determining parental satisfaction. Knoll and Bedford (1989) found that parents were most satisfied with respite care when they maintained maximum control over selection of the provider as well as the time and place for caregiving. The more inflexible, bureaucratic, or geographically remote the services, the less parents were inclined to endorse them.

One potential emerging source of respite for parents is before- and after-school child care. With increased pressures to enter the job market, parents need child-care services for their children with handicaps in addition to school and preschool services (Fink, 1988). In most states, day-care services are scarce. Mandated center-based infant and preschool services often operate for only 2–4 hours a day (Rule et al., 1987). Also, as children age, day care becomes much more difficult to find (Fink, 1988). The absence of reliable after-school child care forces many parents out of the labor force despite their desire for employment. One effort to correct this situation has been an initiative to expand the capacity of generic child-care services to serve children with severe handicaps. The need for such an enlargement of roles can be seen in a study from California (Fink, 1988) showing that although children with severe handicaps made up 1.4% of the K–12 public school population, only .4% were served by subsidized child-care programs.

As day care for children who are nonhandicapped becomes a prominent national issue, it will be important for advocates to work to ensure that expanded day care will be fully integrated and available to *all* children, regardless of their handicapping conditions. The public schools represent one important potential resource for before- and after-school day care for children with severe handicaps. The schools already have the mission of serving these children and represent one of the few public institutions where knowledgeable and skilled personnel can be found. A program in Madison, Wisconsin, offers one promising model. A community-based leisure and recreation program is available to students with severe handicaps after school hours; trained professionals and paraprofessionals staff the program (Fink, 1988). Another school-based means for enlarging the capacity of local day-care services is by expanding access to generic after-school activities such as sports, Scouting, special-interest clubs, and local recreation centers' events. These kinds of voluntary activities provide important social supports to children who are nonhandicapped and require expansion to assist children with severe handicaps as well. Peer tutors, paraprofessionals, trained special recreation workers, and friends can make up part of the resource pool necessary for enlarging the capacity of community organizations to serve all children. Such supported recreation efforts represent a much needed aspect of community integration as well as supports for families.

Educational Services

Effective educational services for children with severe handicaps offer the possibility of reducing caregiver stress by increasing a child's capacity for self-care, communication, and participation in normal family life. Because other chapters in this book address public education issues, we do not review the literature here. However, it is important to keep in mind that effective educational services with functional curricula have the potential to reduce many of the stressors that have been identified as problematic. Effective instruction in self-care, communication, independent play, community mobility, and age-appropriate social skills can all reduce the need for caregiver assistance with routines of daily life. Toward this end, approaches to individualized education program (IEP) development that are focused on skills and issues that concern the family are extremely important (e.g., A.P. Turnbull & Turnbull, 1986). Equally essential are effective educational practices for promoting the generalization and maintenance of skills acquired in school to home and community settings (Horner, Meyer, & Fredericks, 1986). Public schools also potentially offer a child with handicaps access to a variety of after-school interests and activities as well as the possibility of establishing social connections with other children and their families.

Parent Training

An issue that must be resolved concerns the role of parent training in supporting families. Through the 1960s and 1970s it was assumed that parents benefited from training on how to teach and manage their handicapped child's behavior. Under the impetus of this approach, parents have learned to be effective teachers of a variety of daily living skills as well as effective managers of problem behavior and promoters of prosocial behavior. An unspoken assumption in this body of work has been that parents gained coping resources through learning skills as teachers and behavior modifiers (Baker, 1984). In the early intervention literature there has been empirical support for the notion that children benefit the most from infant and preschool programs when they receive them intensively at home and school. Some recent work, however, has provided evidence for possible iatrogenic effects of parent training (Jones, 1980; Wright, Granger, & Sameroff, 1984). Kogan and Tyler (1973) studied parent-infant interactions while parents administered physical therapy to their infants with cerebral palsy. They found that over a 2-year period, the affective interactions in the dyad became increasingly negative. Similarly, special

educators have worried that an excessive emphasis on orienting parents and siblings as teachers may distort family relationships (A.P. Turnbull et al., 1986). For example, parents may learn to value their child only as an achiever, and thereby diminish parental involvement in nongoal-directed activity such as playing, joking, and enjoying being together. Also, parents must fulfill many other essential roles as wage earners, spouses, homemakers, and parents of siblings; too great a demand on a parent to deliver instruction in addition to the many tasks involved in these many roles may overtax a parent and contribute to caregiver stress.

In the long run, the strength and continuity of affective social ties between family members and individuals with disabilities is vital to positive community outcomes. If an undue emphasis on parents as teachers undermines these ties, then reform is needed. When parents are viewed primarily as instructors and therapists, it is plausible that harm can ensue. However, it is probably simplistic to posit achievement and teaching as polar opposites of acceptance, bonding, and unconditional love. It is likely that parents who learn to prevent or control a child's aberrant behavior, or who teach a child to dress him- or herself, or know how to encourage a child to play will have an easier time enjoying their child—provided that the instruction is not at too great a cost in terms of time and energy. Parents who must face difficult behavior without a realistic sense of efficacy or who must dress a child for years without a sense that there are ways to promote greater independence (or cooperative interdependence) are likely to feel less empowered than those who can manage these circumstances.

One likely antidote for an undue emphasis on parents as formal instructors is emerging from changes in pedagogy for children with severe handicaps. In the 1970s, when parents were encouraged to be teachers as much as possible, the prominent model for instruction and therapy for children with severe handicaps had emerged from the operant laboratory. Lessons often involved repeated or massed practice of a skill, data collection, and planned schedules of reinforcement—all delivered at a time and place that were separate from the normal flow of daily activities. As we as special educators have had to deal with the knotty problems surrounding how to teach communication and social skills, and as we have gathered more experience with limited generalization from structured teaching sessions, we have begun to design instruction differently.

More recent approaches to instruction attempt to maintain normal stimulus conditions, task structures, and intrinsic rewards. In early childhood programs, Bromwich (1981) and Mahoney and Powell (1988) have created curricula aimed at making parents more responsive during normal play and caregiving interactions with their infants with handicaps. In the area of communication training, educators have worked to embed instruction into the context of normal chains of behavior (Goetz, Gee, & Sailor, 1983), to use prompting strategies designed to promote rapid transfer of stimulus control from the teacher to the natural stimulus conditions (Schwartz, Anderson, & Halle, 1989), and to build instruction into naturally occurring routines (Warren & Kaiser, 1986). In addition, special educators have endeavored to change the pull-out model of therapy and instead have urged specialists to embed their instruction into functional activities. And, curriculum developers have attempted to anchor instruction in normal home and community activities (Falvey, 1986). Through the use of adaptive technologies and accommodative instructional strategies, educators are now emphasizing the importance of engaging children in activities as fully as possible while learning skills rather than waiting until skills are mastered to gain access.

Taken as a whole, this shift from isolated, laboratory-like instruction to learning embedded in normative activity represents a substantial change in direction. Variously called incidental teaching, teaching in natural settings and times, milieu teaching, and partial participation, these approaches hold promise as a way to assist parents to teach their children with less distortion in normal routines and, possibly, with fewer undesirable side effects (Baker, 1984).

Singer, Irvine, and Irvin (1989) reported on a parent training program in which parents were encouraged to maximize their child's participation in home and community activities. Instructors emphasized the fact that parents play many roles. They were to determine the relative impor-

tance of the role of instruction. All instructional interactions were illustrated with videotapes of parents giving incidental instruction in the course of daily household or community activities. Parents were encouraged to play with children, to allow children to make choices and to lead activities, and to increase positive attention for participation. The study found that the affective tone of observed parent-child interactions improved as a result of the intervention, and that parents reported reductions in problem behavior as well as increases in the number of activities in which their children participated. Further research is needed on the ways in which parents of children who are nonhandicapped conduct incidental teaching while preserving positive affective exchanges, and on how to extend these approaches to children with handicaps.

On the basis of existing research, it is too early to assume that there are inevitable iatrogenic effects of training parents as teachers. While approaches that view parents solely as instructors or behavioral engineers can represent an unfortunate distortion of normative family roles, there are other alternatives that may preserve the benefits of enabling and empowering parents to deliberately teach their children. Research on parent training is needed that examines the impact of different forms of behavioral parent training on parental attributions concerning the child, parent-child affective exchanges, and child development. It is important that we not go beyond the data in deciding the relative merit of parent training. For example, the studies by Kogan and Tyler (1973) and Kogan, Tyler, and Turner (1974) concerned the interactions of mothers and infants around physical therapy. It is a mistake to equate all parent training with the interactions required to administer range-of-motion exercises to a child with cerebral palsy. It is quite possible that longitudinal studies of parent-child interactions around incidental communication, play, or community-living skills may demonstrate improved affect over time.

Fiscal Assistance

Family home caregiving often entails serious financial costs to families. These costs can be direct out-of-pocket expenses for medical care, special equipment, respite care, and other day-to-day needs, or they may be incurred as opportunity costs. That is, if a family member who would otherwise work outside of the home must stay home as a caregiver, his or her potential earnings are sacrificed. The relationship between family income and fiscal assistance needs to be carefully evaluated. Several states have established some form of family support services that require families to meet a means test for eligibility. For example, Georgia, Illinois, and Iowa limit eligibility to families with annual incomes less than $30,000, $50,000, and $40,000, respectively. From one point of view, these eligibility criteria would appear to be a fair way to distribute limited resources. However, Breslau and Prabucki (1987) found that lower middle–class and poor families were the most adversely affected by reduced parental participation in the labor force because of the opportunity costs entailed in home caregiving.

Every state but one now offers some form of services for families of children with developmental disabilities (Knoll et al., 1990). States have created three kinds of family support services: 1) payment for direct services such as respite care, counseling, and case management; 2) cash assistance paid to the family; and 3) a combination of the two (Agosta, 1989b).

Dunst et al. (1988) argued cogently that there is a direct relationship between the extent of a family's unmet needs and its available time and energy for implementing professionally recommended regimens for children with handicaps. In a series of three studies, Dunst and his colleagues found that the greater the number of unmet needs families reported, the greater their emotional and psychological distress, and the lower their commitment of time and energy to implementing child-intervention regimens (Dunst & Leet, 1987; Dunst, Vance, & Cooper, 1986; Trivette & Dunst, in preparation). These findings, along with the Michigan data (Parrott & Herman, 1988), would suggest that some priority should be given to the neediest of families. However, needs can not be catalogued easily through simple standards such as family income. For example, even upper income families can experience hardship when they must meet extraordinary caregiving costs. A family earning $100,000 per year may not be advantaged if

it must meet $85,000 annual medical bills—a sum that is not uncommon for medically fragile children (Agosta & Bergman, 1989). We believe that in the long run this issue will be resolved best by a national policy to support all families at a basic level that will permit them to carry out home caregiving roles. Thus, a low-income family would receive fiscal assistance targeted at a child with disabilities in addition to other kinds of social assistance ranging from job training for parents, housing subsidies, educational grants, and medical care. The special aid for the child with disabilities would not be meant to supplant other basic forms of assistance but rather to supplement them. This policy is emerging as a common approach in western Europe. That is, all families are offered societal assistance to raise children. Those families with additional caregiving demands are provided further supplements.

In a recent survey of 772 families in the states of Arkansas, Massachusetts, Virginia, and Missouri, Agosta (1989a) asked family members to rate their perceived level of need for several kinds of assistance. Two points emerge from reviewing these data: 1) family needs are diverse and vary by individual family, and 2) some resources and services appear to be needed by a majority of families. This core of services would, at least, include fiscal assistance (including medical insurance), a variety of respite options, case management (including planning for the future, service linkage, and information), provision of services focused on the individual needs of the family member with disabilities (e.g., communication training, interventions for challenging behavior, specialized medical and dental services), and contact with other similar families. Along with a core of services that are commonly requested, families have diverse needs that reflect the tremendous variability to be found among families in general and, in particular, reflecting the great heterogeneity in the population of persons with disabilities. Bird (1984) identified over 30 distinct services offered across several states to support caregiving families.

When these services are provided, family members (mostly parents in existing surveys) report satisfaction. For example, the state of Michigan has offered pilot family-support services since 1983 to families of individuals with severe handicaps (under age 18) living at home. The Michigan program (Parrott & Herman, 1988) consists of cash assistance to families as well as provision of services according to individual family needs; these include, in some counties, respite care, behavior management, case work, and counseling. The cash subsidy in 1986 was $267 a month per family. An evaluation conducted in 1986 found that 90% of the recipient families reported that the support subsidy and services were helpful to their family, and 94% reported they were helpful to their child with developmental disabilities. Fifty-two percent said the program greatly improved family life and another 34% said it improved family life somewhat. Sixty percent believed that it greatly improved their family's ability to care for their child with disabilities. Similarly, 60% reported that it greatly eased financial worries due to their child with developmental disabilities. Forty-six percent said it greatly reduced stress in their family's life; 33% said it somewhat reduced family stress. Approximately 15% of the respondents said that the program had only a little impact in each of these areas. Although these findings are encouraging, they are based solely on self-report measures and restrict assessment to global measures of satisfaction. As we discuss later, program evaluation could be improved.

While state-level efforts provide an important laboratory for experimenting with new policies, there are some serious drawbacks to relying solely on the states to support caregiving families. The numbers of families served in these programs, and the dollars spent, vary tremendously from region to region (Braddock et al., 1989). For example, while Michigan offers some families a subsidy of $256 per month, Montana only offers a maximum of $350 per year for respite. Also, a great deal of variability exists within each state so that services are often concentrated in urban areas and scarce in others (Castellani, Downey, Tausig, & Bird, 1986).

Deciding who should receive fiscal assistance for the extra costs of family home caregiving will require further clarification of the goals of family support. A recent evaluation of the state of Michigan's family subsidy program investigated the ways in which families utilized state family-support funds (Herman & Parrott, 1989).

Low-income families utilized the state subsidy for such basic family needs as shelter, food, and clothing. Families with middle levels of income were able to use the funds for respite care and architectural modifications. Only upper income families were able to use the funds to obtain special therapies for their children with handicaps.

Interventions Centering on Appraisal and Coping Skills

The quantity of resources that families receive is only one dimension of effective family support. The right kinds of support must be matched to family needs and they must also be delivered in ways that, in the long run, strengthen the family. Family stress theory as well as intervention research suggests that effective interventions must not only reduce sources of stress but also enhance the ways in which family members think about their situation and the skills that they bring as a family to the ongoing process of coping.

One component of contemporary family stress and coping models consists of the cognitive appraisals as well as the efforts to adapt to troubles that families utilize. Both appraisals and coping skills have been studied by psychologists and recently these approaches have been tested with caregiving families. In this section of the chapter, we present some recent evidence for the efficacy of enhancing family cognitive and active coping strategies.

Cognitive behavioral psychologists have successfully taught people to relabel narrower concepts in order to alter perceptions of difficult events (Beck, 1976; Beck et al., 1961). This process, called *cognitive reframing*, may be one skill that contributes to a wider sense of meaning. In our mutual assistance groups for parents we have taught reframing by asking parents to keep diaries of stressful events and their reactions to them. We have then modeled ways for people to think alternatively about the stressors. Table 16.2 presents some examples of comments from parents' diaries; parents recorded stressful events, negative reactions, and cognitive reframing statements.

Hawkins and Singer (1989) and Singer, Irvin, and Hawkins (1988) explored the efficacy of teaching cognitive and behavioral coping strategies to parents of children with severe handi-

Table 16.2. Examples of reframing from parents' diaries

Stressful events	Negative reactions	Cognitive reframing statements
Tim gets sick in the car.	If I wasn't in such a hurry to leave, this wouldn't have happened.	Just change him. He will be better soon.
Sarah was carrying a bowl with milk to the table. She poured it on the floor.	Why me? Why do I let small things bother me so much?	I need to calm myself. It wasn't that big of a deal.
People are watching while the child has an attack of coughing.	It's never going to quit.	Relax until she's done coughing. Carry on. Don't worry about them.

caps. In one work (Singer et al., 1988) the utility of teaching a set of cognitive-behavioral stress management skills to parents in caregiving families was studied. The stress management intervention consisted of an 8-week class held in the format of a guided support group for parents. Each class was devoted to discussing a specific coping skill, sharing efforts to use skills at home, and rehearsing the use of new skills for the following week. The combination of parent-to-parent support and active skill acquisition has been effective in reducing parental stress and anxiety in repeated evaluations (Singer et al., 1988; Singer, Irvin, et al., 1989). The skills that are taught in the stress management class have been presented in a treatment manual by Hawkins (1989); they include pinpointing sources and symptoms of stress, using brief forms of progressive muscle relaxation, using covert rehearsal, identifying and modifying negative automatic thoughts, seeking social support, and increasing pleasant activities.

Building upon this work, Nixon (1989) expanded the cognitive-behavioral interventions in order to help parents with guilt and self-blame. The literature has indicated that many caregiving parents hold themselves responsible for their child's handicapping condition and that they blame themselves for difficulties that arise in caregiving (e.g., Featherstone, 1982). While the problem has been widely reported, there have been no published studies showing that self-blame and guilt can be alleviated through intervention. Nixon reviewed the burgeoning literature on self-blame in persons who experience challenging life events and developed a group intervention based upon the work of cognitive-behavioral psychologists (Beck, Rush, Shaw, & Emery, 1979; Burns, 1980). He identified paren-

tal attributional style as a pivotal mechanism for creating self-blame as opposed to selecting problem-focused coping styles.

According to attribution theory, a few foundational cognitive stances generate perceptions and affective reactions (S.E. Taylor, 1983). For any given event, a person may attribute its cause to internal or external sources. The trouble may be judged to be either a global or a specific one, and it can be viewed as either temporary or stable. Nixon (1989) found that the parents who attended his support groups tended to blame problems with their child on themselves, to assume that they were unchangeable, and that their failings were global in nature.

Through a combination of group discussion and sharing, lecture on cognitive-behavioral modification, and specific exercises, parents were able to assume alternative points of view (Nixon, 1989). Randomly assigned treatment and waiting list control groups were compared on measures of guilt, depression, attributional style, and self-esteem. The treatment group participated in a 5-week mutual support group led by an experienced counselor. The leader guided discussions of topics of blame, responsibility, control and lack of it, common attributional distortions, and ways to challenge cognitive assumptions. Much of each session was devoted to encouraging parents to talk with one another about these issues. A MANCOVA analysis comparing the treatment and control groups on the dependent measures found statistically significant improvements in the treatment group's reports of situational guilt, self-esteem, depression, and attributional styles.

The above results are encouraging because there appears to be a kind of unspoken assumption in the literature that problems such as guilt and self-blame are not amenable to intervention; they are described typically either as permanent states (Olshansky, 1970) or as somehow changing at their own time and pace without assistance (Simons, 1987). We are concerned that the advances in cognitive behavior therapy of the past 20 years have not been applied to caregiving families even though many of them have been designed for alleviating related problems. Thus, the results of our work (i.e., Singer et al., 1988; Singer, Irvin, et al., 1989) on stress management and Nixon's (1989) findings in regard to treatment of self-blame suggest that a wealth of helping procedures may be made available to families—provided that researchers proceed carefully and base their efforts to transfer psychological interventions to these families in empirically validated strategies. Once again, these strategies are appealing because they do not presume pathology in families but rather that normal coping processes that are helpful to many people in difficult circumstances may be of assistance to caregiving families.

Cognitive reframing around specific stressors is not the same as giving a broad meaning to a more global condition, but it may be one contributory skill. And it may give parents experience with a broader skill of being able to operate upon thoughts and feelings in such a way as to alter perceptions of a difficult situation. We are not suggesting that learning to reframe certain reactions is the same as generally coming to terms with a family member with severe handicaps. Generalized adaptation as described in broad terms such as acceptance and mastery certainly involves much more. It may involve relationships over time with people who have experienced very similar life difficulties and who currently are somewhat less distressed and more accomplished in navigating the specific difficulties posed by a challenging life situation (Thoits, 1986). It is also likely to involve a coherent set of values and meanings that can serve as a guide to thought and action.

Strengthening Intrafamily Support

Parents are the most satisfied with their role as caregivers when they perceive their family as supportive and working together as a team (McCubbin et al., 1983). This satisfaction probably derives in part from the simple practical help that such families offer and also from their supportive set of values and behavioral standards. Decisions about allocation of instrumental support within the family may be enhanced, in some families, through family problem-solving interactions and other forms of communication training (Hawkins & Singer, 1989). Family members can learn to assign work at family meetings, and parents can learn to use various reward systems as ways to motivate siblings to assist with family tasks. Caution is required to respect a family's cultural values around division of labor in the home. Intervention efforts to teach communication skills to distressed couples have been modestly but consistently successful (Hahlweg, Revenstorf, & Schindler, 1984).

Working in our clinic at the Oregon Research Institute, Lichtenstein (1989) recently showed that short-term behavioral marital therapy can improve marital satisfaction in couples who are parents of children with severe handicaps. She worked with four couples who responded to advertisements offering marital counseling. During baseline sessions the couples were observed in brief problem-solving interactions and they completed a battery of assessments designed to pinpoint areas of agreement and disagreement in the relationship. Treatment consisted of brief behavioral marital therapy in which couples received instruction, practice, and homework assignments in various communication and problem-solving skills (Jacobson & Gurman, 1986). Couples showed improvements in observed problem-solving skills as well as in self-reported marital satisfaction. A multiple-baseline design was used to establish experimental control. In some families, the therapy was associated with improvements in parental attitudes toward their children with severe handicaps. Behavioral marital and family interventions appear to hold real promise for assisting families to cooperate, resolve conflicts, and develop shared meanings.

Strengthening Informal Social Ties Outside the Family

Similarly, the social context is an important contributor to a sense of meaning. When a family member says that he or she finds meaning, he or she is in part connecting to a cultural and language community. Religious meanings and religious affiliations play a prominent part in positive adaptation for many families of children with disabilities. Historically, religious institutions have promoted the value of caregiving. In the Middle Ages when parents abandoned their infants with disabilities, the Church was charged with their care. In contemporary America, religious institutions often promote a set of values that transcend both stoic and hedonistic individualism (Bellah, Madsen, Sullivan, Swidler, & Tipton, 1985). Values concerning caring for and supporting vulnerable persons may counter some of the prevalent cultural emphasis on individual pleasure and achievement.

In a similar way, mutual assistance groups can help people to find meaning in challenging circumstances. Estimates suggest that as many as 7 million Americans currently belong to mutual assistance groups for a variety of problems and life circumstances ranging from alcoholism to stuttering to coping with a chronic illness. Several groups support parents of children with disabilities. Organizations such as the Association for Retarded Citizens, Sick Kids Need Involved People (SKIP), United Cerebral Palsy, Autism Society of America (ASA), and TASH, as well as mutual aid groups tied to hospitals and schools, provide a great deal of support to many families. There is a sound psychological reason for the proliferation of groups with highly specific foci. People are more likely to compare themselves and affiliate with others who have faced the same stressful circumstances. Research points out that not just anyone will do for support (Thoits, 1986). People are most likely to seek support from others who have had similar experiences and whose emotional reactions are neither a lot more severe nor a lot more calm. Attempted help from people who are seen as dissimilar is often perceived as controlling and demanding (Thoits, 1986).

A study by Lehman, Ellard, and Wortman (1986) serves as a useful illustration. They interviewed 94 people who had lost a relative within the preceding 4–7 years regarding what kinds of support were helpful and unhelpful. The three most helpful kinds of support were: contact with similar others, opportunities to express feelings, and expressions of concern. The results of this study also point out the dangers of the wrong kinds of helping efforts from the wrong sources, and should serve as a caution against the casual dissemination of cognitive coping approaches. Unhelpful support included advice giving, encouraging statements, and efforts to minimize feelings or to express forced cheerfulness.

In our clinical work we have frequently heard from parents that their feelings of isolation are aggravated by well-meaning but painfully superficial statements of supports from others. For example, the mother of a child with muscular dystrophy said: "I hate it when people tell me how strong I am. They'll say 'I'm so sorry to hear about your boy. You must be very strong.' But inside I feel like I am falling apart and hearing these clichés from people only makes me feel more alone." People who "have been there" and who listen intently with acceptance of another's painful feelings can sometimes help others to overcome this kind of isolation.

There are many emerging alternatives in the way that mutual aid groups can be organized and in their relationships with formal institutions. At one end of the spectrum, some groups have been started, operated, and maintained by professional helpers under the fiscal auspices of hospitals or public service agencies. At the other end, parents and siblings have formed independent groups open only to family members and run solely via voluntary contributions. The boundary between formal services and mutual aid groups, and between professionals and group members, is fruitful ground for examination of a set of emerging policy and professional issues. Two topics lie at the heart of the matter: the relationship between the traditional medical model of aid and the nature of chronic life stressors. The concept of empowerment has recently captured attention in applied and academic concerns about family support services. Dunst, Trivette, Gordon, and Pletcher (1989) defined empowerment as: "the ability to identify needs, deploy competencies to mobilize resources to meet needs, and gain a greater sense of intrapersonal and interpersonal control over life events involving interactions with personal social network members" (p. 126). The opposite of empowerment is helplessness, dependency, and the weakening of supportive social networks. Mutual assistance groups are promising, in part, because they provide opportunities for family members to reciprocate by giving as well as receiving aid. The challenge for professional helpers as well as for those who design support services is to give aid in ways that empower rather than weaken family members.

The research on mutual assistance organizations does point to several successful groups that have been stable and innovative and that have relied upon partnerships between laypersons and professionals and combinations of public and private resources. Maton (1988) studied 144 members of three mutual aid organizations and found that people who reported that they both gave and received social support were most satisfied with the groups. Similarly, Menolascino and Coleman (1980) described a parent-to-parent network in which public resources are used to maintain a directory of parents and a computer system for matching new parents with veterans based upon several similarities. The purpose of parent-to-parent networking is to link inexperienced parents with similar families who have successfully dealt with caregiving problems. The service is deliberately designed to emphasize mutual assistance, nonprofessional helping interactions, and to provide a structure that allows new parents eventually to become helpers to others in the network. Social reciprocity is built into the workings of the parent-to-parent network so that parents are encouraged to think of themselves as emerging experts rather than as long-term dependents. In this kind of semiformal service system, professionals largely play the roles of facilitators, consultants, and resources to the members of the helping network. For example, professionals may be invited to present workshops on communication skills to members of the network or to describe new services or technologies to keep the helping parents up to date.

As just stated, the purpose of a parent-to-parent network is primarily to promote exchange of information between families and also to create opportunities for long-term friendships to arise. A step beyond an informational network adds the exchange of goods and services. Dunst et al. (1989) described a skills bank for family members to exchange supportive services. They established a system in which families could identify their needs and request assistance from others in the network in exchange for some service or good that they provided. All exchanges were reciprocal. When a family had a need that could not be met by other network members, project staff recruited help from outside organizations such as church groups. For example, a parent could acquire needed clothing from a church group in exchange for donating the labor of housepainting.

Dunst and his colleagues' (1989) work is particularly noteworthy because of the careful attention to the way in which help is given by project staff, the way in which family needs are assessed, and the emphasis on mutual reciprocity. A self-report evaluation by participant families demonstrated that families exhibited reduced needs, increased percentages of needs met, and an increase in the number of independent exchanges over a 12-month period. This last variable is exemplary; help-giving research suggests that a possible undesirable effect of some kinds of ineffective help giving is increased dependence upon the helper. The measurement of independent exchanges initiated is a way to index the extent to which families acquired skills at activating social support networks on their own without professional assistance. The role of staff in this project was to assess family needs and strengths, assist family members to activate their existing social networks for help, or to build networks through mutual exchange. In this approach, the professional serves to enhance a community's capacity to provide support to its families and to enable family members to improve their access and use of instrumental social support.

The notion of giving family members skills that enable them to carry on with less professional assistance has been a key idea in the kinds of mutual aid groups organized at the Oregon Research Institute. Hawkins and Singer (1989) described psychoeducational groups for parents that are professionally led but are also designed to encourage mutual sharing and support between parents. The groups are conducted as skills training classes in various coping skills that have been empirically validated, such as self-monitoring, utilizing social support, muscle relaxation, anger control, covert rehearsal, and problem solving. Professionals and parent co-leaders demonstrate these skills during weekly class meetings. Parents then practice the skills as "homework" during the week. Each class session includes extension discussion of the homework. These problem-focused discussions provide the opportunity for parents to exchange information, make comparisons, and provide one another with support. In this model, the professional plays the roles of an empathetic listener, group facilitator, counselor, and instructor. Parents are encouraged to assist one another and to build contacts outside of the class meetings.

Part of the attraction of mutual aid organizations is that they may be better suited to the nature of long-term stressful circumstances than are helping mechanisms based upon the traditional medical model. Medical help is primarily aimed at short-term cures. When translated into helping models for family members, this approach gives rise to short-term classes and programs aimed at delivering intensive but short-term "treatments." However, living with a family member with severe handicaps is not a short-term proposition. The challenges and benefits of the relationship change over the life cycle of the family. Many of the challenges are mundane coping issues that are highly situation specific (e.g., What locker room should an 11-year-old use when he goes to the gym and needs his mother's help to dress? How can the school bus driver be persuaded to let a child off closer to the curb? What should be said to a teenager with severe retardation who says she wants a baby?). Because these challenges are rooted in the changeability of daily life, a one-shot set of classes or short-term training cannot possibly anticipate their diversity and novelty. Mutual aid groups offer the possibility of long-term membership and usage on demand.

We believe that along with mutual aid groups, expert professional services must also be available on demand to meet some of the changing needs of families over time. Professionals can contribute important leadership and group-process skills to mutual aid groups (Jacobs & Goodman, 1989). Services need to be designed in such a way that they take into account the life-long needs of caregiving families as well as the right mixture of professional and lay support. Community psychologists have advocated a model of community services akin to the agricultural extension center. The center is available as a resource for information, problem solving, linkage to other services, and counseling as needed. It is designed as a long-term coping institution on the assumption that many needs are recurrent and that families will have changing needs over time.

Mutual assistance is not simply a tool for achieving social support. In many instances, it is a necessary means for achieving solutions to problems that are larger than any one person can overcome. Many of the concerns that are encountered by parents and siblings of persons with handicaps are not simply personal or familial troubles, but rather are the direct result of societal neglect or of outmoded social institutions. The recognition that an individual problem is shared by others and thus is amendable to collective action may, in itself, promote a sense of community (Mills, 1959). When organized action leads to social change it may lead to a sense of empowerment and control for persons who might otherwise feel helpless (Levine, 1988). If well designed and implemented, the social innovation may promote well-being, prevent unwanted conditions, and alleviate suffering. Despite its shortcomings, PL 94-142 appears in many ways to have been a social reform that resulted from people sharing a common problem and working together to address it as a collective issue. Since the end of World War II, parental advocacy efforts have been the driving force behind the creation of community service options for persons with developmental disabilities. This ongoing social revolution is the product of mutual aid and pooling of resources in order to change a socially created set of unacceptable conditions. The same approach will be necessary to create better living conditions for caregiving families. In fact, major parent and professional organizations are currently at the forefront of efforts to generate state- and federal-level support services for families.

Strengthening Formal Ties

Successful efforts to bridge gaps between parents and professionals have attempted to alter professionals' attitudes (Darling, 1983; Pecora,

Delewski, Booth, Haapala, & Kinney, 1985; Singer, Hawkins, et al., in preparation) and communication skills (Evans, Hearn, Uhlemann, & Ivey, 1984); improve the quality of professionals' training (A.P. Turnbull & Turnbull, 1986); and teach parents skills for communicating with professionals during formal or informal interactions (Walker, 1989), and in situations in which advocacy skills are required (Singer, Hawkins, et al., in preparation). Reform efforts also need to address the lack of design and coordination in the service system, which often forces parents and professionals to wrestle with a maze of confusing eligibility criteria, unclear funding priorities, and obscure regulations.

There is some evidence that parents find public services to be most beneficial when they offer a wide range of individual choice and flexibility. For example, in their recent nationwide survey of respite care, Knoll and Bedford (1989) reported that parents were least satisfied with respite care resources when they had to meet rigid criteria for duration or time of use. Several innovative state family-support programs have relied upon cash assistance, voucher systems, and individualized family plans as means of personalizing support services. These broad program parameters undoubtedly affect the face-to-face interactions of parents and professionals. The one part of our national social system that has most consistently attempted to serve children with handicaps while individualizing services has been the public schools (since the passage of PL 94-142). Although there are many problems, evaluations of school programs for children with severe handicaps have found high levels of parental satisfaction with these services (Blacher & Meyers, 1983).

In our work at the Oregon Research Institute we conducted a set of experimental evaluations of a cluster of family support services for families of school-age individuals with severely handicapping conditions (Singer, Irvin, et al., 1989). We used parental morale and social validation, direct observation of parent-child interactions, as well as the child's participation in community activities as indicators of the program's effectiveness. The model consists of the following services: case management, support

groups focused on stress management skills and behavioral parent training, respite care, volunteers who assist children to join in community activities, and behavioral counseling for individuals and couples. Recently, we extended the model to include cooperation and coordination with the public school program for children with handicaps. Evaluations of the model have shown repeatedly that it reduces parental demoralization, increases children's participation, and earns highly favorable evaluations from parents (Singer, Irvin, et al., in preparation). As in the Michigan study (Parrott & Herman, 1988), we found that a small group of families did not benefit from our interventions. These families usually had multiple presenting problems, often including substance abuse, poverty, and alleged family violence. We believe that much more intensive interventions are required in these dysfunctional caregiving families.

RESEARCH QUESTIONS AND DIRECTIONS

With the growing demand for family support services, there is a large and potentially useful research agenda that needs to be addressed. We have briefly reviewed a small portion of the recent literature on family home caregiving. Each of the many topics touched upon presents questions begging to be answered. We now highlight a few of the questions and approaches we believe might be the most useful in improving the lives of caregiving families.

1. There are a number of basic research questions that need to be resolved concerning families in general. Perhaps the largest and most troublesome of these has to do with how to measure the family as a unit of analysis. Most of what passes for family assessment in the literature consists of one family member's perceptions of the rest of the family. Usually the informant is the mother. Foundational work needs to be done on how to accomplish family assessment as opposed to assessment of the individuals who make up the family.

2. Research needs to break out of the residualist tradition and its accompanying emphasis on pathology in families. We need to ask a set of broad-based questions about what conditions al-

low families to succeed as caregivers: Which families weather crises and how? Which kinds of organization, communication, affective and instrumental exchanges, social networks, coping skills, and formal services are found in successful families? How do these families change in their needs, resources, and coping skills across the family life cycle? Which family and community conditions are associated with positive adjustment by siblings and other extended family members?

3.   The research community would do well to concentrate on intervention research. Enough correlational and descriptive data have accumulated. We believe it is time to test effective means of promoting family cohesion and adaptation, preventing family dysfunction, and ameliorating distress in troubled families. The applied behavior analytic literature on parent training has had an admirable intervention focus. However, its scope has been too limited so that the effect of treatment on the family unit has rarely been assessed. Researchers would do well to team up with innovative social services programs in order to test effective practices for supporting families.

At the moment, social support is not very well understood: while everyone agrees that it is powerful, no one is sure exactly what it is or how it works. Research should address ways to create, sustain, and strengthen intrafamilial support and informal social support, as well as more formal professional supports.

4.   Dunst et al. (1988) have taken the lead in the field of special education in pointing out the potential positive and negative consequences of various approaches to helping families of children with handicaps. They have drawn upon an emerging body of knowledge concerning help seeking and help giving (e.g., DePaulo, Nadler, & Fisher, 1983) to formulate a set of non-residualist guidelines for helping families. These recommendations provide an important agenda for social research as well as public policy in the next decade.

5.   We believe that researchers would do well to explore the commonalities between the needs of caregiving families and other populations under stress. There has been a tendency in the study of families of children with handicaps

to proceed in a vacuum as if the problems of these families are generically different. This approach isolates us from a large body of ongoing work in other complementary fields such as public health, social psychology, community psychology, and applied anthropology. For example, in our recent work (Singer & Irvin, 1989b) we have tried to make research on families of children with handicaps conversant with a wider literature on causes and treatment for demoralization in families in general.

A variety of methodologies will be useful in studying caregiving families. Ethnographic, direct observation, and psychometric methods all have their uses in this endeavor. The complexity of family systems will make multivariate analyses increasingly necessary. The use of linear modeling techniques offers a compelling way to explore the relationships between various ecological levels.

6.   Improved program evaluation research is sorely needed. Several states in the United States began to experiment with modest family support programs in the mid-1970s and some evaluations of these programs have been published (e.g., Slater & Wikler, 1984). Residualist thinking has colored evaluations of support programs for families of children with developmental disabilities, frail elderly persons, and persons with chronic mental illness. The residualist tradition holds that the only legitimate purpose of public assistance is to provide minimal levels of support to vulnerable persons after they have been placed outside of the home. As a result, early evaluation studies (Slater, Bates, & Eicher, 1986) have focused on the question "Do family support services reduce numbers of out-of-home placements?" In these early studies, the outcomes have been negative; out-of-home placement rates have not been significantly reduced. These data should not be interpreted to mean that family support services are not helpful to a majority of recipients. A much broader range of questions needs to be asked in order to determine ways to support families more effectively. Out-of-home placement is only one variable of interest.

7.   Research and demonstration efforts are needed on ways to help families to prevent and to ameliorate crises. Those families most at risk

appear to have multiple stressors, children with severe health problems or behavioral problems, social isolation, and very limited support services. We need to be able to intervene early and effectively in these high-risk homes yet little is known about how to do so. One of the most problematic of the low-incidence responses to family stress, child abuse and neglect in families of children with handicaps requires careful examination.

8. Research should examine ways to increase participation by children and youth with severe handicaps in normal home and community activities. Ways of opening up generic neighborhood and community organizations including day-care providers, youth groups, sports teams, clubs, churches, and so forth need to be developed and tested.

9. We need to define the roles and necessary skills of the personnel who will staff emerging family support programs. We probably need to create a new hybrid profession for this role while avoiding the pitfalls of unhelpful professionalism. Research will be needed to define

these roles and skills and to test effective ways to teach them.

10. Family research needs to encompass the full diversity of families in their contemporary form, including single-parent families, ethnically diverse families, well-adjusted families, and families who experience dysfunction.

The wealth of coping skills that has been tested in other areas of clinical psychology should be applied to these families and field tested. The similarities between caregiving families regardless of the cause of the disability and across various (sub)cultures should also be explored.

11. The relationship between the public schools and emerging family support services needs to be explicated and different models tested. At the present time, the public schools represent one of the few institutions with available expertise concerning children with severe disabilities. The possibilities for extending and coordinating this expertise with family support agencies need to be tested.

REFERENCES

Abramowitz, I.A., & Coursey, R.D. (1989). Impact of an educational support group on family participants who take care of their schizophrenic relatives. *Journal of Consulting and Clinical Psychology, 57,* 232–236.

Agosta, J. (1989a). *Selected state survey findings.* Monmouth: Western Oregon State College, Human Services Research Institute.

Agosta, J. (1989b). Using cash assistance to support family efforts. In G.H.S. Singer & L.K. Irvin (Eds.), *Support for caregiving families: Enabling positive adaptation to disability,* (pp. 189–204). Baltimore: Paul H. Brookes Publishing Co.

Agosta, J., & Bergman, A. (1989, December). *Family support mechanisms.* Presentation to the National Conference of The Association for Persons with Severe Handicaps, San Francisco.

American Association of Retired Persons. (1986). *A profile of older persons: 1986.* Washington, DC: Author.

Anthony-Bergstone, C.R., Zarit, S.H., & Gatz, M. (1988). Symptoms of psychological distress among caregivers of dementia patients. *Psychology and Aging, 3,* 245–248.

Antonovsky, A. (1987). *Unraveling the mystery of health: How people manage stress and stay well.* San Francisco: Jossey-Bass.

Apolloni, A.H., & Triest, G. (1983). Respite services in California: Status and recommendations for improvement. *Mental Retardation, 21,* 240–243.

Bailey, D.B., & Winton, P.J. (1989). Friendship and acquaintance among families in a mainstreamed day care center. *Education and Training in Mental Retardation, 24*(2), 107–113.

Baker, B.L. (1984). Intervention with families with young, severely handicapped children. In J. Blacher (Ed.), *Severely handicapped young children and their families* (pp. 319–375). Orlando, FL: Academic Press.

Baldwin, S. (1985). *The costs of caring: Families with disabled children.* London: Rutledge & Kegan Paul.

Beck, A.T. (1976). *Cognitive therapy and the emotional disorders.* New York: International Universities Press.

Beck, A.T., Rush, A.J., Shaw, B.F., & Emery, G. (1979). *Cognitive therapy of depression.* New York: Guilford Press.

Beck, A.T., Ward, C.H., Mendelson, M., Moch, T.E., & Erbaugh, J.H. (1961). An inventory for measuring depression. *Archives of General Psychiatry, 4,* 561–571.

Beckman, P.J. (1983). Influence of selected child characteristics on stress in families of handicapped infants. *American Journal of Mental Deficiency, 88,* 150–156.

Beckman, P.J., Pokorni, J.L., Maza, E.A., & Balzer-Martin, L. (1986). A longitudinal study of stress and support in families of preterm and full-term infants. *Journal of the Division for Early Childhood, 11*(1), 2–9.

Bellah, R.N., Madsen, R., Sullivan, W.M., Swidler, A., & Tipton, S.M. (1985). *Habits of the heart: Individualism and commitment in American life.* New York: Harper & Row.

Billings, G.G., & Moos, R.H. (1985). Psychosocial stressors, coping, and depression. In W.W. Beckham & W.R. Leber (Eds.), *Handbook of depression: Treatment, assessment and research* (pp. 940–976). Chicago: Dorsey Press.

Bird, W.A. (1984). *A survey of family support programs in 17 states.* Albany: New York State Office of Mental Retardation and Developmental Disability.

Blacher, J., & Meyers, C.E. (1983). A review of attachment formation and disorder of handicapped children. *American Journal of Mental Deficiency, 87,* 359–371.

Boswell, J. (1988). *The kindness of strangers: The abandonment of children in western Europe from late antiquity to the Renaissance.* New York: Pantheon Books.

Braddock, D., Hemp, R., Fujiura, G., Bachelder, L., & Mitchell, D. (1989). *Public expenditures for mental retardation and developmental disabilities in the United States: State profiles* (Working paper, 3rd ed.) Chicago: University Affiliated Program in Developmental Disabilities, University of Illinois at Chicago.

Brady, P.E. (1987, Fall). Coverage for children with catastrophic illness and their families: A federal legislative update. *Family Support Bulletin,* p. 9. (Available from United Cerebral Palsy Associations, 1522 K Street, Suite 112, Washington, DC 20205)

Breslau, N., & Davis, G.C. (1986). Chronic stress and major depression. *Archives of General Psychiatry, 43,* 309–314.

Breslau, N., & Prabucki, K. (1987). Siblings of disabled children: Effects of chronic stress in the family. *Archives of General Psychiatry, 44,* 1040–1046.

Breslau, N., Staruch, K.S., & Mortimer, E.A. (1982). Psychological distress in mothers of disabled children. *American Journal of Disabled Children, 136,* 682–686.

Bristol, M.M. (1987). The home care of children with developmental disabilities: Empirical support for a model of successful family coping with stress. In S. Landesman & P. Vietze (Eds.), *Living environments and mental retardation* (pp. 401–422). Washington, DC: American Association on Mental Retardation.

Bristol, M.M., Gallagher, J.J., & Schopler, E. (1988). Mothers and fathers of young developmentally disabled and nondisabled boys: Adaptation and spousal support. *Developmental Psychology, 24,* 441–451.

Bromwich, R. (1981). *Working with parents and infants: An interactional approach.* Baltimore: University Park Press.

Brown, L., Long, E., Udvari-Solner, A., Davis, L., Van Deventer, P., Ahlgren, C., Johnson, F., Gruenewald, L., & Jorgensen, J. (1989). The home school: Why students with severe intellectual disabilities must attend the schools of their brothers, sisters, friends, and neighbors. *Journal of The Association for Persons with Severe Handicaps, 14,* 1–7.

Burdz, M.P., Eaton, W.O., & Bond, J.B. (1988). Effect of respite care on dementia and nondementia patients and their caregivers. *Psychology and Aging, 3,* 38–42.

Burns, D.D. (1980). *Feeling good: The new mood therapy.* New York: New American Library.

Bush, G.W. (1988). The National Head Injury Foundation: Eight years of challenge and growth. *Journal of Head Injury Rehabilitation, 3*(4), 73–77.

Cantor, M.H. (1983). Strain among caregivers: A study of experience in the United States. *The Gerontologist, 23,* 597–604.

Castellani, P.J., Downey, N.A., Tausig, M.B., & Bird, W.A. (1986). Availability and accessibility of family support services. *Mental Retardation, 24,* 711–719.

Chetwynd, J. (1985). Factors contributing to stress on mothers caring for an intellectually handicapped child. *British Journal of Social Work, 15,* 295–304.

Cohen, S., & Warren, R. (1987). *Child abuse, disability, & family support: An analysis of dynamics in England and the United States with references to practices in other western European countries.* New York: World Rehabilitation Fund.

Cole, D.A. (1986). Out-of-home child placement and family adaptation: A theoretical framework. *American Journal of Mental Deficiency, 91,* 226–236.

Cole, D.A., & Meyer, L.H. (1989). Impact of needs and resources on family plans to seek out-of-home placement. *American Journal on Mental Retardation, 93,* 380–387.

Cummings, S.T. (1976). The impact of the child's deficiency on the father: A study of fathers of mentally retarded and of chronically ill children. *American Journal of Orthopsychiatry, 46,* 246–255.

Cutrona, C.E., & Russell, D.W. (1987). The provisions of social relationships and adaptation to stress. In W.H. Jones & D. Perlman (Eds.), *Advances in personal relationships* (Vol. 1, pp. 37–67). Greenwich, CT: JAI Press.

Darling, R.B. (1983). Parent-professional interaction: The roots of misunderstanding. In M. Seligman (Ed.), *The family with a handicapped child: Understanding and treatment* (pp. 95–124). Orlando, FL: Grune & Stratton.

Davies, R. (1985, November). *Caregiver burden tasks and experiences.* Paper presented at the meeting of the Gerontological Society of America, New Orleans.

Depaulo, B.M., Nadler, A., & Fisher, J.D. (1983). *New directions in helping: Help-seeking* (Vol. 2). New York: Academic Press.

Doernberg, N.L. (1982). Issues in communication between pediatricians and parents of young mentally retarded children. *Pediatric Annals, 11,* 438–444.

Drinka, T.J.K., Smith, J.C., & Drinka, P.J. (1987). Correlates of depression and burden for informal caregivers of patients in a geriatrics referral clinic. *Journal of the American Geriatric Society, 35,* 522–525.

Dunst, C.J., & Leet, H.E. (1987). Measuring the adequacy of resources in households with young children. *Child: Care, Health, and Development, 13,* 111–125.

Dunst, C.J., Trivette, C.M., & Cross, A.H. (1986). Roles and support networks of mothers of handicapped children. In R.R. Fewell & P.F. Vadasy (Eds.), *Families of handicapped children: Needs and supports across the life span* (pp. 167–192). Austin, TX: PRO-ED.

Dunst, C., Trivette, C., & Deal, A. (1988). *Enabling and empowering families: Principles and guidelines for practice.* Cambridge, MA: Brookline Books.

Dunst, C.J., Trivette, C.M., Gordon, N.J., & Pletcher, L.L. (1989). Building and mobilizing informal family support networks. In G.H.S. Singer & L.K. Irvin (Eds.), *Support for caregiving families: Enabling positive adaptation to disability* (pp. 121–141). Baltimore: Paul H. Brookes Publishing Co.

Dunst, C.J., Vance, S.D., & Cooper, C.S. (1986). A social systems perspective of adolescent pregnancy: Determinants of parent and parent-child behavior. *Infant Mental Health Journal, 7,* 34–48.

Dyson, L., Edgar, E., & Crnic, K. (1989). Psychological predictors of adjustment by siblings of developmentally disabled children. *American Journal on Mental Retardation, 94,* 292–302.

Dyson, L. & Fewell, R.R. (1986). Stress and adaptation in parents of young handicapped and nonhandicapped children: A comparative study. *Journal of the Division for Early Childhood, 10*(1), 25–35.

Erickson, M., & Upshur, C.C. (1989). Caretaking burden and social support: Comparison of mothers of infants with and without disabilities. *American Journal on Mental Retardation, 94,* 250–258.

Evans, D.R., Hearn, M.T., Uhlemann, M.R., & Ivey, A.E. (1984). *Essential interviewing: A programmed approach to effective communication.* Pacific Grove, CA: Brooks/Cole.

Falvey, M. (1986). *Community-based curriculum: Instructional strategies for students with severe handicaps.* Baltimore: Paul H. Brookes Publishing Co.

Featherstone, H. (1982). *A difference in the family.* New York: Penguin Books.

Ferguson, P.M., & Asch, A. (1989). Lessons from life: Personal and parental perspectives on school, childhood, and disability. In D. Biklen, D. Ferguson, & A. Ford (Eds.), *Schooling and disability: NSSE 88th Yearbook* (pp. 108–140). Chicago: University of Chicago Press.

Fewell, R.R., & Vadasy, P.F. (1986). *Families of handicapped children: Needs and supports across the life span.* Austin, TX: PRO-ED.

Fink, D.B. (1988). *School-age children with special needs.* Boston: Exceptional Parent Press.

Fitting, M., Rabins, P., Lucas, M.J., & Eastham, J. (1986). Caregivers for dementia patients: A comparison of husbands and wives. *The Gerontological Society of America, 26*(3), 248–252.

Frey, K.S., Greenberg, M.R., & Fewell, R.R. (1989). Stress and coping among parents of handicapped children: A multidimensional approach. *American Journal on Mental Retardation, 94,* 240–249.

Friedrich, W.N., & Friedrich, W.L. (1981). Psychosocial assets of parents of handicapped and nonhandicapped children. *American Journal of Mental Deficiency, 85,* 551–553.

Friedrich, W.N., Wilturner, L.T., & Cohen, D.S. (1985). Coping resources and parenting mentally retarded children. *American Journal of Mental Deficiency, 90,* 130–139.

Gabel, H., & Kotsch, L.S. (1981). *Social characteristics and economic status of the U.S. aged population* (Report No. 81-32EPW). Washington, DC: The Library of Congress, Congressional Research Service.

Gallagher, J.J., Beckman, P., & Cross, A.H. (1983). Families of handicapped children: Sources of stress and its amelioration. *Exceptional Children, 50,* 10–19.

Garbarino, J., Stocking, S.H., Collins, A.H., Gottlieb, B.H., Olds, D.L., Pancoast, D.L., Sherman, D., Tietjen, A.M., & Warren, D.I. (1980). *Protecting children from abuse and neglect.* San Francisco: Jossey-Bass.

Gath, A. (1977). The impact of an abnormal child upon the parents. *British Journal of Psychiatry, 130,* 405–410.

Goetz, L., Gee, K., & Sailor, W. (1983, December). *Using interrupted sequences to establish pictoral communication skills.* Paper presented at the annual meeting of The Association for Persons with Severe Handicaps, San Francisco.

Goldberg, W.A., & Easterbrooks, M.A. (1984). Role of marital quality in toddler development. *Developmental Psychology, 20,* 504–514.

Goldfarb, L.A., Brotherson, M.J., Summers, J.A., & Turnbull, A.P. (1986). *Meeting the challenge of disability or chronic illness: A family guide.* Baltimore: Paul H. Brookes Publishing Co.

Goldman, H. (1982). Mental illness and family burden: A public health perspective. *Hospital and Community Psychiatry, 33,* 557–560.

Goode, D.A. (1980). *Deaf-blind: An examination of*

extraordinary communication and its significance to the sociology of knowledge. Unpublished doctoral dissertation, University of California, Los Angeles.

Grossman, F.K. (1972). *Brothers and sisters of retarded children.* Syracuse, NY: Syracuse University Press.

Hahlweg, K., Revenstorf, D., & Schindler, L. (1984). Effects of behavioral marital therapy on couples' communication and problem-solving skills. *Journal of Consulting and Clinical Psychology, 52,* 553–566.

Haley, W.E., Levine, E.G., Brown, S.L., & Bartolucci, A.A. (1987). Stress, appraisal, coping, and social support as predictors of adaptational outcome among dementia caregivers. *Psychology and Aging, 2,* 323–330.

Hawkins, N. (1989). *Stress management for handicapped children.* Unpublished manuscript, Oregon Research Institute, Eugene.

Hawkins, N.E., & Singer, G.H.S. (1989). A skills training approach for assisting parents to cope with stress. In G.H.S. Singer & L.K. Irvin (Eds.), *Support for caregiving families: Enabling positive adaptation to disability* (pp. 71–83). Baltimore: Paul H. Brookes Publishing Co.

Herman, S.E., & Parrott, M.E. (1989). *Report on the Michigan Family Support Subsidy Program.* Lansing: Michigan Department of Mental Health.

Holroyd, J., & Guthrie, D. (1979). Stress in families of children with neuromuscular disease. *Journal of Clinical Psychology, 35,* 734–739.

Holroyd, J., & McArthur, D. (1976). Mental retardation and stress on the parents: A contrast between Down's syndrome and childhood autism. *American Journal of Mental Deficiency, 80,* 431–436.

Homeward Bound, Inc., et al. v. Hissom Memorial Center et al., WL 27104 (N. D. Okla. 1987).

Horner, R.H., Meyer, L.H., & Fredericks, H.D.B. (Eds.). (1986). *Education of learners with severe handicaps: Exemplary service strategies.* Baltimore: Paul H. Brookes Publishing Co.

Huang, L.N., & Heifetz, L.J. (1984). Elements of professional helpfulness: Profiles of the most helpful and least helpful professionals encountered by mothers of young retarded children. *Perspectives and progress in mental retardation: Vol. 1.* (social, psychological, and educational aspects (pp. 425–433). Baltimore: University Park Press.

Ilfeld, F.W. (1977). Current social stressors and symptoms of depression. *American Journal of Psychiatry, 134*(2), 161–166.

Intagliata, J. (1986). Assessing the impact of respite care services: A review of outcome evaluation studies, In C.L. Salisbury & J. Intagliata (Eds.), *Respite care: Support for persons with developmental disabilities and their families* (pp. 263–287). Baltimore: Paul H. Brookes Publishing Co.

Jacobs, M.K., & Goodman, G. (1989). Psychology and self-help groups: Predictions on a partnership. *American Psychologist, 44*(3), 536–545.

Jacobson, N.S., & Gurman, A.S. (1986). *Clinical handbook of marital therapy.* New York: Guilford Publications.

Jones, O.H. (1980). Prelinguistic communication skills in Down syndrome and normal infants. In T. Field, S. Goldberg, D. Stern, & A. Sostek (Eds.), *High risk infants and children: Adult and peer interactions* (pp. 205–225). New York: Academic Press.

Joyce, K., Singer, M., & Isralowitz, R. (1983). Impact of respite care on parents' perceptions of quality of life. *Mental Retardation, 21,* 153–156.

Kagan, J. (1989, June/July). Investment in children. *Word from Washington.* (Available from United Cerebral Palsy Associations, 1522 K Street, Suite 112, Washington, DC 20205).

Kahn, A.J., & Kamerman, S.B. (1983). *Income transfers for families with children: An eight country study.* Philadelphia: Temple University Press.

Kanner, A., Coyne, J., Schaefer, C., & Lazarus, R. (1981). Comparison of two modes of stress measurement: Daily hassles and uplifts versus major life events. *Journal of Behavioral Medicine, 4,* 1–39.

Karoly, P., & Kanfer, F.H. (1982). *Self-management and behavior change.* Elmsford, NY: Pergamon Press.

Kazak, A.E., & Marvin, R.S. (1984). Differences, difficulties and adaptation: Stress and social networks in families with a handicapped child. *Family Relations, 33,* 67–77.

Kitchen, W.H., Rickards, A.L., Ryan, M.M., Ford, G.W., Lissenden, J.V., & Boyle, L.W. (1986). Improved outcome at two years of very low–birthweight infants: Fact or artifact? *Developmental Medicine and Child Neurology, 28,* 479–588.

Kitchen, W.H., Ryan, M.M., Rickards, R.A., Astbury, J., Ford, G., Lissenden, J.V., Keith, C.G., & Keir, E.H. (1982). Changing outcome over 13 years of very low birthweight infants. *Seminars in Perinatology, 6,* 373–389.

Knoll, J., & Bedford, S. (1989, May/June). Respite services: A national survey of parents' experience. *Exceptional Parent,* pp. 34–37.

Knoll, J., Covert, S., Osuch, R., O'Connor, S., & Blaney, B. (1990). *Family support services in the United States: An end of decade status report.* Cambridge, MA: Human Services Research Institute.

Kogan, K.L., & Tyler, N. (1973). Mother-child interaction in young physically handicapped children. *American Journal of Mental Deficiency, 77,* 492–497.

Kogan, K.L., Tyler, N., & Turner, P. (1974). The process of interpersonal adaptation between mothers and their cerebral palsied children. *Developmental Medicine and Child Neurology, 16,* 518–527.

Lazarus, R.S., & Folkman, S. (1984). *Stress, appraisal, and coping*. New York: Springer.

Lehman, D.R., Ellard, J.H., & Wortman, C.B. (1986). Social support for the bereaved: Recipients' and providers' perspectives on what is helpful. *Journal of Consulting and Clinical Psychology, 54*, 438–446.

Levine, M. (1988). An analysis of mutual assistance. *American Journal of Community Psychology, 16*(2), 167–188.

Lichtenstein, J. (1989). *Behavioral marital therapy for parents of children with severe handicaps*. Unpublished doctoral dissertation, University of Oregon, Eugene.

Livingston, M.G., & Brooks, D.N. (1988). The burden on families of the brain injured: A review. *Journal of Head Trauma Rehabilitation, 3*(4), 6–15.

Lobato, D., Faust, D., & Spirito, A. (1988). Examining the effects of chronic disease and disability on children's sibling relationships. *Journal of Pediatric Psychology, 13*(3), 389–407.

Lubchenco, L.O., Butterfield, L.J., Delaney-Black, V., Goldson, E., Koops, B.L., & Lazotte, D.C. (1989, March). Outcome of very-low-birth-weight infants: Does antepartum versus neonatal referral have a better impact on mortality, morbidity, or long-term outcome? *American Journal of Obstetrics and Gynecology, 160*, 539–545.

Lynch, E.C., & Stalock, N.H. (1988). Parental perceptions of physicians' communication in the informing process. *Mental Retardation, 26*, 77–81.

Mahoney, G., & Powell, A. (1988). Modifying parent-child interaction: Enhancing the development of handicapped children. *Journal of Special Education, 22*, 82–96.

Markman, H.J. (1979). Application of a behavioral model of marriage in predicting relationship satisfaction of couples planning marriage. *Journal of Consulting and Clinical Psychology, 47*, 743–749.

Markman, H.J. (1981). The prediction of marital distress: A five-year follow-up. *Journal of Consulting and Clinical Psychology, 49*, 760–762.

Matheny, K.B., Aycock, D.W., Pugh, J.L., Curlette, W.L., & Cannella, K.A.S. (1986). Stress coping: A qualitative and quantitative synthesis with implications for treatment: *Counseling Psychologist, 14*, 499–549.

Maton, K.I. (1988). Social support, organizational characteristics, psychological well-being, and group appraisal in three self-help group populations. *American Journal of Community Psychology, 16*, 53–77.

McCubbin, H.I., McCubbin, M.A., Patterson, J.M., Cauble, A.E., Wilson, L.R., & Warwick, W. (1983). CHIP—Coping health inventory for parents: An assessment of parental coping patterns in the care of the chronically ill child. *Journal of Marriage and the Family, 45*(2), 359–370.

McCubbin, H.I., & Patterson, J. (1983). The family stress process: The double ABCX model of adjustment and adaptation. *Marriage and Family Review, 6*, 7–37.

Menolascino, F.J., & Coleman, R. (1980). The Pilot Parent Program: Helping handicapped children through their parents. *Child Psychiatry and Human Development, 11*, 41–48.

Mills, C.W. (1959). *The sociological imagination*. New York: Oxford University Press.

Moeller, C.M. (1986). The effect of professionals on the family of a handicapped child. In R.R. Fewell & P.F. Vadasy (Eds.), *Families of handicapped children: Needs and supports across the life span* (pp. 149–166). Baltimore: Paul H. Brookes Publishing Co.

Montgomery, R.J.V., Gonyea, J.G., & Hooyman, N.R. (1985). Caregiving and the experience of subjective and objective burden. *Family Relations, 34*, 19–26.

Moos, R.H., & Moos, B. (1981). *Family Environment Scale manual*. Palo Alto, CA: Consulting Psychologists Press.

Morgan, D.L. (1989). Adjusting to widowhood: Do social networks really make it easier? *The Gerontologist, 29*, 101–107.

Moroney, R.M. (1986). *Shared responsibility: Families and social policy*. New York: Aldine.

Nixon, C. (1989). *The treatment of self-blaming attributions and guilt feelings in parents of developmentally disabled children*. Unpublished doctoral dissertation, University of Oregon, Eugene.

Notarius, C.I., Benson, P.R., & Sloane, D. (1989). Exploring the interface between perception and behavior: An analysis of marital interaction in distressed and nondistressed couples. *Behavioral Assessment, 11*, 39–64.

Olshansky, S. (1970). Chronic sorrow: A response to having a mentally defective child. In R.L. Noland (Ed.), *Counseling parents of the mentally retarded: A sourcebook* (pp. 49–54). Springfield, IL: Charles C Thomas.

Olson, D.H., McCubbin, H.I., Barnes, H., Larsen, A., Muxen, M., & Wilson, M. (1983). *Families: What makes them work*. Beverly Hills: Sage Publications.

Orford, J. (Ed.). (1987). *Treating the disorder, treating the family*. Baltimore: Johns Hopkins University Press.

Pahl, J., & Quine, L. (1987). Families with mentally handicapped children. In J. Orford (Ed.), *Treating the disorder, treating the family* (pp. 39–61). Baltimore: Johns Hopkins University Press.

Parrott, M.E., & Herman, S.E. (1988). *Family support: Subcity program report, FY 1986–87*. Lansing: Michigan Department of Mental Health.

Pearlin, L.T., & Schooler, C. (1978). The structure of coping. *Journal of Health and Social Behavior, 19*, 2–21.

Pearson, J., Verma, S., & Nellet, C. (1988). Elderly

psychiatric patient status and caregiver perceptions as predictors of caregiver burden. *The Gerontological Society of America*, *28*(1), 79–83.

Pecora, P.J., Delewski, C.H., Booth, C., Haapala, D., & Kinney, J. (1985). Home-based, family-centered services: The impact of training on worker attitudes. *Child Welfare League of America*, *64*(5), 529–539.

Poulshock, S.W., & Deimling, G.T. (1984). Families caring for elders in residence: Issues in the measurement of burden. *Journal of Gerontology*, *39*(2), 230–239.

Powers, L. (1989). *Cognitive coping with grief*. Unpublished doctoral dissertation, University of Oregon, Eugene.

Pratt, C.C., Schmall, V.L., Wright, S., & Cleland, M. (1985). Burden and coping strategies of caregivers to Alzheimer's patients. *Family Relations*, *34*, 27–33.

Radloff, L. (1977). The CES-D Scale: A self-report depression scale for research in the general population. *Applied Psychological Measurement*, *1*, 385–401.

Radloff, L.S., & Cox, S. (1981). Sex differences in depression in relation to learned susceptibility. In S. Cox (Ed.), *Female psychology: The emerging self* (2nd ed., pp. 334–350). New York: St. Martin's Press.

Rahe, R.H., & Arthur, R.J. (1978). Life change and illness studies: Past history and future directions. *Journal of Human Stress*, *4*(1), 3–15.

Reiss, D., & Oliveri, M.E. (1983). Family stress as community frame. *Marriage and Family Review*, *6*(1/2), 61–83.

Rimmerman, A. (1989). Provision of respite care for children with developmental disabilities: Changes in maternal coping and stress over time. *Mental Retardation*, *27*, 99–103.

Roach, D.C. (1984). Psychosocial stress in parents of normal, physically handicapped and hyperactive children. *Dissertation Abstracts International*, *46*, 1699B. (University Microfilms No. DER85-10741)

Rodgers, H.R. (1982). *The cost of human neglect*. New York: M.E. Sharpe.

Rosenthal, M., & Young, T. (1988). Effective family intervention after traumatic brain injury: Theory and practice. *Journal of Head Trauma Rehabilitation*, *3*(4), 42–50.

Rule, S., Stowitschek, J.J., Innocenti, M., Striefel, S., Killoran, J., & Swezey, K. (1987). The social integration program: An analysis of the effects of mainstreaming handicapped children into day care centers. *Education and Treatment of Children*, *10*(2), 175–192.

Salisbury, C.L. (1986). Parenthood and the need for respite. In C.L. Salisbury & J. Intagliata (Eds.), *Respite care: Support for persons with developmental disabilities and their families* (pp. 3–28). Baltimore: Paul H. Brookes Publishing Co.

Salisbury, C.L. (1987). Stressors of parents with young handicapped and nonhandicapped children. *Journal of the Division for Early Childhood 11*(2), 154–160.

Salisbury, C.L., & Intagliata, J. (Eds.). (1986). *Respite care: Support for persons with developmental disabilities and their families*. Baltimore: Paul H. Brookes Publishing Co.

Schwartz, I.S., Anderson, S.R., & Halle, J.W. (1989). Training teachers to use naturalistic time delay: Effects on teacher behavior and on the language use of students. *Journal of The Association for Persons with Severe Handicaps*, *14*, 48–57.

Simons, R. (1987). *After the tears: Parents talk about raising a child with a disability*. San Diego: Harcourt Brace Jovanovich.

Singer, G.H.S., Hawkins, N., Walker, B., Irvine, B., & Peters, M. (in preparation). *Advocacy skills for parents of children with handicaps*. Eugene: Oregon Research Institute.

Singer, G.H.S., & Irvin, L.K. (1989a). Family caregiving, stress and support. In G.H.S. Singer & L.K. Irvin (Eds.), *Support for caregiving families: Enabling positive adaptation to disability* (pp. 3–25).

Singer, G.H.S., & Irvin, L.K. (1989b). *Support for caregiving families: Enabling positive adaptation to disability*. Baltimore: Paul H. Brookes Publishing Co.

Singer, G.H.S., Irvin, L.K., & Hawkins, N.J. (1988). Stress management training for parents of severely handicapped children. *Mental Retardation*, *26*, 269–277.

Singer, G.H.S., Irvin, L.K., Irvine, A.B. (in preparation). *The unit of analysis in stress research with parents of handicapped children*. Eugene: Oregon Research Institute.

Singer, G.H.S., Irvin, L.K., Irvine, A.B., Cooley, E.C., Nixon, C., Hawkins, N., & Hegrenes, J. (in preparation). *Replication of a family support model for parents of severely handicapped children*. Eugene: Oregon Research Institute.

Singer, G.H.S., Irvin, L.K., Irvine, A.B., Hawkins, N., & Cooley, E.C. (1989). Evaluation of community-based support services for families of persons with developmental disabilities. *Journal of The Association for Persons with Severe Handicaps*, *14*, 312–323.

Singer, G.H.S., Irvin, L.K., & Yovanoff, P. (in preparation). *Caregiver stress: A meta analysis*. Eugene: Oregon Research Institute.

Singer, G.H.S., Irvine, A.B., & Irvin, L.K. (1989). Expanding the focus of behavioral parent training: A contextual approach. In G.H.S. Singer & L.K. Irvin (Eds.), *Support for caregiving families: Enabling positive adaptation to disability* (pp. 85–102). Baltimore: Paul H. Brookes Publishing Co.

Slater, M.A., Bates, M., & Eicher, L. (1986). Survey: Statewide family support programs. *Applied Research in Mental Retardation*, *7*, 241–257.

Slater, M.A., & Wikler, L. (1984). Normalized family resources for families with a developmentally disabled child. *Social Work, 31,* 385–390.

Stagg, V., & Catron, T. (1986). Networks of social supports for parents of handicapped children. In R.R. Fewell & P.F. Vadasy (Eds.), *Families of handicapped children: Needs and supports across the life span* (pp. 279–295). Austin, TX: PRO-ED.

Sultz, H., Schlesinger, E., Mosher, W., & Feldman, J. (1972). *Long-term childhood illness.* Pittsburgh, PA: University of Pittsburgh.

Summers, J.A., Behr, S.K., & Turnbull, A.P. (1989). Positive adaptations and coping strengths of families who have children with disabilities. In G.H.S. Singer & L.K. Irvin (Eds.), *Support for caregiving families: Enabling positive adaptation to disability* (pp. 27–40). Baltimore: Paul H. Brookes Publishing Co.

Tausig, M. (1985). Factors in family decision-making about placement for developmentally disabled individuals. *American Journal of Mental Deficiency, 89,* 352–361.

Taylor, S.E. (1983). Adjustment to threatening events: A theory of cognitive adaptation. *American Psychologist, 38,* 1161–1173.

Taylor, S.J., Knoll, J.A., Lehr, S., & Walker, P.M. (1989). Families for all children: Value-based services for children with disabilities and their families. In G.H.S. Singer & L.K. Irvin (Eds.), *Support for caregiving families: Enabling positive adapation to disability* (pp. 41–53). Baltimore: Paul H. Brookes Publishing Co.

Tew, B.J., Payne, E.H., & Lawrence, K.M. (1974). Must a family with a handicapped child be a handicapped family? *Developmental Medicine and Child Neurology, 16*(Suppl. 32), 95–98.

Thoits, P.A. (1986). Social support as coping assistance. *Journal of Consulting and Clinical Psychology, 54,* 416–423.

Todis, B., & Singer, G.H.S. (in press). Stress and coping in multiple adoptive families. *Journal of The Association for Persons with Severe Handicaps.*

Toseland, R.W., & Rossiter, C.M. (1989). Group interventions to support family caregivers: A review and analysis. *The Gerontologist, 29*(4), 438–448.

Trivette, C.M. (1982). *The study of role division and stress in families with handicapped children.* Unpublished master's thesis, Appalachian State University, Boone, NC.

Trivette, C.M., & Dunst, C.J. (in preparation). *Notions of constitutional support and its relationship to maternal well-being.*

Turnbull, A.P., Blue-Banning, M., Behr, S., & Kerns, G. (1986). Family research and intervention: A value and ethical examination. In P.R. Dokecki & R.M. Zaner (Eds.), *Ethics of dealing with persons with severe handicaps* (pp. 119–140). Baltimore: Paul H. Brookes Publishing Co.

Turnbull, A.P., & Turnbull, H.R. (1986). *Families, professionals, and exceptionality: A special partnership.* Columbus, OH: Charles E. Merrill.

Turnbull, H.R., Guess, D. & Turnbull, A.P. (1988). Vox Populi and Baby Doe. *Mental Retardation, 26,* 127–132.

Turnbull, H.R., Turnbull, A.P., Bronicki, G.J., Summers, J.A., & Roeder-Gordon, C. (1989). *Disability and the family: A guide to decisions for adulthood.* Baltimore: Paul H. Brookes Publishing Co.

U.S. Department of Commerce. (1987). *Statistical abstract of the United States, 1987.* Washington, DC: Bureau of the Census.

Vadasy, P.F. (1986). Single mothers: A social phenomenon and population in need. In R.R. Fewell & P.F. Vadasy (Eds.), *Families of handicapped children: Needs and supports across the life span* (pp. 221–249). Austin, TX: PRO-ED.

Venters, M. (1981). Familial coping with chronic illness: The case of cystic fibrosis. *Social Science and Medicine, 154,* 289–297.

Versluys, H.P. (1986). Thuishulpcentrale: A Dutch model for practical family assistance. *Rehabilitation Literature, 47*(3–4), 50–59.

Vincent, L.J., & Salisbury, C.L. (1988). Changing economic and social influences on family involvement. *Topics in Early Childhood Special Education, 8*(1), 48–59.

Vitaliano, P.P., Maiuro, R.D., Russo, J., & Becker, J. (1987). Raw versus relative scores in the assessment of coping strategies. *Journal of Behavioral Medicine, 10,* 1–18.

Wahler, R.G. (1988). Skill deficits and uncertainty: An interbehavioral view on the parenting problems of multi-stressed mothers. In R.DeV. Peters & R.J. McMahon (eds.), *Social learning and systems approaches to marriage and the family* (pp. 45–71). New York: Brunner/Mazel.

Walker, B. (1989). Strategies for improving parent-professional cooperation. In G.H.S. Singer & L.K. Irvin (Eds.), *Support for caregiving families: Enabling positive adaptation to disability* (pp. 103–119). Baltimore: Paul H. Brookes Publishing Co.

Waring, M. (1988). *If women counted: A new feminist economics.* San Francisco: Harper & Row.

Warren, S.F., & Kaiser, A.P. (1986). Incidental language teaching: A critical review. *Journal of Speech and Hearing Disorders, 51,* 291–299.

Weiss, R.S. (Ed.). (1973). *Loneliness: The experience of emotional and social isolation.* Cambridge, MA: MIT Press.

Werner, E.E. (1989, April). Children of the garden island. *Scientific American,* pp. 106–111.

Wikler, L.M. (1979, May). *Single parents of mentally retarded children: A neglected population.* Paper presented at the annual conference of the American Association on Mental Deficiency, Miami, FL.

Wikler, L.M. (1986a). Family stress theory and research on families of children with mental retardation. In J.J. Gallagher & P.M. Vietze (Eds.), *Families of handicapped persons* (pp. 167–195). Baltimore: Paul H. Brookes Publishing Co.

Wikler, L.M. (1986b). Periodic stresses of families of

older mentally retarded children: An exploratory study. *American Journal of Mental Deficiency*, *90*, 703–706.

Wilkin, D. (1979). *Caring for the mentally handicapped child*. London: Croom Helm.

Winogrond, I.R., Fisk, A.A., Kirsling, R.A., & Keye, B. (1987). The relationship of caregiver burden and morale to Alzheimer's disease patient function in a therapeutic setting. *The Gerontological Society of America*, *27*(3), 336–339.

Wright, J.S., Granger, R.D., & Sameroff, A.J. (1984). Parental acceptance and developmental handicap. In J. Blacher (Ed.), *Severely handicapped young children and their families: Research in review* (pp. 51–90). Orlando, FL: Academic Press.

Zarit, S.H., Reever, K.E., & Bach-Peterson, J. (1980). Relatives of the impaired elderly: Correlates of feelings of burden. *The Gerontologist*, *20*(6), 649–655.

Zarit, S.H., Todd, P.A., & Zarit, J.M. (1986). Subjective burden of husbands and wives as caregivers: A longitudinal study. *Journal of The Gerontological Society of America*, *26*, 260–266.

CHAPTER 17

Personnel Preparation
Directions for the Next Decade

DIANE BAUMGART
University of Idaho, Moscow, Idaho

DIANNE L. FERGUSON
University of Oregon, Eugene, Oregon

Over the last dozen or so years of mandated education for students with severe handicaps, teachers have had to respond to rapid change. Best practices in 1976, or even in 1980, have been greatly expanded and in some cases replaced. These quick changes demand that teachers both understand and explore their constantly evolving roles while trying to adapt their daily teaching to reflect new research and innovation. Initially, we needed teachers who could demonstrate and document to the educational community that students previously thought "unteachable" could indeed learn. Now we need teachers who can create maximally effective educational environments and experiences for a very heterogeneous and programmatically complex group of students. Those with the most direct experience in this the 1990s' decade of change, the teachers "in the field," face the greatest challenge. Many of the details of emerging best practices will require skills and philosophical orientations that are not readily implemented without training as well as support from within the school systems. Inservice training for many of these veteran teachers must not just update, but also reorient teachers to new roles.

If the plight of teachers "in the field" seems difficult to resolve, one might expect to find hope in the new generation of teachers who leave their preservice preparation programs armed with the ideological foundations and technical details of best practices. Even if the field continues to grow rapidly, surely these newest educators will be prepared to respond, since their training has the benefit of the 1980s as a decade of experience with change and innovation that the vanguard could not have anticipated. However, the expectation that the field's newest teachers arrive better equipped either to provide exemplary programming for students with severe handicaps or to respond to new information and developments in a timely way may be fragile indeed. If, as Steven Taylor (1988) has argued, the field in general seems "caught in the continuum," the preparation of teachers for the field may well be "trapped in tradition." That is, unless the preconceived notions of where students must be educated are reevaluated, the practices of the past will limit future practices. This chapter investigates the relationship between emerging best educational practices for students with severe disabilities and the capacity of preservice training programs to prepare teachers to implement these practices. First, we briefly review critical features of the process and status of reform in schooling services for students with severe disabilities. Second, we review literature that supports and challenges the key tenets of current best practices. Finally, we detail the implications of these reforms for preservice person-

Preparation of this chapter was supported, in part, by U.S. Department of Education Grant #G008630162 and #G008730222-88 to the University of Idaho and Grant #G008635093-01 to the University of Oregon, Specialized Training Program. However, the opinions expressed herein do not necessarily reflect the position or policy of the U.S. Department of Education and no official endorsement should be inferred.

nel preparation together with some recommendations for successful responses by academic educators.

FRAMEWORK FOR REFORM

In the preface of the new edition of *Teacher Preparation: An Unstudied Problem in Education,* S. Sarason, Davidson, and Blatt (1986) review the dramatic reforms that occurred in all of education during the 1960s only to conclude that "during this same period, the preparation of teachers remained unchanged" (p. xviii). This "disjointedness between the substance of teacher training programs and the realities of schools" (S. Sarason et al., 1986, p. xviii) is certainly not new. Some current reform recommendations (e.g., Carnegie Commission, 1986; Holmes Group, 1986) argue for extended teacher preparation programs and increased quality standards, usually documented by national test scores and regulated with new certification approaches that reflect status of knowledge and experience (novice and master teachers) rather than differences in content (regular or special certification). At the same time, others criticize these reform recommendations as simplistic and unlikely to succeed in having an impact on schooling, generally because they are not adequately sensitive to a complexity of historical and cultural forces that affect schools and teachers (see, for example, Aronowitz & Giroux, 1985; Bastian, Fruchter, Gitell, Greer, & Haskins, 1985; Feinberg, 1985; S.B. Sarason, 1983; Tom, 1987). This section provides a brief review of some of the schooling forces that both generated and may well limit current best-practices reforms for students with severe handicaps.

Impact of Law and Policy

The Education for All Handicapped Children Act (PL 94-142) certainly attempted widespread, emancipatory reform in both special and regular education, possessing the potential to challenge the fundamental structures and philosophy of public schooling. The 1974 vision, both implicitly and explicitly, was one of completeness and inclusion. Public education should include and "work" for all of America's schoolchildren. Yet the process of reform implementation

did not abolish inequality and these issues remain paramount today (Office of Special Education and Rehabilitative Services, 1983, 1987; Singer & Butler, 1987). At the same time, current reform analysts in general education charge 1960 reform efforts with the current demise of excellence (National Commission on Excellence in Education, 1983; Twentieth Century Fund Task Force on Federal Elementary and Secondary Education Policy [Twentieth Century Fund], 1983). This indictment of the reform efforts generally takes one of two forms. One position argues that earlier reforms resulted in such substantial changes for such an increased array of students that available resources are now spread too thin, watering down excellence for everyone. Alternatively, some argue that the reforms failed to make any substantive difference for those students they were designed to serve and thus can be safely discontinued in the face of competing demands (Bastian et al., 1985; Bermon, 1985).

There is, of course, some truth to these interpretations. Active efforts to eliminate or at least significantly reduce inequalities in school have not worked. One explanation is that the past efforts have put their emphasis on access to equal opportunities to learn rather than on equal outcomes. Desirable outcomes are defined by successful members of the system and are correlated with membership in this same system. Instances of this correlation between membership and outcomes abound in many areas of education (see, for example, Auerback, 1976, and Brandt, 1989, for a discussion on educational membership and outcomes in the legal profession). As the heterogeneity of students increased with compulsory schooling, students who were different (race, language, citizenship) were provided opportunities to learn, but not with those already in the system. These students were afforded equal opportunities to learn via separate classes, but not equal outcomes via instruction within existing classes. Thus vocational rather than academic preparation became an educational track in the schools. This differentiated educational content has become not a critique of the school's products, but a mandate of educational tracks to be provided.

Similarly, the earliest examples of special education—the "ungraded classes"—collected a variety of students judged not to "fit" the curricular content of the regular class (Ferguson, 1987). What began as a parallel track soon developed into a parallel system, attached to but not integrally entwined with regular education. The reforms of the 1960s reinforced, rather than diminished, the structural segregation of regular and special education. Disproportionate numbers of poor and minority students in the schools' lowest tracks (similar to the disproportionate numbers of poor, non-English speaking immigrant children a half century earlier) this time were said to be in need of a different educational approach and setting, for environmental instead of biological reasons. This time, cultural disadvantage was cited to explain the inequality, but the solution did not differ substantially. Renewed demands for equalized opportunities resulted in a variety of federally supported compensatory programs designed to overcome cultural and racial barriers by helping students to "catch up" or receive a "head start." Not only did special programs remain "add-ons" to the regular system, the fundamental explanation for inequality continued to reside within the student. Thus in the 1960s and 1970s, when reform efforts directly focused on the full range of students with disabilities, the effort to equalize opportunity rather than outcome prevailed. What change did occur was limited to what could be gained within a segregated, add-on system. The best practices reforms of the 1980s are now poised either to recapitulate these earlier patterns or to end them with finality (Lilly, 1989).

Reform for Students with Severe Disabilities

Part of the uniqueness of students with severe disabilities in public schooling lies in the fundamental challenge they present to the meaning of education—a challenge that is only now being resolved in the articulation of exemplary programming practices. Special education's traditional strategy of accommodating "different" students in appropriate tracks falters in the face of overwhelming physiology. On the one hand, it has been more difficult to attribute lack of achievement to lack of interest, motivation, or application if a student clearly has limbs that do not move properly or senses that fail to register

stimuli. On the other, it has been much easier to state explicitly what is only an implicit assumption about students with mild handicaps: This assumption is that students with severe handicaps are unable to learn.

In fact, this latter assumption has historically served as the school's explanation for the almost total exclusion of students with severe handicaps until the late 1970s. With inclusion, however, came the need to clearly articulate answers to all the old questions that had served as the rationale for exclusion: What could education possibly mean for such students? What would be the purpose of schooling; what could be taught; for what future end? The answers generated since 1975 have, like the reform initiatives, sought to find a balance between technical/clinical and social/ideological forces.

Encouraged by the success of the parent-led movement of the 1950s, which achieved a reluctant, but real, inclusion for students with moderate handicaps, the reforms of the 1960s and 1970s depended more on the tools and rhetoric of advocacy, empowerment, and rights than on the cool clinical evidence of learning potential or success. In fact, initial attempts to describe the purposes and content of education for students with severe disabilities more often spoke to redressing the wrongs of exclusion, institutionalization, discrimination, and abuse (Anderson & Greer, 1976; Perske & Smith, 1977; Sontag, 1977; Thomas, 1976) than to any clear articulation of students' future lives or strategies for increasing students' abilities and competence.

The clinical counterweight for the social rights half of the reform agenda gradually emerged as the adoption of a behavioral approach to instructional technology for learners with severe cognitive impairments. The principles of operant learning, underpinned with techniques of shaping, reinforcement, and task analysis, led behavioral psychologists and special educators alike to conclude that careful analysis and instruction could result in skill acquisition regardless of the severity of a student's cognitive disability (Bijou, 1980; Sailor & Guess, 1983; Wilcox & Bellamy, 1982).

Having demonstrated the clinical soundness of "education" in terms of increasing the behavioral repertoire of students with severe handicaps, there remained a need to seek a more secure balance between the technically driven "how to teach" and the socially grounded "what to teach." The field responded to this need to link values and technology in the practice arenas of an applied science with the "functional approach." "Ultimate" and next environments, ecologically inspired categories of curricular content, and a commitment to teaching skills that are functional and would immediately accomplish improvement in a student's life, dominated the professional reform rhetoric of the early 1980s (Baumgart, Brown, et al., 1982; L. Brown, Branston-McLean, et al., 1979; L. Brown, Nietupski, & Hamre-Nietupski, 1976).

New Reform Debates

As an applied social science, education has always struggled to verify its scientific status through rigorous use of scientific methods for developing and testing theory. The comfortableness and appropriateness of a positivist approach to knowledge generation integrated well with special education's dominant behavioral perspective, especially as articulated and refined for understanding the learning of students with severe disabilities. In fact, much of the research supporting current best practices has focused on describing and verifying the details of a complex instructional technology. However, clinical understanding and competence, as defined by a behavioral approach to learning, is only one half of the educational reform initiative on behalf of students with severe disabilities. From the beginning, the reform webbed the need for a firm technical foundation in behavioral technology and engineering with an equally powerful ideological commitment to social justice and participation. It is this second strand, grounded in social and political perspective, that now presents fundamental challenges to special education's understanding of research and evidence. Some authors point out that there is an increasing accumulation of data on the details of how to build functional skill competence for students with severe handicaps, but there are few data available to support the value-based features and outcomes advanced as descriptive of exemplary programming (Wilcox & Bellamy, 1987b). At

the same time, other authors challenge the need or appropriateness of researching some of these value-based features at all, or of using the same research tools as special education has traditionally depended upon (Biklen, 1985; Ferguson, Ferguson, & Bogdan, 1987; S. Stainback & Stainback, 1984): A logic of social justice, civil rights, and social access does not depend on a test of scientific evidence for its power.

Our field has not yet found the new identity that will adequately meld our scientific ability with its social conscience. As a result, we risk at least imbalance: emphasizing program features over instructional competence, as described in a critique by Stoddard (1987). As a consequence, our program may meet all the "checklist" features of a best practice, such as being integrated and data based, but may still fail to teach students anything they can actually use in their lives outside of school. At worst we risk framing our debates and choosing our professional alliances so as to split rather than to integrate the personality of the field. If in the end we fail to find our identity, we risk losing not only the reform impact for students with severe disabilities, but also an opportunity to finally change the structural relationships throughout education (Biklen, Ferguson, & Ford, 1989). In the sections that follow we review the status of best-practices research in terms of this need for coherence. In this way, potential strategies for not recapitulating the errors of special education's past, or perpetuating the conflicts of its present with the newest members of the professional club, can be more succinctly drawn.

BEST PRACTICES: REVIEW OF RESEARCH

As noted above, once applied behavioral analysis succeeded in demonstrating that students with severe cognitive impairments could indeed learn, the best-practices focus shifted to making sure that teachers choose to teach those skills their students need to be active in current and future environments. The literature and research of a decade ago focused primarily on defining this "functional approach" to curriculum and instruction. One category of articles and chapters took the form of position papers that detailed and even operationalized the principles of functionality (e.g., L. Brown, Branston, et al., 1979; L. Brown et al., 1976; Thomas, 1976; Vincent et al., 1980). Once the basic approach had been articulated, a wealth of supporting notions followed, including: teaching skill clusters that cross traditional content domains (Guess & Helmstetter, 1986; Sailor & Guess, 1983), teaching chronologically age-appropriate skills (L. Brown et al., 1980), use of natural and community environments as instructional contexts (Hamre-Nietupski, Nietupski, Bates, & Maurer, 1982; Horner, McDonnell, & Bellamy, 1986; Sailor et al., 1986), and the unique demands of programs for secondary students (Wilcox & Bellamy, 1982).

These largely value-driven descriptions of programming features were supported by another large body of literature that attempted to provide the pragmatic detail necessary to translate principles into practice. Sometimes authors tried to capture these details in a single textbook (Falvey, 1985; Sailor & Guess, 1983; Snell, 1978, 1983, 1986), but more often a series of edited texts provided both narrowly defined interpretations of the most recent best practices and ongoing reports of the status of the reform agenda. For example, the third volume of *Teaching the Severely Handicapped* (N. G. Haring & Bricker, 1978) reported on federal involvement (Sontag & Smith, 1978), the status of "least restrictive educational opportunity" (Kenowitz, Zweibel, & Edgar, 1978), and advice for personnel preparation (Iacino & Bricker, 1978), as well as details on developing instructional programs (Williams & York, 1978) and instructions on completing job-skill inventories (Belmore & Brown, 1978). Similarly, an edited volume only 2 years later by Sailor, Wilcox, and Brown (1980) included detailed information on assessment (W. Bricker & Campbell, 1980), instruction and documentation (L. Brown et al., 1980; N. G. Haring, Liberty, & White, 1980), and program development (Gaylord-Ross, 1980; Guess, 1980). Gradually the list of best-practices features became refined. Table 17.1 represents our summary of the literature and reveals the breadth with which the issue has been addressed. It is clearly not enough to offer the best possible curricula content, without also attending to the manner in which the content is delivered and the

Table 17.1. Best-practices features of programs for students with severe handicaps

CONTENT
  Activity based
  Community referenced
  Family referenced
  Comprehensive
PROCESSES
  Collaboration
  Fairness
  Substantive family involvement
  Negotiation
  Instructional effectiveness
OUTCOMES
  Community participation
  Supportive social networks
  Ordinariness and invisibility

eventual impact on student competence. Thus, our summary organizes best-practices features according to content, process, and outcome. Some of these best-practices features have a supportive research base (e.g., effective instruction), while others stand as ideological guideposts that require more adherence than evidence (e.g., substantive family involvement). The remainder of this section briefly discusses the literature that supports those best-practices features that represent the resolutions on the continuum of services of The Association for Persons with Severe Handicaps and those that have a substantial research base.

Best-Practices Content

When the field had firmly rejected a developmental rationale for determining the curricular content for students with severe disabilities, a new functional rationale replaced it. Students should learn those "things" that represented a contribution to and had immediate impact upon their daily lives (L. Brown, Branston-McLean, et al., 1979; Sailor & Guess, 1983; Sailor et al., 1980). Despite the appeal of this new functional rationale, much was left unclear and unexplained: What exactly constitutes a functional piece of curriculum content? What does the scope and sequence of such a curriculum look like? How will we know this new functional approach is working? Gradually, the answers to such questions produced the host of supporting notions captured in the best-practices content features of Table 17.1. Some of these best-practices features enjoy a stable and growing base of confirmatory research. For example, we now have formal demonstration of students' successful acquisition, generalization, and maintenance of such critical community participation activities as grocery and other forms of shopping (McDonnell, Horner, & Williams, 1984; Nietupski, Welch, & Wacker, 1983; Storey, Bates, & Hanson, 1984), home living skills (Browder, 1987), and community jobs (e.g., Certo, Mezzullo, & Hunter, 1985).

In the process of demonstrating such active, functional outcomes for students, other effective instructional practices emerged. A growing instructional technology advises practitioners in the systematic use of negative teaching examples, pretask rehearsal to improve task compliance, use of self-monitoring and management strategies to improve the quality of performance, and the optimum sequencing of varied learning examples (see, for a comprehensive summary of this research, Albin, Horner, Koegel, & Dunlap, 1987; Rudrud, Rice, Robertson, & Tolson, 1984; Rusch, Martin, & White, 1985). Moving well beyond a simple confirmation that all students can learn, this research base assures the field that students with severe handicaps can learn complex chains of behavior that demonstrably affect their lives both within and outside the school environment.

Together with such advances in instructional technology, a somewhat smaller body of research confirms and directs teachers in the details of program development and planning. The importance of active, if sometimes only partial, participation in activities of daily life began to override narrower interpretations of "functional skills" in favor of an activity-based approach to both curriculum development and daily programming (Baumgart et al., 1982; Sailor & Guess, 1983; Wilcox & Bellamy, 1982, 1987b). Arguing in favor of efficiency in the form of enhanced generalization, and improved opportunities for social contact, the activity-based approach rejects all planning logics that establish any form of prerequisite to actual performance and participation. This abandonment of "test"

results as sole determiners of curricula resulted in an emphasis on selecting those actual activities that are available in the community and enough a part of family lives to be frequently practiced, both within and outside school environments and teacher control.

This shift to an activity-based logic for selecting curricular content requires dependence on strategies for community- and family-referenced curricular content. Activities from among which teachers choose must emerge from students' own lives, not just the teachers' schedule or imagination. Use of environmental inventories (L. Brown, Branston-McLean, et al., 1979; Falvey, 1985) and activity lists or catalogues (Wilcox & Bellamy, 1987a) or individualized curriculum sequences (Bambara, Warren, & Komisar, 1988) provided teachers with the basic tools to move beyond classrooms and developmentally referenced curricular domains.

Much of the support for this articulation of a functional curricular approach emerges not so much from a clinical research base (except, of course, as it builds upon the research on generalization and maintenance) as from the ideological commitments to increase and enhance the visibility and participation of students in their local communities. What research is available is evaluative and socially validating in nature. Follow-up with teachers using such an approach with high school students (Wilcox & Bellamy, 1987b) documented high satisfaction of both teachers and parents. A specific investigation of the contributions parents made to individualized education program (IEP) content using an activity goal nomination and negotiation process (Twain, 1986) revealed that while teachers still selected more goals than parents, a third of all IEP goals were at least commonly nominated by both parents and teachers.

In summary, some of the best-practices indicators of curricular content are grounded in an increasingly solid base of efficacy research. Others depend for support on the values of those who seek to support the learning of students with severe disabilities. Subsequent research faces the challenge of not seeking to prove the obvious and accepted while still developing the details of an instructional technology that can produce durable changes in students' behavior in integrated community environments. A forum for this research should include investigations into the implementation of those practices and barriers that limit practice and expansion.

Best-Practices Processes

Once the scope of what to teach expanded beyond "table-top" performance tasks, the milieu of teaching practices altered and expanded as well. The best-practices processes listed in Table 17.1 are our compilation of the critical strategies that we find supported in the literature and that we expect to continue to have a critical role (see Meyer, Eichinger, & Park-Lee, 1987, and Putnam & Bruininks, 1986, for research studies that support these as best practices). Each of these process strategies is reviewed below and supporting research for some is summarized in Table 17.2. The research on barriers to their implementation is also reviewed and forms a framework for considering the changes for future personnel preparation programs, which we later discuss in the section entitled "Model for Personnel Preparation."

Team Collaboration

Investigations conducted by Inge and Snell (1985), Giangreco (1986), and Campbell (1987a, 1987b) typify the enhancement of learning for students possible with team collaboration. In each study, the collaboration by teachers and physical/occupational therapists resulted in faster acquisition of skills and a decrease in nonhabilitative handling and positioning. These studies epitomize the advantages that accrue with team collaboration, which include the synthesis of expertise for effective diagnosis, intervention, evaluation, and follow-along resulting in sharing and using information and skills to meet the needs of a student and his or her family. Although the advantages of team collaboration have been discussed for at least the past 20 years, frustration and challenges with its implementation have been noted.

The challenges and frustrations with implementing team collaboration are seen at both the service provider and preservice level of personnel preparation. A review of the literature in these practice arenas yields similar problems and difficulties. Courtnage and Smith-Davis (1987) reviewed training practices at 360 higher education institutions and reported that 48% offered no training in team collaboration. R.B. Johnson (1980) noted that those that attempted this process found considerable difficulties across faculty, students, and administrators with roles and responsibilities, philosophical and procedural disagreements, lack of ownership of the process, lack of administrative leadership and support, and ownership of courses within departments rather than to "core" team efforts. Researchers in the service provider arena have documented similar problems. Among the difficulties listed most frequently are: professional turfism; differences and confusion regarding responsibilities and philosophical orientation (including parental expertise); absence of administrative support, structure, or evaluation; and lack of training by university programs. Each of these problem areas has been mentioned as a key element in successful implementation of this best-practices process (Campbell, 1987a; Epanchin & Owen, 1982; Lindsey, O'Neal, Haas, & Tewley, 1983; Wolery & Dyk, 1985). What appears to exist is a process judged as valid and beneficial by parents and other professionals that is not extensively practiced in either the service provider or the preservice arena.

Substantive Family Involvement

Family involvement, as used here, refers to the support of the family or caregivers to ensure that a student has opportunities to practice or perform activities in nonschool hours that are taught or learned during school hours. For instance, if scheduling transportation to a community site or requesting a drink by pointing to a miniature cup is an activity requested by parents and performed during school hours, family involvement might consist of encouraging and/or requiring similar performance on the weekends. Substantive family involvement assumes that the activities incorporated into school instruction were based upon family input or requests, and when changes in support or routines are needed to perform these activities in nonschool hours the family will provide or arrange this support. To a

Table 17.2. Supporting research for best-practices processes

References	Descriptions
Team collaboration	
Inge & Snell (1985) Campbell & Stewart (1986) Giangreco (1986) Campbell (1987b)	Studies outlining the advantages of team collaboration in addressing students' service needs.
Courtnage & Smith-Davis (1987)	Reviews of training practices in 360 higher institutions with regard to team collaboration.
R.B. Johnson (1980)	Reviews of difficulties encountered by those who attempted team collaboration.
Epanchin & Owen (1982) Lindsey, O'Neal, Haas, and Tewey (1983) Wolery & Dyk (1985)	Key elements in successful implementation of team collaboration.
Hart (1977) Campbell (1987a)	Discussions of team collaboration through the multidisciplinary, interdisciplinary, and transdisciplinary models.
Hutchinson (1974) D. Bricker (1976) Beck (1977) Sternat, Messina, Nietupski, & Brown (1977) McCormick & Goldman (1979) Baine & Sobsey (1980) Lyon & Lyon (1980) Nietupski, Scheutz, & Ockwood (1980) Sears (1981) Gullo & Gullo (1984) Rainforth & York (1986) Siders, Riall, Bennett, & Judd (1987)	Authors from various fields of discipline cite the advantage of team collaboration.
Pugach & Allen-Meares (1985)	Failure to bring persons training for professional positions together at preservice levels hampers the implementation of team collaboration in the field.
Bennett (1982) Del Polito (1983) Smith-Davis, Burke, & Noel (1984)	Problems encountered by collaboration teams in regard to philosophy, responsibilities, priorities, support and eval-

(continued)

Table 17.2. *(continued)*

References	Descriptions
	uation, and professional turfism.
Family involvement	
Frith & Kelly (1981) Waldo et al. (1981) Wilcox & York (1982) Twain (1986)	Discussions of family involvement in the educational process.
Wilcox & Bellamy (1982) Baumgart, Filler, & Askvig (in press)	Descriptions of parental participation and satisfaction in the individualized education program (IEP) process.
Snell & Beckman (1984)	Examination of research on the use of family members as interventionists.
Negotiations	
Cohen (1974)	Description of two attempts to use a conflict-resolution approach in an academic setting.
Dostal (1982) Shaw & Emilsson (1984) Savage (1985) Gouran & Guadagnino (1988)	Discussions of best practices in communication, decision making, and negotiation.
Joyce & McNair (1979) B.D. Taylor (1986)	Studied educators to investigate decision-making, conflict-resolution, and negotiation skills.
Donohue (1976) Cross (1977) Dennison & Shenton (1987) Kersten (1987)	Theoretical frameworks or models for negotiation, decision making, or conflict resolution.
Adam (1970) Zartman (1977)	Evaluations of the strengths and weaknesses of particular approaches to conflict resolution or negotiation.
Love, Rozelle, & Druckman (1983) G.C. Whitney & Hunsaker (1983) Pederson (1985)	Descriptions of simulation activities for negotiation and the decision-making process.
Instructional effectiveness 1. *Data-based instruction*	
Lindsley (1964)	Description of precision teaching that emphasizes frequent measures of repetitive behaviors.

(continued)

Table 17.2. (continued)

References	Descriptions
Lynch, McGuigan, & Shoemaker (1977)	Description of systematic instruction with steps for planning, implementing, and using formative data.
Fredericks, Anderson, & Baldwin (1979) Deno & Mirkin (1980)	Advantages of direct and frequent performance measurements for instruction.
Gentry & Haring (1976)	Description of two levels of instructional measures: formative and summative.
Fuchs, Fuchs, & Warren (1982)	Disadvantages of the reliance on summative data to the exclusion of formative measurement.
Jenkins, Mayhall, Peschka, & Townsend (1974) Bohannon (1975) Lovitt (1977) Fredericks, Anderson, & Baldwin (1979) Fuchs, Fuchs, & Warren (1982) Skiba, Wesson, & Deno (1982) Fuchs, Deno, & Merkin (1983b) Idol-Maestas, Ritter, & Lloyd (1983)	Reports on the effectiveness of direct and frequent measures on student performance with the use of data-based programs.
Deno, Mirkin, & Chiang (1982) Wesson, Deno, & Mirkin (1982)	Comparisons of direct and frequent measures of student academic performance with results from standardized tests.

2. Data-based decisions

References	Descriptions
Kunzelman (1970) N.G. Haring & Brown (1976) Fuchs, Deno, & Mirkin (1983a)	Descriptions of approaches that outline frequent data collection with instructional decision making.
N.G. Haring, Liberty, & White (1980)	Use of performative data in making strategy decisions.
Wesson (1984)	Description of performative data as vital to gauging effective instruction.
Liberty (1975) Detwiler (1982)	Teachers who collect frequent data may make incorrect instructional decisions. Separation of data collection from instruction decisions is

Table 17.2. (continued)

References	Descriptions
	likely to lead to inappropriate instruction.
Liberty (1975) White & Liberty (1976)	Graphing and charting methods to assist in decision-making strategies.
Deno & Mirkin (1980) Fuchs, Deno, & Mirkin (1983b)	Completed a 5-year study, which concluded with a data-based program modification model.
Bohannon (1975)	Student performance improved with the use of some form of decision-making strategy.

3. Computer-managed instruction (CMI)

References	Descriptions
Baker (1978) Detwiler (1982) Hofmeister (1982, 1984a, 1984b)	Discussions of the applications, ranges, and limitations of computers in education.
Baker (1978) Behrmann (1984) Tinsley (1984)	Discussions of the use of CMI.
Hasselbring & Crossland (1981) Budoff & Hutten (1982) Wilson & Fox (1982)	Descriptions of the use of CMI as a prescriptive and diagnostic tool.
N.P. Brown (1982) Cruscial & Schimmer (1983) Fuchs, Deno, & Mirkin (1983a) Hasselbring & Hamlett (1983) Wesson (1984)	Developed data-based instructional programs to assist educators in student instruction.
N.G. Haring, Liberty, & White (1980) Detwiler (1982) Miller & Ragghianti (1984) Stowitschek & Stowitschek (1984)	Discussions of the potential time saved using CMI, as well as cost-effectiveness.
Stevens (1980) Wirth, Stile, & Cole (1983) Behrmann (1984)	Discussions of the need for more teacher training in using CMI and suggestions for possible training objectives.
Stallard (1982)	Suggestions that special educators involve themselves in CMI so they can have a part in its development.

(continued)

(continued)

Table 17.2. *(continued)*

References	Descriptions
4. Generalization	
N. Haring, Liberty, Billingsley, Butterfield, & White (1983)	Review of the literature on generalization practices.
Hopkins (1983)	
W. Stainback, Stainback, & Strathe (1983)	
Billingsley, Haring, Liberty, Weisenstein, & White (1984)	
Boer (1984)	
N. Haring (1984)	
N. Haring (1985, 1987)	
Bourbeau, Sowers, & Close (1986)	Examinations of the use of simulated training in producing generalized performance in the real environment.
Shafer & Inge (1986)	
Browder, Snell, & Wildonger (1988)	
Hupp & Mervis (1981)	Descriptions of the acquisition and generalization of skills for students with moderate to profound disabilities.
R. Whitney & Stiefel (1981)	
Nietupski, Welch, & Wacker (1983)	
S. Stainback, Stainback, Wehman, & Spangiers (1983)	
Storey, Bates, & Hanson (1984)	
Tateyama-Sniezek (1989)	Examination of the use of multiple exemplars as a practice to increase generalization.
Horner, Dunlap, & Koegel (1988)	Literature reviews and best-practices recommendations for decision rules and current advances in applied procedures for generalization.
Liberty, Haring, White, & Billingsley (1988)	
McDonnell, Horner, & Williams (1984)	Comparison of three strategies to teach generalized skills to severely handicapped students.

large extent the support for this process is value driven and is contained within the research cited in the section entitled "Best-Practices Content." Examples of some curricula that use this process are contained in Table 17.2.

Negotiation

The process of negotiation, balancing between what is ideal and what is practical or realistic in specific instances, is a critical dimension in the systems-change literature. However, it is only briefly discussed within the writings on teacher preparation. Falvey, Brown, Lyon, Baumgart, and Schroeder (1978) discuss the process of negotiation in reference to selecting content and goals for the instructional plans, and Baumgart and Van Walleghem (1986), Evans and Meyer (1985), and Elias and Clabby (1989) incorporate this process within their decision-making schema for staffing programs, implementing behavior change, and teaching social decision making. Support for this process is seen in the research on teacher burn-out and stress (Fimian, 1984). Problem solving, rectifying discrepancies between optimal and realistic practices, and maintaining a sense of professional worth are vital to the teacher and vital to the students she or he teaches. The relative newness of special education as it pertains to students with severe disabilities coupled with the continued rapid changes and expansions experienced in the past contribute to the need for negotiation skills to be within the repertoire of all educators.

Instructional Effectiveness

A number of instructional strategies have been shown to dramatically enhance the effectiveness of instruction. These include the use of direct and frequent data collection for formative evaluation of pupil learning, and the incorporation of generalization strategies into the long- and short-term goals and objectives on the IEP. The research studies that directly support the implementation of these processes are summarized in Table 17.2. The theoretical underpinnings of direct and frequent data collection were described by Lindsley (1964) under the title of "precision teaching" and were expanded to include strategies for use by various writers including Lynch, McGuigan, and Shoemaker (1977), Fredericks, Anderson, and Baldwin (1979), and Deno and Mirkin (1980).

The research data that support direct, frequent measurement and the corollary, data-based decisions, are extensive (Van Walleghem, 1986). These strategies result in improved student performance across the range of exceptionalities and skill areas. The decision-making implications of not collecting data are also of interest and were clearly shown in a study by Fuchs, Fuchs, and Warren (1982). In this study, teachers' ratings of how they thought students were performing were compared to ratings of student teachers, who followed typical classroom data collection procedures, and to ratings of experimenters, who collected direct performance measurements. The ratings of teachers and student teachers were significantly higher than the actual performance measurements indicated. The implications of using direct and frequent data collection to make data-based decisions seem clear: Student performance increases when the strategies are used and their absence may result in teachers' progressing to more difficult material despite lack of student mastery. Computer-assisted management (CMI) tools are available and successfully assist with these processes. Burello, Tracy, and Glassman (1983) reviewed the status of CMI in special education and Van Walleghem (1986) reviewed the literature and research on the efficiency of these tools. The benefits that can result from the use of these tools are thus well documented. The barriers appear to be lack of access to the technology, lack of time to learn its use, and an avoidance of the technology.

A second major area that affects instructional effectiveness is generalization and maintenance. This area, defined as widespread performance of skills across diverse stimulus conditions, responses, and times without comprehensive programming in each of these conditions (Stokes & Baer, 1977), has been extensively investigated. Initially, generalization was thought to be a skill deficit residing within persons with disabilities. After all, the tasks they were taught (touch the red one, touch the blue one) were simple, and yet a change in the stimulus often resulted in incorrect responses. The extensive investigations, many of which are summarized by Donnellan and Mirenda (1983), N. Haring (1984), Horner, Dunlap, and Koegel (1988), have found that successful strategies for generalization are both individually and environmentally centered. The previous positing of the deficit as residing within a student overlooked, once again, the confining influences of limited stimuli and expectations on instruction. A listing of tactics that have resulted in successful generalization and maintenance of learning were described by Stokes and Baer and

include: teaching useful and adaptive behaviors; modifying environments to reduce or enhance behaviors; using or recruiting naturally present reinforcers; using a range of stimulus and response exemplars; training loosely, using progressively less discriminative contingencies; reinforcing unprompted generalizations; using social and physical stimuli commonly present; and using self-mediated stimuli. These tactics for generalization present information that can greatly enhance the efforts of practitioners. By the same token, the assessment procedures for determining the most appropriate exemplars and tactic or combination of tactics is time consuming and at times clear only after a "try and see if it works" approach. Thus, although the practitioner has numerous tactics to consider, and numerous case histories and group studies to use in the decision-making process, careful deliberation will be required to select strategies and evaluate the result.

Best-Practices Outcomes

What do we want to see upon graduation? Essentially for youth with and without disabilities we want the same things: a job and a place to live in the community, a network of friends and acquaintances, options for recreation/leisure, and access to community services as needed. The content and process components of best practices have been designated to accomplish these results, listed as the outcomes of best practices: community participation, supportive social networks, and ordinariness and invisibility. Can these occur for youth with severe disabilities? The research on integration, mainstreaming, and social skills is reviewed here to respond in part to this query.

Community Participation

The first community in which a child resides is that of the family/caregivers, followed by that of schools. The school community, regardless of its nature (day care, preschool, elementary, middle or high school), has at its core a function to socialize. This function, often called "the hidden curriculum," because it frequently receives only tertiary support in classrooms, has received renewed interest centered around the language of PL 94-142's least restrictive mandate:

To the maximum extent appropriate, handicapped children including children in public and private institutions or other care facilities, are educated with children who are not handicapped . . . and special classes, separate schooling or other removal of handicapped children from the regular educational environment occurs only when the nature or severity of the handicap is such that education in regular classes . . . cannot be achieved satisfactorily. (Education for All Handicapped Children Act of 1975, PL 94-142, Vol. 89, Stat. p. 773)

Over a decade of research has investigated the education of all children with and without disabilities in the contexts of classrooms (mainstreaming) and neighborhood schools (integration). Some research has sought to compare students educated in different environments (segregated versus integrated schools or classrooms) to pinpoint advantages or disadvantages that may accrue in one or both situations. Through these efforts a number of factors have been identified that appear to be indices of positive participation within the community or school. These factors consist primarily of attitudes, contact between peers with and without disabilities, classroom atmosphere and structure, social skills, and social support networks. Many attempts have been made to alter teacher and student attitudes through the provision of information and/or training (L. Brown et al., 1976; Fiedler & Simpson, 1987; Frith & Lindsey, 1981; Kaye, Gruenewald, & Baumgart, 1981). However, changes gained through these methods are reportedly of short duration (Donaldson, 1980; S. Stainback, Stainback, Strathe, & Dedrick, 1983). Improvements in attitudes have also been obtained via direct contact involving peer tutoring, recreational opportunities, play opportunities in preschools, and contacts during the sharing of common school activities and facilities such as recess, lunch, library times, and instructional classroom sessions. The peer tutoring contacts, although resulting in reported positive changes in attitudes on the part of the tutors (Asselin, 1983; Roddy, 1980), have primarily an instructional focus and may limit interactions of a social nature outside of the tutoring situations (Certo & Kohl, 1984; Voeltz, 1980; Voeltz, Wuerch, & Bockhaut, 1982). Investigations of social interactions between students with severe disabilities and tutors have produced mixed

results (Gaylord-Ross, Haring, Breen, & Pitts-Conway, 1987; T.G. Haring, Breen, Pitts-Conway, Lee, & Gaylord-Ross, 1987; Odom, Hoyson, Jamieson, & Strain, 1985). The researchers found that adolescent tutors and special friends may not have differences in attitudes or frequency of interactions, but interactions were relatively short (30 seconds), their maintenance beyond one semester was not determined, and younger students did not interact outside of the training settings without teacher prompts to do so.

The research on contact alone, without the overlay of tutoring or classroom structure, revealed positive changes in attitudes. Voeltz (1980) noted significantly more positive attitudes on the part of nondisabled students as a function of contact, and these results were further supported in her follow-up study (Voeltz, 1982). Esposito and Reed (1986) found similar results with 9 young students integrated with age-peers with severe disabilities in a preschool setting. Her follow-up of these children 2 years later revealed that the changes had maintained and a comparison of these 9 children with age-mates with no contact ($N = 31$) and age-mates with recent or past contact indicated that the contact groups had significantly higher attitudes than the noncontact group.

Research on contact within instructional settings has produced different results. McHale and Simeonsson (1980) and Sandberg (1982) reported no changes in attitudes as a result of contact between students with autism or severe disabilities and their nondisabled peers in instructional settings. Other researchers found that attitude changes were more negative as a result of contact (Goodman, Gottlieb, & Harrison, 1972; Gottlieb & Budoff, 1973). To determine the meaning behind these equivocal results is not a simple task and a more in-depth investigation of the relationship between attitudes and types, variety, and settings of contacts is needed.

Work by D.W. Johnson and Johnson (1975, 1978, 1983, 1984a, 1984b, 1986), as well as by Lyon and Lyon (1980), Rynders, Johnson, Johnson, and Schmidt (1980), Schleien and Ray (1988), and Schleien, Ray, Sodermen-Olson, & McMahon (1987), lends strong support to structuring instructional and other learning situations in a cooperative manner in order to facilitate the goals of mainstreaming and to alleviate the negative results (primarily for students with learning/mild disabilities) reported above. Johnson and Johnson (1986) stated:

> There are three ways in which student-student interaction may be organized for mainstreaming. Of the three, cooperation is the only instructional strategy congruent with the goals of mainstreaming. When cooperative learning is implemented effectively, positive relationships between handicapped and nonhandicapped students result. (p. 223)

The attitudes of professionals as revealed in school district philosophy and orientation or in teacher willingness to serve various students has also been investigated. A recent Office of Special Education Programs report (Danielson & Bellamy, 1989) and investigations by Jacobson and Janicki (1985) and Mallory and Herrick (1987) revealed that from state to state, students with severe disabilities placed within integrated, mainstreamed, or segregated settings did not differ significantly in level of functioning, multiplicity of handicaps, or health-status characteristics. Attitudes of professionals, in large part, were cited as a major indicator of placement. The work of Brinker and Thorpe (1985) and Gans (1987) underscores the relationship between attitudes, state policies, and district placements. The outcome of community involvement is thus related to the enhancement of attitudes and opportunities for contact. Certainly community involvement can be facilitated when the future neighbors, employers, and co-workers of those with disabilities have had a myriad of interactions within the school community. However, this relationship between positive attitudes and actions either during or after school cannot be assumed (Asher & Taylor, 1981; Greenwood, Walker, & Hops, 1977; Peck & Semmel, 1982; Van Hasselt, Hersen, Whitehall, & Bellack, 1979). Research by Ray (1985) noted that although children with disabilities were perceived as less socially acceptable by teachers and peers, the direct observation data revealed no differences in actual social interactions. Thus, the call to investigate the validity of ratings seems paramount. The opportunities afforded through integration, whether in classrooms, schools, neighborhoods, or work sites, are only the first step toward the outcome of community involvement. In order to achieve this outcome, as well as supportive social networks and the ordinariness and invisibility associated with belonging, social skills and social competence must be sought.

Social Support Networks

Researchers in social support networks have not as yet determined if there is a causal relationship between a person's social nature and having or not having a supportive network. However, it is clear that there is a high correlation between the two. Persons who are perceived as socially competent, have high self-esteem, or are rated as socially skilled are reported to have more varied social contacts and more satisfaction with their support system (L. Cohen, McGowan, Fooskas, & Rose, 1984; Hacker, Sarason, Sarason, & Basham, 1984; B.R. Sarason, Sarason, Hacker, & Basham, 1985). Likewise, increases in the support network or satisfaction with the network are related to enhanced ratings of competence, social skills, and/or self-esteem. At this junction with the research it is not clear how to efficiently change a network to supportive or to alter perceptions of satisfaction with a network (I.G. Sarason & Sarason, 1986). Although work by Horner (1987) is currently underway in this area, most work continues to focus on the enhancement of social skills or perceived competence in this area. Interventions that lead to competence in academic performance, classroom academic responses (e.g., being on time), and interpersonal and job-related social behaviors have resulted in being liked, receiving more invitations for interactions with peers or involvement in leisure routines, and increases in obtaining and maintaining employment. The research on social skills interventions is summarized in Table 17.3 and current best practices to achieve the desired outcomes with respect to ordinariness and invisibility are discussed below.

Ordinariness and Invisibility

In order to achieve ordinariness and invisibility for persons with severe disabilities, successful exchanges between those with and without disabilities must occur, and a perception of social competence regarding the interactors must exist.

Table 17.3. Supporting research for mainstreaming and social skills

References	Descriptions
Mainstreaming: Socialization	
Cartledge & Milburn (1978)	Position papers on the role of schools in the socialization process.
Strully & Strully (1985)	
S.W. Taylor, Biklen, & Knoll (1987)	
L. Brown et al. (1988)	
Martin (1988)	
Kaufman, Gottlieb, Agard, & Kukic (1975)	Interpretations of "least restrictive environment."
L. Brown et al. (1983)	
Student and teacher attitudes	
L. Brown, Nietupski, & Hamre-Nietupski (1976)	Changing student and teacher attitudes through information and training.
Naor & Milgram (1980)	
Frith & Lindsey (1981)	
Kaye, Gruenewald, & Baumgart (1981)	
Pumpian (1981)	
Fiedler & Simpson (1987)	
Smelkin & Lieberman (1984)	
Gersten, Walker, & Darch (1988)	
Donaldson (1980)	Information and training produce attitude changes of short duration.
S. Stainback, Stainback, Strathe, & Dedrick (1983)	
D.W. Johnson & Johnson (1975, 1978, 1983, 1984a, 1984b, 1986)	Best practices for structuring learning situations in a cooperative manner to alleviate negative results and promote positive attitude changes.
Lyon & Lyon (1980)	
Rynders, Johnson, Johnson, & Schmidt (1980)	
Odom & Strain (1984)	
Schleien, Ray, Saderman-Olson, and McMahan (1987)	
Schleien & Ray (1988)	
Voeltz (1980, 1982)	Unstructured and structured contact between nonhandicapped students and students with disabilities improved attitudes.
Esposito & Reed (1986)	
Goodman, Gottlieb & Harrison (1972)	Contact between severely handicapped and nonhandicapped peers resulted in no attitude
Gottlieb & Budoff (1973)	

(continued)

Table 17.3. *(continued)*

References	Descriptions
Gottlieb (1974)	changes or negative attitude changes when contact was in instructional settings.
McHale & Simeonsson (1980)	
Sandberg (1982)	
Gresham (1984)	Review of literature concluding that attitudes had primarily become negative as a result of contact in the instructional setting between students with mild and learning handicaps and those without handicaps.
Roddy (1980)	Peer tutoring results in positive attitude changes for tutors.
Asselin (1983)	
Voeltz (1980)	Peer tutoring might limit social interactions outside of the tutoring situations.
Voeltz, Wuerch, & Bockhaut (1982)	
Certo & Kohl (1984)	
Gaylord-Ross, Haring, Breen, & Pitts-Conway (1984)	Peer tutoring produced mixed results for social interactions between students with severe disabilities and their tutors.
Odom, Hoyson, Jamieson, & Strain (1985)	
Haring, Breen, Pitts-Conway, Lee, & Gaylord-Ross (1987)	
Osguthorpe, Eiserman, & Shisler (1985)	When students with mental retardation acted as tutors for their regular-class nonhandicapped peers, free-play interactions increased between the two groups.
C.R. Greenwood, Walker & Hops (1977)	A correlation between attitudes and actions cannot be assumed.
Van Hasseelt, Whitehall, Hersen, & Bellack (1979)	
Asher & Taylor (1981)	
Peck & Semmel (1982)	
Ray (1985)	
Effect of attitudes upon policy	
Brinker & Thorpe (1985)	Attitudes, state policies, and district placement of students are related.
Gans (1987)	
Jacobson & Janicki (1985)	Student placements are due more to school district philosophy and orientation than to a
Mallory & Herrick (1987)	
Danielson & Bellamy (1988)	

(continued)

Table 17.3. *(continued)*

References	Descriptions
	student's type or degree of handicap.
Social skills and social support	
Libet & Lewinsohn (1973)	Definitions of social skills and social competence.
Wine (1981)	
McFall (1982)	
Ray (1985)	
Cohen, McGowan, Fooskas, & Rose (1984)	Research on the relationship of social skills, social support, and self-esteem as well as studies on enhancing social support networks.
Hacker, Sarason, Sarason, & Basham (1984)	
B.R. Sarason, Sarason, Hacker & Basham (1985)	
I.G. Sarason & Sarason (1986)	
Horner (1987)	
Gresham (1984)	Adolescents and adults with disabilities have more deficits in social skills than their peers.
Schumaker & Hazel (1984)	
Walker & Calkins (1986)	
Shores (1987)	
Matson & Andrasik (1982)	Research studies and position papers concluding that job productivity and accuracy of performance are less important than job-related social skills for obtaining and maintaining a job.
Burton & Bero (1984)	
Chadsey-Rusch (1986)	
Sitlington & Easterday (1986)	
Baumgart & Anderson (1987)	
Hops & Cobb (1974)	Increased academic achievement was correlated with development of social behavior.
Walker & Hops (1976)	
Glick (1978)	Rejection by peers correlates to aggressive behavior. Increased social status relates to social competence.
Interventions	
Hartup (1964, 1970, 1976, 1978)	Peers were found to be critical for the social development of children.
Lee (1975)	
Mueller & Lucas (1975)	
Rubenstein & Howes (1976)	
Hecimovic, Fox, Shores, & Strain (1986)	Peers initiated social interactions with 1 of 3 socially withdrawn persons with disabilities in both segregated and integrated free-play situations. Results indicated

(continued)

Table 17.3. *(continued)*

References	Descriptions
	an increase in initiations and interactions for all 3 children with disabilities in both settings. The greatest increase was in the integrated setting.
Guralnick & Groom (1987)	Found higher ratings of peer social behaviors in the mainstreamed setting.
Kohler & Fowler (1985)	This research article describes an intervention aimed at a peer group in an attempt to increase their reciprocations to initiations by a fellow student whose performance of initiations decreased following training. This intervention was successful in increasing and maintaining the student's initiations.
Guralnick (1981)	Peers can be involved in interventions without risk of negative side effects to themselves.
Odom & Strain (1984)	
Strain & Odom (1986)	
Gresham (1984)	Reviews of studies on social skills interventions for children and adolescents. The studies support peer-mediated interventions using competent peers, structured interventions by teachers, and use of environmental opportunities. Maintenance and generalization were described as common problems in research.
Gaylord-Ross & Haring (1987)	
McEvoy & Odom (1987)	
Davies & Rogers (1985)	A review and classification, according to complexity, of social skills studies on interventions for persons with mental retardation. Several observations based on the review are summarized.
W. Stainback, Stainback & Strathe (1983)	Selected social skills research with students with severe handicaps is analyzed by generalization effects. Teaching implications are discussed.

(continued)

Table 17.3. (continued)

References	Descriptions
McConnell (1987) Shores (1987)	Literature reviews of social skills interventions with students with severe disabilities. Maintenance beyond training was found to be a common problem.
Powell & Lindeman (1983)	Outline of several "best-practices" characteristics of programs to teach social interaction skills to young children with handicaps.
Gottlieb & Budoff (1973) Howes & Rubenstein (1978) S. Stainback, Stainback, Courtnage, & Joken (1985) Burstein (1986)	Environmental rearrangement best practices for facilitating mainstreaming and social interaction.
Cartledge & Milburn (1978) Ferguson (1987) Baumgart, Filler, & Askvig (in press)	Position papers supporting breaking down the distinctions between special and regular education and establishing new job descriptions as a prerequisite for implementation of best practices.
Dowrick (1986)	Describes social skills training procedures to various professionals including teachers, psychologists, social workers, and others. Appendices include examples of assessment and training materials.
Schloss, Schloss, Wood, & Kiehl (1986)	A review of research on social skills training with students with behavior disorders. Suggestions for interventions are given.
Scott & Gilliam (1987)	Position paper suggesting that social and behavioral skills be the major emphasis for training students with autism because such skills will affect other areas.

These outcomes are examined by reviewing interventions to enhance social behaviors. The focus for intervention to enhance social behaviors has shifted from a student-centered assessment-intervention-evaluation paradigm to a systems-and-interactors assessment, intervention, evaluation, and follow-along model. In the past, intervention started with determining what a student with disabilities needed to learn, teaching the skill, and requiring the student to perform the skill in numerous settings with a variety of people. This practice was innovative at the time because of the involvement with nondisabled peers. Since most students had very limited opportunities within their educational placements to interact with nondisabled peers, skill performance and generalization were affected by either bringing peers into the setting or taking the student to peers. To a large extent, the history of successes and disappointments in the area of social skills reflects the history of moving from segregated, isolated settings to integrated and interactive settings. A reconceptualization of the failures of the past as an intervention problem rather than a student problem is seen in the reviews of McConnell (1987) and Shores (1987) and the work of Walker et al. (1983), on effective interventions; D.W. Johnson and Johnson (1975, 1978, 1983, 1984a, 1984b, 1986), on cooperative learning environments; Ray (1985), on perception of social competence; McConnell (1987), on entrapment of social skills; and Burstein (1986) and S. Stainback, Stainback, Courtnage, and Joken (1985), on environmental rearrangements.

The consensus of the research to date requires changing the focus of intervention from imparting skills to an individual who has deficits to enhancing the skillfulness of exchanges between individuals in natural settings. This change requires that the individual and the peer target group be involved in the assessment and the intervention processes. The role of peers in assessment is to provide information on the naturally occurring actions involved in being an initiator, recipient, reinforcer, and evaluator of social exchanges within settings. The role of the teacher is to identify where the breakdown occurs in this process; to involve peers in the instruction of skills that will be reinforced/responded to by the peer group in these settings; and to restructure, as needed, the reinforcing contingencies so that naturally occurring contingencies will maintain the skills acquired by children with disabilities. This is clearly not the perceived role of many teachers, regardless of whom they teach. An investigation by Kohler and Fowler (1985) illustrates this point. The researchers followed an elementary student after intervention to ensure that initiation skills taught had generalized and had been maintained in the regular class setting. The student had performed the skills initially but her performance had decreased over time. This decrease was attributed to the lack of response of the peer target group to her initiations. Only after intervention with the peer target group was conducted did the researchers see an increase of initiations to an appropriate level, with maintenance of exchanges observed during follow-up observations.

Conclusions

The research on attitudes, integration/mainstreaming, and social skills indicates that current state-of-the-art practices are capable of producing the outcomes of community participation, supportive social networks, and ordinariness and invisibility. However, these outcomes are not widespread and the practices required necessitate teachers' assuming new roles and responsibilities. Some of the investigations (Baumgart, Filler, & Askvig, in press; Cartledge & Milburn, 1978; Ferguson, 1988) suggest that restructuring and even dissolving the separation between regular and special education is needed along with new "job descriptions" before these state-of-the-art practices can be implemented. The barriers that exist and impede these outcomes, as well as the content and process practices described earlier are harbingers of necessary changes. Their importance in this chapter is viewed not from the vantage of how teachers must perform differently, but rather from the vantage of asking the right questions in response to the data on barriers. That is, given the current system of personnel preparation, we must ask, "Can these state-of-the-art practices become typical practices?" and, "If so, how?"

Do Teachers Succeed in Implementing Best Practices?

Studies conducted in the 1980s have revealed that integration/mainstreaming, team collaboration, functional skills, and activity-based curricula with the new associated roles for teachers are the desired practices for the 1990s. Putnam and Bruininks (1986) conducted a Delphi-like survey to identify the desirability of education services for persons with disabilities as well as their perceived likelihood of occurrence. Of the categories listed, those that were noted as desirable and predicted to occur were: programming in the least restrictive environment, greater coordination among those working with persons with severe disabilities, instruction in the natural environment using natural cues and correction procedures, a research focus on effectiveness of a variety of instructional strategies and groupings, and greater training in functional skills. In a later study, Meyer et al. (1987) polled experts, parents, state administrators, and researchers in the area of severe disabilities to validate program quality indicators in educational services. The authors acknowledged that a mix of empirically validated and socially valued (or devalued) practices often direct the efforts of personnel in the field. The survey results were grouped (based on a factor analysis) to include as best practices the implementation of integration, home-school cooperation, staff development, data-based instruction, and the criterion of ultimate functioning.

The results of the above studies highlight the agreement across experts, parents, and researchers on the overall importance of these practices. Both studies provide strong support for the social validity of the "best practices" as described. The results also indicate a current and more widespread acceptance and, in fact, desirability of issues that had been identified and discussed in the 1970s. It appears that the philosophical information noted as present in university personnel preparation programs by Burke and Cohen (1977) was imparted and accepted as valid in the 1980s. However, it also appears that the discrepancy noted by Burke and Cohen between areas thought to be essential for personnel preparation and those that are actually developed and implemented at university training centers is similar to the discrepancy that exists between desired and actual "best practices" in the field. Numerous other studies attest to this lag in the implementation of best practices.

The research of Helmstetter et al. (1987) was centered on this discrepancy between desired best practices and their implementation. The researchers collected self-report implementation levels of best practices (cited by Meyer et al., 1987) from 78 teachers of students with moderate and severe disabilities in Washington and Idaho. The self-reports of implementation of the practices were verified by on-site visits and observation in the classroom. The mean rating of implementation on a scale from 0 (the practice is not implemented) to 4 (the practice is implemented with all students) across all practices was 2.19, with ratings ranging from 1.61 (for curricular content) to 3.05 (for instructional scheduling). Similar discrepancies between desirable practices and actual practices in the classroom were noted in Alabama (McLean, 1988), Connecticut and Massachusetts (Norman, Brookfield-Norman, & Meyer, 1985), and New Hampshire (Jorgensen & Nisbet, 1987). Hill, Seyfarth, Banks, Wehman, and Orelove (1987) discussed the differences of parents of school-age students and parents of adults in both the state-of-the-art services actually provided and the desirability of these services. Hill and her colleagues surveyed parents of adults with disabilities regarding their attitudes toward best practices and preferences for optimal vocational settings. The authors found that parents of adults with moderate and severe disabilities who responded were satisfied with the placements of their son/daughter consisting of segregated programs, low wages, and a poor work environment. This is in direct contrast to the attitudes and preferences of parents of students as reported by Meyer et al. and Putnam and Bruininks (1986) whose sons/daughters have been served in schools as mandated by PL 94-142 for the past decade.

A review of the information presented above indicates there is, for the most part, agreement among various groups regarding the desirable best practices for children and students with disabilities: That is, the practices are valued by administrators, experts, parents, and teachers of school-age students and the practices are predicted by experts to occur. However, in large part, the practices are not being implemented. Why not? The research on the "best practices" just reviewed indicates that their implementation has advantages for students with and without disabilities. The research also highlights the roles and responsibilities of teachers to implement best practices. The identified challenges to implementing team collaborative efforts were the lack of structure, preservice training, and role release necessary to implement the practice. The role of teachers in the process of integration, mainstreaming, and social skills enhancement has identified strategies for assessment, instruction, and entrapment of attitudes and social skills. The strategies include teachers assessing in the natural setting (recess, classrooms, and so forth—wherever students interact), intervening with students with and without disabilities, and conducting evaluation and follow-along in the natural setting.

These new roles and responsibilities of special education teachers will require the employment of teaching techniques used by other educators to supplement the use of instructional technology. A challenge to the implementation of these roles includes the current separate structures of special and regular education. The implementation of best practices requires access to environments and students that is not possible when the mainstream "belongs" to one classification of students and teachers. A large body of literature exists in which the separation between regular and special education services has been critiqued and more collaborative efforts have been advocated (Bickel & Bickel, 1986; Bogdan, 1983; Dunn, 1968; Gerber, 1988; Lilly, 1987; Pugach, 1987; Reynolds, Wang, & Walberg, 1987; Skrtic, 1987; S. Stainback & Stainback, 1984). The research on implementing best practices highlights the change that may be needed in this structure, one that will prepare all teachers to impart skills/information to "regular" and "special" education students as well as work within school and community systems to make changes. The tools of teaching obtained in part from these preparation programs must enable teachers to be good adaptive learners—teachers who can problem solve as challenges arise. This skill is critical even if the roles of teachers and the structures of schools do not change.

The above issues in the structure of service delivery and training programs, as well as the roles of teachers, have implications for personnel preparation programs. Some of the recommended changes in focus are described in the next section in a model for personnel preparation, which we expect also addresses the preparation needed to implement best practices.

In summary, we wish to acknowledge that programs of excellence exist and have existed in the past and will continue to emerge. However, as the data on implementation illustrate, these sites are limited in their scope of influence. These sites of excellence exist because a few teachers, parents, administrators, and related services personnel, some with university support and external funding, have managed despite the numerous barriers encountered. It would be unfortunate if only these pockets of excellence existed and families of students continued to face vast differences in the quality of educational services.

STATUS OF PERSONNEL PREPARATION

We said earlier that the status of personnel preparation in special education might well be "trapped in tradition." If the development of best practices in special education includes a dual emphasis on social conscience and technical ability, even if not always integrated or balanced, current practices in personnel preparation seem unable to claim any such eclecticism. Perhaps persuaded by the success of a behavioral approach to instruction for learners with severe handicaps, the new personnel preparation speciality born in the 1970s adopted a similar behavioral approach described as *competency based* (Burke & Cohen, 1977; Perske & Smith, 1977). Although other "personalistic," "craft-oriented," and "inquiry-oriented" strategies for teacher preparation exist and generate continuing discussion in regular education (Aronowitz & Giroux, 1985; Zeichner, 1983), special education has continued to rely almost entirely upon the same tools. While having the advantage of being systematic, clear, and behaviorally measurable, a competency-based approach also risks preparing teachers who may succeed in demonstrating specified competencies, while failing to acquire competence. This section reviews the barriers to implementing best practices in the larger context of professional development and reform throughout education. We argue that realizing the best-practices themes of inclusion, collaboration, functional learning,

and activity-based instruction while also overcoming barriers of limited time, resources, opportunity, and authority requires concomitant changes in our university preparation programs. While teachers must be prepared to fill new schooling roles, the reforms once again risk failure if we focus only on restructuring teachers.

Traditions of Professionalization and Personnel Preparation

It is difficult to pinpoint exactly when the teachers who found themselves working in the early ungraded and special classes first thought of themselves as "special" educators. What is clear is that the same forces that created the structural separateness between "special" and "regular" education also demanded parallel strands of professionalization. In a process similar to that of regular educators for professional status, special educators sought the badges of identity that would secure their "special" status within the larger group. Special organizations such as the Ungraded Class Teachers Association (Phillips, 1934/35) and the International Council for the Education of Exceptional Children (formed in 1922), journals such as *Ungraded* or *Training School Bulletin*, and the development of licensing procedures all foretold the birth of a new profession (Etzioni, 1969; E. Greenwood, 1957). It is this "special" aspect of professionalism, creating a market for new and separate services through the development of an "expertise" that challenges the current reform attempts (Lilly, 1989). A unique body of expert knowledge helps to maintain professional status and power through the use of technical jargon, emphasizing areas of special expertise and deemphasizing areas of common expertise and responsibilities, and erecting organizational and administrative barriers such as separate administrative structures and different licensing procedures (Kerr, 1983). Ironically, resolving some of the barriers to implementing practices will require the dismantling of "special" and "regular" education as separate professional categories, both in the field and in university preservice preparation programs. Further, it may well be that some of the forces that serve to inhibit a balanced and coherent articulation of best practices emerge from the continuing practices that seek to maintain a separate *professional* if not *programmatic* identity.

Countering the forces of specialization that isolate and segregate is further complicated by professional fragmentation within special education itself. With each historical influx of increasingly more students with disabilities came calls for yet another category of special education professional, usually delineated by disability category and accompanied by separate certification standards. Thus, while regular education supported elementary and secondary professional distinctions, special education generated categorical specialists (the learning disabilities, mental retardation, or autism teacher), curriculum specialists (vocational teacher), level of disability specialists (mild/severe), and problem-oriented specialists (behavioral consultant).

Meanwhile, the preparation of both regular and special educators experience the same dilemmas and discontinuities. Both remain troubled by the classic dichotomies between theory and practice, becoming competent and acquiring competencies (S. Sarason et al., 1986), and the "deskilling" effects of increasingly "packaged" technology that permit little exercise of creative pedagogy (Apple, 1982; Aronowitz & Giroux, 1985). Over time, following highly detailed, even scripted, published curriculum materials and equally narrow programming approaches can allow teachers' own intellectual creativity to atrophy. As a consequence, teachers may become so dependent upon their teaching "tools" that they are unable to successfully instruct students for whom the packaged curriculum or program was not specifically designed. Students who do not fit once again risk exclusion, if not from the school, at least from the classroom in which only certain "tools" are used.

Reform Efforts

In the midst of efforts to reduce the disjointedness between best educational practices and the reality of most programs and between the substance of teacher preparation programs and the reality of special education within public schools, reform efforts in regular education focus on renewing the profession's status with little mention

of special education. To some, this lack of mention indicates a lack of concern for low-achieving students; for others, the lack of focus signals the separation of special and regular education as part of the problem being addressed (Lilly, 1987; Sapon-Shevin, 1987). Two key national reports, one by the Carnegie Commission (1986) and the other by the Holmes Group (1986), outline a series of recommendations aimed at improving teaching and schools by reforming teacher preparation. As with other reform reports, these, too, have generated a great deal of discussion and dissension (see, for example, the first issue of *Educational Policy*, 1987). Nevertheless, several major themes of teacher preparation reform outlined in these two reports seem to be weathering the storm: 1) teachers should build their professional competence on a foundation of strong liberal arts undergraduate education; 2) the bulk of professional preparation should emulate that of other professions (such as law and medicine) and occur during a graduate degree program offered by professional development schools; 3) teaching staff should be differentiated hierarchically according to their knowledge and advanced training; 4) standards for entry and continuation in the profession should be stiffened, nationally articulated, and universally regulated; and 5) the authority to implement and maintain quality programs should be invested in teachers, the professionalism of the field, and a focus on outcomes at the classroom, school, and district level.

The simple, but powerful, premise underlying the current reform activity is that teacher candidates need more time to acquire necessary knowledge, skills, attitudes, and values. This premise, combined with schooling's tradition of labeling, sorting, and adding on specialized alternatives, offers thin hope for fundamental changes in how special and regular educators communicate and work together. Clearly the challenge is great. Securing the best possible educational experiences for students with severe disabilities demands changes in the content, processes, and outcomes of personnel preparation. Even more, the process of reform itself must, for the first time in special education's history, resist the familiar operation of professionalization in favor of sharing the responsibility for the support of all students with all educators. The final section of this chapter outlines our recommendations for achieving this new shared responsibility.

MODEL FOR PERSONNEL PREPARATION: PRESERVICE AND UNIVERSITY STRUCTURE

The roles of teachers of students with severe disabilities is now much broader than instructing students with categorical labels and managing the resources focused on this task. In order to implement currently articulated best practices, reforms within special and regular education will be necessary. In fact, it is increasingly clear that teachers must be prepared to function within both current and future models of educating students. Personnel preparation must be refocused to successfully impart not just the prevailing ideology, but the knowledge, skills, and judgments needed to implement best practices. At the same time, facilitation and implementation of team collaboration, integration, mainstreaming, social skills enhancement, and attitude changes, as well as durable student learning outcomes, can rarely be accomplished by a single teacher. Instead, teachers must be prepared to create communities of collegial support that can share responsibility for these roles. Personnel preparation programs must begin to train professionals, both conceptually and practically, to seek this balance. This section presents a model for personnel preservice programs that addresses this need for a new focus. Table 17.4 outlines teacher practices that relate directly to the best-practices features for students presented earlier in Table 17.1. Each of the features in Table 17.4 represents a sphere of competence rather than specific teacher competencies and attends to content, processes, and outcomes. At the end of this section we similarly analyze the structure and practices of university preparation programs.

Preservice Best-Practices Features

Best-Practices Teaching Content: Skills, Knowledge, and Judgment

In order for preservice programs to accomplish a shift in focus, training content must be broad-

Table 17.4.   Best-practices features of the preparation of teachers

CONTENT
- Multitheoretical fluency
- School and work teaching tools
- Analytical teaching tools
- Creative problem solving
- Individual ability strengths

PROCESSES
- Simulated and in vivo practice
- Learning experience in exemplary and nonexemplary settings
- Negotiation

OUTCOMES
- Self-evaluation and professional development
- Ability to generate and manage resources
- Professional transferability

ened beyond that of producing technically competent teachers to include at least four other equally important capacities. These are outlined in Table 17.4 and explained below.

First, teachers must have a multitheoretical fluency to enable them to work within the complex structure of schools and with a variety of students and professionals. Teachers will need to utilize theoretical foundations beyond the domains usually covered in the typical diagnostic, assessment, and intervention paradigms. The critical role of peers, other professionals, and community personnel in the implementation of best practices will require skills to produce student learning but also the ability to explain "why," investigate "why not," and utilize and conjure resources to reinforce and maintain best practices.

Second, teachers must possess the skills to design the accommodations and adaptations so critical to the community and school participation of persons with severe disabilities. Successful community presence and participation will be achieved not only through technical instruction, but also through a facilitative and sensitive understanding of the social context and forces that will allow the participation to be valued and as socially enhancing as possible.

Third, preservice programs must systematically build teachers' abilities to problem solve creatively. Resnick's (1987) school tools (paper and pencil) and work tools (objects, people, and situations) are both necessary for the teaching enterprise. It is the imaginative use of all available resources that marks the adaptive learner/ educator who is still able to teach when unexpectedly challenged. It is the responsibility of teacher preparation programs to achieve this goal. No program can provide teachers with the educational solutions for all the student, staff, and school policy challenges they may encounter. Instead, programs must prepare teachers to analyze, brainstorm, negotiate, reflect, and continuously revise their solutions in conversation and interaction with their professional and nonprofessional colleagues. Without this critical appreciation of and commitment to creative change, reflection, and problem solving, teachers can easily become dependent on instructional programming that teaches isolated skills to segregated students.

Fourth, preparation programs should assist teachers to identify the unique personal and professional abilities they bring to teaching, fostering a process of self-evaluation and self-managed professional growth. Personnel preparation programs need to assist teachers to create contexts for collegial sharing through mentoring and networking. Not only do these strategies offer teachers the opportunity to find in others the strengths to complement their own weaknesses, the experience of collegial connectiveness itself may well alleviate the isolation and eventual "burn out" long experienced by many special educators.

This content differs from what is traditionally outlined as best-practices features for teachers in a number of ways. The content incorporates information from other disciplines in lecture, coursework, and discussions typically not offered in teacher training programs. In addition, by helping teachers acquire and use a range of teaching orientations, teachers learn to work comfortably with all students. This broader content extends the role of teachers beyond the child-teacher instructional dyad to encompass other students, other professionals, parents, employers, and the general public. Finally, the content is structured to assist teachers to become good adaptive learners through the use of school and work tools. As a result, they can embark on careers with the self-appreciation and self-confidence to maximize their impact by sharing both their strengths and weaknesses with others. This contrasts markedly with the traditional goal of having all teachers exit with minimal competencies in all areas of teaching and the self-assumed responsibility to fulfill all responsibilities of the job alone.

Best-Practices Teaching Processes: Analysis, Reflection, and Practice

Of course, it is not just *what* you teach, but *how* you teach. If university preparation programs are to impart the skills, knowledge, and judgments just discussed, they must also revise the pedagogical strategies used to impart that content. University instructors' traditional dependence on lecture/testing formats offers little opportunity for future teachers to learn the critical lessons required for team collaboration, negotiation, and the use of work tools. Telling people how to listen to others is not nearly adequate. Instead, programs will need to create experiences as well as opportunities to analyze and reflect on those experiences. Best-practices teaching processes for teachers are listed in Table 17.4 and consist of simulated practice, learning experiences in exemplary and nonexemplary settings, and negotiation. Each is described below.

Simulated practice is considered necessary for a number of reasons. There are some important skills that cannot be "practiced" in a classroom or in a school system for a number of reasons. First, schedules are often in place, aides trained, and parent priorities assimilated into instructional goals. Likewise, practice in areas of enhancing attitudes of nondisabled students or potential employers or working with culturally different families could be more risk than gain. Second, opportunities for systems change are typically not available to temporary members of a system. Third, many university instructors construct course assignments that emphasize retention rather than use. Simulations can help students make the link between course theory and field experiences. Fourth, few classrooms are perfect. Yet students must have guided opportunities to discuss good and poor teaching examples in order to develop the critical judgment skills they will need to create better examples. Simulations offer opportunities for confidential and politically safe discussions of examples. Fifth, the practica may not be numerous enough or geographically accessible to meet the demand for placing students nor offer the range of experiences deemed optimal.

Since the social and technical complexities of classrooms make it impossible to practice all skills, simulated learning experiences offer an important pedagogical tool. These simulations may involve video or written discussions, simulated computer-based apprenticeships, role playing, personal action plans, or problem-solving activities with exemplary and nonexemplary examples (Adler & Goodman, 1986; Ferguson & Storey, 1988; Resnick, 1987; Ross & Hannay, 1986). Simulations can broaden experiences beyond those readily accessible and reduce the time required for actual planning and implementation, permitting more time for critical thinking skills, practical applications, and generating a variety of acceptable strategies. Table 17.5 contains simulation experiences we have used in preservice instruction.

Refocusing the practica experience is also deemed necessary. Traditionally, practica have been viewed by students and university faculty alike as a context for risk-free practice. Students are encouraged to try things learned in coursework, within the constraints set by the cooperating teacher, with the security that if their attempt fails, someone will be available to minimize any lasting deleterious effects on students. Supervisors, whose schedules and commitments are often thinly stretched, can appear relatively infrequently, able to offer only quick support, suggestions, and anecdotal feedback before rushing off to the next student. One consequence of this relatively freely structured approach to practica is that very often students practice and learn errors instead of systematically practicing the better skills and decisions that may have been emphasized in their coursework. Students *may* successfully transfer information acquired in coursework and simulated practice to real classroom experiences, but too often a few things get lost in the process. Instead, we believe that students need carefully orchestrated modeling, coaching, and discussion through a series of practica, each with increasing demands. In early practica, for example, students need to acquire

the critical-thinking skills that allow them to design an appropriate program or lesson for students. They also need to practice the simultaneous reflecting and acting that characterizes the instructional exchange. In subsequent practica, these critical-thinking skills become expanded to include figuring out how to explain a program and instructional plan to another professional who may have very different teaching abilities. Practica must offer the opportunity not only for "receiving feedback," but also for systematically discovering the conceptual *processes* of teaching.

Viewing practica less as practice labs and more as instructional settings requires that students have much more generous support. In some cases, this support may come from the cooperating teacher. In others, the university program may prefer, and have the necessary resources, to offer a rich schedule of supervisory time. In most situations, it will probably be a shared responsibility among cooperating teachers, the field-based program supervisors, university teaching staff, and the students themselves.

Finally, we believe that negotiation is critical to teaching and planning. Our legal and policy processes require that school personnel negotiate individual program plans directly with students and families. During the past decade, as we discussed earlier, we have made some modest improvements as a field in openly negotiating with families. In a similar vein, we have struggled to learn how to employ skills of negotiation with colleagues from other disciplines. Judging from the continued discussions of less-than-perfect team collaboration, negotiation involves a set of skills and judgments that is difficult for teachers to acquire. An even greater concern is that lack of fluency in negotiation may well result in teachers' interpreting challenges and conflicts not as problems that can be solved, but as barriers that defy changes. University preparation programs not only need to teach people about negotiation and all the ways in which it will be critical in their professional lives, programs also need to engage in negotiation with students. Students should be able to negotiate their own individualized programs. Students might negotiate to spend more time with students of certain ages, or to focus part of their

Table 17.5. Simulation experiences

Simulation descriptor	Evaluation criteria
1. Given the integration history of an elementary, junior high, or high school; the layout of the school; and descriptors of students with disabilities; the preservice students will design a plan to maximize integration throughout the school building for each student with disabilities. The plan should include: a. Systematic assessment of the regular education environments where integration might occur b. Opportunities for group as well as individual integrated activities c. Opportunities for social integration as well as academic or other program integration d. A system for implementation of integration	The written plan must target specific children and activities, must include integrated activities for all classroom students, and must be acceptable to the instructor and a building principal or administrative intern.
2. A videotape of recess at an elementary school will be shown. Two students who are nonverbal will be viewed interacting/playing at recess with other students. The preservice students will discuss and then write out: a. Vocabulary used/needed at recess by interactors b. Systems that could be used during recess for each nonverbal child and understood by others c. Strategies for enhancing communication during already existing interactions	The vocabulary and systems described must be judged to be most appropriate by the instructor. Strategies for working with nonhandicapped students will be evaluated as acceptable/not acceptable by a regular education professional.
3. Given formal evaluation results of a student and a videotaped parent interview, the students will view the interview between a teacher and a parent regarding priorities for what to teach. The students will discuss: a. What priorities the parent had b. Whether the teacher acknowledged the priorities Each student will write a long-term goal for each parent priority and meet in small groups to discuss how to teach one of the goals.	The students individually or collectively should list all 10 parent priorities. The plan on how to teach will be presented orally and judged to be acceptable by the instructor.
4. Preservice students will reside with a person with severe handicaps for 48 hours, keeping to the schedule of the person with disabilities in his or her environment. A reaction paper describing the lifestyle and surprises, disappointments, and so forth experienced will be written (instructor permission required).	The written reaction paper will be judged to be well written, coherent, and informative by the instructor.
5. During the course of their program, students will interview at least three teachers of students with severe handicaps (usually encountered in practica) about strategies for maximizing integration. Students will summarize the information generated during interviews into a product that addresses the barriers, resources needed, and school support realized.	The product must address all elements and receive a score equivalent to a B or better, as evaluted by the course instructor.

program on developing skills and knowledge from other disciplines.

Best-Practices
Teaching Outcomes: Stability, Longevity, and Ongoing Development

We believe that shifting the focus of content and pedagogy of university preparation programs along the lines suggested here will result in professionals who are skillful at working within the complex world of American public schooling. They will define their professional experiences as satisfying, succeed in producing desirable learning outcomes for students, and continue to grow as professionals throughout a long career. This kind of stability, longevity, and ongoing development, however, must be grounded in the personnel preparation program that defines desired outcomes that exceed the acquisition of information and skills. We suggest three additional outcomes necessary to support teachers' stability, longevity, and ongoing development: self-evaluation and professional development, an ability to generate and manage resources, and professional transferability. While these currently are required of most teachers, they are often not targeted outcomes. Management skills will help teachers to conduct need evaluations; that is, the process of determining the adequacy of resources/information and targeting where and what assistance is needed and for whom. Professional transferability is defined as the ability of teachers to generate instructional content and strategies for students of various ages and abilities. In essence, the teacher will not perceive two types of students, some being in "special" education and others not. Rather, professional transferability will result in perceiving all students as unique individuals with certain learning characteristics.

University Best-Practices Features

Reforms toward best practices must logically have parallel changes in the structure of training programs, certification, policies, and funding mechanisms. Such efforts will require coordinated efforts of state and local educational agencies as well as college and university personnel. The revisions that will be necessary to implement the best practices of services to students with and without disabilities will require a sharing of responsibility and a time commitment at various levels. As noted by S. Stainback and Stainback (1987) and Lilly (1988), this process can begin within the existing university and college structures and in fact has been addressed at a number of already-strong personnel preparation programs. A number of best-practices features that can be initiated are discussed and illustrated with examples in this section. An outline of the best-practices features of university programs for the 1990s are outlined in Table 17.6 and consist of content, process, and outcome features.

Best-Practices University Content

The content features of university training reflect similar spheres of competence delineated previously for teachers. The program should be structured to provide theoretical content in edu-

Table 17.6. Best-practices features of university programs

CONTENT
Theoretical grounding in history, learning theory, and social theory
An expanded instructional technology milieu
Curriculum design and development
Management of students, adults, and systems
Planning for students, adults, and systems

PROCESSES
Team teaching across disciplines and schools
Practicum instruction as a shared responsibility
Collaboration and negotiation across faculty and departments

OUTCOMES
Joint faculty appointments
Professional transferability
Balance of depth and breadth

cational history, learning theory, social systems theory, and communication strategies. This broad-based foundation is not necessarily a new suggestion (Boyer, 1983; Lilly, 1989; Pugach, 1987) but the provisions of the content across certification areas is a relatively new focus. This content, as well as expanded instructional technology coursework and coursework on classroom and systems management and planning, is a compilation of basic "core" content currently offered to preservice teacher trainees from some certification areas, and in the case of systems management and planning, rarely outside of the administration coursework. The difference here is the provision of core content that is to be provided across areas of at least regular and special education. For example, the instructional technology of direct and systematic instruction is commonly perceived as a tool needed only by special educators while the skills of utilizing the discovery method of teaching are perceived as required only by regular educators (Pugach, 1987). The provision of the broad field of instructional technology as core content for all personnel will emphasize the similarities that exist among learners in classrooms and thus among the perceived roles of all teachers.

Best-Practices University Processes

It would be a mistake to delineate one strategy for organizing the process of reform and the associated personnel preparation. The variety of strategies that could be used must be as varied as the personalities and preferences of the professionals who will utilize them. Faculty and university teaching reform committees are currently utilized to plan and implement changes as are individual faculty meetings, college-wide reform committees, curriculum revision committees, and special education and other individual department committees (Pugach, Waller, & Schug, 1988; S. Stainback, Stainback, & Forest, 1989).

One strategy used to implement changes is discussed here not because it is judged to be superior to other strategies but because the process of revision is often easier to visualize if a particular strategy is discussed and illustrated. (It is also a strategy with which one of us is most familiar.) The strategy is one of delineating content into modules, application sessions, and strands across program areas and involves collectively looking across current content coursework offered within one or more specialization areas or departments and investigating where common areas of content and theory exist. The common content is organized into content modules. Each module consists of information common or similar in focus across the areas being reviewed (e.g., writing behavior objectives is common across all departments within a certain college and instructional strategies and teaching techniques recur with varying emphasis across departments). Each module of information has associated with it certain application sessions. It is in the application sessions that students divide into smaller groups based on the age of students they intend to teach and problem solve regarding the application of the content information and theory across ability levels of students. The discussions offer trainees an opportunity to apply the information across certification areas as they currently exist. In this fashion, potential teachers can discuss teaching theory and content across a wide range of ability levels and instructors can assist in noting the similarities that exist within the instructional process for all students. Content that is specific to only one or a few certification areas is organized into strands. Preservice students would sign up for a certain number of strands that would correlate to an area of initial expertise, which could be expanded at the gradu-

ate level. These strands could include information, theory, and teaching issues such as: fine and gross motor; electronic and manual communication systems; federal wage-and-hour guidelines; phonic skills; reading in the content area; or organizing and managing chemistry, biology, and physics laboratories. An example of this strategy and its contrast with a more traditional approach is presented in Table 17.7.

The advantages of the approach are its provision of core content for students across certification areas, which lends itself to providing an emphasis on similarities of roles and functions of all teachers, and the opportunity to discuss the module theory and information in smaller groups across ability levels where problem solving and team planning can occur. The team effort, so often merely theoretically discussed in lectures, can become an integral part of training via the organization of module content and ensuing class discussions. The fragmentation that can occur across courses and certification areas can be minimized by integrating problem solving into the content areas and through fostering discussion with at least some of the future team members in the training program. The process of delivering the revised training could utilize systems already available within the university structure. Team teaching in departments and colleges could be utilized to ensure, for example, that coursework in instructional technology included content previously taught only in special education, regular education, recreation, or physical therapy departments. Likewise, courses in curriculum development and design could be organized in a similar manner.

This strategy, as are all strategies, is not without disadvantages. Collaboration between faculty from various disciplines on content and competencies as well as negotiation on the emphasis within modules and strands will of necessity become weekly if not daily occurrences. The time factor, the perceived loss of ownership over particular domains of instruction and courses, and a sense of this philosophical orientation being of lower priority than other items on the agenda of faculty and administrators will sufficiently deter many from the process of reform. Certainly many of the barriers reviewed in

Table 17.7. An example of the application of modules, application sessions, and strands to university courses

Traditional courses and structure

Beginning of term — End of term

COURSE A
Early childhood instruction and curriculum

COURSE B
Curriculum and instruction for students with severe disabilities

COURSE C
Special education instruction and curriculum (for students with mild handicaps)

COURSE D
etc.

Revised courses and structure

Beginning of term — End of term

Module A
· Philosophical assumptions underlying instruction and curriculum
· History of special education and services

Application Session A
Discussion about philosophy and future implications

Module B
Strategies for obtaining and verifying parent input and priorities for what to teach

Application Session B
· View parent-teacher interviews on what to teach
· Discuss what priorities parents are stating
· Role play
· Discuss assignments on parent input

Module C
Strategies for curricular assessment

Application Session C
· Examples of uses for a variety of ability levels
· Role Play
· Assignment

Modules D–M
Strands (select at least four)
Fine and gross motor
Transitions
Study skills
Social skills
Computers
Reading

339

the section on team collaboration will be faced by those university leaders striving to meet the challenges in education and many of the same solutions discussed in that section may be beneficial at the higher education level regardless of the strategy used.

Last in the process area of university factors is the provision of practica. The focus of practica will change from solely that of practice to that of an instructional-and-practice course. Few programs are extensive enough to permit one or two faculty members to continuously monitor students' experiences in both practica and coursework. As a result, students may acquire information in class before having an opportunity to apply it in practica, often then forgetting or failing to realize the relevance of the information at the appropriate time. Alternatively, they may try to apply course information, but may fail to receive the necessary coaching to avoid misapplication, or may need additional information or review, which is left to the field supervisor to teach according to his or her own perspective. In order to tie coursework, supervision, and practica experiences together more closely, all supervisors could be required to attend a bimonthly seminar that provides a forum for several critical exchanges; once a month, course instructors could review material covered during the preceding weeks, describe the assignments and exercises practiced, and engage in a dialogue with supervisors regarding the provision of timely and objective feedback to students on selected course content. In this way, students could receive information on their attempts to apply course material as soon as possible in a natural setting and instructors and supervisors could receive feedback on content that may need more emphasis or revision. Alternately, or in addition to the above structuring of supervisors, all practicum students could attend a weekly discussion session dealing with a teaching practice, concerns, and/or heightened awareness of teaching issues they have experienced. Presentations of videotaped examples of teaching experiences could be shared by students and act as catalysts for discussion. Obviously, the more diverse the class is in terms of experience, the more the discussion session can challenge student creativity

and team collaboration skills. Through the process outlined above, universities and colleges can begin to bridge the gulf of separateness that they have been charged with enforcing. As noted by S.B. Sarason and Doris (1979), " . . . school personnel are graduates of our colleges and universities. It is there that they learn there are at least two types of human beings [disabled and nondisabled] and if you choose to work with one of them you render yourself legally and conceptually incompetent to work with the other" (p. 391).

The strategies mentioned above clearly show that changes are possible and in fact are already occurring within some university structures.

Best-Practices University Outcomes

Expected outcomes will include joint faculty appointments across departments and/or areas of expertise, professional ability to provide content to trainees across certification areas (professional transferability), and a balance of both depth of content across ability levels as well as breadth of content across ages of students. The first area will require administrative support and the latter may require task forces and faculty development to study, conceptualize, plan, and deliver the refocus training.

CONCLUSION

The message of this chapter is not only that reform in the area of teacher preparation is needed, but this reform must include all teachers and must result in professionals who are team members and see their roles as that of teaching all students. We have attempted, through an analysis and synthesis of qualitative and quantitative research, to compile new directions to achieve this end. The impetus and the generation of questions that the Holmes Group (1986) and the Carnegie Commission (1986) epitomize must go further. The preparation of teachers at the graduate level only with undergraduate coursework in subject areas may be a viable certification route. However, the primary focus must become the content, processes, and outcomes of the preparation. The best-practices features for students, teachers, and university programs are features we believe will effect the needed restructuring of special and regular education and refocus the direction of all of education upon instructing all students.

REFERENCES

Adam, C.F. (1970). *Alienation and the negotiation process*. Unpublished manuscript.

Adler, D., & Goodman, J. (1986). Critical theory as a foundation for methods courses. *Journal of Teacher Education, 37*(4), 1–8.

Albin, R.W., Horner, R.H., Koegel, R.L., & Dunlap, G. (1987). *Extending competent performance: Applied research on generalization and maintenance*. Eugene: University of Oregon, Specialized Training Program.

Anderson, R.M., & Greer, J.G. (1976). *Educating the severely and profoundly retarded*. Baltimore: University Park Press.

Apple, M. (1982). Curriculum and the labor process: The logic of technical control. *Social Text, 5*, 108–125.

Aronowitz, S., & Giroux, H.A. (1985). *Education under siege: The conservative liberal, and radical debate over schooling*. South Hadley, MA: Bergin & Garvey Publications.

Asher, S.R., & Taylor, A.R. (1981). Social outcomes of mainstreaming sociometric assessment and beyond. *Exceptional Education Quarterly, 1*(4), 13–30.

Asselin, S.B. (1983). Peer tutoring inservice program: Effects on home economics teachers' knowledge and attitudes. *Home Economics Research Journal, 11*, 352–358.

Auerback, J.S. (1976). *Unequal justice*. London: Oxford University Press.

Baine, D., & Sobsey, R. (1980). Implementing transdisciplinary services for severely handicapped persons. *Special Education in Canada, 58*(1), 12–14.

Baker, F.B. (1978). *Computer managed instruction: Theory and practice*. Englewood Cliffs, NJ: Educational Technology Publications.

Bambara, L.M., Warren, S.F., & Komisar, S. (1988). The individualized curriculum sequencing model: Effects on skill acquisition and generalization. *Journal of The Association for Persons with Severe Handicaps, 13*, 8–19.

Bastian, A., Fruchter, N., Gitell, M., Greer, C., & Haskins, K. (1985). Choosing equality: The case for democratic schooling. *Social Policy, 15*(4), 34–41.

Baumgart, D. (1990). *Career exploration: A curriculum for students with handicaps*. Rockville, MD: Aspen.

Baumgart, D., & Anderson, J. (1987). *Assessing and teaching job related social skills: A curriculum manual for students with mild handicaps*. Unpublished manuscript, University of Idaho, STEP Project, Moscow.

Baumgart, D., Brown, L., Pumpian, I., Nisbet, J., Ford, A., Sweet, M., Messina, R., & Schroeder, J. (1982). Principle of partial participation and individualized adaptations in educational programs for severely handicapped students. *Journal of The Association for the Severely Handicapped, 7*(2), 17–27.

Baumgart, D., Filler, J., & Askvig, B. (in press). Perceived importance of social skills: A survey of teachers, parents, and other professionals. *Journal of Special Education*.

Baumgart, D., & Van Walleghem, J. (1986). Staffing strategies for implementing community based instruction. *Journal of The Association for Persons with Severe Handicaps, 11*, 92–102.

Beck, R. (1977). Interdisciplinary model: Planning and distribution and ancillary input to classrooms for the severely/profoundly handicapped. In E. Sontag (Ed.), (pp. 397–404). *Educational programming for the severely and profoundly handicapped*, Reston, VA: CEC Publications.

Behrmann, M.M. (1984). *Handbook of microcomputers in special education*. San Diego: College-Hill Press.

Belmore, K., & Brown, L. (1978). A job skill inventory strategy designed for severely handicapped potential workers. In N.G. Haring & D.D. Bricker (Eds.), *Teaching the severely handicapped* (Vol. 3, pp. 223–252). Seattle: American Association for the Education of the Severely/Profoundly Handicapped.

Bennett, F.C. (1982). The pediatrician and the interdisciplinary process. *Exceptional Children, 48*, 306–314.

Bermon, E. (1985). The improbability of meaningful educational reform. *Issues in Education, 3*, 99–111.

Bickel, W.E., & Bickel, D.D. (1986). Effective schools, classrooms and instruction: Implications for special education. *Exceptional Education, 52*(6), 489–501.

Bijou, S. (1980). Behavioral teaching of young handicapped children: Problems of application and implementation. In S. Bijou & R. Ruiz (Eds.), *Contributions of behavior modifications to education* (pp. 97–110). Hillside, NJ: Lawrence Erlbaum Associates.

Biklen, D. (1985). *Achieving the complete school: Strategies for effective mainstreaming*. New York: Teachers College Press.

Biklen, D.P., Ferguson, D.L., & Ford, A. (Eds.). (1989). *Schooling and disability*. Chicago, IL: National Society for the Study of Education Yearbook.

Billingsley, F., Haring, N., Liberty, K., Weisenstein,

G., & White, O. (1984). *Investigating the problem of skill generalization* (2nd ed.). Unpublished manuscript, University of Washington, Washington Research Organization, Seattle.

Boer, M. (Ed.). (1984). *Investigating the problem of skill generalization: Literature review I.* Unpublished manuscript, University of Washington, Washington Research Organization, Seattle.

Bogdan, R. (1983). 'Does mainstreaming work?' is a silly question. *Phi Delta Kappan, 64*, 427–429.

Bohannon, R.M. (1975). *Direct and daily measurement procedures in the identification and treatment of reading behaviors of children in special education.* Unpublished doctoral dissertation, University of Washington, Seattle.

Bourbeau, P.E., Sowers, J., & Close, D.W. (1986). An experimental analysis of generalization of banking skills from classroom to bank settings in the community. *Education and Training of the Mentally Retarded, 21*, 98–107.

Boyer, E.L. (1983). *High school: A report on secondary education in America.* New York: Harper & Row.

Brandt, E. (1989). *Discipline and the shape of the modern legal profession.* Unpublished doctoral dissertation, Case Western University, Cleveland, OH.

Bricker, D. (1976). Educational synthesizer. In A. Thomas (Ed.), *Hey, don't forget about me!: Education's investment in the severely, profoundly and multiply handicapped* (pp. 84–97). Reston, VA: Council for Exceptional Children.

Bricker, W., & Campbell, P. (1980). Interdisciplinary assessment and programming for multihandicapped students. In W. Sailor, B. Wilcox, & L. Brown (Eds.), *Methods of instruction for severely handicapped students* (pp. 3–45). Baltimore: Paul H. Brookes Publishing Co.

Brinker, R.P., & Thorpe, M.E. (1985). Some empirically derived hypotheses about the influence of state policy on the degree of integration of severely handicapped students. *Remedial and Special Education, 6*(3), 18–26.

Browder, D.M. (1987). *Assessment of individuals with severe handicaps: An applied behavior approach to life skills assessment.* Baltimore: Paul H. Brookes Publishing Co.

Browder, D.M., Snell, J.E., & Wildonger, B.A. (1988). Simulation and community-based instruction of vending machines with time delay. *Education and Training in Mental Retardation, 23*, 175–185.

Brown, L., Branston, M., Hamre-Nietupski, S., Johnson, F., Wilcox, B., & Gruenewald, L. (1979). A rationale for comprehensive, longitudinal interaction between severely handicapped students and nonhandicapped students and other citizens. *AAESPH Review, 4*, 3–14.

Brown, L., Branston-McLean, M., Baumgart, D., Vincent, L., Falvey, M., & Schroeder, J. (1979).

Using characteristics of current and subsequent least restrictive environments in the development of curricular content for severely handicapped students. *AAESPH Review, 4*(4), 407–424.

Brown, L., Falvey, M., Vincent, L., Kaye, N., Johnson, F., Ferrara-Parrish, P., & Gruenewald, L. (1980). Strategies for generating comprehensive, longitudinal, and chronological-age-appropriate individualization education programs for adolescent and young-adult severely handicapped students. *Journal of Special Education, 14*, 199–215.

Brown, L., Ford, A., Nisbet, J., Sweet, M., Donnellan, A., & Gruenewald, L. (1983). Opportunities available when severely handicapped students attend chronological age appropriate regular schools. *Journal of The Association for the Severely Handicapped, 8*(3), 16–24.

Brown, L., Long, E., Solner, A.U., Davis, L., Van Deventer, P., Ahlgren, C., Johnson, F., Gruenewald, L., & Jorgensen, J. (1988). *The home school: Why students with severe intellectual disabilities must attend the schools of their brothers, sisters, friends and neighbors.* Unpublished manuscript, University of Wisconsin–Madison and Madison Metropolitan School District.

Brown, L., Nietupski, J., & Hamre-Nietupski, S. (1976). Criterion of ultimate functioning. In A. Thomas (Ed.), *Hey, don't forget about me! Education's investment in the severely and profoundly handicapped* (pp. 2–15). Reston, VA: Council for Exceptional Children.

Brown, N.P. (1982). CAMEO: Computer assisted management of educational objectives. *Exceptional Children, 49*, 151–153.

Budoff, M., Hutten, L.R. (1982). Microcomputers in special education: Promises and pitfalls. *Exceptional Children, 49*, 123–128.

Burke, P.J., & Cohen, M. (1977). The quest for competence in serving the severely/profoundly handicapped: A critical analysis of personnel preparation programs. In E. Sontag (Ed.), *Educational programming for the severely and profoundly handicapped*, (pp. 445–465). Reston, VA: CEC Publications.

Burrello, L.C., Tracy, M.L., & Glassman, E.J. (1983). A national report on the use of electronic technology in special education management. *Journal of Special Education, 17*, 341–354:

Burstein, N.D. (1986). The effects of classroom organization on mainstreamed preschool children. *Exceptional Children, 52*, 425–434.

Burton, L., & Bero, F. (1984). Is career education really being taught? *Academic Therapy, 19*, 389–395.

Campbell, P.H. (1987a). Integrated programming for students with multiple handicaps. In L. Goetz, D. Guess, & K. Stremel-Campbell (Eds.) *Innovative program design for individuals with dual sensory impairments* (pp. 159–188). Baltimore: Paul H. Brookes Publishing Co.

Campbell, P.H. (1987b). The integrated programming

team: An approach for coordinating professionals of various disciplines in programs for students with severe and multiple handicaps. *Journal of The Association for Persons with Severe Handicaps, 12,* 107–117.

Campbell, P.H., & Stewart, B. (1986). Measuring changes in movement skills with infants and young children with handicaps. *Journal of The Association for Persons with Severe Handicaps, 11,* 153–162.

Carnegie Commission (1986). *A nation prepared: Teachers for the 21st century.* New York: Carnegie Forum.

Cartledge, G., & Milburn, J.F. (1978). The case for teaching social skills in the classroom: A review. *Review of Educational Research, 1,* 133–156.

Certo, N., & Kohl, F.L. (1984). A strategy for developing interpersonal interaction instructional content for severely handicapped students. In N. Certo, N. Haring, & R. York (Eds.), *Public school integration of severely handicapped students: Rational issues and progressive alternatives* (pp. 221–244). Baltimore: Paul H. Brookes Publishing Co.

Certo, N., Mezzullo, K., & Hunter, D. (1985). The effects of total task chain training on the acquisition of bus person job skills at a full service community restaurant. *Education and Training of the Mentally Retarded, 20,* 148–156.

Chadsey-Rusch, J. (1986). Identifying and teaching valued social behaviors. In F.R. Rusch (Ed.), *Competitive employment issues and strategies* (pp. 273–287). Baltimore: Paul H. Brookes Publishing Co.

Cohen, L., McGowan, J., Fooskas, S., & Rose, S. (1984). Positive life events and social support and relationships between life stress and psychological disorder. *American Journal of Community Psychology, 12,* 567–587.

Cohen, S.P. (1974, August). *International conflict resolution workshops.* Paper presented at the annual convention of the American Psychological Association, New Orleans.

Courtnage, L., & Smith-Davis, J. (1987). Interdisciplinary team training: A national survey of special education teacher training programs. *Exceptional Children, 53,* 451–460.

Cross, J.G. (1977). Negotiation as a learning process. *Journal of Conflict Resolution, 21*(4), 581–606.

Cruscial, B., & Schimmer, J. (1983). *Data handler.* (Available from B. Cruscial, Oregon State School for the Deaf, 999 Locust St., Salem, OR 93703)

Danielson, L.C., & Bellamy, G.T. (1989). State variations in placement of children with handicaps in segregated environments. *Exceptional Children, 55,* 448–455.

Davies, R.R., & Rogers, E.S. (1985). Social skills training with persons who are mentally retarded. *Mental Retardation, 23,* 186–196.

Del Polito, C.M. (1983, April). *Multidisciplinary education: Core competencies for meeting the needs of youngsters with disabilities.* Paper presented at

the Interprofessional Health Leadership Symposium for the Southeast Region, Gainesville, FL. (ERIC Document Reproduction Service No. ED 233 518).

Dennison, W.F., & Shenton, K. (1987). *Challenges in educational management: Principles into practice.* (Available from Nicholos Publishing Co., P.O. Box 96, New York, NY).

Deno, S., & Mirkin, P. (1980). Data based IEP development: An approach to substantive compliance. *Teaching Exceptional Children, 12*(3), 92–98.

Deno, S.L., Mirkin, P.K., & Chiang, B. (1982). Identifying valid measures of reading. *Exceptional Children, 49,* 36–45.

Detwiler, R. (1982). *Effects of computer managed instruction on pre-instructional decisions of teachers of severely handicapped pupils.* Unpublished doctoral dissertation, University of Washington, Seattle.

Donaldson, J. (1980). Changing attitudes toward handicapped persons: A review and analysis of research. *Exceptional Children, 46,* 504–514.

Donnellan, A.M., & Mirenda, P.L. (1983). A model for analyzing instructional components to facilitate generalization for severely handicapped students. *Journal of Special Education, 17,* 317–332.

Donohue, W.A. (1976). *A reconceptualization of negotiation: Test of an empirical framework.* Unpublished doctoral dissertation, Ohio State University, Columbus.

Dostal, L. (1982). *Team development manual: Family nurse practitioner/physician assistant program.* Davis: University of California at Davis, Department of Family Practice.

Dowrick, P.W. (1986). *Social survival for children: A trainer's resource book.* New York: Brunner/Mazel.

Dunn, L.M. (1968). Special education for the mildly retarded: Is much of it justifiable? *Exceptional Children, 35,* 5–22.

Education for All Handicapped Children Act of 1975, PL 94-142, Vol. 89, Stat. p. 773.

Elias, M.J., & Clabby, J.F. (1989). *Social decision-making skills: A curriculum guide for the elementary grades.* Rockville, MD: Aspen.

Epanchin, B.C., & Owen, M. (1982, April). *Facilitating multi-disciplinary conferences: Requisite skills.* Paper presented at the Annual International Convention of the Council for Exceptional Children, Houston, TX. (ERIC Document Reproduction Service No. ED 219 896)

Esposito, B.G., & Reed, T.M. (1986). The effects of contact with handicapped persons on young children's attitudes. *Exceptional Children, 53,* 224–230.

Etzioni, A. (Ed.). (1969). *The semi-professions and their organization.* New York: Free Press.

Evans, I.M., & Meyer, L.H. (1985). *An educative approach to behavior problems: A practical decision model for intervention with severely handicapped learners.* Baltimore: Paul H. Brookes Publishing Co.

Falvey, M.A. (1985). *Community-based curriculum: Instructional strategies for students with severe handicaps*. Baltimore: Paul H. Brookes Publishing Co.

Falvey, M., Brown, L., Lyon, S., Baumgart, D., & Schroeder, J. (1978). Strategies for using cues and correction procedures. In W. Sailor, B. Wilcox, & L. Brown (Eds.), *Methods of instruction for severely handicapped students* (pp. 109–135). Baltimore: Paul H. Brookes Publishing Co.

Feinberg, W. (1985). Fixing the schools: The ideological turn. *Issues in Education*, *3*(2), 113–138.

Ferguson, D. (1987). *Curriculum decision-making for the students with severe handicaps: Policy and practice*. New York: Teachers College Press.

Ferguson, D.L. (1988). *Severity of need and educational excellence: Public school reform and students with disabilities*. (Available from Diane L. Ferguson, University of Oregon, Specialized Training Program, Eugene, OR 97403).

Ferguson, D.L. (1989). Severity of need and educational excellence: Public school reform and students with disabilities. In D.P. Biklen, D.L. Ferguson, & A. Ford (Eds.), *Schooling and disability* (pp. 25–58). Chicago, IL: National Society for the Study of Education Yearbook.

Ferguson, D., Ferguson, P., & Bogdan, R. (1987). If mainstreaming is the answer, what is the question? Perspectives on integrating students with special needs. In V. Kiehler (Ed.), *Educator's handbook: Research into practice* (pp. 394–419). New York: Longmons.

Ferguson, D., & Storey, K. (1988). *Rethinking the preparation and practice of teachers of severely handicapped students*. Unpublished manuscript, University of Oregon, Eugene.

Fiedler, C.R., & Simpson, R.L. (1987). Modifying the attitudes of nonhandicapped high school students towards handicapped peers. *Exceptional Children*, *53*, 342–351.

Fimian, M.J. (1984). Organization variables related to stress and burnout in community-based programs. *Education and Training of the Mentally Retarded*, *19*, 201–209.

Fredericks, H.D., Anderson, R., & Baldwin, V. (1979). Identifying competency indicators of teachers of the severely handicapped. *AAESPH Review*, *4*, 81–95.

Frith, G.H., & Kelly, P. (1981). The parent/paraprofessional relationship in programs for severely and profoundly retarded children. *Education and Training of the Mentally Retarded*, *16*, 231–234.

Frith, G.H., & Lindsey, J.D. (1981). The effects of in-service training on regular educators' attitudes toward handicapped students. *Education Unlimited*, *3*(3), 29–31.

Fuchs, L.S., Deno, S.L., & Mirkin, P.K. (1983a). Data-based program modification: A continuous evaluation system with computer software to facilitate implementation. *Journal of Special Education Technology*, *6*(2), 50–57.

Fuchs, L.S., Deno, S.L., & Mirkin, P.K. (1983b). *The effect of alternative data-utilization rules on spelling achievement: An N of 1 study* (Research report No. 120). Minneapolis: University of Minnesota, Institute for Research on Learning Disabilities.

Fuchs, L.S., Fuchs, D., & Warren, L.M. (1982). *Special education practice in evaluating student progress toward goals* (Research report No. 81). Minneapolis: University of Minnesota, Institute for Research on Learning Disabilities.

Gans, K.D. (1987). Willingness of regular and special educators to teach students with handicaps. *Exceptional Children*, *54*, 41–45.

Gaylord-Ross, R. (1980). A decision model for the treatment of aberrant behavior in applied settings. In W. Sailor, B. Wilcox, & L. Brown (Eds.), *Methods of instruction for severely handicapped students* (pp. 135–158). Baltimore: Paul H. Brookes Publishing Co.

Gaylord-Ross, R., & Haring. T. (1987). Social interaction research for adolescents with severe handicaps. *Behavioral Disorders*, *12*, 264–275.

Gaylord-Ross, R.J., Haring, T.G., Breen, C., & Pitts-Conway, V. (1987). The training and generalization of social interaction skills with autistic youth. *Journal of Applied Behavior Analysis*, *17*, 229–247.

Gentry, D., & Haring, N.G. (1976). Essentials of performance measurement. In N.G. Haring & L. Brown (Eds.), *Teaching the severely handicapped* (Vol. I, pp. 209–236). New York: Grune & Stratton.

Gerber, M.M. (1988). Tolerance and technology of instruction: Implications for special education reform. *Exceptional Children*, *54*, 309–316.

Gersten, R., Walker, H., & Darch, C. (1988). Relationship between teachers' effectiveness and their tolerance for handicapped students. *Exceptional Children*, *54*, 433–439.

Giangreco, M.F. (1986). Effects of integrated therapy: A pilot study. *Journal of The Association for Persons with Severe Handicaps*, *11*, 205–209.

Glick, J. (1978). Cognition and social cognition: An introduction. In J. Glick & K.A. Clarke-Stewart (Eds.), *The development of social understanding* (pp. 1–10). New York: Gardner Press.

Goodman, H., Gottlieb, J., & Harrison, R.H. (1972). Social acceptance of EMRs integrated into a nongraded elementary school. *American Journal of Mental Deficiency*, *76*, 412–417.

Gottlieb, J. (1974). Attitudes toward retarded children: Effects of labeling and academic performance. *American Journal of Mental Deficiency*, *79*, 268–273.

Gottlieb, J., & Budoff, M. (1973). Social acceptability of retarded children in nongraded schools differing in architecture. *American Journal of Mental Deficiency*, *78*, 15–19.

Gouran, D.S., & Guadagnino, C.S. (1988). *Small group communication: An annotated bibliography*. (Available from Speech Communication Association, 5105 Blackbird Rd., Suite E, Annandale, VA 22003)

Greenwood, C.R., Walker, H.M., & Hops, H. (1977). Issues in social interaction/withdrawal assessment. *Exceptional Children, 43*, 490–499.

Greenwood, E. (1957). The attributes of a profession. *Social Work, 2*, 44–55.

Gresham, F.M. (1984). Social skills and self-efficacy for exceptional children. *Exceptional Children, 51*, 253–261.

Guess, D. (1980). Methods in communication instruction for severely handicapped persons. In W. Sailor, B. Wilcox, & L. Brown (Eds.), *Methods of instruction for severely handicapped students* (pp. 195–226). Baltimore: Paul H. Brookes Publishing Co.

Guess, D., & Helmstetter, E. (1986). Skill cluster instruction and the individualized curriculum sequencing model. In R.H. Horner, L.H. Meyer, & H.D.B. Fredericks (Eds.), *Education of learners with severe handicaps: Exemplary service strategies* (pp. 221–248). Baltimore: Paul H. Brookes Publishing Co.

Gullo, P.H., & Gullo, J.C. (1984). An ecological language intervention approach with mentally retarded adolescents. *Language Speech and Hearing Services in Schools, 15*(3), 182–191.

Guralnick, M.J. (1981). Programmatic factors affecting child-child social interactions in mainstreamed preschool programs. *Exceptional Education Quarterly, 1*(4), 71–91.

Guralnick, M.J., & Groom, J.M. (1987). Peer interactions in mainstreamed settings and specialized classrooms: A comparative analysis. *Exceptional Children, 54*, 415–425.

Hacker, T.A., Sarason, I.G., Sarason, B.R., & Basham, R.B. (1984). *Social skills, attractiveness, and gender: Factors in perceived social support.* Seattle: University of Washington, Psychology Department.

Hamre-Nietupski, S., Nietupski, J., Bates, P., & Maurer, S. (1982). Implementing a community-based educational model. *Journal of The Association for the Severely Handicapped, 7*(4), 38–43.

Haring, N. (1984). *Investigating the problem of skill generalization: Literature review I.* Seattle: University of Washington, Washington Research Organization. (ERIC Document Reproduction Service No. ED 234 573)

Haring, N. (1985). *Investigating the problems of skill generalization* (3rd ed.). Unpublished manuscript, University of Washington, Washington Research Organization, Seattle.

Haring, N. (1987). *Investigating the problem of skill generalization: Literature review III.* Unpublished manuscript, University of Washington, Washington Research Organization, Seattle.

Haring, N.G., & Bricker, D.D. (Eds.). (1978). *Teaching the severely handicapped* (Vol. 3). Seattle: American Association for the Education of the Severely/Profoundly Handicapped.

Haring, N.G., & Brown, L.J. (Eds.). (1976). *Teaching the severely handicapped.* (Vol. 1). New York: Grune & Stratton.

Haring, N., Liberty, K., Billingsley, F., Butterfield, E., & White, O. (1983). *Investigating the problem of skill generalization.* Unpublished manuscript, University of Washington, Washington Research Organization, Seattle.

Haring, N.G., Liberty, K.A., & White, O.R. (1980). Rules for data-based strategy decisions in instructional programs: Current research and instructional implications. In W. Sailor, B. Wilcox, & L. Brown (Eds.), *Methods of instruction for severely handicapped students* (pp. 159–192). Baltimore: Paul H. Brookes Publishing Co.

Haring, T.G., Breen, B., Pitts-Conway, V., Lee, M., & Gaylord-Ross, R. (1987). Adolescent peer tutoring and special friend experiences. *Journal of The Association for Persons with Severe Handicaps, 12*, 280–286.

Hart, V. (1977). The use of many disciplines with the severely and profoundly handicapped. In E. Sontag, J. Smith, & N. Certo (Eds.), *Educational programming for the severely and profoundly handicapped* (pp. 391–396). Reston, VA: Council for Exceptional Children.

Hartup, W.W. (1964). Friendship status and the effectiveness of peers as reinforcing agents. *Journal of Experimental Child Psychology, 1*, 154–162.

Hartup, W.W. (1970). Peer interaction and social organization. In P.H. Mussen (Ed.), *Carmichael's manual of child psychology* (pp. 361–456). New York: John Wiley & Sons.

Hartup, W.W. (1976). Peer interaction and the behavioral development of the individual child. In E. Schopler & R.J. Reichler (Eds.), *Psychopathology and child development* (pp. 203–217). New York: Plenum.

Hartup, W.W. (1978). Peer interaction and the processes of socialization. In M.J. Guralnick (Ed.), *Early intervention and the integration of handicapped and nonhandicapped children* (pp. 27–52). Baltimore: University Park Press.

Hasselbring, T., & Crossland, C. (1981). Using microcomputers for diagnosing spelling problems in learning-handicapped children. *Educational Technology, 21*(4), 37–39.

Hasselbring, T.S., & Hamlett, C.L. (1983). *AIMSTAR.* Portland, OR: ASIEP Education Co.

Hecimovic, A., Fox, J.J., Shores, R.E., & Strain, P.S. (1986). An analysis of integrated and segregated free play settings and generalization of newly acquired social behaviors. *Behavioral Assessment, 7*, 367–388.

Helmstetter, E., Baumgart, D., Curry, C., Donaldson, B., Lynch, V., & Peck, C. (1987, October). *The Inland Northwest Consortium for Severely Handicapped/Deaf-Blind Inservice Training: Results of needs assessments of teachers.* Paper presented at the meeting of The Association for Persons with Severe Handicaps, Chicago.

Hill, J.W., Seyfarth, J., Banks, P.D., Wehman, P., &

Orelove, F. (1987). Parent attitudes about working conditions of their adult mentally retarded sons and daughters. *Exceptional Children, 54*, 9–23.

Hofmeister, A.M. (1982). Microcomputers in perspective. *Exceptional Children, 49*, 115–121.

Hofmeister, A.M. (1984a). *Microcomputer applications in the classroom.* New York: Holt, Rinehart and Winston.

Hofmeister, A.M. (1984b). The special education in the information age. In M.M. Behrmann & L. Lahm (Eds.), *Proceedings of the National Conference on the Use of Microcomputers in Special Education* (pp. 2–14). Reston, VA: Council for Exceptional Children.

Holmes Group. (1986). *Tomorrow's teachers: A report of the Holmes Group.* East Lansing, MI: Author.

Hopkins, K.D. (1983). Estimating reliability and generalizability in coefficients in two-facet design. *Journal of Special Education, 17*, 371–375.

Hops, H., & Cobb, J.A. (1974). Initial investigations into academic survival skill training, direct instruction, and first-grade achievement. *Journal of Educational Psychology, 66*, 548–553.

Horner, R.H. (1987). *Community network project: Research on strategies for supporting social networks* (Available from University of Oregon, Dept. of Education, 135 Education Building, Eugene, OR 97403).

Horner, R.H., Dunlap, G., & Koegel, R.L. (Eds.). (1988). *Generalization and maintenance: Life-style changes in applied settings.* Baltimore: Paul H. Brookes Publishing Co.

Horner, R.H., McDonnell, J.J., & Bellamy, G.T. (1986). Teaching generalized skills: General case instruction in simulation and community settings. In R.H. Horner, L.H. Meyer, & H.D.B. Fredericks (Eds.), *Education of learners with handicaps: Exemplary service strategies* (pp. 289–314). Baltimore: Paul H. Brookes Publishing Co.

Howes, C., & Rubenstein, J. (1978). *Peer play and the effect of the inanimate environment.* Paper presented at the 49th annual convention of the Eastern Psychological Association, Washington, DC (ERIC Document Reproduction Service No. ED 163 323)

Hupp, S., & Mervis, C. (1981). Development of generalized concepts by severely handicapped students. *Journal of The Association for the Severely Handicapped, 6*(1), 14–21.

Hutchinson, D.A. (1974). *A model for transdisciplinary staff development. A nationally organized collaborative project to provide services to atypical infants and their families* (Technical report #8). New York: United Cerebral Palsy.

Iacino, R., & Bricker, D. (1978). The generative teacher: A model for preparing personnel to work with the severely/profoundly handicapped. In N. Haring & D. Bricker (Eds.), *Teaching the severely handicapped* (Vol. 3, pp. 62–76). Seattle: American Association for the Education of the Severely/Profoundly Handicapped.

Idol-Maestas, L., Ritter, S., & Lloyd, S. (1983). A model for direct, data-based reading instruction. *Journal of Special Education Technology, 6*(3), 61–77.

Inge, K.J., & Snell, M.E. (1985). Teaching positioning and handling techniques in public school personnel through inservice training. *Journal of The Association for Persons with Severe Handicaps, 10*, 105–111.

Jacobson, J.W., & Janicki, M.P. (1985). Functional and health status characteristics of persons with severe handicaps in New York State. *Journal of The Association for Persons with Severe Handicaps, 10*, 51–61.

Jenkins, J., Mayhall, W., Peschka, C., & Townsend, V. (1974). Using direct and daily measures to increase learning. *Journal of Learning Disabilities, 7*, 605–608.

Jenkins, J.R., Speltz, M.L., & Odom, S.L. (1981). *The effects of integrated special education preschool on child development and social interaction.* Unpublished manuscript, University of Washington, Seattle.

Johnson, D.W., & Johnson, R. (1975). *Learning together and alone: Cooperation, competition, and individualization.* Englewood Cliffs, NJ: Prentice-Hall.

Johnson, D.W., & Johnson, R. (1978). Cooperative, competitive, and individualistic learning. *Journal of Research and Development in Education, 12*, 3–15.

Johnson, D.W., & Johnson, R. (1983). The socialization and achievement crisis: Are cooperative learning experiences the solution? In L. Bickman (Ed.), *Applied social psychology annual 4* (pp. 119–164). Beverly Hills: Sage Publications.

Johnson, D.W., & Johnson, R. (1984a). Building acceptance of differences between handicapped and nonhandicapped students: The effects of cooperative and individualistic problems. *Journal of Social Psychology, 122*, 257–267.

Johnson, D.W., & Johnson, R. (1984b). Classroom learning structure and attitudes toward handicapped students in mainstream settings: A theoretical model and research evidence. In R.L. Jones (Ed.), *Special education in transition: Attitudes toward the handicapped.* Reston, VA: ERIC Clearinghouse on Handicapped and Gifted Children, Council for Exceptional Children.

Johnson, D.W., & Johnson, R.T. (1986). Mainstreaming and cooperative learning strategies. *Exceptional Children, 52*, 553–561.

Johnson, R.B. (1980). *A guide to interdisciplinary training.* Baltimore: AAUAP National Training Director's Council, University of Maryland.

Jorgensen, C., & Nisbet, J. (1987). *A review of special education certification in the state of New Hampshire.* Durham: University of New Hampshire, Center for Health Promotion and Research.

Joyce, B., & McNair, K. (1979). *Teaching styles at South Bay School: The South Bay Study, part I.*

(Research Series No. 57). East Lansing: Michigan State University, East Lansing Institute for Research on Teaching.

Kaufman, M., Gottlieb, J., Agard, J.A., & Kukic, M.B. (1975). Mainstreaming: Toward an explication of the construct. In E.L. Meyen, G.A. Vergason, & R.J. Whelan (Eds.), *Alternatives for teaching exceptional children* (pp. 35–54). Denver: Love Publishing.

Kaye, N., Gruenewald, L., & Baumgart, D. (1981). Strategies for interaction with severely handicapped students. In L. Burrello & N. Kaye (Eds.), *Initiating change through inservice education: A topical instruction module series* (pp. 1–36). Bloomington, IN: National Inservice Network.

Kenowitz, L., Zweibel, D., & Edgar, E. (1978). Determining the least restrictive educational opportunity for the severely and profoundly handicapped. In N. Haring & D. Bricker (Eds.), *Teaching the severely handicapped* (Vol. 3, pp. 49–61). Seattle: American Association for the Education of the Severely/Profoundly Handicapped.

Kerr, S.T. (1983). Teacher specialization and the growth of a bureaucratic profession. *Teachers College Record, 84*, 629–651.

Kersten, G.E. (1987). On two roles decision support systems can play in negotiations. *Information Processing and Management, 23*(6), 605–614.

Kohler, F.W., & Fowler, S.A. (1985). Training prosocial behaviors of young children: An analysis of reciprocity with untrained peers. *Journal of Applied Behavior Analysis, 18*, 187–200.

Kunzelman, H.P. (Ed.). (1970). *Precision teaching: An initial training sequence.* Seattle: Special Child Publications.

Lee, L.C. (1975). Toward a cognitive theory of interpersonal development: Importance of peers. In M. Lewis & L.A. Rosenblum (Eds.), *Friendship and peer relations* (pp. 204–223). New York: John Wiley & Sons.

Liberty, K.A. (1975). *Decide for progress: Dynamic aims and data decisions* (Working paper No. 56). Seattle: University of Washington, College of Education Child Development and Mental Retardation Center.

Liberty, K.A., Haring, N.G., White, O.R., & Billingsley, R. (1988). A technology for the future: Decision rules for generalization. *Education and Training in Mental Retardation, 23*(4), 315–326.

Libet, J.M., & Lewinsohn, P.M. (1973). Concept of social skill with special reference to the behavior of depressed persons. *Journal of Consulting and Clinical Psychology, 40*, 304–312.

Lilly, M.S. (1987). Lack of focus on special education in literature on educational reform. *Exceptional Children, 53*, 325–326.

Lilly, M.S. (1988). *The regular education initiative: A force for change in general and special education.* Unpublished manuscript, Washington State University, College of Education, Pullman.

Lilly, M.S. (1989). Teacher preparation. In D.K.

Lipsky & A. Gartner (Eds.), *Beyond separate education: Quality education for all* (pp. 143–158). Baltimore: Paul H. Brookes Publishing Co.

Lindsey, D., O'Neal, J., Haas, K., & Tewey, S. (1983, April). *A cooperative adventure: The integration of physical therapy services into North Carolina's Schools.* Paper presented at the Annual International Convention of the Council for Exceptional Children, Detroit. (ERIC Document Reproduction Service No. ED 229 976)

Lindsley, O.R. (1964). Direct measurement and prosthesis of retarded behavior. *Journal of Education, 147*, 62–81.

Lipsky, D.K., & Gartner, A. (1989). *Beyond separate education: Quality education for all.* Baltimore: Paul H. Brookes Publishing Co.

Love, R., Rozelle, R., & Druckman, D. (1983). Resolving conflicts of interest and ideologies: A simulation of political decision-making. *Social Behavior and Personality, 11*(2), 23–28.

Lovitt, T.C. (1977). *In spite of my resistance, I've learned from children.* Columbus, OH: Charles E. Merrill.

Lynch, V., McGuigan, C., & Shoemaker, D. (1977). An introduction to systematic instruction. In N.G. Haring (Ed.), *The experimental education training program: An inservice training program for personnel serving the severely handicapped: Vol. I. Systematic instruction.* Seattle: University of Washington, College of Education.

Lynch, V., McGuigan, C., & Shoemaker, D. (1983). An introduction to systematic instruction. *B.C. Journal of Special Education, 7*(1), 1–13.

Lyon, S., & Lyon, G. (1980). Team functioning and staff development: A role release approach to providing integrated educational services for severely handicapped students. *Journal of The Association for the Severely Handicapped, 5*(3), 250–263.

Mallory, B.L., & Herrick, S.C. (1987). The movement of children with mental retardation from institutional to community care. *Journal of The Association for Persons with Severe Handicaps, 12* 297–306.

Martin, R. (1988). Review of recent court decisions. *Proceedings of the Ninth National Institute on Legal Problems of Educating the Handicapped.* Alexandria, VA: CRR Publishing Co.

Matson, J.L., & Andrasik, F. (1982). Training leisure time social skills to mentally retarded adults. *American Journal of Mental Deficiency, 86*, 533–542.

McConnell, S.R. (1987). Entrapment effects and the generalization and maintenance of social skills training for elementary school students with behavioral disorders. *Behavioral Disorders, 12*, 252–263.

McCormick, L., & Goldman, R. (1979). The transdisciplinary model: Implications for service delivery and personnel preparation for the severely and profoundly handicapped. *AAESPH Review, 4*, 152–161.

McDonnell, J.J., Horner, R.H., & Williams, J.A. (1984). Comparison of three strategies for teaching generalized grocery purchasing to high school students with severe handicaps. *Journal of The Association for Persons with Severe Handicaps, 9,* 123–133.

McEvoy, M.A., & Odom, S.L. (1987). Social interaction training for preschool children with behavioral disorders. *Behavioral Disorders, 12,* 242–251.

McFall, R.M. (1982). A review and reformulation of the concept of social skills. *Behavioral Assessment, 4,* 1–33.

McHale, S.M., & Simeonsson, R.J. (1980). Effects of interaction on nonhandicapped children's attitudes toward autistic children. *American Journal of Mental Deficiency, 85,* 18–25.

McLean, M. (1988). [Priority training needs from personnel preparation survey]. Unpublished raw data.

Meyer, L.H., Eichinger, J., & Park-Lee, S. (1987). A validation of program quality indicators in educational services for students with severe disabilities. *Journal of The Association for Persons with Severe Handicaps, 17,* 251–263.

Miller, R., & Ragghianti, S. (1984). A soft sell for hardware: The use of microcomputer technology for cost effective special education management. In M.M. Behrmann & L. Lahm (Eds.), *Proceedings of the National Conference on the Use of Microcomputers in Special Education* (pp. 46–54). Reston, VA: Council for Exceptional Children.

Mueller, E., & Lucas, T. (1975). A development analysis of peer interaction among toddlers. In M. Lewis & L.A. Rosenblum (Eds.), *Friendship and peer relations* (pp. 223–259). New York: John Wiley & Sons.

Naor, M., & Milgram, R. (1980). Two preservice strategies for preparing classroom teachers for mainstreaming. *Exceptional Children, 47,* 126–129.

National Commission on Excellence in Education. (1983). *A nation at risk: The imperative for educational reform.* Washington, DC: Author.

Nietupski, J., Scheutz, G., & Ockwood, L. (1980). The delivery of communication therapy services to severely handicapped students: A plan for change. *Journal of The Association for the Severely Handicapped, 5*(1), 13–24.

Nietupski, J., Welch, J., & Wacker, D. (1983). Acquisition, maintenance and transfer of grocery item purchasing skills by moderately and severely handicapped students. *Education and Training of the Mentally Retarded, 18,* 279–286.

Norman, M.E., Brookfield-Norman, J., & Meyer, L.H. (1985). *A professional development needs assessment: A discrepancy model.* Syracuse, NY: Syracuse University Division of Special Education and Rehabilitation.

Odom, S.L., Hoyson, M., Jamieson, B., & Strain, P.S. (1985). Increasing handicapped preschoolers' peer social interactions: Cross setting and component analysis. *Journal of Applied Behavior Analysis, 18,* 3–16.

Odom, S.L., & Strain, P.S. (1984). Peer-mediated approaches to promoting children's social interaction: A review. *American Journal of Orthopsychiatry, 54,* 544–557.

Office of Special Education and Rehabilitative Services. (1983). *Fifth annual report to Congress on the implementation of the Education of the Handicapped Act.* Washington, DC: Words & Pictures Corp.

Office of Special Education and Rehabilitative Services. (1987). *Ninth annual report to Congress on the implementation of the Education of the Handicapped Act.* Washington, DC: U.S. Department of Education.

Osguthorpe, R.T., Eiserman, W.D., & Shisler, L. (1985). Increasing social acceptance: Mentally retarded students tutoring regular class peers. *Education and Training of the Mentally Retarded, 20,* 235–240.

Peck, C.A., & Semmel, M.I. (1982). Identifying the least restrictive environment (LRE) for children with severe handicaps: Toward an empirical analysis. *Journal of The Association for the Severely Handicapped, 7*(1), 56–63.

Pedersen, P.B. (1985). Decision making in a multicultural group. *Journal for Specialists in Group Work, 10*(3), 164–173.

Perske, R., & Smith, J. (1977). *Beyond the ordinary: The preparation of professionals to educate severely and profoundly handicapped persons.* Parsons, KS: Words & Pictures Corp.

Phillips, H.C. (1934/35). Elizabeth E. Farrell: 1870–1932. *International Council for Exceptional Children Review, 1,* 73–76.

Powell, T.H., & Lindeman, D.P. (1983). Developing a social-interaction teaching program for young handicapped children. *Exceptional Children, 50,* 72–75.

Pugach, M. (1987). The national education reports and special education: Implications for teacher preparation. *Exceptional Children, 53,* 308–315.

Pugach, M.C., & Allen-Meares, P. (1985). Collaboration at the preservice level: Instructional and education activities. *Teacher Education and Special Education, 8*(1), 3–11.

Pugach, M., Waller, S., & Schug, M. (1988, February). *A study of interdisciplinary change in teacher education: The University of Wisconsin–Milwaukee Center for Teacher Education.* Paper presented at the Annual Meeting of the American Association of Colleges for Teacher Education, New Orleans.

Pumpian, I. (1981). *Variables affecting attitudes toward the employability of severely handicapped persons.* Unpublished doctoral dissertation, University of Wisconsin–Madison.

Putnam, J.W., & Bruininks, R.H. (1986). Future directions in deinstitutionalization and education: A Delphi investigation. *Exceptional Children, 53,* 55–62.

Rainforth, B., & York, J. (1986). *The role of related services in community-referenced instruction.* Unpublished manuscript. (Available from B. Rainforth, Division of Education, State University of New York, Binghamton, NY 13901)

Ray, B.M. (1985). Measuring the social position of the mainstreamed handicapped child. *Exceptional Children, 52,* 57–62.

Resnick, L.B. (1987). The 1987 presidential address: Learning in school and out. *Educational Researcher, 16*(9), 13–20.

Reynolds, M.C., Wang, M.C., & Walberg, H.J. (1987). The necessary restructuring of special and regular education. *Exceptional Children, 53,* 391–399.

Roddy, J. (1980). *Integrating normal and severely handicapped children using a peer tutoring approach.* Unpublished doctoral dissertation, University of Wisconsin–Madison.

Ross, W.E., & Hannay, L.M. (1986). Towards a critical theory of reflective inquiry. *Journal of Teacher Education, 37*(4), 9–15.

Rubenstein, J., & Howes, C. (1976). The effects of peers on toddler interaction with mother and toys. *Child Development, 47,* 597–605.

Rudrud, E.H., Rice, J.M., Robertson, J.M., & Tolson, N.M. (1984). The use of self-monitoring to increase and maintain production rates. *Vocational Evaluation and Work Adjustments, 17*(1), 14–17.

Rusch, F.R., Martin, J.E., & White, D.M. (1985). Competitive employment: Teaching mentally retarded employees to maintain their work behavior. *Education and Training of the Mentally Retarded, 20,* 182–189.

Rynders, J.E., Johnson, R.T., Johnson, D.W., & Schmidt, B. (1980). Producing positive interaction among Down syndrome and nonhandicapped teenagers. *American Journal of Mental Deficiency, 85,* 268–273.

Sailor, W., & Guess, D. (1983). *Severely handicapped students: An instructional design.* Boston: Houghton-Mifflin.

Sailor, W., Halvorsen, A., Anderson, J., Goetz, L., Gee, K., Doering, K., & Hunt, P. (1986). Community intensive instruction. In R.H. Horner, L.H. Meyer, & H.D.B. Fredericks (Eds.), *Education of learners with severe handicaps: Exemplary service strategies* (pp. 251–288). Baltimore: Paul H. Brookes Publishing Co.

Sailor, W., Wilcox, B., & Brown, L. (Eds.). (1980). *Methods of instruction for severely handicapped students.* Baltimore: Paul H. Brookes Publishing Co.

Sandberg, L.D. (1982). Attitudes of nonhandicapped elementary school students toward school-aged trainable mentally retarded students. *Education and Training of the Mentally Retarded, 17,* 30–34.

Sapon-Shevin, M. (1987). The national education reports and special education: Implications for students. *Exceptional Children, 53,* 300–306.

Sarason, B.R., Sarason, I.G., Hacker, A.T., & Basham, R.B. (1985). Concomitants of social support: Social skills, physical attractiveness, and gender. *Journal of Personality and Social Psychology, 49,* 469–480.

Sarason, I.G., & Sarason, B.R. (1986). Experimentally provided social support. *Journal of Personality and Social Psychology, 50,* 1222–1225.

Sarason, S.B. (1983). *Schooling in America: Scapegoat and salvation.* New York: Free Press.

Sarason, S., Davidson, K., & Blatt, B. (1986). *Teacher preparation: An unstudied problem in education* (rev. ed.). New York: John Wiley & Sons.

Sarason, S.B., & Doris, J. (1979). *Educational handicaps, public policy, and social history: A broadened perspective on mental retardation.* New York: Free Press.

Savage, G.T. (1985, May). *A critical theory of dialogue: A review and critique of Habermas' theory of universal pragmatics and implications for theories of decision making and negotiation.* Paper presented at the annual meeting of the International Communication Association, Honolulu.

Schleien, S., & Ray, M.T. (1988). *Community recreation and persons with disabilities: Strategies for integration.* Baltimore: Paul H. Brookes Publishing Co.

Schleien, S.J., Ray, M.T., Soderman-Olson, M.L., & McMahon, K.T. (1987). Intergrating children with moderate to severe cognitive deficits into a community museum program. *Education and Training in Mental Retardation, 22,* 112–120.

Schloss, P.J., Schloss, C.N., Wood, C.E., & Kiehl, W.S. (1986). A critical review of social skills research with behaviorally disordered students. *Behavioral Disorders, 12,* 1–14.

Schumaker, J.B., & Hazel, J.S. (1984). Social skills assessment and training for the learning disabled: Who's on first and what's on second? Part II. *Journal of Learning Disabilities, 17,* 492–499.

Scott, B.S., & Gilliam, J.E. (1987). Curriculum as a behavior management tool for students with autism. *Focus on Autistic Behavior, 2,* 1–8.

Sears, C.S. (1981). A process of compliance with P.L. 94-142. *Journal of The Association for the Severely Handicapped, 6*(1), 22–29.

Shafer, M.S., & Inge, K.J. (1986). Acquisition, generalization, and maintenance of automated banking skills. *Education and Training of the Mentally Retarded, 21,* 265–272.

Shaw, A.M., & Emilsson, E. (1984, June). *Negotiation, strategies, and whose fault was it anyway?* Paper presented at the Conference of Mexico Teachers of English to Speakers of other Languages, Mexico City.

Shores, R.E. (1987). Overview of research on social interaction: A historical and personal perspective. *Behavioral Disorders, 12*, 233–242.

Siders, J.Z., Riall, A., Bennett, T.C., & Judd, D. (1987). Training leadership personnel in early intervention: A transdisciplinary approach. *Teacher Education and Special Education, 10*(4), 161–170.

Singer, J.D., & Butler, J.A. (1987). The Education for All Handicapped Children Act: Schools as agents of reform. *Harvard Educational Review, 57*(1), 125–152.

Sitlington, P.L., & Easterday, J.R. (1986). *Analysis of employer incentive rankings relative to employment of retarded persons. COMPETE: Community-based model for public school exit and transition to employment.* Bloomington: Indiana University, School of Education.

Skiba, R., Wesson, C., & Deno, L.L. (1982). *The effects of training teachers in the use of formative evaluation in reading: An experimental-control comparison* (Research report No. 88). Minneapolis: University of Minneosta, Institute for Research on Learning Disabilities.

Skrtic, T.M. (1987, April). *An organizational analysis of special education reform.* Presented at the Annual Meeting of the American Educational Research Association, Washington, DC.

Smelkin, L.P., & Lieberman, L.L. (1984). Educating students' awareness of mainstreaming concerns: Implications for improving training programs. *Education, 104*, 258–263.

Smith-Davis, J., Burke, P.J., & Noel, M. (1984). *Personnel to educate the handicapped in America: Supply and demand from a pragmatic viewpoint.* College Park: University of Maryland.

Snell, M. (Ed.). (1978). *Systematic instruction of the moderately and severely handicapped.* Columbus, OH: Charles E. Merrill.

Snell, M.E. (Ed.). (1983). *Systematic instruction of the moderately and severely handicapped* (2nd ed.). Columbus, OH: Charles E. Merrill.

Snell, M.E. (1986). *Systematic instruction of the moderately and severely handicapped* (3rd ed.). Columbus, OH: Charles E. Merrill.

Snell, M.E., & Beckman, B.S. (1984). Family involvement in intervention with children having severe handicaps. *Journal of The Association for Persons with Severe Handicaps, 9*, 213–230.

Sontag, E. (Ed.). (1977). *Educational programming for the severely and profoundly handicapped.* Reston, VA: Council for Exceptional Children.

Sontag, E., & Smith, J. (1978). BEH and S/PH: The interface and the impact. In N. Haring & D. Bricker (Eds.), *Teaching the severely handicapped* (Vol. 3, pp. 34–48). Seattle: American Association for the Education of the Severely/Profoundly Handicapped.

Stainback, S., & Stainback, W. (1984). Broadening the research perspective in special education. *Exceptional Children, 50*, 400–408.

Stainback, S., & Stainback, W. (1987). Integration versus cooperation: A commentary on "Educating Children with Learning Problems: A Shared Responsibility." *Exceptional Children, 54*, 66–69.

Stainback, S., Stainback, W., Courtnage, L., & Joken, T. (1985). Facilitating mainstreaming by modifying the mainstream. *Exceptional Children, 52*, 144–153.

Stainback, S., Stainback, W., & Forest, M. (Eds.). (1989). *Educating all students in the mainstream of regular education.* Baltimore: Paul H. Brookes Publishing Co.

Stainback, S., Stainback, W., Strathe, M., & Dedrick, C. (1983). Preparing regular educators for the integration of severely handicapped students: An experimental study. *Education and Training of the Mentally Retarded, 18*, 205–209.

Stainback, S., Stainback, W., Wehman, P., & Spangiers, L. (1983). Acquisition and generalization of physical fitness exercises in three profoundly retarded adults. *Journal of The Association for the Severely Handicapped, 8*(2), 47–55.

Stainback, W., Stainback, S., & Strathe, M. (1983). Generalization of positive social behavior by severely handicapped students: A review and analysis of research. *Education and Training of the Mentally Retarded, 18*, 293–299.

Stallard, C.K. (1982). Computers and education for exceptional children: Emerging applications. *Exceptional Children, 49*, 102–104.

Sternat, J., Messina, R., Nietupski, J., Lyon, S., & Brown, L. (1977). Occupational and physical therapy services for severely handicapped students. In E. Sontag, J. Smith, & N. Certo (Eds.), *Educational programming for the severely and profoundly handicapped* (pp. 263–278). Reston, VA: Council for Exceptional Children.

Stevens, D. (1980). How teachers perceive computers in the classroom. *AEDS Journal, 13*(3), 221–232.

Stoddard, D.W. (1987). The Oregon High School secondary education model for students with Down syndrome. In S.M. Pueschel, C. Tingey, J.E. Rynders, A.C. Crocker, & D.M. Crutcher (Eds.), *New perspectives on Down syndrome* (pp. 225–232). Baltimore: Paul H. Brookes Publishing Co.

Stokes, T.T., & Baer, D.M. (1977). An implicit technology of generalization. *Journal of Applied Behavior Analysis, 10*, 349–367.

Storey, K., Bates, P., & Hanson, H.B. (1984). Acquisition and generalization of coffee purchase skills by adults with severe disabilities. *Journal of The Association for Persons with Severe Handicaps, 9*, 178–185.

Stowitschek, J.J., & Stowitschek, C.E. (1984). Once more with feeling: The absence of research on teacher use of micro-computers. *Exceptional Education Quarterly, 4*(4), 23–29.

Strain, P.S., & Odom, S.L. (1986). Peer social initiations: Effective intervention for social skills development of exceptional children. *Exceptional Children, 52*, 543–551.

Strully, J., & Strully, C. (1985). Friendship and our children. *Journal of The Association for Persons with Severe Handicaps, 10*, 224–227.

Tateyama-Sniezek, K.M. (1989). The effects of stimulus variation on the generalization performance of students with moderate retardation. *Education and Training in Mental Retardation, 24*, 89–94.

Taylor, B.O. (1986, April). *Metasensemaking: How the effective elementary principal accomplishes school improvement.* Paper presented at the annual meeting of the American Educational Research Association, San Francisco.

Taylor, S.J. (1988). Caught in the continuum: A critical analysis of the principle of least restrictive environment. *Journal of The Association for Persons with Severe Handicaps, 13*, 41–53.

Taylor, S.J., Biklen, D., & Knoll, J. (1987). *Community integration for people with severe disabilities.* New York: Teachers College Press.

Thomas, M.A. (Ed.). (1976). *Hey, don't forget about me!* Reston, VA: Council for Exceptional Children.

Tinsley, T.E., Jr. (1984). Data base management systems. In M.M. Behrmann & L. Lahm (Eds.), *Proceedings of the National Conference on the Use of Microcomputers in Special Education* (pp. 64–72). Reston, VA: Council for Exceptional Children.

Tom, A.R. (1987). A critique of the rationale for extended teacher preparation. *Educational Policy, 1*, 43–56.

Twain, K.R. (1986). *Parental participation in IEP conferences.* Unpublished master's thesis, University of Oregon, Specialized Training Program, Eugene.

Twentieth Century Fund Task Force on Federal Elementary and Secondary Education Policy. (1983). *Making the grade.* New York: Author.

Van Hasselt, V.B., Hersen, M., Whitehall, M.B., & Bellack, S.S. (1979). Social skill assessment and training for children: An evaluation review. *Behaviour Research and Therapy, 17*, 413–437.

Van Walleghem, J. (1986). *The effect of learning to use a computer data management program on special education teachers' measurement practices.* Unpublished doctoral dissertation, University of Idaho, Moscow.

Vincent, L., Salisbury, C., Walker, G., Brown, L., Gruenewald, L., & Powers, M. (1980). Program evaluation and curriculum development in early childhood/special education: Criteria of the next environment. In W. Sailor, B. Wilcox, & L. Brown (Eds.), *Methods of instruction for severely handicapped students* (pp. 303–328). Baltimore: Paul H. Brookes Publishing Co.

Voeltz, L. (1980). Children's attitudes toward handicapped peers. *American Journal of Mental Deficiency, 84*, 455–464.

Voeltz, L.M. (1982). Effects of structured interactions with severely handicapped peers on children's attitudes. *American Journal of Mental Deficiency, 86*, 380–390.

Voeltz, L.M., Wuerch, B.B., & Bockhaut, C.H. (1982). Social validation of leisure activities training with severely handicapped youth. *Journal of The Association for the Severely Handicapped, 7*(4), 3–13.

Waldo, L.J., Wulz, S., Klien, D., Hall, M., Meyers, S., & Carpenter, S. (1981). *A comprehensive communication curriculum for the education of severely multiply handicapped school children: Handicapped children's model program: Final report.* Topeka: Kansas Neurological Institute. (ERIC Document Reproduction Service No. ED 221 964).

Walker, H.M., & Calkins, C.F. (1986). The role of social competence in the community adjustment of persons with developmental disabilities: Process and outcome. *Remedial and Special Education, 7*(6), 46–53.

Walker, H.M., & Hops, H. (1976). Increasing academic achievement by reinforcing direct academic performance and/or facilitative nonacademic responses. *Journal of Educational Psychology, 68*, 218–225.

Walker, H.M., McConnell, S., Walker, J.L., Clarke, J.Y., Todis, B., Cohen, G., & Rankin, R. (1983). Initial analysis of the ACCEPTS curriculum: Efficacy of instructional and behavior management procedures for improving the social adjustment of handicapped children. *Analysis and Intervention in Developmental Disabilities, 3*, 105–127.

Wesson, C. (1984). Data based program modification: A disk for monitoring student progress. In M.C. Behrmann & L. Lahm (Eds.), *Proceedings of the National Conference on the Use of Microcomputers in Special Education* (pp. 55–61). Reston, VA: Council for Exceptional Children.

Wesson, C., Deno, L.L., & Mirkin, P. (1982). *Research on developing and monitoring progress on IEP goals: Current findings and implications for practice* (Monograph No. 18). Minneapolis: University of Minnesota, Institute for Research on Learning Disabilities.

White, O.R., & Liberty, K.A. (1976). Behavioral assessment and precise educational measurement. In N.G. Haring & R.L. Schiefelbusch (Eds), *Teaching special children* (pp. 31–71). New York: McGraw-Hill.

Whitney, G.C., & Hunsaker, P.L. (1983). Learning negotiation skills through simulation. *Simulation and Games, 14*(4), 391–399.

Whitney, R., & Striefel, S. (1981). Functionality and generalization in training the severely and profoundly handicapped. *Journal of Special Education Technology, 4*(3), 33–39.

Wilcox, B., & Bellamy, G. (1982). *Design of high school programs for severely handicapped students.* Baltimore: Paul H. Brookes Publishing Co.

Wilcox, B., & Bellamy, G.T. (1987a). *The activities catalog: An alternative curriculum for youth and adults with severe disabilities.* Baltimore: Paul H. Brookes Publishing Co.

Wilcox, B., & Bellamy, G.T. (1987b). Secondary education for students with Down syndrome: Implementing quality services. In S.M. Pueschel, C. Tingey, J.E. Rynders, A.C. Crocker, & D.M. Crutcher (Eds.), *New perspectives on Down syndrome* (pp. 203–224). Baltimore: Paul H. Brookes Publishing Co.

Wilcox, B., & York, R. (Eds.). (1982). *Quality education for the severely handicapped*. Falls Church, VA: Counterpoint Handcrafted Books.

Williams, W., & York, R. (1978). Developing instructional programs for severely handicapped students. In N.G. Haring & D.D. Bricker (Eds.), *Teaching the severely handicapped* (Vol. 3, pp. 124–152). Seattle: American Association for the Education of the Severely/Profoundly Handicapped.

Wilson, M.S., & Fox, B.J. (1982). Computer administered bilingual language assessment and intervention. *Exceptional Children, 49,* 145–149.

Wine, J.D. (1981). From defect to competence models. In J.D. Wine & M.D. Smye (Eds.), *Social competence* (pp. 3–36). New York: Guilford Press.

Wirth, P.A., Stile, S.W., & Cole, J.T. (1983). The need for inservice training in instructional technology for special education personnel in small rural school districts. *Journal of Special Education Technology, 6*(1), 25–29.

Wolery, M., & Dyk, L. (1985). Arena assessment: Description and preliminary social validity data. *Journal of The Association for Persons with Severe Handicaps, 9,* 231–235.

Zartman, W. (1977). Negotiation as a joint decision-making process. *Journal of Conflict Resolution, 21*(4), 619–638.

Zeichner, K.M. (1983). Alternative paradigms on teacher education. *Journal of Teacher Education, 34,* 3–9.

CHAPTER 18

Integrated Related Services

WINNIE DUNN

University of Kansas Medical Center, Kansas City, Kansas

In the 1970s and 1980s, significant cultural and political events have occurred that have altered the demands placed on the professional disciplines involved in the provision of related services to individuals with severe disabilities. Prior to this time, these professionals routinely provided services within hospitals or other clinical settings, using a medical model to address client needs. Persons requiring services were most frequently seen individually to work on those skill components that were considered the expertise of each discipline. When various professionals met to discuss a case, a large portion of time was spent with each discipline reporting their findings and treatment plans, and little time was spent determining methods for collaboration or intervention outside the clinic setting. Children with significant impairments were frequently placed in special schools, hospitals, or agencies, and the same model of discipline-specific services was carried into these settings. The passage of Section 504 of the Rehabilitation Act in 1973 and PL 94-142 in 1975 can be cited as significant events that marked the turn from this model of services toward more inclusionary, interdependent, and team-oriented models. As the traditional medical model does not apply to this framework, therapists have encountered both a new role and new environments within which to provide services (Dunn, 1988; Ottenbacher, 1982).

Much progress has been made in creating effective strategies for therapeutic intervention. As in any dynamic system, however, the demands of the educational environment have also changed at a rapid pace; many strategies considered "best practices" in the late 1970s are not considered so today. Professionals have sometimes struggled to keep pace as changes in expectations have occurred. As all professionals become more familiar with the unique contributions made by each discipline on the interdisciplinary team, there will be a confluence of ideas so that growth and change can be synchronized. This chapter is intended as a contribution to that process of synchronization.

The chapter has two purposes. The first is to review work in the related services that supports the goal of integrating these services with the services of other professionals and into natural settings. This integration requires that assessment, planning, intervention, and program evaluation are: 1) performed within natural environments, and 2) designed in collaboration with others to address functional skills development and generalization of behavior to all relevant settings. The second purpose of the chapter is to recommend directions for future administrative, research, and intervention practices in the related services.

There are many professional disciplines that are considered related services, including occupational therapy, speech/language pathology, physical therapy, psychology, recreation, and audiology. Although any of these professional disciplines could be integral to a comprehensive array of services, the present chapter focuses on occupational therapy, physical therapy, and speech/language services; these are the services most commonly provided to individuals with severe disabilities as part of a free and appropriate public education in the United States.

MULTIPLE DIMENSIONS OF INTEGRATION

A discussion of integrated related services is complicated by the fact that the literature addresses several types of integration without clarification of their similarities and differences. At least four aspects of integration may be described: peer integration, functional integration, practice integration, and comprehensive integration. These categories can exist separately or in concert with each other as diagrammed in Figure 18.1.

Peer integration occurs when typical children and children with special needs are placed together. The most common example of peer integration occurs when a child with a disability is placed in a regular education classroom during the school day. However, peer integration also includes social and recreational activities and vocational opportunities.

Functional integration occurs when professionals apply therapeutic strategies to an individual's life environments. Figure 18.1 demonstrates the relationship between related services expertise and work, school, living, and/or leisure environments. Functional integration is increasingly being recognized as an important goal within therapeutic disciplines:

Physical therapists in educational environments should consider utilizing the classroom as a therapeutic environment in order to ensure the functional usefulness of skills being taught and the generalization of skills to environments in which they are needed. (American Physical Therapy Association [APTA], 1980, p. 42)

Arrow A on Figure 18.1 represents those situations that combine peer and functional integration. Therapeutic strategies are applied to those life environments that are age appropriate and contain typical children alongside children with special needs. For example, when a therapist teaches peers to reinforce language attempts during free play, combined peer and functional integration occur.

Practice integration occurs when professionals from more than one discipline (e.g., teachers and therapists) collaborate to design a combined approach to meet a child's needs. In

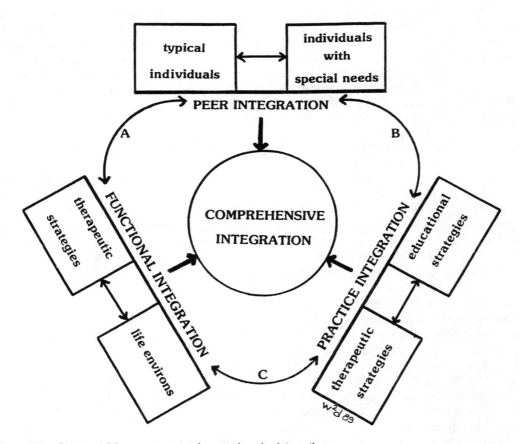

Figure 18.1. Diagram of the components of comprehensive integration.

order to implement practice integration successfully, professionals must be knowledgeable about the unique contributions of their own discipline and the potential contributions of others. For example, a teacher and therapist may design an activity that requires reaching and pointing. The teacher may contribute ideas about the concepts to be addressed, while the therapist may design facilitation techniques that would support muscle and joint actions during the reaching portion of the activity. Practice integration strategies cannot be designed by using single-discipline knowledge. Practice integration most fequently occurs between special education teachers and therapists, but may also occur between related services disciplines.

Arrow B on Figure 18.1 represents those situations that combine the collaborative efforts of teachers and therapists (practice integration) with peer integration. Regular classroom teachers are more likely to be involved in this pattern of integration, since they direct these age-appropriate life environments. Collaborative efforts with regular classroom teachers may be different from collaboration with special educators. For example, regular education teachers may have received very different training than special education teachers have received, demanding a shift in the approaches taken by related personnel.

Arrow C on Figure 18.1 represents those situations in which collaborative efforts and functional considerations within life environments are combined. Although not optimal, this combination can occur in a segregated environment, such as a self-contained special education classroom in a regular school. For example, the therapist could move furniture around in the special education classroom so that a child independently manipulates the wheelchair to the computer station (functional integration), and the teacher and the therapist might collaborate to design the proper computer input device and choose appropriate software for the child's reading level.

Comprehensive integration combines all three areas of integration, and thus is the optimum situation. Children with special needs are served in age-appropriate environments with peers who do not have disabilities. Therapeutic expertise is applied to the needs of the child within the peer environment to optimize independence and participation during activities. Therapists and teachers collaborate to make instructional activities therapeutic.

There are presently many situations in which only one or perhaps two types of integration are occurring. Professionals must create strategies for incorporating other types of integration into learning, working, and living environments. The work of related services professionals should involve all of the types of integration just described.

PROVIDING THERAPEUTIC SERVICES IN NATURAL CONTEXTS

The concept of integrating therapeutic interventions into daily life tasks is not a new one to most related services fields. For example, the philosophical constructs of occupational therapy are based on the concept of purposeful activity or those tasks that have meaning for the individual, believing that this characteristic provides intrinsic motivation to persist in reaching goals (Breines, 1984; P.N. Clark, 1979; Fidler & Fidler, 1978; Hinojosa, Sabari, Rosenfeld, & Shapiro, 1983; Kircher, 1984; W.L. West, 1984). Kircher and Steinbeck found that persons without disabilities persisted significantly longer on an identical task of exertion when the task had an identifiable purpose, rather than when perceived merely as an exercise. Gliner (1985) proposed that professionals create normal life events within which to learn or relearn motor skills, suggesting that actor and environment are inseparable.

These concepts have been reflected in changes in practice across disciplines. Physical therapy emphasizes the biological and mechanical support necessary to enable independent movement and activity (Harris, 1981; Hulme, Gallacher, Walsh, Niesen, & Waldron, 1987; Nakaoka, Ishida, Nishiwaki, & Manabe, 1984; Taylor & Harris, 1986). However, physical therapists are recognizing that people do not transfer new motor skills from isolated practice situations to everyday movements like walking (Gonnella, Hale, Ionta, & Perry, 1981). Although technical aspects of speech and language have been part of the speech/language pathology literature, a greater emphasis is now being placed on the context of communication (Halle, 1982; Oliver & Halle, 1982; Warren & Kaiser, 1986). There is an emphasis on establishing natural environments that cue, support, direct, and reinforce spontaneous communication. And so the conceptual groundwork is present; the task becomes one of discovering successful strategies for making these philosophies apparent in the provision of services in natural settings.

MODELS OF
RELATED SERVICES PROVISION

The evolution in practice from an isolated therapeutic model to an integrated one has been a long, sometimes difficult process that remains incomplete. Early arguments for integrated services were advanced by Sternat, Messina, Nietupski, Lyon, and Brown (1977). These authors described an isolated therapy model as reflecting the following underlying assumptions: 1) the motor skills manifested in the therapy room are also manifested in other settings, 2) the normal sequence of skill acquisition can be applied as intervention with persons with disabilities, 3) intervention once or twice a week will substantially affect overall motor skill development, and 4) skills developed in the isolated environment will then be observed in other environments. The corresponding assumptions of integrated therapy were described as follows: 1) motor assessment is most useful in natural environments, 2) clusters of functional skills are the best therapeutic goals, 3) longitudinal and contextual intervention will be most successful, and 4) skills are only useful when they are demonstrated in the necessary life task. Although this contrast may suggest that the only way service provision occurs is via one extreme or the other, a wider array of service models is actually available.

For example, the American Occupational Therapy Association (AOTA) (1987, 1989) has recommended a broad model of service provision appropriate for the public schools. A comprehensive program of services to the full range of students in a school district includes all types of service provision. Several specific models were described.

Direct Therapy

Direct therapy includes both individual and small-group activities between the student(s) and the therapist focused on meeting individualized student needs. Direct therapy is reserved for those student needs that require specialized therapeutic interventions that cannot be safely carried out by others (Dunn & Campbell, in press). For example, some sensory integration and neurodevelopmental treatment strategies might activate autonomic nervous system responses, such as quick changes in heart rate or breathing, sweating, or eye dilation. These reactions suggest a significant change in the nervous system's level of responsivity, and signal a need to alter the level of arousal or input. Direct therapy would be the choice in these cases, because the therapist would know how to alter the stimuli quickly in response to needs.

Monitoring

Monitoring is a service provision strategy that acknowledges the importance of both specialized expertise and the need for consistent application of strategies across environments. The therapist uses specialized knowledge to evaluate and develop program strategies but trains persons in the individual's life environments to carry out activities with therapeutic goals in mind. The therapist remains responsible for the outcomes of these specific intervention strategies and remains in regular contact with the person(s) carrying out the program to ensure that: 1) the health and safety of the student are protected at all times, 2) the individual implementing the strategies demonstrates correct use of the procedures without cues, and 3) the implementor identifies all precautions and signs of failure and takes appropriate action without cues. Since the therapist cannot be with the implementor and student at all times, the two "without-cues" criteria are vital to the first criterion of safety. The American Physical Therapy Association (1980) and Connolly and Anderson (1978) also supported the concept of monitored programs for physical therapists. Monitored programs with ongoing contact have been suggested by Rainforth and York (1987) and P.H. Campbell (1987b) as a means to ensure continued quality programming. Reichle and Keogh (1985) noted that therapists must be skilled at training classroom personnel in what to look for and how to carry out interventions. They also noted the need for empirical data relative to the effectiveness of this service strategy.

Consultation

Consultation, the third service provision category (AOTA, 1989), differs from direct therapy and monitoring in that the responsibility for outcomes rests with the consultee, usually the teacher. The therapist serves as a consultant, provides therapy-based expertise and collaborates with the consultee to solve problems (e.g., for knowledge of developmental or sensorimotor principles that support adaptive behaviors, see Dunn, 1988, 1990; Sternat et al., 1977). The APTA (1980) and Connolly and Anderson (1978) suggested that consultation expands the effectiveness of physical therapy expertise.

Three types of consultation have been discussed as relevant to public school service provision (AOTA, 1989). *Case consultation* focuses attention on the specific needs of an individual student. For example, the teacher and the therapist might collaborate to design a strategy for positioning that facilitates group participation of a student with poor social interaction skills. *Colleague consultation* involves activities that improve the skills of a peer (e.g., classroom teacher) and frequently occurs along with case consultation. For example, the therapist and the teacher might collaborate to design techniques that maintain an appropriate level of arousal in the students during morning activities. *System consultation* addresses problems or issues that affect the agency, school district, and so on. For example, the therapist may participate in a preschool parent-education program, conduct an architectual barriers assessment, or serve on a district-level curriculum committee.

Consultation models similar to those just described have been advanced in the language intervention literature. Marvin (1987) described the combination of case and colleague consultation as the teacher approaches the speech/language pathologist to seek assistance for program development and implementation on a specific case. The teacher remains the actual service provider, but can create more effective strategies because of this input. C.R. Campbell, Stremel-Campbell, and Rogers-Warren (1985) discussed three models of service provision that can be used to meet the needs of students with severe disabilities. In the first, the teacher serves as the facilitator, while the speech/language pathologist serves as the primary trainer; this model utilizes direct intervention and functional integration to meet children's needs. The second model assigns the teacher to the role of primary trainer, but the speech/language pathologist is available as a consultant; this description is compatible with the consultant roles described by AOTA (1989). The third model refers to situations where no direct support from related services professionals is available to the teacher.

Stremel-Campbell and Campbell (1985) commented that with models such as these a shift in professional goals has to occur. Whereas therapists previously emphasized helping a student to meet a set of performance criteria through direct therapy, now therapists must work toward the attainment of spontaneous language use in a variety of contexts. Since the speech/language pathologist cannot be in all of those environments, new professional skills must also be acquired. Now the therapist must know how to train other adults, embed interventions within natural environments, and identify or create natural consequences within those environments (Halle, 1982).

In the language domain, Reichle and Keogh (1985) advocated for a combination approach to addressing the related services needs of children with severe disabilities. When a child is severely disabled, he or she may not generate enough opportunities to practice language. Reichle and Keogh (1985) suggested that more structured strategies may be effective to produce the language components, while monitoring and consultation may be more effectively chosen for generalization and spontaneous use. A flexible approach such as this one, which is based on differentiation of needs, is likely to be most effective.

Consultation Strategies

Consultative strategies have been discussed extensively in the organizational psychology, school psychology, mental health, and, more recently, special education literature (e.g., Idol, Paolucci-Whitcomb, & Nevin, 1986; Pryzwansky & White, 1983; West & Idol, 1987). Although several models of consultation have been investigated (e.g., expert, medical, mental health), the consensus is that *collaborative consultation* is the most preferred and has the potential to yield the most productive outcomes (Babcock & Pryzwansky, 1983; Pryzwansky & White, 1983). Idol et al. (1986) defined collaborative consultation as "an interactive process that enables people with diverse expertise to generate creative solutions to mutually defined problems. The outcome is enhanced, altered, and produces solutions that are different from those that the individual team members would produce independently" (p. 1). In this model of consultation, both the consultant and the consultee share responsibility for identifying the problem, planning strategies, evaluating effectiveness, and altering plans as necessary (Idol et al., 1986). In addition to solving the current educational problem, a second goal of collaborative consultation is to increase the consultee's skills for dealing with similar problems in the future (Gutkin & Curtis, 1982; Marvin, 1987; J.F. West & Idol, 1987).

There are a number of advantages to collaborative consultation when it is applied to services for individuals with severe disabilities. Communication among team members is required, and specialized expertise becomes a tool of the team rather than an end in itself. Student needs are the focus of attention; the educational label or medical diagnosis does not drive the decision-making process. The team owns the problems and the solutions; therefore all members take both credit and responsibility for successes and failures. Students get more opportunities to develop essential skills because the team members are collaborating on an integrated approach. Because team members are all involved in the planning process, decisions are more likely to be based on data and functional analyses of behaviors to determine both direction and priorities (Idol et al., 1986).

A number of authors have summarized the core principles of collaboration (Damico, 1987; Idol et al., 1986; Marvin, 1987). Basic communication skills underlie all of the principles.

First of all, team members must demonstrate mutual respect. From this premise emerges an ability to determine leadership by situational demands, and to participate in conflict resolution. Team members must also utilize active listening, productive interviewing techniques, jargon-free oral and written communication, and positive nonverbal language when collaborating. Damico suggested that therapeutic professionals establish "consulting office hours" to establish the equivalent importance for consultation among the other professional duties and to provide flexibility within the work schedule for meeting with school personnel. Furthermore, strategies such as careful documentation of how consultation time is spent will validate its productivity to teachers, principals, and school district administrators.

Although the literature has discussed collaboration in relation to the consulting model of service provision, it seems that collaborative principles apply to all integrated service provision strategies. Direct therapy can be part of a collaborative plan by being provided within educational, work, leisure, or living environments. The hallmark of both collaboration and integrated related services is communication and mutual respect.

Research on Consultation

Research on outcomes of consultative service provision to students with severe disabilities is sparse. Dunn (1990) compared the use of direct intervention and consultation in preschool programs for children with developmental delays. Findings revealed that although both service provision models yielded the same percentage of goals being met (approximately 70%), when teachers collaborated in a consultation model, they reported that the occupational therapist contributed to 24% more of the goal attainment. Peck, Killen, and Baumgart (1989) reported on a "nondirective" consultation technique used to increase implementation of language intervention in mainstream preschools. Using an intrasubject design replicated across 5 subjects in two independent experiments, they demonstrated that consultation could effectively facilitate teachers to develop effective intervention strategies for simple language goals. Importantly, teachers generalized use of the techniques they had developed to situations that had not been the focus of consultation. This "spread" of effects from collaborative consultation is, of course, one of its most important goals.

DECIDING AMONG MODELS

Decisions regarding the amount and type of related services provision should be made by the interdisciplinary team. Dunn and Campbell (in press) suggested that service provision models are selected according to the level of interference of the problem in relation to targeted outcomes. Rourk, Dunn, Wendt, Stephens, and Andrews (1987) recommended that several parameters be used to determine the most appropriate complement of related services provision strategies.

A thorough discussion of these parameters can be found in the AOTA (1989) document; some examples are provided here.

1. *Potential for functional improvement* A therapist must determine the necessary level of related services involvement in order for the student to make functional gains. For example, a student who moves from tube feeding to mouth feeding may require more intense related services involvement initially to make this functional change successfully; after the new pattern of behavior is established, a shift in service provision strategies would be appropriate.

2. *Expertise of other professionals in the educational environment* A related services professional may need more frequent on-site contact with a regular classroom teacher who has just received his or her first student with moderate disabilities for integrated placement. A therapist may spend less time with an experienced special educator with whom a productive collaborative relationship has already been established.

3. *Age of the student* This does not involve assigning priority for services to any particular age, but rather refers to the relationship between the student's chronological age and the natural cultural expectations for persons of that age group. Related services are provided in relation to the student's ability to meet age-appropriate

expectations. For example, a 10-year-old student who is meeting the challenges of his or her elementary classroom may not presently require high-intensity related services involvement. That same student may require an increase in related services involvement when he or she is 13 years old and is preparing to enter a middle school involving a whole new set of demands.

The above parameters and others (see AOTA, 1989), serve as a mechanism to remind professionals of the active relationship between the student's needs and the integrity of environmental variables. Integrated programming thus requires constant evaluation to determine the delicate balance of strategies that will produce life independence.

WORKING AS TEAM MEMBERS

A critical aspect of comprehensive integration is teamwork among the professionals serving the child and his or her family. Munson, Nordquist, and Thuma-Rew (1987) summarized three major types of teams often described in the literature. *Multidisciplinary teams* contain a range of professionals who work individually to provide evaluation and intervention from each of their own perspectives. Meetings among the team members are not routine, and may even occur rarely. *Transdisciplinary teams* contain several professionals, each of whom evaluates the child, but then the team members contribute to one program plan that has components from each discipline. One team member serves as the primary intervention agent to carry out the plan on behalf of the team. *Interdisciplinary teams* also contain a varied group of professionals. The team works with the child, family, and other agencies to develop a comprehensive program; the emphasis is on the total needs of the child. A core team provides the total care plan, with input from routinely scheduled meetings.

Issues Affecting Team Functioning

Team structure obviously affects the functioning of the team. However, no one team structure may be best for all situations; some authors have maintained that the needs of particular clients and the characteristics of particular settings should dictate the team structure (Musselwhite & St. Louis, 1982). For example, a transdisciplinary team approach may not work well initially in a special education classroom led by a teacher with very little knowledge of the related services. Group dynamics among the persons serving on the team must also be considered; an interdisciplinary team model may function more smoothly after the members have worked together for a period of time.

A number of characteristics have been associated with the success of team interactions. Yoshida (1980) found that team member participation was positively correlated to satisfaction with the decisions made. More decisions are carried out when team members are part of making the decisions, and when clear assignments of responsibility are made during the team meeting (Yoshida, 1980). Kaiser and Woodman (1985) suggested that team decision making is more effective when structured group strategies are used to formulate decisions.

Team members can find it stimulating and satisfying to work together (Abelson & Woodman, 1983). However, teams are not always effective in these ways. Attendance without involvement in the group process leads to negative attitudes. Members may feel pressured to conform, leading to support of poor decisions and reduction of problem solving. Teams can be time consuming, and if outcomes do not seem to be effective, resentment can build.

Building Effective Teams

P. H. Campbell (1987b) and Rainforth and York (1987) discussed strategies for developing *integrated programming teams*. Several principles seem to form the foundation for this process. First, team goals and objectives form a picture of a student performing successfully within the appropriate environment; they are not recognizable as specific discipline strategies (P. H. Campbell, 1987b; Dunn, 1987; Rainforth & York, 1987). Second, each team member contributes specialized knowledge to the problem-solving process to meet the student's needs (P. H. Campbell, 1987b; Dunn, 1988; Rainforth & York, 1987). Third, team members design assessment, inter-

vention, data-collection, and supervision strategies that incorporate all areas of expertise into selected functional life tasks, while maintaining a safe learning environment for the student (AOTA, 1989; P. H. Campbell, 1987b; Rainforth & York, 1987). Ongoing strategies for training and monitoring both team member implementation and student progress reduce risks that might be associated with integrated programming (AOTA, 1989; P. H. Campbell, 1987b). In order for integrated programming to be successful, discipline specialists recognize that their value to the team is not in designing an elaborate direct service treatment plan, but rather in drawing upon their unique frames of reference to assess environmental variables, consider the impact of student abilities and needs on functional performance in chosen environments, and create ways to weave effective strategies into a collaborative instructional sequence.

Scheduling is a pragmatic consideration, and must be more flexible for integrated programming than traditional approaches allow. Rainforth and York (1987) suggested that related services personnel arrange a weekly schedule that contains blocks of time for classrooms focused on integrated and community-based instruction. This would allow the teacher and related services professional to plan according to individualized needs for each week. Other times are blocked for direct services in regular education (Rainforth & York, 1987).

Effective task analysis is a cornerstone of integrated team programming (P. H. Campbell, 1987a; P. H. Campbell & Wetherbee, 1988). P. H. Campbell (1987a) discussed the performance of essential skills to enable independent functioning; these are simple forms of behavior with inherent value that also provide the basis for more complex behavior. Looking, vocalizing, reaching, and manipulation are examples of essential skills (P. H. Campbell, 1987a). Integrated programming teams design appropriate interventions by organizing information they acquire about essential skills into functional outcomes. Occupational and physical therapists are likely to contribute information to help control and generate movement; speech/language pathologists contribute information regarding communication; and educators provide information regarding teaching strategies, behavioral management, and functional use of needed skills (P. H. Campbell, 1987a). A number of authors have provided detailed examples of task analyses that have been successful for planning with students with multiple disabilities (e.g., P. H. Campbell, 1987a; P. H. Campbell & Wetherbee, 1988).

The individualized education program (IEP) is the official document recording the educational plan for the student. If an integrated programming team approach is utilized, IEPs reflect this by having functional and generalizable outcomes addressed in the goals and objectives (Dunn, 1987). Recently, P. H. Campbell and Wetherbee (1988) conducted a study using Hunt, Goetz, and Anderson's (1986) IEP analysis technique. They analyzed the IEPs in one school year, and then initiated integrated programming teams for the next school year. Therapists were assigned to specific classrooms, teachers became team leaders for the student programs, inservice training for teachers and therapists was provided, and professionals were given release time for team planning. Results of IEP analysis following this intervention revealed a significant improvement in functionality, use of appropriate settings, and age appropriateness of objectives. Smaller changes were noted in generalizability and use of interactional objectives. The authors thus recommended formal planning and inservice time for successful implementation of integrated programming teams.

Summary

Services for individuals with severe disabilities evolved a great deal in the 1980s, moving from segregated, exclusionary models toward integrated, inclusionary ones. This has stimulated development of new approaches to provision of therapeutic services. Team members such as related services professionals have made gains in their efforts to fulfill their roles successfully within this dynamic environment. A number of authors have demonstrated the utility of specific team strategies for integrating related services into the life activities of students with special needs (e.g., P. H. Campbell & Wetherbee, 1988; Dunn, 1990; Peck et al., 1989). However, this is

an area of professional practice that is in need of substantial research and program development.

RECENT RESEARCH ON RELATED SERVICES INTERVENTION STRATEGIES IN SPECIFIC DOMAINS

Since the implementation of PL 94-142, related services research has been designed to create and refine isolated intervention procedures and determine their effects on various developmental outcomes. These studies have identified potentially useful strategies, but the task is not complete until successful techniques are applied to functional tasks within life environments. A number of authors have taken this next step and have investigated the use of related services expertise to achieve functional, practice, and comprehensive integration. This section summarizes related services research that reflects some aspect of the integration of related services (see Figure 18.1).

Sensorimotor Development and Postural Control

Occupational and physical therapy's disciplinary contributions to functional outcomes are most easily recognized in the postural control and sensorimotor development areas. Studies in the therapy literature have frequently investigated the postural or motor outcomes from specified procedures. There has been an assumption that changes in postural or motor outcomes would affect functional skills development. However, it is clear that functional outcomes will most likely occur when effective therapeutic strategies are incorporated into the performance of life tasks.

Sensory and Neuromotor Procedures

P. H. Campbell, McInerney, and Cooper (1984) reported on an intervention illustrating both functional and practice integration. They studied the interaction between neuromotor procedures and motivation for task with a preschooler with multiple disabilities. The team determined that reaching for objects was an important objective for this child, and established a neuromotor facilitation procedure to be used throughout the school day. All persons coming in contact with this child were trained to implement this procedure correctly and document the results. Across all activities the child attained only 65% competence by session 44. However, there were differences in performance for different activities. When trials were plotted for opening circle—an activity that seemed more motivating to the child—performance was 100%. P. H. Campbell et al. (1984) concluded that there is an interaction between facilitation procedures and interest in the task, stating, "Therapists must be attentive to both the neuromotor and motivational components of movement to develop maximally effective treatment programs for severely handicapped children" (p. 599). The study also pointed out the potentially powerful impact that therapeutic procedures can have when incorporated into activities across the daily routine.

Giangreco (1986) conducted a study to compare isolated therapy services with practice integration strategies for a student with multiple disabilities. During baseline, the physical and occupational therapists provided exercises in joint range of motion, movement facilitation, and tone reduction and the teacher provided separate instruction on engaging a microswitch. The intervention phase involved collaboration between the teacher and therapists to design a switch-activation program that safely incorporated facilitation and tone-reduction techniques prior to each activation trial. The child performed significantly better during the collaboration phase, supporting the effectiveness of practice integration in comparison to isolated direct therapy (Giangreco, 1986). In a situation such as this, isolated services did not seem to be the best use of either the student's or the professionals' time. The author also pointed out that without the expertise of therapists, educators have a tendency to draw on their own professional resources to alter the reinforcement, change the objective, and so on. While these alterations may be appropriate, equally viable changes to improve performance might instead involve postural adjustments, tone changes, creation of an adaptive device, and so forth; these are more likely to be attempted and successful with the therapist's input (Giangreco, 1986).

Occupational and physical therapists have a great deal of expertise in the sensory and neuromuscular substraits of performance. It has been most common in the past for this expertise to be applied in isolated contexts, limiting our knowledge of their potential power to influence daily life tasks more directly. Although much more study is needed on sensory and neuromuscular procedures, measures of functional performance should be included to address both functional and practice integration questions. Since measurement of sensory and neuromuscular components of performance is difficult, functional outcome measures may also be more fruitful.

Oral-Motor Control

Oral-motor dysfunction can have serious effects on life tasks such as eating, communication, physical and emotional development, and even survival (Ottenbacher, Bundy, & Short, 1983). Related services personnel have knowledge about oral-motor development and therefore can address these problems with effectively designed intervention strategies within all components of comprehensive integration.

The normal process of oral-motor development has been related to sensory stimulation; overall physical development; integration of reflexes; patterns of tongue, lip, and throat movement; and hand-to-mouth motor patterns (P.H. Campbell, 1979; Morris, 1977; Ottenbacher, Bundy, & Short, 1983; Schmidt, 1976). Any or all of these areas can be affected in children with physical or multiple handicapping conditions, and various methods have been designed to deal with these needs (P.H. Campbell, 1979; Morris, 1977; Ottenbacher, Bundy, & Short, 1983; Schmidt, 1976).

A number of studies have addressed the effects of different oral-motor procedures within functional integration contexts (Ottenbacher, Hicks, Roark, & Swinea, 1983; Ottenbacher, Scoggins, & Wayland, 1981; Sobsey & Orelove, 1984). For example, Ottenbacher, Hicks, et al. (1983) used facilitation and inhibition techniques to prepare persons with eating problems for mealtime. Analysis of subject characteristics in relation to results revealed that the subjects' initial characteristics affected the outcome (e.g., ratio of weight to age). Perhaps during functional and practice integration, the child's individual characteristics must be included in collaborative discussions in order to yield the most fruitful outcomes.

Sobsey and Orelove (1984) investigated functional integration by studying the effects of neurophysiological facilitation on the eating skills of children with severe disabilities. A reversal design was used to identify changes in oral-motor control. Lip closure improved and spilling of food and drink from the mouth decreased after intervention. Rotary chewing was dependent on food type, but this result is not interpretable since foods were chosen according to the children's individual needs (i.e., puréed foods for children who were more at risk for choking). Jones (1983) addressed practice integration issues by combining desensitization, facilitation, jaw and lip control, and behavioral contingencies to investigate eating problems in children with mental retardation without neuromotor involvement. Outcomes revealed that a combination of sensory and neuromotor procedures, paired with immediate use of solid foods and ignoring avoidance behaviors, was most effective (8 of 10 accepting solid food after 15 meals). In a comparison group, the sensory and neuromotor procedures were withdrawn when avoidance was displayed and a sequence of increasing food textures was employed (2 of 10 accepting solid foods). The alteration of two major variables makes interpretation of these results difficult; however, it is promising to see positive outcomes from a practice integration approach that utilized a combination of sensory, neuromotor, and behavioral techniques.

Some studies have suggested that facilitation techniques applied in a functional integration context strengthen the oral-motor control of children with severe disabilities. Maintenance and generalization of these initially obtained skills to eating, talking, and socialization remains in question. It is also not yet clear whether oral-motor skills are sustained without the continuation of facilitation techniques. If ongoing use of facilitation is necessary, this could interfere with peer integration: The use of a daily 10–15 minute preparation period or the application of techniques during eating can be quite intrusive to peer interactions. The cost-benefit ratio of an intrusive intervention such as oral-motor facilitation in relation to integration priorities may lead to appropriate decisions to restrict such procedures to certain settings, times, portions of meals, and so on. In this way, the child would have the benefit of therapeutic techniques without being compelled to sacrifice all opportunities for more normalized peer and family interactions in public environments.

Gross and Fine Motor Development

Many of the gross and fine motor investigations that have been reported in the therapy literature address developmental changes from isolated approaches. When changes are reported, it still is not known whether skill acquisition will affect functional performance. Only a few authors have expanded the question of effectiveness of these isolated approaches to include intervention frequency issues: These studies point out that more is not necessarily better. For example, Jenkins et al. (1982) studied the outcomes from two levels of intensity of a 15-week occupational and physical therapy intervention program. Children with developmental disabilities were placed in three groups. One group received individual therapeutic intervention once a week, another group received therapy three times a week, and the third group served as controls. Jenkins and his colleagues found that the two treatment groups differed significantly from the control group on gross motor skills, but did not differ from each other. There were no significant differences across groups in fine motor scores. The authors concluded that therapy has a significant impact, but that multiple weekly sessions may not be necessary for this outcome.

Miedaner and Renander (1987) also investigated frequency of service provision but with children who were nonambulatory. They used passive stretching programs as the intervention and passive range of motion for the measurement over a 10-week period. Baseline measurements were taken, after which one group received intervention five-times weekly while the other group received the program two times weekly for 5 weeks. Interim measurements were taken, and then the intervention frequency was switched for another 5-week phase to investigate order effects. There were no differences in the joint range of motion for six of seven tested joints when comparing twice a week to five times a week. One might question the usefulness of measuring intervention outcomes with a technical measurement device as was done in this study. If functional performance was the desired outcome, the functional performance should be observed and measured. The authors also reported that bracing and positioning strategies were used as functional integration for all children; these integrated strategies may have accounted for the children's status, so that the small difference in frequency of the range-of-motion exercises added nothing of significance.

A few authors have investigated the components of practice integration in relation to gross and fine motor development. Talbot and Junkala (1981) conducted a study to determine whether auditory feedback significantly improved eye-hand coordination of children with normal intelligence who had cerebral palsy. Posttest comparisons revealed that auditory feedback from tracing (a light-sound pen) significantly enhanced performance in comparison to regular tracing. Talbot and Junkala concluded that eye-hand activities that produce immediate external feedback may have a greater impact on future performance; they hypothesized that auditory feedback may be preferable for children whose other sensory systems process ineffectively (e.g., in the case of children with cerebral palsy, perhaps somatosensory and proprioceptive feedback is less useful due to abnormal tone). As delayed posttesting revealed no maintenance of effect after 3 months, the authors suggested that effective procedures (such as the one they investigated) should be incorporated into daily routines through functional integration rather than being reserved for specific intervention periods.

P.H. Campbell et al. (1984) conducted a study on practice integration with a 15-year-old girl with severe disabilities. A reach-and-open movement sequence was chosen as an appropriate functional behavior, because the student encountered many opportunities during the day that required this skill (e.g., locker door, microwave oven door, cake mix box, food containers).

Demonstration and physical guidance for task completion revealed a steadily increasing rate of success. When P.H. Campbell et al. (1984) extended the procedure to include object permanence, the child demonstrated an increase in performance but not at predicted rates, suggesting that demonstration and physical guidance did not constitute a sufficient practice integration strategy for this higher level task. In a study using similar procedures, Ilmer, Rynders, Sinclair, and Helfrich (1981) investigated the effects of practice integration by combining verbal prompts and physical prompts to teach cognitive concepts to children with motor impairments. They found that the combined approach had a positive effect on children with higher levels of motor skills, but was no more or less effective for the children with poorer motor skills. One might hypothesize that either the children with higher motor skills profited from this practice integration strategy by being able to demonstrate their cognitive skills when physical guidance procedure was added, or that the physical guidance procedure was only effective with milder motor problems.

The P.H. Campbell et al. (1984) study also illustrated practice integration by combining various behavioral consequences with upper extremity reaching patterns and activation of a microswitch. Rock music was more effective at increasing use of that motor movement than a fan, vibrator, or other music. The authors concluded that the consequences of movement are critical variables to consider when designing intervention programs.

Play is a motivating contextual life task for children; it incorporates many aspects of development into functional performance. Embracing these concepts, Anderson, Hinojosa, and Strauch (1987) discussed functional integration of neuromotor handling techniques into play experiences. They suggested that the interweaving of these techniques provides a mechanism for teaching new motor skills in a natural context, facilitating more independent exploration. Peganoff (1984) employed functional integration of therapeutic techniques into an 8-week aquatics program with an adolescent with cerebral palsy and found not only improved joint range of motion during the leisure task, but also identified generalization of upper extremity use in other environments during life tasks such as self-care skills and learning.

Summary and Conclusions

Occupational and physical therapists contribute sensorimotor development expertise to the interdisciplinary team. Most studies of gross and fine motor development have been conducted within an isolated model of service provision, leaving one to wonder whether changes in motor skills acquisition will indeed affect performance of functional life tasks. The motor systems represent one of the major mechanisms through which the nervous system acts on the environment, so they must not be ignored. Rather, therapists must begin to recognize the contextual nature of motor skills usage and take advantage of the naturally occurring events that stimulate a person to move and reinforce one for having moved. It is only when frequently occurring environmental conditions support or control the use of motor movements that they will have any meaning.

Assistive and Adaptive Devices

Related services personnel have expertise to support functional skills development and increase independence through the design and application of adaptations. Adaptations are not outcomes themselves; rather, they prevent or minimize the effects of deformities or support more independent forms of behavior, and enable individuals with moderate to severe handicapping conditions to have access to natural environments and more normal life experiences (P.H. Campbell, Green, & Carlson, 1977; Garner & Campbell, 1987).

Functional integration has been reflected in the application of adaptive devices to children's needs in daily life situations. Hulme, Schulein, Hulme, Poor, and Pezzino (1983) surveyed caregivers of individuals who were nonambulatory to determine the usefulness of adaptive equipment for improving performance in selected life activities. Caregivers reported both significantly improved performance and a high degree of satisfaction with the adaptive devices. In a follow-up study, Hulme et al. (1987) directly observed individuals in their homes both before and after

providing an adaptive seating device for 19 preschool children with multiple disabilities. Observations revealed that posture, head control, and grasp were significantly improved after provision of the seating device, and families reported increased ability to engage in home and community activities. Trefler, Nickey, and Hobson (1983) identified specific needs of preschool children and assembled appropriate technological aids. Effectiveness of the devices was measured through observation of head and trunk control, purposeful gross motor movements, mobility and eating efficiency, with improvements noted in all areas (Trefler et al., 1983).

Switch mechanisms are also valuable tools for functional integration. When effectively designed, a switch enables the child to gain access to many learning experiences—but they must be chosen carefully. York, Nietupski, and Hamre-Nietupski (1985) outlined several issues to consider when applying functional integration through the use of microswitches in educational programs for students with severe disabilities. First, the use of microswitches is only relevant as its action facilitates functional, educationally relevant outcomes. Age appropriateness, use in peer integration environments, and personal preference are all variables that contribute to relevance of tasks. Educational goals and objectives incorporate adaptations; separate goals for microswitch use are inappropriate. Second, direct skill performance without the use of adaptive devices should be the preferred option. Third, microswitches are only one form of adaptation; other adaptations must also be considered to meet children's needs.

The importance of combining functional and practice integration strategies has been illustrated by several microswitch application studies. Two studies illustrated functional integration by applying microswitches and auditory feedback to improve head control in children with multiple handicaps (Maloney & Kurtz, 1982; Walmsley, Crichton, & Droog, 1981). However, results were inconclusive in both studies. Although contingent auditory feedback provides a purpose for head control, it may not provide a strong enough linkage to head-erect behavior for the child; in this case, functional integration alone may be inadequate. Everson and Goodwyn (1987) combined functional and practice integration to compare the effectiveness of four types of microswitches for a vocational readiness task. Of 3 adolescent subjects with cerebral palsy, 2 demonstrated a clearly higher productivity level with one switch. Interestingly, the researchers reported a related but indirect outcome from participation in this project. The intrinsically motivating features of this functional vocational task seemed to enhance the student's physical control over extraneous athetoid movements. Everson and Goodwyn suggested that wider use of vocationally relevant tasks in combination with therapeutic interventions might better prepare students for employment options, while providing a vehicle for improving physical control.

Leiper, Miller, Lang, and Herman (1981) also combined practice and functional integration to cue children with cerebral palsy to self-monitor head position while engaging in learning activities in the classroom. Three children who were able to work independently on classroom activities also learned to monitor head position independently. Horn and Warren (1987) combined functional and practice integration to intervene with 2 toddlers with severe and multiple disabilities. These researchers carefully combined neuromotor principles with behavioral contingencies by selecting switches that required correct position and movement to activate the mechanical toy. The children developed and maintained new adaptive sensorimotor behaviors with this approach.

As more adaptations and technological advances become available, team members will consider new instructional possibilities, especially for students with severe and multiple disabilities (Garner & Campbell, 1987). Life tasks that require complex physical or cognitive skills may now be relevant activities for students as professionals apply technology through functional and practice integration.

Garner and Campbell (1987) described three areas that need attention before students will be able to benefit optimally from adaptations and technological devices. First, obstacles must be overcome; these include perceived costs of de-

vices, lack of knowledge to operate and troubleshoot the equipment, and lack of resources to fabricate devices. Garner and Campbell suggested that training efforts for all team members, systematic procedures for student assessment, and clear guidelines for selection, design, and use of adaptations will remove these obstacles. Incorporation of adaptations into educational environments through functional and practice integration is another area needing attention. Garner and Campbell described the successful use of an interdisciplinary technology team to match student needs with available devices. Finally, these authors discussed the need to attend to values that promote personal dignity and provide opportunities for both personal choice and increased access to natural environments. For example, indiscriminant use of technological devices could lead to increased isolation and decreased opportunities to interact with other persons, working against comprehensive integration.

Language Intervention

Since the late 1970s, a notable shift in the theoretical orientation of language research has resulted in increased attention to the social factors affecting language development and use (Bates, 1976; Bruner, 1977). These developments have had great impact on current conceptualizations of best practices in the field of speech/language therapy (Prutting, 1982; Snow, Midkiff-Borunda, Small, & Proctor, 1984). Many authors have discussed the importance of integrating language into children's daily life routines (e.g., Hamre-Nietupski et al., 1977; Hart & Rogers-Warren, 1978; Kopchick & Lloyd, 1976; Williams & Fox, 1977). Warren and Rogers-Warren (1985) stated that traditionally isolated models are no longer acceptable intervention strategies; the child must learn how to control his or her own environment with communication. Comprehensive integrated related services focus on the contextual aspects of the intervention process.

Paul (1985) also described basic dimensions of communication that highlight its contextual nature. First, there must be a reason for using language; second, one must consider where language is being used; and third, one must consider to whom language is being addressed.

> Language training should be conducted by those who spend the most time communicating with the child . . . . It simply makes no sense from the perspective of facilitating acquisition and generalization for a therapist who sees a child once or twice a week to be entirely responsible for teaching language. (Warren & Rogers-Warren, 1985, p. 7–9)

The recommended approach to teaching language skills in everyday contexts has typically been termed "functional" or "naturalistic" (Warren & Rogers-Warren, 1985).

This naturalistic approach to language intervention also provides a greater opportunity for family members to become involved as intervention agents with their children (Musselwhite & St. Louis, 1982). However, Warren and Rogers-Warren (1985) cautioned professionals to remember that parents have multiple roles, and so program design must be carefully constructed to maintain family flexibility and not contribute additional stress.

Musselwhite and St. Louis (1982) considered generalization a critical outgrowth of naturalistic language intervention. They described two components of generalization that must be addressed: generalization of the stimulus to new situations and expansion of learned responses to new language opportunities. When either the stimuli or the responses are bound by restricted conditions, they are not useful to the child in everyday functional situations. The child continues to be dependent on therapists or teachers to provide the proper conditions for communication. Functional integration efforts must incorporate varied settings, stimuli, examples, and expected responses in order to maximize generalization possibilities. Peer integration provides naturally occurring opportunities to enrich and expand communication skills. Practice integration allows professionals to work together to make specific alterations in the environmental conditions so that children with language deficiencies can learn from naturally occurring interactions (Warren & Rogers-Warren, 1985).

It is also important for professionals to establish the effectiveness of integrated language opportunities empirically. This is not only necessary for comparisons between isolated and integrated interventions, but also for investigations of various forms of integrated language intervention.

Research on Naturalistic Language Intervention

Although highly structured prompting and reinforcement techniques have been used successfully to teach form and structure of language, spontaneous and functional language use frequently have not been demonstrated as an outcome from these strategies (Guess, Keogh, & Sailor, 1978; Halle, 1987). A number of authors have investigated methods for teaching language using more naturalistic techniques (Halle, Marshall, & Spradlin, 1979; Haring, Neetz, Lovinger, Peck, & Semmel, 1987; Hart & Risley, 1975). The authors generally concluded that language activities within the natural environment have a greater impact on usefulness and generalizability of communication skills.

Researchers working with persons with moderate and severe disabilities have applied similar principles to language acquisition (Halle et al., 1979; Haring et al., 1987; Peck et al., 1986). For example, Halle et al. used a naturalistic strategy (delaying anticipated delivery of a food tray) to prompt communication from 6 children with severe mental retardation. The technique produced rapid and generalized increases in communicative behavior in the context of naturally occurring daily routines. Peck (1985) demonstrated functional integration of communication interventions through a similar procedure, including providing choices of tasks and materials to students with autism and severe disabilities, resulting in increased spontaneous communications in daily classroom activities.

In another illustration of functional integration, Haring et al. (1987) taught incidental teaching techniques to 3 teachers of preschool children with moderate to severe disabilities in an attempt to increase spontaneous communication opportunities during regular classroom routines. A self-instructional packet was provided to introduce the teachers to four procedures: giving choices, placing objects out of reach, blocking access to materials and activities, and providing noncontextual objects for events. There was a significant increase in opportunities for communication in each classroom.

Hunt, Goetz, Alwell, and Sailor (1986) used a functional integration approach to create a method for interrupting well-established behavior patterns in 3 children with severe disabilities in an attempt to elicit communication. They hypothesized that the children would be motivated to complete the familiar activity, and would therefore use communication skills to reach their goal. This procedure was successful both for establishing this communication pattern and in generalizing it to other activities that were interrupted.

Augmentative Communication

The selection of augmentative communication systems has been a large focus of attention in recent literature (Chapman & Miller, 1980; Nietupski & Hamre-Nietupski, 1979; Reichle & Karlan, 1988; Reichle & Keogh, 1986; Sailor et al., 1980). The authors did not agree about the criteria for the selection of augmentative devices, but similar parameters seemed to emerge (Reichle & Karlan, 1988). All the parameters involve practice integration, since expertise from multiple disciplines is necessary. Cognitive status, level of severity of handicapping condition, and communication status are consistent areas of focus, but it is unclear exactly what status is necessary in each case or how the criterion is to be evaluated (Reichle & Karlan, 1988; Romski, Lloyd, & Sevcik, 1988).

Some research has indicated the importance of naturalistic context for nonspeech communication interventions. For example, Kohl, Wilcox, and Karlan (1978) found that children with severe disabilities learned signs faster within the classroom than in individual therapy. Generalization to a new teacher was noted by Oliver and Halle (1982). Findings such as these led Romski et al. (1988) to conclude that "instruction within natural communicative settings seems to be the method of choice when the end goal of intervention is functional use of the nonspeech symbol system" (p. 357).

Summary and Conclusions

Provision of integrated language intervention must be considered the alternative of choice. Functional communication is only possible when embedded in the natural stimuli and consequences that present themselves during age-appropriate life tasks. Further study might focus on which strategies are most effective within each phase of language intervention. For example, peer integration might prove to be the most productive context for developing language competence once language components are acquired and have begun to generalize.

Effects of Combined Interventions

A series of studies has investigated practice integration between occupational therapy and language development (Ayres & Mailloux, 1981; F. A. Clark & Steingold, 1982; Kantner, Kantner, & Clark, 1982; Magrun, McCue, Ottenbacher, F.A., & Keefe, 1981; Reilly, Nelson, & Bundy, 1983). Ayres and Mailloux provided weekly occupational therapy intervention for 1 year to 4 children diagnosed as aphasic, and compared rate of language acquisition before and after the onset of occupational therapy. Language comprehension increased at a faster rate in all 4 children during the year they received occupational therapy intervention; 2 children with specific neurodevelopmental patterns also demonstrated significantly larger gains in expressive language (Ayres & Mailloux, 1981). For all children, individual speech therapy was reduced or discontinued sometime before or during the first quarter of the study, but they were placed in a public school aphasia classroom (2 placed before and 2 after the initiation of this study). Perhaps the combination of occupational therapy treatment and contextual language opportunities contributed to the positive outcome.

The Ayres and Mailloux (1981) study illustrated the interdependent contributions that related services personnel make to the educational process through practice integration. Future investigations must address the incorporation of these principles into direct investigations of functional outcomes in natural environments.

IMPLICATIONS FOR POLICY, PRACTICE, AND RESEARCH

The challenges of integrating related services into the natural life environments of persons with moderate and severe disabilities are numerous and complex. Successful implementation requires policy shifts that provide support for integrated services, philosophical and behavioral adaptations in practice, and careful and innovative research.

Policy Directions

A critical policy issue that must be addressed is the establishment of administrative mechanisms that support integrated programming. Even if research and practice produce overwhelming evidence that integrated services work, administrative procedures must be available to enable professionals to carry out such programs. For example, scheduling flexibility would enable professionals to combine multiple areas of expertise into learning tasks (Rainforth & York, 1987); teams would be able to establish regular meeting times throughout the year for integrated planning (P.H. Campbell & Wetherbee, 1988), and natural environment schedules would be designed to accommodate a heterogeneous group of learners rather than the elusive "average" ones. Presently, IEPs contain a written declaration regarding the portion of time spent in a mainstreamed setting and the type and duration of other services that make up the school week. This is generally interpreted to mean that the therapist must meet directly with a student for the specified time. Such policies need to be reinterpreted to include integrated programming options. Related to scheduling are caseload and payment for related services professionals. Frequently, schools contract with therapists to provide services, and specify those activities that are reimbursable such as direct service to a student. In these situations, therapists who choose to meet with teachers or work with students in classrooms or community settings do so at their own expense. Practices such as these attach unnecessary costs to integrated services; policy shifts would contribute to changes in these types of practices.

Flexibility in our concept of the educational environment is also vital to the success of integrated related services. Flexible policies are needed that describe where services might take place and how those environments may look (Brown et al., 1983). Resources must be structured so that students have access to the environments that are age and task appropriate; this includes supplies, transportation, and equipment to support integration in general. Related services personnel have expertise in the development and adaptation of environments to support functional outcomes. They should be included in the design and selection of those environments.

A second necessary policy shift concerns the preservice and continuing education experiences of professionals serving individuals with severe disabilities (York, Rainforth, & Dunn, 1990). Too commonly, each professional is trained solely in the philosophy and approaches of the singular profession, with only brief information provided regarding the roles of other team members or how to work on teams. Interaction among professionals to practice interdisciplinary problem solving is uncommon, yet this skill is at the core of integrated service provision. This pattern is perpetuated in continuing education, with each profession attending workshops focused on that specific profession's concerns. Although specialty knowledge is an important component of effective service provision, it does not serve a more systemic purpose. Policies must not only encourage, but require, training in interdisciplinary teamwork in order for the next generation of professionals to consider integrated service provision a basic assumption rather than a goal to attain.

A third policy issue regards maintaining an *array* of choices available to practitioners for providing services. Clearly, integrated approaches to provision of related services are consistent with the valued outcomes of supporting individuals with severe disabilities in natural school and community settings. The research reviewed in the present chapter illustrated the promise of this approach, and supports it as the intervention model of choice. However, this is a complex set of issues, and rigid definition of acceptable practices can be a barrier to progress. Careful study is required before professionals will know the safest and most effective means for integrating related services into learning, work, leisure, and living situations.

There must also be a policy commitment directed at dissemination activities to support the growth of collaborative professional knowledge. Research findings, theory development, and practice innovations should be published and presented collaboratively and across discipline lines. Therapists must be made aware of special education issues if they are to contribute intelligently to designing solutions to problems. Educators must be willing to learn about the specialized expertise and philosophies of related services personnel in order to request this type of consultation correctly and carry out integrated procedures safely. Collaborative debate through forums such as these is likely to produce action that could not have been created in isolation.

Philosophy and Practice

Therapists and teachers who serve school-age children made significant advances in the 1970s and 1980s toward more integrated approaches to programming. A renewed commitment to this construct must be an integral part of the related services' philosophies, with an accompanying commitment to investigating strategies for intervention in natural environments. Related services personnel must actively explore practice options that facilitate independence, and must be willing to abandon therapeutic strategies that do not yield functional or generalizable outcomes. Therapists must adopt a position that incorporates integrated strategies as the usual practice and requires justification for segregated, isolated approaches—rather than the other way around (Dunn & Campbell, in press). All professionals must value the product of collaborative practice as more powerful than any separate strategies that might be designed.

One of the reasons for a lack of research on integrated related services may be that professionals are trained to practice their profession, not study its effects. The evolution of clinician to clinical researcher is a difficult one, and one that has not been supported by the agencies within which services are provided. As demands for "proof of effects" increase in a productivity-driven environment, this attitude is changing.

Therapists must embrace the need to document their effects systematically and seek assistance to do so.

To that end, measurement issues must be examined. Research and intervention outcomes are difficult to interpret when the methods used for measurement of the target behaviors are tenuous. There is an intimacy between intervention and measurement of outcomes that causes one to affect the other in a variety of ways. Good interventions that are viewed through poor measurements may be discarded; poor interventions evaluated with poor measurements may continue to be used. Improvement of measurement methods must be a priority as part of the study of integrated related services. Several strategies may be useful.

Peck et al. (1986) discussed the inherent problems with traditional measurement methods when used with persons who have moderate or severe disablities. Norm- and criterion-referenced measures compare the student's behavior to a set of "normal" or expected behaviors. With this approach, differences are commonly interpreted as deficits, and idiosyncratic competencies can be overlooked. Data are typically collected in isolated, one-to-one interactions, which may result in the individual's demonstrating different behaviors than are elicited in natural environments.

Peck et al. (1986) offered three primary strategies for functional assessment in the area of communication. First, the evaluation must include both the form and use of the communication behaviors; this includes verbal, nonverbal, device-oriented, and even aberrant behaviors that communicate a message. Second, multiple methods should be employed in the assessment, including free-field observation and interviews with caregivers focused on description of situations and functions of communicative behaviors. Finally, a set of contrived situations may be used to simulate natural situations, enabling the professional to identify behaviors a student uses to control the social environment.

Parette and Hourcade (1984) discussed the problems associated with traditional instrumentation in the motor domain. They commented that measurement of motor milestones does not enable documentation of qualitative differences in movement. Additionally, because a person with a severe disability has, by definition, significant performance deficits, developmental skills checklists do not present sufficient refinement to measure and change (P.H. Campbell & Stewart, 1986).

In an attempt to deal with this problem, P.H. Campbell and Stewart (1986) created a method for measuring the qualitative aspects of posture and movement during activity, hypothesizing that these measures would more adequately reflect the performance changes of children with severe disabilities. One example of functional performance measurement involved a toddler with hemiplegia who had difficulty with functional arm use. While the child engaged in self-selected play activities involving scooping with an object, data were collected on the movement components required to perform this task, including humeral flexion, internal rotation, elbow movement, wrist position, forearm movement, finger position, and object contact. Over the course of the changing criterion design, successive approximations were reinforced to move the child toward the correct movement pattern. Procedures such as this one, incorporating functional activities with observations of the components of performance, are likely to yield important data regarding description of effective intervention approaches.

Unfortunately, even those studies that have developed useful measurement strategies (e.g., P.H. Campbell et al., 1984; P.H. Campbell & Stewart, 1986; Talbot & Junkala, 1981) have not been replicated, which would strengthen the evidence for the use of those procedures.

Research Needs

The study of integrated related services is in its infancy. Many needs exist, related to both methodological issues and study of specific policy and intervention problems.

Methodological Issues

It may be particularly useful for researchers to broaden their views regarding what constitutes a valid methodological approach. Traditional group experimental designs, intrasubject designs, and naturalistic approaches all yield useful but different information.

Classic group experimental designs are partic-

ularly useful for many policy questions, including, for example, those of the relative cost-effectiveness of alternative service provision models. Some of the pertinent questions regarding integrated related services for individuals with severe disabilities do not easily lend themselves to group research designs. Intrasubject designs, however, may be more compatible with research questions focused on direct service to persons with severe disabilities. These designs allow each individual to serve as his or her own control to evaluate whether an intervention strategy is effective. Multiple subjects can serve as replications to evaluate the generalizability of effects for a technique, rather than grouping individuals together and masking important individual effects.

Naturalistic inquiry provides yet another means of gathering valuable information related to some research questions. When formally designed and carried out, naturalistic inquiry allows the researcher to analyze complex patterns of behavior systematically. The richness of the original data enables the researcher to use pertinent anecdotes to illustrate particularly important phenomena. This research methodology provides the opportunity to analyze patterns of performance without ignoring or controlling the context within which they occur. One might investigate those intervention-related activities most interesting to the child by recording the amount, type, and descriptions of attending behaviors in various settings. Qualitative comparisons across behaviors, environments, and interventions would be possible with such data.

Specific Policy and Intervention Issues for Study

First, there is a need for studies that describe how persons with severe disabilities successfully carry out life tasks, providing baseline data to guide the design of integrated procedures. These studies should include thorough descriptive information regarding the procedures, statements clarifying how persons were trained and monitored in conducting the procedures, and data recording the outcomes of the procedures so that effectiveness might be assessed. Anecdotal data would also be helpful to identify additional variables that may be contributing to outcomes, such as the child's motivation to participate in various environments or time of day the procedures were employed.

Second, research is needed to formulate a decision-making process for service provision. Presently, professionals rely on personal experience or agency tradition to decide which therapeutic strategies and which service models might be applied in any given situation. The studies reviewed in this chapter provide preliminary evidence that there are successful applications of present knowledge within this framework (e.g., P.H. Campbell, 1987b; P.H. Campbell & Stewart, 1986; Giangreco, 1986), but the available evidence is not sufficient to recommend a particular decision-making process. Studies with multiple dependent measures or those that use factorial comparisons could clarify decision processes that optimize student outcomes.

A third critical area for research in the related services is measurement and instrumentation. Much of the research presently available has generated equivocal findings partially related to the outcome measurement chosen for the study (Ottenbacher et al., 1981). In order to establish their validity, measurement systems must be tested, refined, and replicated by others (e.g., Gisel, Lange, & Niman, 1984a, 1984b). Operational definitions for functional performance should be a major focus of attention in this endeavor.

Experimental research using both single-subject and group designs must be directed at identification of effective therapeutic procedures (Connell & Thompson, 1986; Kearns, 1986; McReynolds & Thompson, 1986; Ottenbacher & York, 1984; Siegel & Young, 1987). Although pilot investigations may occur in an isolated manner to identify a useful technique, the primary focus of these studies should be on identifying techniques that can be integrated into learning, living, leisure, and work tasks. Collaborative studies will be more useful than single-discipline studies. During this process, effectiveness should be judged in relation to contribution to functional skills development or performance.

There is a great need for studies to examine the length of time and the amount and type of resources needed to acquire, maintain, and generalize skills. For example, perhaps skill acquisition occurs faster in a more isolated intervention strategy, but generalization is more easily attained in a peer integration environment. The interaction among these variables is a critical area of knowledge to develop, because it is not likely that one intervention model will be the best choice to serve all needs.

Research efforts must also focus on effective ways to train teachers, paraprofessionals, and other nontherapy staff to carry out safe therapeutic components of tasks. There must also be an emphasis on the motivational components of practice and functional integration, so that classroom personnel continue to feel committed to the process. Some initial work in this area has been carried out by those who have studied collaborative consultation, but this body of literature needs to be extended to integrated related services strategies.

Although the team literature provides many explanations and examples of transdisciplinary and interdisciplinary practice, there is not an adequate data base to allow professionals to make confident decisions regarding the best team structure for specific integrated therapy situations. It is likely that there is a relationship between the needs of a child and family and the team structure that is used to create the intervention strategy and carry it out. Furthermore, research on the attitudes of professionals and families about teaming approaches seems likely to contribute to decisions about teaming strategies.

Given choices between using several potentially effective approaches, cost-effectiveness is also an issue that is best addressed through research. Analyses of the direct and indirect costs of integrated and isolated approaches must be undertaken. There will certainly be situations within an integrated environment when it is more cost-effective to provide one or another service provision model, but presently there are not adequate data to guide any decisions that are made.

Many of the policy shifts that are necessary will be clearer when the above issues have been investigated more thoroughly. It is not responsible for systems to alter policies each time a new idea is brought to the table for discussion. Therefore it is imperative that research efforts take as the highest priority those issues that, when addressed, will facilitate the necessary cultural, policy, and political shifts to support comprehensive integration.

SUMMARY AND CONCLUSIONS

The integration of related services strategies into natural environments is evolving rapidly as the participation and the inclusion of people with severe disabilities in normalized school and community settings expand. Occupational and physical therapists and speech/language pathologists have specialized knowledge that can enhance functional performance and increase independence, but this knowledge has frequently been used in isolation from functional life tasks, thereby limiting its effects. Researchers have shown that it is possible to incorporate related services strategies safely and have demonstrated positive functional outcomes from these strategies. Existing research, however, is limited and needs to be expanded to extend the appropriate use of therapeutic procedures in natural environments. Progress in these areas is dependent on shifts in policy and professional philosophy that fully embrace the principles underlying comprehensive integration.

REFERENCES

Abelson, M.A., & Woodman, R.W. (1983). Review of research on team effectiveness: Implications for teams in schools. *School Psychology Review, 12,* 125–136.

American Occupational Therapy Association. (1987). *Guidelines for occupational therapy services in school systems.* Rockville, MD: Author.

American Occupational Therapy Association. (1989). *Guidelines for occupational therapy services in school systems* (2nd ed.). Rockville, MD: Author.

American Physical Therapy Association. (1980). *APTA guidelines for PT practice in educational environments.* Washington, DC: Author.

Anderson, J., Hinojosa, J., & Strauch, C. (1987). Integrating play in neurodevelopmental treatment. *American Journal of Occupational Therapy, 41,* 421–426.

Ayres, A.J., & Mailloux, Z. (1981). Influence of sensory integration procedures on language development. *American Journal of Occupational Therapy, 35,* 383–390.

Babcock, N.L., & Pryzwansky, W.B. (1983). Models of consultation: Preferences of educational professionals at five stages of service. *School Psychology, 21,* 359–366.

Bates, E. (1976). *Language in context.* New York: Academic Press.

Breines, E. (1984). An attempt to define purposeful activity. *American Journal of Occupational Therapy, 38,* 543–544.

Brown, L., Nisbet, J., Ford, A., Sweet, M., Shiraga, B., York, J., & Loomis, R. (1983). The critical need for nonschool instruction in educational programs for severely handicapped students. *Journal of The Association for the Severely Handicapped, 8*(3), 71–77.

Bruner, J. (1977). Early social interaction and language acquisition. In H.R. Schaffer (Ed.), *Studies in mother-infant interaction* (pp. 271–290). London: Academic Press.

Campbell, C.R., Stremel-Campbell, K., & Rogers-Warren, A.K. (1985). Programming teacher support for functional language. In S.F. Warren & A.K. Rogers-Warren (Eds.), *Teaching functional language: Generalization and maintenance of language skills* (pp. 251–288). Baltimore: University Park Press.

Campbell, P.H. (1979). Assessing oral-motor skills in severely handicapped persons: An analysis of normal and abnormal patterns of movement. In R.L. York & E. Edgar (Eds.), *Teaching the severely handicapped* (Vol IV, pp. 39–63). Seattle: American Association for the Severely and Profoundly Handicapped.

Campbell, P.H. (1987a). Integrated programming for students with multiple handicaps. In L. Goetz, D. Guess, & K. Stremel-Campbell (Eds.), *Innovative program design for individuals with dual sensory impairments* (pp. 159–188). Baltimore: Paul H. Brookes Publishing Co.

Campbell, P.H. (1987b). The integrated programming team: An approach for coordinating professionals of various disciplines in programs for students with severe and multiple handicaps. *Journal of The Association for Persons with Severe Handicaps, 12,* 107–116.

Campbell, P.H., Green, K.M., & Carlson, L.M. (1977). Approximating the norm through environmental and child-centered prosthetics and adaptive equipment. In E. Sontag (Ed.), *Educational programming for the severely/profoundly handicapped* (pp. 300–322). Reston, VA: Division on Mental Retardation.

Campbell, P.H., McInerney, W.F., & Cooper, M.A. (1984). Therapeutic programming for students with severe handicaps. *American Journal of Occupational Therapy, 38,* 594–602.

Campbell, P.H., & Stewart, B. (1986). Measuring changes in movement skills with infants and young children with handicaps. *Journal of The Associa-*

tion for Persons with Severe Handicaps, 11, 153–161.

Campbell, P.H., & Wetherbee, R., Jr. (1988). The integrated programming team: A process for integrating therapy services. Occupational Therapy News, 42(5), 13.

Chapman, R., & Miller, J. (1980). Analyzing language and communication in the child. In R.L. Schiefelbusch (Ed.), Nonspeech language and communication: Acquisition and intervention (pp. 159–196). Austin, TX: PRO-ED.

Clark, F.A., & Steingold, L.R. (1982). A potential relationship between occupational therapy and language acquisition. American Journal of Occupational Therapy, 36, 42–44.

Clark, P.N. (1979). Human development through occupation: Theoretical frameworks in contemporary occupational therapy practice, Part 1. American Journal of Occupational Therapy, 33, 505–514.

Connell, P.J., & Thompson, C.K. (1986). Flexibility of single-subject experimental designs. Part III: Using flexibility to design or modify experiments. Journal of Speech and Hearing Disorders, 51, 214–225.

Connolly, B.H., & Anderson, R.M. (1978). Severely handicapped children in the public schools: A new frontier for the physical therapist. Physical Therapy, 58, 433–438.

Damico, J.S. (1987). Addressing language concerns in the schools: The SLP as consultant. Journal of Childhood Communication Disorders, 11(1), 17–40.

Dunn, W. (1987). Development of the individualized education program and occupational therapy intervention plans. In American Occupational Therapy Association, Guidelines for occupational therapy services in school systems (pp. 8-1–8-14). Rockville, MD: American Occupational Therapy Association.

Dunn, W. (1988). Models of occupational therapy service delivery in public schools. American Journal of Occupational Therapy, 42, 718–723.

Dunn, W. (1990). A comparison of service provision models in school-based occupational therapy services. Occupational Therapy Journal of Research.

Dunn, W., & Campbell, P.H. (in press). Designing pediatric service provision. In W. Dunn (Ed.), Pediatric occupational therapy: Facilitating effect service provision. Thorofare, NJ: Charles B. Slack.

Everson, J.M., & Goodwyn, R. (1987). A comparison of the use of adaptive microswitches by students with cerebral palsy. American Journal of Occupational Therapy, 41, 739–744.

Fidler, G.S., & Fidler, J.W. (1978). Doing and becoming: Purposeful action and self actualization. American Journal of Occupational Therapy, 32, 305–310.

Garner, J.B., & Campbell, P.H. (1987). Technology for persons with severe disabilities: Practical and ethical considerations. Journal of Special Education, 21(3), 122–132.

Giangreco, M.F. (1986). Effects of integrated therapy: A pilot study. Journal of The Association for Persons with Severe Handicaps, 11, 205–208.

Gisel, E.G., Lange, L.J., & Niman, C.W. (1984a). Tongue movements in 4- and 5-year-old Down's syndrome children during eating: A comparison with normal children. American Journal of Occupational Therapy, 38, 660–665.

Gisel, E.G., Lange, L.J., & Niman, C.W. (1984b). Chewing cycles in 4- and 5-year-old Down's syndrome children: A comparison of eating efficacy with normals. American Journal of Occupational Therapy, 38, 666–670.

Gliner, J.A. (1985). Purposeful activity in motor learning theory: An event approach to motor skill acquisition. American Journal of Occupational Therapy, 39, 28–34.

Gonnella, C., Hale, G., Ionta, M., & Perry, J.C. (1981). Self-instruction in a perceptual motor skill. Physical Therapy, 61(2), 177–184.

Guess, D., Keogh, W., & Sailor, W. (1978). Generalization of speech and language behavior: Measurement and training tactics. In R.L. Schiefelbusch (Ed.), Bases of language intervention (pp. 373–396). Baltimore: University Park Press.

Gutkin, T.B., & Curtis, M.J. (1982). School-based consultation. In C.R. Reynolds & T.B. Gutkin (Eds.), The handbook of school psychology (pp. 796–826). New York: John Wiley & Sons.

Halle, J.W. (1982). Teaching functional language to the handicapped: An integrative model of natural environment teaching techniques. Journal of The Association for the Severely Handicapped, 7(4), 29–37.

Halle, J.W. (1987). Teaching language in the natural environment: An analysis of spontaneity. Journal of The Association for Persons with Severe Handicaps, 12, 28–37.

Halle, J., Marshall, A., & Spradlin, J. (1979). Time delay: A technique to increase language use and facilitate generalization in retarded children. Journal of Applied Behavior Analysis, 12, 431–439.

Hamre-Nietupski, S., Stoll, A., Holtz, K., Fullerton, P., Ryan-Flottum, M., & Brown, L. (1977). Curricular strategies for teaching selected nonverbal communication skills to nonverbal and verbal severely handicapped students. In L. Brown, J. Nietupski, S. Lyon, S. Hamre-Nietupski, T. Crowner, & L. Grunewald (Eds.), Curricular strategies for teaching functional object use, nonverbal communication, problem solving and mealtime skills to severely handicapped students (Vol. II, part 1, pp. 94–250). Madison, WI: Department of Specialized Educational Services, Madison Metropolitan School District.

Haring, T.G., Neetz, J.A., Lovinger, L., Peck, C., & Semmel, M.I. (1987). Effects of four modified incidental teaching procedures to create opportunities for communication. *Journal of The Association for Persons with Severe Handicaps, 12*, 218–226.

Harris, S.R. (1981). Effects of neurodevelopmental therapy on motor performance of infants with Down's syndrome. *Developmental Medicine and Child Neurology, 23*, 477–483.

Hart, B., & Risley, T.R. (1975). Incidental teaching of language in the preschool. *Journal of Applied Behavior Analysis, 8*, 411–420.

Hart, B., & Rogers-Warren, A. (1978). A milieu approach to teaching language. In R.L. Schiefelbusch (Ed.), *Language intervention strategies* (pp. 193–235). Baltimore: University Park Press.

Hinojosa, J., Sabari, J., Rosenfeld, M.S., & Shapiro, M.S. (1983). Purposeful activities. *American Journal of Occupational Therapy, 37*, 805–806.

Horn, E.M., & Warren, S.F. (1987). Facilitating the acquisition of sensorimotor behavior with a microcomputer-mediated teaching system: An experimental analysis. *Journal of The Association for Persons with Severe Handicaps, 12*, 205–215.

Hulme, J.B., Gallacher, K., Walsh, J., Niesen, S., & Waldron, D. (1987). Behavioral and postural changes observed with use of adaptive seating by clients with multiple handicaps. *Physical Therapy, 67*, 1060–1067.

Hulme, J.B., Schulein, M., Hulme, R.D., Poor, R., & Pezzino, J. (1983). Perceived behavioral changes in multihandicapped individuals using adapted equipment. *Physical and Occupational Therapy in Pediatrics, 3*(3), 63–73.

Hunt, P., Goetz, L., Alwell, M., & Sailor, W. (1986). Using an interrupted behavior chain strategy to teach generalized communication responses. *Journal of The Association for Persons with Severe Handicaps, 11*, 196–204.

Hunt, P., Goetz, L., & Anderson, J. (1986). The quality of IEP objectives associated with placement on integrated versus segregated school sites. *Journal of The Association for Persons with Severe Handicaps, 11*, 125–130.

Idol, L., Paolucci-Whitcomb, P., & Nevin, A. (1986). *Collaborative consultation*. Rockville, MD: Aspen.

Ilmer, S., Rynders, J., Sinclair, S., & Helfrich, D. (1981). Assessment of object permanence in severely handicapped students as a function of motor and prompting variables. *Journal of The Association for the Severely Handicapped, 6*(3), 30–40.

Jenkins, J.R., Sells, C.J., Brady, D., Down, J., Moore, B., Carman, P., & Holm, R. (1982). Effects of developmental therapy on motor impaired children. *Physical and Occupational Therapy in Pediatrics, 2*(4), 19–28.

Jones, T.W. (1983). Remediation of behavior-related eating problems: A preliminary investigation. *Journal of The Association for the Severely Handicapped, 8*(4), 62–71.

Kaiser, S.M., & Woodman, R.W. (1985). Multidisciplinary teams and group decision-making techniques: Possible solutions to decision-making problems. *School Psychology Review, 14*, 457–470.

Kantner, R.M., Kantner, B., & Clark, D.L. (1982). Vestibular stimulation effect on language development in mentally retarded children. *American Journal of Occupational Therapy, 36*, 36–41.

Kearns, K.P. (1986). Flexibility of single-subject experimental designs. Part II: Design selection and arrangement of experimental phases. *Journal of Speech and Hearing Disorders, 51*, 204–214.

Kircher, M.A. (1984). Motivation as a factor of perceived exertion in purposeful versus nonpurposeful activity. *American Journal of Occupational Therapy, 38*, 165–170.

Kohl, F., Wilcox, B., & Karlan, G. (1978). Effects of training conditions on the generalization of manual signs with moderately handicapped students. *Education and Training of the Mentally Retarded, 13*, 327–335.

Kopchick, G.A., & Lloyd, L.L. (1976). Total communication for the severely language impaired: A 24-hour approach. In L.L. Lloyd (Ed.), *Communication assessment and intervention strategies* (pp. 501–522). Baltimore: University Park Press.

Leiper, C.I., Miller, A., Lang, J., & Herman, R. (1981). Sensory feedback for head control in cerebral palsy. *Physical Therapy, 61*, 512–518.

Magrun, W.M., McCue, S., Ottenbacher, K., & Keefe, R. (1981). Effects of vestibular stimulation on spontaneous use of verbal language in developmentally delayed children. *American Journal of Occupational Therapy, 35*, 101–104.

Maloney, F.P., & Kurtz, P.A. (1982). The use of a mercury switch head control device in profoundly retarded, multiply handicapped children. *Physical and Occupational Therapy in Pediatrics, 2*(4), 11–17.

Marvin, C.A. (1987). Consultation services: Changing roles for SLPs. *Journal of Childhood Communication Disorders, 11*(1), 1–15.

McReynolds, L.V., & Thompson, C.K. (1986). Flexibility of single-subject experimental designs. Part I: Review of the basics of single-subject designs. *Journal of Speech and Hearing Disorders, 51*, 194–203.

Miedaner, J.A., & Renander, J. (1987). The effectiveness of classroom passive stretching programs for increasing or maintaining passive range of motion in non-ambulatory children: An evaluation of frequency. *Physical and Occupational Therapy in Pediatrics, 7*(3), 35–43.

Morris, S.E. (1977). *Program guidelines for children with feeding problems*. Edison, NJ: Childcraft Education.

Munson, J.H., Nordquist, C.L., & Thuma-Rew, S.L. (1987). *Communication systems for persons with*

severe neuromotor impairment: An Iowa interdisciplinary approach. Iowa City: University of
Iowa (Division of Developmental Disabilities, Uni-
veristy Hospital School).

Musselwhite, C.R., & St. Louis, K.W. (1982). Com-
munity programming for the severely handicapped:
Vocal and non-vocal strategies. San Diego: College-
Hill Press.

Nakaoka, Y., Ishida, S., Nishiwaki, M., & Manabe,
K. (1984). Relation between head control and loco-
motor ability in athetoid children. Physical and Occupational Therapy in Pediatrics, 4(2), 29–35.

Nietupski, J., & Hamre-Nietupski, S. (1979). Teaching auxiliary communication skills to severely
handicapped learners. AAESPH Review, 4(2), 107–
124.

Oliver, C.B., & Halle, J.W. (1982). Language training in the everyday environment: Teaching functional sign use to a retarded child. Journal of The
Association for the Severely Handicapped, 7(3),
50–62.

Ottenbacher, K. (1982). The effect of a controlled program of vestibular stimulation on the incidence of
seizures in children with severe developmental delay. Physical and Occupational Therapy in Pediatrics, 2(2/3), 25–33.

Ottenbacher, K., Bundy, A., & Short, M.A. (1983).
The development and treatment of oral-motor dysfunction: A review of clinical research. Physical
and Occupational Therapy in Pediatrics, 3(2), 1–
13.

Ottenbacher, K., Hicks, J., Roark, A., & Swinea, J.
(1983). Oral sensorimotor therapy in the developmentally disabled: A multiple baseline study. American Journal of Occupational Therapy, 37, 541–
547.

Ottenbacher, K., Scoggins, A., & Wayland, J. (1981).
The effectiveness of a program of oral sensory-
motor therapy with the severely and profoundly developmentally disabled. Occupational Therapy
Journal of Research, 1, 147–160.

Ottenbacher, K., & York, J. (1984). Strategies for
evaluating clinical change: Implications for practice
and research. American Journal of Occupational
Therapy, 38, 647–659.

Parette, H.P., Jr., & Hourcade, J.J. (1984). A review
of therapeutic intervention research on gross and
fine motor progress in young children with cerebral
palsy. American Journal of Occupational Therapy,
38, 462–468.

Paul, L. (1985). Programming peer support for functional language. In S.F. Warren & A.K. Rogers-
Warren (Eds.), Teaching functional language: Generalization and maintenance of language skills (pp.
289–308). Baltimore: University Park Press.

Peck, C.A. (1985). Increasing opportunities for social
control by children with autism and severe handicaps: Effects on student behavior and perceived
classroom climate. Journal of The Association for
Persons with Severe Handicaps, 10, 183–193.

Peck, C.A., Killen, C.C., & Baumgart, D. (1989).
Increasing implementation of special education instruction in mainstream preschools: Direct and
generalized nondirective consultation. Journal of
Applied Behavioral Analysis, 22, 197–210.

Peck, C.A., Schuler, A.L., Haring, T.G., Willard,
C., Theimer, R.K., & Semmel, M.I. (1986).
Teaching social/communicative skills to children
with autism and severe handicaps: Issues in assessment and curriculum selection. Child Study Journal, 16, 297–313.

Peganoff, S.A. (1984). The use of aquatics with cerebral palsied adolescents. American Journal of Occupational Therapy, 38, 469–473.

Prutting, C. (1982). Pragmatics as social competence.
Journal of Speech and Hearing Disorders, 47,
123–134.

Pryzwansky, W.B., & White, G.W. (1983). The influence of consultee characteristics on preferences for
consultation approaches. Professional Psychology
Research and Practices, 14, 457–461.

Rainforth, B., & York, J. (1987). Integrating related
services in community instruction. Journal of The
Association for Persons with Severe Handicaps, 12,
190–198.

Reichle, J., & Karlan, G. (1988). Selecting augmentative communication interventions: A critique of
candidacy criteria and a proposed alternative. In
R.L. Schiefelbusch & L.L. Loyd (Eds.), Language
perspectives (2nd ed., pp. 321–342). Austin, TX:
PRO-ED.

Reichle, J., & Keogh, W.J. (1985). Communication
intervention: A selective review of what, when, and
how to teach. In S.F. Warren & A.K. Rogers-
Warren (Eds.), Teaching functional language: Generalization and maintenance of language skills (pp.
25–62). Baltimore: University Park Press.

Reichle, J., & Keogh, W.J. (1986). Communication
instruction for learners with severe handicaps:
Some unresolved issues. In R.H. Horner, L.H.
Meyer, & H.D.B. Fredericks (Eds.), Education of
learners with severe handicaps: Exemplary service
strategies (pp. 189–219). Baltimore: Paul H.
Brookes Publishing Co.

Reilly, C., Nelson, D.L., & Bundy, A.C. (1983). Sensorimotor versus fine motor activities in eliciting
vocalizations in autistic children. Occupational
Therapy Journal of Research, 3(4), 199–212.

Romski, M.A., Lloyd, L.L., & Sevcik, R.A. (1988).
Augmentative and alternative communication is-
sues. In R.L. Schiefelbusch & L.L. Lloyd (Eds.),
Language perspectives (2nd ed., pp. 343–366).
Austin, TX: PRO-ED.

Rourk, J., Dunn, W., Wendt, E., Stephens, L., & Andrews, J. (1987). Setting priorities for providing services. In American Occupational Therapy Association, Guidelines for occupational therapy services
in school systems (pp. 9-1–9-8). Rockville, MD:
American Occupational Therapy Association.

Sailor, W., Guess, D., Goetz, L., Schuler, A., Utley,

B., & Baldwin, M. (1980). Language and severely handicapped persons: Deciding what to teach to whom. In W. Sailor, B., Wilcox, & L. Brown (Eds.), *Methods of instruction for severely handicapped students* (pp. 71–105). Baltimore: Paul H. Brookes Publishing Co.

Schmidt, P. (1976). Feeding assessment and therapy for the neurologically impaired. *AAESPH Review*, *I*(8), 19–27.

Siegel, G.M., & Young, M.A. (1987). Group designs in clinical research. *Journal of Speech and Hearing Disorders*, *52*, 194–199.

Snow, C., Midkiff-Borunda, S., Small, A., & Proctor, A. (1984). Therapy as social interaction: Analyzing the contexts for language remediation. *Topics in Language Disorders*, *4*, 72–85.

Sobsey, R., & Orelove, F.P. (1984). Neurophysiological facilitation of eating skills in children with severe handicaps. *Journal of The Association for Persons with Severe Handicaps*, *9*, 98–110.

Steinbeck, T.M. (1986). Purposeful activity and performance. *American Journal of Occupational Therapy*, *40*, 529–534.

Sternat, J., Messina, R., Nietupski, J., Lyon, S., & Brown, L. (1977). Occupational and physical therapy services for severely handicapped students: Toward a naturalized public school service delivery model. In E. Sontag (Ed.), *Educational programming for the severely and profoundly handicapped* (pp. 263–278). Reston, VA: Division on Mental Retardation.

Stremel-Campbell, K., & Campbell, C.R. (1985). Training techniques that may facilitate generalization. In S.F. Warren & A.K. Rogers-Warren (Eds.), *Teaching functional language: Generalization and maintenance of language skills* (pp. 251–288). Baltimore: University Park Press.

Talbot, M.L., & Junkala, J. (1981). The effects of auditorily augmented feedback on the eye-hand coordination of students with cerebral palsy. *American Journal of Occupational Therapy*, *35*, 525–528.

Taylor, C.L., & Harris, S.R. (1986). Effects of ankle-foot orthoses on functional motor performance in a child with spastic diplegia. *American Journal of Occupational Therapy*, *40*, 492–494.

Trefler, E., Nickey, J., & Hobson, D.A. (1983). Technology in the education of multiply-handicapped children. *American Journal of Occupational Therapy*, *37*, 381–387.

Walmsley, R.P., Crichton, L., & Droog, D. (1981). Music as a feedback mechanism for teaching head control to severely handicapped children: A pilot study. *Developmental Medicine and Child Neurology*, *23*, 739–746.

Warren, S.F., & Kaiser, A.P. (1986). Generalization of treatment effects by young language-delayed children: A longitudinal analysis. *Journal of Speech and Hearing Disorders*, *51*, 239–251.

Warren, S.F., & Rogers-Warren, A.K. (1985). Teaching functional language: An introduction. In S.F. Warren & A.K. Rogers-Warren (Eds.), *Teaching functional language: Generalization and maintenance of language skills* (pp. 3–24). Baltimore: University Park Press.

West, J.F., & Idol, L. (1987). School consultation (Part I): An interdisciplinary perspective on theory, models, and research. *Journal of Learning Disabilities*, *20*, 388–408.

West, W.L. (1984). A reaffirmed philosophy and practice of occupational therapy for the 1980s. *American Journal of Occupational Therapy*, *38*, 15–23.

Williams, W., & Fox, T. (1977). Communication. In W. Williams & T. Fox (Eds.), *Minimum objective system for pupils with severe handicaps: Working draft number one* (Vol. 1). Burlington: University of Vermont, Center for Special Education.

York, J., Nietupski, J., & Hamre-Nietupski, S. (1985). A decision-making process for using microswitches. *Journal of The Association for Persons with Severe Handicaps*, *10*, 214–223.

York, J., Rainforth, B., & Dunn, W. (1990). Training needs of physical and occupational therapists who provide services to children and youth with severe disabilities. In A.P. Kaiser & C.M. McWhorter (Eds.), *Preparing personnel to work with persons with severe disabilities* (pp. 153–179). Baltimore: Paul H. Brookes Publishing Co.

Yoshida, R.K. (1980). Multidisciplinary decision making in special education: A review of issues. *School Psychology Review*, *9*, 221–227.

CHAPTER 19

Community School
An Essay

WAYNE SAILOR

San Francisco State University, San Francisco, California

My two young children, both students in our town's local, regular public schools, still don't really quite understand just what it is their daddy does for a living. They sit with me in our living room and watch training tapes that I bring home from time to time, such as *Regular Lives,* and comment on the fact that they never see kids "like those" in their schools, let alone in their classrooms. We live in a progressive community, known widely for its early efforts in school desegregation and for being the birthplace of the Center for Independent Living, among other things. So why can't my children associate educationally with children who happen to have disabilities? I, like many parents, want my children to grow up with tolerance and sensitivity for people whose lifestyles are more restricted and challenged than theirs. But something about the way we are educating our children, *all* of them, is preventing this possibility.

Hope, however, springs eternal. Educational change is most definitely in the wind in my town, and in the rest of the United States as well. My sense is that there is a glimmering of a back-to-school movement underway in this country, and if this proves indeed to be the case, then I wish to add my shoulder to the task. By "back to school," I mean the ding-dong school, of course; and it is to the cause of resurrection of that mainstay institution from our nation's development that I write this essay.

DEMISE OF SPECIALIZATION

For the ding-dong school to return to America, the death of the age of educational specialization must be imminent. I believe that the educational specialization movement reached its zenith in the publication of the Holmes Group report (1986). Before the recommendations of this report could be implemented, however, colleges and universities have increasingly had to deal with the implications of the new values-based education movement in our society. We have, in fact, reached a point of struggle now in educational policy and its stepchild, reform, between the forces of test-based outcome in educational practice and values-based outcome. The test-based people argue for yet more extensive and highly specialized teacher training programs. Such programs will, the argument goes, enhance the status and prestige of the teaching profession; justify and lead to high salaries; attract smarter, more capable people into the teaching profession; and result in higher achievement test scores for the recipients of the effort. Emphasize their professionalism, the argument goes, make them more like doctors and lawyers.

The values-based folks seem to have a somewhat different set of specifications in mind, although a position comparable to the Holmes Group report (1986) has yet to surface from this emerging camp. The values-based position argues that increased educational specialization has led to a corresponding sense of educational isolation among the recipients. Specialization has been manifest in categorization of children, by special need, and the categorization has resulted in placement and grouping configurations that are out of the mainstream. As public pressure from an increasingly aging U.S. population has mounted toward greater accountability from educators, the specialization movement has fostered the achievement test–outcome standard in

[1]Supported in part by Cooperative Agreement #G0087C3056-88, U.S. Department of Education. No official endorsement is intended or should be inferred.

the hopes of providing a means to evaluate success in the aggregate. As classes, schools, school districts, and whole states clamor to show better bang for the buck through higher test scores, the pressure has mounted to remove increasing numbers of "categorical" populations from the mainstream so that they don't drag down the scores.

The values-outcome people argue that the more pressure generated by test-score evaluation, the more teachers must necessarily teach what the tests measure, and that this process is devoid of values. So we have two legacies of the test-outcome movement that would seem to suggest that the time is ripe for an alternative to emerge. The first is the increasingly fractionated and bureaucratic forms of educational service delivery that have emerged, with concomitant special groupings that occur at some time during the educational day for practically everyone who deviates at all from an upper middle–class norm of standardized performances. The second is an educational curriculum at all ages that is increasingly bereft of value-laden instruction of the kind that used to be the hallmark of an American education.

So what is at the root of the values-outcome movement? Is it, as many seem to believe, the rantings of an increasingly vociferous minority of born-again Neo-Christians, clamoring for religiosity in the schools? My feeling is that while that group is likely to be a bedfellow in the values-outcome movement, the origins of the movement stem from some much broader issues than than those that are implied by the simple notion of a separation of church and state.

For one thing, the schools are increasingly coming under attack for failing to solve a growing number of social problems, including drugs, teenage pregnancies, youth crime, and AIDS. The argument goes something like this. There is a breakdown in American society of its sense of community and of the basic "nuclear" family structure. Because of the dissolution of these mainstays of our social system, other institutions must step in and instill the basic Judeo-Christian moral ethic in our citizenry that was formerly the prerogative of the family and community (including the church or synagogue).

The institutions that have been nominated to fulfill this role are education and, later on, business and industry. One hears increasingly at present about the need for ethics in the industrial marketplace, and how Japan, for example, exemplifies a program of industrial participation in the transmission of ethics and moral behavior to its citizens, a factor that may, the argument goes, help to explain its productivity gains relative to U.S. manufacturing and industry.

The schools, however, are increasingly blamed for everything. If the family and community cannot instill values, then the schools must. If the schools fail, then their tax base should be reevaluated, so the argument goes. Extreme school blamers push the ideology of "vouchers," by which students can get a parochial, private education at public expense.

Here is the locus of the struggle for school policy reform. If schools are to teach values, then the outcomes of this teaching must themselves be valued and positively sanctioned. To be so sanctioned, they must be evident and to be evident implies measurement. But if we are committing all of our resources to achievement test outcomes based upon academic content, and all available resources to educational systems are geared to these relative outcomes, then how can schools afford to take the time and trouble to teach something for which no measurement systems exist, the nature of which is bereft of any real consensus and agreement, and for which no resources are to be provided contingent upon success?

The state of California, for example, evaluates the adequacy of its myriad secondary schools on the percentage of graduates who achieve academic eligibility for admission to the various campuses of the University of California and the California State University systems. The taxpayers of California are confronted each year with the dilemma of comparing the positive statistic of an academic eligibility for higher education gain, statewide, of 0.5%, with the depressing statistic of a 2% increase in the high school drop-out rate.

Specialization has pretty much run its course, I think. It was probably necessary to evolve a categorical nexus in order to generate the kinds of technologies needed to render the educational system at least applicable to the complex and diverse populations entering the nation's schools from the post–World War II period to the present time. Such technologies probably evolve best in the relative sanctuary of separate subsystems. Teachers and educational researchers have probably benefited from the close-up view and understanding gained about distinct, categorical "problem" populations when those populations could be isolated and removed from the mainstream. Perhaps no one could have anticipated the extent to which such isolation, to whatever extent it was considered to be temporary, would become institutionalized. It is now axiomatic that once a child is removed from the regular classroom, for whatever reason, the greater the likelihood that such a child will never regain that lost position. Referral out of the mainstream has pretty much become a one-way street.

Have these technologies to benefit special populations proven beneficial to their recipients? The data here appear to be confounded by their application in isolated circumstances. Many now argue, for example, that in the case of populations of persons with disabilities, the outcomes of teaching technologies are largely dependent upon the nature of the educational environments wherein they are imparted. Techniques to improve reading among children with specific learning disabilities, for example, which were developed in categorical "resource room" environments, now appear to have the most demonstrable success when applied in the context of a regular, mainstream classroom. Similarly, many techniques for improving educational outcomes among students with severe disabilities that were developed by teachers and others in "special" schools and classrooms now appear to have their relative success augmented under conditions of application in more fully integrated circumstances.

Perhaps we don't need any more specialization, at least for a time. Perhaps what we need now is a design to apply our specialized teaching technologies under a more generic set of educational conditions. If our various populations of students with special or exceptional education needs can do better when educated with their "normal" peers, then perhaps a window of opportunity exists for those concerned with value-outcomes. That is, perhaps the populations of different children will add something of innate value to an educational process that is concerned

with the transmission of values as educational outcomes.

SCHOOL AS COMMUNITY

In the earlier period of our evolution as a rich and powerful nation, the public school was an "integral" part of something we called "the community." The principal institutions (components) of the community were the church, the neighborhood school, and the general store. Today, the concept of a community has become an academic issue. Entire books are being written about it. There are many vagaries about what a community is now, but what is clear is that it is something that once existed but has been lost. The general store has been replaced by shopping malls, McDonald's, and Toys Я Us. Churches have seen their congregations turn gray and disappear. Schools have fallen victim to specialization and racial busing. Neighborhoods are still there, but they usually don't provide much of an opportunity to meet and exchange information and values. Sometimes "neighborhood watch" committees formed to combat crime in the area approximate a sense of community, but participation tends to dwindle rapidly to a handful of neighborhood representatives.

With the demise of community came the demise of traditional American values. The stresses on families, particularly in urban areas, have become acute. The family as a unit has become dissolute to an alarming extent, particularly in culturally disadvantaged sectors of our society.

If traditional, humanistic values such as caring for one another, respecting the rights of others, and so forth, are not transmitted through the family because it has dissolved and are not transmitted through the community because there is none, then the value structure itself dissolves— and there are indications that this may be happening on a distressingly large scale. In the absence of traditional communities, microcommunities form with their own value structures. The "drug culture" that is present in some form in practically every city and town in America is an example of such a subculture or microcommunity.

Much of the blame for the mess that our society has gotten itself into is placed on the door-step of the school system. Racial busing, for example, was supposed to result in a pluralistic, egalitarian society. The argument, which was well ventilated in the Los Angeles *Times* in the 1960s, was this: if blacks can attend schools in white neighborhoods and vice versa, then the quality of education available to them, coupled with social legislation such as the "fair housing" acts of the period, will lead to economic parity and the neighborhoods will become integrated. Then, cross-town busing can be discontinued. But it didn't happen. Black neighborhoods have grown larger and poorer, and white neighborhoods more affluent. Now the schools are asked to solve the drug problem. New schools are being designed to resemble prisons. Walls and fences are in evidence, bars on the windows and electronic sensing devices are coming into place—not to keep the school population in, but to keep everyone else out. And then there is the "Just say no" campaign. Do you believe these measures will solve the drug problem? Neither do I.

What is needed is to re-create the traditional community, so that once again a mainstream for the societal transmission of cultural values is in place and operational. Perhaps this is a viable role for the schools after all. Certainly the nation's politicians have made much of demanding such a role. While former Secretary of Education William Bennett suggested that school funding should be tied to evidence of *values instruction,* he made this suggestion at exactly the same time the schools under his jurisdiction were receiving their resource allotments partly on the basis of performance indicators geared to *academic content instruction.*

Incorporating a curriculum of values-based instruction to be taught to children at their public school is probably not the way to go. Perhaps there is another alternative, however, and that is to use the existence of the school in our society to create a *community.* If traditional values are transmitted by participating in and belonging to a community, and this function of a community can offset to some degree the damage to values transmission that accrues from the dissolution of the family and the demise of organized religion, then re-creation of a community through the

mechanism of the school could prove a worthwhile social experiment.

Schools, as we know them today, will have to undergo some fairly major changes in order to form the basis for communities. For schools to serve as the vehicles for the transmission of cultural values, they must represent those values. This means that all of those special needs populations that have been referred out of school must be brought back. For a school to form the basis of a community, it must meet the educational needs of all of the students who make up this community. If it segregates some or discriminates against others, then these are the values that it transmits.

If current trends were to persist much into the future, our schools would become like factories with tightly regulated labor forces and a product (children's education) entirely driven by formulas and standardized productivity measures. As pressures to increase test scores increasingly drive the allocation of school resources, teacher advancement and pay, and so forth, the more children who score below the norm will be referred out of the process to separate and unequal but parallel systems of special, compensatory, migrant, bilingual, and other educational groupings.

It is, perhaps ironically, the most unlikely population of all of those who have been excluded from the regular classroom that is now knocking on the door to be reinstated, the population of children with severe disabilities. It was undoubtedly necessary to create special education. It was probably necessary to create it in a relatively separate set of environments, just as chemists isolate elemental compounds to synthesize natural substances. But now the technology is extant and the time has come to rejoin the party, certainly for children with severe disabilities, because it is demonstrably and inarguably better for them, and probably also for all of the other special needs populations as well. The question is how best to rethink the American educational process.

THE COMMUNITY SCHOOL

At a brainstorming session, which occurred as part of a meeting called in Washington, D.C., by the U.S. Office of Education and sponsored by Syracuse University, I had the pleasure of working with a particularly creative group of parents and professionals who delineated, at that meeting, the rough form of an idea called "supported education." This rubric really describes a process for education that has parallels to the supported employment initiative. In the idea of supported education, there is a single process called "education" and it is delivered through the vehicle of the local school. If there are children who, in order to be served at their local school, need particular supports to be in place, then those supports are entered into the process at the school site. Specialized educational services (special education) can be one of those supports offered to the regular educational program. Supported education should thus be the hallmark of the community school. The educational program for the school's students is driven by a system of shared values in addition to an academic content curriculum. Outcomes for evaluative purposes are multiple rather than uniformly driven by standardized test scores. But for a community school to deliver supported education, some changes are needed in several important areas.

Administration

A community school needs to have a site-based administrative structure. This means that the principal has responsibility for the provision of appropriate educational services for all of the students. There is not a separate special education department or program at the school that reports to a separate administrative structure downtown. To do the job of providing support to the child in the regular program, the needs of support services staff at the school are met by the principal, who negotiates with the district central administration for these resources. Obviously, such site-based administrators need to learn about special populations and their resource personnel.

Funding

Funds now come tied to categorical programs. This is probably the mechanism that allowed education to become so fractionated in the first place. Supported education at the community school requires coordinated revenue utilization at the school site. This is not "co-mingling" of funds, which is illegal. Funds must be spent to educate the categorical population for which they are intended. However, planning for the utilization of various revenues at the school site can result in a coordinated effort that best meets the needs of all students. Special educators need to remember that there is nothing in PL 94-142 or PL 99-457 or in their regulations that calls for the delivery of special educational services in a separate environment. Rather, the reverse is true. The laws require keeping pupils in the regular classrooms unless it can be shown that such a placement would work to the students' detriment.

Teacher Training

Regular teachers need more competencies in effective practices with special needs populations to implement a supported education model. Inservice and preservice efforts will be needed to support the effort. Support personnel need to have a more generic set of competencies than is presently the case under categorical specialization models. Teachers of students labeled as "autistic," "deaf," "blind," "behaviorally disabled," "learning disabled," "severely handicapped," and so on and so forth will need to become resource specialists with capabilities of assisting regular teachers to meet the needs of more diverse populations, both in and out of the regular classroom, and in a variety of community settings as needed. Teacher licensing and credentialing systems will need to evolve to fit the changing competencies of instructional personnel at the community school.

Nonteaching Support Services

To educate all children at the community school will require a team of various professionals, some of whom will serve only the school in question, while others may provide itinerant services to a number of schools in the region. Support personnel are planned and budgeted for each year to fit the particular needs of the children to be served in the school that year. Effective supported education requires an integrated transdisciplinary approach, characterized by role release, role sharing, consultation, and inservice training.

Educational Groupings

Supported education implies support to the regular program, so separate groupings are discouraged. If children with disabilities need instruction outside of the regular classroom, as when students with severe disabilities are instructed in community settings, the support personnel manage those aspects of each student's individualized education program (IEP). When the student is in the regular classroom, support personnel assist the regular teacher to the extent necessary to maximize the educational advantage for all the students in the class. Class sizes must be adjusted for supported education. A class size of 25 students maximum is recommended when 1 or 2 students in the class have disabilities or other special service needs. Such class sizes become possible under supported education because of more efficient use of categorical resources at the school site. Regular students are accepting of their disabled peers and there is even some recent evidence to suggest that the performance of regular education students under supported education models tends to be enhanced on a variety of outcome measures, including standardized achievement tests. When regular teachers realize benefits for their instructional programs from the participation of the specialized support personnel, they become enthusiastic about the supported education model. The critical factor on the part of both regular teachers and administrators is an attitude of viewing *all* children as needing and being entitled to a free and appropriate public education in the environment that maximizes their social and communicative development in addition to their other educational needs. Regular teachers in supported education become acutely aware of the importance of motivation in the education of all students, including those with even the most severe disabilities.

Responsibility and Monitoring

Schools, at present, remain aloof from the society. Elected, or worse, appointed, boards of education "represent" the members of the population at large. Parent input into the system is sanctioned only through "back-to-school night" and meetings of the PTA to raise funds for new playground equipment.

Supported education at the community school implies a different level of participation. The school defines the community. It is, at once, the community meeting place and the educational resource of the community. Community schools solicit direct parent involvement through site representation teams and curriculum councils. The site teams are groups that include elected parents, teachers, and student representatives who advise the principal, and indirectly, the district board of education on the needs and resources of their community school. Curriculum councils are teams of parents, teaching and support staff, and kids who assume responsibility for planning the curricular needs of groups of students at the school. Typical curriculum councils each have up to 100 students within their jurisdiction, including all ages, and special needs, as well as regular, students. Sometimes a community school's curriculum councils will compete with each other in a friendly and spirited way, to see whose group of students will reflect the best educational outcomes from their efforts. Curriculum councils advise the site representation team, and through it the teachers, principal, and other staff of the school. Just about everyone gets into the act and that is what makes a community. From such a hodgepodge of humanity at the community school may evolve some pretty harebrained schemes. It is unlikely, however, that such schemes will be any less functional than those that characterize typical schools where instruction is categorized and specialized. How about "attention deficit disorder (ADD)" for a harebrained scheme award?

Community schools become accessible for meetings in the evening and on weekends when necessary. In the days when there were communities, there were town halls where people met to solve problems and improve life in their communities. The community school is a return to the town hall model and serves a broader constituency than the parents of its kids.

Final Remarks

Finally, and most importantly, community schools exist in various forms now around the country, and have already demonstrated the validity of the concept. It has not, thus far, been revealed to be a harebrained scheme. The results appear to be positive, for all its participants. Schools once served an important mission in the transmission of values that made our nation the envy of the Western world. Those days are over and gone, but the persistent idea of a community school and values-based education may yet constitute the reformation in American education.

◇ **CHAPTER 20** ◇

Social Policy, Social Systems, and Educational Practice

Douglas P. Biklen

Syracuse University, Syracuse, New York

MYTHS

It is difficult to change education beliefs and practices if they are clouded by false assumptions. Such is the case with efforts to change from segregated to integrated education. Certain assumptions about special and regular education make change difficult.

One such assumption is that before schools can adopt an integrationist approach, researchers must accumulate evidence that integration will be more educationally profitable than segregation for the students involved. This assumption contradicts the language of PL 94-142, which places the burden of proof on those who would segregate. Further, this assumption suggests that the decision to pursue integration is a question for research to answer rather than being a moral issue, as, for example, whether to educate males and females together or students of color with white students.

A second commonly held assumption is that individual placement of students into programs is more or less precise, with the proper program being matched to the students' needs. Public Law 94-142, The Education for All Handicapped Children Act, helps to create this assumption (see Biklen, Ferguson, & Ford, 1989). In fact, placement has proven to be imprecise; one review found no real distinctions between students who are and are not labeled as learning disabled and those who are or are not served in learning disability programs (Algozzine, 1985). A study of placements for students with severe disabilities demonstrated that the type and location of a student's placement is determined more by the type of programs available than by the perceived needs of the student (Biklen, 1988). This latter study demonstrated that students with a particular type of disability (e.g., multiple handicaps or emotional disturbance) are more than 25 times more likely to attend separate schools for students with disabilities in some states than in others.

When Congress passed PL 94-142, it could have prohibited segregated schooling. Obviously, private schools and some public separate school leaders pressured Congress not to preclude their continuance or even expansion. Congress chose to circumvent this politically sensitive issue. It incorporated a presumption that "integrated schooling is best" into the law:

> . . . procedures to assure that . . . handicapped children . . . are educated with children who are not handicapped, and that special classes, separate schooling, or other removal of handicapped children from the regular educational environment occurs only when the nature or severity of the handicap is such that education in regular classes with the use of supplementary aids and services cannot be achieved satisfactorily. (The Education for All Handicapped Children Act of 1975, Section 612 [5] [B])

This language was expected to spawn an incremental change process. Placement committees are empowered under the law to assess students, to determine their needs, and to recommend the appropriate, individualized education program (IEP), including the location of the program. Parents can participate in the classifica-

Preparation of this chapter was partially supported by the U.S. Department of Education, Office of Special Education and Rehabilitative Services, National Institute on Disability and Rehabilitation Research (NIDRR), under Cooperative Agreement #G0085CO3503 awarded to the Center on Human Policy, Division of Special Education and Rehabilitation, Syracuse University, Syracuse, New York. The opinions expressed herein are solely those of the author and no official endorsement of the U.S. Department of Education should be inferred.

tion/placement committee meeting and decision and may challenge a classification, placement, or program with which they disagree.

The problems with such a process are that: 1) it ignores the fact that there will always be a tendency to replicate established, past practices (e.g. segregation); 2) it does not address the fact that nonclinical factors such as educational financing methods influence the availability of choices to professionals and parents alike; and 3) it places the burden for changing educational practice on individual students and the individual case review process.

FINANCING METHODS

Throughout this book, a number of authors identify and describe barriers to integrated schooling (e.g., dual administrative hierarchies, inappropriate curricula, handicapist attitudes, and an absence of social/educational planning). One factor that looms large and that also deserves careful consideration is *educational financing*. By focusing on school finance as a barrier to integrated schooling, we move beyond the traditional assumptions about student placements.

Local property taxes provide the primary source of revenue for public education in America. State revenues generally supplement the local contributions; state funds typically serve two goals, to sponsor special services (e.g., special education, transportation, community education, inservice training) and to foster equity across school districts of unequal wealth. In the latter case, proportionally more funds are allocated to poorer districts than to wealthier ones. When states expend state revenues on the education of students labeled as disabled, they do so through one or a combination of strategies:

Specific purposes funding (e.g., counseling, transportation, resource programs)

Personnel funding (e.g., resource teacher salaries, consulting teacher salaries, special class teacher salaries)

Per capita funding (e.g., an amount of money or percentage of cost of serving students with particular disabilities)

Within any of these funding types, a state may provide a percentage of the total cost, a set dollar amount, a weighted amount depending on the purpose (e.g., type of program, type of personnel, or type of disability), or total cost over a certain initial local expenditure level. In addition, states may adjust allotments to account for the relative wealth of a school district, providing more funds to poorer than to wealthier districts.

While each of the funding mechanisms can target funding for the education of students with disabilities, each also has the potential to encourage segregated services and increased labeling of students. Funding by categories of students tends to influence the numbers of students identified in particular categories. Funding for types of service tends to force districts into establishing discrete services (i.e., segregated services such as special classes, separate schools, and resource rooms), for accountability. Funding of personnel could facilitate teachers, consultants, and aides working where the students are (e.g., in typical classes), although states usually want to limit the special educator to working only with labeled students in order to ensure that special funding is not siphoned off for the education of nonclassified students. None of these funding methods encourages districts to adopt a unified approach to developing programs for *all* students; each calls for differentiating and separating educational services to students classified as disabled.

Another approach would be special funding for a unit or personnel involved in the integration process. This approach would reject the idea that integrated services do *not* cost more than educating nondisabled students alone. It would reject the assumption that the only students who can be integrated are those who can succeed despite their disabilities, indeed as if they did not have disabilities that affected their learning. The problem with this form of special funding, even though it fosters integration, is that it singles out integration and integration teachers as special (i.e., unusual).

The preferred approach would be unitary funding (funds emanate from a single or sole source) of all programs. This approach is reasonable only if three conditions prevail:

1.   All classes are refashioned to accommodate smaller class sizes; all classes serve a het-

erogeneous group; schools utilize diverse models of organizing staff, including team teaching, consulting teaching, teaching assistance, and multidisciplinary teaming.

2. Schools and the public share a basic commitment to the belief that the education of students with the most profound disabilities is as important as the education of students with great academic skill; such schools therefore expect to devote financial resources in a fashion that maximizes the opportunities available to all students.

3. States monitor school expenditures to ensure a continuing commitment to students of varying abilities.

CONCLUSION

It is unfair and ultimately self-defeating to place the responsibility for achieving integration on parents and on individual case conferences. Integration will occur more certainly and rapidly when state governments and local school districts make integrated schooling a task for policy planning and implementation.

REFERENCES

Algozzine, B. (1985). Low achiever differentiation: Where's the beef? *Exceptional Children, 52,* 72–75.

Biklen, D. (1988). The myth of clinical judgment. *Journal of Social Issues, 44*(1), 127–140.

Biklen, D., Ferguson, D., & Ford, A. (Eds.). (1989). *Schooling and disability* (88th Yearbook, Part 2). Chicago: National Society for the Study of Education.

The Education for All Handicapped Children Act of 1975, (Public Law 94-142), 20 U.S.C. §§ 1401–1420 (1975).

◇ **CHAPTER 21** ◇

Preparation of Personnel to Educate Students with Severe and Multiple Disabilities
A Time for Change?

Doug Guess
Barbara Thompson
University of Kansas, Lawrence, Kansas

In 1977, Burke and Cohen published what is likely the first description and analysis of competencies that were then used by a relatively small number of existing personnel training programs to prepare teachers to provide educational services to students with severely handicapping conditions. Their analysis reviewed 11 special personnel projects that had been funded by the Bureau of Education for the Handicapped (now the Office of Special Education and Rehabilitative Services). The competency areas addressed in the mid-1970s reflected a strong behavioral, environmental approach to the education of students with severe handicaps, and do not differ significantly from what the much larger number of university training programs today would likely consider to be state-of-the-art practices in the severely handicapped area of special education. Exceptions and additions would be a deemphasis on the use of aversive procedures to decelerate unwanted behavior, a much stronger effort to provide educational services in community and other integrated settings, and the utilization of advanced computer technology—all of which, of course, reflect positive changes in our field of specialization.

It could be argued, of course, that many of these progressive changes (e.g., community integration, competitive employment, acknowledgment of choices and preferences) could, or even would, have emerged independent of the behavioral orientation that was adopted in the early 1970s; and that many of the gains achieved

for this population are more a result of sociopolitical activism and advocacy, rather than adherence to a specific educational philosophy or orientation. In this respect, one can speculate on whether advances in our field were the result of the prevailing educational model, a greater advocacy effort by professionals and parents, or possibly both.

There is in our field, nevertheless, a continuation of the diagnostic-prescriptive model of intervention and education that is based on a rational approach that has been extracted from the natural sciences—an approach that attempts to limit knowledge to the facts of experience and that eschews speculation on the ultimate and possible unobserved nature of things or reality. As pointed out by Winzer (1986), current practices in special education are consistent with the French *philosophes* that emerged during the Enlightenment period, particulary the second half of the 18th century. The *philosophes* extended the speculations of Locke that knowledge is experienced through sensation and reflection, and that humans have no innate ideas or primary notions. The application of the rational positivism approach to the field of special education was further strengthened by the contributions of the emerging psychology of applied behavior analysis that was based heavily on the principles of Skinnerian operant conditioning (Skinner, 1971) although, as pointed out by Edgar and Sulzbacher (1983) many of the practices of special educators today (e.g., task-analysis, discrimination learning, errorless learning) are not new, but just refinements of the work of earlier educators such as Itard.

A significant contribution of behaviorism to current practices in special education was an attempt to provide a more scientific methodogy—one designed to emulate more the natural and, especially, the physical sciences (Skinner, 1971). This has included the requirement for observable and reliable data reflecting instructional procedures and student outcomes, and the introduction of single-subject research designs (cf. Baer, Wolf, & Risley, 1968) to analyze the manipulation of independent variables that were derived primarily from the principles of applied behavior analysis. Consistent with the basic tenets of the rational positivism approach, the advancement of the technology, and hence of special education, has been perceived as the gradual accumulation of knowlege producing ever further and more microscopic refinements of instructional procedures—refinements that have attempted to address acknowledged problems in current practices (e.g., generalization and maintenance of learned skills, limited spontaneous repertoires, and, for many students with profound handicaps, a general failure to learn). The data-based approach of current practices in special education and the accompanying efforts to use observable data as a critical component of the accumulated technology are derivations of a broader *paradigm* that has been strongly embraced by the field for well over 20 years.

DIAGNOSTIC-PRESCRIPTIVE-REMEDIAL PARADIGM IN SPECIAL EDUCATION

A paradigm, generally defined, encompasses a model or pattern by which researchers, educators, and practitioners operate. It provides, in many respects, an orientation and philosophy by which new knowledge is assimilated into a theoretical perspective on the nature of observed phenomena. A paradigm offers a central organizing gestalt for the identification of new research questions, the interpretation of wide and often varying research findings, and, impor-

tantly, a possible framework for a larger world view. As we discuss subsequently, paradigms and paradigm shifts are integral components of scientific inquiry, and have significant influences on the values and behaviors of both professional communities and society at large. As noted, the prevailing paradigm in special education, and especially the severely handicapped area of this field, has deep roots in the philosophical concepts of environmental determinism merged with the manipulation of antecedent and consequence events associated with the psychology of behaviorism. At the applied level, the paradigm operates to identify among persons with disabilities areas of deficits and "deviancies," as determined by the consensus of those persons who assume responsibility (and control) over their behavior, and buttressed by an array of diagnostic instruments and surveys that depict either expected "normal" development or assumed community standards for behavior and conduct. The assumption is, of course, that once having identified the problems associated with the disability, the environment can be arranged, controlled, or otherwise manipulated to bring about the desired change in the student. This orientation, variously referred to as "prescriptive teaching," "remedial," "let's fix it," and so on, always carried with it the (at least) implicit assumption that persons with disabilities are somehow less than normal or, at its worst, "deviant."

What we fail to consider is that while the diagnostic-prescriptive-remedial paradigm has produced numerous instances in which discrete behaviors have been taught or modified, the emphasis of the paradigm essentially equates mental retardation with "deviancy"; and this equation might well project to both professionals and society at large such a negative image of these persons that true acceptance (and optimal integration) will never be fully achieved.

Additionally, the heavily emphasized "scientific" orientation of the paradigm might similarly create an atmosphere in which persons with handicapping (and especially severely handicapping) conditions are perceived in a depersonalized manner that obscures both their positive human qualities and perceived value. As pointed out by Iano (1986), "the natural science–

technical model promotes a conception of students as 'objects' to be technically manipulated in the interest of achieving given and externally imposed objectives" (p. 56).

Most persons would acknowledge, however, that the paradigm currently embraced by the severely handicapped area of special education is well entrenched and highly resistant to radical change. It occupies the greatest attention of researchers, the bulk of what is disseminated in teacher training programs and textbooks, and the primary content and curriculum orientation of practitioners in the field. It presents itself not as an alternative or option to other paradigms or models, nor even as a significantly modifiable educational approach (other than further refinement of its procedures); it is, to the contrary, offered as the sine qua non for the education of students with severe disabilities. We later address this observation with respect to the issue of personnel training. First, however, it is useful to discuss some general observations on the nature of paradigms and how they are changed, and some small, yet significant indications in our field that might signal the beginnings of a crack in the dominance of the present paradigm in the severely handicapped area of special education.

WILL THE MODIFIERS BE MODIFIED?

Thomas Kuhn's classic book *The Structure of Scientific Revolutions* (1970) is having an increasing influence on at least a small number of persons in the field of special education who perceive the need for change in how we both perceive and intervene with persons with disabilities. Although Kuhn's book addresses the natural sciences, his analysis would appear to have similar importance for the positivist, natural-science orientation of the paradigm that has been embraced by the field of special education. Kuhn's analysis addresses, in large part, paradigms and paradigm *shifts* that have occurred in the natural sciences. Shifts refer to changes in paradigms that result from new research findings or even dramatically alternative interpretations of the same data base. Significantly, Kuhn's analysis shows that in the natural sciences major breakthroughs (or paradigm shifts) occur not

from accumulated knowledge within an existing paradigm (as assumed by the rational positivists), but as the result of major discoveries or reinterpretations from an alternative or competing paradigm. Additionally, the newer paradigms are often the product of recognized anomalies (i.e., unexpected outcomes or difficult-to-reconcile data) or a crisis within an older and popularly accepted paradigm.

In discussions of current practices in special education, Skrtic (1986, 1988) posited that the knowledge in our field has evolved primarily from the disciplines of biology and psychology, resulting in intervention approaches that are grounded in diagnostic-prescriptive teaching and behaviorism. Within this context, he further maintains that special education, both in theory and practice, operates within an exceedingly small portion of just one possible paradigm of social scientific thought (referred to as "functionalist; micro-objective," which emphasizes both rational positivism and determinism). Skrtic (1986, 1988) argued that our field must expand its disciplinary base to include various other social, political, and cultural sciences, to adopt multiple paradigms for special education practices, and generally to break away from the narrow theoretical thinking that currently dominates our field.

In addressing the needs of persons with the most profoundly handicapping conditions, Ferguson (1987) called for substantive reforms in current attitudes and policies. His reform recommendations, similar to many of the suggestions of Skrtic (1986, 1988), offered a sociopolitical perspective (and change in societal and professional attitudes) that presupposes a radically different view on the nature of mental retardation and how it should be addressed. One might also include with the positions of Skrtic (1986, 1988) and Ferguson (1987) the recommendations for the field of special education that were presented recently by Gartner and Lipsky (1987). They called for major changes on how the field of special education perceives students with disabilities, and the public policies and professional conduct that limits their acceptance and accommodation into integrated school and community settings. It is noteworthy that the various types of social reforms emerging in our field are in basic conflict with many of the assumptions of the diagnostic-prescriptive-remedial model that dominates our field today—a model that stresses "deviant" individuals as an outcome of mental retardation, rather than biased societal perceptions and attitudes that are based on stereotypes and comparisons with assumed "normal" standards for behavior. These reform recommendations, in essence, point to the need to reevaluate how we both perceive and behave toward persons with disabling conditions—a development that Kuhn (1970) might identify as a *crisis* in our field.

In addition to the emerging social reform recommendations for our field that conflict with many of the broader attitudinal assumptions of the prevailing rational positivism paradigm in special education, Edgar (1988) recently questioned even the eventual success of our current, environmentally based technology, at least as it applies to the early intervention efforts for preschool children with handicapping conditions. Edgar, who also alluded substantially to the writings of Kuhn (1970), pointed out that "a major sign of an aged paradigm is when the questions being asked by the scientists are so minute that the answers are of no importance to anyone save themselves" (p. 68). Edgar also stated that the current environmental paradigm used in early childhood education for children with handicaps has arrived at the point where very few new answers will be found, yet we have not reached our goal. He maintained further that "our technology has peaked and new advances will only come from radically different ways of viewing the world" (p. 70). Edgar suggested, however, that until a new paradigm is found, we must continue to use, and do the best with, what we have currently available to us.

Even given the emergence of some professionals who now are seriously questioning the continuation of the present paradigm, a shift to a new paradigm, if indeed needed, does not appear on the immediate horizon—or at least a "revolution" is not likely to come from the researchers, policymakers, and teacher trainers who now are the recognized leaders in our field. As observed by Kuhn (1970) in the natural sciences, major breakthroughs, and those that lead to paradigm shifts, are typically made by persons of a young age or those who are relatively new to the field. Even with the occurrence of new discoveries, however, the established paradigms are resistant to change and, as often noted, must await the actual demise of the old guard. As noted by Edgar and Sulzbacher (1983), "the behavioral paradigm has become an accepted part of the special education psyche. Many professionals are not even aware that they are operating within the general behavioral paradigm" (p. 4). In support of this statement, Edgar and Sulzbacher conducted interviews with prominent special educators who had, in earlier years, been instrumental in establishing the behavioral paradigm in our field. The interviews indicated that these leaders had changed very little over the years in their commitment to, and defense of, the paradigm that yet today represents the prevailing orientation in the field of special education.

The observations of Edgar and Sulzbacher (1983) were further supported by a questionnaire survey sponsored by TASH to identify, among teacher trainers at major U.S. universities, competencies needed by classroom teachers to provide educational services to students with the *most profoundly handicapping* conditions (Rainforth, Siegel-Causey, Thompson, & Guess, 1988). The overwhelming majority of respondents indicated that behavioral (operant) theory and techniques were both highly important for training teachers and very strongly emphasized in teacher training curricula. Potentially competing positions (e.g., Piaget's cognitive theory and van Dijk's movement-based approach) were perceived by the majority of university teacher trainers both as unimportant for classroom teachers to know and as being addressed little, if any, in the personnel preparation programs. Interestingly, several respondents appeared not to even recognize the name of van Dijk. It would seem that any major paradigm shift or revolution in our field is unlikely to come from university teacher trainers when they are not inclined to introduce even potentially competing "theories" to future classroom teachers. It is also very possible that, when alternative or competing theories are presented, they are done so as negative contrasts to the virtues of the prevailing paradigm.

MESSAGES FROM THE FIELD?

For some of us at least, Alan Bloom's (1987) best-selling critique of higher education in the country, *The Closing of the American Mind*, rings a more urgent alarm when we confront our even further specialized area of special education for students with severe and profound handicaps. We need to ask ourselves, if indeed our present paradigm is found wanting or, even worse, detrimental to the lives of persons with handicaps in ways that are not now apparent to us, from where will the changes come? As pointed out by Skrtic (1986), our present paradigm is based on theoretical assumptions that "demonstrate no recognition of the possibility of alternate frames of reference" (p. 14).

Iano (1986), in discussing a separation of theory and practice in both regular and special education, suggested that two class systems are in operation. The lower class consists of practitioners and teachers in the public schools, while the upper class comprises researchers and professors who have the assumed responsibility for the scientific and professional development of the field. He suggested that the positivist ideology works in concert with an institutionalized separation of theory and practice and that both, together, have impaired our ability to study and develop education models other than the prevailing natural science–technical model. With respect to the severely handicapped area of special education, Iano (1987) maintained that behavioral practices have achieved predominance "by default rather than healthy competition with other approaches" (p. 59).

Yet, it is our opinion that, in the long run, it might be a minority of teachers and practitioners in real-life classroom settings who will encourage, if not demand, both the need to pursue in earnest new and likely multiple paradigms and practices in the field of special education, and the need for more inclusive university-based teacher training curricula to accompany a multiple-paradigm approach. We emphasize "minority of

teachers" because most teachers exiting from existing university personnel preparation programs are, as a result of their training, unconvinced (or more likely unaware) that there might ever be other ways and systems to educate students with disabilities. Interestingly there are, however, many teachers of students with severe handicaps who, after facing the realities of the classroom, seek out, or at least recognize, the need to identify and use educational approaches that were likely not presented in their formal teacher training programs. Two, although admittedly modest, examples serve to emphasize this point.

The first example is derived from a written questionnaire that one of us administered to a graduate-level class of advanced and, for the most part, experienced teachers who served students with severely handicapping conditions. They were requested to rate, on a Likert-type scale, the importance to them as classroom teachers of four educational orientations/theories: 1) Behavioral, 2) Cognitive (Piaget), 3) Maturational, and 4) Eclectic. Results indicated a very strong preference for the Eclectic category. A distant second was the Cognitive approach, followed closely by the Behavioral orientation. The Maturational approach was rated last in importance. These results, although representing a small sample of teachers, are quite surprising and appear to conflict with the prevailing paradigm embraced by the majority of university programs in this country that prepare teachers for educating students with severely handicapping conditions.

The second example comes from a qualitative study on the perceptions of teachers who provide educational services to students with profoundly handicapping conditions (Thompson & Guess, 1989). The 6 teachers who participated in this investigation were selected because of their recognized expertise in working with these types of students, in combination with their extensive classroom experiences. All had been certified from the training program at the University of Kansas. What emerged from the findings of this study is that these teachers adopted a "clinical style and eclectic approach" that differs in some significant ways from their formal university-based training program, and that certainly deviates from the type of curriculum and content that would typify the majority of teacher training programs in the severely handicapped area of special education. Their teaching style resembles a clinician who relies on sensitive observational skills and intuition in combination with a broad base of information and instructional techniques and procedures. This stands in marked contrast to a heavy reliance on the applied behavior analysis perspective that has dominated our field.

> These participants have not abandoned procedures based on a behavioral approach. All take data and value skills as those involved in shaping, task analysis, program writing, and the effective application of positive reinforcement. However, they view these procedures as a small part of a larger array of techniques that come from a wide range of disciplines and theoretical approaches. (Thompson & Guess, 1989, p. 13)

IMPLICATIONS FOR PERSONNEL TRAINING PROGRAMS: "DO AS I DO" OR "THINK FOR YOURSELF"?

The type of clinical and eclectic approach observed among the experienced teachers just noted is contrasted with the "technician" label that some have used in describing the products of our personnel training programs that have followed the dominant behavioral paradigm in our field (cf., for example, the exchange between Heshusius, 1982, 1986, and Ulman & Rosenberg, 1986). Of special interest is that the teachers in the Thompson and Guess study (1989) were using and advocating techniques and procedures (e.g., van Dijk's movement-based approach) that had not, at the time of their formal training, been included in our university curriculum for preparing teachers to serve students with severe and profound handicaps. Nor had we earlier included other procedures that were being used by these teachers—procedures such as vestibular stimulation and systematic sensory stimulation that have been traditionally perceived as "suspect" by many leading teacher trainers and researchers in our field. As noted by Edgar (1988), one of the many indicators of an aging paradigm is the proliferation of nontraditional interventions—an observation that appears consistent with the examples provided

above. It is our opinion that *some* teachers, and probably the better ones, are trying to tell us something about how they are being prepared to intervene with students who have severely and multiply handicapping conditions; as teacher trainers, we need to be more sensitive to what they are trying to convey to us.

Our opinions are underlined by observations made by Skrtic (1988) relating to professional training in special education. He noted that induction into a profession is accomplished through *training*, involving the internalization of presumably objective knowledge, and *indoctrination*, which is the internalization of values and norms. Skrtic (1988) maintained that this knowledge is actually "subjective" because it represents the accepted and unquestioned practices of a tradition. Nevertheless, the process of professional induction requires the student to submit to the authority of the instructor, as well as to the institutional legitimacy of the profession. "As such, professional education tends to be dogmatic and authoritarian, as well it might be, given its institutional context and the fact that the inductee lacks enough of the profession's specialized knowledge and skills to be able to evaluate it on its own terms" (Skrtic, 1988, p. 423).

Skrtic's (1988) critique of professional training in special education, combined with our own observations of teacher behavior once they have exited from the university, is important, we think, to both teacher certification and doctoral-level training programs in the severely handicapped area.

At the certification level, both graduate and undergraduate, it would seem important to systematically and thoroughly present to prospective teachers a variety of educational approaches, theories, and orientations that have at least potential applicability for intervention with students who have severe and multiple disabilities. Each approach should be presented in a fair and honest manner that includes not only the procedural or technical application of the theory, but also the basic assumptions about human learning and behavior that are indigenous to that particular orientation. Importantly, a discussion of each orientation should include a presentation about the values (both personal and educational) associated with each theory, and how these values might either support or conflict with those of the prospective teachers.

In essence, we are advocating that teachers be provided with *choices* for the type of learning theory and pedagogy that they might adopt, wholly or in part, in their future roles as educators for students with severe and multiple handicaps. For those university professors who would argue that prospective teachers will make the "wrong" choices in selecting a theory of learning (or paradigm), we need only remind them that the same concern has long been expressed in allowing the recipients of special education (i.e., students with handicapping conditions) the opportunities to make choices—and, unfortunately, for many of the same reasons. We confirm also the capacity of teachers to critically evaluate varying and often unconventional theories, techniques, and procedures advocated for intervening with students who have handicapping conditions. We further submit that both the opportunity to critically evaluate differing, and often opposing, theories and approaches is a fundamental tenet of higher education; the process of doing so will produce teachers with a more accurate perspective on the complexities of human behavior, and on the educational interventions that are offered on behalf of students with handicapping conditions.

At the level of doctoral training in the field of special education, especially including the severely and multiply handicapped area, we recommend an even more concerted effort to move away from the narrowness that has come to characterize our personnel training programs. This recommendation is based on the concern that our professional "in-breeding" has reached the point where new and innovative paradigm shifts in our field are less likely to occur due, in part, to our own overspecialized, but limited knowledge base—a condition that is perpetuated by many university professors in special education who, themselves, operate *exclusively* from the behavioral paradigm.

Preparation of doctoral students in the field of special education should include, as a basic competency, a thorough knowledge of varying and competing theories and approaches to learning and child development—at least at a level commensurate to what we have recommended for the teacher certification level. Beyond this, however, doctoral-level students should be provided with a strong interdisciplinary training program that traverses a variety of fields of human inquiry such as sociology, philosophy, anthropology, biology, and history; or even some of the more technical fields and disciplines such as business and computer science. This recommendation is based on the assumption that mental retardation is a total societal problem that is best approached through a better understanding of those many fields of inquiry that have an impact on community life, and on the possibility that knowledge in other fields of academic study might, for a creative and bright doctoral student, lead to a future, innovative paradigm shift in our field of all too "special" education.

Admittedly, our recommendations for changes in both teacher certification and doctoral-level training programs are likely to be met with skepticism or even hostility by many professors and researchers in our field of special education and, certainly, we do not pretend to have all or even the right answers. We do, nevertheless, perceive a need for change in our field that does not compromise our basic values toward a fuller and more productive life for all persons with handicapping conditions, but that does question the status quo and overall future gains of the existing paradigm. We would hope that the 1990s will represent a time in our area of special education in which professionals are rewarded for truly new and innovative practices that will, over time, significantly improve not only the lives of children and adults who experience severe and multiply handicapping conditions, but the societal perceptions of these individuals as well.

REFERENCES

Baer, D.M., Wolf, M.M., & Risley, T.R. (1968). Some current dimensions of applied behavior analysis. *Journal of Applied Behavior Analysis, 1*, 91–97.

Bloom, A. (1987). *The closing of the American mind.* New York: Simon & Schuster.

Burke, P., & Cohen, M. (1977). The quest for competence in serving the severely/profoundly handicapped: A critical analysis of personnel preparation programs. In E. Sontag, J. Smith, & N. Certo (Eds.) *Educational programming for the severely and profoundly handicapped* (pp. 445–465). Reston, VA: Council for Exceptional Children.

Edgar, E. (1988). Policy factors influencing research in early childhood special education. In S. Odom & M. Karnes (Eds.), *Early intervention for infants and children with handicaps: An empirical base* (pp. 63–73). Baltimore: Paul H. Brookes Publishing Co.

Edgar, E., & Sulzbacher, S. (1983, March). *Influence and effects of the behavioral paradigm in special education.* Paper presented at the Banff Behavior Modification Conference, Banff, Alberta, Canada.

Ferguson, P. (1987, Summer). The social construction of mental retardation. *Social Policy*, pp. 51–56.

Gartner, A., & Lipsky, D.K. (1987). Beyond special education: Toward a quality system for all students. *Harvard Educational Review*, 57, 367–395.

Heshusius, L. (1982). At the heart of the advocacy dilemma: A mechanistic world view. *Exceptional Children*, 49, 6–13.

Heshusius, L. (1986). Paradigm shifts and special education: A response to Ulman and Rosenberg. *Exceptional Children*, 52, 461–465.

Iano, R. (1986). The study and development of teaching: With implications for the advancement of special education. *Remedial and Special Education*, 7(5), 50–61.

Iano, R. (1987). Rebuttal: Neither the absolute certainty of prescriptive law nor a surrender to mysticism. *Remedial and Special Education*, 8(1), 52–87.

Kuhn, T. (1970). *The structure of scientific revolutions* (2nd ed.). Chicago: University of Chicago Press.

Rainforth, B., Siegel-Causey, E., Thompson, B., & Guess, D. (1988). *Preparation of personnel to educate students with profound and multiple handicaps.* Unpublished report prepared for The Association for Persons with Severe Handicaps, Seattle.

Skinner, B.F. (1971). *Beyond freedom and dignity.* New York: Alfred A. Knopf.

Skrtic, T. (1986). The crisis in special education knowledge: A perspective on perspective. *Focus on Exceptional Children*, 18(7), 1–16.

Skrtic, T. (1988). The crisis in special education knowledge. In E. Meyen & T. Skrtic (Eds.), *Exceptional children and youth: An introduction* (3rd ed., pp. 415–447). Denver: Love Publishing Co.

Thompson, B., & Guess, D. (1989). Students who experience the most profound disabilities: Teacher perspectives. In F. Brown & D.H. Lehr (Eds.), *Persons with profound disabilities: Issues and practices* (pp. 3–41). Baltimore: Paul H. Brookes Publishing Co.

Ulman, J., & Rosenberg, M. (1986). Science and superstition in special education. *Exceptional Children*, 52, 459–460.

Winzer, M.A. (1986). Early developments in special education: Some aspects of enlightenment thought. *Remedial and Special Education*, 7(5), 42–49.

CHAPTER 22

It's About Relationships

MARSHA FOREST, ED.D.
Frontier College, Toronto, Ontario, Canada

To the old ones
of my childhood
who taught me
the most important
lesson of all:
That I did not need
to be perfect to
be loved.
That no one
does.

—Alice Walker (1967, p. 1)

The above message in Alice Walker's (1967) beautiful children's book *To Hell With Dying* speaks volumes to me personally. All I really ever wanted in my own life was a group of people around me and especially one central person in my life who would just love me totally as I am.

For years the people in my own life and family said they loved me, but I felt they never really knew me. The men in my life said they loved me, but all the while they tried to change me, criticize me, or pick at me. I tried and tried to be perfect and I felt worse and worse.

I was successful at work. Nobody knew when my heart was breaking. I thought this was good. I could control my feelings. I'd be tough at work and crack up at home. I, who love life so dearly, thought about death, dying, suicide—I lost weight, I cried in hidden places.

And then at the age of 34 something snapped. I visited another culture in Asia and the distance from home and the strangeness of the land and people opened my heart and soul. I decided I wanted to "fly"—that is, to be free of the past, and I opened myself to love.

At this very time of change I met two people who changed my life both personally and professionally—Jack Pearpoint and Judith Snow. They are both entwined with me on this journey to create a world where people are loved for who they are and cherished for the gifts they have to offer.

I have started this essay with a bit of my own journey as I feel it is important to stress the universality of my theme and that universality must begin with myself. I did not get involved in the movement to integrate children with disabilities into regular schools because I am a saint, a martyr, or a Christian. I am indeed far from being a saint, I despise martyrs, and I'm not a Christian—my own heritage is in the Jewish tradition.

I am not at all interested in disability, mental retardation, or special education. I am, however, passionately interested in being part of building a just and humane society where each human being can live in dignity and have his or her needs met—whatever that may involve.

I strongly believe we have the money and resources to do just that.

FORCE ONE

Picture for a moment a sleek, white airplane called Force One. Its nose is pointed, sharp, and black. This plane has three 15-foot (4.57m) one-weapon bays. Each can carry an eight-round drum of strategic air missiles (SAMs) plus other cruise missiles. In addition, 14 cruise missiles can be hung on the external pylons.

In 1981, U.S. President Ronald Reagan announced a force of 100 B-1B Bombers—a prototype of the B-1—to enter service in 1988 at a cost of $28 billion.

This, to me, is not only insane but obscene. The cost is beyond my wildest notions of money. I know Judith Snow needs $60,000 to run a decent attendant care system. I know that $5,000 would go a long way to help the Frank family. Let's be honest . . . money in the trillions is there for weapons that kill, maim, and destroy the human race. Can you imagine if we used that money to help people?

To talk about integration without looking at the wider social issues of war, poverty, illiteracy, and so on is foolish. The school systems in the United States and Canada are falling apart at the seams for at least 75% of the population. There are grave social and political problems that face us.

We are looking at and for major social change, and the movement to bring children back into real classes where they belong is simply one part of a wider social movement to create a just society that is fit for human existence. Is this possible? YES! Will it happen tomorrow or without an enormous amount of hard work? NO.

THE CHALLENGE

Bringing people who have been excluded on the basis of race, class, sex, or handicapping condition back into the mainstream is an exciting, controversial, and dynamic process, for it challenges the basic assumptions of each of us and at the same time introduces us to new ways of thinking and seeing.

I was not born thinking like I do today. I accepted the notion that people with disabilities needed institutions, special care, special education, special housing. I, however, was open to being challenged (at times yelled at) by friends who saw another way.

As I got to know my friend Judith Snow and as I became involved in her struggle to get out of a chronic care nursing home, I learned about the reality of life for most people with disabilities. I was angry and disgusted at the injustice of it all.

Judith was my friend. How could she stand to live in a prison—or, as she called it, a "concentration camp"? How could she put up with all that disrespect and pain? At the time, she had two choices—live there or die.

I learned that loving friends means that you stand with them and fight with them and laugh and cry with them. You don't try to change, adjust, or cure them. You want the best for your friends and in return those friends want the best for you.

You won't take the "least restrictive environment"—you want the BEST, the MOST. You never want the "least" for those you love.

But the attitudes of wanting perfection start at birth (or today even before, with the trend to abort all unborn children diagnosed with Down syndrome through amniocentesis). Just this week a friend of ours gave birth 1 month prematurely to a 3-pound baby who is said to be "profoundly" brain damaged. She was supposed to die. But this tough little girl didn't die.

The advice given by physicians to the family in 1989 in a supposedly progressive hospital in Vancouver, British Columbia, is "Don't bond with the baby—she will probably die, or at best be a burden to you for the rest of your lives."

The young couple is told daily by medical experts and family members not to LOVE their child. What kind of world is this where we tell parents not to love a child? No one has any idea what this baby will become. She may be dead in a week or live to be the oldest woman on record. No one can predict.

The message NOT TO LOVE is insane, mean, cruel, and horrible. Love the baby if it's perfect. Hate the baby if it's imperfect in any way. Love me if I live the life you want. Hate me if I am not perfect in your eyes. Throw me away if I am different. Get rid of me if I am unique.

The implication is horrible—I will love you as long as you are perfect—but if you are in a car accident, if you lose a leg, if you become hard of hearing, and if you become old and unattractive then I will stop loving you. I will put you away and I will reject you.

It starts in the hospital—it too often ends in a nursing home.

Luckily, most families fall in love with their babies and love them despite the best advice from doctors (these great fortune tellers of the future of a newborn).

And so the child is loved and welcomed to the family and then the child hits school age and the curtain drops again.

The child is not welcomed in his or her neighborhood school; rather, he or she is sent to that SPECIAL place where SPECIAL people do SPECIAL things to the SPECIAL person and in reality absolutely nothing special is going on at all. Segregated schooling is a holding action until adulthood, when more SPECIAL places called group homes or sheltered workshops or day programs do more of nothing special and the only unspecial place that child ever ends up in is the regular cemetery where he or she is as we all will be one day—dead.

But while we are alive we have the right to live, to love, to have fun, to make mistakes, and to fly in our own direction with our own friends.

THE KARATE CLASS

Why can't the school system act more like my karate class?

I recently joined the Northern Karate Club on St. Clair Avenue in Toronto. Terrified, I went to my first class dressed in an old sweatsuit and feeling terribly out of place among all the "karateites" decked out in crisp white suits with colorful belts.

It was the all-belts class—this means all levels of ability (including me, with absolutely no ability at all). I was afraid. I felt foolish and out of place. I was motivated, however, by my age, 5 extra pounds I wanted to shed, and the knowledge that I better practice what I preach—that is, take better care of myself.

I also have high tolerance for making a total fool of myself knowing full well most people are not looking at me anyway. The Sensai (head teacher, Ceasar Borowkowski) told me that I was to work at my own speed and push myself and not worry about others. I liked that.

The woman teaching the class that day assigned Patty Piletti to be my "tutor." Now she didn't say that—she just asked Patty to make sure I didn't kill myself in my first lesson and to keep an eye on me.

Patty is a black belt—the top. She is 23 years old, a pro. She gently guided me through the exercises, helping place my feet in the right position and always making me feel I was doing okay.

I went home elated. I had lived through a karate class at the age of 46. I punched and kicked and screamed Japanese-sounding phrases. I was sore in body but elated in spirit!

Most of all, as I dashed into my house, I was brimming over with the idea that integration is alive and well out there in the world—in families, in karate studios, in health clubs, in workplaces. WHY NOT IN OUR SCHOOLS??

In subsequent karate classes I have always been the white belt (the lowest level) and my goal is to get a yellow belt. I plan to invite the entire neighborhood to my yellow belt party because for me, that will be as great an achievement as getting a black belt!

The moral of the story is that I experienced integration/inclusion first hand and I loved it. I was not the best in the class (I can honestly say I was the worst); however, I work diligently at my own pace, I have tutors, I am making friends (much younger than myself), and I am improving with each class I take.

I was welcomed and included from the first moment I walked into the studio. There was no pressure, only much support. I know schools can do this too, for I am privileged to work in schools and systems where all children are fully welcomed. If one place can do it, so can every place. It is matter of will, choice, and values. It is our future.

THE WEDDING

On July 23, 1988, about 300 people celebrated the marriage of Judith Snow and Laurence Hunt at the Eglinton United Church in Toronto, Ontario. It is a day etched in my heart and in my mind. I have now known Judith Snow for over 10 years—years of change and years of struggle. When we met, did we dare dream that 10 years later Judith would be living in an apartment of her own, with an attendant care system designed and managed by her circle of friends and advocates (the Joshua Committee), and married? Inclusion into community doesn't begin with a blueprint, but often with a simple dream, a desire, a hope, a yet unspoken cry for freedom. Judith's dream was not spelled out in detail—it was more a scream of despair that said, "Get me out of this institutional hell hole and let me see the light. I want to be free!"

That light, that anger, that drive and determination, and her courage radiated with clarity and brilliance as Judith, dressed in a white cotton dress from Thailand, came up the specially built ramp at the church to meet her husband-to-be at the altar. The hush in the church was thunderous as everyone watched love roll up the ramp that day. The musicians played the song "Power of Love" by Jennifer Rush. Tears of joy flowed.

Judith was followed by her four attendants

(myself included) dressed in identical dresses of different colors and Laurence (also dressed in white) was attended by his four friends. A male and a female minister officiated at the ceremony, designed and written by Judith and Laurence themselves—designed to dedicate their new life together to the service of others and to bring their community into that mission with them. This was a wedding that involved the participants in building the vision of the new community that Judith and Laurence plan to build.

At the beginning of the service all the children were invited to come forward and sit on the steps of the stage area while Judith and Laurence explained to them why they were getting married. They asked the children for their support and assistance in building a world where no one would be shut out in jails, hospitals, segregated schools, segregated classes, and institutions of any kind.

There wasn't a dry eye in the house as Judith and Laurence spoke to the assembled children— many of them in wheelchairs, many of them rejected by their own neighborhood churches and schools. Today, all were accepted—today, all were welcome.

The music through the ceremony, played by a small band, was chosen to accent the proceedings. It was uplifting as they sang with their young and vibrant voices.

As Judith and Laurence spoke their vows, the community was asked to join in and pledge their support for the newly joined couple. A rousing "WE WILL!" was the answer to the traditional wedding question.

Instead of the traditional Communion the wedding party took baskets of bread and grapes out to the over 300 guests as music played and all shook hands or hugged or laughed and cried together.

Judith and Laurence beamed as the entire congregation became a community, sharing love and commitment with one another.

This was no ordinary service. It was not simply joining two people in marriage—it was joining an entire community into true communion and dedication, not to self, but to building community and service to others.

Everyone present could not help but be touched by the symbolic nature of the event. Ev-

eryone present in some way had been part of Judith's struggle to reach this day.

Through planning this day, Judith and her parents came to a new and deeper appreciation of one another. Judith's mother (Rita Snow) presented a tapestry that had taken her almost a year to sew that represented Judith's journey. The biological family had come together with Judith's "friendship" family. Laurence's mother was also present, and kept wondering how she could possibly describe this event to her friends back in Missouri.

The wedding was integration in action. Everyone was represented—young and old, men and women, rich and poor, black and white, gay and straight. It was a celebration of diversity, but most of all it was a celebration of the possible. It was a kaleidoscope in full and living color.

For those of us who remembered the "Judy" of 9 years earlier, it was a triumph of courage, cooperation, partnerships, and circles. "Judy" had truly become Judith, and as her namesake in the Old Testament, she was a noble and courageous mother of a community.

"Judy and Larry" had become Judith Snow and Laurence Hunt and together they will be even stronger than each has been alone. This is the wedding that, according to all the medical experts, human services policymakers, and so forth, could and should never have happened. But it did happen. And once again, it happened because of a dream and the hard work needed to make that dream a reality. The wedding was planned by a circle—a committee of friends, and church and family members. As with all of Judith's life, the wedding was planned by a circle and it became a celebration of life.

Guests came from all over North America and Europe. Of the many speeches after the dinner, for me it was the image of the "two Bobs" that stands out in my mind.

Bob Perske and Bob Williams had flown up from the United States. They stood together and as Bob Williams pointed to letters on his letter board, Bob Perske translated loud and clear: "This wedding is the true meaning of community."

After wedding toasts and food, more tears, and lots of laughter, everyone partied and joyously danced the night away. If you ask, maybe Judith and Laurence will show you their photo album. The photographs, taken not by a professional photographer but by a friend, reflect the magic and love of this celebration.

Once, "Judy" decided she would rather die than live alone in an institution. Ten years later, Judith Snow got married and proved once again that dreams indeed can become reality.

When you dream alone it is only a dream, but when you dream together it is the beginning of reality.

—Dom Helder Camera, 1987
(from a speech given in Toronto at a
Youth Corps meeting)

THE EMPEROR IS NAKED:
THE MYTH OF SPECIAL EDUCATION

I think we've lost our hearts to a myth of special education. We've created a new breed of magician or witch doctor, a teacher/car mechanic who we believe can "fix" children like we "fix" cars. But children aren't cars, they are flesh and blood. They bleed real blood and cry real tears when hurt.

I, too, came from this "magician" mode of thinking. I am a trained special educator. I taught in segregated schools and classes and I did the best I could at the time given what I then knew. But I changed!

I realized that the power of the segregated environment was teaching negative messages daily. The environment said, "You are not good enough to be part of the real school. You need 'special education'—and this really means, 'We don't want you with us'." I realized that no matter how good a teacher I was, I couldn't give my students what they needed most—real experiences and real relationships in a real school, a real classroom.

I saw that the emperor (special education) was naked (not working). I didn't think I was bad or evil or horrible—I just saw that there was something better out there not only for my students but for me and my own family.

We need to shout this news from the rooftops

—ALL CHILDREN NEED TO LEARN WITH AND FROM OTHER CHILDREN. . . . ALL CHILDREN NEED TO BELONG AND FEEL WANTED AND LOVED. . . . ALL CHILDREN NEED TO HAVE FUN AND ENJOY NOISE AND LAUGHTER IN THEIR LIVES. . . . ALL CHILDREN NEED TO TAKE RISKS AND FALL AND CRY AND GET HURT. . . . ALL CHILDREN NEED TO BE IN REAL FAMILIES AND REAL SCHOOLS AND REAL NEIGHBORHOODS.

Recently, I was at a meeting enthusiastically telling stories of children I know who are fully included in regular schools and classrooms. A young teacher interrupted me.

"But what about getting Melanie to the bathroom?" she asked. "How can she go to the bathroom—she has no arms. It's just not practical."

I have always suspected that what drives most of special education is a preoccupation with bathrooms, with toilet training and bowel movements. Now I was sure this was true. "But what was really underlying this teacher's preoccupation with the bathroom?" I asked myself. My answer: fear.

The teacher was afraid of the unknown. She was afraid to admit her fear. She was afraid she might not know what to do with Melanie. She, as most of us, feared anything new and different. But instead of talking about fear, she talked about the bathroom.

I wanted to scream at this teacher, "How can you be so ignorant—how can you be so cruel—how can you think of bathrooms when this kid needs friends, love, education?! How can you be so out of it?"

Instead of screaming, however, I took a deep breath and asked her what she wanted for her own son. I said, "God forbid your son was in a car accident today and he had to have a wheelchair to walk and a communication device to speak with from today on. Where would you want him to go to school when he gets out of the hospital? Where do you think he'd want to live and work and play?"

"Well, of course I'd want him to live at home and go back to his class," she answered without hesitation. "Oh, I see what you're getting at," she said, with a wise smile.

I then more calmly went on, "You see how we move to all the wrong issues out of our own ignorance, prejudice, and fear and we lose sight of the real needs of children."

Let's look at some of the ridiculous things we do:

If a child needs more relationships, we give him less: We will with good intentions assign an educational assistant and build a one-to-one dependency.

If a child needs more time, we give her less hours at school and more hours riding around town to "segregation land" in a "special bus."

If a child needs normal behavior models, we give him six other kids, who scream, as his "pals" and then we wonder why he doesn't improve.

If a child needs more communication, we put her in a room with 10 other kids who don't communicate well and again we wonder why she won't learn.

THE ABOVE IS CALLED CRAZY-MAKING BEHAVIOR AND IT HAS TO STOP—*NOW*!!

Children don't need segregated community-based experiences in supermarkets. They need to go shopping with their classmates when the need arises. Children at age 10 don't need jobs outside of the school, they need to do errands in the school that are typical for 10-year-olds. High school kids don't need work experience that's different from their typical peers. They need to build relationships so that their friends and the mothers and fathers of their friends who own stores or work in factories will encourage their co-workers to hire their son's friend. Most people get jobs through personal networks, not simply job experience programs.

Surely if we can put people on the moon, we can figure out how to get a 5-year old to the washroom and how to get a 21-year-old a job! It is all pure nonsense that we can't do it. It is simply a matter of will.

GRADE 7/8
ST. FRANCIS SCHOOL:
MY GREAT TEACHERS OF 1989!!

Integration is happening. Several school systems in Canada and the United States are proving that true inclusion can work. These school boards are good places for ALL children. They have policies of equality on issues involving racial minorities, women, and so on. They believe that EACH BELONGS.

Once one system can do it, everyone else needs to prove why they can't. It is no longer up to us to show why integration can work. We know it can. It is up to others to show why they can't do it.

We know the blocks aren't money or staff. We know it is strong leadership and clear values that make the difference. We need to applaud those who believe in love and inclusion and expose those who would create a new elite in our schools.

When the staff decided to welcome all children back into their regular classes at St. Francis Elementary School (Waterloo Region Separate School Board) we simply went to talk to the children and ask them what they thought about this issue.

Their questions and responses touched everyone involved. (The reader can watch and hear these children in the video tape "With A Little Help From My Friends.") [(Forest, 1988)]. Some of their questions were:

Why did we segregate May in the first place?
What was Jason learning in the "life-skills" room anyway? Nothing, I think.
How would you feel if you weren't with kids your own age and had to go on "special" trips to the circus, bowling and that stuff?

We had to answer these and other questions. Entering into honest dialogue with children wasn't always easy for the teachers. "I know how to teach these kids, but I've forgotten how to talk to them," one teacher admitted. We also asked the children how they would feel if they had no friends, if no one ever called them, and if they never could go to parties, sports events, or other places with their friends. We explained that most people with disabilities had few people in their lives other than those *paid* to be in their lives. "How would that make you feel?" we asked.

I'd feel old.
I'd want to die.
I'd feel like I was in jail.

I'd think only the teachers were my friends.
I'd commit suicide.

And so, all the children previously in segregated classes were "welcomed home."

Everyone was nervous, no one knew what individual programs would look like, but with teamwork and support everyone survived and indeed thrived. Today, the Waterloo Region of the Separate School Board is a model. People flock to Kitchener from all over the world to see inclusion in process.

If you visit, you won't see the perfect school or system. It is far from perfect but it is on the road. It is, after all, just a school system and has the problems that beset most schools today—but there's a real difference . . .

IN THE WATERLOO REGION, IT'S NOT FOR "THEM"—IT'S FOR "US"!

Too often *integration* or *mainstreaming* has been seen as a placement issue. It is something we do for or to "them." But integration isn't another "charity ball for the disabled." Integration in the true sense of the word, meaning "making whole," is for *all of us*. It truly takes the philosopher Martin Buber's (1937) concept of "I-Thou" and puts it into action.

All too often I see "I-It" relationships in schools between pupils or between pupil and teacher and too often between teacher and teacher.

Bringing back children who have been historically "left out" also brings back our humanity. You can't teach the value of love or diversity or tolerance by preaching or lecturing *at* people— we all have to live these values and have real situations to test our morality and humanity.

"But, tell me *how* to do it," teachers in frustration say to me. Those who truly understand the *why* seem to easily do the *what*. *What* to do comes out of a team problem-solving process of adults and children who *together* come up with creative solutions to unique challenges.

There is no way to do an inservice for this "new way of thinking," except to have the children present and discuss values and attitudes, cry and laugh together, and work cooperatively as problems arise. It is no longer the sole "Lone

Ranger" teacher having to come up with the answer. It is the whole school and community, parents, consultants, and, most of all, the children who can help.

A True Story

About a year after May had been fully included in Grade 7/8, she and some of her friends went to a neighboring schoolyard to play. Some Grade 8 boys from the other school started teasing a child in a wheelchair. The girls, smaller by far than these boys, hesitated for a moment before they took on these "bullies."

Amy, the leader of the girls, told the boys to stop. They didn't. She persisted. Amy was, by this time, furious. When they got back to school they stormed into the principal's office and wanted him to take immediate action against these "bullies" at School X.

I visited the class soon after the incident and asked everyone to tell me what had happened. A lively debate ensued about whether Amy and her friends should have gotten involved.

Some of the children felt Amy had been "foolish," "stupid," "naive," and so on to take on boys much bigger and stronger than she. "She could have been hurt," some felt.

Amy was indignant. "You have to stand up for what's right," she argued. Her friends (including May) chimed in, arguing for what was right and decent according to them.

I widened the conversation by asking what they thought the role of students in South Africa today is and what they thought happened in Nazi Germany when non-Jewish children befriended Jewish children. The room was in an uproar of incredible philosophical debate. I was struck that the level of discussion was far more sophisticated than among several of my graduate seminars at the university. The discussion was thoughtful, deep, and passionate.

The issue in the Waterloo region has gone far beyond "integration" and ranges into the real meaning of community, social justice, and the integrity of each individual. I was impressed, moved, and thrilled to see this ordinary group of working-class children handling the "big" ideas that we so infrequently allow children to discuss.

This was beyond curriculum guides on individual differences. This was *real*. This wasn't an abstract discussion about wooden puppets with different disabilities—this was about the meaning of life itself.

Microwave Thinking and Feeling

Society today wants the quick fix, the quick high. Teachers seek out the "answer." Well, we mustn't give in. Good teachers know that real learning takes time and that education is a journey and a process.

Inclusion won't cook fast in the microwave. Inclusive education means commitment and energy of a different kind. It needs teachers who can talk to children, touch them, teach them, and laugh and cry with them.

The learning going on in the Waterloo Region under the gutsy and able leadership of George Flynn, the director of education, is like a jewel. It shines and it lasts. Amy and Becky and May and Susie and the crew in Grade 8 don't know anything about special education. I hope they never will.

What We Need to Make This Happen

We need more leadership with the guts and courage displayed by Amy, May, Becky, and the other kids. We need more educational leaders who take the time to read and think and who know the research on what makes an effective school. We need more leaders who still love and care about *all* kids. We need leaders who will dare to expose special education as an empty shell and who have the courage to move ahead into the year 2000.

Special education is an idea whose time is up. It is now time to build inclusive communities where together we can teach everyone to love as well as to read and write. We need most of all to fully and finally believe that *all* truly means *all*.

We now need to put that *all* into practice and bring our children home to where they can all learn from one another. We need to do it right now so we won't have to publish another book like this 20 years from now!

We need to act now because, as Amy said, "It's not fair to treat some people like they don't belong."

CONCLUSION

Working with hurt and rejected people is not always easy. It takes time, energy, and the power of love. There are no simple answers except that we *must* do it—because if we don't, the human cost to us and our children will be enormous.

The greatest diseases in North America today are loneliness and meaninglessness. Bringing back the least powerful into our schools is an incredible antidote to suicide, alcoholism, and drugs. Helping one another is a beautiful thing, but it's not something you simply talk about—it is something you *do*.

About 8 years ago Sherry arrived at my husband's and my home when we had just discovered we could not have biological offspring. Through a series of strange events, this lost and lonely teenager came through our front door, not to leave again for many years.

Sherry had been neglected and abused by her father, and her mother was deceased. She trusted no one, least of all herself. She tested my very soul.

I was good with kids who were physically or mentally handicapped, but Sherry, who presented no outward manifestation of handicap, drove me crazy. I learned that she had the most terrible handicap of all—self-hate.

Through the years we stuck it out. It wasn't easy or nice but it was honest and real at all times.

The story has a happy ending. Sherry was married in our home 3 years ago to a wonderful young lawyer and they now have a beautiful daughter named Sarah. As I was writing this chapter, Sherry gave me a letter that I will end with. She, who withstood years of abuse by the child welfare system, is now standing up to the same human services system that almost killed her as a child.

Sherry is now working with parents of children with disabilities and getting in trouble for taking on the bureaucrats. She is proud of herself and we are proud of her. She (with her enthusiastic permission) gets the last word in this chapter. She and I and Jack and Judith and Laurence and our circle of friends are what it's all about:

Tonight when I spoke to the Board of my organization, I was calm and confident because you were all with me—Lorne and Carrie and David and Marsha and Jack and Tanya and Judith and Vanessa, and Andrea and Barb and most of all my dear sweet Sarah, my living breathing link with the future.

I wasn't defensive. I didn't yell or cry. I spoke with my heart and each word seemed to bring with it some healing.

People were listening to me—me, this useless nothing that the social service system saw fit to abuse and abuse, and who wished would just go away and die, because I had nothing to offer, no gift, no nothing.

Tonight this nothing just became something. For the first time in sixteen years I know I am going to make it. For sixteen years I still accepted their vision of me. Now finally, after sixteen years, I am putting all the labels they put on me where they belong—in the garbage! I am going to make it with a little help from my friends. I am going to put the power back where it belongs—with me—with us!

Tonight I sit here overflowing with love and gratitude for all of you and all you have done for me—

for your friendship and caring. For sixteen years I have been walking around with a knife stuck in my back—you have all helped me to pull it out. The sharp pain is subsiding, slowly the skin will regenerate and the scar will fade—never completely though. But now what I will remember is not just the wound but the friends who helped me heal.

This is your victory too and I want all my friends to share it with me. I hope someday to make a difference in somebody else's life like you have all made in mine.

I hope my beautiful Sarah and her children and friends will grow up without ever knowing the awful pain of being excluded and of being utterly and totally alone. I want to help build a loving community out there that will embrace every child. I want the community to see the lovely gifts all our children have to offer.

If only all children and parents could receive the love I feel today then the world would truly be a better place for us all.

Thank you all. I love you. (Sherry, personal communication, March, 1989)

REFERENCES

Buber, M. (1937). *I and thou.* Edinburg: T. and T. Clark.

Forest, M. (1988). *With a little help from my friends* [Videotape]. Available in the U.S. from Expectations Unlimited, P.O. Box 655, Niwot, CO 80544.

Available in Canada from the Center for Integrated Education, 24 Tome Cresent, Toronto, Ontario, Canada M6H 255.

Walker, A. (1967). Introduction. In *To Hell with dying* (p. 1). New York: Harcourt Brace Jovanovich.

CHAPTER 23

Achieving Integration during the Second Revolution

FRANK J. LASKI

Public Interest Law Center of Philadelphia, Philadelphia, Pennsylvania

CURRENT STATUS OF INTEGRATION: UNMET OBLIGATIONS

Persons with disabilities of all ages, along with their families and their advocates, for over 20 years have devoted their substantial talents and energies to securing their civil rights. In the national and state legislatures, in the city and town councils, and in the courthouses throughout the United States, they have been notably successful in achieving declaration of their civil rights and affirmation of their worth as equal citizens.

It is now widely established in the public consciousness that children with disabilities have a right to education; that adults with severe disabilities can be productive workers; that public transportation and public facilities should be accessible to all persons, including those whose mobility is impaired; and that community services and participation of children and adults with disabilities in all aspects of community life are preferred to their isolation and segregation in institutional schools, hospitals, workshops, and rehabilitation facilities. The national awareness and attention to disability rights was recently captured in President Bush's address to a joint session of Congress, where he proclaimed that persons with disabilities belong in the "mainstream": "Disabled Americans must become full-time partners in America's opportunity society" (1989, p. H266).

"Disabled Americans," particularly those with the most severe disabilities and who are most disadvantaged, have their declarations of civil rights. But they have yet to receive those rights and the creation of the civil reality. In the face of substantial achievement:

Nearly 200,000 persons with developmental disabilities are still unnecessarily institutionalized or are living in substandard nursing facilities (Braddock, Hemp, Fujiura, Bachelder, & Mitchell, 1990).

Over 1 million children with disabilities are in separate, unnecessarily segregated, special education programs (*Eleventh Annual Report to Congress on the Implementation of the Education of the Handicapped Act,* 1989).

Thousands of students with disabilities are graduating from school each year without jobs or job training (*Federal Register,* 1990, p. 7970).

Over 2.6 million persons with physical disabilities live near public mass transit but cannot use it (1980 U.S. Census).

In the face of a permanent chasm between the declaration of rights and the reality, many people with disabilities and their families lose hope, their sense of their own worth, and the possibilities of productive and meaningful lives.

Central to the achievement of a civil reality for children and adults with the most severe disabilities is *community integration*—not only the regular and routine presence of individuals with disabilities in the schools, workplaces, and shopping malls of the nation, but ongoing reciprocal interactions among peers, with and without disabilities, equal and effective access to all public services and accommodations, and full participation in the life of the community. Each and every step in this country taken to advance the status of persons with severe disabilities has been grounded in and faithful to the community integration imperative.

Community integration has consistently been both the first value and the final objective of our national policy for persons with disabilities. In 1974, before enactment of the federal education acts, the Congress found and declared it essential to assure that all individuals with handicaps are able to live their lives independently and with dignity, and that the complete integration of all individuals with handicaps into normal community living, working and service patterns be held as the final objective. (Rehabilitation Act of 1973, §701n.)

The Rehabilitation Act of 1973 yielded the requirement that all federally assisted service be provided "in the most integrated setting appropriate to the person's needs" (*Code of Federal Regulations*, 1987, §104.4[b][2]). The plain language of PL 94-142, the Education for All Handicapped Children Act (1975), required the states and local school districts to "assure that, to the maximum extent appropriate, handicapped children . . . are educated with children who are not handicapped" (§1412[5][B]). Also, the Supreme Court, led by Chief Justice William Rehnquist, has more than once pinpointed the integration language along with the appropriate education requirement as the two substantive federal mandates in PL 94-142 (*Board of Education of the Hendrick Hudson Central School District v. Amy Rowley*, 1982).

Now and in the near future, the integration obligation will extend to infants and toddlers eligible for early intervention services. Those services, as appropriate, "must be provided in the types of settings in which infants and toddlers without handicaps would participate" (*Federal Register*, 1989, p. 26312). In the same vein, Congress, in its amendment and reform of vocational rehabilitation, has made clear that the primary purpose of the federal vocational rehabilitation and independent living programs for individuals with disabilities is "integration into the workplace and community" (Rehabilitation Act of 1973, §701).

In federal law, the integration imperative is most clearly elaborated in the Developmental Disabilities and Bill of Rights Act (DD Act). There, Congress's finding that "it is in the national interest to offer persons with developmental disabilities the opportunity . . . to live in typical homes and communities" and recognizing "the capability of persons with developmental disabilities to be engaged in competitive work in integrated settings" set as the explicit purpose of the law "to enable such persons to

achieve their maximum potential through increased independence, productivity, and integration into the community" (DD Act, 1989, §6000). As set forth in the DD Act: Definitions, the meaning and impact of integration is clear:

> [Integration includes] participation by persons with developmental disabilities in the same community activities in which nondisabled citizens participate, together with regular contact with nondisabled citizens, . . . and the residence by persons with developmental disabilities in homes or in home-like settings which are in proximity to community resources, together with regular contact with nondisabled citizens in their communities. (1989, §6001[8])

Our strong and unambiguous public policy promoting total community integration in public education and the rest is grounded in and reflects a broad-based professional consensus and growing expectation and demands of individuals with disabilities and their families. The resolve of the professions to achieve community integration across the entire range of disability is well established. Research and practice, particularly in the areas of education, community living, and work, are effectively confirming the professional judgment about integration and moving it into the public arena.

Recently, a 45-member task force representative of the diverse interests in education, appointed by the secretary of education in Pennsylvania to consider how best the state could integrate the education of students with and without disabilities, reported:

> Task Force research has located throughout the country programs that successfully integrate every classification of handicapped students. Educators have planned and implemented high quality programs in which students with disabilities are integrated into regular schools, into classrooms, and the community with non-handicapped peers. These programs have four elements in common: individualization, curricular reform, research-based practices, and teacher supports. (Task Force on the Education of Students with Disabilities [Task Force], 1988, p. 17)

Although not without dissent and dissension, the organized parent advocacy movement and organizations of people with disabilities are now unequivocal about the community integration objective. As Barbara Sackett, the president of the Association for Retarded Citizens of the United States stated:

> *All* children with mental retardation should be in regular school settings preferably in their own neighborhoods. They should participate in the regular daily flow of activities with specialized services provided during portions of the day on an individualized need basis within or without a regular classroom setting. How can we meet the goal of integrated adult opportunities when we are still segregating our children? (1989, p.2)

Despite well-established policy, accumulating professional teachings, and experience for children and adults with severe disabilities, community integration is at best a chance event. Inconsistency both within states and across the country is well known and has been well documented (Biklen, 1988; Danielson & Bellamy, 1989) In certain localities—for example, Fairfax County, Virginia, St. Louis County, Missouri, and Bucks County, Pennsylvania—segregation in school and adult life is the reality now. And if the local decision makers have their way, it will be the reality for the near, if not the long-term, future. In the area of schooling, the U.S. Department of Education's annual report on implementation noted that the last 10 years reveal no substantial change in the proportion of students with disabilities educated in handicapped-only facilities (Viadero, 1989). In some states, 35%–40% of all students labeled retarded are in handicapped-only facilities. In certain regions, the designation of a student as severely impaired or multiply disabled automatically leads to placement in a private school or segregated center.

Given the variation in integration practices and the presence of singularly good programs in otherwise segregated districts, it is perhaps unfair to cite particular districts. However, examples help us understand the depth and staying power of segregation in our schools.

1. In St. Louis County, Missouri, the 23 local school districts assume no responsibility for the education of their 16,000 children with disabilities. A Special School District (SSD) of St. Louis County evaluates such children and assigns them to one of four possible placements, depending on the severity of their disabilities.

The segregated classrooms provide little or no contact with non-SSD teachers and students, and no access to counseling, library, or interscholastic athletics. Cooperation between the special education teachers and regular classroom teachers is practically impossible.

For example, William Shawcross attends River Bend Elementary School, far from his home in the Parkway School District. All of his classmates are labeled mentally retarded. His disabilities mean that he is barred from attending the elementary school closest to his home, and is not even assured of attending the same school from one year to the next. His segregation from children who are not disabled includes riding a bus with other students with disabilities. He is together with nondisabled students for physical education only, and that experience is taken away from William as a punishment for behavior that relates to his disabilities. Because he has disabilities, he receives no grades or report cards, and is unlikely to complete his high school education and receive a diploma. Since the local school district has nothing to do with William's education, except provide space to the special school district, his parents have no effective way to challenge the practices of the Parkway School District.

2. Some of the richest school districts in the country are the most segregated. Virginia's Fairfax County school district, with a special education budget approaching $100 million, has a de facto policy and practice of exclusion of whole categories of students with severe disabilities. In the 1988 school year, in all of Fairfax County, not a single school-age student categorized as autistic attended his or her home base school, and students classified as mentally retarded or multiply disabled also were systematically excluded from their home schools. Of 286 students with multiple disabilities in the county, 6 (2%) attended their home school. Of 598 students in the county classified as mentally retarded, less than 30 actually attended their home school.

Of the 20 high schools in Fairfax County, only 6 have students with severe disabilities; the remaining 14 high schools, some with as many as 2,000 students, have none.

3. Crossing the city line can preclude inte-

gration opportunity. In the city of Philadelphia, Pennsylvania, the fourth largest school district in the country, virtually all children with severe disabilities, including those labeled multiply disabled, attend their neighborhood schools. In the adjacent and affluent county of Montgomery, the Cheltenham Township school district serves no children with disabilities except for those designated as learning disabled. Becky O'Toole, a child with Trisomy 18 who just came of school age, cannot attend school anywhere in her district or close to her home. Her parents' choice would be to have Becky attend a class with nondisabled children in the same school her older sister attends and receive assistance as needed in the classroom.

However, Becky receives a homebound program simply because the only school program available to her is a segregated center operated by the Intermediate Unit, an hour's bus ride away from her home. For medical reasons, the long transit to the center's school is harmful.

For Becky O'Toole and many other children and adults, the first disabled rights revolution has had little meaning, despite its success in dismantling some of the most regressive and dehumanizing institutions and creating a multitude of special services. The first revolution has passed them by; in the Jeffersonian tradition, they need their own second revolution.

FORCES AND VALUES OF THE SECOND REVOLUTION

In the early 1970s, when the Constitutional underpinnings of a right to education seemed to be in place, those persons with severe disabilities and their families who were successful in ending school exclusion were *viewed* as the advance guard of a "quiet revolution"—a revolution that would transform education not only for children with disabilities but for all children disadvantaged by the educational system (Dimond, 1973). In the tradition of the strategists in *Brown v. Board of Education* (1954), advocates for children with disabilities saw equality in education as the fulcrum for equal respect and full admission to society for all persons with disabilities (Gilhool, 1989).

While the "quiet revolution" created opportunities for significant educational reform and made drastic changes in the rules for special education, the long-term impact of those reforms on the quality of life for all persons with disabilities and others disadvantaged (beyond those formerly excluded from schooling), may be too subtle to be noteworthy. The gap between the principles of the revolution and present practices, particularly on the dimensions of equal respect and full admission to society, is fully illustrated in the accounts of students and adults with disabilities (Asch, 1989; Hahn, 1989). It is nice and necessary to debate and analyze the extent to which the first revolution succeeded or fell short, but it is better to focus on whether the conditions necessary for the second revolution are sufficiently vital and how they can be nourished to the end that full integration can be achieved in this century.

The second revolution is not sparked by radically new ideas or principles; nor is it narrowly based in access to special education or other special services. It links the existent integration imperative with the now mature disabilities rights movement and is grounded in a powerful combination of values and forces that depend less on special interest advocacy and more on the national social and political trends that have strong potential to break down longstanding as well as recently created barriers to integration. These forces and values include:

All children, including those children with severe disabilities, belong in their local school, specifically their home school.

All children with learning problems, whether they be "special education" students, "at-risk" students, or otherwise regarded as disadvantaged in schooling, belong in regular classroom environments.

All persons, including those with severe disabilities, should be paid and supported to work in typical, integrated employment settings.

Infants and toddlers who require early intervention belong in community-based or school-based settings with maximum contact and interaction with nondisabled children.

The measure of effectiveness and appropriateness of integrated education, early intervention, community living, and work is the state-of-the-art standard.

All persons with disabilities belong first in their own homes and natural, family-scale community settings.

In all aspects of community life, non-discrimination and effective accommodation of persons with disabilities is expected and that expectation is to be enforced.

Home School

Although the integration imperative in education has been with us now for nearly 20 years (*Pennsylvania Association for Retarded Citizens v. Commonwealth of Pennsylvania,* 1971) and is stated quite clearly in federal law (Education for All Handicapped Children Act of 1975, §1412 [5] [B]), its interpretation by educators, advocates, and federal policymakers—and sometimes the courts—has created a confusion that allows for the perpetuation of segregated schools and educational programs that condone minimal interaction with nondisabled children. The requirements as to placement (the school the child would attend if not disabled) and the requirement for setting (regular classes unless education in those classes with the use of supplementary aids and services cannot be satisfactorily achieved) have not been taken as seriously by most educators as they have been by most courts (*Campbell v. Talladega County Board of Education,* 1981; *Roncker v. Walter,* 1983). Instead, in day-to-day practice as individualized education programs (IEPs) are framed, the requirements of the law have been transmuted into the issues of mainstreaming and least restrictive environment (LRE).

Neither LRE nor mainstreaming—terms devoid of objective standards—have any basis in law. Thus, they can be dealt with superficially or ignored outright (*Ninth Annual Report,* 1987). The concept of least restrictive environment is closely related to the pre–right to education concept of a continuum of educational placements (Reynolds, 1962). The long outmoded notion that some restrictive placements are acceptable and movement from more restrictive to less restrictive represented educational progress, somehow survived and displaced the strong presumption against segregation from the local school and against separation within the school building.

The conceptual flaws in the LRE model for education and other human services have been exposed by Taylor (1988). Among its other evils, Taylor showed that LRE legitimizes restrictive environments, reifies the readiness model, and effectively confers all decisions to professional judgments couched in terms of appropriateness. Hahn (1989) identified LRE as a pure professional ploy that avoids the integration imperative:

> The somewhat negative concept of "a least restrictive environment" was developed as a standard . . . rather than the distinctly positive goal of creating an environment adapted to the needs of everyone. Integration, . . . appeared to become a secondary or distant purpose instead of an urgent or primary objective. (p. 237)

In practice, LRE has been shown to be of no significance in placing students with severe disabilities (Brown et al., 1983; Lipsky & Gartner, 1989b) or of any current relevance to special education reform (Lipsky & Gartner, 1989b; Will, 1984).

Three generations of children subject to LRE are enough. Just as some institution managers and their organizations—both overt and covert—seek refuge in the continuum and LRE, regional, intermediate unit, and special school administrators and their organizations will continue to defend the traditional and professionally pliable notion of LRE. The continuum is real and represents the status quo. However, the morass created by it can be avoided in the design and implementation of reformed systems by focusing all placement questions on the local school and routinely insisting on the home school as an absolute and universal requirement. In terms of placement, the home-school focus renders LRE irrelevant and the continuum moot.

The local school is now and in the future the real and concrete embodiment of the PL 94-142 placement presumption. The last director of the Office of Special Education acknowledged that a decade of advances in educational technology and what we now know about effective schools have virtually eliminated the past justifications for removal of children from regular education (Irwin & Wilcox, 1987).

Local schools should be for *everyone*. . . . It is better for children; it is better for parents; it is better for communities; it is better for future employees; it is better for peers; and it is better for teachers when children with disabilities attend and are served well by the regular schools in their neighborhood. (Irwin & Wilcox, 1987, p. 3)

Brown and his Madison, Wisconsin, colleagues have put the local-school preference where it belongs in terms of the law and experience by defining the home school as the school the student with disabilities would attend if he or she were not disabled (Brown et al., 1989; *Code of Federal Regulations,* 1986). Their professional rationale for insisting on the home school tracks the congressional purpose in requiring integration in the first instance (Gilhool, 1989; Gilhool & Stutman, 1978). They demonstrated that in the home school all children can be prepared to function in a pluralistic society, the most meaningful instructional environment can be used, family members can have access to school and services, and the widest range of social relationships can be developed and maintained over the long term (Brown et al., 1989). In sum, "any important skill, attitude, or value that can be developed in a clustered school" (Brown et al., 1989, p. 2) also can be developed in a home school.

However, the inverse does not hold true: That is, there are many important skills, attitudes, and values that can be developed in a home school that cannot be developed in a clustered school. It is that proposition that should be tested; and a heavy burden of proof should be imposed if a child is to be sent away from his home school and separate from his brothers, sisters, and neighborhood peers. Such a test, if properly made, will serve nicely to replace and make unnecessary any reference to LRE, and will result in home-school placement for virtually all.

Regular Class

Just as the unwavering focus on the home school resolves most placement issues, the same focus on regular education and the regular classroom is necessary to avoid LRE and mainstreaming ambiguities concerning educational setting and the quality of peer interactions children with disabilities experience. Use of the regular education classroom as the base for education of students with severe disabilities has been shown to be effective and sufficient to meet the "Rowley test" of real educational benefits (Biklen, 1985; Forest, 1984; Gaylord-Ross, 1987; Gilhool, 1989). The power of the specification of the regular class focus, however, rests in its impact on those students not usually considered severely disabled. It is somewhat ironic that over the past 10 years as students with severe disabilities left segregated centers for neighborhood schools—for the purpose of facilitating interaction with non-disabled students—many other special education students present in those schools remained effectively segregated and isolated in self-contained classes and various pull-out programs (Lipsky & Gartner, 1989b). In Pittsburgh, Pennsylvania, for example, although students labeled mildly to moderately disabled were found clustered in 38 of the district's 56 elementary schools, over 90% of those students were never assigned to a regular education academic class. Fewer than 10% of those students with mild disabilities participated in regular education classes and less than half of that number participated in any class on a full-time basis (Lipsky & Gartner, 1989b; Sansone & Zigmond, 1986). With consistency, the Pittsburgh district also excluded students with severe disabilities, leaving them in intermediate unit centers (Task Force, 1988).

While we know there is a wide variation among states and even within states on integration measures, and that within the same district integration can be advanced differentially among different categories of students, it is essential that those advocating for and working to integrate students with severe disabilities examine the opportunities for interaction and participation in regular education for all children presently excluded and caught in the second system of special remedial and compensatory programs (Wang, Reynolds, & Walberg, 1987). There are four main reasons why efforts to integrate any one student should be grounded in concern for the integration of all students. First, the consequences of segregation are the same for all: no preparation, no educational benefit, and marginal and dependent postschool careers. Lipsky and Gartner (1989b) reported that review and meta-analysis of the large number of special education efficiency studies show little or no effect for students at all levels placed in special education. Thus, they concluded "there is no compelling body of evidence demonstrating that segregated special education programs have significant benefits for students" (Lipsky & Gartner, 1989b, p. 19).

Second, the conceptual framework used to defend and maintain separate programs of little or no benefit is the same for all students: the continuum and least restrictive environment. The same process, structure, and readiness barriers embodied in LRE that serve to keep students with severe disabilities out of local schools also keep other students out of regular education. For those students in the second system of remedial programs not in special education, the tracking placement process substitutes for the LRE process, but the result is the same. Track placements segregate, stigmatize, and deny individuality and variability in learning (Goodlad, 1984). The Committee on Policy for Racial Justice (1989), recommending the elimination of tracking and ability groupings, concluded:

> The inflexibility of track placements, ... represents a problem of paramount proportions. Black and other low-income students are often imprisoned in the bottom tracks, shunted away from mainstream classroom instruction. . . . [M]ost frequently, black students are dropped into low-ability groups, sometimes at a very early age, with little possibility of movement upward. James Rosenbaum, in *Making Inequality,* likens inflexible tracking to a sports tournament: "When you win, you win only the right to go on to the next round; when you lose, you lose forever." (p. 18)

Third, for students with severe disabilities, for those students labeled as mildly handicapped, and for those children considered "at risk," there are states of the art in education that are proven methods that work best when children are integrated and interact significantly in regular education. Lipsky and Gartner (1989b) provided numerous examples of cooperative learning activities, peer learning, mastery learning and adaptive learning environments, and other effective methods. As they are developed and vali-dated, successful techniques can be introduced into integrated settings. The Adaptive Learning Environment Model, for example, provides "a built in mechanism to incorporate on an ongoing basis the best practices that have a strong research base for improving instruction and learning on a year-round basis" (Wang & Walberg, 1988, p. 132).

Fourth, the close association between the conditions to achieve integration of any single student and the conditions necessary for effective schooling for all students compels a strong focus on the regular class and the school as a whole. Over the last decade, an accumulation of research has identified and elaborated the characteristics of schools that are effective (Edmonds, 1979). The effective schools literature and practice form the keystone of reform in general education (Council of Chief State School Officers, 1988; U.S. Department of Education, 1986). Some of the characteristics that make schools effective are longstanding basic mandates and obligations in education for students with disabilities (e.g., parent involvement, frequent monitoring, periodic assessment of performance). Moreover, a review of the effective schools' principles leads to the conclusion that "these same principles are outlined in virtually every special education text as the hallmark of a good 'special' education program" (Knoll & Meyer, Undated, p. 3).

At least three central characteristics of effective schools bear directly on the integration of any student, severely disabled or not. They are: 1) a positive climate of expectations that embraces all children; 2) an orderly and disciplined school atmosphere; 3) a clear focus on pupils' acquisition of skills; and 4) strong administrative leadership, especially at the principal level.

Schools that are effective by general education measures should prove conducive places for integration of students with severe disabilities into regular class settings. Indeed, they may be the only places that such integration can be achieved on a systematic and enduring basis. Such close interdependence for reform of special education and general education supports the concept of a merged or unitary system of education (Stainback, Stainback, & Forest, 1989).

One need not fully embrace the single-system idea to appreciate the power of aligning the interests of the effective school movement, the regular education initiative, and the integration imperative. The combination of research, practice, and advocacy brought by such an alliance represents the critical mass to sustain a good part of the second revolution.

Employment and Productivity

For as long as we have included persons with disabilities in our educational system, and long before "special education" as we now know it was invented, we have pretended that the education provided is for the purpose of postschool employment and/or productive activities (*White House Conference on Child Health Protection*, 1930). The evolution and the experience of the 70-year-old state-federal vocational rehabilitation program is both testament to our adherence to employment as a worthy goal for all persons with disabilities and to the tokenism with which that goal has been pursued.

Adult Americans with disabilities have the highest rates of unemployment, poverty, and welfare dependency in the country (Bowe, 1978, 1980). Incredibly, high unemployment statistics simply reflect the fact that as long as there is a surplus labor pool, persons with substantial disabilities are excluded from the labor market. Public provision for persons with disabilities, including income maintenance programs, living arrangements, and day activity programs, virtually require that beneficiaries with disabilities be poor and remain dependent. The very system of supports and services intended to assist persons with disabilities serves to separate and segregate them from all others seeking employment (National Council on the Handicapped, 1986).

Given the rigid and pervasive segregation structure of adult services, it is not surprising that the great majority of students who "age out" of special education are neither employed nor engaged in further education or productive activity (Edgar, 1987; Zollers, Conroy, & Newman 1984). Nor is it unexpected that thousands upon thousands of adults with moderate to severe disabilities are in or waiting to get in long-term sheltered workshops and segregated day activity centers (Buckley & Bellamy, 1985). Without

substantial changes in the structure and direction of adult services, it is predictable that costly, segregated day treatment will continue to be one of the most rapidly expanding program models in the future (Laski & Shoultz, 1987).

There are, however, widely noted powerful developments in policy and educational technology that can reverse the pattern of segregation when coupled with the demographics. The demographics of the 1990s will create a labor shortage that will provide employment opportunities to those currently excluded in greater numbers than anytime since World War II. In the future, it will be more difficult than ever, and much more costly, to treat persons with serious disabilities as a surplus population and to disregard and discard their productive capacity. The demographics and their economic consequences are stark. "In 1952, there were 17 people working for each retiree. By 1992, there will be only three" (Gilhool, 1987, p. 2). Of these three, one will be black or Hispanic or disabled; 50% will come from low-income families. As we enter the next century, the increasing number of students with special learning needs in the "second system" of education (Wang et al., 1987) will become the dominant share of the labor force in many regions of the country (Levin, 1988).

The decline in youthful workers and the labor shortage, particularly in lower paying jobs, will focus the attention of private-sector employers on persons with severe disabilities as potential workers. However, it is the expansion and extension of supported employment policy and the technology-forcing aspects of that policy that will ultimately translate employer attention into decent jobs for adults with severe disabilities.

Supported employment, as defined and authorized by Congress in 1986 (PL 99-506), and as put in place by the Rehabilitation Service Administration in the past 4 years (Wehman, Kregel, & Shafer, 1989), has the potential not only to supply jobs but to end systematic segregation of adults with severe disabilities. Supported employment is now commonly understood to mean paid work that occurs in integrated places of business for persons with severe disabilities and to secure and maintain employment without long-term support during employment.

The revolutionary dimensions of supported

employment cannot be overstated. First, it completely redefines employability in a way that makes everyone eligible for and possessed of the potential for work (Laski, 1986). Second, in unprecedented fashion, it gives equal standing to and requires both integration and productivity. Thus, it challenges the current segregated workshops and activity centers more directly than PL 94-142 implementation has challenged segregated schools. The supported employment movement has no tolerance for, and does not allow for, the perpetuation of dual systems of segregated and integrated employment.

During its brief existence, supported employment has had remarkable success (Wehman et al., 1989). In the 27 states with most experience, about 1,400 supported employment projects have been established since 1986. Funding increased from $25 million in 1986 to over $215 million in 1988. The number of individuals working—most for the first time— and earning significant wages increased by 250% over 2 years (Kregel, 1989). Supported employment is also beginning to have an impact on segregated adult services. In the 27 states surveyed in 1986, 96% of all clients were in traditional sheltered workshop or day activity settings with less than 4% in supported employment. In 1988, participation in supported employment reached nearly 10% of all clients served (Shafer, 1989).

Even in this early stage of implementation, there has been insistence that the integration imperative be strictly interpreted (Callahan, 1986) and a great deal of advanced thinking to avoid the physical setting and LRE focus that has plagued school integration. Shafer and Nisbet (1988) reported on the development of the following outcome-and-capacity indicators of integration in employment:

Acceptance: Integration occurs when workers are accepted by other members of the work force.

Interdependence: Vocational integration occurs when work tasks of the supported employee are interdependent with work operations of other employees.

Interaction: Integration requires opportunities for interaction with fellow employees or customers.

Opportunity for relationships: Integration in the workplace occurs when there is opportunity for friendships and other relationships with non-disabled employees.

Opportunity for decision making: Integration occurs when the supported employee has the same decision-making powers and opportunity to affect working conditions as other employees.

Although these indicators are preliminary, their content and direction, together with an understanding that integration must be planned and facilitated throughout the supported employment process, reinforce the proposition that the continued development of integrated employment will transform completely the role of adults with disabilities in our society.

Early Intervention

Just as integration in the workplace is most easily accomplished upon a foundation of integrated education (Brown et al., 1987), integrated elementary and secondary schooling may be accomplished fully and most completely when infants and toddlers experience integration in the preschool years. The chances that those children will have such experiences as early in life as possible have been augmented greatly by PL 99-457. That act mandated preschool education and intervention for children with handicaps ages 3–5 and created programs to assist states in implementing statewide systems of early intervention services for the youngest children, from birth to 3 years of age.

A review of the legislative history and purposes of the 1986 Education Amendments (PL 99-457) reveals a renewed Congressional concern to minimize, if not completely eliminate, the separation of regular and special education. Wang (1989), annotating the several objectives of the law, concluded:

P.L. 99-457 and the programmatic and administrative developments being implemented as a result, may be viewed as important precursors of systemwide improvement in the provision of state-of-the-art, integrated education for children of all ages. (p. 52)

Indeed, in its findings, Congress declared the ultimate integration objective to "minimiz[e] the need for special education and related services after handicapped infants and toddlers reach school age, to minimize likelihood of institutionalization" (PL 99-457, §671[a]). While LRE is already prevalent in discussions of early intervention and the federal regulations are susceptible to being muddled, experience in implementing PL 94-142 should be sufficient to avoid the creation of a parallel second system for preschoolers.

Sailor (1989) lent clarity to the integration requirement. Early intervention should be provided in day-care and preschool settings that serve primarily nondisabled children: "No matter how severely or multiply disabled a child is, there is no aspect of his or her educational needs that cannot be met in a private day care or pre-school context" (p. 63). There are a multitude of sound educational reasons for integration at an early age relating to acceptance, acquisition of socialization skills, and preparation for home-school placement. However, the most powerful reason is directly related not to child development in the early years, but rather to the effect on the family and society in later years. As Sailor explained:

> This process has to do with the effect on the family as a whole of not having their child kept apart from normal children as a consequence of disability. When their child is in [an integrated] program, parents seem to see themselves as a part of general education and day care rather then as unique people faced with a lifetime of separate structures (Hanline & Halvorsen, 1988). The potential for greater acceptance, . . . is obvious. . . . The developmental question for later ages becomes: "What is the difference between being a special child with unique needs versus being just another child who happens to have some special requirements to facilitate learning?" The public ethos appears to be changing, and for good reason, from accentuating the specialness to accentuating inclusion. (p. 64)

The point is perhaps not so subtle. Families who experience real and effective integration will not accept segregated kindergarten or special education in the second system. What works for them in the early years is what they will demand, thus fulfilling the Congressional expectation.

State-of-the-Art Requirements

In work, community living, and schooling (preschool, elementary, secondary, and adult), the integration imperative is advanced and integration made possible when state and local officials are required to pay attention to the state of the art, that which is known to work effectively. In PL 94-142, Congress imposed the first state-of-the-art requirement in education. Section 1413 (a) (3) of the law required of each local and state education authority:

> (A) the development and implementation of a comprehensive system of personnel development which shall include the in-service training of general and special educational instructional and support personnel, detailed procedures to assure that all personnel necessary to carry out the purposes of this chapter are appropriately and adequately trained, and effective procedures for acquiring and disseminating to teachers and administrators of programs for handicapped children significant information derived from educational research, demonstration, and similar projects, and (B) adopting, where appropriate, promising educational practices and materials. (Education for All Handicapped Children Act of 1975, §1413 [a] [3] [A] & [B])

Courts have used the state-of-the-art requirement to order or otherwise secure integrated school programs (*Campbell v. Talladega County Board of Education*, 1981; *Roncker v. Walter*, 1983).

The legislative mandate and court orders enforcing state of the art make clear it is not professional consensus that controls, but rather what works. By that standard, properly applied separate education, work, or living arrangements cannot survive scrutiny. As to schools,

> we know that separate special education does not work. . . . And its failure is costly . . . in dollars, in public confidence, and, most importantly in students' lives. . . . We know that integrated programs work. We know that preparation for full lives can only occur in integrated settings. (Lipsky & Gartner, 1989a, p. 281)

The knowledge base as to work and community living and early intervention is the same. Thus, strong state-of-the-art criteria should be imposed in all programs having an impact on adults and toddlers as well as school-age children. To say we know what works and have the strength of our convictions is not to say no further research is necessary or to minimize the important role that research will play in achieving integration. In fact, the state-of-the-art requirement, by focusing on promising practices, enhances the role of relevant research on promising practices. However, we now have hundreds of examples of exemplary integrated programs in all program areas. Persons with severe disabilities should not have to wait for integration until professionally devised solutions are universally accepted. Children and adults who do not have access to integrated programs that work should be able to gain access to those programs by invoking a state-of-the-art obligation.

REFERENCES

Asch, A. (1989). Has the law made a difference?: What some disabled students have to say. In D.K. Lipsky & A. Gartner (Eds.), *Beyond separate education: Quality education for all* (pp. 181–205). Baltimore: Paul H. Brookes Publishing Co.

Biklen, D. (1985). *Achieving the complete school.* New York: Teachers College Press.

Biklen, D. (1988, November). Integrated education. In S. Taylor, J. Racino, & B. Schultz (Eds.), *From being in the community to being part of the community:The proceedings of the Leadership Institute on community integration for people with developmental disabilities.* Syracuse, NY: Syracuse University, Center on Human Policy.

Board of Education of the Hendrick Hudson Central School District v. Amy Rowley, 102 S.Ct. 3034 (1982).

Bowe, F. (1978). *Handicapping America: Barriers to disabled people.* New York: Harper & Row.

Bowe, F. (1980). *Rehabilitating America: Toward independence for disabled and elderly people.* New York: Harper & Row.

Braddock, D., Hemp, R., Fujiura, G., Bachelder, L., & Mitchell, D. (1990). *The state of the states in developmental disabilities.* Baltimore: Paul H. Brookes Publishing Co.

Brown v. Board of Education, 347 U.S. 483 (1954).

Brown, L., Ford, A., Nisbet, J., Sweet, M. Donnellan, A., & Gruenewald, L. (1983). Opportunities available when severely handicapped students attend age appropriate regular schools. *Journal of The Association for the Severely Handicapped, 8*(1), 16–24.

Brown, L., Long, E., Udvari-Solner, A., Davis, L., Van Deventer, P., Ahlgren, C., Johnson, F., Gruenwald, L., & Jorgensen, J. (1989). The home school: Why students with severe intellectual disabilities must attend the schools of their brothers, sisters, friends, and neighbors. *Journal of The Association for Persons with Severe Handicaps, 14,* 1–7.

Brown, L., Rogan, P., Shiraga, B., Zanella Albright, K., Kessler, K., Bryson, F., Van Deventer, P., & Loomis, R. (1987). A vocational follow-up of the 1984-1986 Madison Metropolitan School District graduates with severe intellectual disabilities. *Monograph of The Association for Persons with Severe Handicaps, 2*(2).

Buckley, J., & Bellamy, G.T. (1985). National survey of day and vocational programs for adults with severe disabilities: A 1984 profile. In P. Ferguson (Ed.), *Issues in transition research: Economic and social outcomes* (pp. 1–12). Eugene: University of Oregon, Specialized Training Program.

Bush, G. (1989, February 8). [Address to joint session of Congress]. *Congressional Record, 135,* H266.

Callahan, M. (1986). Systematic training strategies for integrated workplace. In *Accommodating individual abilities in the workplace: Jobs for people with special needs* [Draft]. Omaha, NE: The Center on Applied Urban Research.

Campbell v. Talladega County Board of Education, 518 F.Supp. 47 (N.D. Ala. 1981).

Code of Federal Regulations. (1986, July). Education for All Handicapped Children Act, *34,* §300.552.

Code of Federal Regulations. (1987, July). Discrimination prohibited, *34,* §104.4 [b][2].

Committee on Policy for Racial Justice. (1989). *Visions of a better way: A black appraisal of public schooling.* Washington, DC: Joint Center for Political Studies Press.

Council of Chief State School Officers. (1988). *School success for students at risk: Analysis and recommendations of the Council of Chief State School Officers.* Orlando, FL: Harcourt Brace Jovanovich.

Danielson, L.C., & Bellamy, G.T. (1989). State variation in placement of children with handicaps in segregated environments. *Exceptional Children, 55,* 448–455.

Developmental Disabilities Assistance and Bill of Rights Act, 42 U.S.C. §6000 (1989).

Developmental Disabilities Assistance and Bill of Rights Act: Definitions, 42 U.S.C. §6001 [8] (1989).

Dimond, P. (1973). The constitutional right to education: The quiet revolution. *Hastings Law Journal, 24,* 1987.

Edgar, E. (1987). Secondary programs in special education: Are many of them justifiable? *Exceptional Children, 53,* 555–561.

Edmonds, R. (1979). Some schools work and more can. *Social Policy, 9*(5), 26–31.

Education for All Handicapped Children Act of 1975, 20 U.S.C. §1412 [5][B].

Eleventh Annual Report to Congress on the Implementation of the Education of the Handicapped Act (1989). Washington, DC: U.S. Office of Special Education and Rehabilitation Services.

Federal Register. (1989, June 22). Early Intervention Program for Infants and Toddlers with Handicaps, *54*(119), 26312.

Federal Register. (1990, March 6). Handicapped Special Studies Program, *55*(44), 7970.

Forest, M. (1984). *Integration/education: A collection of readings on the integration of children with mental handicaps into regular school systems.* Downsview, Ontario: National Institute on Mental Retardation.

Gaylord-Ross, R. (1987). School integration for students with mental handicaps: A cross-cultural perspective. *European Journal of Special Needs Education, 2*(2), 117–129.

Gilhool, T.K. (1987, March 5). *Pennsylvania State Senate Committee on Education: Confirmation hearing.*

Gilhool, T.K. (1989). The right to an effective education: From *Brown* to PL 94-142 and beyond. In D.K. Lipsky & A. Gartner (Eds.), *Beyond separate education: quality education for all* (pp. 243–253). Baltimore: Paul H. Brookes Publishing Co.

Gilhool, T.K., & Stutman, E.A. (1978). Integration of severely handicapped students: Toward criteria for implementing and enforcing the integration imperative of PL 94-142 and Section 504. In *Developing criteria for the evaluation of the least restrictive environment provision* (pp. 193–227). Washington, DC: U.S. Office of Education, Bureau of Education for the Handicapped, Division of Innovation and Development, State Program Studies Branch.

Goodlad, J.I. (1984). *A place called school.* New York: McGraw-Hill.

Hahn, H. (1989). The politics of special education. In D.K. Lipsky & A. Gartner (Eds.), *Beyond separate education: Quality education for all* (pp. 225–241). Baltimore: Paul H. Brookes Publishing Co.

Irwin, M., & Wilcox, B. (1987). *Proceedings of the National Leadership Conference. Least restrictive environment: Commitment to implementation.* Bloomington: Indiana University, Institute for the Study of Developmental Disabilities.

Knoll, J., & Meyer, L. (undated). *Principles and practices for school integration of students with severe disabilities: An overview of the literature.* Syracuse, NY: Center on Human Policy.

Kregel, J. (1989). Opportunities and challenges: Recommendations for the future of the national supported employment initiative. In P. Wehman, J.

Kregel, & M.S. Shafer, *Emerging trends in the national supported employment initiative: A preliminary analysis of twenty-seven states* (pp. 128–137). Richmond: Virginia Commonwealth University, Rehabilitation Research and Training Center.

Laski, F. (1986). *Vocational rehabilitation services for severly handicapped persons: Rights and reality.* Unpublished document, Philadelphia.

Laski, F., & Shoultz, B. (1987, June). Supported employment: What about those in Medicaid funded day treatment and day activity centers? *Word from Washington,* pp. 11–14.

Levin, H. Accelerating Elementary Education for Disadvantaged Students, In Counsel of Chief State School Officers. (1988). *School success for students at risk: Analysis and recommendations of the Council of Chief State School Officers* (p. 210). Orlando, FL: Harcourt Brace Jovanovich.

Lipsky, D.K., & Gartner, A. (1989a). Building the future. In D.K. Lipsky & A. Gartner (Eds.), *Beyond separate education: Quality education for all* (pp. 255–290). Baltimore: Paul H. Brookes Publishing Co.

Lipsky, D.K., & Gartner, A. (1989b). The current situation. In D.K. Lipsky & A. Gartner (Eds.), *Beyond separate education: Quality education for all* (pp. 3–24). Baltimore: Paul H. Brookes Publishing Co.

National Council on the Handicapped. (1986). *Toward independence: A report to the President and to the Congress.* Washington, DC: Author.

Ninth annual report to the Congress on the implementation of the Education of the Handicapped Act. (1987). Washington, DC: U.S. Department of Education.

Pennsylvania Association for Retarded Citizens v. Commonwealth of Pennsylvania, 334 F. Supp. 1257 (E.D. Pa. 1971), 343 F. Supp. 279 (E.D. Pa. 1972).

PL 99-457, *the Education of the Handicapped Act Amendments of 1986.*

Rehabilitation Act of 1973, 29 U.S.C. §701 *et seq.*

Reynolds, M.C. (1962). A framework for considering some issues in special education. *Exceptional Children, 28,* 367–370.

Roncker v. Walter, 700 F.2d 1058 (6th Cir. 1983), *cert. denied,* 104 S.Ct. 196 (1983).

Rutter, M., et al. (1979). *15,000 hours: Secondary schools and their effects on children.* Cambridge, MA: Harvard University Press.

Sackett, B. (1989). To Ann with love, Mom: An open letter to my daughter LeeAnn. *Newspaper of ARC of the U.S., 38*(2), 2.

Sailor, W. (1989). The educational, social, and vocational integration of students with the most severe disabilities. In D.K. Lipsky & A. Gartner (Eds.), *Beyond separate education: Quality education for all* (pp. 53–74). Baltimore: Paul H. Brookes Publishing Co.

Sailor, W., Gee, K., Goetz, L., & Graham, N. (1988). Progress in educating students with the most severe disabilities: Is there any? *Journal of The Association for Persons with Severe Handicaps, 13,* 87–99.

Sansone, J., & Zigmond, N. (1986). Evaluating mainstreaming through an evaluation of students' schedules. *Exceptional Children, 52*(5), 455–456.

Shafer, M.S. (1989). The implementation of supported employment: A national status report. *Avant Garde: The National Newsletter on Integrated Services, 3*(4).

Shafer, M., & Nisbet, J. (1988). Integration and empowerment in the workplace. In *Supported employment implementation issues.* Richmond: Virginia Commonwealth University, Rehabilitation Research and Training Center.

Stainback, S., Stainback, W., & Forest, M. (Eds.). (1989). *Educating all students in the mainstream of regular education.* Baltimore: Paul H. Brookes Publishing Co.

Task Force on the Education of Students with Disabilities. (1988). *Quality education, preparation for life.* Harrisburg: Bureau of Special Education in the Pennsylvania Department of Education.

Taylor, S.J. (1988). Caught in the continuum: A critical analysis of the principle of least restrictive environment. *Journal of The Association for Persons with Severe Handicaps, 13,* 41–53.

U.S. Department of Education. (1986). *What works: Research about teaching and learning.* Washington, DC: Author.

Viadero, D. (1989, June 21). States found still using private-placement "option." *Education Week, 7*(39), 4.

Wang, M.C. (1989). Implementing the state of the art and integration mandates of PL 94-142. In J.J. Gallagher, P.O. Trohanis, & R.M. Clifford (Eds.), *Policy implementation & PL 99-457: Planning for young children with special needs* (pp. 33–57). Baltimore: Paul H. Brookes Publishing Co.

Wang, M.C., Reynolds, M.C., & Walberg, H.J. (1987). *Repairing the second system for students with special needs.* Paper presented at the Wingspread Conference, Racine, WI.

Wang, M.C., & Walberg, H. (1988). Four fallacies of segregationism. *Exceptional Children, 55*(2), 132.

Wehman, P., Kregel, J., & Shafer, M.S. (1989). *Emerging trends in the national supported employment initiative: A preliminary analysis of twenty-seven states.* Richmond: Virginia Commonwealth University, Rehabilitation Research and Training Center.

White House Conference on Child Health Protection: Committee Report. (1930, November). (Section IV, The handicapped, pp. 316–317).

Will, M. (1984). Educating children with learning problems: A shared responsibility. *Exceptional Children, 52,* 411–416.

Zollers, N., Conroy, J., & Newman, E. (1984). Transition from school to work: A study of young adults and their families in Pennsylvania. In *Report to the Administration on Developmental Disabilities.* Philadelphia: Temple University Developmental Disabilities Center/UAF.

EXTENSIONS OF THE PUBLIC LAW AND EDUCATIONAL SERVICES

Public Law 94-142 guaranteed a free and appropriate public education to all students with disabilities during the school years. In fact, this legislation also allowed for the extension of that right to publicly support preschool (from birth to school age) and postsecondary (for ages 18–21) educational services as the states permitted. Thus, while there now existed mandated educational and related services for a child with a disability once he or she reached school age. There was no requirement that any services be provided to that child before or beyond the school years. "Permissive" educational and other support services might be provided by particular states or agencies working within specific regions in any given state, but the extent to which such services were available to children and their families varied greatly across the country.

This section of the book—as does the previous section—focuses heavily upon developments in the United States to extend the concept of an individually appropriate education to better meet the needs of students with severe disabilities. Thus, the resolutions in this section advocate for extensions of PL 94-142 throughout the child's developmental years—before and after traditionally defined "school age" as well as throughout the year and thus beyond the traditional "school year." Educational best practices and legal precedents are comprehensively reviewed in the chapters in this section. Finally, several authors raise some serious questions regarding remaining issues, our priorities, and the impact of these extensions of educational services upon the family and the relationship of professionals to the family. For example, what is the risk that the provision for the individualized family services plan mandated by PL 99-457 could ultimately function primarily as yet another professional intrusion into the ability of these families to adjust and blend into their communities? And how might our practices be altered to ensure that preschool and extended school year programs do not carry with them yet another potential for segregation and isolation from children's peer groups and the family's community support network?

Resolution in Support of the Education of the Handicapped Act and Section 504 of the Rehabilitation Act of 1973

Part 1—Introduction

WHEREAS, The Executive Board of The Association for Persons with Severe Handicaps and its membership affirm the rights of persons who experience handicaps to an education and other human services in order to achieve fuller participation in community life. We also advocate for the United States Congress to continue their role of passing, sustaining, and supporting legislation that authorizes federal agencies to act in a leadership role to assure those rights. The role of federal agencies in assuring the rights of persons with handicaps has contributed to attitudinal changes over the last two decades and to the many examples of successful programming now in existence.

Part 2—Response to withdrawal of federal leadership

WHEREAS, The historical belief that local entities alone would adequately serve persons with severe handicaps has been erroneous. There has been little evidence of effective and efficient local initiative without federal leadership. Until recently, the paucity of consistent, appropriate, and relevant patterns of educational programs and services led professionals and parents to use the courts, state legislature, and Congress for remedying these problems. The passage and implementation of the Education of the Handicapped Act (EHA) and Section 504 of the Rehabilitation Act has resulted in significant accomplishments relative to the number of students served and the quality of programs and services offered. A reason for this success has been strong federal leadership. This leadership fosters full service goals and through various means encourages and cajoles local entities to fulfill these goals; and

WHEREAS, Another area of concern is the human services system. The journey toward full participation in the community for individuals with severe handicaps is arduous, lacks coherence, and is often expensive. The individual at each level of development requires many and varied services. To be effective we must coordinate and streamline the service delivery model used. We pay homage to the ideal of coordination and cooperation, but rarely, if ever, achieve it without clear leadership. We submit that the best method to achieve this goal is for our government, especially Congress and the Executive Branch, to take an active leadership role. Both examples emphasize the issue facing us in the 1980's and 90's: identification and implementation of the most effective and efficient means for providing education and other human services to persons with handicaps; and

WHEREAS, The exigencies of the 1980's and 90's demand changes. It is our belief that the federal government's role and responsibilities must include acting as a catalyst for change and providing guidance to the school districts and human services agencies so that the best practice can be developed. The perspective of the federal government is needed to generate, initiate, and coordinate services to persons with handicaps—especially in light of social, economic, and political realities. Sixteen thousand independent school districts cannot begin to meet the myriad needs of persons with handicaps; and

WHEREAS, Persons who experience severe handicaps must achieve full integration into our society. TASH believes that the present social legislation contributes to the goal of integration. The EHA and Section 504 of the Rehabilitation Act of 1973 and their regulations must be maintained and enforced. It is especially important that the Executive Branch continue and intensify its efforts to enforce the presumption of these laws for ensuring opportunities for people with severe disabilities to receive education, leisure, community living, transportation, work, and other aspects of living in integrated settings where they can routinely interact with people who are not disabled.

RESOLVED, In summary, TASH urges the United States Congress, Executive Branch, and all federal agencies to continue their important coordinative and leadership role in promoting education and other human services which foster the full integration for persons with severe handicaps into community life. TASH also urges that the laws and regulations continue as a concrete manifestation of the federal commitment to persons with severe handicaps.

ORIGINALLY ADOPTED OCTOBER 1981
REVISED OCTOBER 1987

* * * * *

DOCUMENT IV.2

Resolution on Extended School Year

WHEREAS, Public Law 94-142 guarantees children with handicapping conditions the right to a "free appropriate public education"; and

WHEREAS, Public Law 94-142 designates the school the lead agency for identifying children's needs and coordinating I.E.P. programs; and

WHEREAS, The I.E.P must include a statement of the child's needs, long- and short-term instructional goals, related services and extent of participation of persons who do not have handicaps for a "full calendar year"; and

WHEREAS, In litigation, the limiting of special education and related services, on the basis of a 180-day school year, has been found to be a violation of Public Law 94-142; and

WHEREAS, We believe that the acquisition and generalization of many crucial community, vocational, domestic, and recreational/leisure skills are facilitated by year-round programming; and

WHEREAS, We believe that the acquisition and maintenance of such skills are necessary to ensure successful integration into the community by children with disabilities when they reach adulthood; and

THEREFORE BE IT RESOLVED, THAT The Association for Persons with Severe Handicaps urges local and state educational agencies and community agencies to include year-round programming as part of the range of educational opportunities for children with handicaps. These programs should be functional, integrated, and meet individual needs.

ORIGINALLY ADOPTED NOVEMBER 1986

* * * * *

CHAPTER 24

Early Childhood Services for Children with Severe Disabilities
Research, Values, Policy, and Practice

Carol R. Westlake
Ann P. Kaiser
Peabody College of Vanderbilt University, Nashville, Tennessee

Systematic provision of early childhood services is a relatively new development in the field of special education. Most of the progress in service provision and research related to early childhood services for children of all ability levels has occurred since 1960 (Linder, 1983). Only in the last decade have services for young children with severe disabilities become available in community-based programs. And, only as recently as 1986 with the passage of PL 99-457 has support for early childhood services been mandated through federal legislation. As a result of recent legislation and as a result of continuing commitment by parents, practitioners, policymakers, and researchers, early childhood services is one of the fastest growing aspects of special education and services for persons with disabilities.

HISTORICAL PERSPECTIVES

In the 25-year history of early childhood intervention, the language used to describe this aspect of special education has changed several times, reflecting not only the state of the art for services but also current theoretical and political thinking upon which the provision of these services is based. Thus, most early research and program development were described as "early intervention" and focused on the provision of specific interventions to the child for the purpose of preventing further deficits in development. As the prominent models of child development

shifted to more complex, interactive, dynamic ones, and the understanding of multiple influences on the child's development became clearer in theory and practice, multiple disciplines became associated with intervention programs and interdisciplinary training and service delivery emerged as implicit standards for quality early interventions. The expansion of the interactionist model of child development (Sameroff & Chandler, 1975) and subsequent shift in theoretical focus to include the family as a critical context and co-actor in the intervention process was accompanied by further shifts from child-centered to family-focused interventions (D.B. Bailey & Simeonsson, 1988). Only recently has the phrase "early childhood services" emerged, finally acknowledging that such services are part of the expected and, to some extent, institutionalized aspects of education in the United States.

DEFINING AND TRACKING AN EMPIRICAL BASE

While the changes in language describing early childhood intervention programs are cues to the shifting perception of these types of services, such changes make identification of the relevant empirical base somewhat difficult. Because services, per se, have existed for only a few years, research in support of "services" (defined as a multicomponent, stable program of intervention, available in community settings) is almost nonexistent. What does exist is a number of studies examining components of early childhood services (e.g., investigating the effects of specific interventions, involvement of parents, and applications of curricular models). In addition, there are program evaluations, typically of less scientific rigor, that examine the effects of interventions that are similar to services currently available in communities. The methodological and conceptual limitations of the research base are discussed in more detail in subsequent sections. Changes in terminology, in service configuration, and conceptualization of the treatment targets and the desired outcomes of early intervention make determination of the appropriate empirical base supporting early childhood services difficult.

Research has not always led practice in this area of special education. More often, practice and research have proceeded together, sometimes mediated by the actions of policymakers. The history of factors influencing early childhood services is long and the relationship between these factors and empirical knowledge is complex and dynamic.

In this chapter, we propose four axioms that represent the knowledge base upon which early intervention services have been constructed. These axioms derive from three sources of knowledge: cultural/political knowledge and values, empirical or scientific knowledge, and the conventional wisdom derived from practice. These sources of knowledge concomitantly influence the development of services and they act upon one another. Cultural values are influenced by both conventional wisdom and empirical knowledge. The research conducted in search of empirical knowledge is to a large extent guided by the values of the culture and the parameters of current, conventional wisdom (Lincoln & Guba, 1985). Thus, while we describe three knowledge domains separately, it is impossible to determine the separate influences of any single type of knowledge on the development of early childhood services.

Cultural/Political Knowledge and Values

Early childhood services for children with severe handicaps derive, to a considerable extent, from the social, cultural, and political events that occurred during the 1960s. During this period of relative economic prosperity, the social values related to the elimination of poverty and the building of a more equitable society in terms of civil rights and educational opportunity were articulated through social action and through federal legislation. Early childhood services for children "at risk" for developmental disabilities were established as a means of breaking the poverty cycle and as a preventive measure against mental retardation (Gray & Klaus, 1969). These services were intended to compensate for the impoverished environments of at-risk children. Providing enriched early experience was a means of giving children a "head start" on education and increasing the probability of their success in later educational experiences.

Two clear cultural values were articulated in the policies developed to ameliorate poverty through educational intervention: first, compensatory interventions designed to ensure equity or equality of opportunity for people who are disadvantaged relative to the general population; and second, education as a primary means of intervention.

Although many of the first federally supported programs for children with handicaps were proposed on the basis of ultimately improving the economic outcomes of individuals and benefiting the larger society by limiting the costs to be incurred in supporting these children, the cost-benefit argument was paralleled by increasing attention to the rights of all children to have access to an appropriate and free education. For children with severe disabilities, the emergence of a strong civil rights approach to the provision of educational services was critical because the cost-benefits arguments were least tenable with children who have continuing needs for services and support.

In sum, the values base from which services for children with severe disabilities emerged was similar to the base from which education was extended to children who were members of minority groups: equality of educational opportunity. In addition, services for children with severe handicaps were built from a logic of prevention of further effects of their disabilities through early intervention. While the civil rights basis was derived almost entirely from the cultural value base, the logic of prevention was more directly tied to theoretical and empirical knowledge emerging concurrently with the social movements of the period.

Empirical Knowledge

Concurrent with the social action movements of the 1960s and 1970s was a resurgent interest in the role of early experience in child development. Theories of child development forwarded by Hunt (1961), Bloom (1964), and others emphasized the critical impact of early environment and experience on intellectual development. The writings of Gesell (1928), Skinner, (1953), Piaget (1952), and others were considered as potential models of environmental influence that might be applied to predict or enhance the developmental outcomes for children. Child development became a central focus in mainstream psychology and most child psychologists of the time adopted a relatively strong stand favoring the role of environment in determining developmental outcomes (e.g., Horowitz & Paden, 1973). Theoretical models of environmental influence initially postulated a direct and strong influence of early experience on social and cognitive development (Yarrow, 1978). These models of development formed the backdrop for early intervention with disadvantaged and environmentally deprived children (e.g., Gray & Klaus, 1969; Karnes, Hodgins, & Teska, 1969; Lazar & Darlington, 1982). Although, ultimately, the data resulting from these experimental applications of early interventions required reconceptualization of the direct causal model of influences on child development (Bronfenbrenner, 1975), the immediate effect of the Head Start programs was to introduce the logic for and feasibility of early intervention into both scientific inquiry and conventional wisdom.

Concurrent with the renewed interest in early child development was a growing focus on applied behavior analysis and the development of technology for teaching specific skills to persons with disabilities (cf. Bijou & Baer, 1963, 1978). The rapidly expanding set of applied, experimental research studies demonstrating that persons with a range of disabilities could be systematically taught a broad array of skills brought new energy to the field of special education (Ysseldyke & Algozzine, 1984). Early studies demonstrating that changes in social, academic, and adaptive behavior could be accomplished through the application of operant conditioning principles functionally changed the definition of educability for persons with severe handicaps. From the beginning, domain-specific investigations of specific teaching strategies included young children with handicapping conditions (cf. Hart & Risley, 1968; Stokes, Fowler, & Baer, 1978); however, relatively few studies included children who were young and *severely* handicapped.

The empirical knowledge base has grown in several different directions, as is discussed later in this chapter. In addition to studies of domain-specific intervention, studies in which the effects of programs, curricula, family involvement, and policies have been evaluated from the empirical base upon which services for young children with disabilities were proposed and developed.

Rarely have programs been designed on the basis of specific research findings—for a variety of reasons. First, relatively few studies have actually been conducted with young children with severe handicaps; second, the methodological characteristics of the existing studies limit their applicability to actual programs; and third, the linkage between research and practice is not linear. Practice has sometimes preceded research and often research has not been rapidly translated into practice.

Conventional Wisdom and Knowledge of Practice

Conventional wisdom is the folklore of teaching and program development that is communicated informally through practitioner-oriented workshops and inservice and preservice training, and realized in functioning early intervention programs. While conventional wisdom may have linkages to empirical knowledge, it is the "street-level" version of that knowledge, and the linkages may not be immediately apparent or even known to the practitioner or the observer. Sometimes, conventional wisdom is the application of a principle that is tied to empirical knowledge derived in limited experimental conditions. For example, as we discuss later, there is some limited empirical evidence supporting the tenet that "earlier is better," but the conventional wisdom surrounding this tenet is a much more general rule derived from practice than from a specific empirical base.

The exact path by which conventional wisdom influences practice and development of services is difficult to trace. Sometimes, commonly held beliefs will become the basis for research or will be rediscovered in the context of research findings (e.g., "Grandmother's Rule," reconceptualized in the context of the Premack [1959] principle). More often, effective practices are passed along through informal observations and training without specifically being investigated in research studies. To the new professional in the field, it may not be readily apparent which of the current "best practices" derive from conventional wisdom and which are grounded in empirical knowledge.

Conclusion

These three sources of knowledge—cultural, empirical, and practical—have shaped the development of services for young children with handicaps. In the following section, we introduce four axioms that undergird current services:

Axiom I: Young children with severe handicaps have a right to services that improve the quality of life and maximize their developmental potential.

Axiom II: Early childhood services for children with severe handicaps are effective in improving quality of life and maximizing developmental potential.

Axiom III: Intervention services that begin earlier in a child's life will be more effective than services that begin later.

Axiom IV: Early childhood services that involve families are more effective than those that do not.

These axioms derive from all three sources of knowledge and in discussing each of them, we attempt to identify how each is grounded in these sources.

AXIOM I

Young children with severe handicaps have a right to services that improve the quality of life and maximize their developmental potential.

This tenet is the basis upon which services to young children with severe handicaps have been built. It is the foundation of the three axioms that follow. The notion of a right to services derives from a fundamental societal value. Historically and contemporaneously, society has implicitly defined education as a shared cultural responsibility that is undertaken to enhance the development of children. Both the child and society are presumed to benefit from the enhancement of individuals' development through education. Our society further presumes that opportunities for education and development should be available equally to all persons regardless of gender, race, or developmental status.

To a considerable extent, PL 94-142 and PL 99-457 have operationalized the cultural valuing of education as a right for all children. PL 94-142, the Education for All Handicapped Children Act of 1975, specified that the "right to a free appropriate public education" should be extended to all children, including those with handicaps. Further, the law defined an appropriate education for children with handicaps as one that is "designed to meet their unique needs" (*Code of Federal Regulations,* 1978, § 300.1). Individualized education programs (IEPs) were mandated as the mechanism to be used in formalizing and delivering appropriate educational services. Thus, equality of educational opportunity for children with disabilities was further defined to include provision of special conditions and extraordinary efforts to enhance development and learning by children with disabilities.

One of the special conditions required to enhance learning and development is the provision of services at a younger age. PL 99-457 amends the Education for All Handicapped Children Act to extend the provision of a free, appropriate public education to children with handicaps who are 3–5 years old and establishes a program for the development of comprehensive services for infants and toddlers with handicaps. Lowering the age at which services may begin was based on arguments that there is an "urgent and substantial need" to enhance the development of infants and toddlers with handicaps, enhance the capacity of families to meet the needs of their children, and maximize the potential for individuals with handicaps to live independently in society (U.S. Department of Education, 1986).

The definition of the right to equal educational opportunity and the right to services in order to maximize developmental potential for young children with severe handicaps has evolved across the last 25 years, paralleling the development of the services themselves. Early intervention services as a means of enhancing development and equalizing opportunity were first provided to children at risk for developmental delays due to social and environmental reasons. Prevention of mental retardation and realizing the potential for normal development were the implicit rationales for efforts to enhance development in young children during the 1960s and early 1970s. The original early intervention programs were designed to ameliorate the negative effects of biological and environmental risk and to enable children to become functioning, autonomous, competent adults (Anastasiow, 1986). Improvements in educational and medical technology, along with a growing social commitment to the rights of children with more severe handicaps, resulted in changes in the population being served in early intervention programs. Subsequently, changes in the goals and practices of early intervention have occurred. There has been a subtle shift from a focus on prevention and achieving normal developmental outcomes to a focus on maximizing the developmental potential of individual children through appropriate intervention services. In early intervention for children with severe handicaps, maximizing developmental potential is a means to enhance the quality of their lives—not just an end in itself. Maximizing developmental potential is observed in the positive changes in the individual's ability to lead a life that includes friends, personal choice making, independence, and dignity in living circumstances and in work. Measures of intellectual functioning or simple descriptions of adaptive behavior may or may not correlate with these positive, functional changes in developmental potential.

The social and cultural values that provide a foundation for the right to services do not emerge from an empirical base, but to some extent they have been shaped by research findings and have provided critical incentives for research. The extension of rights to appropriate educational services to young children with severe handicaps has accelerated research exploring strategies to effectively enhance individual development.

If Axiom I is accepted as a cultural value, then the question "Should services be provided to young children with severe disabilities" is no longer an appropriate focus for empirical investigation (Anastasiow, 1986; Meisels, 1985). As a culture, we have agreed implicitly and mandated explicitly that such services are a right. There remain, however, many questions about the efficacy of early childhood services. The issue of effectiveness is addressed in the second axiom.

AXIOM II

Early childhood services for children with severe handicaps are effective in improving quality of life and maximizing developmental potential.

The assumption that early childhood services are effective for young children with handicaps has been held since the beginning of these services. In addition to theoretical arguments supporting effectiveness (Anastasiow, 1986; Meisels, 1985), the rapid expansion of services and growing public commitment over the last 20 years have been an explicit statement of the common assumption of effectiveness (Beckman & Burke, 1984; Simeonsson, Cooper, & Scheiner, 1982; Swan, 1981).

Empirical Evidence of Effectiveness: A Critical View

Much scientific inquiry has been directed toward answering the question "Is early intervention effective?" Although the first generation of research supported the conclusion that early intervention services have positive impact on young children with handicaps and their families (White, Bush, & Casto, 1985), this research has been subject to considerable criticism. In recent years, critics have pointed out that research in this area is seriously limited by its inadequate methodology, the poor or incomplete conceptualization of research questions, and the constraints on generalizability that must be considered when the population is extremely heterogeneous

(Bricker, Bailey, & Bruder, 1984; Dunst & Rheingrover, 1981; Simeonsson et al., 1982). Although these criticisms are valid from a scientific perspective, it is important to recognize that the social context from which this body of literature emerged was one in which the general effectiveness of and need for early childhood intervention was assumed. Thus, while researchers conducted studies examining the effects of various treatment procedures and intervention programs, increasingly large numbers of children with immediate needs for services were being identified. Often, research was conducted in conjunction with a service program that had the primary function of providing interventions to children and families. In some cases, the tension created between sound research methods and concurrent service delivery has been resolved by choosing compromise designs that allowed some evaluation of the intervention while still ensuring service delivery to the children involved in the evaluation. Such compromises may be criticized on empirical grounds but not on ethical grounds.

Critiques of early childhood intervention research have identified three issues of scientific concern: 1) conceptual considerations, 2) methodological issues, and 3) issues related to population. In the following section, we briefly examine each of these issues before turning to an overview of the research literature on the effectivness of early intervention with children who have severe handicaps.

Conceptualization

Efforts to evaluate the effectiveness of early intervention have been constrained by incomplete conceptualization of early intervention services and their intended effects (Dunst, 1986). The theoretical frameworks guiding research, conceptualization of the intervention, and choice of outcome measures are not well articulated in most published studies. When frameworks for intervention are identified, they generally have been extrapolated from research and principles in related domains rather than developed specifically for comprehensive interventions for young children with handicaps (Guralnick & Bennett, 1987).

Researchers' choices of research questions and measures have varied widely. Early intervention has been defined to include short-term specific interventions as well as longer term, multiple-component interventions. Outcome measures also vary widely and, apparently, unsystematically. In the absence of a conceptual framework guiding the evaluation of the intervention, the choice of outcome measures has been affected more directly by the available or easily applied instruments than by an understanding of ideal outcomes related to a specific intervention. The result is a research literature that is incomplete and difficult to integrate into a cohesive analysis of effectiveness.

Methodology

The effectiveness research in early childhood services also has been criticized on methodological grounds (Bricker et al., 1984; Dunst, 1986; Dunst & Rheingrover, 1981; Odom & Fewell, 1983; Simeonsson et al., 1982; White & Casto, 1985). Critics have argued that serious methodological inadequacies limit the scientific conclusions that can be drawn from the existing data base. At the least, methodological limitations must be considered carefully in interpreting the reported findings.

The choice and application of research design has been a particularly problematic issue. Scientific arguments that early childhood services are effective must be based on evidence of a causal relationship between interventions and outcomes: When children are provided with services, they will demonstrate change or progress that would otherwise not occur. The extent to which the outcomes can be attributed to the intervention provided and not to extraneous factors depends to a large degree on the design used for evaluation (D. Campbell & Stanley, 1966). Early childhood research designs generally have been limited by the inability to randomly assign subjects to treatments in group-design studies (White & Pezzino, 1986). Other design flaws include lack of an adequate control group, inadequate description of subjects and treatments, limited documentation of fidelity of treatment, limited assessment of reliability, and incomplete or incorrect statistical analysis.

While some of these design limitations have been the result of poorly designed studies, more often the designs have been limited by the availability of suitable control groups and the ethical considerations related to withholding treatment for the sake of experimental control. Research designs have often been selected in order to balance the ethical considerations surrounding treatment with the desire to evaluate the effectiveness of those treatments.

Population

Heterogeneity of population presents a challenge when conducting research to assess the effectiveness of early childhood services. Children receiving services vary according to their organic, environmental, and developmental status. Children studied in early intervention research include those who are at risk for developmental delays, children with identified handicaps of different types and severity, and children with multiple handicaps. Most program evaluations and many experimental analyses of intervention procedures have included children with varying characteristics. Rarely are the effects of programmatic interventions reported separately for subgroups of children with a specific characteristic such as severe handicaps.

Frequently, efficacy arguments for children with handicaps are built on the foundation of data from studies of at-risk children. Most of the large-scale research on the efficacy of early intervention has been conducted with disadvantaged or at-risk children (e.g., Berrueta-Clement, Schweinhart, Barnett, Epstein, & Weikart, 1984; Lazar & Darlington, 1982) rather than children with identified handicaps. Analytical reviews designed to characterize the effectiveness of early childhood services also have been based, at least in part, on at-risk populations (Casto & Mastropieri, 1986; White & Mott, 1987). Generalizing the findings from studies involving at-risk children to children with severe handicaps is inappropriate for at least three reasons: 1) critical differences in subject populations, 2) related differences in program variables, and 3) the goals and intended outcomes of interventions for different populations. These three are now discussed.

First, the populations are not equivalent. The characteristics and needs of at-risk children and children with severe handicaps differ substantively. The presence of a disability, its type and severity, related secondary problems, and functional characteristics, in addition to social/environmental variables, are all factors that affect the provision and outcomes of early services (Guralnick, 1988). While most children classified as at risk are organically intact, children with severe handicaps are likely to have chronic disabilities and genetic anomalies that contribute to their condition and its prognosis for remediation. Because environmental conditions are a primary source of their developmental status, at-risk children should be the most amenable to the effects of altered social and physical environments as well as direct teaching. Children with severe handicaps typically show developmental patterns that are not primarily influenced by the environment. Although physical and social contexts may play a role in their development, the degree of influence is mediated by their physiological status. Thus, while children with severe disabilities do benefit from environmental interventions, the effects are likely to be more limited and less direct than the effects expected for children who are classified as at risk.

Second, because the needs and characteristics of the subject populations differ, the nature of services and programs that constitute appropriate intervention must also differ. For example, program content for children with severe handicaps is more likely to include special therapeutic services (Parette & Hourcade, 1983) and specialized approaches for sensory impairments or other specific handicaps (Snell, 1986). Models of service delivery, type and level of parent involvement, and program intensity may also vary.

Finally, the purposes and goals of early childhood services differ by subject population. Program outcome measures should be closely related to program goals. Outcomes of programs that are designed to prevent developmental delays in young children who are environmentally at risk differ substantively from those programs for young children who are experiencing severe mental retardation and multiple handicaps. For example, changes in cognitive measures, such as IQ, might be argued to be an appropriate outcome for children at risk in an early intervention program. More appropriate outcomes for children with severe handicaps are increases in functional skills and development of early motor, social, and communicative behavior. Such changes may or may not be reflected by changes in IQ, but nonetheless represent valid and important outcomes for this population. The implicit logic of "increasing normalcy" or remediating the handicapping condition to the extent that a child will function "at age level" is generally inapplicable in designing and evaluating interventions for young children with severe handicaps—even when intervention is intended to enhance their abilities to meet environmental demands in as normal a manner as possible. When populations, interventions, and goals and outcomes differ, generalization from findings with one population to another must be done with care.

Research with Heterogeneous Populations

Arguments for the effectiveness of early childhood services have relied heavily on program evaluation research (Casto, 1988). Since most early intervention programs serve heterogeneous groups of young children, the result has been a body of research conducted with mixed-subject populations. Some studies have combined children who are at risk and children with identified handicaps (e.g., E.J. Bailey & Bricker, 1984; Hutinger, 1978) when evaluating the effects of interventions. Other studies present data for subject samples that represent a variety of handicapping conditions: for example, 50 children, ages 7–54 months, 35 severely or profoundly retarded, 13 moderately retarded, 1 mildly retarded, and 1 not retarded (Bricker & Dow, 1980); or 30 children, ages 1–36 months, 1% mildly handicapped, 54% moderately handicapped, and 38% severely, multiply handicapped (Hanson, 1985). Studies may or may not report results for subject subgroups. While general conclusions regarding the effectiveness of treatment may be drawn from mixed-subject samples, the generalization of these findings to children with severe handicaps must be done with great caution.

Typically, studies with heterogeneous samples will include relatively few children with severe handicaps and the results obtained with these children may or may not be similar to those reported for the larger group. While this criticism may be applicable for any individual subject

when a group design is used and means for the total group are reported, special care in drawing conclusions regarding children with severe handicaps is probably warranted given the learning characteristics of this population.

Issues related to population arise even among those studies including a population whom researchers define as exhibiting severe handicaps. For example, there are no standard criteria for defining severe handicaps among young children. Individual studies may apply very different standards for "severity," and frequently researchers do not adequately report the standards or definition used. Changing trends in the classification of children with handicaps must also be considered. For example, 10 years ago children with Down syndrome were routinely classified as having severe handicaps; today, most children with Down syndrome are not so classified.

Research Base

Research on the effectiveness of early intervention can be placed into five categories: 1) evaluations of specific intervention techniques, 2) evaluations of early intervention programs, 3) reviews and secondary analyses of existing data, 4) policy studies and large-scale program evaluation, and 5) economic analyses. Research on the effectiveness of early intervention for young children with *severe* handicaps and their families is a small subset of the body of early intervention research and can be found within the first three categories.

In reviewing research for inclusion in this section, the following criteria were applied. First, subjects were less than 5 years old. Second, the subjects were described as meeting contemporary criteria for severe handicaps. We applied the current TASH definition, to the extent possible (see Document I.1, this volume). Third, the author of the research described the subjects as severely handicapped and we could discern no evidence that the subjects would *not* meet contemporary definitions. The latter criterion was necessary because adequate subject description is frequently absent. Finally, in general, only research conducted within the last 10 years was included unless subject descriptions were specific enough to accurately determine if subjects were severely handicapped. This criterion limits potential problems with outdated classifications of severe handicaps. Studies that identified only children with severe handicaps, reported results for children with severe handicaps separately, or addressed a mixed population but did not report results for children with severe handicaps separately were included in the analysis.

In the following sections, three categories of effectiveness research are described and the limitations of research in each area are discussed. Specific studies involving children with severe handicaps that exemplify these categories of research are cited.

Studies of Specific Intervention Techniques

There is a small body of literature describing the effects of applications of specific interventions, curricular approaches, or treatment models to preschool children with severe handicaps. Studies investigating the effects of motor skills training, social interaction intervention, language or communication training, and general instructional interventions are found in this literature. As in other areas of early childhood special education research, research involving only children with severe handicaps and who are under the age of 5 years is relatively infrequent. In this section, studies in four domains are described and the findings of these investigations are related to services for young children with severe handicaps.

Motor interventions

For most young children with severe handicaps, motor skills training, including physical and occupational therapy, is a component of early childhood services. There are a number of examples of research related to this area. Research has been conducted to test the effects of neurodevelopmental training (P. Campbell & Stewart, 1988) and sensory integration therapy (Harris, 1988).

Laskas, Mullen, Nelson, and Willson-Broyles (1985) examined the effects of four specific neurodevelopmental training activities on the motor development of young children with multiple handicaps using an A-B-A design. Two dependent measures were identified: physiological (dorsiflexor muscle activity during a posterior equilibrium reaction as measured through a biofeedback instrument) and behavioral (frequency of heel contact during "rising to stand"). Significant changes during the treatment phase were reported in both dependent measures as compared to the two baseline phases.

Horn and Warren (1987) studied the effects of using a microcomputer-mediated teaching system on the acquisition of sensorimotor behavior by 2 children with severe multiple handicaps, ages 24 and 17 months. A microcomputer-mediated system (a computer, individually adapted switches, positioning equipment, and battery-operated toys) was used to teach three basic motor skills to each of the subjects. The computer monitored and activated reinforcers for child movements and recorded data on teacher prompts and child behavior. The effects of motor training were evaluated using a multiple-probe design across behaviors. For both children, the implementation of training resulted in substantial increases in performance of motor tasks when compared to baseline. In addition, both children demonstrated high levels of generalization and maintenance of each skill.

Research on motor interventions has direct applicability to preschool services. Evidence of the modifiability of early motor behavior in young children has reinforced a continued emphasis on physical and occupational therapy as services for this population. Because the motor development needs of preschoolers with severe handicaps may be extensive, research that focuses on efficiency in training new responses and on the linkage of critical motor responses into a developmental system resembling that observed in normally developing children continues to be an area for critical research. Problems in measurement and reliability of assessment prior to and following intervention is another area of concern in both research and intervention (P. Campbell & Stewart, 1988).

Social skills

Interventions to improve social interactions are of interest to researchers and practitioners because almost all children with severe handicaps lack these skills. In particular, the use of peers as intervention agents has been an innovation in services to young children with severe handicaps directly resulting from research in this area (Odom & Strain, 1986).

Studies by Weisen, Hartley, Richardson, and Roske (1976) and Young and Kerr (1979) were among the first to demonstrate that social skills of preschool children with severe handicaps could be enhanced. Wisen and his colleagues applied operant techniques to train 6 young children with severe mental retardation to be reinforcing agents for their peers. Young and Kerr trained a child with mild mental retardation to prompt social interaction in classmates with more severe mental retardation and to provide tangible reinforcers when interactions occurred. Positive changes in the social interaction of both the tutor and the subjects with severe handicaps were observed.

Two studies of peer training were conducted by Peck, Apolloni, Cooke, and Raver (1978). In their first experiment, 3 children with mental retardation, ages 36, 37, and 38 months, and 3 normally developing peer models were identified. The effects of direct peer-imitation training in a naturalistic setting were assessed using a combined multiple baseline across subjects and a multielement baseline design (Ulman & Sulzer-Azaroff, 1975). Rates of social interaction increased for 2 of the subjects with mental retardation subsequent to implementation of training procedures.

In the second study (Peck et al., 1978), 1 normally developing child, age 44 months, served as a peer model for 2 children with mental retardation, ages 25 months and 34 months. Both subjects with mental retardation had low rates of parallel and solitary play at the outset of the study. In this experiment, data were collected on the affective nature of the interactions between the subjects with mental retardation and the peer model. Using a multielement baseline design to assess the effects of training, the authors found that rates of positive social interaction increased for both subjects with mental retardation during the intervention.

Evidence from these studies and others involving children with autism (McHale, 1983; Strain & Kerr, 1979) suggest that social interactions of young children with severe handicaps can be enhanced through environmental arrangement and social interaction trainers. Two caveats should be noted: first, the skills that have been taught have been relatively simple early social skills such as nonverbal initiations and parallel play; second, a very small number of children with severe handicaps have been involved. The studies were intensive, relatively long term, and included a training of peers by a skilled intervenor. Although these findings generally indicate that social skills intervention can be effective for preschool children with severe handicaps, additional research is needed to examine the facilitative effects of such interventions on the development of more complete social repertoires and on the day-to-day use of new skills with untrained peers (Odom & Strain, 1986).

Language and communication

The development of early communication skills is also a frequent concern for children with severe handicaps (Kaiser, Alpert, & Warren, 1986). There has been a considerable amount written about the need for very early communication intervention with this population (cf. McLean & Snyder-McLean, 1978); however, there is a relatively small body of empirical literature. In part, the limited empirical base for preschool children with severe handicaps is a function of the delayed language development of these children. Until relatively recently, language intervention research has involved primary-age children who exhibited a capacity for verbal imitation. For many children with severe handicaps, the emergence of verbal imitation occurred after the age of 5. Thus, the research base on didactic and naturalistic instruction with students with severe handicaps has involved mostly students age 6 or older. For similar reasons, the preschool language intervention research literature has included mostly subjects who are not classified as severely handicapped.

Interventions that involve teaching single words or alternative modes of communication have been the most frequent example of communication research with young children with severe handicaps. For example, Kaiser, Alpert, Hemmeter, and Ostrosky (1988) trained three preschool special education teachers to use milieu language-teaching strategies to teach small nonvocal (communication board and signing) repertoires to three 3-year-old boys with severe handicaps, using a multiple-baseline design across teacher-child dyads. Use of the naturalistic language teaching procedures during a small-group period in the preschool classroom resulted in increased responsiveness to teacher communication, increased imitation of signs and communication board for all 3 subjects, and increases in spontaneous communication for 1 of the subjects.

Other evidence of modifiable learning in children with severe handicaps

In addition to examples of interventions in specific domains, there are studies that have demonstrated that very young children with severe handicaps can learn new skills in various instructional contexts. At one end of a continuum from simple to complex demonstrations of learning is a study by Dunst, Cushing, and Vance (1985) examining response-contingent learning by 6 infants with profound mental retardation and multiple handicaps. The 6 infants acquired head turns to specific stimuli as a function of prompting, reinforcement, and massed trials. Dunst, Cushing, and Vance's findings suggest that simple learning strategies are available to even the very youngest children with severe handicaps and thus, that reinforcement-based instruction with this population is potentially a means to enhance performance during the first 2 years of life.

At the other end of the continuum is an experimental analysis of the application of a curriculum model that involved learning multiple skills in naturalistic classroom contexts. Bambara, Warren, and Komisar (1988) demonstrated that the Individualized Curriculum Sequencing (ICS) model could be used as an effective instructional strategy for preschool children with severe handicaps. The effects of the ICS model on the acquisition and generalization of skills by 2 preschoolers were evaluated using a within-subject probe design across different target responses. Target motor, communication, and self-help skills were taught across three classroom activities and in routines during the school day. One of the 2 subjects showed clear acquisition and generalization of the newly taught skills

while the other subject showed acquisition of one skill and a trend toward acquisition of a second skill.

While it is commonly assumed that young children with severe handicaps can and will learn simple skills during instruction, the empirical evidence is limited but generally positive. One notable aspect of the studies across domains is the length of time required to demonstrate systematic changes in child behavior and the degree of support needed to ensure generalization of the newly learned behaviors. While this finding has implications for the intensity, duration, and effects of intervention, there is no evidence that would contraindicate instructional interventions.

Program Evaluations

This category of research includes evaluations of the effectiveness of specific programs of services to young children with handicaps. Early intervention programs represented in this category most often are demonstration or model projects. While there are many studies in this category of early intervention research, most program evaluations have been done with at-risk, mildly handicapped, or heterogeneous populations. Few program evaluations have focused exclusively on children with severe handicaps.

E.J. Bailey and Bricker (1984) reviewed 13 evaluations of early intervention programs described as serving children with severe handicaps. Two aspects of the evaluation studies reviewed are striking. First, none of the studies evaluated outcomes for children with severe handicaps separately. In most of the studies, the population was heterogeneous with a few children with severe disabilities. (Studies by Bricker and Dow [1980] and Safford et al. [1976] are exceptions. The majority of children in both studies were severely handicapped.) Results for children with severe disabilities were not analyzed separately, except in a study by Bricker and Sheehan (1981). Thus, it is difficult to determine if the results reported in most of these 13 studies can be generalized to children with severe handicaps. Second, with one exception (Brassell & Dunst, 1978), none of the studies included an adequate experimental design. Most studies did include multiple measures of outcomes and reported pre- and posttreatment changes that were statistically significant. However, without appropriate experimental controls, these changes cannot be interpreted as strong evidence of effective intervention.

Three examples of studies included in the E.J. Bailey and Bricker (1984) review exemplify the existing program evaluation data base for children with severe disabilities. In an ex-post facto study of 191 children with moderate to severe handicaps, Moore, Anderson, Fredericks, Baldwin, and Moore (1979) compared children who had 1, 2, or more years of early intervention with those who had no early intervention experience. Results indicated that child-performance levels in specific areas at ages 9, 10, and 11 differed significantly between children who had 2 years or more of intervention and those who had no early intervention or 1 year of early intervention.

Hanson (1985) used a pretest/posttest design to evaluate a 2-year model program for children with mental retardation, including children with Down syndrome. The program was both center and home based and used a transdisciplinary approach. Pretest and posttest measures of child development and parent behavior for 24 infants and toddlers (38% with severe handicaps) were collected. Statistically significant changes in both children and parents were reported as resulting from the intervention.

Hoyson, Jamieson, and Strain (1984) also used a single-group, pretest/posttest design to evaluate the effects of a curriculum model in a program for 6 preschool children with severe handicaps (i.e., children with autistic-like characteristics). Their results indicated that the subjects' mean rate of development was higher at the end of the program participation than at the entry. Comparing each child's rate of developmental program entry to rate of development after the child had been in the program for a period of time allows children to serve as their own controls (Irwin & Wond, 1974; Rosenberg, Robinson, Finkler, & Rose, 1987; Wolery, 1983), but it is not an adequate substitute for the use of a control group.

Secondary Analyses

Secondary analyses are a means of integrating findings across multiple studies. There are two types of analyses used to discern a pattern in research findings and address global questions regarding effectiveness. In research overviews and critical reviews of research, evaluations of effectiveness are formulated by informally reviewing, comparing, and synthesizing research from multiple studies. A more formalized secondary analysis is the use of meta-analysis. Meta-analysis is a comprehensive statistical approach that creates a common metric that may be used to compare the effect size resulting from individual studies (Glass, 1976). In a meta-analysis, the emergent trends and sizes of effects obtained for a particular class of treatments are examined statistically.

Integrative reviews

Many critical reviews of early childhood research are available (Bricker et al., 1984; Dunst, McWilliam, & Trivette, 1985; Dunst & Rheingrover, 1981; Gibson & Fields, 1984; Guralnick & Bennett, 1987; Simeonsson et al., 1982). Critical reviews generally identify studies on the basis of a specific set of criteria and analyze them according to relevant dimensions of the research. In addition to providing information on the data base that supports early intervention, critical reviews often focus on important methodological issues related to the work that has been done in the field of early childhood services.

In the first comprehensive review of early intervention research, Dunst and Rheingrover (1981) analyzed the methodology and findings of 49 evaluation studies conducted between 1970 and 1980. Criteria for selection required that intervention begin before the age of 3; that the majority of the children in each program had one or more organic impairments; and that child progress data were provided. This review included studies that reported interventions with children then (in 1981) classified as severely handicapped. Inadequate subject descriptions in most studies limit the confidence with which outcomes from these studies can be generalized to children currently considered severely handicapped. While many of the studies reported positive child outcomes, Dunst and Rheingrover concluded that the methodological limitations of most studies posed sufficiently serious threats to internal validity to prevent drawing conclusions about the effectiveness of early intervention.

E.J. Bailey and Bricker (1984) described 13 evaluations of programs that served young children with severe handicaps. As discussed earlier, the actual percentage of children with severe handicaps varied from possibly 0% (Bagnato & Neisworth, 1980) to 70% (Bricker & Dow, 1980). In many studies, it was not possible to determine how many children were severely handicapped. A wide variety of measures were used to characterize child outcomes including standardized tests, anecdotal written records, and curriculum-referenced and criterion-referenced tests. The models of intervention, as well as the length of the intervention period (range 2 months to 3 years), varied. Bailey and Bricker pointed out the methodological limitations of the research base and the conceptual problems in aggregating results across program models and diverse measures. However, Bailey and Bricker emphasized the consistent pattern of positive outcomes as indexed by a range of child performance gains across studies. They supported "the conservative conclusion that early intervention can produce changes in the behavioral repertoire of a wide range of severely handicapped children" (E.J. Bailey & Bricker, 1984, p. 49).

In general, integrative reviews have proven extremely valuable in identifying the data base on children with severe handicaps and in drawing attention to the repeated methodological and conceptual limitations of research in early intervention. The analysis of the aggregated evidence only modestly enhances the empirical knowledge of effectiveness.

Meta-analysis

Meta-analysis provides a means of assessing a range of outcomes of early intervention by applying statistical procedures. It allows the development of a comprehensive picture of the results of primary studies across a range of programs, measures, and subjects (Pillemer & Light, 1980). And, the aggregation of effects helps in the identification of patterns of findings across studies. The inherent limitation of a meta-analysis, however, is that it can be no better than the data base that it uses (Dunst & Snyder, 1986; Shonkoff & Hauser-Cram, 1987). If the primary studies are flawed, the meta-analysis will share the weaknesses. Furthermore, if inappropriately applied to disparate studies, meta-analysis can have the effect of "mixing apples and oranges" (Strain & Smith, 1986). Without strict conceptualization and specific definitions, there is a risk of computing effect sizes that have no referent in reality. Casto and Mastropieri (1986) analyzed 74 studies of early intervention with young children with handicaps. Most of the children in the studies were characterized as mentally retarded or multiply handicapped. The outcomes and characteristics of each study were analyzed using a 98-item coding system. Using a "standardized mean difference effect size" measure (Glass, McGaw, & Smith, 1981), 215 effect sizes were computed from the individual study data. The overall conclusion of the study was that early intervention programs do result in moderately large immediate benefits across a wide variety of children, conditions, and types of programs. Casto and Mastropieri noted in their analysis that the study contains "only a few effect sizes for children with the most severe handicaps" (1986, p. 420); however, they did not discuss these findings specifically.

Shonkoff and Hauser-Cram (1987) selected a subset of 31 studies from those in the Casto and Mastropieri (1986) meta-analysis. These studies met more rigorous methodological standards and were coded for 87 variables. The data from the studies yielded 91 effects. Seventy-five percent of those effects could be classified in three groups; IQ/DQ, motor skills development, or language development. Shonkoff and Hauser-Cram concluded that early intervention services are effective in promoting developmental progress for many children with handicaps, but pointed out that "data-base limitations preclude any meaningful conclusions regarding the influence of severity of disability on child outcomes" (1987, p. 653).

When applying the techniques of meta-analysis or conducting a critical review of research with populations of children with severe handicaps, the limitations of the methodologies are compounded. Small sample sizes, mixed populations, and studies of mixed design all complicate and weaken the integrative analysis. For example, meta-analyses generally do not include findings from single-subject research, a method often employed for studying young children with severe handicaps. Findings from studies with heterogeneous populations make aggregation of data potentially meaningless in terms of drawing conclusions for any population subgroup.

Conclusions

It is possible to conclude that early intervention is effective with children who have severe handicaps. Across the three categories of research considered in this section, there is consistent evidence that modest effects are typically observed when systematic interventions are applied to these preschool children. The actual empirical evidence is modest, however. The overall number of studies that involved children with severe handicaps under the age of 5 years is less than 25. In most cases, children with severe handicaps were included in a heterogeneous sample and the data on this subgroup were not reported separately. In studies where specific interventions were applied, the number of subjects in each study was typically less than six. In these studies, intersubject variability and modest gains resulting from extensive interventions were modal findings. In no study is there evidence to suggest that intervention with this population was not or could not be effective. However, problems in measurement, experimental design, and classification of subjects make any interpretation of positive or negative findings a tentative one.

Axiom II proposes that early intervention is effective for children with severe handicaps. A critical examination of the research base provides parameters that must qualify this axiom. Within a small data base, with its particular limitations, it appears that there is modest evidence that early intervention can be effective with preschool children with severe handicaps. There are many unanswered questions regarding the extent, generalization, and maintenance of the effects of early interventions. Furthermore, effectiveness must be considered in terms of the intensity of treatment required to facilitate relatively small developmental changes. There is a continuing need for systematic analyses of interventions for this population that focus on effective and efficient interventions and on strategies for enhancing service delivery of proven interventions.

AXIOM III

Intervention services that begin earlier in a child's life will be more effective than services that begin later.

The notion that the earlier intervention is started, the more effective it will be, is a popularly held belief about the provision of services to young children with handicaps. In a study of introductory textbooks in special education, Mastropieri, White, and Fecteau (1986) found that eight of the nine texts reviewed made statements consistent with the position that intervention should start as early as possible. In "reviewing reviews" of early intervention research, Casto and Mastropieri (1986) reported that 18 of 24 reviewers cited "age at start" as an important variable, concluding that an earlier start is better.

Initial arguments for "earlier" intervention were formulated in support of interventions for preschool children at risk (during the preschool period [ages 3–6]), as discussed in Axiom I. Beginning around 1975, "early" intervention with handicapped children and children biologically or environmentally at risk increasingly referred to the application of teaching, therapy, stimulation, or family-based interventions during the first 2 years of life. Currently, early interventions may begin immediately after birth, sometimes occurring in the neonatal intensive care unit or in the context of parent-child interactions at home during infancy.

The continuing move toward earlier intervention is rooted in developmental theory and research. Theoretical models of infant development posit that the first few years of life are the period in which the most rapid neurological, physical, and cognitive growth occurs (Bower, 1977). For example, Bloom (1964) reported that "50 percent of [the variance in intellectual] development takes place between conception and age four" (p. 88). The work of Bloom; and Hunt (1961) articulated developmental principles that support the importance of this period for intellectual, social, and emotional growth, and thus, for interventions to enhance developmental outcomes.

In recent years, a shift in developmental theory has provided an even stronger premise for very early intervention drawn from "bi-directional" models of child development (Anastasiow, 1986; Meisels, 1985). Interactionist models of development such as Sameroff and Chandler's (1975) transactional model; Bronfenbrenner's (1975) ecological model; and the general systems model described by Ramey, MacPhee, and Yeates (1983) posit a psychobiological view of development. This view holds that infant development results from a complex interaction of genetic and environmental variables. The resulting models of development are bi-directional in the sense that mutual transactions between the child and the social and caregiving environments help to shape not only the child's development, but also aspects of the child's environment, specifically the behavior of caregivers. The mutually influential aspects of caregiver-child interaction enhance the impact the child's current developmental status has on his or her future development. Thus, very early environmental intervention for children at risk and for those with handicaps is essential to maximize positive development outcomes (Anastasiow, 1986).

Developmental interventions during infancy have taken two general forms: interventions that provide additional sensory stimulation to compensate for presumed sensory deficits and interventions to enhance caregiver-child interactions (Bricker, 1986). There is evidence to suggest that the outcomes for high-risk preterm infants can be improved by those interventions that improve the child's interactions with the environment (Cornell & Gottfried, 1976; Kopp, 1983). There is also evidence from interventions with handicapped children, particularly children with Down syndrome (Gibson & Fields, 1984), to suggest that positive changes in social-communicative behavior (Mahoney, 1988) and motor development (Hanson & Schwarz, 1978) can be achieved during the first 2 years of life.

Age-At-Start Research

Although the special education literature has reported that the earlier a child is involved in services, the more effective the program will be in producing positive developmental outcomes (Bronfenbrenner, 1974; Garland, Stone, Swanson, & Woodruff, 1981; Smith & Strain, 1984), the empirical base is more equivocal. The research is very limited, and like other research in early childhood, the population samples generally comprised children who are at risk or who have less severe handicaps. White and Casto (1985), in an integrative review of research, identified only five studies that made direct comparisons of starting children in interventions at two different ages while holding other variables constant. None of these studies included children with severe handicaps. Further, the aggregated results of these five studies did not indicate a clear advantage for earlier age of start.

There have been a few studies that tested for and reported a positive correlation between age of start and outcomes. For example, Fenske, Zalenski, Krantz, and McClannahan (1985) conducted a retrospective study of children with autism. All 18 children had received the same treatment; half of the children had entered the treatment program prior to 60 months of age, half later. While 6 of the 9 children who entered prior to 60 months achieved positive outcomes, only 1 of the 9 children who entered after 60 months of age achieved a positive outcome.

Similarly, Strain, Steele, Ellis, and Timm (1982) reported results of a follow-up study with children who had severe behavior problems including a possible diagnosis of autism. All children had received comparable interventions. Three to 9 years later, those who had begun the program prior to 36 months of age tested more similarly behaviorally to their same-sex peers in current classroom placements than those who had begun later.

In a complex analysis of the effects of early intervention, LeLaurin (1985) correlated age at onset of intervention with degree of developmental rate change for 12 nonhandicapped children and 16 children with handicaps participating in a model early intervention program. One of the children with handicaps was described as "severe/profound"; 9 others were "trainable." All children entered the program between 3 and 31 months of age. For the group with handicaps, the results showed the later the onset of intervention, the smaller the amount of developmental progress.

Clunies-Ross (1979) compared the trends in

mean developmental quotients observed for three groups of children with Down syndrome who began intervention at three different ages (0–11 months, 12–23 months, and after the age of 24 months). The 8 children who began intervention at the earliest age entered the program with the highest developmental quotients and showed the highest quotients at the fourth assessment period. Children beginning intervention at all three ages showed an upward trend in developmental quotients between period 1 and period 4. Since it is generally reported that the developmental quotient of children with Down syndrome declines with age, Clunies-Ross's findings suggest that early intervention may be especially effective for this population and that very early intervention may be most effective. It is not apparent that any of the children in the Clunies-Ross study were severely handicapped at the outset of the study. However, since the population of children with Down syndrome is diverse, the findings in this study might be suggestive of the conclusion that very early intervention for some children in this population may reduce the possibility of their becoming severely handicapped.

Other studies involving children with Down syndrome have compared very early intervention with no treatment or minimal treatment. For example, Hanson and Schwarz (1978) reported that infants with Down syndrome who were enrolled in an intensive early intervention program achieved developmental milestones consistently earlier than similar infants not involved in an intervention program. The differences reported were large, with the experimental group lagging only slightly behind a comparison group of normally developing infants. Somewhat conflicting results were reported by Piper and Pless (1980), who found no significant differences between intervention and control groups of children with Down syndrome. The intervention in this study was less intense than in other studies investigating the effects of very early intervention with children with Down syndrome and some methodological limitations are evident in the analysis (see Bricker, 1986, for a discussion of these limitations).

The direct empirical evidence for the axiom

"earlier is better" as applied to children with severe handicaps is modest and largely derived from results of interventions with children at risk, with Down syndrome, with behavior disorders, or with other less severely handicapping conditions (e.g., hearing impairments) (Horton, 1976). Relatively few studies have directly compared the effects of intervention prior to age 2 in comparison to intervention beginning in the later preschool years (after age 3). Those studies that have made direct comparisons present somewhat disparate results, suggesting that other factors such as type of intervention, intensity and duration, and possibly the specific etiology of the child's handicap may mediate the advantage offered by earlier intervention. There is no evidence to recommend against very early intervention.

One additional caution should be noted. Two interpretations are possible for any study comparing the effects of treatments with relatively early and late onsets. One interpretation of the finding that children who began treatment earlier had better outcomes is that the early onset of the intervention was responsible for the observed outcome. Another equally plausible interpretation is that children who begin intervention earlier received more treatment. For example, children beginning at age 2 and observed at age 6 would have received 4 years of treatment, while children beginning at age 4 would have received only 2 years of treatment by age 6. Studies by Clunies-Ross (1979), Bagnato and Neisworth (1980), and LeLaurin (1985) that described rates of changes are less subject to alternative interpretations related to total amount of intervention, but the results such as those reported by Strain et al. (1982) and Fenske et al. (1985) should be interpreted more cautiously.

Conclusions

There are many specific questions that might reasonably be raised in regard to this axiom (e.g., What constitutes an intervention? How early may intervention actually begin? Are effects different across domains of development for children of varying entry-level abilities?) In light of PL 99-457, which provides for intervention beginning at birth, research efforts might best be focused on comparing alternative strategies for very early intervention with children with identified handicaps. In particular, empirical analyses of the effects of specific very early interventions for children with severe handicaps will be of both practical and theoretical importance in understanding if, when, and why earlier is better.

AXIOM IV

Early childhood services that involve families are more effective than those that do not.

Since the mid-1970s, family involvement in early intervention has emerged as a common component of services to young handicapped children (Rosenberg & Robinson, 1988). Emphasis on involvement has resulted both from the prevailing models of child development and from the mandated participation of parents in educational decision making contained in PL 94-142 and PL 98-199. The value and the effectiveness of family involvement in enhancing child developmental gains is generally accepted in the professional literature (Mastropieri et al., 1986). In this section, we examine the empirical evidence in support of the axiom that early childhood services that involve families are more effective than those that do not. We begin by considering four related assumptions that support the argument for a central role for families in early intervention:

1. Families are the natural developmental context for young children.
2. A family is an interactive social system that influences and is influenced by its members.
3. Support to families of children with handicaps affects both family and child.
4. Family members can fulfill many of the roles and functions traditionally in the domain of the early intervention professional.

Families are a natural and critical developmental context for young children, including those with handicaps. For all infants and toddlers, much learning occurs in caregiving interactions. Family members are the first and primary influence on the development of young children (Maccoby & Martin, 1983). Research on aspects of parent-child interaction, including attachment, maternal responsiveness, maternal involvement, and affect, provides evidence that parents serve an important role as facilitators of social and cognitive development in young children (Sibler, 1989).

In recent years, family systems theory has been used as a basis for the development of models for services to families including young children with handicaps. According to this theory, families are social systems in which individual members affect and are affected by their interactions and mutual ecological circumstances (Minuchin, 1974). In a systems model of families, interactions and relationships are reciprocal (Barber, Turnbull, Behr, & Kerns, 1988; Bell, 1968; Sameroff & Chandler, 1975). Child development is ecologically based and transactional —the family influences the child's development and the child's development influences the family. Changes in individuals, interaction patterns, settings, and circumstances have an impact upon the behavior of system members individually and on the system as a whole.

When intervention proceeds from this perspective, "the objective is not merely to change or improve the child, but to make the system work" (Hobbs, 1975, p. 15). Thus, there are multiple purposes of family involvement in early intervention, including enhanced positive outcomes for both children and families. While traditional early childhood special education focused almost exclusively on child outcomes (Dunst & Rheingrover, 1981; Simeonsson et al., 1982), adopting a family systems framework has moved contemporary intervention programs toward enhancing family outcomes as well (D.B. Bailey & Simeonsson, 1984; D.B. Bailey et al., 1986; Dunst, 1985). The full impact of the field's acceptance of the systems approach is best exemplified in the PL 99-457, Part H directive to provide services to families through the development of an individualized family service plan.

Families are presumed to benefit from involvement in early childhood services in several ways. First, involvement may help families enhance the natural developmental context for their children with handicaps. Second, involvement may assist families in developing specific skills for interacting with their children and involve family members as agents in their children's interventions. Third, involvement may enhance the family system and provide specific services to support family members.

In examining the evidence supporting Axiom IV, research on families with children of varying disabilities was reviewed. Inclusion of these studies was justified on two bases. First, when the effects of family involvement are considered in terms of impact on the family, there does not appear to be either logical arguments or specific data suggesting that differential effects would be observed for families of children with more severe handicaps. Second, when family involvement is examined in terms of outcomes for the child (e.g., the effects of parent training on child behavior), there may be arguments suggesting differential outcomes for children with more severe handicaps. However, there are few studies that include only children with severe handicaps or compare outcomes for children with different ability levels. Since many studies focus on changes in parent behavior exclusively or in combination with changes in child behavior, it seemed fair to include these studies with some caution about interpreting the changes in child behavior as being generalizable to children with severe handicaps.

In the current context, family involvement was defined to include: 1) family participation in planning and decision making, 2) family members acting as interveners, and 3) family support services. Research related to each of these types of family involvement is now discussed.

Family Participation in Planning and Decision Making

Family participation in the planning process for early education services is the most basic form of family involvement. There are several common arguments for family participation in planning and decision making: 1) parents are the natural advocates and decision makers for their young children in other contexts and are given that right by law (PL 94-142, PL 99-457) in special education, 2) parents have valuable information about their child to contribute to the process (D.B. Bailey & Simeonsson, 1984), and 3) services are

most effective when parents are included in the process of planning (Bryant & Ramey, 1984). These arguments for family participation have strong face validity, but empirical information on the effects of including parents in the planning process on the outcomes of intervention is lacking. Research on the planning process has largely focused on examining parent involvement in planning team meetings. The results of this research suggest that parent involvement is often limited. When parents attend such meetings, they do not generally contribute significantly to the decision-making process (Gilliam & Coleman, 1981; Goldstein, Strickland, Turnbull, & Curry, 1980). When parents do participate, they typically give and receive direct input into the instructional planning (Goldstein et al., 1980). Interestingly, Walker, Slentz, and Bricker (1985) found evidence that parents can accurately identify their children's developmental problems during planning.

Although an empirical base demonstrating the effectiveness of family involvement in planning, information sharing, and decision making is lacking, family involvement is apparently valued in the field. This value is reflected in policy (PL 94-142 and PL 99-457) and in practice as well. Professionals are increasingly interested and willing to include parents of young children with handicaps in the planning, assessment, and delivery of services (Bricker, 1986).

Family Members as Interveners

The rationales proposed for training family members as interveners are largely child focused. First, families represent the natural context for early learning and young children spend more time with family members than with anyone else (Bricker, 1986). Family interactions are potentially useful as teaching opportunities. Second, the family home setting may provide opportunities to train skills that are less easily or less appropriately taught in educational settings. For example, use of functional skills for daily living such as bathing and dressing occur primarily in the home environment. Opportunities for learning functional communication skills also occur regularly in the home. Third, training family members as interveners may facilitate generalization across settings. Finally, for children with severe handicaps, the need for intense treatment may require the involvement of several interveners.

Effectiveness of
Family-Implemented Intervention

Research involving families and young children with handicaps has demonstrated that, through training, parents and siblings can acquire and apply instructional skills (Rosenberg, Robinson, & Beckman, 1984; Schreibman, O'Neil, & Koegel, 1983; Shearer & Shearer, 1976). Parents can also be trained to change their patterns of parent-child interaction to enhance their own child's responsiveness (Affleck, McGrade, McQueeny, & Allen, 1982; Mahoney, Powell, Finnegan, Fors, & Wood, 1986).

A substantive body of literature related to parent training has documented the effectiveness of such training. It is beyond the scope of this chapter to thoroughly review this research; excellent reviews can be found elsewhere (Cowart, Iwata, & Poynter, 1984; Daurelle, Fox, MacLean, & Kaiser, 1987; Moreland, Schwebel, Beck, & Wells, 1982; Rosenberg & Robinson, 1988). In general, studies have shown that parents can be trained to address effectively a wide variety of child behaviors and to teach new skills using behavioral techniques (Filler & Kasari, 1981; Snell & Beckman-Brindley, 1984), to improve social interactions (McCollum, 1984, 1986; McCollum & Stayton, 1985), and to provide specific therapeutic interventions (Gross, Eudy, & Drabman, 1982; Howlin, 1984).

The Portage Project is the best known early education program that included behavioral parent training in its intervention system (Shearer & Shearer, 1976). As a part of that project, Boyd (1978) conducted a study investigating the acquisition and generalization of teaching and child management behaviors in parents of preschool children. The study involved 48 families randomly selected from project caseloads; at-risk children and children with identified handicaps were included. Parents were assigned to one of two treatment groups or a control group. One treatment group received home-based early intervention services. The other received those services and, in addition, a parent training component. Both treatments lasted 34 weeks, and included components in which parents delivered programming to the child. Baseline data were collected using a Parental Behavior Inventory (Boyd, Stauber, & Bluma, 1977), and observational data on parent-child interactions were collected every 2 weeks. Within the treatment groups, families with at least one other child were observed for generalization of treatment effects. Data were analyzed using a repeated-measures analysis-of-variance design to determine whether parental antecedents, child behaviors, and parental consequences changed as a function of the treatment. Results showed positive effects of both treatment groups over the control group; however, there were limited differences between the two treatment groups. Generalization of treatment was found for both groups and performance was maintained at the 10-week follow-up visit.

In an investigation of the effects of different formats for training parents to intervene with their children who had mental retardation, Baker, Heifetz, and Murphy (1980) studied 160 families. Families were assigned to one of four treatment groups or a control group. Each treatment group received a different training format designed to assist parents in the acquisition of behavior management skills. Treatment lasted 20 weeks. Formats included provision of a training manual only, and provision of the manual with assistance by telephone, group meetings, or home visits. The control group received delayed training. Changes in parent knowledge were assessed on the Behavioral Vignettes Test (Baker & Heifetz, 1976) using a pre-test/posttest design. All mothers in the study demonstrated significant improvement on the test compared to the control group. Results for the fathers in the study were related to the training format used. The skill acquisition of children in all treatment groups was significantly improved over the control as determined from parent reports. Baker and Heifetz suggested that child change was directly related to parental skill acquisition; however, a causal relationship between parent skill and child change was not established in this study.

Other studies, using both single-subject and group designs, have also reported successfully training parents and siblings of children with handicaps in the use of specific intervention procedures and techniques. These studies reported that family members are able to use the instructional skills acquired to work effectively with a child with handicaps (cf. Filler & Kasari, 1981; Schriebman et al., 1983; Snell & Beckman-Brindley, 1984).

Some caution should be used in generalizing the conclusions of studies with children with moderate mental retardation to families including children with severe handicaps. The extent of child gains and ease of parent application of behavioral and instructional strategies reported in the parent training literature may overestimate what is possible and likely to result from interventions involving children with severe handicaps. For example, Kaiser et al. (1988) reported that among a group of 8 parent-child dyads trained in milieu language teaching, the results were least positive for the families including the youngest children and those with the most severe handicaps. A longer period of training for parents, more difficulty in applying the intervention, and smaller child gains were observed for the three families with 2-year-old children with severe handicaps. The effects of parent-based intervention may be more modest with this population of children for the same reasons any environmental intervention is somewhat less powerful when the sources of the child's behavioral deficits are both physiologically and environmentally based.

Social Interaction Interventions

Wright, Granger, and Sameroff (1984) distinguished between early intervention approaches that involve families by training family members to teach and those that focus on effecting change in patterns of social interaction among family members. To the extent that a child's handicap may negatively affect patterns of family interaction, interventions that enhance parents' interactional skills can have a positive influence on interactions, and ultimately the child (Rosenberg & Robinson, 1988).

Mahoney (1988) investigated the effects of an interactional intervention strategy with 41 families who had a child with moderate to severe mental retardation. At the beginning of the 2-year study, the children with handicaps were between 2 and 32 months of age. The Transactional Intervention Program (TRIP) was used to teach parents general interactional strategies and to train them to implement specific strategies to improve their interactions with their infants and toddlers. Data were collected from pretreatment/posttreatment video observations of parent-child interactions and assessments of child developmental status. The results indicated significant changes in parent implementation of interactional strategies following training and related changes in some aspects of parental interactional style. Changes in parental interactional strategy were correlated positively with developmental gains in children.

Rosenberg and Robinson (1985) conducted a similar study with 16 families who had young children with handicaps. Treatment consisted of individualized instructional sessions with parent and child. Pre/post videotaped observations of parent-child interactions were rated using the Teaching Skills Inventory (Rosenberg et al., 1984). Instruction focused on interactive teaching style and sensorimotor tasks. Results showed that ratings of parents' interactional skill increased significantly at the posttest and were maintained at a follow-up check. Interestingly, Rosenberg et al. (1984) reported that the degree of improvement in parent-child interaction did not differ according to the severity of the handicap of the child.

Maintenance and Generalization of Child Treatment Gains

Another rationale for family involvement is to facilitate the maintenance of treatment gains made by the child and to facilitate generalization to multiple settings and people. Bronfenbrenner (1975) and Karnes et al. (1969) concluded that early intervention programs that have parent involvement components produce gains in children that are maintained longer than those from programs that do not. Shearer and Shearer (1976) also suggested that generalization appears to be a more likely benefit of programs when families are involved. The only large-scale analysis of the effects of parent involvement does not support this conclusion, however. Casto and Mastropieri (1986) interpreted the finding of their meta-analysis as indicating that "parents can be effective interveners but they are probably not essential to intervention success, and those intervention programs which utilize parents are not more effective than those that do not" (p. 421). As discussed earlier, the findings of this meta-analysis must be interpreted with caution. In this case, translation from child gain to evidence of generalization and maintenance is particularly tentative. Nonetheless, there is not strong evidence of enhanced effectiveness resulting from parent involvement in the program evaluation literature on which the meta-analysis is based.

Studies that have specifically examined maintenance and generalization offer some counter-evidence. For example, Lovaas, Koegel, Simmons, and Long (1973) compared follow-up results for two groups of children with autism. One group had received 1 year of behavior therapy treatment by trained clinicians. The other group had received the same treatment, but in addition their parents had been trained to carry out behavior therapy. Follow-up measures were obtained 1–4 years after termination of treatment. Results indicated that children whose parents had been trained maintained their treatment gains and improved, while those who were returned to nontrained parents or to an out-of-home placement lost the gains they had made. Lovaas et al. concluded that the effects of clinic treatment alone did not appear to be successful in producing results that are maintained over time or aid in the transfer of these gains to new situations, persons, and behaviors. This conclusion was replicated by Koegel, Schreibman, Britten, Burke, and O'Neill (1982).

Family Support Services

The presence of a child with handicaps in a family has been noted to increase the stress experienced by the family and the family members' needs for social support (Blacher, 1984; Gallagher, Beckman-Bell, & Cross, 1983). Potentially, social support can mediate the effects of stressors on families, thus enabling parents and siblings to interact more effectively with the child with handicaps, as well as to continue to fulfill their roles and developmental tasks as family members. Social support for families can take a variety of forms: information, instrumen-

tal, or socioemotional. The critical aspect of effective social support is that it meets the individual needs experienced by family members. The quality of the social support, as perceived by family members, may be more important than the size of the social support network; informal support appears to be of greater value to many families than formal support provided through social services and intervention agencies (Dunst & Trivette, 1988).

The provision of social support and its relationship to stress and coping in families with a member who is handicapped is a complex theoretical and practical issue (D.B. Bailey & Simeonsson, 1984; D.B. Bailey et al., 1986; Barrera & Ainlay, 1983; Dunst, 1985; McCubbin & Patterson, 1983; Schilling, Gilchrist, & Schinke, 1984; Thiots, 1982). While many benefits have been attributed to social support, the exact mechanism by which these benefits are achieved is not yet well understood. Social support has been postulated to directly and indirectly influence the behavior, attitudes, expectations, and knowledge of parents and their children (Dunst, Trivette, & Cross, 1986). Social support has been shown to mediate stress, and possibly to facilitate building coping skills in families (McCubbin et al., 1980). Personal well-being, parental attitudes toward children, family integrity, and child behavior and development may also be positively affected by social support (Dunst et al., 1986).

Extensive research on the influence of social support on families of preschool children with handicaps has been conducted by Dunst and his colleagues (Dunst, 1985; Dunst et al., 1986). Dunst's data provided evidence that the provision of social support to families can have a positive influence on child behavior and development and on family functioning.

Dunst et al. (1986) studied 137 parents enrolled in a program that provided broad-based social support to families. The children in the study were grouped in three classifications: at risk, mentally retarded, or physically handicapped. Parents rated 18 sources of support on a 5-point scale, and completed the Questionnaire on Resources and Stress (Holroyd, 1974) and a parent-child interaction rating scale. Families and children were described in terms of families' socioeconomic status (SES) and income and children's sex, age, developmental quotient, and diagnosis. A multiple regression analysis assessed the variance of the 12 dependent measures according to: 1) satisfaction with social support and 2) number of sources of support. Dunst et al. (1986) concluded that there are complex relationships between social support and personal, family, and child outcomes. However, they suggested that social support is a mediating influence on stress and coping—that it may influence child outcomes, parent-child interactions, and family functioning.

Although severity of handicapping condition was not a specific focus in the Dunst et al. (1986) study, they reported that child developmental quotient predicted a number of family functioning variables. For children with lower developmental quotients, families reported more stress, more use of community resources, and smaller support networks. There was a tendency toward support having a somewhat more limited influence when the child's developmental level was lower. Dunst et al. (1986) did not describe their population in terms of the percentage of children with severe handicaps; thus, any conclusions based on their findings related to this population specifically should be made with caution.

Conclusions

Research examining the effects of family involvement in early childhood services on children with handicaps and their families indicates some types of parent involvement are effective in enhancing child outcomes and family adjustment. However, the empirical base is limited. While the effects of training family members as interveners have been well documented, effects of other family-based interventions have yet to be researched adequately (D.B. Bailey & Simeonsson, 1988). There are few studies investigating the effects of assessment, implementation, and evaluation of family-focused services. There is very modest evidence to support enhanced positive effects for children as a result of parent involvement in their children's preschool intervention. The limited research on family participation in planning does not allow an empirically based conclusion about the benefits of this type of family involvement, although policy and best practices suggest that participation is valued by

the field. Research on social support, both with families of preschool handicapped children and with other populations, indicates that support is also valued by families. The particular linkages between provision of support and specific outcomes for families and children has not been clearly demonstrated in experimental analyses, although there is correlation evidence relating support and outcomes for families and children. Only one study cited in this section (Kaiser et al., 1988) analyzed data separately for children with severe handicaps and most of the conceptual papers reviewed did not make specific reference to children with varying handicapping conditions. Thus, the specific effects of various types of family involvement for families with a young child with severe handicaps is unknown. However, in the case of the other axioms, there is no empirical evidence that contraindicates involving parents and families in early intervention.

RECOMMENDATIONS FOR FUTURE RESEARCH

Any research agenda in special education is guided by the values of the investigators and of the field in general. In this chapter, we have identified common values, research findings, and practices that shape the services for young children with severe handicaps. In proposing a research agenda for the future, we again begin with the values that underlie the education and treatment of these children. These values and their associated assumptions form a set of caveats that shape our research agenda.

Four basic assumptions underlie our research agenda:

1. All children with severe handicaps have a right to treatment.
2. The goal of treatment is to maximize the developmental potential of the child.
3. Effective treatments promote independence, dignity, caring and friendship, and quality of life.
4. The scientific study of children with severe handicaps must be both methodologically rigorous and value based.

These assumptions lead to the following general recommendations. First, treatment versus no treatment comparisons are not appropriate research designs because this population of children has a right to treatment. Second, any treatment that is being investigated must be a potentially effective intervention, and must meet the criteria of promoting development, dignity, and quality of life. These assumptions bear particularly on investigations of aversive treatment strategies, but also encourage research focused on the health of the whole child and not simply the targeted increase of a single behavior. While research within a domain such as motor development or language is important, we urge that domain-specific research be linked to the overall development of the child and that the impact of domain-specific research on the child's day-to-day and longer term functioning be assessed with respect to independence and quality of life. Keeping the whole child in view, even as we investigate discrete aspects of the child's behavior, is essential to affecting the treatment of children with severe disabilities in positive ways.

The tension between scientific rigor and values-based approaches to treatment is readily evident in the area of severe handicaps. It is essential that future research agendas acknowledge both. There is a very small set of scientifically rigorous research studies that include children with severe disabilities. It is apparent that practice has developed based on generalizations from research with other populations and from the values held by practitioners in the field.

In retrospect, it seems entirely appropriate to draw from related research and the extant values as the basis for initiating services to young children with severe disabilities. These sources of scientific and common practice knowledge are not sufficient, however, for determining which particular strategies are most effective for this population. While research about the general appropriateness of early intervention is no longer needed, careful, rigorous research that investigates alternative specific interventions is critical. The criteria for sound experimental analyses, whether based in single-subject or group design, specify the conditions under which knowledge about an intervention can be considered dependable and replicable. The need for dependable, replicable knowledge to guide practice is greater than ever before because we have made a commitment to the provision of effective services for this population of children. It is apparent in the preceding portions of this chapter that we have little dependable, replicable knowledge about effective treatments for young children with severe handicaps. Thus, our research agenda is both substantive and urgent.

In addition to these assumptions, four additional considerations shape the research agenda: 1) considerations related to theory and conceptual framework, 2) considerations related to the population, 3) considerations regarding documentation of treatment, and 4) considerations related to research design and methodology. Each of these considerations is now discussed; then, recommendations for specific investigations are offered.

Considerations Related to Theory and Conceptual Framework

Most research with young children with severe handicaps has been nontheoretical. To some extent, this has occurred because there is no specific dominant theory of development that has appeared to be reasonably adequate to guide intervention. Research has been largely conducted in a behavior analytical framework within specific domains, and the problems of concern were pressing practical ones rather than theoretical ones. The result has been fragmented information with few attempts to understand the overall development of children with severe handicaps. As our values lead us to concern for the healthy development of the whole child, we must begin to formulate a conceptual framework for interventions and to integrate empirical information into that framework and into a broader understanding of the development of children with severe disabilities.

Considerations Related to Population

Children with severe handicapping conditions are an extremely diverse population with varying etiologies and complex, multiple needs. Generalizations regarding effective treatment from investigations with children with less severe disabilities cannot be made automatically to this population of children. Further, generalizations of findings across children with severe disabilities must be made with great caution. It is extremely important that research involving children with severe disabilities routinely includes careful descriptions of the child subjects.

In reviewing the existing literature, it was often impossible to determine if child subjects were severely handicapped by current definitions. Almost never would it have been possible to determine if the treatments being investigated could have been applied to a particular child with severe handicaps because the subject descriptions were never sufficient to allow such a generalization. Two recommendations follow. First, subject descriptions included in published reports of research should be as detailed as possible and include standardized information, etiological description, and specific behavioral description. Second, archives of research on young children with severe handicaps are needed. Such archives would provide a data base of research in this area and would allow inclusion of more detailed subject descriptions than are typically published. The purpose of the archives would be to allow researchers access to more complete data when attempting to integrate research findings for children with specific characteristics or needs within the population of children identified as severely handicapped. Such archives would be especially valuable because this is a low-incidence, highly heterogeneous population. Dependable, replicable scientific knowledge could be increased through the sharing of data. Further, placing data for individual children in studies utilizing child subjects with varying levels of disabilities in archives would allow much more meaningful aggregate analyses of the effects of interventions on children with severe handicaps.

Considerations Regarding Documentation of Treatment

The third obvious limitation of the existing research base is the limited description of the experimental interventions. Since a large portion of research in early intervention has been conducted in the tradition of program evaluation, many studies do not describe the specific content, intensity, or duration of treatment for individual subjects. Investigations conducted within specific domains (e.g., language or motor development) are better described, but rarely are the descriptions sufficient that the treatment could be easily replicated. Description of prerequisite or preexisting skills are also infrequent. Inclusion of such descriptions would facilitate gener-

alization to other children and would place the intervention in a much more complete treatment perspective.

As the focus in early intervention has shifted from a general analysis of the effectiveness of early intervention to a more focused analysis of specific interventions, the documentation of the exact intervention becomes critical. Further, in the absence of such description, translation of research into practice while maintaining the integrity of the intervention is impossible.

Considerations Related to Research Design and Methodology

While values may constrain us from certain research designs (such as the use of a nontreatment control group), it is more often the case that the limited number and heterogeneous characteristics of young children with severe handicaps are the functional constraints on choice of research design. In part, the paucity of research with young children with severe handicaps may be the result of the difficulty in selecting appropriate research designs. While single-subject analyses would appear to be the design of choice in many cases, variability across subjects can limit replicability, and therefore compromise the interpretation of results. Within-subject analyses are often promising alternatives. It is important, however, that whatever specific research design is selected that the investigation relate its finding to the whole child. Measures of generalization and maintenance are one way in which this may be done; longitudinal evaluations of treatment are another. Including general measures of development as well as the specific acquisition measures used in the particular design may be useful when appropriate measures can be found. Assessing the response of family members to the intervention may also provide perspective on the perceived and valued effects of the treatment. Developing taxonomies of early behaviors that are indicative of our valued outcomes of interventions and assessing specific interventions in relationship to this taxonomy is a promising alternative for relating specific interventions to the healthy development of the whole child. Exploring these alternatives may assist us not only in developing better scientific knowledge and expanding our conceptual framework for understanding the development of children with severe handicaps, it will also assist us in focusing our empirical investigations in ways that will inform best practices and have a significant impact on the lives of children.

Critical Areas for Research

Research is needed on almost every aspect of intervention with young children with handicaps. The research base is extremely limited. Research within domains of development is needed to address how functional skills can be best established, maintained, and integrated into more complex developmental repertoires. For example, research is needed on the development of both early social interaction skills and communication. Research should address how these two skill areas can be integrated into a social communication repertoire that allows the child with severe handicaps to interact most effectively with caregivers and peers. Research within domains might also focus on comparisons of alternative intervention strategies with emphasis on contrasting the outcomes of interventions along multiple dimensions including rapidity of initial skill acquisition, generalization, skill integration, and facilitation of sequential related skills. The examination of multiple outcomes should be guided by a conceptual framework based in an integrated view of child development and reference to that framework. Similarly, careful longitudinal studies examining the impact of multiple interventions such as those provided in an early intervention program are needed to understand better the scope of impact on the development of young children with handicaps that is possible. Within that area of research, consideration of the learning histories created by specific interventions and the effects of these interventions on subsequent interventions is an area for future development. As services for children with severe handicaps become widely available from birth through the school years, the impact of multiple interventions and the analysis of how sequences of interventions can best be structured becomes an important conceptual and practical issue.

In addition to research focusing specifically on the development of the child, there is a continuing need to examine how families can best be supported. The perspective of research directed toward the goal of strengthening families, to promote healthy development of the family unit, and to support positive interactions among its members is recommended. Families of children with severe handicaps are not themselves severely handicapped: They are *normal* families in difficult situations. Aside from research on parent training, there is very little empirical support for the effectiveness of interventions with families.

Similarly, there is little research on training teachers and other professionals and paraprofessionals to effectively implement interventions with young children with severe handicaps. Since the implementation of PL 94-142, studies of teacher training appear to have decreased. Research on innovative, efficient means for training teachers with special skills required to work with children with severe handicaps and examination of the maintenance, generalization, and integration of these skills into teachers' repertoires is both necessary and important to the providing of high-quality services. Such research need not be limited to studies training specific skills. Examination of naturalistic interactions and strategies for enhancing social and affective interactions are important areas for systematic inquiry. Research on both families and professionals as they interact with young children with severe handicaps should be informed by our understanding of social systems and reciprocity in interactions. Both the child with disabilities and the adult with whom he or she interacts may need special training for those interactions to be the basis for learning and for social-affective development.

CONCLUSION

While the challenge for the 1980s was to build a rationale for providing services to young children with severe handicaps, the challenge for the 1990s is to ensure that those services are effective. As a field, we have drawn on arguments from a civil rights perspective, research on children at risk, limited domain-specific research, and the knowledge of practice as a basis for formulating early intervention services for this population. With the basic conditions for services mandated by law, we must turn our attention to examination of specific interventions and their effects on children with severe handicapping conditions. Both the costs and the benefits are considerable. While intervention services are expensive, early intervention may be most critical to the children with severe disabilities. Research to guide, to refine, to improve, and to support best practices is critical.

REFERENCES

Affleck, G. McGrade, B., McQueeny, M., & Allen, D. (1982). Promise of relationship-focused early intervention in developmental disabilities. *Journal of Special Education*, *16*, 413–430.

Anastasiow, N.J. (1986). The research base for early intervention. *Journal of the Division for Early Childhood*, *10*(2), 99–105.

Bagnato, S., & Neisworth, J. (1980). The intervention efficiency index: An approach to preschool program accountability. *Exceptional Children*, *46*, 264–269.

Bailey, D.B., & Simeonsson, R.J. (1984). Critical issues underlying research and intervention with families of young handicapped children. *Journal of the Division for Early Childhood*, *9*, 38–48.

Bailey, D.B., & Simeonsson, R.J. (1988). Assessing needs of families with handicapped infants. *Journal of Special Education*, *22*(1), 117–127.

Bailey, D.B., Simeonsson, R.J., Winton, P.J., Huntington, G.S., Comfort, M., Isbell, P., O'Donnell, K.J., & Helm, J.M. (1986). Family-focused intervention: A functional model for planning, implementing and evaluating individualized family services in early intervention. *Journal of the Division for Early Childhood*, *10*(2), 156–171.

Bailey, E.J., & Bricker, D. (1984). The efficacy of early intervention for severely handicapped infants and young children. *Topics in Early Childhood Special Education*, *4*(3), 30–51.

Baker, B., & Heifetz, L. (1976). The Read Project: Teaching manuals for parents of retarded children. In T. Tjossem (Ed.), *Intervention strategies for high risk infants and young children* (pp. 351–370). Baltimore: University Park Press.

Baker, B., Heifetz, L., & Murphy, D. (1980). Behavioral training for parents of mentally retarded children: One year follow-up. *American Journal of Mental Deficiency*, *85*, 31–38.

Bambara, L.M., Warren, S.F., & Komisar, S. (1988). The Individualized Curriculum Sequencing model: Effects on skill acquisition and generalization. *Journal of The Association for Persons with Severe Handicaps*, *13*, 8–19.

Barber, P.A., Turnbull, A.P., Behr, S.K., & Kerns, G.M. (1988). A family systems perspective on early childhood special education. In S.L. Odom & M.B. Karnes (Eds.), *Early intervention for infants and children with handicaps: An empirical base* (pp. 179–198). Baltimore: Paul H. Brookes Publishing Co.

Barrera, M., & Ainlay, S. (1983). The structure of social support: A conceptual and empirical analysis. *Journal of Community Psychology*, *11*, 133–134.

Beckman, P.J., & Burke, P.J. (1984). Early childhood special education: State of the art. *Topics in Early Childhood Special Education*, *4*(1), 19–32.

Bell, R.Q. (1968). A reinterpretation of the direction of effects in studies of socialization. *Psychological Review*, *75*, 85–91.

Berrueta-Clement, J.R., Schweinhart, L.J., Barnett, W.S., Epstein, A.S., & Weikart, D.P. (1984). Changed lives. *Monographs of the High/Scope Educational Research Foundation*, *8*.

Bijou, S., & Baer, D. (1963). *Behavior analysis of child development*. Englewood Cliffs, NJ: Prentice-Hall.

Bijou, S., & Baer, D. (1978). *Behavior analysis of child development*. Englewood Cliffs, NJ: Prentice-Hall.

Blacher, J. (1984). Sequential stages of parental adjustment to the birth of a child with handicaps: Fact or artifact? *Mental Retardation*, *22*, 55–68.

Bloom, B.S. (1964). *Stability and change in human characteristics*. New York: John Wiley & Sons.

Bower, T.G.R. (1977). *A primer of infant development*. San Francisco: W.H. Freeman.

Boyd, R. (1978). *Final report—acquisition and generalization of teaching and child management behaviors in parents of handicapped children: A comparative study*. Portage, WI: Cooperative Educational Service Agency 12.

Boyd, R., Stauber, K., & Bluma, S. (1977). *Portage Parenting Program*. Portage, WI: Cooperative Educational Service Agency 12.

Brassell, W.R., & Dunst, C.J. (1978). Fostering the object construct: Large scale intervention with handicapped infants. *American Journal of Mental Deficiency*, *82*, 507–510.

Bricker, D. (1986). *Early education of at-risk and handicapped infants, toddlers, and preschool children*. Glenview, IL: Scott, Foresman.

Bricker, D., Bailey, E., & Bruder, M. (1984). The efficacy of early intervention and the handicapped infant: A wise or wasted resource. *Advances in Developmental and Behavioral Pediatrics*, *5*.

Bricker, D., & Dow, M. (1980). Early intervention with the young severely handicapped child. *Journal of The Association for the Severely Handicapped*, *5*(2), 130–142.

Bricker, D.D., & Sheehan, R. (1981). Effectiveness of an early intervention program indexed by child change. *Journal of the Division for Early Childhood*, *4*, 11–27.

Bronfenbrenner, U. (1974). *Is early intervention ef-

fective? A report on longitudinal evaluations of preschool programs (DHEW Publication No. OHD75-25, Vol. 2). Washington, DC: Department of Health, Education, and Welfare.

Bronfenbrenner, U. (1975). Is early intervention effective? In M. Guttentag & E. Stevening (Eds.), *Handbook of evaluation research* (pp. 519–603). Beverly Hills: Sage Publications.

Bruner, J., Roy, C., & Ratner, N. (1980). The beginnings of requests. In K.E. Nelson (Ed.), *Children's language* (Vol. 3, pp. 91–138). New York: Gardner Press.

Bryant, D.M., & Ramey, C.T. (1984). Prevention-oriented infant education programs. *Journal of Children in Contemporary Society, 17*(1), 17–35.

Campbell, D., & Stanley, J. (1966). *Experimental and quasi-experimental designs for research.* Chicago: Rand-McNally.

Campbell, P., & Stewart, B. (1988). Measuring change in movement skills with infants and young children with handicaps. *Journal of The Association for Persons with Severe Handicaps, 11,* 152–162.

Casto, G. (1988). Research and program evaluation in early childhood special education. In S.L. Odom & M.B. Karnes (Eds.), *Early intervention for infants and children with handicaps: An empirical base* (pp. 51–62). Baltimore: Paul H. Brookes Publishing Co.

Casto, G., & Mastropieri, M. (1986). The efficacy of early intervention programs: A meta-analysis. *Exceptional Children, 52,* 417–424.

Clunies-Ross, G.G. (1979). Accelerating the development of Down syndrome infants and young children. *Journal of Special Education, 13*(2), 169–177.

Code of Federal Regulations. (1978). *34,* §300.1.

Cornell, E., & Gottfried, A. (1976). Intervention with premature human infants. *Child Development, 47,* 32–39.

Cowart, J.D., Iwata, B.A., & Poynter, N. (1984). Generalization and maintenance in training parents of the mentally retarded. *Applied Research in Mental Retardation, 5,* 233–244.

Daurelle, L.A., Fox, J.J., MacLean, W.M., & Kaiser, A.P. (1987). An interbehavioral perspective on parent training for families of developmentally delayed children. In D.H. Rube & D.J. Delprato (Eds.), *New ideas in therapy: Introduction to an interdisciplinary approach* (pp. 159–168). New York: Greenwood Press.

Dunst, C.J. (1985). Rethinking early intervention. *Analysis and Intervention in Developmental Disabilities, 5,* 165–201.

Dunst, C.J. (1986). Overview of the efficacy of early intervention programs: Methodological and conceptual considerations. In L. Bickman & D. Weatherford (Eds.), *Evaluating early intervention programs for severely handicapped children and their families* (pp. 79–148). Austin, TX: PRO-ED.

Dunst, C.J., Cushing, P., & Vance, S. (1985). Response-contingent learning in profoundly handicapped infants: A social systems perspective. *Analysis and Intervention in Developmental Disabilities, 5,* 33–47.

Dunst, C., McWilliam, R., & Trivette, C. (1985). Early intervention [Special Issue]. *Analysis and Intervention in Developmental Disabilities, 5*(1–1).

Dunst, C.J., & Rheingrover, R.M. (1981). An analysis of the efficacy of early intervention programs with organically handicapped children. *Evaluation & Program Planning, 4,* 287–323.

Dunst, C.J., & Snyder, S. (1986). A critique of the Utah State University early intervention meta-analysis research. *Exceptional Children, 53,* 269–276.

Dunst, C.J., & Trivette, C. (1988). A family systems model of early intervention with handicapped and developmentally at-risk children. In D.P. Powell (Ed.), *Parent education and support programs: Consequences for children and families* (pp. 131–179). Norwood, NJ: Ablex.

Dunst, C., Trivette, C., & Cross, A. (1986). Mediating influences of social support: Personal, family, and child outcomes. *American Journal of Mental Deficiency, 90,* 403–417.

Fenske, E.C., Zalenski, S., Krantz, P.J., & McClannahan, L.E. (1985). Age at intervention and treatment outcome for autistic children in a comprehensive intervention program. *Analysis and Intervention in Developmental Disabilities, 5*(1–2), 49–58.

Filler, J., & Kasari, C. (1981). Acquisition, maintenance, and generalization of parent taught skills with two severely handicapped infants. *Journal of The Association for the Severely Handicapped, 6*(1), 30–38.

Gallagher, J., Beckman-Bell, P., & Cross, A. (1983). Families of handicapped children: Sources of stress and its amelioration. *Exceptional Children, 50,* 10–19.

Garland, C., Stone, N.W., Swanson, J., & Woodruff, G. (1981). *Early intervention for children with special needs and their families: Findings and recommendations* (Westar Series Paper #11, pp. 207–278). Seattle: University of Washington.

Gesell, A. (1928). *Infancy and human growth.* New York: Macmillan.

Gibson, D., & Fields, D.L. (1984). Early infant stimulation programs for children with Down syndrome: A review of effectiveness. *Advances in Developmental and Behavioral Pediatrics, 5,* 331–371.

Gilliam, J., & Coleman, M. (1981). Who influences IEP committee decisions? *Exceptional Children, 47,* 642–644.

Glass, G.V. (1976). Primary, secondary and meta-analysis of research. *Educational Researcher, 5,* 3–8.

Glass, G.V., McGaw, B., & Smith, M.L. (1981). *Meta analysis in social research.* Beverly Hills: Sage Publications.

Goldstein, S., Strickland, B., Turnbull, A.P., & Curry, L. (1980). An observational analysis of the

IEP conference. *Exceptional Children*, *46*, 278–286.

Gray, S.W., & Klaus, R.A. (1969). *The early training project: A seventh year report*. Nashville, TN: George Peabody College, Demonstration and Research Center in Early Education.

Gross, A.M., Eudy, C., & Drabman, R.S. (1982). Training parents to be physical therapists with their physically handicapped child. *Journal of Behavioral Medicine*, *5*, 321–327.

Guralnick, M.J. (1988). Efficacy research in early childhood intervention programs. In S.L. Odom & M.B. Karnes (Eds.), *Early intervention for infants and children with handicaps: An empirical base* (pp. 75–88). Baltimore: Paul H. Brookes Publishing Co.

Guralnick, M.J., & Bennett, F.C. (1987). *The effectiveness of early intervention for at-risk and handicapped children*. New York: Academic Press.

Hanson, M.J. (1985). An analysis of the effects of early intervention services for infants and toddlers with moderate and severe handicaps. *Topics in Early Childhood Special Education*, *5*(2), 36–51.

Hanson, M.J., & Schwarz, R.H. (1978). Results of a longitudinal intervention program for Down syndrome infants and their families. *Education and Training of the Mentally Retarded*, *13*, 403–407.

Harris, S. (1988). Early intervention: Does developmental therapy make a difference? *Topics in Early Childhood Special Education*, *7*(4), 20–32.

Hart, B.M., & Risley, T.R. (1968). Establishing the use of descriptive adjectives in the spontaneous speech of disadvantaged preschool children. *Journal of Applied Behavior Analysis*, *1*, 109–120.

Hobbs, N. (1975). *The futures of children*. San Francisco: Jossey-Bass.

Holroyd, J. (1974). The Questionnaire on Resources and Stress: An instrument to measure family response to a handicapped family member. *Journal of Community Psychology*, *2*, 92–94.

Horn, E., & Warren, S. (1987). Facilitating the acquisition of sensorimotor behavior with a microcomputer-mediated teaching system: An experimental analysis. *Journal of The Association for Persons with Severe Handicaps*, *12*, 205–216.

Horowitz, F.D., & Paden, L.Y. (1973). The effectiveness of environmental intervention programs. In B.M. Caldwell & H.N. Ricciuti (Eds.), *Review of child development research* (Vol. 3, pp. 331–482). Chicago: University of Chicago Press.

Horton, K. (1976). Early intervention for hearing-impaired infants and young children. In T. Tjossem (Ed.), *Intervention strategies for high risk infants and young children* (pp. 371–379). Baltimore: University Park Press.

Howlin, P. (1984). Parents as therapists: A critical review. In D.J. Miller (Ed.), *Remediating children's language: Behavioral and naturalistic approaches* (pp. 197–229). San Diego: College-Hill Press.

Hoyson, M., Jamieson, B., & Strain, P. (1984). Individualized group instruction of normally develop-

ing and autistic-like children: The LEAP curriculum model. *Journal of the Division for Early Childhood*, *8*, 157–172.

Hunt, J.M. (1961). *Intelligence and experience*. New York: Ronald Press.

Hutinger, P. (1978). *Program performance report for handicapped children's early education program: Macomb 0–2 regional project*. Macomb: Western Illinois University.

Irwin, J., & Wond, G. (1974). Compensation for maturity in long-range intervention studies. *Acta Symbolica*, *5*, 33–46.

Kaiser, A.P., Alpert, C.L., Hemmeter, M.L., & Ostrosky, M.M. (1988, October). *Social linguistic interactions of very young handicapped children and their caregivers: Implications for early intervention*. Paper presented at the annual meeting of the AAUAP-MRRC Directors Conference, Denver, CO.

Kaiser, A.P., Alpert, C.L., & Warren, S.F. (1986). Teaching functional language: Strategies for language intervention. In M.E. Snell (Ed.), *Systematic instruction of persons with severe handicaps* (3rd ed., pp. 247–272). Columbus, OH: Charles E. Merrill.

Karnes, M.B., Hodgins, A.S., & Teska, J.A. (1969). *Earlier intervention: Effects of the ameliorative program initiated with three year old children and maintained for two years*. Washington, DC: Department of Health, Education, and Welfare.

Koegel, R., Schreibman, L., Britten, K., Burke, J.C., & O'Neill, R.E. (1982). A comparison of parent training to direct child treatment. In R.L. Koegel, A. Rincover, & A.L. Egel (Eds.), *Educating and understanding autistic children* (pp. 260–279). San Diego: College-Hill Press.

Kopp, C. (1983). Risk factors in development. In M. Haith & J. Campos (Eds.), *Infancy and developmental psychobiology*, *2*. In P. Mussen (Ed.), *Manual of child psychology* (pp. 1081–1088). New York: John Wiley & Sons.

Laskas, C., Mullen, S., Nelson, D., & Willson-Broyles, M. (1985). Enhancement of two motor functions in the lower extremity of a child with spastic quadriplegia. *Physical Therapy*, *65*, 11–16.

Lazar, I., & Darlington, R.B. (1982). Lasting effects of early education. *Monographs of the Society for Research in Child Development*, *47*, (1–2 Serial No. 195).

LeLaurin, K. (1985). Early intervention. *Analysis and Intervention in Developmental Disabilities*, *5*, 129–150.

Lincoln, Y.S., & Guba, E.G. (1985). *Naturalistic inquiry*. Beverly Hills: Sage Publications.

Linder, T.W. (1983). *Early childhood special education: Program development and administration*. Baltimore: Paul H. Brookes Publishing Co.

Lovaas, I.O., Koegel, R., Simmons, J., & Long, J. (1973). Some generalizations and follow-up measures on autistic children in behavior therapy. *Journal of Applied Behavior Analysis*, *6*, 131–166.

Maccoby, E., & Martin, J. (1983). Socialization in the context of family: Parent-child interactions. In E.M. Hetherington (Ed.) & P.H. Mussen (Series Ed.), *Handbook of child psychology: Vol. 4. Socialization, personality and social development* (pp. 1–101). New York: John Wiley & Sons.

Mahoney, G. (1988). Maternal communication style with mentally retarded children. *American Journal of Mental Retardation, 92*(4), 352–359.

Mahoney, G., Powell, A., Finnegan, C., Fors, S., & Wood, S. (1986). The transactional intervention program, theory procedures, and evaluation. In D. Gentry & J. Olson (Eds.), *The family support network series: Individualizing family services* (Monograph 4, pp. 8–21). Moscow: University of Idaho, Warren Center on Human Development.

Mastropieri, M.A., White, K.R., & Fecteau, F. (1986). Introduction to special education textbooks: What they say about the efficacy of early intervention. *Journal of the Division for Early Childhood, 2*(1), 59–66.

McCollum, J. (1984). Social interaction between parents and babies: Validation of an intervention procedure. *Child Care, Health, and Development, 10*, 301–315.

McCollum, J. (1986). Charting different types of social interaction objectives in parent-infant dyads. *Journal of the Division for Early Childhood, 11*, 28–45.

McCollum, J., & Stayton, V. (1985). Infant-parent interaction: Studies and intervention guidelines based on the SAIA model. *Journal of the Division for Early Childhood, 9*, 125–135.

McCubbin, H., Joy, C., Cauble, A., Comean, J, Patterson, J., & Needle, R. (1980). Family stress and coping: A decade review. *Journal of Marriage and the Family, 42*, 855–871.

McCubbin, H., & Patterson, J. (1983). Family transitions: Adaptation to stress. In H. McCubbin & C. Figley (Eds.), *Stress and the family: Vol. 1. Coping with marmative transitions* (pp. 5–25). New York: Brunner/Mazel.

McHale, S.M. (1983). Social interactions of autistic and nonhandicapped children during free play. *American Journal of Orthopsychiatry, 53*, 81–91.

McLean, J.E., & Snyder-McLean, L.K. (1978). *Transactional approach to early language training.* Columbus, OH: Charles E. Merrill.

Meisels, S.J. (1985). The efficacy of early intervention: Why are we still asking this question? *Topics in Early Childhood Special Education, 5*(2), 1–11.

Minuchin, S. (1974). *Families and family therapy.* Cambridge, MA: Harvard University Press.

Moore, M.G., Anderson, R.A., Fredericks, H.D., Baldwin, V.L., & Moore, W.G. (1979). *The longitudinal impact of preschool programs on trainable mentally retarded children.* Monmouth: Oregon State System of Higher Education, Exceptional Child Department, Teaching Research Division.

Moreland, J.R., Schwebel, A.I., Beck, S., & Wells, R. (1982). Parents as therapists: A review of the behavior therapy parent training literature: 1975–1981. *Behavior Modification, 6*, 250–276.

Odom, S.L., & Fewell, R.R. (1983). Program evaluation in early childhood special education: A meta-analysis. *Educational Evaluation and Policy Analysis, 5*, 443–460.

Odom, S.L., & Strain, P.S. (1986). A comparison of peer-initiation and teacher-antecedent interventions for promoting reciprocal social interaction of autistic preschoolers. *Journal of Applied Behavior Analysis, 19*, 59–72.

Parette, H.P., & Hourcade, J. (1983, June). *The effectiveness of therapeutic intervention with infants who have cerebral palsy or motor delay.* Paper presented at the 107th annual meeting of the American Association on Mental Deficiency, Dallas, TX.

Peck, C.A., Apolloni, T., Cooke, T., & Raver, S. (1978). Teaching retarded preschoolers to imitate the free-play behavior of nonretarded classmates: Trainee and generalized effects. *Journal of Special Education, 12*(2), 196–207.

Piaget, J. (1952). *The origins of intelligence in children.* New York: International University Press.

Pillemer, D.B., & Light, R.J. (1980). Benefiting from variations in study outcomes. In R. Rosenthal (Ed.), *New directions for methodology of social and behavior science: Quantitative assessment of research domains* (pp. 1–12). San Francisco: Jossey-Bass.

Piper, M., & Pless, I. (1980). Early intervention for infants with Down's snydrome: A controlled trial. *Pediatrics, 65*, 463–468.

Premack, D. (1959). Toward empirical behavior laws: Positive reinforcement. *Psychological Review, 66*, 219–233.

Ramey, C., MacPhee, & Yeates, K. (1983). Preventing developmental retardation: A general systems model. In L. Bond & J. Joffe (Eds.). *Facilitating infant and early childhood development* (pp. 343–401). Hanover, NH: University Press of New England.

Rosenberg, S.A., & Robinson, C.C. (1985). Enhancement of mothers' interactional skills in an infant educational program. *Education and Training of the Mentally Retarded, 20*, 163–169.

Rosenberg, S.A., & Robinson, C.C. (1988). Interactions of parents with their young handicapped children. In S.L. Odom & M.B. Karnes (Eds.), *Early intervention for infants and children with handicaps: An empirical base* (pp. 159–178). Baltimore: Paul H. Brookes Publishing Co.

Rosenberg, S., Robinson, C., & Beckman, P. (1984). Teaching skills inventory: A measure of parent performance. *Journal of the Division of Early Childhood, 8*, 107–113.

Rosenberg, S., Robinson, C., Finkler, D., & Rose, J. (1987). An empirical comparison of formulas evaluating early intervention program impact on development. *Exceptional Children, 54*, 213–219.

Safford, P., Gregg, L., Schneider, G., & Sewell, J. (1976). A stimulation program for young sensory-impaired, multihandicapped children. *Education and Training of the Mentally Retarded*, *11*, 12–17.

Sameroff, A.J., & Chandler, M.J. (1975). Reproductive risk and the continuum of care-taking casualty. In F.D. Harowitz, M. Hetherington, S. Scarr-Salapatek, & G. Siegel (Eds.), *Review of child development research* (Vol. 4, pp. 187–244). Chicago: University of Chicago Press.

Schilling, R., Gilchrist, L., & Schinke, S. (1984). Coping and support in families of developmentally disabled children. *Family Relations*, *33*, 47–54.

Schreibman, L., O'Neil, R., & Koegel, R. (1983). Behavioral training for siblings of autistic children. *Journal of Applied Behavioral Analysis*, *16*, 129–138

Shearer, D., & Shearer, M. (1976). The Portage Project: A model for early childhood intervention. In T. Tjossem (Ed.), *Intervention strategies for high risk infants and young children* (pp. 335–350). Baltimore: University Park Press.

Shonkoff, J.P., & Hauser-Cram, P. (1987). Early intervention for disabled infants and their families: A quantitative analysis. *Pediatrics*, *80*(5), 650–657.

Sibler, S. (1989). Family influences on early development. *Topics in Early Childhood Special Education*, *8*(4), 1–23.

Simeonsson, R.J., Cooper, D.H., & Scheiner, A.P. (1982). A review and analysis of the effectiveness of early intervention programs. *Pediatrics*, *69*, 635–651.

Skinner, B.F. (1953). *Science and human behavior*. Englewood Cliffs, NJ: Prentice-Hall.

Smith, B., & Strain, P. (1984). The argument for early intervention. *ERIC Digest*. Reston, VA: ERIC.

Snell, M.E. (1986). *Systematic instruction of persons with severe handicaps* (3rd. ed.). Columbus, OH: Charles E. Merrill.

Snell, M.E., & Beckman-Brindley, S. (1984). Family involvement in intervention with children having severe handicaps. *Journal of The Association for Persons with Severe Handicaps*, *9*, 213–230.

Stokes, T.F., Fowler, S.A., & Baer, D.M. (1978). Training preschool children to recruit natural communities of reinforcement. *Journal of Applied Behavior Analysis*, *11*(2), 285–303.

Strain, P., & Kerr, M. (1979). Effects of peer medicated social initiations and prompting/reinforcement procedures on the social behavior of autistic children. *Journal of Autism and Developmental Disorders*, *9*(1), 41–54.

Strain, P., & Smith, B. (1986). A counter interpretation of early intervention effects: A response to Casto and Mastropieri. *Exceptional Children*, *53*, 260–265.

Strain, P.S., Steele, P., Ellis, T., & Timm, M.A. (1982). Long term effects of oppositional child treatment with mothers as therapists and therapist trainees. *Journal of Applied Behavior Analysis*, *15*, 163–169.

Swan, W. (1981). Efficacy studies in early childhood special education: An overview. *Journal of Development of Early Childhood*, *4*, 1–4.

TASH Newsletter. (1988, March). *14*(3).

Thiots, P. (1982). Conceptual, methodological, and theoretical problems in studying social support as a buffer against life stress. *Journal of Health and Social Behavior*, *23*, 145–159.

Ulman, J., & Sulzer-Azaroff, B. (1975). Multielement baseline design in educational research. In E. Ramp & G. Semb (Eds.), *Behavior analysis: Areas of research and application* (pp. 377–392). Englewood Cliffs, NJ: Prentice-Hall.

U.S. Department of Education. (1986). *Eighth annual report to Congress on the implementation of the Education of the Handicapped Act*. Washington, DC: Office of Special Education and Rehabilitative Services, Division of Special Education Programs.

Walker, B., Slenz, K., & Bricker, D. (1985). *Parent involvement in early intervention* [Rehabilitation Research Review]. Washington, DC: National Rehabilitation Information Center, The Catholic University of America.

White, K., Bush, D., & Casto, G. (1985). Let the past be prologue: Learning from previous reviews of early intervention efficacy research. *Journal of Special Education*, *19*(4).

White, K.R., & Casto, G. (1985). An integrative review of early intervention efficacy studies with at-risk children: Implications for the handicapped. *Analysis and Intervention in Developmental Disabilities*, *5*, 3–31.

White, K.R., & Mott, S.E. (1987). Conducting longitudinal research on the efficacy of early intervention with handicapped children. *Journal of the Division for Early Childhood*, *12*(1), 13–22.

White, K., & Pezzino, J. (1986). Ethical, practical, and scientific considerations of randomized experiments in early childhood special education. *Topics in Early Childhood Special Education*, *6*(3), 100–116.

Weisen, A., Hartley, G., Richardson, C., & Roske, A. (1976). The retarded child as reinforcing agent. *Journal of Experimental Psychology*, *5*, 109–113.

Wolery, M. (1983). Proportional change index: An alternative for comparing child change data. *Exceptional Children*, *50*(2), 167–170.

Wright, J., Granger, R., & Sameroff, A. (1984). Parental acceptance and developmental handicap. In J. Blacher (Ed.), *Severely handicapped young children and their families* (pp. 51–90). Orlando, FL: Academic Press.

Yarrow, L.U. (1978). Historical perspectives and future directions in infant development. In J.D. Osofsky (Ed.), *Handbook of infant development* (pp. 897–917). New York: John Wiley & Sons.

Young, C.C., & Kerr, M.M. (1979). The effects of a retarded child's social initiations on the behavior of severely retarded school-aged peers. *Education and Training of the Mentally Retarded*, *14*, 185–190.

Ysseldyke, J.E., & Algozzine, B. (1984). *Introduction to special education*. Boston: Houghton-Mifflin.

CHAPTER 25

Extended Year
Special Education Programming
A Legal Analysis

CARROLL L. LUCHT
Yale Law School, New Haven, Connecticut

SONDRA B. KASKA
University of Iowa College of Law, Iowa City, Iowa

The Education for All Handicapped Children Act, PL 94-142, provides neither specific reference nor criteria regarding the provision of extended year special education programming to children with disabilities. As a result, advocates and parents are all too frequently waged in battle against administrators when a determination must be made regarding whether a child with disabilities requires extended year special education programming in order to receive a "free appropriate public education." Because each child's special education program must be individualized, it is difficult to establish guidelines specific enough to address each child's unique needs.

This chapter and Chapter 26 are intended to clarify the issues involved in determining the need for the provision of extended year special education programming from both a legal and an educational perspective. It is hoped that they will provide guidance to parents, educators, and advocates to ensure that special education students receive programming that is truly meaningful.

OVERVIEW

The length of school year necessary to provide children with disabilities with a free appropriate public education is fast becoming one of the most controversial issues arising under the Education for All Handicapped Children Act. A child with handicapping conditions makes progress that, in comparison to the rapid development of his or her nonhandicapped peers, may appear to be painstakingly slow. Additionally, the gains made by the child with disabilities may be in areas previously viewed as being outside the realm of the traditional educational system, including such areas as self-help skills, rudimentary communication, and the acquisition of appropriate social responses. On the one hand, educational administrators argue that the effort and expense that goes into the teaching of such basic skills are neither cost nor time efficient. Parents and advocates, on the other hand, urge that, regardless of how rudimentary these skills and how painstaking their development may seem, the effort and expense that go into the acquisition of these skills by children with disabilities pay off in financial, educational, and humanitarian terms—because the result, increased self-sufficiency and sense of self-worth, is the goal of the educational system. These conflicting viewpoints have led to the controversy over extended year special education programming.

The courts have attempted to address the question of the necessity of extended year programming for children with disabilities through a more objective analysis. In order to understand the analysis used, it is helpful to begin with an examination of the basic components of the Education for All Handicapped Children Act, as well as case law that has attempted to interpret its various provisions.

EDUCATION FOR ALL HANDICAPPED CHILDREN ACT

The Education for All Handicapped Children Act (1978) was the culmination of an increased awareness throughout the United States of the need for and the right of children with disabilities to have a public education. Two landmark district court cases, *Mills v. Board of Education of the District of Columbia* (1972) and *Pennsylvania Association for Retarded Citizens v. Commonwealth* (1972), holding that children with disabilities are guaranteed certain fundamental rights under the United States Constitution, provided impetus for the passage of the act. In 1974, realizing the need for more comprehensive legislation to address the educational needs of children with disabilities, Congress undertook an interim study to examine more closely the problems of persons with disabilities. Results of the study indicated that in 1975 there were more than 8 million children with disabilities in the United States whose special education needs were not being met (*Senate Report No. 168, 1975*). One million of those children were completely excluded from the public schools and thus would not participate with their peers in the educational system. In 1975, more than half of the children with handicaps did not receive educational services appropriate to meet their special needs or to permit them equality of opportunity (*Senate Report No. 168, 1975*). These findings laid the foundation for the purpose of PL 94-142, which, as codified, is:

> to assure that all handicapped children have available to them, within the time periods specified . . . , a free appropriate public education which emphasizes special education and related services designed to meet their unique needs, to assure that the rights of handicapped children and their parents or guardians are protected, to assist States and localities to provide for the education of all handicapped children, and to assess and assure the effectiveness of efforts to educate handicapped children. (Education for All Handicapped Children Act, 1988, 20 U.S.C. §1400[c].)

As observed by the the Third Circuit Court of Appeals in *Kruelle v. New Castle County School District* (1981), the three interlocking goals of PL 94-142 are: 1) to ensure through legislation the educational opportunities guaranteed persons with handicaps in *Mills v. Board of Education of the District of Columbia* (1972) and *Pennsylvania Association for Retarded Citizens v. Commonwealth* (1972), 2) to increase the personal independence and productivity of persons with handicaps through the provision of educational programming, and 3) to expand the federal fiscal role in order to assure state compliance with court decisions and to guarantee that the rights of children with handicaps are protected. Congress's rationale for the passage of PL 94-142 included a cost-benefit analysis that supported the underlying goals of the act. Congress reasoned that legislation and federal financial assistance to promote the education of persons with disabilities would assist those individuals to become productive members of society, rather than limiting them to a minimally acceptable life of dependence on society.

Procedural Requirements of PL 94-142

PL 94-142 provides federal financial incentives to states demonstrating that they have in effect policies and procedures, made in accordance with a state plan, that guarantee that all children with disabilities will receive a free appropriate public education. Because Congress believed that utilization of the act's due process guarantees, combined with the input of concerned parties, would best ensure that each child with disabilities receives special education and related services tailored to meet his or her individual needs, the act's requirements are more procedural than substantive in nature. Consistent with this country's traditional policy of decentralizing decisions regarding education, the act leaves many of the substantive and policymaking decisions to state and local educational agencies. This approach also allows states some flexibility in developing methods by which children with disabilities are provided a free appropriate public education.

PL 94-142 requires participating states to develop plans by which all children with disabilities between the ages of 3 and 21 receive special education and related services, unless such a requirement conflicts with applicable state law. States are free to expand coverage beyond the ages mandated by the act.

It is clear that the key operative feature of the

procedural requirements of PL 94-142 is the individualized education program (IEP), a comprehensive statement of the educational needs of a child with disabilities and the specially designed instruction and related services utilized to meet those needs. The development of the IEP is the means by which PL 94-142's mandate is "tailored to the unique needs of the handicapped child" (*Rowley v. Board of Education*, 1982, 458 U.S. at 181).

Substantive Requirements of PL 94-142

The eligible population of children with handicaps is defined in PL 94-142 as those children who are "mentally retarded, hard of hearing, deaf, speech or language impaired, visually handicapped, seriously emotionally disturbed, orthopedically impaired, or other health impaired children, or children with specific learning disabilities, who by reasons thereof require special education and related services" (Education for All Handicapped Children Act, 1988, 20 U.S.C. §1401(a)(1)). The plan required of each state must give first priority to children with handicaps who are not receiving any educational programming. Second priority is given to children with the most severe handicaps, within each disability category, who are receiving inadequate educational programming (Education for All Handicapped Children Act, 1978, 20 U.S.C. §1412[3].). Thus, under the provisions of the act, eligible students with handicaps are entitled to a "free appropriate public education," defined as:

> special education and related services which (A) have been provided at public expense, under public supervision and direction, and without charge, (B) meet the standards of the State educational agency, (C) include an appropriate preschool, elementary, or secondary school education in the State involved, and (D) are provided in conformity with the individualized education program required under section 1414(a)(5) of this title. (Education for All Handicapped Children Act, 1978, 20 U.S.C. §1401[8])

For the purposes of PL 94-142, "special education" is defined as "specially designed instruction, at no cost to parents or guardians, to meet the unique needs of a handicapped child, including classroom instruction, instruction in physical education, home instruction, and instruction in hospitals and institutions" (Education for All

Handicapped Children Act, 1988, 20 U.S.C. §1401(a)(16)). The act defines "related services" as:

> transportation, and such developmental, corrective, and other supportive services (including speech pathology and audiology, psychological services, physical and occupational therapy, recreation, and medical and counseling services, except that such medical services shall be for diagnostic and evaluation purposes only) as may be required to assist a handicapped child to benefit from special education, and includes the early identification and assessment of handicapping conditions in children. (Education for All Handicapped Children Act, 1988, 20 U.S.C. §1401[a][17])

In contrast to the precise definitions given much of PL 94-142's terminology, the question of what constitutes an "appropriate" education is not provided a functional definition in the act. The U.S. Supreme Court first attempted to clarify the meaning of appropriate education under PL 94-142 in the landmark case of *Rowley v. Board of Education* (1982). At issue in *Rowley* was the nature of the services that the school was required to provide a deaf child of normal intelligence in order to ensure that she received a free appropriate public education. Rather than listing specific criteria that an educational program appropriate for all children with disabilities must include, the Supreme Court set forth a two-part analysis for determining whether the requirements of PL 94-142 have been met:

> First, has the State complied with the procedures set forth in the act? And second, is the individualized educational program developed through the act's procedures reasonably calculated to enable the child to receive educational benefits? If these requirements are met, the State has complied with the obligations imposed by the Congress and the courts can require no more. (*Rowley*, 1982, 458 U.S. at 207)

Educational Benefit Test

In its examination of the substantive requirements of PL 94-142, the *Rowley* (1982) Court turned to the legislative history of the act and found that the intent behind PL 94-142 was "more to open the door of public education to handicapped children on appropriate terms than to guarantee any particular level of education once inside" (458 U.S. at 192). The Court elucidated further:

Implicit in the congressional purpose of providing access to a "free appropriate public education" is the requirement that the education to which access is provided be sufficient to confer some educational benefit upon the handicapped child. It would do little good for Congress to spend millions only to have the handicapped child receive no benefit from that education . . . [T]he "basic floor of opportunity" provided by the Act consists of access to specialized instruction and related services *which are individually designed* [italics added] to provide educational benefit to the handicapped child. (*Rowley*, 1982, 458 U.S. at 200–01)

Under *Rowley* (1982), educational agencies are not required to provide the best possible educational program, nor are equality of opportunity for children with and without disabilities and the basis for determining "appropriateness" under the act discussed. Instead, a special education program for a child with handicaps is "appropriate" under the act if it provides for access to services reasonably calculated to confer educational benefit on the child. Amy Rowley, the student whose education was at issue in *Rowley*, was a child of normal intelligence with a hearing impairment who was being educated in a regular classroom with the assistance of special education and related services. The Court's determination that Amy was receiving educational benefit was based on the fact that she was achieving passing marks and advancing from grade to grade. The Court was quick to point out, however, that achieving passing marks and advancing from grade to grade were important, but were not the only criteria for determining whether a child was receiving educational benefit (*Rowley*, 1982).

In discussing the "educational benefit" test, the *Rowley* (1982) Court emphasized that it was not attempting to define a level of educational benefit adequate for all children with disabilities. Clearly, any attempt to formulate a fixed standard of educational benefit applicable to all children with disabilities is inconsistent with the act's emphasis on individual consideration of each child's unique needs. The Court noted that "benefits obtainable by children at one end of the spectrum will differ dramatically from those obtained by children at the other end, with infinite variations in between (*Rowley*, 1982, 458 U.S. at 202). As observed by the Court in *Hall v. Vance City Board of Education* (1985), "Clearly, Con-

gress did not intend that a school system could discharge its duty under the act by providing a program that produces some minimal academic advancement, no matter how trivial" (774 F.2d at 636).

The level of educational benefit required by the act was at issue in *Board of Education of East Windsor Regional School v. Diamond* (1986), a case distinguishable from *Rowley* (1982) in that the child in question was not being educated in the regular classroom. Andrew Diamond was born with several congenital physical abnormalities and was classified as neurologically impaired and moderately mentally retarded. A dispute arose between his parents and the school district over an appropriate educational placement. Andrew's parents contended that the placement recommended by the school district would deny him a free appropriate public education because it failed to provide him with educational benefit. The school district argued that it was required by the act to provide no more for Andrew than would be "of benefit" to him. In holding against the school district, the Third Circuit Court found that PL 94-142 "clearly imposes a higher standard" than simple benefit (*Board of Education*, 1986, 808 F.2d at 991). The court stated that it was unlikely that the criteria for determining educational benefits applied in *Rowley* (i.e., that of achieving passing marks and advancing from grade to grade) could ever be applied to Andrew. The court went on to hold that "*Rowley* makes it perfectly clear that the act requires a plan of instruction under which educational *progress* [italics added] is likely . . . . *The act* . . . *requires a plan likely to produce progress, not regression or trivial educational advancement* [italics added]" (*Board of Education*, 1986, 808 F.2d at 991).

In a recent interpretation of the educational benefit test, the Third Circuit Court of Appeals in *Polk v. Central Susquehanna Intermediate Unit 15* (1988) analyzed *Rowley* (1982) in conjunction with the text of PL 94-142 and the legislative history concerning the 1975 amendments. The court pointed out that the self-defined purpose of the act is to provide "*full* educational opportunity to all handicapped children" (*Polk*, 1988, 853 F.2d at 181). Although the court conceded that it is clear in light of *Rowley* that this language cannot be relied on for the proposition that the act requires the states to *maximize* a child's education, it held that it is equally clear that Congress did not intend that the educational process confer merely trivial benefit to students with handicaps.

In attempting to define the meaning of appropriateness, it is helpful to examine the underlying intent of PL 94-142. Certainly one of the central purposes of the act was to "increase the personal independence and enhance the productive capacities of handicapped citizens" (*Kruelle v. New Castle County School District*, 1981, 652 F.2d at 691). The sponsors of the act placed emphasis on increasing skills that contribute to personal independence for two reasons. First, "they advocated dignity for handicapped children" (*Polk*, 1988, 853 F.2d 181). Second, one of the major selling points in the passage of the act was that although it is initially costly to provide the expensive individualized assistance necessary early in life to teach basic life skills and self-sufficiency, this initial outlay of funds eventually benefits the public fisc by making these children into productive members of society rather than forcing them to remain burdens dependent (*Polk*, 1988, 853 F.2d at 181–182).

The *Polk* court (1988) examined this purpose of the act in its analysis of the appropriateness of the educational program offered to a child with severe disabilities. The court stated that such an emphasis in the legislative history indicates that what Congress had in mind was not mere access to the schoolhouse door, but some type of meaningful education once students with handicaps were inside. The *Polk* court went on to hold that although it is obvious that self-sufficiency cannot serve as the substantive standard by which to measure the appropriateness of the child's education under the act, "the heavy emphasis in the legislative history on self-sufficiency as one goal of education, where possible, suggests that the 'benefit' conferred by the EHA [PL 94-142] and interpreted by *Rowley* must be more than *de minimus*" (853 F.2d at 182).

The *Polk* (1988) court elaborated on this interpretation in light of *Rowley*, noting that the *Rowley* (1982) court described the education that must be provided under PL 94-142 as "meaningful," unquestionably indicating that the court ex-

pected children with handicaps to receive more than *de minimus* educational benefit under the act. Obviously, a bright child with mild disabilities may well receive a *substantial* amount of benefit from her or his education.

The needs of a child with severe disabilities are certainly far different than those of a child with mild handicapping conditions, though of no less importance. The progress of a child with severe disabilities cannot be measured by advancement from grade to grade or progress in academics. Progress is often slow and gains are often small. It must be remembered, however, that the needs of children with severe disabilities were seen as paramount to the sponsors of PL 94-142, who provided that the children with the most severe disabilities should be the first served.

The decision in *Board of Education of East Windsor Regional School v. Diamond* (1986) is frequently cited for the proposition that a child who has demonstrated regression is not receiving sufficient educational benefit to meet the requirements of the act. The *Polk* (1988) court also examined the Diamond decision and expanded upon its interpretation of educational benefit. The court noted that progress for some children with severe disabilities may require optimal benefit. Because children with severe disabilities have a tendency to regress, a program calculated to lead to nonregression might actually impose a greater burden on the school than one that requires a program designed to lead to merely "more than trivial progress." The *Polk* court described the educational progress of a child with handicaps whether it be in the acquisition of life skills or in a more sophisticated academic program, as a continuum in which the point of regression versus progress is less relevant than the conferral of benefit. Thus, the court concluded that the Diamond holding should not be construed solely as an issue of progress or regression but also as requiring that any educational benefit be more than *de minimus*. Following this detailed analysis of legislative history, the landmark *Rowley* (1982) decision, and subsequent case law, the *Polk* court concluded:

> Just as Congress did not write a blank check, neither did it anticipate that states would engage in the idle gesture of providing special education designed to confer only trivial benefit. Put differently,

and using *Rowley's* own terminology, we hold that Congress intended to afford children with special needs an education that would confer *meaningful* benefit [italics added]. (853 F.2d at 184)

EXTENDED YEAR PROGRAMMING UNDER PL 94-142

A federal court first addressed the question of extended year programming in the pre-*Rowley* (1982) decision of *Armstrong v. Kline* (1979). The issue before the court was whether the state's policy and practice of refusing to provide students with handicaps with an educational program in excess of 180 days satisfied the act's requirement that eligible children receive a "free appropriate public education." The court analyzed the definition of special education set forth in the legislative history in an attempt to determine what is meant by appropriate. Although the terms of the act seem to mandate that the state provide instruction "designed to meet all of the handicapped child's 'unique needs' without limitation", *Rowley* and subsequent case law clearly impose some restrictions on the needs to be met under PL 94-142. In order to determine which of the unique needs of the children with disabilities must be met by the special education provided pursuant to PL 94-142, the *Armstrong* court examined the goal to be achieved. An examination of the legislative history revealed a heavy emphasis on the importance of the acquisition of self-sufficiency and independence from caregivers by children with disabilities. The court concluded that the state is not required to provide children with disabilities with educational programs designed to allow them to reach their maximum potential in every respect, but rather to provide an educational program that would permit children with disabilities, upon completion of their program, to be "as independent as possible from dependency on others, including the state, within the limits of handicapping condition" (*Armstrong,* 1979, 475 F.Supp. at 604).

After analyzing the 180-day rule applied by the state of Pennsylvania, the *Armstrong* (1979) court held that such a rule violated the right of the children involved to a free appropriate public education. The court found that such a rule was in violation of the due process procedures outlined in the act. "For certain handicapped children . . . , a program in excess of 180 days is required if they are to attain the level of self-sufficiency that is otherwise possible given an appropriate education" (*Armstrong,* 1979, 476 F. Supp. at 605).

Although its rationale was slightly different, on appeal the Third Circuit Court of Appeals emphasized the need for individualization under the act and affirmed *Armstrong* (1979) in *Battle v. Commonwealth* (1981). The circuit court held that the "inflexible application of a 180-day maximum prevents the proper formulation of appropriate educational goals for individual members of the plaintiff class" (*Battle,* 1981, 629 F.2d at 281), and stated:

> Rather than ascertaining the reasonable educational needs of each child in light of reasonable educational goals, and establishing a reasonable program to attain those goals, the 180-day rule imposes with rigid certainty a program restriction which may be wholly inappropriate to the child's educational objectives. This the Act will not permit. (629 F.2d at 280)

Other pre-*Rowley* (1982) cases with similar holdings include *Georgia Association for Retarded Citizens v. McDaniel* (1981) (affirmed in 1983, after *Rowley*), *Hilden v. Evans* (1980), *Lee v. Clark* (1981), and *Moore v. Roberts* (1981). These pre-*Rowley* cases uniformly held that state administrators were required by PL 94-142 to consider the needs of children with disabilities in excess of the traditional 9-month school year. The single court decision upholding the application of a policy limiting the education of children with disabilities to a 180-day school year was subsequently reversed by the Fifth Circuit Court of Appeals in *Crawford v. Pittman* (1983).

Following the Supreme Court's decision in *Rowley* (1982), other federal courts analyzed the extended year programming question by applying the two-part test outlined in *Rowley.* The courts addressing this issue have uniformly found that a policy that prevented consideration of an educational program in excess of the traditional 180-day school year violated both prongs of the test set forth in *Rowley.* In *Georgia Asso-*

ciation for Retarded Citizens v. McDaniel (1983), *Crawford v. Pittman* (1983), and *Yaris v. Special School District of St. Louis* (1983), such a policy was held to ignore the procedural requirement of PL 94-142 demanding that each child's needs must be determined on an individualized basis. Additionally, such a policy has been found to violate the core substantive mandate of the act, which requires that the educational program of a child with disabilities confer educational benefit upon that child. As stated by the Fifth Circuit Court of Appeals in *Crawford:*

> A policy of refusing to consider or provide special education programs of a duration longer than 180 days is inconsistent with [the state]'s obligation under the Act. Rigid rules like the 180-day limitation violate not only the Act's procedural command that each child receive individual consideration but also its substantive requirements that each child receive some benefit and that lack of funds not bear more heavily on handicapped than nonhandicapped children. (708 F.2d at 1035)

In *Alamo Heights Independent School District v. State Board of Education* (1986), the Fifth Circuit Court elaborated on the substantive standard required under the act in a case addressing the extended year programming issue. The court analyzed the educational benefit provided in accordance with each child's unique needs and found that, in relation to the provision of extended year programming:

> The some-educational-benefit standard does not mean that the requirements of the Act are satisfied so long as a handicapped child's progress, absent summer services, is not brought "to a virtual standstill." Rather, if a child will experience severe or substantial regression during the summer months in the absence of a summer program, the handicapped child may be entitled to year-round service. (*Alamo Heights*, 1986, 790 F.2d at 1158)

The challenge then becomes one of converting the educational benefit standard from its legal definition into practical implementation.

REFERENCES

Armstrong v. Kline, 475 F. Supp. 604 (E.D. Pa. 1979), *aff'd sub nom.* Battle v. Commonwealth, 629 F.2d 280 (3rd Cir. 1981).

Alamo Heights Independent School District v. State Board of Education, 790 F.2d 1153 (Fifth Cir. 1986).

Board of Education of East Windsor Regional School v. Diamond, 808 F.2d 987 (Third Cir. 1986).

Crawford v. Pittman, 708 F.2d 1028 (Fifth Cir. 1983).

Education for All Handicapped Children Act, 20 U.S.C. §§1400 *et seq.* (1988).

Georgia Association for Retarded Citizens v. McDaniel, 511 F. Supp. 1263 (1981), *affm'd,* 716 F.2d 1565 (Eleventh Cir. 1983).

Hall v. Vance City Board of Education, 774 F.2d 629 (Fourth Cir. 1985).

Hilden v. Evans, No. 80-511-RE (D. Or-R, Nov. 5, 1980).

J.G. v. Board of Education of Rochester, 648 F. Supp. 1452 (W.D.N.Y. 1986).

Kruelle v. New Castle County School District, 642 F.2d 687 (3rd Cir. 1981).

Lee v. Clark, No. 80-0418 (D. Hawaii, Jan. 30, 1981).

Mills v. Board of Education of the District of Columbia, 348 F. Supp. 866 (D.C. 1972).

Moore v. Roberts, No. LR-C-81-419 (E.D. Ark., July 24, 1981).

Pennsylvania Association for Retarded Citizens v. Commonwealth, 334 F. Supp. 1257 (E.D. Pa. 1971) and 343 F. Supp. 279 (E.D. Pa. 1972).

Polk v. Central Susquehanna Intermediate Unit 15, 853 F.2d 171 (Third Cir. 1988).

Rowley v. Board of Education, 458 U.S. 175 (1982).

Senate Report No. 168. (1975). 94th Congress, 1st Session, 9. (Reprinted in *U.S. Code Cong.* and *Admin. News* 1425).

Yaris v. Special School District of St. Louis County, 558 F. Supp. 545 (E.D. Mo. 1983).

CHAPTER 26

Extended Year
Special Education Programming
Educational Planning

DIANE BROWDER

Lehigh University, Bethlehem, Pennsylvania

The litigation supporting extended school year (ESY) for some children with handicaps as part of their appropriate education has influenced the increasing provision of these services. Alper and Noie's (1987) survey indicated that 49 states now have statutes and policies that permit ESY on a statewide basis or permit it to be provided as a local district option. However, the type of service provided varies widely across and within states. This variation is due in part to the lack of research and written guidelines on how to plan extended school year programs. Three issues must be addressed in this planning, including: 1) determing eligibility, 2) developing services to maintain targeted skills, and 3) incorporating features of current best practices for students with severe handicaps in ESY programs.

DETERMINING ELIGIBILITY

ESY is a service that must be determined for students on an individual basis. However, the criteria for eligibility and the method for determining an individual student's eligibility have not been well developed in the literature or in state policies. In a survey of state policies, Alper and Noie (1987) found variation in both the criteria for eligibility and the method for determining eligibility. The survey revealed that most states have no specific criteria for eligibility, but rather base eligibility on an individual review and decision provided by the individualized education program (IEP) team. By contrast, eight states use the criteria of significant summer regression with inadequate recoupment in the subsequent year. Problems arise in both of these methods for determining eligibility. When ESY is decided on

an individual basis with no explicit criteria, idiosyncratic patterns may emerge in students who do and do not receive services. Also, parents may find it difficult to advocate for these services when the rationale for their provision is not explicit. However, stating criteria such as regression and inadequate recoupment, with no clear method of measurement, is equally problematic. The literature on skill maintenance is not yet sophisticated enough to identify methods to assess "significant regression" (Browder, Lentz, Knoster, & Wilansky, 1988). Thus, idiosyncratic eligibility patterns may also emerge when criteria are stated that have not been operationalized.

Three methods have been used or suggested in the literature to measure regression-recoupment patterns. The first is to use a global measure or published instrument, such as an adaptive behavior scale, at three intervals—in the spring, the early fall, and the late fall (Barton, Johnson, & Brulle, 1986; Edgar, Spence, & Kenowitz, 1977; McMahon, 1983). A comparison of the spring to the early fall scores is purported to demonstrate regression, whereas the early fall to the late fall comparison of scores would demonstrate recoupment. Given the global nature of adaptive behavior scales, it would be unusual to see differences in scores across a 3-month period. Also, some students with severe handicaps would have few to none of the skills listed on these scales. Most important, these scales are not directly linked to IEP objectives and thus, cannot demonstrate regression on the student's individualized plan. In most of the studies in which global measures were used, the purpose was to demonstrate the effectiveness of the extended school year program. Since regression on a global measure such as an adaptive behavior scale would not be likely given the nature of this type of measurement, its use for demonstrating program effectiveness is also questionable.

A second method to assess eligibility is to use teacher-made tests of the IEP objectives with repeated testing across months. Tilley, Cox, and Stayrook (1986) used teacher-made assessment with testing conducted in June, July, September, October, November, and December. Tilley et al. also evaluated the regression-recoupment of non-handicapped students by using the California Achievement Test and found regression to be 4%. Based on a comparison of students with and without handicaps, they developed "cutoff scores" based on the spring-to-fall regression for each category of students. Students with severe handicaps were eligible if their regression was 10% on cognitive skills; 26% on language; or 18% on self-help, gross motor, or fine motor. For students with behavior disorders, a regression on the raw score of 3 points on a behavioral checklist for aggression/disruption qualified them for services. As a result of this policy on eligibility, 11% of the students with severe handicaps qualified for services. While Tilley et al. have made a notable contribution in defining eligibility with explicit criteria, the difficulty of determining whether the standards are applicable in other locales limits their generalizability to those other districts. Also, it is uncertain whether Tilley et al.'s results would have been the same if more frequent measures than monthly tests had been used.

A third method to measure regression-recoupment is possible if teachers take ongoing data (Browder & Lentz, 1985). In this method, the data trend and mean level of performance can be compared for the months before and after the summer. The number of days for progress to fully recoup can also be defined and compared to initial acquisition. The weakness of this approach is that no clear standards exist for the drop-in performance that should be considered "significant regression," nor is it clear what period of time is acceptable for recoupment. Also, teachers may not be able to collect data on all IEP objectives. The data that are collected may indicate skill maintenance across the summer, even though the parents and the teacher note substantial regression in some critical behaviors that were not targeted for data collection during the previous year.

To make ESY eligibility more explicit, Browder et al. (1988) recommended using multiple assessment from parents and teachers. These sources of assessment would include: 1) ongoing data on high-priority IEP objectives, 2) repeated testing on a broader range of skills (e.g., all objectives), and 3) anecdotal notes made by the teacher and/or parents on regression and recoupment. Regression might be noted for a summer when the child does not receive services or over a brief break in services such as winter vacation. Additionally, Browder at al. recommended considering the feasibility of parents maintaining skills taught during the school year based on the complexity of the teaching or behavior management procedures and the family's current level of stress. Much more research is needed to further delineate how regression-recoupment can be measured for making decisions for assignment of ESY services.

PLANNING SERVICE DELIVERY

Alper and Noie (1987) found that only three states set a standard for the duration of ESY services. Most states allow the IEP team to determine both the duration of service (i.e., number of days) and the length of the day. At the time of the survey, the duration of services ranged from 2 to 10 weeks, and the length of the day ranged from 2 hours to the full school day.

The variation in service delivery also reflects how little is known about the type and duration of services required for skill maintenance. In fact, the concept of teaching toward maintenance, and not skill acquisition, requires further thought. To qualify for ESY, regression need not be for mastered skills only, but may be demonstrated for partially mastered skills. In applied behavior analysis, maintenance strategies and measurement are typically applied to mastered skills or problem behavior that has been eliminated or reduced to acceptably low rates. ESY services, if purely to prevent skill regression, might target maintenance of partial acquisition. Since the concept of "maintenance of partial mastery" is different from the concept of maintenance in applied behavior analysis, no literature exists on how to achieve this goal. Rather, it is likely that in an extended school year program, if instruction is continued, the student will continue to progress in acquisition of the targeted skills.

Thus, planning the duration and length of services for "maintenance" only may not be feasible. As an alternative, planning might focus on the number of objectives and the instructional time invested in these objectives to determine the length of service. For example, if regression is notable for the student's eating skills during a previous summer or winter break, but no other IEP area reflects regression, it would be logical to provide a daily lunch-time program to maintain and continue to improve these skills for most weeks of the summer. By contrast, if a student shows regression in most skill areas, a full school day for 10 weeks may be essential. Also, if the skill that reflects regression requires teaching across most of the school day, such as teaching alternatives to aggression or the acquisition of a picture communication system, a full-day program may be essential. For students receiving job training in community settings, full-time provision of a job coach with a student in the site may be essential to meeting an employer's expectations for performance. The job coach would be assigned during the summer for the same number of hours as during the school year to prevent job regression.

Selection of the teachers and therapists, or other professionals, who provide the service also needs careful consideration. In some school districts, seniority is the criterion for receiving summer support for ESY. In states where teacher certification is noncategorical, such as Pennsylvania, it is possible for a teacher who instructs students with mild handicaps in academics during the school year to be an ESY teacher for students with severe physical handicaps in the summer. Staff turnover might negatively affect skill maintenance unless staff receive explicit training in the instructional protocols for the IEP objectives targeted for ESY. However, this critical need for staff training has been overlooked in the ESY literature. Procedures for conducting this staff training, such as the use of manuals and feedback sessions, can be found in the staff training literature as described by Demchak (1987).

CONTINUATION OF PROGRAM QUALITY IN ESY SERVICES

Another critical issue for planning ESY services is that they maintain the program quality offered in the school year. Meyer, Eichinger, and Park-Lee (1987) defined quality indicators for programs for students with severe handicaps. These include, for example, integration with nonhandicapped students, community-based instruction, data-based systematic instruction, and parental involvement. Unfortunately, ESY services sometimes sacrifice these components of quality by segregating students in buildings where no summer school is offered for nonhandicapped students, eliminating community-based instruction, and failing to keep parents updated. Several models of service delivery might maintain skills and ongoing program quality.

The first, and most typically used, is to provide services in a school building similar to school year services. To maintain quality, the school selected should include a summer session for nonhandicapped students so that integration can be fostered. Instruction across school sites and in the community should also be maintained. A second option is to provide homebound instruction. This option sacrifices the secondary benefit of ESY, which is to give parents respite during the summer. However, if the skills to be maintained relate to the home domain, this option may be the most appropriate. A third option is to use the varied, normalized experiences children pursue in the summer as sites for ESY instruction. For example, a student whose regression problem is social behavior might be enrolled in a day camp that serves nonhandicapped children. The ESY service would consist of a teacher providing support to help the student display positive social behavior in the context of the myriad of experiences of the camp. A fourth option, which is most applicable to students near transition, is to focus ESY on the student's job-training and transition-related objectives. A school site probably would not be necessary since training could be provided on the job and in the community. Whichever of these four options is selected, parents should be involved in the decision.

CONCLUSIONS AND RECOMMENDATIONS

Extended school year has been established by a history of litigation that supports all children's right to an appropriate education that, for some children with special needs, may include a program in excess of 180 days. Since ESY is a service provided to a subpopulation of special children based on their individual education needs, it is critical to establish clear eligibility guidelines and to include parents in the decision-making process. The duration and type of service should also clearly relate to the IEP objectives targeted for ESY.

The planning guide provided in Form 26.1 illustrates one possible format to organize this essential information in support of educational decisions regarding ESY services. Clearly, a needs summary such as this could be most helpful as documentation of the kinds of ESY services needed by each individual student. Ultimately, the accumulation of these kinds of data across children could assist in overall program design and the continued development of ESY services most likely to meet the needs for which they were intended.

FORM 26.1

PLANNING GUIDE FOR EXTENDED SCHOOL YEAR (ESY) SERVICES

Student's Name _____   School _____

Evaluator _____   Date _____

I. *Eligibility Considerations* (Check all that apply and attach supporting data or anecdotal reports from teachers and parents. If attachments support ESY, proceed to Part II. If not, so state below.)

_____ 1. Regression for mastered and partially mastered skills occurred in the previous summer when ESY was not provided.

_____ 2. Regression occurred after a school-year break (e.g., winter holiday).

_____ 3. Current instructional strategies are too complex for family maintenance (attach written strategies).

_____ 4. Student is not maintaining mastered skills once instruction ends.

_____ 5. Other considerations support ESY (e.g., family stress level; recent behavioral or medical problems of student support summer regression risk).

Does documentation support ESY eligibility? _____

II. *Service Provision Considerations*

1. Attach a list of each individualized education program (IEP) objective for which ESY is proposed and the daily instructional time currently devoted to each. Note if instructional time for each objective is in one time block or distributed across the day.

2. Based on the IEP list, what is your recommendation for the duration of service (i.e., number of days; number of hours per day)?

3. Based on the type of objectives proposed for ESY, what is your recommendation for the location of services (e.g., school based, home based, or alternative service such as summer camp)?

4. What other educational services need to be provided to maintain the quality of the student's instruction (e.g., community-based instruction, therapy, social integration)?

REFERENCES

Alper, S., & Noie, D.R. (1987). Extended school year services for students with severe handicaps: A national survey. *Journal of The Association for Persons with Severe Handicaps, 12,* 61–66.

Barton, L.E., Johnson, H.A., & Brulle, A.R. (1986). An evaluation of the effectiveness of an extended school year program. *Journal of The Association for Persons with Severe Handicaps, 11,* 136–138.

Browder, D., & Lentz, F.E. (1985). Extended school year services: From litigation to assessment and evaluation. *School Psychology Review, 14,* 188–195.

Browder, D., Lentz, F.E., Knoster, T., & Wilansky, C. (1988). Determining extended school year litigation. From esoteric to explicit criteria. *Journal of The Association for Persons with Severe Handicaps, 13,* 235–243.

Demchak, M. (1987). A review of behavioral staff training in special education settings. *Education and Training of the Mentally Retarded, 22,* 205–217.

Edgar, E., Spence, W., & Kenowitz, L. (1977). Extended school year for the handicapped: Is it working? *Journal of Special Education, 11,* 441–447.

McMahon, J. (1983). Extended school year programs. *Exceptional Children, 49,* 457–461.

Meyer, L.H., Eichinger, J., & Park-Lee, S. (1987). A validation of program quality indicators in educational services for students with severe disabilities. *Journal of The Association for Persons with Severe Handicaps, 12,* 251–263.

Tilley, B.K., Cox, L.S., & Stayrook, N. (1986). *An extended school year validation study* (Report No. 86-2). Seattle, WA: Seattle Public Schools.

CHAPTER 27

An Essay on Preschool Integration

PHILIPPA H. CAMPBELL

Children's Hospital Medical Center of Akron, Akron, Ohio

As far as we know, no anthropologist, or embriologist, or astrologer has announced discovery of the great cosmic clock that supposedly predetermines and controls the growth pattern of humanity. If so, all children at the precise age of 3 years, 2 months, 1 week, 4 days, 18 hours, and 31 seconds would be able to say "Rumpelstiltskin." Well, that doesn't seem to be nature's way. Instead, each individual develops as an individual, some faster, some slower, some more rapidly in particular motor skills, some in particular cognitive skills. Since all youngsters develop at different rates, it doesn't seem feasible to segregate children into calendars and categories of growth capability. Instead, let them help each other in their own peculiar growth potentials and let the educators maximize each person as an individual.

—W.A. Bricker (1972)

So begins a film made in 1972 at the Kennedy Center, George Peabody College, Nashville, Tennessee. The opening scene shows preschool children on a playground—some are running, some are sliding. One child is trying to climb a jungle gym. A second child, guided by an adult, is showing the first child how to do it—where to put hands and feet to get up onto the first rung. As the camera focuses in on the children, we see two young boys, each with different abilities, smiling, laughing, and enjoying the challenge of the activity. Looking closer, we see two children, two friends, one with Down syndrome and one who appears typical. We are watching *Time To Learn,* a documentary of Bill and Diane Bricker's innovative Toddler Research and Intervention Project (W.A. Bricker & Bricker, 1971).

One wonders why, so many years after this precedent-setting program, integration of preschool-age children of varying abilities and disabilities remains such a controversial issue. Certainly, the limited nationwide adoption of integrated preschool education models is not due to lack of efficacy data (Odom & McEvoy, 1988). More than in any area of special education, the benefits of noncategorical programming where young children with disabilities are educated with those with typical development has been empirically supported (Guralnick, 1978a; Strain, Guralnick, & Walker, 1986.)

A potpourri of different approaches for providing integrated education and related services for preschool-age children has been validated. Various models of reverse mainstreaming where a small number of typical children are educated with children with disabilities have been described (e.g., D. Bricker, Bailey, & Bruder, 1984; W.A. Bricker & Bricker, 1976; Guralnick, 1978b; Safford & Rosen, 1981; Vincent et al., 1980.) True mainstreamed models that place a small number of children with disabilities within day-care or public or private preschool programs for children who are not handicapped have been reported (Apolloni & Cooke, 1978; Galloway & Chandler, 1978; Hanline, 1988; Klein & Sheehan, 1987.) Integrated preschools and kindergarten programs with approximately equal ratios of children with and without disabilities have also been validated (Odom & Speltz, 1983; Walter & Vincent, 1982). In each instance, effects of interactions among young children with various disabilities and their nonhandicapped peers have been measured in terms of positive change in the developmental competence of the children with disabilities.

Research efforts have not only defined various integrated service delivery options but have also provided clear definitions of activities necessary to facilitate social, communicative, and cognitive growth among preschool children (Apolloni & Cooke, 1978; Beckman & Kohl, 1984; Guralnick, 1980; Strain & Cordisco, 1983.) Physical placement of children with and without disabilities together in classrooms or day-care settings, without specific attempts to facilitate interactions, is insufficient to alter the developmental growth of children with disabilities (Strain & Odom, 1986). Inconsistent and periodic contacts between children with and without disabilities, such as during lunch or recess, result in "cosmetic" approaches to integration that are not likely to influence the social or communicative competence of children with disabilities (Smith & Strain, 1988.)

Competent children can act as "teachers" or models of appropriate behavior for children who are less competent when provided *structured* opportunities to do so. These opportunities occur when teachers structure the physical environment to promote meaningful interactions among children (Bailey, Clifford, & Harms, 1982; Beckman & Kohl, 1984; Guralnick, 1980), use specific strategies to teach typical children to function as models (Apolloni & Cooke, 1978; Raver, Cooke, & Apolloni, 1978), or employ instructional methods that facilitate meaningful social and instructional interactions (Campbell & Stanley-Bryson, 1987; Jenkins, Speltz, & Odom, 1985). A decade of research makes clear that normally developing young children will choose to interact with similar children in unstructured situations, such as free play, and that structure and teacher interventions are necessary to ensure social and communicative interaction among children with and without disabilities (Odom & McEvoy, 1988).

One realizes that scientific support of a particular educational practice is insufficient to institutionalize that practice on a nationwide basis. Incentives and disincentives—some real, some believed—function to facilitate or inhibit adoption (D.D. Bricker, 1978). Primary among these are the influence of federal and state legislative policy on local public and private service delivery systems as well as social and ethical considerations about people with disabilities (Hayden, 1979). Federal educational legislation and policy for children with handicaps have been weak historically in their incentives for early intervention and preschool services (Smith, 1984). Ten years after enactment of the Education for All Handi-

capped Children Act (PL 94-142) and support through discretionary incentive programs such as the Handicapped Children's Early Education Program (HCEEP) and the State Planning Grants (authorized under the Education Amendments of 1983, PL 89-313), statewide adoption of early intervention and preschool services remained sparse. Six states had adopted legislation to serve children from birth through 2 and fewer than one third of the states mandated preschool education for children age 3–5 years (Weiner & Koppelman, 1987). It was within this climate of limited state commitment to the needs of the nation's young children that Congress passed the Education Amendments of 1986, PL 99-457, and established clear public policy supporting service provision for children with disabilities from 3 to 5 and birth through 2 years of age. This legislation created the Preschool Grant Program and extended all rights and provisions of PL 94-142 to children from 3 years of age.

We enter the next decade of special education with substantial scientific and policy support for integrated program options for young children with disabilities but with little reassurance that integrated programs will become a reality for all eligible children nationwide. Why is it that many program administrators, service delivery providers, and parents are likely to continue debates about whether to provide intervention for young children in integrated settings? The obvious bottom-line reality is that life is an integrated experience. A better debate than whether children with disabilities benefit from integrated program options is whether we can justify removing them from the normal life experiences to which they are entitled by virtue of being young children.

The purpose of education is to prepare our nation's children and youth for a quality life as adults. One dimension of school success is the extent to which a student has achieved the adopted curriculum by the time of high school graduation. Other outcomes, such as employability, income, and self-sufficiency following graduation, are less frequently used but are of equal or greater importance. The purpose of early childhood education is to prepare young children for kindergarten and elementary school experiences (Edgar, McNulty, Gaetz, & Maddox, 1984). We have made an assumption in early childhood special education that later success is related to developmental competence, measured in terms of positive change in the development of children with disabilities. Our concept in readying children for life has been to enhance their development of preschool readiness skills. Less consideration has been given to other expectations and outcomes.

Adults with disabilities have contended that the single most important thing that can happen in the life of a child with disabilities is for that child to become an adult. When children are young, the adults in their lives focus on skill acquisition and performance of essential skills using only conventional means. Early childhood specialists emphasize perfection in motor skills and in patterns of motor coordination, only to resort to a motorized chair after a child has "proven" beyond a doubt that walking is impossible. Young children are given any number of opportunities and specific interventions to teach them to speak in words and sentences and are taught total communication or use of communication devices only after failure to speak and "proof" that no amount of intervention will result in intelligible speech. Guided by well-trained interventionists and a standard knowledge of normal child behavior, parents are encouraged to "practice" conventional developmental milestone skills with their children at home. Denied access to interventions that would facilitate participation in regular classroom environments, successful achievement of those skills that have their greatest value in early childhood years becomes a primary vehicle for coming one step closer to regular preschool or elementary class placement. Yet, we applaud with true amazement and respect the adult with disabilities who wins a marathon in a wheelchair or who works using a computer operated by eye movement or who manages to shop in a grocery store successfully without being able to see. The very interventions and devices used as a "last resort" with young children earn our respect when used by an adult.

At what point in a person's life is it acceptable to have disabilities? Turnbull and Turnbull (1986) proposed a principle of empathetic reciprocity to focus on each individual's uniqueness and judge "the rightness or wrongness of our professional decisions in terms of the impact of our decisions on meeting a person's needs for love, fulfillment, and respect" (p. 106). The impact of measuring program effectiveness in terms of developmental normality (rather than uniqueness), witholding intervention practices that allow nonconventional skill performance until a child has proven that "fixing" is impossible, and providing opportunities for interaction only with other children with disabilities have the potential of adding additional disabilities to the one(s) that qualified a child for early intervention. We must question program practices not solely in terms of their capacity to "fix" children developmentally but also on the basis of their impact on children's self-esteem, acceptance by other children, and life experiences.

As professionals, we perhaps have lost sight of the value of maintaining young children with disabilities in the mainstream of society in the myriad of debates and arguments around issues such as empirical support, efficacy, or legislative and program regulations. It is hoped that we have not established expectations that define the use of particular practices solely in terms of positive change in individual children's developmental or behavioral outcomes. Rather, we must balance these debates with values that respect children's individual growth patterns and practices that promote each child as an individual with needs for love, fulfillment, and respect.

As an infant, my son Ryan's development was not normal. He fussed a lot and did not seem to do things that other babies were doing. At 5 months of age, his pediatrician confirmed Ryan's multiple handicaps and suggested that we enroll in an early intervention program. We had no idea what the future held for our son. He was 7 months old by the time I had the courage to visit an early intervention program. I went to the school and was taken on a tour by a staff member. What I saw were classrooms for infants and preschoolers. The children were playing in one classroom. In another, they were at a table doing an art project. I knew this was a special program for children with handicaps, but everything looked so normal. The experience was the most reassuring thing that had happened to me—to know that our son could have the same experiences as other children his age.

It hurts to watch your child struggle so hard to do the things that come naturally to other children. A year and a half after Ryan's enrollment in the program, he was unable to even sit alone by himself, and sometimes activities that were perfect for the rest of his infant/toddler class seemed inappropriate for Ryan. One day I came in and found his teachers had laid him on the floor on his back and formed a circle around him with all the children. They sang "Ring-a-Round-the-Rosie" as they skipped around him. Ryan loved it, watching each face as it passed and squealing happily to the music. As I watched him, I realized that while Ryan's handicaps were severe, they didn't need to limit him. He was as much a part of the class that day as any other child in the room. I will always be grateful for the opportunity to see that Ryan didn't have to sit back and watch life go by—he could be a part of it. (Hunt, 1988 pp. 4–5)

REFERENCES

Apolloni, T., & Cooke, T.P. (1978). Integrated programming at the infant, toddler and preschool levels. In M.J. Guralnick (Ed.), *Early intervention and the integration of handicapped and nonhandicapped children* (pp. 147–165). Baltimore: University Park Press.

Bailey, D.B., Clifford, R.M., & Harms, T. (1982). Comparison of preschool environments for handicapped and nonhandicapped children. *Topics in Early Childhood Special Education, 2*(1), 9–20.

Beckman, P.J., & Kohl, A.K. (1984). The effects of social and isolate toys on the interactions and play of integrated and nonintegrated groups of preschoolers. *Education and Training of the Mentally Retarded, 19*, 169–174.

Bricker, D.D. (1978). A rationale for the integration of handicapped and nonhandicapped preschool children. In M.J. Guralnick (Ed.), *Early intervention and the integration of handicapped and nonhandicapped children* (pp. 3–26). Baltimore: University Park Press.

Bricker, D., Bailey, E., & Bruder, M. (1984). The efficacy of early intervention and the handicapped infant: A wise or wasted resource. *Advances in developmental and behavioral pediatrics*. Greenwich, CT: JAI Press.

Bricker, W.A. (Producer). (1972). *Time to learn* [Film]. Nashville, TN: Kennedy Center, George Peabody College.

Bricker, W.A., & Bricker, D.D. (1971). *Toddler research and intervention project report: Year I* (IMRID Behavioral Science Monograph 21). Nashville, TN: Institute on Mental Retardation and Intellectual Development, George Peabody College.

Campbell, P.H., & Stanley-Bryson, K. (1987). *The outcomes of children with Down syndrome following discharge from an integrated early childhood intervention program*. Manuscript submitted for publication.

Edgar, E., McNulty, B., Gaetz, J., & Maddox, M. (1984). Educational placement of graduates of preschool programs for handicapped children. *Topics in Early Childhood Special Education, 4*(3), 19–29.

Galloway, C., & Chandler, P. (1978). The marriage of special and generic early education services. In M.J. Guralnick (Ed.), *Early intervention and the integration of handicapped and nonhandicapped children* (pp. 261–287). Baltimore: University Park Press.

Guralnick, M.J. (1978a). *Early intervention and the integration of handicapped and nonhandicapped children*. Baltimore: University Park Press.

Guralnick, M.J. (1978b). Integrated preschools as educational and therapeutic environments: Concepts, design, and analysis. In M.J. Guralnick (Ed.), *Early intervention and the integration of handicapped and nonhandicapped children* (pp. 115–146). Baltimore: University Park Press.

Guralnick, M.J. (1980). Social interaction among preschool handicapped children. *Exceptional Children, 46*, 248–253.

Hanline, M.F. (1988). Making the transition to preschool: Identification of parent needs. *Journal of the Division for Early Childhood, 12*(2), 98–107.

Hayden, A.H. (1979). Handicapped children birth to age 3. *Exceptional Children, 45*, 510–516.

Hunt, M. (1988, Summer). A mother's story. *Children's Progress*, pp. 4–6.

Jenkins, J.R., Speltz, M.L., & Odom, S.L. (1985). Integrating normal and handicapped preschoolers: Effects on child development and social interaction. *Exceptional Children, 52*, 7–17.

Klein, N., & Sheehan, R. (1987). Staff development: A key issue in meeting the needs of young handicapped children in daycare settings. *Topics in Early Childhood Special Education, 7*(1), 13–27.

Odom, S.L., & McEvoy, M.A. (1988). Integration of young children with handicaps and normally developing children. In S.L. Odom & M.B. Karnes (Eds.), *Early intervention for infants and children with handicaps: An empirical base* (pp. 241–267). Baltimore: Paul H. Brookes Publishing Co.

Odom, S.L., & Speltz, M.L. (1983). Program variations in preschools for handicapped and nonhandicapped children: Mainstreamed vs. integrated special education. *Analysis and Intervention in Developmental Disabilities, 3*, 89–104.

Raver, S.A., Cooke, T.P., & Apolloni, T. (1978). Developing nonretarded toddlers as verbal models for retarded classmates. *Child Study Journal, 8*, 1–8.

Safford, P.L., & Rosen, L.A. (1981). Mainstreaming: Application of a philosophical perspective in an integrated kindergarten program. *Topics in Early Childhood Education, 1*(1), 1–10.

Smith, B.J. (1984). Expanding the federal role in

serving young special-needs children. *Topics in Early Childhood Special Education, 4*(1), 33–42

Smith, B.J., & Strain, P.S. (1988). Implementing and expanding P.L. 99-457. *Topics in Early Childhood Special Education, 8*(1), 37–47.

Strain, P.S., & Cordisco, L.K. (1983). Child characteristics and outcomes related to mainstreaming. In J. Anderson & T. Black (Eds.), *Issues in preschool mainstreaming* (pp. 47–64). Chapel Hill, NC: TADS Publication.

Strain, P.S., Guralnick, M.J., & Walker, H.M. (Eds.). (1986). *Children's social behavior: Assessment, development, and modification.* New York: Academic Press.

Strain, P.S., & Odom, S.L. (1986). Peer social initiations: An effective intervention for social skills deficits of exceptional children. *Exceptional Children, 52,* 543–551.

Turnbull, A.P., & Turnbull, H.R. (1986). *Families and professionals: Creating an exceptional partnership.* Columbus, OH: Charles E. Merrill.

Vincent, L.J., Salisbury, C., Walter, G., Brown, P., Gruenwald, L.J., & Powers, M. (1980). Program evaluation and curriculum development in early childhood/special education: Criteria of the next environment. In W. Sailor, B. Wilcox, & L. Brown (Eds.), *Methods of instruction for severely handicapped students* (pp. 303–328). Baltimore: Paul H. Brookes Publishing Co.

Walter, G., & Vincent, L. (1982). The handicapped child in the regular kindergarten classroom. *Journal of the Division for Early Childhood, 6,* 84–95.

Weiner, R., & Koppelman, J. (1987). *From birth to 5: Serving the youngest handicapped children.* Alexandria, VA: Capitol Publications.

◇ **CHAPTER 28** ◇

Ensuring Quality of Early Intervention for Children with Severe Disabilities

PHILLIP S. STRAIN

University of Pittsburgh, Pittsburgh, Pennsylvania

In this chapter I address three questions related to the quality of early intervention for preschool children with disabilities:

1. Why is there such a profound variance in the quality of service delivery?
2. What are some specific indicators of quality?
3. How can we institutionalize quality services?

However, it is first necessary to put some very general boundaries around what we mean by "quality." Realizing that this task is a highly personal enterprise, and that other conceptualizations are equally valid, I suggest that quality presupposes the following basic ingredients. First, the scope of the intervention should reflect the scope of the problem. That is to say that a family with a history of mental illness, financial hardship, a child with severe disabilities, and four other children should be afforded a comprehensive range of services—services that do not stop with even the most sparkling of educational interventions for the child with disabilities. Second, the intervention procedures should yield measurable gains in those areas targeted for change. If not, the procedures should be changed. Third, the changes brought about by the intervention should be perceivable to the clients. They should like the interventions and the outcomes.

WHY IS THERE SUCH A PROFOUND VARIANCE IN THE QUALITY OF SERVICE DELIVERY?

There are many easy answers to this question, including shortages in qualified staff, too few validated instructional procedures that are known to direct services personnel, and oppositional administrators. My suspicion, however, is that these answers account collectively for only a small fraction of the variance in program quality. In my opinion, there are three other factors that more profoundly influence the quality of early intervention service delivery.

The first of these factors is the existence of what we might call "early intervention piranhas." These early intervention flesh eaters come disguised as commercial publishers, curriculum development moguls who choose the quick royalty check over validation data, intervention practitioners who diagnose everyone the same and treat them accordingly, and myopic zealots for any number of views on human behavior. These views have one thing in common: They seldom get contaminated by data. The piranhas feed on our integrity and the quality of what we do by promoting and perpetuating ill-conceived, nonempirical, and therefore ineffective forms of early intervention. This situation will continue to plague our field until we develop the fortitude to scrutinize, license, and, on occasion, delicense the members of our profession.

Support for this paper was provided by Grants NIMH37110-05, G008730076, and G008730526. However, opinions expressed herein do not necessarily reflect the position of the National Institute on Mental Health or the U.S. Department of Education.

The second factor contributing to the disparity in quality of programming is the scarcity of truly powerful models of early intervention. In a sense, early intervention has seldom been tried. What I mean to point out is that just because one invoked the name "early intervention," it does not follow that early intervention got delivered. Several years ago, Diane Sainato and I did an observational assessment of 20 prominent early childhood centers in Pennsylvania. On average, these 3-hour-per-day programs had children actively involved in instruction for about 15 minutes *each* day. Now that is early intervention below the threshold of meaningfulness and sanity. It may also be typical of early intervention in the majority of cases.

The third factor contributing to a decrement in quality of programming is the perpetual conflict between early intervention and some strongly held beliefs in our society. For example, we have the belief in the "supremacy of mom and the home" as the seat of early growth and development. Never mind that a majority of moms are not at home, forget about dear old dad, and condemn any service system that purportedly supplants the home. Curious, is it not, that the supposed left-wing of our profession and the right-wing of society share this perspective? Consider also the belief in the child's sovereign right to be left alone, to let the winds of maturation blow over the developmental landscape and do their thing. Manifestations of this belief system include the phantom "hurried child," the debate over the morality of day care, and the prevalence of "readiness" in our professional vocabulary. However, the most powerful conflicting belief rests upon greed. Mostly there is a quality problem in early intervention because people want society's resources for something else. Of course, that something else need not be cost-effective, popular, or necessarily prudent. "Star Wars" comes to mind as an alternative that meets all these criteria. Parenthetically, it is interesting to note that the planned funding for this national effort would have to be brutally slashed by 0.004% to fund the new early intervention legislation, PL 99-457, at its maximum level for a decade!

In some respects, we might argue that diversity is a strength. Certainly, diversity of curric-ula, diversity of validated teaching tactics, and diversity of ancillary services can be real strengths. Yet diversity on the dimension of basic quality only detracts from our best efforts. It also perpetuates mediocrity and excludes children and families from truly beneficial services.

WHAT ARE SOME SPECIFIC INDICATORS OF QUALITY?

Given the general parameters of quality enumerated earlier, the question now becomes "How can we best design service delivery systems that ensure quality?" If we focus on the effectiveness-driven model of quality previously presented, several dimensions of service delivery emerge. These dimensions, or program characteristics, are depicted in Table 28.1.

To briefly summarize the indicators of quality shown in Table 28.1, we would have an early intervention program that enrolls children as soon as possible from the point of problem identification. We would have a program with goals and procedures that are sensitive to family interests, needs, strengths, and weaknesses. We would have a program that is intensive, providing all participants with many opportunities to learn and practice critical skills. We would have a program with goals that are derived, in part, from an analysis of future placement demands and expectations. We would have a program that individualizes instruction while still affording children the opportunities to learn from one another. We would have a program where children with and without disabilities participate daily in planful instructional and social interaction. Finally, we would have a program that is carefully sequenced to allow all participants the chance to advance developmentally in the most expeditious fashion.

At a more fine-grain level of analysis, let us

Table 28.1.   Characteristics of effective intervention programs

1. Early screening, referral, and programming
2. Family-focused intervention
3. Time in active instruction
4. Next-environment criteria for programming
5. Group-individualized instruction
6. Social and academic integration
7. Precise scope and sequence of instruction

FORM 28.1

FAMILY-FOCUSED INTERVENTION

Procedural Checklist

____ Are parents participants in the governance of the program?
____ Are parent priorities considered in the development of the individualized education program (IEP)?
____ Are measures of family strengths and weaknesses utilized?
____ Is there intervention planning that is sensitive to family strengths and weaknesses?
____ Do parents assist in the evaluation of the program?
____ Are family supportive services (babysitting, advocacy support groups) provided on an individualized basis?
____ Is family functioning utilized as a program outcome?
____ Is individualized skill training provided to parents in home and community settings?
____ Is there a routine communication system in place between home and intervention site?

consider two of the features identified in Table 28.1: family-focused intervention and precise scope and sequence of instruction. What are the indicators of family-focused intervention and a precise scope and sequence of instruction? In Forms 28.1 and 28.2 I have indicated, by way of a procedural checklist, upon what we might base an evaluative opinion. These procedural checklists are merely illustrative of some points that we might consider to be indicative of high quality vis-à-vis these two program features. For some of these checklist items, data are available to support their efficacy. Other items simply hold considerable face validity, and await empirical analysis. (The interested reader may contact me for sample checklists for all the program features in Table 28.1.)

HOW CAN WE INSTITUTIONALIZE QUALITY SERVICES?

Assuming a working definition of quality, a monumental objective for the field of early intervention is to institutionalize the dimensions of high-quality programs. To accomplish such an objective requires a broad-based and multilevel assault on a "herd of sacred cows." Our sacred cows of early intervention include:

1. A long-standing tradition of "paying-off" programs for service provision, not *quality* service delivery
2. The promotion of entrepreneurial, private-sector, and highly diversified models of early intervention

FORM 28.2

PRECISE SCOPE AND SEQUENCE OF INSTRUCTION

Procedural Checklist

____ Has an early childhood curriculum been adopted?
____ Are specific child objectives individualized within the curriculum structure?
____ Are child outcomes in the curriculum assessed repeatedly throughout the year?
____ Is it clear that children move quickly to the next curriculum step when mastery is achieved?
____ Is the curriculum based in part on "next-environment" demands and expectations?
____ Is there a daily time allotted for teachers to plan instruction?
____ Is there a strategy noted by which children are not subjected to repeated failure experiences with new material?
____ Does the curriculum include social skill objectives, not just cognitive ones?

3. The unaccountability of training institutions
    for the products they produce

How might we gently do away with each of these sacred cows, and thereby promote the best service programs? Considering first the equating of service provision with quality service delivery, we might consider our first job one of "de-institutionalization." Currently, both public and private (implying some gain for the provider at some cost to clients) modes of early intervention are wrapped in a numbers-first, numbers-only mentality. It can be no other way, given the status quo. Clients generate dollars. The contingency is simple, and misplaced. Good client outcomes, in this system, can mean even fewer dollars. The numbers-based contingency exists at local, state, and federal levels. It exists not just in early intervention but in all education, health, welfare, mental health, and developmental disabilities bureaucracies. To alter such a pay-off system will require money, time, and a fundamental reorientation to human services. It will take money necessary to make counts of clients obsolete—that is, obsolete in the sense that services become *universally available* and at *no cost* to clients. It will take time to generate the political awareness and power to mount such an effort. It will take a radically different perspective on human services delivery, one that rejects the notion that any service is appropriate service and embraces the notion that service *outcomes* are the sine qua non of service delivery.

Let us consider next the elimination (or perhaps just harnessing) of our second sacred cow —the promotion of entrepreneurial, private-sector, and highly diversified models of early intervention. At one level, it is fair to say that this sacred cow gives the vital milk of innovation to our field. It also promotes a lack of scrutiny and regulation, "slick" packaging but substanceless content, and a resource-wasteful reinvention (*ad nauseam*) of the basic foundations of early intervention. There is no need to point the finger directly. Suffice it to say that we all know of programs that are never monitored in a fashion facilitative of children's development. We all know of, and receive regularly in the mail, the latest early intervention breakthroughs with no validation data in sight. And we all know that unplanned heterogeneity is the superordinate characteristic of early intervention service models. In my local area, for example, one young child with autism might recieve "equine therapy," another might receive "insight-oriented therapy," another might receive "play therapy," and still another might receive school- and home-based behavioral therapy. What children receive at this gross level of service description is dictated solely by which program they by chance enter.

To harness this sacred cow of diversity will require, for the most part, bold steps by the professional organizations that make up the early intervention enterprise. Where bizarre, empirically refuted, and developmentally trivial programs exist, we must apply, via our professional organizations, appropriate censure. At the same time, we must take the necessary steps to certify educational procedures and service delivery dimensions, not just people. Finally, our professional organizations must be willing to invest in retraining, technical assistance, and all manner of services that encourage professionals to grow, learn, and stay abreast in their fields.

Finally, let us turn to our final sacred cow— the unaccountability of training institutions for the products they produce. By and large, institutions of higher education have adopted a convenient caveat emptor approach to their products—namely, teachers and administrators. The consumer, in the form of school district or some other service delivery entity, has no guarantee, no warranty, and no redress against faulty products. As long as certification, hiring criteria, and degree requirements are linked to coursework rather than competence, the status quo is inevitable.

This sacred cow of unaccountability is protected, more than adequately, by a fully developed system of educational philosophy and practice that is basically incompatible with the very concept of accountability. Accountability implies: 1) performance, 2) criteria for judging performance, 3) corrective remedies, and 4) accessibility to producers on the part of consumers. By contrast, the prevailing focus on coursework and time served *presupposes* that competence is synonymous with these indices. This supposition is made without risk of any negative consequence since consumers do not directly "purchase" (and thus may not purchase or take their business elsewhere) personnel from institutions of higher education.

How might we rearrange the contingencies in this personnel preparation system in order to secure accountability? First, it seems clear that the administrative and bureaucratic distance between institutions of higher education and consumers of their products must be narrowed. We might do this by placing a significant fraction of consumers on curriculum planning committees and by allowing consumers to "order" or "purchase" a certain number and quality of personnel. Of course, this implies a radical change in terms of who now pays for faculty and staff to engage in personnel preparation activities. We should also allow consumers to differentially reinforce exceptional performance on the part of personnel preparation specialists.

A second tactic for rearranging the existing contingencies is to extend schooling for professionals. Presently, this is a concept that is gaining momentum nationwide. However, I suggest that the extension of schooling might well be on the job rather than in preparation for the job. Many logistical nightmares come to mind when we entertain such an idea. Yet, if we move to competency-based higher education, then logistical problems in supervision should be minimized, even on an interstate basis.

SUMMARY AND CONCLUSIONS

For many years, the fundamental issue in the early intervention field was one of *access*. While we are far from universal service delivery, our emerging issue is now one of *quality*. In this chapter I have offered a personalized definition of quality service delivery, suggested what some of the roadblocks are, and outlined some strategies for making quality universal. The strategies outlined are admittedly resource bound. Yet, we should not be immobilized by transient shortfalls in monetary resources. Making institutions of higher education accountable, making professionals more accountable, and rewarding service providers for good work must begin with a sincere commitment from individual professionals and the organizations representing those professionals. I believe the past accomplishments of early intervention professionals bode well for such a commitment and the corollary resources to support the best in service delivery for all.

REFERENCE

Strain, P.S., & Sainato, D. (undated). [Observational assessment of early childhood centers in Pennsylvania]. Unpublished raw data.

CHAPTER 29

Family Assessment and Family Empowerment
An Ethical Analysis

ANN P. TURNBULL
H. RUTHERFORD TURNBULL, III

*The Beach Center on Families and Disability
and the University of Kansas, Lawrence, Kansas*

Several years ago, popular attention focused on the movie *Whose Life Is It Anyway?* (Badham, 1981). There, one issue was the right of a person with severe physical disabilities to refuse life-saving medical treatment. But the title of the movie raised yet another issue: the ethics of professional intervention in face of autonomous decision making by competent people who decline what the professionals offer.

Also many years ago, Elizabeth M. Boggs (1978) cautioned us all to take the "shoes test" as we think about what we—as parents and other family members, professionals, and advocates —want done for, to, with, and by people with disabilities. She asked us to perform a sort of psychic transplant, ceasing to make decisions on the basis of our own experiences, capabilities, and choices; and instead make them as though each of us were the person with disabilities. She asked us to eschew what we ourselves would decide and the basis for those decisions and to adopt instead what the person would decide and the basis for those decisions.

Whether life imitated art in Boggs's (1978) chapter or art imitated life in the movie, there is a common theme. It is that ethical behavior must include respect for and action based on the respect for the perspective of the person whose life it is. Certainly TASH itself, in its recent resolutions on choice, has moved in the direction of ethical decision making based on the principle of empathic reciprocity. This principle admonishes that the ethical course of conduct is that that is

reciprocal with the person whose life is most directly affected by the proposed action, and that the reciprocal consideration is empathic (i.e., congruent and harmonious with that person).

This "golden rule" approach can shed interesting and sometimes unexpected light on professional interventions. TASH's monograph on aversives (Guess, Helmstetter, Turnbull, & Knowlton, 1986) and the accompanying chapter on the ethics of aversive interventions (Turnbull et al., 1987) showed how the principle of empathic reciprocity can be the basis for prohibiting certain otherwise widely practiced interventions.

In this chapter, we seek to show how that same principle can change rather dramatically how professionals assess family strengths and needs as they implement Part H of the Education of the Handicapped Act (infants and toddlers programs under PL 99-457). Our approach is to create an artificial "debate" or "point-counterpoint" in which the advocacy for the traditional position (which we construct to exclude empathic reciprocity) is followed by a rejoinder (which, of course, clearly involves empathic reciprocity). We conclude by stating our own position, which attempts to encompass both the ethical position and the nonconflicting state-of-the-art professional practice.

DISCUSSION

Point One of the critical new components of the individualized family services plan (IFSP) is the assessment of family strengths and needs. In the individualized education program (IEP), only students were assessed. The IFSP, however, adds a requirement to assess families' strengths and needs. This is an exciting opportunity for the professional team to apply their sophisticated assessment instruments to pinpoint how the family functions and how the family might best be served by the program. Assessment should focus on the quality of the home environment, parent-child interaction, knowledge of child development, sources of family stress, coping skills, stage of parental acceptance, and overall family well-being. By obtaining a profile on each family of its strengths and needs in each of these areas, the program can best individualize its services according to what would be most helpful to families.

Counterpoint Taking a family perspective, my first reaction is, "You've got to be kidding!" For starters, I even find the language you are using quite offensive. You talk about assessment instruments. Is it really necessary to administer an "assessment instrument"? Beyond the language issue, I find the whole concept threatening and intimidating. Would you want an assessment instrument administered by a stranger to your family? How eager would you be to disclose all of your family's strengths and needs and to have scores summed up and entered into someone's computer? Why is that even necessary? Finally, the fundamental question is this: Will the administration of assessment instruments help families or will these assessment instruments even do harm by invading the family's privacy, identifying family weaknesses and needs, and creating more problems than they solve? Why must assessment instruments be administered at all?

Point Assessment of the family provides the basis for family-focused intervention. It is impossible to individualize according to the unique strengths and needs of families unless those strengths and needs are identified. It is clear from family theory and research that family assessment is an essential component of an effective early intervention program. In fact, researchers have developed family functioning instruments and scales with impressive validity and reliability. These instruments provide an ob-

jective and precise basis for intervention planning. Families can complete these instruments, and professionals can score them to get a clear profile of each family's strengths and needs. It is important for you to understand that such assessment instruments are highly respected in the professional journals.

Counterpoint It is just as important for you to understand that these assessment instruments may be highly respected in the professional journals, but they are not nearly as respected by the families who must complete them. I can understand that it is important to individualize for families and that every family has different strengths and needs. But I beg to differ with you on the appropriateness of using these instruments and scales that have been developed more from the perspective of professionals than from families. When families are first working in early intervention, and even throughout the whole process of early intervention, they are vulnerable. Perhaps the last thing that they need is the completion of tests and scores compiled on how they are functioning. Their vulnerability may be increased, not decreased.

I can envision a process that would be very "family friendly" in which a parent of an older child—let's call that person a veteran parent— might sit down with new parents and talk with them about what they want for their child and about what they see as their particular needs and strengths. This would be done within the context of having a real, genuine *relationship* with the family where the family has confidence in the support and concern of another person who knows what it's like to "stand in their shoes." This is particularly important for minority parents who may be highly distrustful of professionals in the first place. If parents are suspicious and are thinking that a professional is just out to make one more devaluing and demeaning judgment about them, they may never participate at all if you start out the process by administering a bunch of tests to them. I'm suggesting that you develop the whole concept of *expressing* family strengths and needs (and I want to underscore that I said *express* rather than *assess*) from the context of what is the most comfortable and family-friendly way you can think of to share relevant information.

Point I've never really thought about this so much from the family's point of view, but I can see your point that I don't really think I would want to fill out a whole bunch of assessment instruments on my family. Maybe we have gone a bit overboard in trying to get everything so objective and precise that we have not thought as much about what it is like for the family. Perhaps we ought to be thinking more about conducting interviews with families and asking questions to elicit information on strengths and needs. These interviews should even be conducted in the family's home. By doing this, there could be other members of the family there, including brothers and sisters, and it might be far more family friendly, as you say.

Counterpoint I think you are moving in the right direction, but there are still some things that you don't seem to understand from a family's point of view. Some families may be very comfortable with interviews; in fact, some families may even be comfortable with the scales and instruments that we discussed earlier. But you can't assume that every family will even like interviews. Think about times in the past when you have been interviewed. Have there been instances where you felt uncomfortable because the person interviewing you knew all of the questions that he or she wanted to ask, but each one, perhaps, caught you a little by surprise? Did you ever give answers that you regretted later? Did you ever look back on what you said and feel foolish? In interviews, families are expected to disclose personal information, but the interviewer does not tell the family anything about himself or herself. Also, professionals often make observations during interviews of the nonverbal behavior of the family. They might even make notes in a file about things such as eye contact, any kind of tension they might have perceived between the parents, or other sorts of observations that are never made explicit to the family.

One option for you to consider is that it might even be possible to collect information on families' strengths and needs from having *conversations* with families rather than *interviews*. What if two people sat down together and just visited with each other about what was important for the child and how the family could bring their own

resources to bear to help the child and what kind of special needs the family might have? Isn't it possible to do something that is more informal and more family friendly? If the real purpose of family assessment is to *help* the family, let's look at the process from *their* point of view. Conversations, and even interviews, may not be as objective and precise, and there may not be any numbers to enter into service providers' forms and records, but an informal approach characterized by a trusting and caring relationship might actually result in more accurate (reliable) and relevant (valid) information.

OUR VIEW

We hear from families over and over again that they are most interested in an approach to the expression of family strengths and needs that is as low key and informal as possible. Minority families have emphasized how much the lack of credibility and trust factors serves as barriers to assessment and how important it is for the family to establish a relationship with the person collecting information and to feel that person's support and respect for them. In fact, one recommendation from families is that the most supportive context would be for the expression of family strengths and needs to occur within a *relationship* in which the family who has an infant with disabilities is matched with a veteran family who shares the same cultural background and socioeconomic circumstances. We might think about hiring family members as staff in early intervention programs and utilizing the parent-to-parent model in which a veteran parent provides emotional support and information to a new parent. This same approach could be used in the expression of family strengths and needs. An important point here is that this particular option will not work for all families, because many families will prefer a more professionally directed, more formal approach. Individual options are essential. As a field, however, we must conceptualize the process of expressing strengths and needs from the perspective of what is respectful to the family, including minority families, and not just from the point of view of researchers and specialists in family assessment. Such a process is the essence of empathic reciprocity.

REFERENCES

Badham, J. (Director). (1981). *Whose life is it anyway?* [Film]. Culver City, CA: MGM/UA.

Boggs, E.M. (1978). Who's putting whose head in the sand? (Or in the clouds, as the case may be). In H.R. Turnbull & A.P. Turnbull (Eds.), *Parents speak out: Then and now* (pp. 39–54). Columbus, OH: Charles E. Merrill.

Guess, D., Helmstetter, E., Turnbull, H.R., & Knowlton, S. (1986). *Use of aversive procedures with persons who are disabled: An historical review and critical analysis.* Seattle: The Association for Persons with Severe Handicaps.

Turnbull, H.R., Guess, D., Backus, L., Barber, P., Fiedler, C., Helmstetter, E., & Summers, J.A. (1987). A model for analyzing the moral aspects of special education and behavioral interventions: The moral aspects of aversive procedures. In P.R. Dokecki & R.M. Zaner (Eds.), *Ethics of dealing with persons with severe handicaps: Toward a research agenda* (pp. 167–210). Baltimore: Paul H. Brookes Publishing Co.

◇ SECTION V ◇

ADULT SERVICES REFORM AND OMNIBUS LEGISLATION ISSUES

Do we need an omnibus legislation package to guarantee that persons with disabilities will be provided with appropriate services to meet their individualized needs across the life span? In the mid-1970s, PL 94-142 was heralded as landmark legislation that guaranteed school-age youngsters a place in school, no matter how severe their disabilities. In the 1980s, PL 99-457 extended this right to educational services and family supports for the preschool years, beginning at birth. Are we now ready for comparable guarantees for postschool-age individuals to receive the assistance they may need for continued personal growth and development as adults?

The TASH resolution on adult service reform (1983) (Document V.1, this volume) called for a new perspective on the services needed by adults with severe disabilities to support their right to live, work, and recreate in the community, alongside their nondisabled families, friends, neighbors, and co-workers. The Social Security Resolution (1987) (Document V.2, this volume) was promulgated as a result of growing concerns that traditional funding policies and practices were not designed to support integrated lifestyles—in fact, they worked against integration—and that changes were essential if community participation was to be a reality rather than a distant goal or slogan for persons with disabilities. The 1988

Resolution on Choices (Document V.3, this volume) represented yet another revelation that simply continuing "business as usual" as we moved into the community would not do, nor could we continue to treat persons with disabilities as perennial children across their life span. Professionals have for too long been accustomed to telling people with disabilities what they need and what's good for them. True community integration would surely have to involve empowerment and choices—people with disabilities deciding for themselves. And where those opportunities for choice making and personal autonomy have never before been regarded as possible or made possible, it would be the professionals' responsibility to test the limits. Can we learn to provide services to people that enable them to succeed in and adapt to their communities? And can we do so in a manner that supports those individuals in their attainment of a meaningful lifestyle, but does not make them dependent upon professionals and paid staff in the process? The challenge of the next few years will be to translate our goals for community living and personal autonomy into a new reality that enables persons with disabilities to be what *they* want to be . . . with choices and control. The chapters in this section address these issues.

TASH Calls for Adult Service Reform

When children with severe handicaps leave the educational system, TASH: The Association for Persons with Severe Handicaps affirms their right to live full adult lives, free of the restrictions imposed by rigid service hierarchies and historical patterns of isolation. TASH believes that the task of adult services should be, not to develop readiness for adult roles, but to provide the support needed by individuals to work, live, and recreate in the mainstream of community life. Toward this end TASH endorses the following features of adult services:

1. INTEGRATION. The constellation of services available to a person with a severe disability should result in an integrated adult lifestyle. This means that each individual's life should be characterized by physical proximity to the social mainstream, access to generic resources available to other citizens, regular and personal contact with individuals who are not paid caregivers, and full citizenship status. Integration depends, not on the features of any single service, but on the overall pattern of an individual's interaction with the community.

2. COMMUNITY LIVING. All citizens with severe disabilities should have the opportunity to live in family-scale, home-like residences that support full participation in normal work, leisure, and personal management activities. Toward this end TASH supports the rapid and planful termination of large and small public and private residential facilities that separate, isolate, and restrict persons with disabilities from full community integration. This will require changes in state and local zoning ordinances and program financing policies, as well as the development and broad dissemination of alternatives to complement current residential models.

3. EMPLOYMENT. The opportunity to work, the process of working, and the community opportunities created by the resulting income are all critical to integrated adult lives in our society. Adults with severe disabilities should have the same work opportunities as others in the community. Further, the quality of employment and related day and vocational services for individuals with severe disabilities should be judged by the same criteria used to evaluate the employment of others in our society: income level and the resulting opportunities created by that income; quality of working life, including integration of the workplace, safety, and access to challenging work; and security benefits, including job mobility, advancement opportunities, and protection from lifestyle disruptions due to illness or accident. While many individuals with severe disabilities may well need ongoing support to perform in work situations, this does not mean that they should be excluded from work. TASH calls for the rapid development of supported employment programs that provide the full range of employment outcomes, and the rapid replacement of day and vocational programs that: (1) provide pre-vocational training and readiness activities rather than employment opportunities; (2) segregate workers with disabilities from those without disabilities; and (3) involve performing work without pay.

4. CONSUMER ACCOUNTABILITY. Program management and resource allocation decisions in adult services should be based on information regarding the benefits that consumers receive from those services. An adequate constellation of services will result in performance of activities valued by the individual, contact with others in the community, income from work, individual exercise of choice, and maintenance of health status. Evaluation or accreditation on the basis of service procedures alone does

not provide a sufficient index of accountability. Financial, policy, program, and management decisions should be linked directly to benefits received by consumers with disabilities.

5.   STAFFING.   The entry of individuals with severe disabilities into adult service programs will necessitate changes in staffing. Providing the ongoing support required by many individuals with severe disabilities without creating segregated or devalued lives will require new professional roles and different competencies than those typically found in adult service programs. Parity of pay between staff in community programs and staff of restricted institutional programs is necessary to attract and maintain qualified staff. New training programs are needed to combine competencies developed in existing teacher training programs with those needed for supporting employment, community residence, and other situations. TASH calls for the definition of professional roles, so that individuals with severe disabilities can be better included in adult services; the development of competency standards for those roles; and the initiation of training programs that produce qualified personnel.

ORIGINALLY ADOPTED NOVEMBER 1983

*   *   *   *   *

Social Security Resolution

WHEREAS, Serious inequities exist across Social Security programs affecting individuals with intellectual impairments, especially in SSI and SSDI, and

WHEREAS, Serious inequities exist in standards within programs administered by Social Security for populations with different lifelong impairments, and

WHEREAS, Serious inequities exist in the standards for Applicants versus Recipients in programs of the Social Security Administration, and

WHEREAS, SGA as a concept is outmoded, inadequate, and inequitable at present levels for persons with intellectual impairments, and provides a serious disincentive to work, and

WHEREAS, Forthcoming Medical Reviews are not defined nor their ultimate effect known and they may present a serious problem for those attempting work even through Supported Employment, and

WHEREAS, Eligibility for the proposed Medicaid Home and Quality Community Services Amendments is limited to individuals who meet the eligibility requirements SSI, and

WHEREAS, Many state programs have and will increasingly adopt federal criteria (SSI eligibility) to determine eligibility for state supported programs,

THEREFORE BE IT RESOLVED, THAT TASH shall give appropriate priority to and publicly support the removal of all present inequities within programs, across programs, and those which discriminate against applicants.

THEREFORE BE IT FURTHER RESOLVED, THAT TASH shall propose and/or support reform of present inequities through the elimination of the concept of SGA and/or the increase of SGA levels to reasonable and equitable levels for all programs, all populations, and for applicants as well as recipients.

THEREFORE BE IT ALSO RESOLVED, THAT TASH shall monitor the application of Medical Reviews and their effects on recipients with intellectual impairments.

AND BE IT FINALLY RESOLVED, THAT TASH allocate resources to effect positive changes in these programs.

ORIGINALLY ADOPTED OCTOBER 1987

* * * * *

DOCUMENT V.3

Resolution on Choices

WHEREAS, All people have preferences and express those choices in all aspects of their lives; and

WHEREAS, the natural opportunity for making choices begins early in life; and

WHEREAS, increased opportunities to express everyday preferences and choices can heighten an individual's sense of self-esteem and self-direction; and

WHEREAS, freedom of expression and choice are fundamental human rights which should be shared with all people worldwide; and

WHEREAS, historically some families, professionals, and policy-makers have erroneously believed that persons with severe cognitive or intellectual deficits are unable to communicate, compare, or consciously direct their own thoughts; and

WHEREAS, some families, professionals, and policy-makers have incorrectly assumed that people with severe disabilities are not capable of making choices in their own best interests; and

WHEREAS, in the past, decisions have often been made by professionals, families, policy-makers, and others, based primarily on the assumption of what is in the best interest of the person with severe disabilities; and

WHEREAS, programs and activities that relegate individuals with severe disabilities to a passive role do not encourage or allow a full range of choices that exist; and

WHEREAS, active attempts by people with severe disabilities to exercise choice or modify programs designed by professionals and families have often been interpreted as non-compliance, resulting in development of behavior programs to decrease the presumed "maladaptive" behavior;

THEREFORE BE IT RESOLVED: The Association for Persons with Severe Handicaps affirms the right of persons with severe handicaps to freedom of choice in all types of settings; families and professionals should systematically work toward development of real opportunities and programs across all ages, for choice; and individuals with severe handicaps should be encouraged and supported to make choices through such activities as exposure, awareness, interaction, and instructional opportunities; and research should be supported on successful methods that empower people with severe handicaps to make choices.

ORIGINALLY ADOPTED DECEMBER 1988

* * * * *

A Comprehensive Analysis of Federal Statutes and Programs for Persons with Severe Disabilities

MARTIN H. GERRY
Stanford University, Stanford, California

CELANE M. MCWHORTER
TASH, Alexandria, Virginia

Persons with severe disabilities have historically been excluded from active participation in the social, economic, and political mainstream of American society. The productivity of a large segment of our citizens has been restricted and even precluded—their talents, skills, and contributions ignored or undervalued by our social, economic, and political institutions. The inequity and injustice in our treatment of persons with disabilities have compromised the basic principles and integrity of our national heritage.

While policymakers have begun to come to grips with the various programmatic legacies of past attitudes and policies toward persons with disabilities, even a cursory review of the circumstances still surrounding disabilities in America confirms the continued existence of profound social and economic inequities. This pattern is especially true for persons with more severe and challenging disabilities.

It is the purpose of this chapter to review the current federal programs affecting the lifestyle of persons with severe disabilities with an eye toward legislative changes that could be made to reverse and overcome the effects of over 200 years of social and economic injustice. The chapter is divided into two main sections. The first describes the basic tenets of American social policy toward persons with severe disabilities as that policy has emerged over the past 200 years, and proposes a new social policy framework within which to assess the effectiveness of

federal disability programs. The next part of the chapter utilizes this inclusive social policy framework to assess the effectiveness of federal disability (and disability-related generic) programs for individuals of all ages with more challenging disabilities, including: 1) infants; 2) toddlers; 3) children; 4) young adults attempting to "transition" from school to work and community life; and 5) adults, both employed and unemployed. Also, specific recommendations are outlined for new federal legislation to establish effective programs in each of the five basic areas.

AMERICAN SOCIAL POLICY TOWARD PERSONS WITH SEVERE DISABILITIES

Rather than establishing common social policy goals for *all* Americans, a separate American social policy toward persons with disabilities that is both paternalistic and failure oriented emerged during the first 200 years of this nation's history. The assumptions of this policy have influenced the design and operation of federal programs that, in turn, have minimized the social and economic opportunities for persons with disabilities and squandered their productive energies and talents.

Any serious review of the current design and operation of federal disability-related programs must, thus, start with a careful examination of those social policy goals and an articulation of new, common social policy goals for all Americans, regardless of the nature and extent of any disabilities they may have.

Evolution of Federal Disability Policy

The history of American social policy toward persons with severe disabilities and their families appears centered around three interconnected tenets: 1) dehumanization, 2) an inferior social and legal status, and 3) mandatory segregation.

Dehumanization

The principle of *dehumanization* required that each individual in society be viewed in "relational" rather than "holistic" terms. Within this context, persons with "handicaps" are seen not as whole and intact persons, but rather as "defective" or "subhuman" creatures whose difficulties or "handicaps" are *internal,* created by their own innate disabilities and not by societal attitudes and responses.

As a direct consequence of this principle, social and economic institutions, such as schools, vocational training programs, unions, and employers, were conditioned to view every person with a challenging disability (e.g., student, trainee, member, employee) as "uneducable," "untrainable," "unemployable," and generally unable! These views, of course, also served to relieve the various social and economic institutions of American society of any responsibility to create educational, training, employment, and other "community" environments that maximized rather than minimized each person's inherent possibilities.

Inferior Social and Legal Status

Following logically from the dehumanization of people with disabilities, such persons were assigned a "special" social and legal status that automatically placed them on a different footing from all other citizens with respect to law, government agencies, and other political, social, and economic institutions. One of the most important consequences of the imposition of this separate and inferior status was systematic exclusion (usually created through the enactment of "special" laws pertaining only to persons with disabilities) from many of the basic educational, social, and health programs designed to serve

the general population. For example, the provision of basic preschool, elementary, and secondary education for children with disabilities is governed by "special" federal and state laws that are separate from those governing preschool, elementary, and secondary education for nondisabled children (e.g., the Education for All Handicapped Children Act). A similar, dual legislative approach has also characterized the evolution of discrete housing, transportation, and employment and training programs for individuals with disabilities and their families.

Persons with disabilities were, and still are, the only class of American citizens (other than convicted felons) routinely and categorically deprived by state law of important civil liberties, including the right to marry, the right to procreate, and the right to contract.

Segregation

As "special" laws (as described above) were enacted first to classify and label and then to govern the treatment of persons with disabilities within residential care facilities, special schools, special transportation systems, adult day-care centers, and "sheltered" workshops, a series of rigidly segregated social and economic institutions for persons with severe disabilities was created and expanded. The outcomes of these segregated structures have proven to be "inferior" in virtually every regard—low self-concept and vastly restricted personal autonomy, extraordinarily high levels of unemployment and unproductive activity, and a limited and often nonexistent range of choices in terms of vocation, avocation, friends, lifestyles, housing, and mobility.

Articulation of a New Comprehensive American Social Policy

In contrast to current practice, government policy toward persons with disabilities should be viewed in the context of an overall and *inclusive* American social policy. Rather than creating a separate set of policies for persons with disabilities, legislative and judicial strategies must be developed to ensure that the same basic goals of American social policy established for all of our nondisabled citizens are pursued with equal vigor for citizens with disabilities.

The formulation of an American social policy must be based on a clear vision of the opportunities and choices available to individuals of all ages, interests, and abilities within American society, its families, neighborhoods, schools, workplaces, communities, and social, economic, and political institutions. From this social policy vision, incorporating both the desires and values of our citizens, general social policy goals can be articulated and used for the dual purposes of determining the proper role of government and for measuring the effectiveness of its programs with respect both to the society as a whole (i.e., the social "community") and the individuals within the society.

Community Goals

A careful review of the history of this country—its beginnings at the Constitutional Convention, its reunification following the Civil War, and its revitalization following the Great Depression—leads inevitably to the identification of several clear American social policy goals as viewed from the societal or community perspective. These community goals include: 1) to maximize the economic, social, cultural, and political productivity of all citizens; 2) to maximize the choices for personal freedom and independence (interdependence) of all citizens; 3) to assure the integration and participation of all citizens within the social, economic, and political fabric of American communities; 4) to ensure fairness and equity (justice) within the operation of the social, economic, and political institutions of the society; and 5) to ensure governmental decision making at the smallest unit of government, consistent with fairness and equity goals, so as to facilitate citizen access.

Individual Goals

The cultural, religious, and moral history of this country—its early role as a haven from religious persecution, its focus on individual liberty and economic opportunity, its support of universal education and adoption of universal suffrage, and its commitment to social justice and fairness—has led inevitably to the evolution of several clear American social policy goals as viewed from the individual perspective. These individual goals include maximizing the *opportunities* and *choices* realistically available to each individual with respect to: 1) personal autonomy, independence, self-respect, and freedom from caretakers; 2) economic self-sufficiency, through sustained, integrated, and compensated employment; 3) social integration and participation; and 4) lifestyles, family, and peer association. Together, these community and individual goals should form the basic framework of an American social policy for citizens of any color, either gender, any age, or with any type of disabilities.

Legislative Recommendations

Having defined the community and individual goals that underlie social policy in this country, and having arrived at the conclusion that the current operation of federal disability programs has not been effective in supporting the attainment of these goals for persons with severe disabilities in all age groups, it is conceivable that we could lay out a single legislative measure designed to encompass policies for all persons (from birth through old age) with severe disabilities. Such a measure would most likely be accompanied by a recommendation for a single agency within the federal government with responsibility for all federal disability programs. While this is an intriguing concept, in practice it would reinforce rather than reform the three principal tenets of the historical approach to federal disability policy: dehumanization, inherently different status, and segregation.

It is even more conceivable, in light of our strong concerns about the isolation of people with severe disabilities, that we would recommend the dissolution of all current policies and replace them with the insertion of disability policy in all appropriate authorizations for federal programs addressing the social and economic needs of the general population. Under such an approach, for example, we would recommend that Part B of the Education of the Handicapped Act be included within the Elementary and Secondary Education Act and, further, that the House Subcommittee on Select Education and the Senate Subcommittee on the Handicapped be collapsed into other subcommittees with jurisdiction over elementary and secondary education. Similarly, such an approach might dictate that the Office of Special Education and Rehabilitative Services be collapsed into other existing agencies within the Department of Education and other locations within the federal government with jurisdiction over more generic educational services. While such an approach clearly would represent the purist form of "normalization" and "integrationist" policy, we do not believe that at this time such a strategy would realistically be in the best interest of the individuals it would be intended to benefit.

A more workable approach, within the framework of current laws and policies, would be to identify specific changes in current governmental management and program operations that, taken together, would result in the evolution of an overall program that would be effective in supporting persons with disabilities in the attainment of both individual and community goals. It is our opinion that federal directives most often lag far behind accepted best practices in the field. Monumental challenges are before us in the following discussion of amendments to current authority, directing services into regular schools, real work, integrated leisure, and community living.

With these challenges as a starting point, let us leave the integration at the statutory/policy level to a time in the future when implementation of effective service planning and delivery approaches in all programmatic areas has been widely documented and when concomitant advances in the awareness of policymakers concerning the potentialities of persons with severe disabilities will have occurred. Accordingly, recommendations for specific legislative changes are presented in the following sections in connection with the discussion of the effectiveness of each of the principal program areas.

EFFECTIVENESS OF FEDERAL DISABILITY PROGRAMS

Individuals with severe disabilities and their families currently receive a wide range of educational, health, mental health, diagnostic, habilitative, therapeutic, vocational, housing, transportation, and employment services under several existing federal and state service programs. Given the common and inclusive American social policy goals (community and individ-

ual) articulated in the previous section, two fundamental questions logically may be explored regarding the overall effectiveness of these federally funded services for persons with disabilities: How successful have current programs been in supporting the attainment by society and individual citizens, respectively, of community and individual goals? What factors have contributed most significantly to the lack of program success?

One of the recurring problems in the analysis of federal disability programs is the lack of consistency in defining the term *disability* across federal education, rehabilitation, benefit assistance, employment, and health programs. The National Council on Disabilities (NCD) reported that, as a result of these differing definitions, somewhere between 20 and 50 million Americans are within the social category of disability (NCD, 1986). Approximately 15%–20% of these persons (or anywhere from 3 to 10 million) may be classified as "severely disabled." To provide a degree of consistency in our analysis of current federal disability programs, the population of persons with severe disabilities is divided into four basic categories: 1) infants and toddlers (ages 0–2), 2) school-age children (ages 3–18), 3) the "transition" population (ages 19–25), and 4) adults above the initial transition age (ages 26 +).

EFFECTIVENESS OF PROGRAMS SERVING INFANTS AND TODDLERS

Service delivery to infants and toddlers with disabilities and their families requires multidisciplinary, multiagency involvement in a complex process involving screening, identification, referral, evaluation, diagnosis, intervention, and tracking.

Results of Research Activities

There is substantial evidence that under certain conditions early intervention programs accelerate the development of infants and toddlers with disabilities and reduce the effects of disabilities (Castro & Mastropieri, 1986; Weiss, 1981; White & Greenspan, 1987). Four types of factors appear to dictate or strongly influence whether a child or an infant is likely to require early childhood education services: 1) biological factors (e.g., inherited or congenital characteristics), 2) medically related factors (e.g., prematurity, illness), 3) physical environmental factors (e.g., malnutrition, exposure), and 4) social environmental factors (e.g., child abuse, parental substance abuse) (Donst, Snyder, & Mankinen, 1986). The factors themselves illustrate the need for multiple-agency, interdisciplinary involvement in the provision of services. In reality, professionals from medicine, allied health, education, psychology, and social services are all required to provide infants and toddlers with disabilities and their families with a wide array of needed services, including ongoing medical care, physical therapy, family counseling, education, and parental training (U.S. Department of Education [DOE], 1987). Further, an increasing number of public and private organizations are involved in expanding the availability of early childhood services and the knowledge base that supports them (DOE, 1987).

Overview of Federal Disability Programs

Several federal disability programs, as well as some important federal "generic" service programs, support the provision of early childhood services. Appendix 30.1 (at the end of this chapter) contains a listing of the most important of these programs. Prior to 1986, a discretionary grant program of modest size (the Handicapped Children's Early Education Program) supported the provision of educational services to a subset of infants and toddlers with disabilities within a state participating in demonstration projects. Under this program, there was little coordination among the myriad services for infants and toddlers within a state. Without such coordination, a serious question persisted as to how effective any early intervention approach could be in providing comprehensive, quality care to all infants and toddlers who need services.

Part H Infant and Toddler Program

In long-overdue recognition of the importance of early intervention services and the dangers inherent in the fragmentation of these services, Congress amended the Education of the Handicapped Act in 1986 (PL 99-457) to include a new

Part H program of comprehensive services to infants and young children (ages birth through 2). After a 4-year period that states were given to develop their programs, the new law requires that all infants and young children who meet the state definition of "developmentally delayed" (and their families) be provided services specified in an individualized family services plan (IFSP) that is developed for each child and family, much like the individualized education program (IEP) for older students, under Part B of PL 99-457.

The Part H program requires the establishment of a statewide system of comprehensive, coordinated, multidisciplinary early intervention for all handicapped infants and toddlers and their families. To ensure early intervention services would occur, Congress required that this statewide system include a single line of authority in a "lead agency" designated or established by the governor to carry out the general administration and supervision of all activities, identify and coordinate all available federal, state, and local resources, and establish procedures for the resolution of interagency disputes.

In addition to this legislative centralization and consolidation of state program management responsibility and authority, the new program also requires, as part of the new statewide early intervention program, that "case management" services be provided to the families of infants and toddlers with handicaps in order to: 1) ensure that each family gains access to early intervention (and other needed) services and that services are delivered in a timely fashion; and 2) coordinate the provision of early intervention services and other services that each infant or toddler needs. This case management process is viewed as an ongoing process of identifying, planning, and overseeing the provision of the appropriate services or situations to benefit the development of each infant and toddler.

Implementation of these new requirements has been uneven as states exercise their authority to define for themselves the eligible infants and toddlers and struggle with an interpretation of case management services that will be responsive to the unique needs of very young children and their families. Effective implementation also depends on the achievement of what heretofore has been unachievable: ongoing interagency co-operation at the state and local levels to coordinate the financing of a wide variety of services from numerous state and federal funding sources. Perhaps most challenging, implementation of the new Part H requirements requires the successful balancing of interests: the interests of the family in privacy and strong procedural safeguards, and the interests of the service providers in streamlined decision making and cost-effectiveness.

Legislation to Improve Programs Serving Infants and Toddlers

Part H of PL 99-457 became fully operational in 1990, with an optional 1991 date for states with reasonable requests for an implementation delay of 1 year. However, significant barriers to its effective implementation have already become apparent and can and must be removed. These barriers include the lack of sufficient financial resources, the absence of effective parental participation and case advocacy, and the programmatic isolation of participating children.

Expanded Federal Financing of Part H Program

The Part H mandate places an expensive demand on states for quality services to every infant and toddler who meets the state eligibility requirements. Without enough money to fund the mandate, it is highly possible that states will opt out of this federal grant-in-aid program. We recommend that legislative changes be made to increase both the direct federal funding of the Part H program and the indirect funding of the program through the use of Medicaid funds.

To meet the need that initially led to the passage of this legislation (i.e. the recognition that individuals with disabilities generally require fewer services later and enjoy a higher level of independence if they are identified and receive services from a very early age), the federal share of Part H funding must be dramatically increased to provide states with adequate assistance to meet the federal mandate that all eligible infants and toddlers receive quality services. The distribution of the federal money should be based on a per-child entitlement, as is the Part B entitlement for school-age children; this support should be increased to 40% of the

excess cost (over and above federal contributions) of the program.

We also propose an expansion of Part H services through amendments to basic Medicaid "eligibility" provisions that now treat the family income as "available" to the infant and, thereby, deny needed services to infants with severe disabilities in families of working poor or middle-income taxpayers. The present system places undue burdens on families with infants and toddlers with expensive service needs, discouraging their efforts to care for a child with severe disabilities at home.

To address this inequity, we propose the establishment of a new standard of "medical indigence" under Title XIX of the Social Security Act to include children under age 5 with disabilities under the basic Medicaid program *if* they are members of a family unit that has been required to expend in excess of 10% of gross family income for child medical expenses during any fiscal quarter.

Ensuring Effective Parental Participation and Case Advocacy

Crucial to the success of the early intervention services are a strong commitment to meaningful parent participation and the development and implementation of an effective case advocacy system (including necessary staff training). In order to ensure that an effective case advocacy system is operating within each state, the current level of financial support for case management (advocacy) under the Part H program should be separately expanded. If parents are to participate effectively in the Part H program, they must have a realistic opportunity to challenge those decisions that they believe to be inappropriate to the needs of their infant or toddler. To address these concerns, we recommend that Part H be amended to incorporate a stronger system of procedural safeguards, taking into consideration the need for strict and short timelines because of the short duration of the infant years. In addition, a new authority and responsibility for the State Protection and Advocacy Agency to assist parents who challenge such decisions should be created, with appropriate increases in the federal financial support provided to these agencies under the Developmental Disabilities Act. Expanded federal financial support for both preservice and inservice training of "case advocates" would complete this portion of the legislative package.

Reducing Programmatic Isolation in the Early Years

Current law does not foster integrated early childhood programs. Part H is largely silent on this issue, although the emphasis on the family presumes natural family settings for infants and toddlers. Implementation of family supports bears watching to ensure against service delivery that is intrusive or isolating for the family. The mutual benefits of early interactions between young children with and without disabilities point to the need for an even stronger emphasis on integration during the earlier years. Difficulties in establishing integrated infant and toddler programs are inherent in the Part H program because most states do not have comparable, publicly funded programs for children without disabilities.

In order to strengthen the likelihood of early programmatic integration, we recommend that both Part H and the various federally financed child-care proposals now before Congress be amended to require that participating states and localities work with the myriad of day-care centers and private preschools (now expanding to accommodate the growing number of working families) on the development of consolidated and integrated programs for infants and toddlers. In addition, Part H should be amended to mandate that each IFSP include a plan to foster interaction between the infant and toddler with disabilities and nonhandicapped peers. For the same reasons, parallel changes should be made in the Part B program with respect to the effective integration of children with severe disabilities of preschool age in the range of community day-care and preschool educational activities.

EFFECTIVENESS OF PROGRAMS FOR SCHOOL-AGE CHILDREN

For school-age children with severe disabilities and their families, a formidable array of health, mental health, diagnostic, rehabilitative, therapeutic, residential, and social services are potentially available under several existing federal disability and "generic" service programs.

Appendix 30.1 (at the end of this chapter) contains a listing of the most important of these programs. Under these programs, state and local agencies may provide needed services directly to the child and the child's family ("direct services") or may pay for the provision of services by a third party through a reimbursement procedure ("indirect services").

Extraordinary Accomplishments of PL 94-142 Program

The most important federal disability program providing educational services to children and youth with severe disabilities is the Education of the Handicapped Act (EHA). In 1975 Congress amended the EHA (through passage of the Education for All Handicapped Children Act or PL 94-142) to guarantee to each school-age child with disabilities in the United States the availability of a free, appropriate public education.

The regulations issued to implement PL 94-142 require that each child with disabilities be offered, at no cost to the child or the parents, a free, appropriate public education, including those special education and related services needed by the child. These services, which are identified on the basis of a comprehensive individual evaluation also mandated by the act, are described in an IEP developed jointly by school officials and parents. "Related services" are defined in the statute as transportation and those "developmental, corrective, and other supportive services as are required to assist a handicapped child to benefit from special education" (Education of the Handicapped Act, 1975, Part B, §602[17]). In addition to transportation, PL 94-142 lists several categories of services (e.g., physical therapy, occupational therapy, psychological services) that, prior to the passage of state and federal special education laws, had been provided to children with disabilities and their families by other state and local agencies. Screening and comprehensive individual evaluation incorporated in the PL 94-142 requirements also overlapped with or directly duplicated responsibilities assigned to other state and local agencies under earlier, and in some cases, more expansive legislation (e.g., Titles V and XIX of the Social Security Act).

The 1986 amendments to PL 94-142 (PL 99-457) provide for educational and related services with the same free and appropriate education guarantees for preschool children (i.e., ages 3 to 5) that were mandated for older students (i.e., ages 3 to 18, and up to age 21 by state option) by PL 94-142. While PL 94-142 contains no direct mandate specifically regarding transition from school to work and adult life, Congress has established a discretionary grant program to promote the successful transition from school to work and adult life.

In slightly more than a decade, the PL 94-142 program has been successful in dramatically expanding and improving the educational and support services available to children with severe disabilities in the United States. In 1975, Congress estimated that over 1 million children, most with severe disabilities, were excluded from public education. Today, the opportunities exist for a wide variety and high quality of special education programs for children with severe disabilities. Functional, community-based curricula, successful placements in instructional and work settings with nondisabled peers, and tremendous advances in teacher training and instructional methodology have transformed the potential of the school-age years of children with severe disabilities from ones of inactivity and growing dependence to ones of active learning and ever-expanding independence.

Problems Impairing
Effectiveness of PL 94-142 Program

Against this background of success, however, three serious problems continue to undercut the effectiveness of educational programs for children with severe disabilities: 1) the inadequacy of current arrangements for interagency financing and service coordination, 2) the failure to link school-based programs to the demands of postschool employment and community life, and 3) continued and unnecessary segregation of a substantial percentage of children with severe disabilities.

Inadequacy of Interagency
Financing and Service Coordination

When PL 94-142 was enacted in 1975, the federal share for financing the costs of the special education and related services mandated by the act for each child with disabilities (as de-

scribed in each child's IEP) was set at 40% of the average per-pupil expenditure for such services within public elementary and secondary schools nationwide. In fact, since the passage of the legislation the federal financial contribution has been well under 10% (U.S. Congress, 1983). A 1981 study conducted by the Rand Corporation reported that out of an average total expenditure for special education and related services of $3,500 per child, the federal contribution was slightly less than $250 (7%); the average state expenditure was $900 (26%) (Kakalik & Furry, 1982). The balance of $2,350 (67%) was provided by local funds (Kakalik & Furry, 1982). On the average, over 50% of the per-child expenditure reported was allocable to related service costs, and, in virtually every case studied, the federal, state, and local funds identified were *education* funds (Kakalik & Furry, 1982). More recent studies conducted by the Department of Education have shown a gradual *increase* during the current decade in the federal contribution (from approximately $250 to $270 per child) but a gradual *decrease* in the share of overall costs represented by the federal contribution from 7% to 5% (DOE, 1987).

As the legal and programmatic responsibilities of state and local education agencies have expanded rapidly since 1975, the willingness of other public agencies to provide evaluation and related services (or even to continue the level of services provided prior to the passage of PL 94-142) has declined. Both the 1983 report of a special Congressional commission created to study the financing of special education programs (U.S. Congress, 1983) and a 1986 U.S. General Accounting Office (GAO) study of the financing of health services for children with disabilities noted that various state and local health and social welfare agencies have taken the position that education agencies must bear the costs for all "related services" despite the availability of funding under other federal programs.

The 1986 EHA amendments (PL 99-457) contained several interrelated provisions designed to substantially lessen the financial burden currently borne by state and local education agencies in connection with the broad range of special education and related services required for school-age children with disabilities by the EHA and its amendments and companion state special education legislation. New provisions repudiated the position that public health and social services agencies may limit their financial responsibilities to children with disabilities participating in public special education programs; states were directed not to reduce or deny assistance available under the Social Security Act to these children through either Title V (Maternal and Child Health) or Title XIX (Medicaid) programs because of the children's concurrent right to services under the EHA (PL 99-457, §203 [b] [3]). To ensure compliance with the new mandates, the 1986 EHA amendments also required the state educational agency to include in its EHA State Plan:

> . . . policies and procedures for developing and implementing interagency agreements between the State educational agency and other appropriate State and local agencies to (A) define the financial responsibility of each agency for providing handicapped children and youth with free appropriate public education, and (B) resolve interagency disputes, including procedures under which local educational agencies may initiate proceedings under the agreement in order to secure reimbursement from other agencies or otherwise implement the provisions of the agreement. (PL 99-457, §203 [b] [2])

The goal of the several new "financing" provisions in the 1986 amendments was clearly to ensure that the responsibility of health, mental health, social services, and vocational rehabilitation agencies to provide screening, individual evaluation, related services, and residential services (including room and board and nonmedical care) is not reduced, limited, or abdicated as a result of concurrent participation in the EHA Program B. To date, the Department of Education has not issued regulations designed to implement the new financing provisions, and few local education agencies have actually been able to access the funds available under Title XIX and other federal health programs to supplement the PL 94-142 contribution.

Ineffective Linkage between School Goals and Objectives and Postschool Demands

In light of both the community and individual social policy goals articulated earlier in this chapter, a major objective of the PL 94-142 program must be the provision of whatever educational, vocational, and support services are necessary to the development of skills and abilities required to achieve the maximum degree of personal autonomy, economic self-sufficiency, and social integration possible within the postschool period. In order to attain these goals, experience both in the United States and in other countries has demonstrated the crucial importance of individualized and flexible educational and supportive service arrangements that require the use of curricula and instructional methodologies geared toward the preparation of the student for postschool employment and community demands.

Both the National Council on Disabilities (1986) and the Disability Advisory Council (DAC) (Social Security Administration [SSA], 1988) in recent reports to Congress have identified four specific problems that directly and significantly contribute to the ineffectiveness of special education programs in terms of preparation for the postschool world:

1. The absence of comprehensive individual transition planning (during school years) and the resulting reliance on fragmented, unfocused planning procedures
2. Inadequate secondary school preparation, illustrated chiefly by the failure to establish postschool goals that form the basis for the establishment of both annual goals and short-term instructional objectives within the IEP
3. The abrupt discontinuation of the PL 94-142 entitlement approach at a crucial developmental point
4. The absence of parent and family involvement and the failure to incorporate (and to support the development of the skills necessary to permit) effective self-advocacy and self-determination in the identification of work and community life goals

Adequate secondary preparation of students with severe disabilities from school to work necessarily includes the use of both a comprehensive individual transition planning process and a flexible and individualized instructional and ongoing support system. Individual educational planning recognizes that the provision of effective educational, vocational, and support services to young persons with severe impairments requires both a holistic approach to client needs and the availability of a flexible, client-centered array of service options that permits services to be provided based on individual needs.

If needed skills are to be acquired, generalized, and maintained by young persons with severe impairments, curriculum and instructional methodologies must be used that effectively support the acquisition of skills and abilities needed for maximum choice of, and successful functioning in, postschool employment and community living environments. As part of this process, "learning by doing" within natural community settings must be the centerpiece of a "functional skills" curriculum that addresses not only the "vocational" skills needed for a particular job or job type but also the "learning" competencies, and the social interaction and communication skills necessary to function successfully in a variety of community settings and in any workplace, regardless of specific job assignment. It is important to recognize, however, that no mechanism currently exists within either the EHA or its implementing regulation to ensure that the annual goals and short-term instructional objectives that must be included in the annual IEP of each child with disabilities are linked to postschool employment and community life goals.

Because the attainment of a truly "adult" status necessarily involves the exercising of real choices with respect to the major decisions to be made in the various domains of adult life (e.g., friends, lifestyle, housing, employment), self-advocacy and decision-making components also must form an important part of the overall functional skills curriculum. Positive psychosocial environments within the school, work, and other community settings in which education occurs must be established and maintained, and the ongoing support of family members, employers, and other community members must be actively sought.

Unnecessary Segregation within Education Programs

PL 94-142 contains both a basic presumption in favor of integration of each school-age child with a disability in the regular educational environment and a mandate that, where placement outside of the regular classroom can be justified, public education agencies must place a child with disabilities in the least restrictive alternative setting (PL 94-142, §612 [5] [b]). The plain language of the statute, thus, creates a presumption in favor of regular classroom placement that may only be overcome by demonstrable evidence that education cannot be provided successfully in a regular class and in a typical school. During the 1980s, research demonstrated convincingly that it is possible for all students with severe disabilities, whether tethered to respirators or dependent on "clean intermittent catheterization," to attend regular schools (Biklen, 1988). Classroom integration at both the primary and secondary level has also become increasingly feasible for a substantial percentage of these students (Sailor et al., 1989). The concept of "integration" of students with severe disabilities within regular schools and classrooms clearly involves three separate aspects: physical integration, programmatic integration, and social integration (Sailor et al., 1989).

Successful integration most frequently has been the result of a conscious plan with strong leadership and administrative support (Biklen, 1988). Most successful integration efforts have incorporated all or most of the following elements: 1) teacher collaboration, including team teaching and consultant teaching; 2) high teacher expectations; 3) skilled teaching and technically sophisticated educational methods; 4) parent participation; and 5) opportunities for experiential learning (Biklen, 1988).

Research has also demonstrated that school and classroom integration yields a variety of positive educational results. The attitudes of students (both with and without disabilities) toward each other improve through exposure and interaction, and opportunities for friendships are created (Biklen, 1988; Sailor et al., 1989). The effective implementation of functional curricula for students with severe disabilities requires regular school placement.

National leaders in the field of education for children with severe disabilities agree that our system is a long way from "making the promise of integrated schooling universally available"

(Biklen, 1988, p. 3; see also Sailor, Gerry, & Wilson, in press). During the 1989 legislative reauthorization of the EHA and its amendments, the Education Task Force of the Consortium for Citizens with Disabilities (CCD) (a coalition of disability groups with representation in Washington) presented written testimony to Congress summarizing the principal problems encountered in the implementation of PL 94-142 (CCD, 1988). Ineffective implementation of the integrated placement or "least restrictive environment" provisions of the statute was cited by the task force as a major problem area. Likewise, in testimony before the Subcommittee on Select Education of the Committee on Education and Labor of the U.S. House of Representatives, Fred Orelove (1989), a noted researcher in the area, challenged Congress to address the discriminatory practices currently isolating students with severe disabilities in separate schools and classrooms.

A recent analysis of data collected annually by the U.S. Department of Education (1989) on students with disabilities reported by each state educational agency under PL 94-142 revealed that there has been little change in the use of separate facilities for students with disabilities since the passage of this act. Approximately 6% of special education students are in segregated day or residential schools; another 24% are placed in separate classes (DOE, 1989). These figures have remained stable over the past decade, indicating little progress in the nationwide understanding of placement in the least restrictive environment for students with severe disabilities. The state-by-state variation in figures is high, verifying the view expressed by Biklen (1988) that "one of the lessons to be learned from the situations of [individual students] is that where a student lives has a lot to do with whether he or she attends a regular school . . . " (p. 41). Other predictors of regular school attendance are state and local educational policy and the incentives or disincentives created by state special education funding formulas (Biklen, 1988). By the 1985–1986 school year, a few states, notably Oregon, Hawaii, Arkansas, and Iowa, had eliminated the segregation in separate schools of virtually all students with disabilities (Biklen, 1988).

In response to the continuing pattern of educa-

tional isolation for students with severe disabilities in most states and school districts, and reflecting recent trends in social policy, a strong integration movement, involving both parents and professionals, has emerged throughout the United States. This movement has as its primary objective the creation of an effective system of educational supports that will allow all students to attend school together, regardless of any disabilities. In many parts of this country, however, parents still must rely on administrative hearing officers and the courts to secure integrated educational opportunities for their sons and daughters with severe disabilities.

Legislation to Improve Programs Serving School-Age Children and Youth

As discussed earlier in this section, a large number of students with severe disabilities continue to be isolated from their nonhandicapped peers. Because an education in isolation does not best prepare an individual for an integrated adulthood, a number of amendments to PL 94-142 are recommended to mandate the development and implementation of *complete schools*. Specifically, we recommend that the statutes be revised to include a guarantee that individual students be provided whatever appropriate supports are necessary for them to function successfully in the natural school environment and to achieve and sustain gainful employment and to live as independently as possible in integrated, community settings in the postschool world.

The concept of a complete school is based on the presumption that all students, including those with severe disabilities, can attend the same public schools that they would attend if they were nondisabled. In addition, it is predicated on the assumptions that children learn from each other and that the skills needed for success in integrated community life and gainful employment are inevitably those needed for success in integrated school life.

Three important characteristics of the overall program of services that would be offered by a complete school are:

1. Individual evaluation (and periodic re-evaluations) of all students, which includes an appropriate assessment of personal autonomy

and self-advocacy, social skills and competencies, and work skills and competencies within integrated settings.

2. Individualized service programs (ISPs) would be developed for each student. For students over the age of 11, the ISP would be integrated within an annual individualized transition plan that also contains specific postschool employment and community living goals. These postschool goals (e.g., community living, competitive employment, supported employment, postsecondary education) would be used as the basis for defining both the annual goals and the short-term instructional objectives established by the ISP (SSA, 1988).

3. Parents would play an important role in the development of complete school models, and extensive parent training on the benefits of and strategies for achieving the integration of all students within the complete school would be provided.

Implementation of the new complete school concept would be accomplished through a series of interrelated administrative steps. First, an expanded research-and-demonstration program will be established under the EHA to identify, implement, and evaluate the range of educational support strategies necessary to provide quality services within the complete school. These research-and-development activities should include qualitative case studies of successful integration, research on student outcomes, research on funding strategies to remove fiscal barriers and to create fiscal incentives for integrated programming, and studies on the impact of integration on students with and without disabilities.

Second, based on these research activities, indepth technical assistance and consultation to states and school districts on integration and conversion to the complete school concept would be provided by federally funded, university-based, technical assistance centers.

Third, personnel preparation funds (Part D of EHA) will be earmarked for the training of both regular and special education policymakers, administrators, and teachers. Current preservice and inservice training efforts under the Comprehensive System of Personnel Development

now in effect under PL 94-142 within each state will be expanded. New training activities will focus on the training of experienced special educators to become "master teachers" in the complete school setting, and on the training for regular educators, educational administrators, related services personnel, and hearing officers on the special educational characteristics of individuals with severe disabilities and their integration into the complete school.

Finally, the new legislation will contain a specific prohibition against the use by states of educational financial systems that create financial incentives to place children in inappropriately restrictive environments, including residential placements, and in separate schools.

EFFECTIVENESS OF TRANSITION PROGRAMS

The absence of effective coordination among federal disability programs has had a severe, adverse impact on the transition of school-age children with severe disabilities from school to gainful employment. Extraordinary developments in medical and vocational rehabilitation programs and in education, habilitation, and employment transition strategies during the 1980s have demonstrated convincingly that a very high percentage of persons with even the most severe disabilities can reach or be restored to work capacity sufficient to achieve gainful employment.

One reason for the dramatic expansion of our awareness of the work potential of persons with severe disabilities has been the extraordinary success of *supported employment* and *independent living* strategies. Supported employment is a system of job training and support for persons with disabilities for whom competitive employment at or above the minimum wage without supports is unlikely. Supported employment involves the provision of intensive ongoing support (including supervision, training, and transportation) to individuals to perform in work settings in which nondisabled persons are employed. This range of services has included: direct job support and supervision during initial on-the-job training and orientation; intensive job coaching services as employee responsibilities are expanded; intervening support/coaching, if work performance problems are encountered; counseling; and transportation. While many different and successful supported employment programs have been demonstrated, there is general agreement that for persons participating in these programs, job-focused, community-based teaching should be initiated as early as possible, preferably prior to the beginning of secondary school.

Outcomes of Current Transition Programs

Only one third of youths with disabilities leaving school graduate to a job or some form of advanced education. This high rate of unemployment has been attributed to "the lack of an effective transition process from school to work for youths with disabilities" (NCD, 1986, p. 22). A dramatically lower rate of transition success (less than 5%) for young persons with severe disabilities has also been reported (SSA, 1988).

The ineffectiveness of the current transition process has been attributed to the absence of a systematic vocational transition process (NCD, 1986; SSA, 1988). It has been recommended that Congress direct the Department of Education to require state and local education agencies to initiate and carry out the transition process, "including contacting the appropriate personnel in regular and special education, vocational education, vocational rehabilitation, community colleges, developmental disabilities and other agencies from whom each student receives services" (NCD, 1986, pp. 22–23).

The 1988 report of the Disability Advisory Council to Congress also addressed the issue of the ineffectiveness of federal disability programs serving school-age children with severe disabilities attempting to transition from school to gainful employment and community living:

> Many children with developmental disabilities now leaving secondary school have significantly benefited from the passage of Federal and State equal opportunity laws, but few make a successful transition from school to sustained, gainful employment. It is estimated that in 1986, over 90 percent of these special education graduates left school for one form of dependency or another. (SSA, 1988, pp. 28–29)

Other indicators of the severity of current program fragmentation include (SSA, 1988):

1. Young persons with disabilities leaving Supplemental Security Income (SSI) and Disability Insurance (DI) benefit status as a result of gainful employment: fewer than 0.05%
2. Young persons with disabilities referred by SSA for vocational rehabilitation services (i.e., determined to have "rehabilitation potential"): fewer than 13%
3. Young persons with disabilities referred by SSA for vocational rehabilitation services who actually receive such services as a result of referral: fewer than 2%

Reasons for Ineffectiveness of Transition Programs

The direct link between these outcome measures and the ineffectiveness of current transition strategies appears well documented. Three specific problems that directly and significantly contribute to the ineffectiveness of special education programs in terms of preparation for the postschool world have been identified (SSA, 1988):

1. The absence of comprehensive individual transition planning (during the transition years) and the resulting reliance on fragmented, unfocused planning procedures
2. The absence of effective case advocacy and service coordination systems that maximize service continuity, coupled with the "selective" nature of vocational rehabilitation and developmental disabilities services
3. The absence of parent and family involvement in the determination of transition goals, service strategies, and service providers

The current lack of coordination among these programs in terms of support for the transition goal is exemplified by several characteristics of current program structure and operations. First, as is discussed above, PL 94-142 makes no direct reference to transition from school to work and adult life, and only a few states passed legislation during the 1980s designed to create comprehensive and coordinated (among the variety of responsible agencies) transition services. Second, the Developmentally Disabled Assistance and Bill of Rights Act (PL 98-257) established a nationwide program of assistance to states in developing comprehensive plans for meeting the needs of persons with developmental disabilities within the state but left control over the financial resources to implement such plans with the state Medicaid agency—not the state mental retardation and developmental disabilities agency. Finally, while Congress created a priority within the federal/state vocational rehabilitation (VR) system for serving persons with severe disabilities, the basic eligibility criterion for VR services (i.e., the ability of individuals to achieve gainful employment as a result of the provision of VR services) continues to inherently disadvantage those clients who have been least well served by the public schools (i.e., those in need of long-term services who are least likely to be quickly "rehabilitated").

Legislation to Support Transition, Employment, and Community Living

Because of the need of many persons with severe disabilities for long-term employment and community living support services, and the incompatibility of those service needs with the traditional VR program (Title I of the Rehabilitation Act of 1973, as amended), we recommend that Congress create a new comprehensive transition, employment, and independent living support program for persons with severe disabilities over the age of 13 and below the age for regular eligibility for SSA retirement benefits (i.e., 65). Under this program each eligible person will be entitled to receive whatever habilitative, training, and support services are necessary to maximize his or her economic self-sufficiency, personal autonomy and independence, and social integration and participation. Covered services would include: habilitation, including the development of social, self-advocacy, and work skills; vocational and job preparation; training and retraining; employment support services, such as attendant care and transportation; supported employment services, including job modification and restructuring, job sharing and pooling, job coaching, and co-worker support; and indepen-

dent living services, including housing and housing support services, health and mental health services, and recreation and social services.

This new, long-term support service program would be located at the federal level within the Office of Human Development Services of the Department of Health and Human Services. At the state level, the program would be under the overall supervision of a single state agency designated by the governor. Local administration would be assigned to a local transition council composed of representatives of state and local education agencies, developmental disabilities protection and advocacy programs, state Medicaid agencies, and state developmental disabilities/mental retardation programs.

Planning and delivery of all covered services to each eligible participant would be the responsibility of a case advocate appointed by the state protection and advocacy agency. Required procedures would include the development of annual individualized transition plans by an interagency committee that includes the participant with disabilities, other family members (where appropriate), the case advocate, employers, and co-workers. With training and support from the case advocate, eligible persons and their families would make all final decisions regarding plan goals, service strategies, and service providers.

The financing of this new entitlement program would be revenue neutral (i.e., derived from existing sources) and would include: 1) all of the funds appropriated under current supported employment authorities, 2) a substantial percentage of the funds (federal and state) appropriated under Title I of the Rehabilitation Act, 3) funds equal to a percentage (up to 25% of reductions over first 10 years; 10% of reductions over second 10 years) of the actual SSI/Medicaid and DI/Medicare benefit reductions that occur as a direct result of program-supported employment transition and employment support activities, and 4) Medicaid funds for community-based services available under Section 2176 of PL 100-203.

We also believe consideration should be given to the creation of a new "group advance" program within SSI, which would allow groups of beneficiaries to draw out capital from the SSA Trust Fund to finance entrepreneurial activities.

EFFECTIVENESS OF PROGRAMS FOR ADULTS

Persons with severe disabilities pursue the same personal goals as do persons without disabilities: a comfortable home, a meaningful job, and a social network of family members and friends. Where underlying social policies in a community have reflected a social philosophy of "inclusion," persons with disabilities have successfully achieved these goals and have emerged as valuable members of the overall community.

Unlike their nondisabled fellow citizens, however, persons with severe disabilities pursuing these goals must often overcome a series of unique barriers erected within social and economic institutions by a philosophy of "exclusion." These barriers are most frequently manifested through: the design of housing and transportation systems that are inaccessible to persons with physical, sensory, and communication disabilities; the development of employment training programs that fail to include job categories suitable for young persons with diverse skills and competencies; the organization of work in a manner that unnecessarily precludes the employment of persons with certain impairments; the creation of income and medical assistance programs that penalize or prevent integrated community life and gainful employment; the inaccessibility of appropriate health insurance coverage within the private sector; and the inflexible and categorical (rather than individualized) nature of personal and family support systems (NCD, 1986; SSA, 1988).

In fact, many of the federal programs designed to ensure equal opportunity contribute to the establishment or maintenance of these barriers rather than to their elimination; in many instances, the current ineffectiveness of the system has led directly to the unemployment and institutionalization of large numbers of individuals with severe disabilities. Our analyses of these problems suggest that each of the following factors have contributed significantly:

1. The absence of an appropriate range of community-based services (including personal assistance services) under the Medicaid program

2. The inadequate financing and lack of coordination between the Department of Housing and Urban Development programs and other federal disability programs, such as the Independent Living Centers program administered by the Department of Education

3. The ineffectiveness of income maintenance and rehabilitation programs in assisting persons with severe disabilities to enter or reenter the labor market

4. The failure of the responsible federal agencies (i.e., SSA, Department of Labor, Department of Justice) to ensure that persons with disabilities are not unlawfully terminated from work

Absence of Community-Based Medicaid Services

In 1978, Congress incorporated a program of Comprehensive Independent Living in Title VII of the Rehabilitation Act, a program administered by the Department of Education. Independent living is also a major program goal of the Developmental Disabilities programs administered by the Department of Health and Human Services. Also, the Developmental Disabilities Act of 1984 established "employment related activities" as one of four priority services to be provided under the basic support grant program. The Intermediate Care Facility/Mental Retardation (ICF/MR) program, however, represents the major source of federal support for the ongoing care of adults with severe disabilities.

ICF/MR Program

The ICF/MR program is well known for its institutional care bias and has been strongly resistant to the establishment and expansion of community-based care alternatives. As a direct result of this bias, relatively few opportunities have been created for individuals to receive Medicaid-reimbursed services provided in community-based settings. In 1981, Title XIX of the Social Security Act was amended to allow the Secretary of Health and Human Services to grant waivers to states to use Medicaid funds to pay for nonmedical services (outside of the ICF/MR program) to persons who are elderly or who

have disabilities and who would otherwise require institutionalization. The Home and Community Based Waivers program was explicitly
designed to promote the development and provision of community-based care and to avoid nee-
dless institutionalization.

In practice, the program has been ineffective
due primarily to the difficulty in demonstrating
that persons to receive community-based services would, in fact, be institutionalized in the
absence of such services. Indeed, the "institutional bias" of the ICF/MR program has continued to dominate overall funding patterns. For
example, the federal share of expenditures for
institutional services under the program has
increased from 23% to 45% during the last decade, whereas the federal share of community-
based services has increased from 6% to only
21%. State general funds account for 70% of
community care services (Conley & Noble,
1988). The institutional program bias of the ICF/
MR program is also strengthened by incentives
linked to prior capital investment practices.
Since 1975, states have "sunk" substantial sums
of state money in the improvement of large residential facilities (Conley & Noble, 1988), which
they are reluctant to abandon for several reasons:

1. "Sunk" costs can only be recovered through
    continued use of residential facilities.
2. The capital cost of developing community
    residential facilities that are not ICF/MR
    certified must be entirely financed by state
    and local funds.
3. State and local agencies must pay all of the
    operating costs of "noncertified" facilities.
4. The ICF/MR medical decision-making
    model greatly simplifies administration al-
    though it is completely incompatible with
    any work orientation.
5. The open-ended character of the ICF/MR
    program allows states to "pass along" wage
    and benefit increases demanded by em-
    ployee unions.

NCD (1986) summarized the current situation
as follows: "If community-based independent
living is to become a realistic goal for Americans
with severe disabilities, institutional bias within
Medicaid and other programs funded under the
Social Security Act must be replaced by a prefer-

ence for community-based services" (pp. 43–
44). Current Title XIX requirements mandating
the involvement of medical professionals in the
delivery of all services hinder the ability of persons with disabilities to live independently by
preventing the delivery of needed personal assistance services, including attendants, readers, in-
terpreters, and advocates (NCD, 1986).

Legislation to Establish a Program of Community-Based Services under Medicaid

Several excellent legislative proposals to reform
the current institution-biased Medicaid structure
have been before the Congress in recent years.
We believe that Congress should enact the Medicaid Home and Community Quality Services
Act of 1987, or similar legislation, to allow states
more flexibility to fund community and family
support services for persons with severe disabilities who are living with their own families; in
their own homes; or in community-based, integrated, family-scale environments. Any appropriate legislative reform of the current Medicaid
system encompasses the following elements:

1. A shift should occur in the underlying ideol-
    ogy of the current federal Medicaid policy
    from one embracing large institutional set-
    tings as the residence of choice for people
    with mental retardation and related condi-
    tions to one embracing an array of small,
    family-type residential options in the com-
    munity and services that foster a full inter-
    pretation of productivity, independence,
    and integration. Federal funding for ser-
    vices in large institutional settings should be
    phased out (or down) over a 10-year period
    with an immediate freeze on an increased
    funding of services provided in institutional
    settings.
2. Medicaid eligibility standards should be
    modified to include any child who meets the
    nonincome-related SSI eligibility standards
    (described earlier), through a special "dis-
    regard" of family income for children with
    severe disabilities.
3. A required group of core community-based
    services should be mandated within each
    state Medicaid plan, including: 1) indepen-
    dent case advocacy and management, 2)

respite care and personal assistance, 3) protective intervention, and 4) supported employment and other vocational services resulting in maximal vocational opportunities.

4. As a prerequisite to Medicaid funding, each state should be required to prepare and submit an implementation strategy to the Secretary of Health and Human Services including: 1) a description of the community and family support services that will be provided; 2) a 5-year plan for the expansion of these services; 3) a procedure for ensuring that each individual currently living in an institution be given a real option to move into the community any time he or she chooses, consistent with the standards and procedures described in a written, individualized transfer plan that is in place before the actual transfer occurs; and 4) a quality assurance system.

5. An independent system of protection and advocacy for persons residing in community settings and a private right-of-action to enforce the guarantees of the program directly in federal district court should be established.

Access to Health Care

In 1987, approximately $443 billion were expended for personal health care in the United States. Of this total, hospital care accounted for approximately $194 billion, physician services for approximately $102 billion, and nursing home care for approximately $41 billion. Expenditures for other professional services, including home health care, nurses, and rehabilitation therapists during the same year amounted to slightly more than $16 billion; expenditures for other personal care were approximately $12 billion (Griss, 1989; Health Care Financing Administration [HCFA], 1988).

The primary government financier of personal health care is the Medicare program, established in 1965 under Title XVIII of the Social Security Act. Medicare is a federally administered and financed health insurance program, which in 1984 enrolled over 30 million Americans: 27 million over the age of 65, including both persons with and persons without disabilities; and 3 million

persons under the age of 65, with disabilities (HCFA, 1988).

The second largest government financier of personal health care is the Medicaid program, established in 1965 under Title XIX of the Social Security Act. Unlike Medicare, Medicaid is a social welfare–based (rather than insurance-based) approach to health care. It is administered by state agencies and jointly financed from federal and state governments, and serves over 23.2 million poor persons. This total includes over 2.5 million persons with disabilities eligible for cash assistance under the SSI program (HCFA, 1988; *Social Security Bulletin,* 1988).

Of the total amount ($443 billion) spent for personal health care in 1987, approximately $177 billion (40%) was contributed by government, approximately $139 billion (31%) was collected from private health insurance, and approximately $127 billion (29%) was paid directly by patients and their families (Griss, 1989). The percentage of personal health care payments derived from each of these sources is not uniform across different personal health care service categories. For example, government is the largest payer of hospital costs, with Medicare alone providing over 27% of all payments and Medicaid providing over 9%. In contrast, government pays approximately 31% of the total cost of physician services, with Medicare contributing almost 22%. Because of the presence of deductibles and co-insurance requirements in private health insurance and Medicare, patients and their families bear almost 26% of the costs of physician services (Griss, 1989).

Due to the acute care–oriented design of the Medicare program, only 1.4% of the costs of nursing home care are borne by the Medicare program despite the average age of beneficiaries; private insurance sources contribute less than 5%. In contrast, Medicaid covers both acute care and long-term care and contributes approximately 44% of the funds supporting nursing home care. Patients and their families currently bear the remaining 49 + % of the costs of nursing home care and an even greater share of the costs of items such as nondurable medical supplies and drugs (74.8%) and durable medical equipment (66.3%) (Griss, 1989).

Within this general health care system, persons with severe disabilities and their families have experienced a number of important problems relating to access to private health insurance and to appropriate health care services under both the Medicare and Medicaid programs.

Access to Private Health Insurance

Experience has shown that many private insurers react strongly to a request by an employer for health insurance to cover a small group if it includes any persons whom the private insurer considers to have a "high risk." In some instances, private insurers have demanded a substantially higher premium for such coverage; in others, private insurers have simply refused to provide such group coverage (U.S. Congress, Office of Technology Assessment [OTA], 1988).

At present, while there are laws in several states prohibiting discrimination against persons with disabilities by insurers, no clear definition of what constitutes insurance discrimination has emerged (OTA, 1988). In the absence of both a national nondiscrimination standard and an employer mandate to provide private health insurance, many employers, particularly small employers, have elected either not to hire persons with severe disabilities or not to provide group health care coverage to employees (Griss, 1989). Both results have had serious adverse consequences for adults with severe disabilities seeking employment and access to private health insurance. The general unavailability of private health insurance coverage that includes long-term support for chronic health care conditions (including a range of health, social services, and long-term care options) also creates a major disincentive for people with severe disabilities considering reentry into the labor market (Griss, 1989).

Access to Appropriate Health Care under Medicare

The current design of the Medicare program creates four important barriers for persons with severe disabilities seeking access to appropriate health care. First, individuals with severe disabilities seeking DI benefits must wait 5 months from the onset of the disabling conditions before

filing a benefit application. Once that application is approved (which takes from 90 days to 3 years), a DI beneficiary must wait an additional 2 years from the time that his or her DI eligibility is established before applying for Medicare benefits. Taken together, these waiting periods impose at least a 3-year delay in access to Medicare benefits (regardless of whether the prospective applicant has private health insurance) at a time where medical intervention is most important in terms of potential reemployment (SSA, 1988).

Second, the Medicare program is patterned on the acute care–orientation of private health insurance and, therefore, does not cover preventive or wellness care, or ongoing maintenance services. In fact, the personal assistance and self-care services needed by a substantial number of persons with severe disabilities are generally excluded from reimbursement under Medicare on the theory that they are "custodial" in nature (Griss, 1989).

Third, Medicare provides only very limited coverage of outpatient mental health services, thus preventing persons with mental impairments from receiving primary care to any meaningful degree, creating a major incentive for unnecessary institutionalization, and denying other persons with severe disabilities the mental health support that may be crucial to sustaining employment and community living.

Fourth, the current structure of the Medicare program creates major problems of economic access for many persons with severe disabilities and their families. Unlike Medicaid, Medicare imposes premium, deductible, and co-payment requirements that are difficult for low-income persons to satisfy (Rowland & Lyons, 1987).

Access to Appropriate Health Care under Medicaid

The current design of the Medicaid program creates two important barriers for persons with severe disabilities seeking access to appropriate health care. First, individuals with severe disabilities under the age of 18 seeking SSI benefits must demonstrate that the family's income and assets are below a certain prescribed level. This requirement has created an incentive for families, particularly those composed of persons in the "working poor" category just above the prescribed level, to place a child in an institution in order to create eligibility for Medicaid coverage. Congress has responded to this problem by allowing (but not mandating) states to disregard the family income ceiling where a child is at risk of institutionalization (Griss, 1989).

Second, many state Medicaid agencies have been allowed under the present program to establish inappropriately low reimbursement rates that have a punitive effect on Medicaid beneficiaries seeking services in various categories (GAO, 1987).

In 1989, Congress created a new Medicare-eligible category entitled "disabled and working," for DI beneficiaries who return to work and earn above the permissible level of monthly earnings ($500, effective January 1, 1990) (Omnibus Budget Reconciliation Act of 1989). Persons in this new category are permitted to "purchase" Medicare coverage so long as the impairment continues that originally qualified them for DI benefits. Payment of the Medicare premium for such individuals will be made by the state Medicaid agency or by the beneficiary, depending on income level and countable assets.

Legislation to
Improve Access to Health Care

We believe that Congress should consider the enactment of new Medicare legislation to include coverage of long-term home care, to eliminate the Medicare waiting period for DI beneficiaries, and to establish a special Medicare "buy-in" procedure. Several legislative proposals have been introduced to add a long-term care component to the Medicare program. While we are not prepared to endorse any of these proposal in toto, we believe that any long-term care program to be added to the Medicare program should include the following elements:

1. Eligibility should be based on functional, cognitive, and behavioral limitations, or the need for supervision because of risk to safety or health, and should not be limited by age or income.
2. Long-term care services should be available in both facility-based and community-based

alternatives; should assist families and informal caregivers; and should include a range of health, social, and individual and family support services.
3. Financing of long-term care should be progressive and the financial risk should be spread as broadly as possible, with both cost-containment mechanisms and protection for persons of low and moderate income from excessive out-of-pocket costs.
4. The program should incorporate an independent care coordination component with aggressive strategies for ensuring full access and acceptable quality of care.

The problems posed for DI beneficiaries by the current 2-year waiting period for Medicare eligibility have been discussed earlier in this chapter. In fact, a recent study shows that 27% of new DI beneficiaries were without any health insurance during the last 6 months of the Medicare waiting period (Griss, 1989). We recommend that Congress eliminate the current waiting period, reduce the current DI waiting period from 5 to 3 months, and establish a concurrent DI and Medicare application and eligibility process similar to that used for the SSI/Medicaid program.

We believe that Congress should consider the enactment of new Medicaid legislation to permit several categories of persons who have difficulty purchasing private health insurance and are not currently eligible for Medicaid benefits to "buy in." These categories include: 1) persons whose income is less than 200% of the poverty level, 2) persons with "pre-existing conditions" who are rejected by private insurers, 3) persons who exhaust the benefit levels of their private insurance coverage, and 4) small employers who cannot purchase affordable health insurance in the private market for their employees. The amount of the buy-in premium would be determined by community-rated experiences of all covered persons; the percentage of the premium (from 0% to 100%) paid by an individual would be based on his or her income level.

Barriers in Housing and Transportation

Persons with severe disabilities are currently subject to discrimination in housing (both private residential and commercial) and by public transportation systems. Examples of housing discrimination include restrictive zoning practices of localities, refusal to provide reasonable accessibility to multiunit residential property, and denial of access to public accommodations. While discrimination against persons with disabilities in housing (public and most private) has been prohibited by recent amendments to Title VIII of the Civil Rights Act of 1968, the unavailability of accessible housing and transportation and the denial of access to many public accommodations (e.g., restaurants, theatres, arenas) continue to pose major problems for persons with severe disabilities seeking to obtain or maintain gainful employment and participate fully in community life.

The Department of Housing and Urban Development administers two housing programs of particular importance to persons with severe disabilities. The first of these, the Section 202 program, provides federal construction and rehabilitation loans to support the development of accessible housing. The second, the Section 8 rent subsidy program, provides housing assistance for eligible tenants with handicaps in rent-subsidized housing. In fact, the Section 8 subsidies have encouraged housing developers to construct Section 202 housing units because they create assured rent revenues. Unfortunately, in practice, the administration of these programs has often resulted in the inappropriate social isolation of persons with severe disabilities (NCD, 1986).

To address the "bricks-and-mortar" issues of community living, we recommend that Congress enact legislation to lower interest rates on FHA financing for the construction and/or remodeling of fully "accessible" single- and multiple-family dwellings. Similarly, we believe Congress should consider the establishment of a new tax credit for private lenders who finance the construction or remodeling costs of homes for individuals with severe disabilities.

Ineffectiveness of Income Maintenance and Rehabilitation Programs

As discussed earlier, the vast majority of adults with severe disabilities are precluded from gain-

ful employment by current policies and practices. Most of these individuals receive cash benefits under the SSI program and medical assistance under the Medicaid program; a significant number of children and a rapidly growing number of young adults with severe disabilities (particularly those with severe mental health problems) receive cash benefits under the DI program and medical assistance under the Medicare program.

Congress has established three basic criteria for determining individual eligibility under both the DI and SSI programs (SSA, 1988): 1) the presence and anticipated long-term continuation of a severe physical and/or mental impairment, 2) the incapacity for gainful employment, and 3) the lack of income (DI) and financial resources (SSI only). A review of the underlying legislation (and its legislative history) indicates that Congress has established two basic goals for both the DI and the SSI programs (SSA, 1988): 1) provide cash and related medical benefits to persons with disabilities, without undue delay or expense but only so long as those disabilities are present (i.e., maximize the efficiency and effectiveness of the eligibility determination and review process); and 2) ensure the provision of services necessary to assist as many beneficiaries as is possible to achieve and sustain gainful employment (i.e., maximize the effectiveness of current strategies in assisting beneficiaries to work).

Three major problems appear to contribute directly and significantly to the ineffectiveness of income maintenance and related rehabilitation programs in providing appropriate services to persons with severe disabilities (NCD, 1986; SSA, 1988):

1. The unavailability of effective job training and supported employment services within the universe of programs (disability specific and generic) administered by a variety of federal agencies

2. The ineffectiveness of the VR system and the vocational rehabilitation referral procedures mandated by Congress under the SSI and DI programs ("the SSA/VR referral process")

3. The adverse effect of remaining work disincentives within several federal disability programs

Unavailable Job Training and Supported Employment Services

The Job Training and Partnership Act (JTPA) program administered by the Department of Labor supports the operation of local job training projects (directed by local Private Industry Councils) to increase the employment of persons who are unemployed. At present, no formal coordination arrangements exist between local JTPA programs and state VR systems or the regular or special vocational education programs administered by local school districts. As a result of the absence of program coordination and the use of income eligibility criteria, which penalize persons with disabilities (because of the receipt of cash benefit payments), the JTPA program does not adequately serve persons with disabilities (NCD, 1986). One solution to this problem would be for JTPA programs to expand to include vocational education and vocational rehabilitation components appropriate to the needs of persons with disabilities and for Private Industry Councils to place a priority upon the participation of persons with disabilities in JTPA programs.

As discussed earlier, supported employment initiatives have concentrated on the community-based development of job skills (including basic job-related behavior and co-worker interaction) and related independent living skills and have presented employers with a range of separately funded postemployment support services. The provision of supported employment services may be financed under several different federal disability and "generic" programs, including Titles I and VI of the Rehabilitation Act, the ICF/MR program, and Title XX of the Social Security Act. At present, the funds available for supported employment under each and all of these programs are totally inadequate and little coordination exists among these programs regarding the planning and provision of supported employment services. Because the major source of ongoing funding for adults with developmental disabilities remains the Title XIX program, the absence of community-based habilitation services is a direct result of the continuing institutional bias of that program, as discussed in detail earlier.

Without changes in the overall structure of current services programs, comparatively few individuals who are now dependent on the SSI system for income are likely to reach a point at which they are confronted by realistic opportunities to enter the competitive labor market.

Ineffectiveness of Current Vocational Rehabilitation Systems

The VR program, established by Congress under Title I of the Rehabilitation Act, is operated and administered through a combination of state agencies (which receive 80% of their funds from federal appropriations and 20% from state appropriations) and private entities (which receive funding from special project grants). The Title I program requires that vocational rehabilitation and related support services be provided to individuals who have physical or mental disabilities that substantially impede employment potential *if* this potential may reasonably be expected to increase through rehabilitation services. The Title I program is not, however, an entitlement program; substantial numbers of eligible persons (estimated to exceed 75% of the total eligible population of persons with disabilities) in most states do not receive services under the program because of limitations imposed by funding levels (SSA, 1988).

Current law also establishes an order of priority that must be followed in selecting participants for the Title I program, the first priority being persons with severe disabilities. The definition of severe disability within the VR system includes lesser disabilities than the definition adopted by TASH; historically, persons falling within the TASH definition have been excluded from the system due to the severity of their disabilities. In fact, the effectiveness of the VR system in successfully rehabilitating clients with severe disabilities has actually decreased during the last decade (SSA, 1988).

As discussed earlier in this chapter, in 1986 Congress added supported employment and independent living objectives to the overall rehabilitation program through the creation of a new Title VI, but did not alter the basic features of the short-term intervention model governing the basic Title I program. However, expanded employment-related support services are available to persons with more severe disabilities who participate in the newly established supported employment programs.

Ineffectiveness of the SSA/VR System

In furtherance of the employment-related goals of the DI and SSI programs, Congress enacted legislation requiring the Social Security Administration to "refer" all DI and SSI applicants and beneficiaries who it determined might achieve substantial gainful employment to the state VR agency for vocational rehabilitation and related employment services. SSA studies reveal that when such services have actually been provided to DI and SSI applicants and beneficiaries, the results both for the individuals involved and for the SSA Trust Fund (or general revenues) have been positive and impressive. A benefit recidivism rate of less than 8% has occurred for DI and SSI beneficiaries who achieve gainful employment, with substantial savings in SSA cash and medical benefit payments (SSA, 1988).

Under SSA's current VR referral programs, however, only a small percentage of disability applicants and beneficiaries are referred for VR services by state disability determination service (DDS) units, and few of those referred ever receive such services. In 1986, nationwide, only 12.1% of all persons submitting allowed DI and SSI applications were referred by DDS units for employment services, and fewer than 15% of those referred for services ever actually entered the VR system (SSA, 1988). The criteria currently used by DDS units to "screen" applicants and beneficiaries for "referral" effectively preclude the identification and referral of many persons with severe disabilities (SSA, 1988).

SSA reimburses state VR agencies for a portion of the expenditures made by those agencies for services successfully provided to referred applicants or beneficiaries who achieve substantial gainful employment (as defined by SSA standards) for a period of 9 months. The traditional standard of program success under the VR program differs substantially, however, from the standard established for reimbursement from SSA. In fact, the state VR agency does not serve as a direct service provider but utilizes a wide variety of public and private agencies to actually deliver services.

The Disability Advisory Council, in analyzing the current operation of the SSA/VR referral system, concluded that for SSI beneficiaries "appropriate and timely VR services, including habilitation services for SSI recipients who may never have worked, can help move such beneficiaries into the workforce" (SSA, 1988, p. 27). Despite uniform SSA referral guidelines, a highly variable DDS referral rate exists among states and much of this variation appears to be attributable to differences in VR service capacity and service priorities. Current information collected by SSA strongly indicated that many DDS units refer substantially more applicants for employment services than could be accommodated within the existing VR system (particularly with respect to counselor caseload capacity) on the expectation that only a small percentage of persons served will ever pursue VR services (SSA, 1988). In fact, some DDS units only refer DI and SSI applicants for employment services who fall within certain disability categories (SSA, 1988). The ineffectiveness and frequently arbitrary nature of this referral process is particularly troubling, because in many states the DDS unit and the state VR agency are organizational components of the same agency.

Program coordination between SSA and the Department of Education and the federal/state VR system is virtually nonexistent, despite the apparently "coordinated" nature of the referral process (SSA, 1988). At present, SSA does not track persons referred by DDS units for employment services in order to see if such services are actually requested and/or provided. SSA also does not attempt to evaluate, either periodically or on an ongoing basis, the "quality" of employment services provided (in terms of their actual contribution to restored work capacity or subsequent gainful employment) or their cost-effectiveness.

In sum, despite the fact that more than sufficient funds currently exist within the SSA Trust Fund to finance all needed habilitation and rehabilitation services, four specific program coordination and administration factors (SSA, 1988) appear to have contributed to the ineffectiveness of the SSA/VR referral system:

1. The failure to provide rehabilitation services to clients at the earliest possible time, including the serious underidentification of DI and SSI applicants and beneficiaries in need of VR services (including short-term intervention); the extraordinarily low percentage of persons needing such services who actually receive them; and the understandable reluctance within the DDS units to refer persons who are never served

2. The absence of ongoing case management and the lack of beneficiary participation in the establishment of job goals and the selection of direct service providers

3. The lack of competition among services planners and providers and the frequent absence of direct employer involvement in the establishment of job goals and in the actual provision of employment services

4. The absence of effective program coordination or supervision by SSA, including both tracking and quality control functions, to support the employment goals of both the DI and the SSI programs

Work Disincentives

Work disincentives of several kinds currently operate within the structure of federal disability programs to defeat the attainment of economic independence for persons with severe disabilities not currently in the work force (NCD, 1986). In 1986 NCD reported that "some Federal programs under current Social Security laws not only fail to promote employment and independence for citizens with disabilities, but actually penalize and discourage people with disabilities if they seek to become employed" (p. 27) and identified several types of work disincentives operating within the SSI and Medicaid programs, including: 1) the inability of employed persons with disabilities to obtain adequate health insurance at an affordable cost, 2) the net reduction in income to SSI beneficiaries that would result if they sought employment in many entry-level and low-paying service jobs, and 3) the loss of medical and other benefits that would also result from such employment.

However, in 1988 Congress made permanent several important provisions contained in Section 1619 of the Social Security Act that dramatically reduce the impact of these work disincentives. Section 1619(a) allows an SSI beneficiary, whose impairment continues, to earn above a fixed minimum level (now at $500 per month) and continue to receive both cash benefits and Medicaid coverage. Until the enactment of Section 1619, any earned income above this fixed amount could result in immediate termination of benefits under both programs. Under the new provisions, SSI benefits are reduced gradually as earned income increases, and eligibility for medical benefits (under Section 1619[b]) may continue even after SSI benefits have been terminated. Persons receiving extended medical benefits under the Section 1619(b) program, however, must still have an annual income below the threshold level for SSI eligibility.

While these changes will be of great value to those SSI beneficiaries who are currently able (or who become able) to choose sustained gainful employment, parallel changes need to be made in the original eligibility standard of "not engaging in substantial gainful activity." That standard is currently set at $500 per month— well below the federally defined poverty level! Moreover, the ineffectiveness of the federal/state VR program will continue to frustrate overall effectiveness because comparatively few young persons eligible for SSI benefits are likely to reach a point at which they are confronted by a realistic choice of whether to enter the competitive labor market (SSA, 1988). Many SSI beneficiaries may also be reluctant to take advantage of the Section 1619 incentives because the effect of these provisions on continuing disability review determinations remains unclear. In this regard, the SSA observed:

Based on the very limited use of SSA's existing work incentives thus far, it is reasonable to assume that work incentives alone are not likely to bring about significant behavioral change for DI and SSI beneficiaries who are disabled or blind. To increase return to work significantly, a comprehensive approach is required, including effective work incentives which are clearly communicated, timely referral to service providers, and efficient and effective job training and placement methods. (1988, p. 75)

The second and third elements in this comprehensive approach clearly depend on improvement in the training and habilitation programs funded by the Departments of Education, Health and Human Services, and Labor.

Legislation to Improve Income Maintenance and Rehabilitation Programs

Changes in the tax code could provide incentives for employers to absorb directly the fiscal impact of employment programs aimed at increasing the participation of persons with severe disabilities in the competitive labor market. Specifically, we recommend that income tax deductions and/or credits be established for employers to encourage employer support for work training, trial work, and permanent employment of persons with severe disabilities, including the costs of: ongoing supported employment, job modification and restructuring, short-term declines in productivity, fringe benefits, facility and equipment modification, counseling, and employee training.

We also believe careful consideration should be given to the establishment of a Federal Insurance Contributions Act (FICA)–based employer incentive for the hiring of persons with severe disabilities. Such an incentive could be established by permitting employers who employ a certain number or percentage of persons with severe disabilities within the employer's work force to reduce the employer's biweekly or monthly DI contribution (paid as part of the current 7.65% FICA contribution). A tax credit should also be established for a portion of the employer's cost of health insurance provided for part-time or full-time employees with severe disabilities.

Legislation to Prevent Unlawful Employment Practices

The major problem undercutting the effectiveness of federal efforts to prevent unlawful employment discrimination against persons with disabilities is the absence of a general federal statutory ban against such discrimination, comparable in scope to Title VII of the Civil Rights Act of 1972 (which bans employment discrimination against persons on the basis of race, national origin, sex, and religion by all employers

of 15 or more persons). Even absent such a statute, active enforcement of two current statutory provisions (Section 503 and 504 of the Rehabilitation Act of 1973), which ban employment discrimination against persons with disabilities by federal contractors and grantees, would have a positive impact in preventing the unnecessary unemployment of persons with disabilities (SSA, 1988). A significant number of persons with severe disabilities who ultimately enter the DI population are employed prior to the onset of the disabling condition (or its increased severity); in many instances, employers, using reasonable modifications to existing job structures, facilities, equipment, and training programs, could reasonably accommodate these employees with severe disabilities within their work forces (SSA, 1988). These accommodations could be sufficient either to permit an employee to retain his or her current job, on either a full-time or part-time basis, or to allow the employer to assign the employee to a different job (existing or newly created) within the overall work force, consistent with the employer's overall work force needs.

We recommend that Congress enact legislation to extend to persons with physical or mental disabilities the equal employment opportunity guarantees contained in Title VII of the Civil Rights Act of 1964 and the nondiscrimination in public accommodations requirements of Title II of that act. Such legislation should also include a specific requirement that employers make reasonable accommodations to avoid the termination of employees with disabilities when such termination is related to a physical or mental impairment.

CONCLUSION

Despite major legislative and programmatic accomplishments of the past 20 years, significant changes in the current design of federal programs serving persons with severe disabilities must be made if we are to overcome the legacy of over 200 years of social and economic injustice. We believe that these changes are likely to occur only if a new inclusive American social policy is adopted that employs a common set of both individual and community goals governing the impact of federal programs upon all of our citizens —including those with severe disabilities and their families. Within this context, legislation in a wide variety of areas, including education, health, human services, housing, and transportation, must be reviewed and, where necessary, revised to ensure a "normalized" and integrative impact upon all segments of our population.

In the preparation of this analysis, we have concentrated our attention on those federal programs of general applicability with which we are most familiar, and within which we believe change to be most urgent. However, because persons with severe disabilities should benefit from all such federal programs, this effort must necessarily be regarded as incomplete.

Specifically, we recommend changes, including expansion of federal financial support, increased parent participation and case advocacy, and decreased social isolation in the operation of current programs serving infants and toddlers. For school-age children and youth, we propose the passage of new federal legislation to support the development and implementation of "com-

plete schools" serving all children, including those with severe disabilities. This legislation would complement, rather than replace, the equal educational opportunity guarantees of PL 94-142.

For young persons with severe disabilities seeking to "transition" from school to work, we propose the establishment of a new comprehensive transition, employment, and independent living support program under the auspices of the Department of Health and Human Services. We further believe that comprehensive federal legislation is needed to establish a program of community-based services under Medicaid. In our view, significant changes should also be made in the structures of both the Medicaid and Medicare programs to ensure the equal access of persons with severe disabilities to the full range of health benefits provided by those programs. Finally, we propose changes in income maintenance and rehabilitation programs to eliminate work disincentives and other inequities within the existing structures, and we recommend expansion of current civil rights laws to ensure equal opportunity.

REFERENCES

Biklen, D., (1988, November 21). [Paper for the Leadership Institute on Community Integration]. Unpublished manuscript, Alexandria, VA.

Castro, G., & Mastropieri, M. (1986). The efficacy of early intervention programs for handicapped children: A meta-analysis. *Exceptional Children, 52*(5), 417–424.

Conley, R.W., & Noble, J. (1988). Americans with severe disabilities: Victims of outmoded policies. In J. Goodgold (Ed.), *Handbook of rehabilitation medicine* (pp. 924–941). St. Louis, MO: C.V. Mosby.

Consortium for Citizens with Developmental Disabilities. (1988). *Analysis of the President's FY 1989 budget proposals and recommended appropriation levels relating to programs for people with developmental disabilities.* Washington, DC: Author.

Donst, C.W., Snyder, S.W., & Mankinen, M. (1986). *Efficacy of early intervention.* Chapter prepared for the Research Integration Project Final Report, University of Pittsburgh, PA (U.S. ED Grant #GO08400748).

Education of the Handicapped Act, Part B, §§602(17), 612(5)(b) (1975).

Griss, B. (1989). Strategies for adapting the private

and public health insurance systems to the health related needs of persons with disabilities or chronic illness [Special Issue]. *Access to Health Care, 1*(3–4).

Health Care Financing Administration. (1988). *Health care financing: Program statistics, Medicare and Medicaid data book* (HCFA Publication No. 03270). Washington, DC: U.S. Government Printing Office.

Kakalik, J.S., & Furry, W.S. (1982). *The cost of special education.* Santa Monica, CA: Rand Corporation.

National Council on Disabilities. (1986). *Toward independence.* (Library of Congress Catalog Number 85-082605). Washington, DC: U.S. Government Printing Office.

Orelove, F. (1989, April 4). [Testimony before the Subcommittee on Select Education of the Committee on Education and Labor of the U.S. House of Representatives].

Rowland, D., & Lyons, B. (1987). *Medicare poor: Filling the gaps in medical coverage for low-income elderly Americans.* Baltimore: Commonwealth Fund Commission on Elderly People Living Alone.

Sailor, W., Anderson, J.L., Halvorsen, A.T., Doering, K., Filler, J., & Goetz, L. (1989). *The comprehensive local school: Regular education for all students with disabilities*. Baltimore: Paul H. Brookes Publishing Co.

Sailor, W., Gerry, M., & Wilson, W. (in press). Policy implications of full inclusion models. In M. Wang, H. Walberg, & M. Reynolds (Eds.), *The handbook of special education* (Vol. IV). Oxford, England: Pergamon Press.

Social Security Administration. (1988). *Report of the Disability Advisory Council*. Baltimore: Author.

Social Security Bulletin, Annual Statistical Supplement. (1988). pp. 55–57.

U.S. Congress. (1983). *The Report from the Commission on the Financing of a Free Appropriate Education For Special Needs Children*. Philadelphia: Research for Better Schools.

U.S. Department of Education. (1987). *Ninth annual report to Congress on the implementation of the Education of the Handicapped Act*. Washington, DC: U.S. Government Printing Office.

U.S. Department of Education. (1989). *Eleventh annual report to Congress on the implementation of the Education of the Handicapped Act*. Washington, DC: U.S. Government Printing Office.

U.S. General Accounting Office. (1986). *Financing health and educational services for handicapped children*. Washington, DC: U.S. Government Printing Office.

U.S. General Accounting Office. (1987). *Medicaid interstate variations in benefits and expenditures* (Publication No. GAO HRD-87-67BR). Washington, DC: U.S. Government Printing Office.

Weiss, R. (1981). INREAL intervention for language handicapped and bilingual children. *Journal of the Division for Early Childhood*, *4*, 40–51.

White, K.R., & Greenspan, S.P. (1987). An overview of the effectiveness of preventive early intervention programs. In I.R. Berlin & J. Noshpitz (Eds.), *Basic handbook of child psychiatry* (pp. 541–553). New York: Basic Books.

Appendix 30.1. Federal Resources for Programs Affecting Individuals with Severe Disabilities

Agency	Program	Authority	Description
Dept. of Education OSEP	Basic State Grant	EHA, Part B	Formula grants to states to partially cover cost of free and appropriate education to all students with handicaps; includes two mandates: preschool (3–5) and school age (5–18/22)
Dept. of Education OSEP	Regional Resource Centers	EHA, Part C	Grants to establish and operate centers providing advice and technical assistance to special educators and administrators
Dept. of Education OSEP	Services for Deaf-Blind Children & Youth	EHA, Part C	Discretionary grants or cooperative agreements and contracts to assist state educational agencies in the education of students with deafness-blindness (technical assistance, preservice, inservice, program replication, facilitation of parent involvement)
Dept. of Education OSEP	Handicapped Children Early Education Program	EHA, Part C	Discretionary grants for projects that focus on services for children with handicaps from birth to 8 (research, demonstration, outreach, training, and technical assistance)
Dept. of Education OSEP	Innovative Programs for Severely Handicapped Children	EHA, Part C	Discretionary grants or cooperative agreements and contracts for projects with innovative approaches to the education of students with severe handicaps (research, demonstration, technical assistance, inservice training, information, and material dissemination)
Dept. of Education OSEP	Postsecondary Education	EHA, Part C	Discretionary grants or contracts for postsecondary program development, operation, and information dissemination (vocational, postsecondary, technical, continuing or adult education)
Dept. of Education OSEP	Secondary Education and Transitional Services	EHA, Part C	Discretionary grants and cooperative agreements for projects focusing on student transition from school to adult activities (postsecondary programs, vocational training, competitive work, continuing education, adult services)
Dept. of Education OSEP	Grants for Personnel Training	EHA, Part D	Grants to institutions of higher education or other nonprofit agencies to train special education/related services personnel

(continued)

Appendix 30.1. *(continued)*

Agency	Program	Authority	Description
Dept. of Education OSEP	Parent Training Centers	EHA, Part D	Grants to nonprofit organizations to provide information and training for parents of students with disabilities and to persons who work with these parents
Dept. of Education OSEP	Clearinghouses	EHA, Part D	Three national clearinghouses: 1) education of children and youth with handicaps, 2) postsecondary services for individuals with handicaps, and 3) special education personnel recruitment
Dept. of Education OSEP	Research & Demonstration	EHA, Part E	Discretionary grants for research, demonstration, and related activities to strengthen special education
Dept. of Education OSEP	Instructional Media & Captioned Film	EHA, Part F	Discretionary grants or contracts to support instructional media and captioned film activities
Dept. of Education OSEP	Technology, Educational Media, & Materials	EHA, Part G	Discretionary grants or contracts/cooperative agreements to advance the use of new technologies, media, and materials used in the education of students with disabilities
Dept. of Education OSEP	Handicapped Infants & Toddlers	EHA, Part H	State grants to assist in the development of statewide, comprehensive interagency services for infants and toddlers with disabilities
Dept. of Education OSEP	State-Operated Programs	ECIA, PL 89-313	Assistance to the states for supplementary supports for students who are or have been enrolled in state-operated programs; includes authority to transfer funds from state program to LEA
Dept. of Education	Vocational Education	Carl Perkins Vocational Education Act	Assistance to states for vocational education programs including students with disabilities
Dept. of Education RSA	Basic Federal-State Vocational Rehabilitation	Rehabilitation Act of 1973, amended	Formula grants to state vocational rehabilitation agencies for services to individuals with disabilities
Dept. of Education RSA	CAP	Rehabilitation Act of 1973, amended	Grants to states' system of protections in assessing rehabilitation services; includes assistance in securing legal/administrative remedies, when needed
Dept. of Education RSA	Innovation & Expansion Grants	Rehabilitation Act of 1973, amended, Title I	Research grants to develop, initiate, and expand rehabilitation services to persons with severe disabilities

(continued)

Appendix 30.1. *(continued)*

Agency	Program	Authority	Description
Dept. of Education RSA	Special Projects & Supplementary Services: Severely Disabled Project; Handicapped Youth Job Training; Supported Employment Special Demonstration; Recreation.	Rehabilitation Act of 1973, amended, Title III, Sec. 311	Discretionary grants for research and demonstration to assist in the rehabilitation of persons with severe disabilities
Dept. of Education RSA	Supported Employment	Rehabilitation Act of 1973, amended, Title VI	Grants to states to assist the development of collaborative, interagency supported employment
Dept. of Education RSA	Comprehensive Services for Independent Living; Centers for Independent Living	Rehabilitation Act of 1973, amended, Title VII	Grants to agency within the state to provide independent living services for persons with severe disabilities
Dept. of Education RSA	National Institute for Disability and Rehabilitation Research	Rehabilitation Act of 1973, amended, Title II	Grants for research, demonstration, and related activities focusing on improved methods for rehabilitation; Rehabilitation Research & Training Centers
Dept. of Labor	JTPA	Job Training Partnership Act	Formula funding for training and placement for persons who are economically disadvantaged, including individuals with disabilities; also, job training research, demonstration, and development projects; Job Corps Program for ages 14–22 (beyond 22 if there is a disability)
IRS	Targeted Jobs Tax Credits	Tax Reduction and Simplification Act	Special tax credit for businesses who hire workers, including persons with disabilities
Dept. of HHS MCH	Maternal & Child Health Services Block Grant	Social Security Act, Title V	Block grants to states to assist in improving the system of health care for mothers and children who have no access to adequate health services (includes prenatal care)
Dept. of HHS MCH	Maternal & Child Health Services, SPRANS	Social Security Act, Title V	Set-aside of 15% of MCH Block Grant for personnel training and research in a number of specific areas, including genetic disease projects, UAPs, and special projects for children with special health needs: primary health care, community service networks, and case management
Dept. of HHS NIH	NICHD	Public Health Services Act, Title IV	Research, training, information dissemination, and related activities regarding maternal and child health, mental retardation, and human development

(continued)

Appendix 30.1. *(continued)*

Agency	Program	Authority	Description
Dept. of HHS ADD	Developmental Disabilities: Basic Grants to States for Planning & Services	DD Assistance and Bill of Rights Act, Part B	Formula grants to states to establish and operate state planning councils to help develop, review, and oversee state plans for systems of service for people with developmental disabilities (identify existing service gaps and set service priorities)
Dept. of HHS ADD	Protection & Advocacy Systems	DD Assistance and Bill of Rights Act, Part C	Formula grants to states for a system of rights protections
Dept. of HHS ADD	University Affiliated Programs	DD Assistance and Bill of Rights Act, Part D	Grants to support administration and operation of UAP interdisciplinary personnel training
Dept. of HHS SSA	SSI	Social Security Act, Title XVI	Direct monthly cash payments to provide minimum income for individuals who meet financial needs test and who are elderly, blind or disabled; major income source for many people with severe handicaps
Dept. of HHS SSA	Old Age Survivors & Disability Insurance Benefits, Adult Disabled Child Program	Social Security Act, Title II	Direct monthly cash payments to surviving children of workers who are retired, deceased, or disabled who were eligible to receive Social Security benefits, if the age of onset for the disability was prior to 22
Dept. of HHS SSA	Social Security Experimental & Demonstration Projects	Social Security Act, Sec. 702	Grants for research studies on the nature of disabilities and the impact on the ability of an individual to function in society; alternative work strategies
Dept. of HHS HCFA	Medicaid	Social Security Act, Title XIX Medical care	Federal-state matching funds for medical care for individuals meeting needs test (AFDC, SSI, or other state-determined criteria; medically needy; or SSI §1619 [a] & [b]; certain more generic medical care services are mandated for state delivery—others are optional
Dept. of HHS HCFA	ICF/MR; HCBW	Social Security Act, Title XIX	Long-term care for individuals with mental retardation and related conditions who need active treatment; traditional funding for large institutional care—used in some states to create small community residences; states may apply for waiver allowing services to a limited number of people in the community
Dept. of HHS OHDS	Social Services Block Grant	Social Security Act, Title XX	Block grant to states for social services, services that states determine; in some states a major source of community services for people with severe handicaps

(continued)

Appendix 30.1. *(continued)*

Agency	Program	Authority	Description
Dept. of HUD	Lower Income Housing; Housing Vouchers	Housing Act of 1937, amended Sec. 8	Direct payments and vouchers providing rental subsidies for housing costs of eligible persons; eligibility based on income and may include individuals with handicaps
Dept. of HUD	Congregate Housing	Housing Act of 1937, amended Sec. 7	Contracts with local authorities to provide social services to "frail elderly and handicapped individuals"; at a minimum the services include two meals a day—may also include transportation, personal care, and housekeeping
Dept. of HUD	Rural Housing	Housing Act of 1949, amended	Guaranteed loans and rent subsidies for low-income rural housing (includes people with disabilities)
Dept. of HUD	Section 202 Direct Loans	Housing Act of 1959, amended	Long-term direct federal loans to private nonprofit corporations and consumer cooperatives to provide housing for persons who are elderly or handicapped
Dept. of HUD	Supportive Housing Demonstration Program	Housing Act of 1959, amended	Transitional and permanent housing for people who are homeless and have disabilities; includes some services such as nutritional counseling, job training, child care, and transportation
Dept. of Transportation UMTA	Urban Mass Transit Grants; Rural & Small Community Transit Grants; Urban Mass Transportation Technology Research and Demonstration; Transportation Technical Studies	Urban Mass Transportation Act Amendments	Numerous programs in the Dept. of Transportation provide transportation resources for: assisting persons with disabilities to enhance access to transportation (separate rural and urban programs); projects focusing on national transportation priorities, including transportation for persons with disabilities; demonstration of innovative techniques and methods; demonstration of identification and training for transit operators and individuals with disabilities

ADD = Administration on Developmental Disabilities
AFDC = Aid to Families with Dependent Children
CAP = Client Assistance Program
dd or DD = Developmental disability(ies)
ECIA = Education Consolidation and Improvement Act
EHA = Education of the Handicapped Act
HCBW = Home and Community Based Waiver
HCFA = Health Care Finance Administration
HHS = Health and Human Services
HUD = Housing and Urban Development
ICF/MR = Intermediate Care Facility/Mental Retardation
IRS = Internal Revenue Service
JTPA = Job Training Partnership Act

LEA = Local education agency
MCH = Maternal and Child Health
NICHD = National Institute on Child Health and Human Development
NIH = National Institutes of Health
OHDS = Office of Human Development Services
OSEP = Office of Special Education Programs
RSA = Rehabilitation Services Administration
SPRANS = Special Projects of Regional and National Significance
SSA = Social Security Administration
SSI = Supplemental Security Income
UAP = University Affiliated Program
UMTA = Urban Mass Transportation Administration

CHAPTER 31

Community Services for Adults with Disabilities
Policy Challenges in the Emerging Support Paradigm

MICHAEL W. SMULL
University of Maryland at Baltimore, Baltimore, Maryland

G. THOMAS BELLAMY
U.S. Department of Education, Washington, D.C.

More than 20 years ago the President's Committee on Mental Retardation (PCMR) reviewed the services of the time and reported that "there is little good news in writing about residential facilities in the United States. . . . Typically, public residential facilities have been plagued by a triple problem: overcrowding, under-staffing, and underfinancing" (Kugel, 1969, p. 1). PCMR recommended a two-part solution that included the development of small community programs as well as institutional reform. As these recommendations were implemented nationally, the concepts of normalization and deinstitutionalization became the foundation for a new paradigm of services that emphasized a continuum of small residential and day programs dispersed throughout the community.

CRISIS IN THE COMMUNITY

By most measures, the community programs that resulted from this paradigm shift have been successful. From 1976 to 1986, the number of people living in institutions nationally declined by one third (Braddock, Hemp, & Fuijiura, 1986) while the percentage of people living in relatively small (15 or fewer beds) community residences increased from 16.3% to 41.3% of the total served (Lakin, Hill, White, & Wright,

1987). As states moved to serve people in smaller and smaller groups, researchers repeatedly demonstrated the benefits of community programs for individuals with disabilities (Conroy & Bradley, 1985; Eastwood & Fisher, 1988; Haney, 1988).

Despite these successes, a crisis threatens the foundations of the community program movement, and has led to proposals for an alternative conceptual framework for services (Minnesota State Planning Council on Developmental Disabilities, 1987). The symptoms of the crisis are problems of scarcity and quality. There are insufficient funds, staff, and program alternatives. Demands and expectations have risen far faster than resources. The slack in the system that was used to cope with unanticipated problems is gone. While most state institutions are operating at capacity with plans to reduce their census (Lakin et al., 1989), many community programs are unable to attract staff at current salaries and they have few vacancies and no plans to expand (New York Office of Mental Retardation and Developmental Disabilities, 1987). Waiting lists for services are growing rapidly, and the families and individuals who are waiting have little hope for assistance (Smull, Sachs, Cahn, & Feder, 1988).

Problems of quality in the community exacer-

This chapter is based in part on a paper, *Crisis in the Community* (1989), by Michael W. Smull, distributed by the National Association of State Mental Retardation Program Directors, Alexandria, Virginia. Dr. Bellamy's contribution to the chapter was undertaken in his private capacity. No official support or endorsement by the Department of Education is intended or should be inferred.

bate the scarcity of services. One investigator found that the abuse of psychotropic medications was more common in community programs than in the institution (Conroy, in press). Newspapers have reported a few community programs where the quality of services is so abysmal that state agencies have forced management changes or closure. While success is still the rule, there is increasing concern that the social segregation of the institution has been traded for social isolation in the community (Bercovici, 1983).

The needs to improve the quality of community programs, expand services to accommodate individuals on waiting lists, and reduce the size of institutions constitute a set of mutually reinforcing pressures on available resources. Yesterday's solution has become today's crisis.

Need for a New Paradigm

The challenge to those responsible for public policy is to reconceptualize how services are designed and developed. Continuing present policies will not work. Projections of funding, staffing, and housing required to alleviate current problems are staggering. A substantial increase in federal financing of community services would be required to solve current problems with staff salaries and to expand the system for those waiting. Even if these funds were available, the pool of potential qualified residential staff may not be adequate, given the demographics of a shrinking labor force and the competition with business for entry-level employees (Smith, 1988). And, if staff could be recruited, the community program model offers too few lifestyle alternatives for the diverse individuals it seeks to serve.

As the expansion of community programs was a response to a crisis in institutional services, the answer to a crisis in the community is not a return to the institution. Institutions have experienced a continuous crisis in attempts to meet evolving interpretations of the minimally acceptable quality of services. To reach quality standards imposed by courts and federal agencies, many states continue efforts to reduce the size of institutions by expanding community programs. The irony is that the institutional crisis we were to solve 20 years ago and today's community crisis have remarkable parallels. The problems of

underfinancing and understaffing cited by the PCMR (Kugel, 1969) are the same problems that face community programs today.

The present can be made better. Better management, more training, and increased funding could make marked improvements in community services. But these are interim solutions. They postpone, but do not prevent, looming disasters in community services. If we are to ensure quality in the existing system and provide a reasonable array of services to those people who are waiting, a more fundamental change in service design is required. We need another paradigm shift.

Support Paradigm

In Kuhn's (1962) formulation, a paradigm shift occurs when so many anomalies have arisen in an existing conceptualization that it is replaced by a new conceptual framework. Under the current paradigm, programs are developed on the basis of a few shared characteristics of the persons served (e.g., severe mental retardation). Even when organized in a continuum of services of varying intensity, the program paradigm has only been partially successful in meeting the diverse needs and preferences of individuals who happen to share some of the same labels. The program paradigm has had difficulty in assisting people to participate fully in the community or to make use of available informal resources. The needed alternative begins with the individual, looks to the resources of the individual's community, and then develops flexible supports that allow participation in the community in response to individual choices. The needed shift is from a paradigm of community programs to a paradigm of individual supports.

The support paradigm is based on several shifts in thinking about disability and public services. While many of these concepts have been present for some time in the professional and advocacy literature, they combine to form an important new basis for thinking about services. The shifts in thinking include:

1. *Shifting view of disability, from an emphasis on individual limitations to a focus on environmental constraints* In 1980, the World Health Organization captured profound changes

in the view of disability in its definitions of impairment, disability, and handicap. In this formulation, an impairment refers to a loss or abnormality of anatomical, psychological, or physiological function. A disability is any restriction of ability (resulting from an impairment) to perform an activity in the manner or within the range considered normal for a human being. A handicap is the disadvantage that results for an individual as a result of an impairment or disability that limits or prevents the fulfillment of a role that is normal for the individual. For example, an injury to the spinal cord (an impairment) may result in the loss of the ability to walk independently (a disability); depending on the accessibility of the community, this may or may not affect the individual's ability to get to work, sports events, and stores (a handicap). It is the interaction between the disability and the environment that is the focus. Rather than labeling the person as "handicapped," it is possible to ask what is needed in the environment to prevent a disability from becoming a handicap. What would the environment need to be like so that no disadvantage results for the individual who experiences a disability? When this question is asked, attention is shifted to eliminating barriers in the physical and social environment, rather than assuming that the entire problem lies in the person (Hahn, 1989).

2. *Shifting emphasis in the public role, from providing community readiness programs to guaranteeing access and providing support* The view that disability and environmental constraints interact to produce handicaps is reflected in changes in advocacy for public programs. In general, there has been a shift from remediation of an individual's deficits and toward environmental changes that enable his or her participation in regular community life. This change is evident in two recent developments. The first is the effort to establish rights of access to regular environments through legal and legislative action. The Americans with Disabilities Act now pending in the Congress exemplifies this approach. The second has been the effort to establish ongoing support services that allow all individuals to participate successfully in community settings. The federal supported employment program is an example of this strategy of shifting from remedial programming to the provision of support in regular settings.

3. *Shifting emphasis in the individualized assessment and planning process from diagnostic-prescriptive approaches to choice-based approaches* Practically all federal programs for individuals with disabilities now involve a formal, individualized mechanism for assessing service needs and planning services to meet those needs. What is changing is the way individual goals are set. Rather than identifying deficits that a program should remediate through treatment or training goals, the alternative is based on identification of people's aspirations and choices about the settings they want to participate in and the roles they wish to emphasize (e.g., Wilcox & Bellamy, 1987). Supporting adults with disabilities in regular adult roles and circumstances means allowing and assisting them to make the same kinds of choices that others make. Where someone lives and works and with whom he or she spends time are matters of personal choice and resources, not matters of diagnosis, disability label, or professional judgment.

4. *Shift in service location, from separate programs to integrated settings* Accompanying the focus on supporting people in natural settings is an increasing emphasis on the social characteristics of those settings. Regular contact and friendships with others in the community is a choice that most people make. Achieving these social outcomes, however, involves not just a change in location, but also an adjustment in service content. Sustaining regular contacts and developing friendships often requires planned opportunities for people to be together, support for initial interactions, and advocacy on behalf of individuals who have difficulty meeting others (e.g., Strully & Strully, 1989).

5. *Shifting emphasis in service strategy, from formal to informal supports* There is an increasing interest in using informal supports to implement individual choices and connect people with the community. When they are available, natural, informal networks of support—family members, co-workers, friends, neighbors, and so on—offer a more flexible and less intrusive means to reach the goal of preventing a disability from becoming a handicap. Several

authors (Forest & Lusthaus, 1988; Mount & Zwernik, 1988; O'Brien, 1987) describe planning strategies designed to assess and expand the informal support resources that can support an individual's lifestyle choices. Program development is underway to replace previously paid staff support functions with paid and unpaid informal supports of co-workers, family members, and friends (Nisbet & Callahan, 1987; Rusch & Hughes, 1988).

These changes in thinking combine to provide a new framework for serving individuals with developmental disabilities. The new framework—the support paradigm—defines the goal of public services as supporting each individual in achieving his or her chosen lifestyle by offering supports to supplement those that are available informally (Froland, Pancoast, Chapman, & Kimboko, 1981).

Elements of the emerging support paradigm are already visible in many community services and a few government programs. One example is the supported employment services that have emerged as alternatives to separate community vocational programs. While these vocational programs emphasized preparation for later employment by helping individuals overcome disabilities, supported employment looks for immediate employment opportunities in regular settings with ongoing support (Bellamy, Rhodes, Mank, & Albin, 1987).

Many supported living programs reflect a similar view: that individuals should live in their own homes, and receive enough support to do so successfully—not to be prepared for later independent living through training in specialized community residences (Bellamy & Horner, 1988; Taylor, Biklen, & Knoll, 1987). Efforts to enhance the functioning of natural supports, rather than replace these with formal programs, are also apparent in the emerging strategies to provide family support and develop friendship networks (Taylor, Racino, Knoll, & Lutfiya, 1987).

As these support services continue to develop, no doubt the distinctions among residential, employment, and leisure services, which reflect constraints of the earlier program paradigm, will blur. Support in the community need not be bound by traditional program distinctions. More generic services may emerge as formal and informal supports are effectively blended. An interesting possibility for service development is analogous to the "cafeteria" models adopted for employee benefit (support) plans in industry. In these plans, employers provide a variety of benefits from which an employee chooses a customized package within a specified total cost.

POLICY CHALLENGES

While current governmental policies have been sufficiently flexible in some areas to allow initial development of support services, it is the creativity and effort of local service providers that must be given most of the credit for the success to date. The challenge for government is to sustain these gains, encourage further development, and make the benefits of the support paradigm more widely available.

The support paradigm is a set of ideas, not a policy blueprint. It can help to clarify policy goals, and by extension, define the policy development challenges that must be addressed if it is to be fostered through government action. Specific solutions to the policy challenges must be developed in the political context of existing state and federal programs.

The policy goals in the support paradigm are not unlike those of earlier approaches to serving persons with developmental disabilities. Differences in emphasis do, however, have important implications for policy and program development. The public's interests in services in the support paradigm might be summarized in the following goals:

1. That adults with disabilities have opportunities to enjoy lifestyles of their own choosing with a quality of life as similar as possible to others in the community
2. That government policies and actions support individuals in relying on their own skills and resources in achieving their chosen lifestyles
3. That, as needed, publicly funded support be available to foster individual quality of life in accordance with individual choices and aspirations

4. That, whenever possible, public resources be used to augment, not replace, the informal assistance desired by the individual from families, friends, and others
5. That public resources providing this support be used efficiently and equitably

Significant policy development challenges exist in at least four major areas if these goals are to be reached: 1) allocation of public resources for support services, 2) administration of services to achieve results, 3) coordination of the local provision of supports, and 4) building the community capacity to provide formal and informal supports.

Allocation of Public Resources

Given the continuing gap between pressing service needs and available resources, the way public agencies allocate and control funding is central to the effectiveness and stability of any social service. The policy development challenge in the support paradigm is to determine what services are to be purchased, who will receive those services, and how much is to be paid.

In the program paradigm, funds are typically used to purchase a category of program (group home, supported apartment, intensive training home, etc.) for individuals who are accepted for those services. Program categories typically are defined by intensity of supervision or other services, and by categories of staff roles. Within this structure, allocation of resources is typically controlled in three ways:

1. *Determining who receives services* In most states, the number of individuals who meet eligibility requirements far exceeds the number who actually receive services. Others are on waiting lists for services until funding becomes available.
2. *Determining which programs these individuals receive* When programs are available that offer different levels of service, there is a bias to place individuals in the program that meets their labeled needs at the lowest cost to the level of government making the placement decision.
3. *Funding programs below the cost of operation* This practice relies on nonprofit pro-

gram providers to generate revenue from the community to meet the cost of services.

Despite efforts to differentiate several types and levels of program categories, this general strategy of program-based funding creates inequities and inefficiencies in the distribution of resources. Inefficiencies result because program categories do not reflect the complexity of the individuals who are served, and because programs are not structured to make use of informal supports. Individuals whose support needs could be met with a combination of informal supports and technology may find themselves in far more expensive group living situations where support needs are met entirely with paid staff. A number of other individuals may be labeled as having maladaptive behavior and receive excess supervision in an effort to compensate for a poor match between the individuals and their environment. Much of the inequity is the result of judging individuals' readiness for community programs by asking whether their needs appear to fit the services that are already offered. The availability and utilization of informal supports is rarely considered. The result is that many are not served at all, some are underserved, and others are overserved.

The support paradigm challenges government agencies to replace program-based funding and rate setting with *individual* decisions about the level of funding required to supplement informal assistance and reach chosen goals. The policy goal is to tailor the level of funding to the individual and his or her existing support resources, thereby eliminating the inequities and inefficiencies of the current pattern of overservice for some and underservice for others. This necessarily means that resource allocation decisions will be made locally, by persons knowledgeable about the individuals with disabilities and their particular circumstances.

The support paradigm is not a panacea for the overall funding problems in the service system. As long as the demand for services exceeds the resources available to meet the demand there will be continuous pressure to find cheaper ways to deliver the services and stretch the finite resources to meet more of the demand. Regardless of the service paradigm used, the costs of serv-

ing all of those waiting will be substantial. There
is no answer to meeting the needs of those waiting that does not require a significant increase in
funding.

There are insufficient data to determine whether
the support paradigm will be cheaper than the
program paradigm. The available information
indicates that a broadly applied support paradigm is likely to provide mixed results. For those
individuals whose programs provide more services than they need, the support paradigm will
be cheaper. For those individuals for whom extensive formal supports are required, the support
paradigm could be no cheaper and could be more
expensive. For those individuals already being
served, the change from a program paradigm to
a support paradigm could result in better services but there is insufficient information to argue that it will be significantly cheaper. Greater
efficiencies in staff utilization may allow providers to increase pay without an increase in
funding but it is unlikely that they will achieve
efficiencies sufficient to raise salaries to the levels required to attract and retain qualified staff.

If the costs of serving everyone waiting for
services is projected, a support paradigm is
likely to be cheaper than the comparable cost of
the program paradigm. Some out-of-home services will be deferred, a number of people will
make use of informal supports at no cost, creative living situations will be developed, and
employment using co-workers for support will
become more frequent. More expensive situations will be common as well. There will be a
number of people living by themselves or with
one other person with extensive support needs.
On balance it seems likely that the efficiencies of
the support paradigm would make it less costly
when looking at the service requests of everyone
but not necessarily cheaper for any individual.

Administering for Results

Public agencies that administer services for
adults with developmental disabilities are responsible for ensuring that funds are used for the
purposes for which they were appropriated, that
individual rights are protected, and that the services purchased address the problems for which
funds were provided. The issue of effectiveness is becoming more and more prominent. A

crowded agenda of service problems makes it
necessary for those responsible for budget decisions to consider not just the need, but also the
likelihood of impact on that need in making
funding decisions (e.g., Walter & Choate,
1984). Consequently, the policy challenge is to
design a system that ensures not just that services are provided as planned, but also that consumers of those services enjoy the intended results.

In the program paradigm, accountable administration was typically sought through program
regulations and requirements for program accreditation. The result was to further standardize
the services available in any particular type of
program, and to create burdensome requirements to document the process of service delivery.

The flexibility of services to be provided in the
support paradigm and the range of people who
provide those supports precludes conventional
program regulation and accreditation approaches.
Because of the varying roles of formal and informal helpers, and because it is unreasonable to
expect that providers of informal assistance will
document their activities, there is little utility in
requiring a set of program activities with particular participants and documentation at each step.

The central challenge to policymakers is to
develop accountability systems that give maximum local flexibility in support procedures to
be used, while ensuring that the goals for which
funds were appropriated remain the focus of the
program. With creative development, measures
of outcomes for people with disabilities—their
lifestyles, quality of life, earnings, social networks, living environments, and so on—could
provide the focal point for public administration
of support services, replacing much of the current process regulation of programs. While this
approach will require development of practical
measures of valued outcomes, it reflects a growing trend toward results-based management of
social services by state and local governments
(Millar & Millar, 1981).

While important quality improvements can
result from outcome monitoring, reasonable
oversight is still required. Not all providers of
support will perform as they should. And, common concerns for health, safety, and protection

of individual rights necessitate some process regulation. These regulations should include requirements that: 1) support plans be developed that document the choices of the individual, the input of others significant to the person's life, the choices that are to be implemented, and the actions and responsibilities for implementation; 2) the implementation of the plans be documented through oversight/monitoring by the relevant professionals; 3) the outcome specified in the plan is achieved; 4) regular assessment of consumer satisfaction be completed; and 5) reasonable standards of safety for the person are met.

Carefully drawn regulations that address these areas should encourage the use of supports and allow for the flexibility and responsiveness required. They should also provide for a determination of outcomes and activities sufficient to maintain minimum standards and serve as the basis for evaluation of effectiveness.

Local Management

The actual implementation of most social services is guided by "street-level bureaucrats" (Weatherly & Lipsky, 1977), the individuals who interact directly with consumers of services as the public agency's representative. How this role is structured is an important policy development issue that can affect the nature of the assistance provided. In the program paradigm, individuals hired as case managers or service coordinators have generally filled this role, with widely varied responsibilities for actual program implementation.

The local management role assumes considerably more importance under the support paradigm because of the flexibility for local decision making. Flexible and responsive services that are individually developed and implemented require that there be individuals who have the requisite skills and authority, and who also know the persons being supported, their circumstances, and the available resources. The real task of local managers is to prevent or diminish the degree to which an individual's disability becomes a handicap. These people should know how to find, nurture, and involve informal supports while assisting the formal support providers to fill gaps in the least intrusive manner.

The policy development challenge is to structure this "support coordinator" role so that it is sufficiently flexible, accountable, protected from local distortion, and attractive to competent professionals.

There are four critical components of the support coordinator's role. The first is identification of individuals who meet eligibility requirements for services. Funds for support services likely will continue to be available only to individuals who meet criteria specified in law or regulation. Determining whether someone meets these standards usually means ascertaining that he or she experiences a disability of a certain type or level. Such a determination may have little or no relevance to decisions about actual delivery of services, but is an essential aspect of the agency's accountability for public funds.

The second component of the support coordinator's role is to ensure that individual support plans are developed. The support coordinator may be the facilitator or leader as this plan is developed, depending on the choices and resources of the individual. Regardless of the role, the support coordinator must have an understanding of the individual that goes beyond standard assessments and includes the preferences, desires, and dislikes of the individual. Development of the plan should include the input of other persons significant to the individual. The support plan should reflect: 1) a broad assessment of the current lifestyle of the individual, 2) the individual's choices about how that lifestyle should change, 3) a description of the individual's resources for self-reliance and informal support to achieve the chosen changes, and 4) a description of the publicly funded supports that will be provided to assist in realizing these choices.

The opportunities and choices available to any individual, with or without disabilities, depend on the individual's skills, financial resources, and support network, as well as the availability of public support. Public support is constrained by local, state, and federal budget allocations, and by the purposes for which various programs are established and funded. One of the challenges for the support coordinator is to assist the individual effectively within the limitations imposed by available resources. An effective policy structure will give the support coordinator a framework for making the resource allocation decisions that financial constraints necessitate, but will maintain sufficient flexibility for the coordinator to address unique needs.

The lifestyle choices available to an individual are also constrained by an inherent bias in the use of public funds. People with disabilities seek to have lives of their own choosing with the highest quality of life. Their objectives are to maximize choice and opportunities without regard to cost. The publicly funded service system seeks to serve the largest number of people, for the smallest number of tax dollars, with each person achieving a reasonable quality of life. The implementation of the support paradigm, using public funding, will result in a bias toward self-reliance and reliance on informal supports. Adequately funded, this will produce minimal conflicts between the choices of the person and the goals of the public system. However, some tension between the public service system and the advocacy community should be anticipated.

The third component of the support coordinator's role is to purchase the formal supports that are needed to implement an individual's plan. Under the program paradigm, residential- and day-program providers typically receive funding for slots. In effect, they are funded for maintaining a service capacity. Under the support paradigm, discrete components of support are provided based on choice and the informal supports available. Both the choices and the available informal supports will change over time. To meet the demand for responsiveness and flexibility, the support coordinator acts as the agent of the individual to secure the needed supports. This fiscal role for the support coordinator makes it difficult for him or her to serve any other support or program function without debilitating conflicts of interest. Appropriate safeguards, such as the establishment of standard rates or the approval of support plans by the funding agency, should provide for local control of individual funding within the context of budget allocations.

The fourth component of the support coordinator's role is documentation. Not only must there be sufficient information to assess whether the public's interest is served by the support coordinator's decisions, but there must also be records that prevent discontinuity of service when personnel changes occur. Information should be available to determine the quality of support coordination in relation to such expectations as: 1) the extent to which the individual is satisfied with the support and its results; 2) the extent to which individual support plans are implemented, so that chosen futures are actually realized; 3) the extent to which informal supports are located and used, so that public resources fund only the necessary formal support; and 4) the relationship between the overall expenditure of public funds and the quality of life of the individuals for whom the support coordinator is responsible. While these criteria serve to highlight the need for practical measures, they nevertheless offer a direction for outcome accountability for support coordination.

Developing Capacity

Public funds result in adequate support only when people are present who care and who have expertise to provide the support. Without systematic investment in the capacity of communities to provide support, little can be expected from public funds allocated for this purpose. Needed public investments in capacity are of three kinds: knowledge development, personnel development, and public information.

New knowledge is continually needed to meet the challenges that arise as new opportunities, new populations, new aspirations, and new barriers are encountered in providing support. Developing and communicating that knowledge requires an active program of applied research and dissemination. There has been research funding from the Administration on Developmental Disabilities, the National Institute on Disability and Rehabilitation Research, and the Rehabilitation Services Administration that address issues of providing ongoing support in community settings. However, a coordinated research effort is needed. Research needs include, for example, efforts to address practical and theoretical issues in assessing choice and quality of life, to establish a decision framework for combining public and private supports, and to solve treatment and training problems that arise as individuals with more and more challenging disabilities aspire to increasingly integrated and productive lives.

The second aspect of capacity building is personnel development designed to ensure a sufficient supply of adequately trained individuals to offer professional assistance where needed. There are currently some efforts to train individuals for community support roles, such as job coaches and community guides. To implement the support paradigm, federal leadership will be needed to build consensus on job roles in the support paradigm, and then to invest in the recruitment and preparation of individuals for those roles. As support roles are analyzed, it is likely that many of the distinctions between job coaches, community guides, community support specialists, and support coordinators will be discarded as remnants of the program paradigm. If this is true, then the outline of a more general support professional role is badly needed, so that federal investments in personnel training can be more focused on the emerging needs.

The third aspect, public information, is seldom viewed as a capacity-building investment, but it is critical to the support paradigm. It is highly unlikely that individuals with disabilities can enjoy a high quality of life without active support from family members, friends, neighbors, co-workers, and others. Public information efforts that assist community members in recognizing opportunities to provide assistance and support, and that increase the likelihood that they will do so, are a critical part of building the capacity to provide support in the community.

The policy challenge is to create a mechanism for systematic investment in the development of knowledge, professional staff, and public awareness so that communities will have the capacity to use to the best advantage the funds that are appropriated for support services.

CONCLUSION

Whether one views the development of flexible, individual supports as an evolutionary development from community programs or as a more radical shift away from those programs, the goals of supporting individuals in chosen community settings creates significant challenges for government agencies. Examples of the support paradigm are in place across the country, but most of these exist because of the skill and enthusiasm of staff, parents, or agency boards. Many of the emerging examples have the encouragement of public agencies, but few of those agencies have approached the task of making similar services available to all individuals with disabilities in a state or region. As this is done, the support paradigm will be associated not just with the innovative services and outcomes of pioneers, but also with the results of underfunded supports, cosmetic attempts to reform existing agencies, inadequate local administration, and other difficulties that can be anticipated but not prevented. The policy development challenge is to achieve implementation of the support paradigm in the face of these challenges, with adequate safeguards for individuals with disabilities, family members, and support providers, and with clearly defined roles for public agencies at the various levels of government.

REFERENCES

Bellamy, G.T., & Horner, R.H. (1988). Beyond high school: Residential and employment options after high school. In M.E. Snell (Ed.), *Systematic instruction of the moderately and severely handicapped* (3rd ed., pp. 491–510). Columbus, OH: Charles E. Merrill.

Bellamy, T., Rhodes, L., Mank, D., & Albin, J. (1987). *Supported employment: A community implementation guide.* Baltimore: Paul H. Brookes Publishing Co.

Bercovici, S.M. (1983). *Barriers to normalization: The restrictive management of mentally retarded persons.* Baltimore: University Park Press.

Braddock, D., Hemp, R., & Fujiura, G. (1986). *Public expenditures for mental retardation and devel-opmental disabilities in the United States: State profiles* (2nd ed.). Chicago: Institute for the Study of Developmental Disabilities, University of Illinois at Chicago.

Conroy, J.W. (in press). Philadelphia's community residential service system: Indicators of quality. In S. Gant, D. DiMichele, R. Melzer, & W. Henderson. *Expert team report* (Civil Action #74-1345).

Conroy, J.W., & Bradley, V.J. (1985). *The Pennhurst longitudinal study: A report of five years of research and analysis.* Philadelphia: Temple University Developmental Disabilities Center.

Eastwood, E., & Fisher, G. (1988). Skills acquisition among matched samples of institutionalized and community-based persons with mental retardation.

American Journal on Mental Retardation, 93, 75–83.

Forest, M., & Lusthaus, E. (1988). *The kaleidoscope: Each belongs—quality education for all.* Unpublished manuscript, Frontier College, Toronto.

Froland, C., Pancoast, D., Chapman, N., & Kimboko, P. (1981). *Helping networks and human services.* Beverly Hills: Sage Publications.

Hahn, H. (1989). The politics of special education. In D.K. Lipsky & A. Gartner (Eds.), *Beyond separate education: Quality education for all* (pp. 225–242). Baltimore: Paul H. Brookes Publishing Co.

Haney, J.I. (1988). Empirical support for deinstitutionalization. In L.W. Heal, J.I. Haney, & A.R. Novak Amado (Eds.), *Integration of developmentally disabled individuals into the community* (2nd ed., pp. 37–58). Baltimore: Paul H. Brookes Publishing Co.

Kugel, R.B. (1969). Why innovative action? In R.B. Kugel & W. Wolfensberger (Eds.), *Changing patterns in residential services for the mentally retarded* (pp. 1–13). Washington, D.C.: President's Committee on Mental Retardation.

Kuhn, T.K. (1962). *The structure of scientific revolutions.* Chicago: University of Chicago Press.

Lakin, K.C., Hill, B.K., White, C.C., & Wright, E.A. (1987). *Longitudinal change and interstate variability in the size of residential facilities for persons with mental retardation.* (Brief Report No. 28) Minneapolis: University of Minnesota, Minnesota University Affiliated Program

Lakin, K.C., Jaskulski, T.M., Hill, B.K., Bruininks, R.H., Menke, J.M., White, C.C., & Wright, E.A. (1989). *Medicaid services for persons with mental retardation and related conditions.* Minneapolis: University of Minnesota Center for Residential and Community Services.

Millar, R., & Millar, A. (Eds.). (1981). *Developing client outcome monitoring systems: A guide for state and local social service agencies.* Washington, DC: The Urban Institute.

Minnesota State Planning Council on Developmental Disabilities. (1987). *A new way of thinking.* St. Paul: Author.

Mount, B., & Zwernik, K. (1988). *It's never too early, it's never too late: A booklet about personal futures planning* (Publication No. 421-88-109). (Available from Metropolitan Council, Mears Park Center, 630 E. Fifth St., St. Paul, MN 55101)

New York Office of Mental Retardation and Developmental Disabilities. (1987). *Future of the workforce: Report of the panel on the future of the workforce serving persons with developmental disabilities.* Albany: Author.

Nisbet, J., & Callahan, M. (1987). Achieving success

in integrated workplaces: Critical elements in assisting persons with severe disabilities. In S.J. Taylor, D. Biklen, & J. Knoll (Eds.), *Community integration for people with severe disabilities* (pp. 184–201). New York: Teachers College Press.

O'Brien, J. (1987). A guide to life-style planning: Using *The Activities Catalog* to integrate services and natural support systems. In B. Wilcox & G.T. Bellamy, *A comprehensive guide to* The Activities Catalog: An alternative curriculum for youth and adults with severe disabilities (pp. 175–189). Baltimore: Paul H. Brookes Publishing Co.

Rusch, F., & Hughes, C. (1988). Supported employment: Promoting employee independence. *Mental Retardation, 26*(6), 351–356.

Smith, G. (1988, October). *Issues in human resources.* Paper presented at the annual meeting of the American Association of University Affiliated Programs, Denver, CO.

Smull, M.W. (1989). *Crisis in the community.* Alexandria, VA: National Association of State Mental Retardation Program Directors.

Smull, M.W., Sachs, M.L., Cahn, L.E., & Feder, S. (1988). *Service requests: An overview.* Baltimore: University of Maryland at Baltimore, Applied Research and Evaluation Unit.

Strully, J.L., & Strully, C.F. (1989). Friendships as an educational goal. In S. Stainback, W. Stainback, & M. Forest (Eds.), *Educating all students in the mainstream of regular education* (pp. 59–68). Baltimore: Paul H. Brookes Publishing Co.

Taylor, S., Biklen, D., & Knoll, J. (Eds.). (1987). *Community integration for people with severe disabilities.* New York: Teachers College Press.

Taylor, S.J., Racino, J., Knoll, J., & Lutfiya, Z. (1987). Down home: Community integration for people with the most severe disabilities. In S.J. Taylor, D. Biklen, & J. Knoll (Eds.), *Community integration for people with severe disabilities* (pp. 36–63). New York: Teachers College Press.

Walter, S., & Choate, P. (1984). *Thinking strategically: A primer for public leaders.* Washington, DC: Council of State Planning Agencies.

Weatherly, R., & Lipsky, M. (1977). Street level bureaucrats and institutional innovation: Implementing special education reforms. *Harvard Educational Review, 47*(2), 171–197.

Wilcox, B., & Bellamy, G.T. (1987). *A comprehensive guide to* The activities catalog: An alternative curriculum for youth and adults with severe disabilities. Baltimore: Paul H. Brookes Publishing Co.

World Health Organization. (1980). *International classification of impairments, disabilities, and handicaps.* Geneva: Author.

CHAPTER 32

An Exchange on Personal Futures and Community Participation

An Interview with John McKnight and Ronald Melzer

SUSAN BRODY HASAZI
University of Vermont, Burlington, Vermont

The dialogue in this chapter presents the personal perspectives of two individuals who have made significant contributions to the conceptualization and development of community supports for individuals with severe disabilities. John McKnight and Ronald Melzer were selected to participate in this dialogue in part because of the similar views they hold regarding the improvement of community integration and participation for people with severe disabilities. They were selected as well because of their varied experiences in working to transform the ways in which services and supports are provided to individuals with disabilities and their families. Both Mr. McKnight and Dr. Melzer were asked to respond to three questions regarding their visions of the ways in which communities and services can assist individuals with disabilities to become valued participants in community life.

How would services be planned, organized, delivered, and evaluated if community participation and the development of friendship and support networks were valued outcomes for individuals with severe disabilities?

McKnight: I think that we don't need to plan services if we want to achieve community participation. That really is the wrong question. A more appropriate question is: "What should policymakers do to redirect funding resources in ways which would allow people with disabilities to be incorporated as totally as possible into the community?" When that is the question, then it seems to me that services are not very important in achieving the solution.

If we want to have policies that direct the dollars and authority in ways that enhance the ability of communities to incorporate individuals with disabilities into the mainstream of life, our first goal would be to reduce dependence on human services by increasing the income of labeled people and decreasing the number of dollars we decide to prespend by purchasing services for them.

Throughout the Western world there has been a gradual increase over the last several decades in the amount of money allocated for services as opposed to income. Studies demonstrate over and over that the relative increase in public and private expenditures for labeled people has been in the provision of service dollars rather than income. Yet, cash income is the key to choice making in communities, especially in consumer societies such as ours. Therefore, it seems to me that the first decision is not how to improve or change services but how to improve and expand choice making and cash income for labeled people. This usually means that there must be a reduction in predefined spending of service dollars and this then results in a decrease in contracted services and other "systems" allocations. Instead, money should be in the hands of people who are labeled so that they or their associates can make choices as to whether they want services or whether they want to use their money in other ways.

After achieving an equitable distribution of

dollars directed at increasing individual income rather than services, we need to focus next on providing special funding that would enable individuals with disabilities to fully participate in community life. This funding would help to guide people with disabilities into communities and keep them there.

It seems to me that few agencies or governments spend significant amounts of money helping to identify the gifts and capacities of labeled people and introducing those gifts to community groups and associations. One of the primary reasons we don't have people incorporated into community life is that we don't have people who see that as their task. There are some people within human services systems who say they would like to do this, but it seems to me that generally they are the wrong people for the job. The people who *are* best prepared to incorporate people with disabilities into community life are those who are now active in community life. Therefore, the second question should be: "What kind of incentives are provided to people who are community leaders and activists outside the service field so they will become active in increasing the involvement of people with labels in community life?"

Rather than investing in more services, we need to ask how resources and authority can be used to provide incentives for community members to become active in bringing people out of the service world and into association with individuals, groups, organizations, clubs, and activities that are expressive of community life.

In summary, I believe that we don't need services for community participation; rather, we need a new policy that sounds like this: We will reduce dependence on human services by increasing interdependence in the community through a focus on the contributions, capacities, and gifts of people who have been excluded because of their label. To achieve this end we will neither improve nor expand services. Rather, we will increase income and invest in incentives for community members to incorporate those who have been excluded in the world of services.

Melzer: Traditional service systems have been built around constructs that promote ac-

countability, professionalism, and formal interventions over participation, friendship, and natural support networks. Not surprisingly, the resulting structure and content of service delivery are, to a great extent, now controlled by funding patterns and regulations which reflect those established values. Making the transformation to services that are more consistent with the outcomes we would now like to stimulate will require fundamental changes at all levels of the system.

Without question, the role of the federal government has been a significant one in shaping the nature of current services to persons with severe disabilities, and has produced much of what is both right and wrong with today's system. The emphasis on active treatment, sufficient therapeutic services, and protection from harm has clearly done much to eliminate the neglect and inhumane conditions to which so many children and adults had been subjected over the years. At the same time, federal funding, especially through the Medicaid program, has encouraged service models and settings which are overly rigid, self-contained, and essentially removed from normal patterns of community living.

In recent years, much effort has been devoted to reforming those aspects of Medicaid which result in a bias toward services which are either institutionally based, or institutional in nature, even when they are provided in community settings. Without such changes, it is difficult to imagine how the goals to which we aspire can be met in a system that is so heavily dependent on federal dollars.

At the state and regional level, we need to examine whether current regulations, standards, and contracting mechanisms shape services in ways that discourage the support of natural networks and settings. Especially within the last decade, the primary responsibility of state government has shifted from one of direct service to the purchase of services from private community-based agencies. These relatively new relationships are often governed by elaborate policies and procedures which, from government's perspective, constitute the necessary means of safeguarding the welfare of clients and the taxpayers' funds. Provider agencies, on the other hand, see many of government's rules as annoyances at best, or as actual barriers to appropriate service delivery. There is, no doubt, some justification for both points of view. The future of service delivery, however, is very much dependent on the ability of the public and private sectors to come to some reasonable accommodations which balance what are coming to be seen as opposing interests. If regulatory procedures and reimbursement methodologies continue to favor rigid program models—which is often now the case —there is little likelihood that services will be able to evolve in the direction of greater participation in community life. Simultaneously, mechanisms must be developed to ensure that increasing flexibility at the provider level will be used in the interest of providing those services and supports which individuals and families truly need to maintain and enhance their independence. One excellent way to accomplish this is through careful attention to the composition and training of citizen boards which govern the operation of local agencies.

Finally, at the consumer level, attention must be given to the fundamental structure and operation of organizations which now provide the majority of community-based services. Do those who make program and fiscal decisions that affect the lives of people know them as individuals or simply as a group of clients? Does the organization encourage integration by linking its consumers with others in the community, or are most of people's interactions with paid staff of the agency? Does the provider attempt to have people use generic community resources (e.g., physicians, transportation, normal recreational events), or does it establish its own parallel community? And, are service recipients and their families true participants in the planning process or simply attendees at meetings that do little more than confirm decisions which have already been made, or worse, which explore options that don't actually exist?

Widespread systems change does not occur easily or quickly. I am convinced, though, that there are significant numbers of people who have come to see and understand the limitations of traditional service approaches. If given the opportunity through changes in funding and reg-

ulatory practices, I honestly believe they would move energetically toward models which promote greater integration and lessened dependency on the formal service system.

With the above ideas in mind, what suggestions do you have for modifying the present service system in order to achieve meaningful community participation for individuals with severe disabilities?

McKnight: It seems to me that the major action necessary for a service system to ensure community incorporation of people with disabilities is for the service system to get out of the way. Service systems represent an economic and psychic wall between the community and individuals who are disabled.

A serious question that must be asked by people in the service world is: "How can we stop being the boundary for the lives of people with disabilities?" Once we understand this is the critical question, then the issue is how to get out of the way. This requires some serious thought about the impact on community perceptions of the notion that if you are disabled, you are owned by service professionals. Many community members believe that people with disabilities cannot survive in the community and must be surrounded by relationships with human services professionals. These ideas have to be changed if people with disabilities are going to be effectively incorporated into community life. Therefore, the primary requirement is for service systems to invite the community to effectively incorporate people with disabilities into its affairs.

Melzer: So much of our current emphasis in service planning has come to revolve around clinical issues, it sometimes appears we view recipients as little more than a collection of deficits. To be sure, today's individualized habilitation plans, with their measurable goals and objectives, are a vast improvement over conditions of not long ago when persons with severe handicaps were thought to be incapable of learning and often were destined to lives of isolation and custodial care. However, in our zeal to identify and ameliorate specific areas of developmental delay, we have lost sight of the fact that some very basic human needs do not readily lend themselves to formal human services solutions. Increasing attention span, improving mobility, and learning how to communicate are goals which interdisciplinary teams handle very well. Unfortunately, they are not nearly as effective in dealing with objectives like making friends, building relationships, and enjoying community resources in normal, everyday ways. This is not a criticism of the traditional approach to service planning; it is merely a recognition that not all aspects of life can be reduced to human services interventions. We also know that the design and location of program settings do not always produce the outcomes we had intended. A small residential environment is not automatically "homelike" and physical integration is no guarantee of meaningful involvement with nonhandicapped community members.

Most people would regard human services systems as being more inclined to supplant natural family and community structures than they are to support them. Historically, special people were sent to special places because this was thought to be best for everyone. There, in protected environments which shielded them from the cruelties of others, it was believed persons with severe handicaps could receive those unique interventions that were simply unavailable elsewhere. More recently, the notion that all people belong in the community has gained increasing support but, to some extent, we've done more to alter the venue of services than we have to changing the fundamental ways we view the role of human services in the lives of persons who are disabled. We still think very much more in terms of *residential programs* than we do about *homes, employment programs* instead of *work,* and *social/recreational programs* rather than *just having fun.* Though not explicitly stated, these human services analogues of normal places and activities help to reinforce old stereotypes that people with disabilities don't (or can't) have a place in the nonhandicapped world. For them, it would seem, carefully planned and controlled simulations of life are more appropriate than the real thing.

Though some have suggested the formal service system may itself be the greatest barrier to community integration, I am not persuaded of this inevitability. Because we haven't yet determined the "right mix" of structured professional intervention and naturally occurring supports for everyone is no proof that such middle ground does not or could not exist. Indeed, just about all of the examples we have of programs and services which truly encourage integration and community participation have sprung from formal service networks. The real challenge, it seems, is to think about ways existing systems can be altered to value, promote, and achieve those outcomes.

Our entry into a period which may come to be known as the "age of disillusionment"—a time when we actually began to acknowledge the very real possibility that the *system* might not be capable of doing everything for everyone—may well provide the impetus for serious reconsideration of service strategies. Now, when parents and families find themselves on growing waiting lists for service, when provider organizations experience personnel shortages at all levels, and when the cost of care continues to escalate much more rapidly than the rate of inflation, the notion of supporting people in natural settings is assuming pragmatic as well as philosophical appeal.

In conceptualizing the fundamental role of the formal service system, I always find it helpful to think about a decision process based on a two-dimensional analysis of need. One axis represents the extent to which a recipient is capable of self-direction (or can be assisted in making decisions by family or friends), while the other deals with the complexity of the required intervention. In the quadrant where self-direction is high and service complexity is low, probably the most useful role that the service system can play is to provide the resources—cash—which people need to get what they want. Participant-directed attendant care is an excellent example of this. At the opposite extreme, where capacity is most limited and the intervention is highly complex, the system's role is much more directive; but that alone does not preclude service strategies which are responsive to issues of integration and community participation. Here, an example might be the facilitation of an individualized, shared living arrangement for someone who might ordinarily be served in a very specialized group home.

As a rule, the goal of maximizing community participation can be greatly advanced simply by limiting the nature and extent of formal responses when simpler actions will meet the underlying need. Even when the required service is a very specialized one, finding ways of bringing the intervention to the recipient will most always be preferable to moving the person. We probably won't stray very far from the mark if we keep in mind that it is far easier to introduce special services and supports into natural settings than it is to create opportunities for inclusion after people have been removed from the mainstream of community life.

What would the role of professionals be in a service system designed to achieve community participation and citizen empowerment? In addition, what kinds of educational and experiential preparation should professionals have to fulfill the responsibilities associated with their roles?

McKnight: I believe that professionals in a service system that allows community participation would be people who are primarily attendants. I distinguish attendants from most people who provide professionalized human services. Attendants are humane people with common abilities rather than people with special expertise and advanced educational training.

In order to maximize the potential for people to remain in or be incorporated into community life, the great majority of people with disabilities need others who will assist them in transportation, the preparation of meals, or in performing bodily functions. Those are roles that are usually understood to be the work of attendants. Since most people with disabilities need attendants, rather than services, training in universities is unnecessary. Rather, preparation for the role of an attendant should be achieved through apprenticeships. Therefore, we need to reduce investments in professional training for human services and increase allocations for attendants for those individuals who are vulnerable and require supports if they are to be effective in the community.

Melzer: Professionals will have a different, but far from diminished role in service systems that stress community participation and citizen empowerment. Most parents, family members, and friends of persons with severe disabilities acknowledge the importance of competent services and therapies in ameliorating the effects of handicapping conditions and building a repertoire of useful skills. Indeed, were it not for the tremendous advances in teaching technology, I seriously doubt the human rights movement alone would have brought us to our current thinking of what persons with disabilities can really do. At the same time, a growing emphasis on professionalism may have inadvertently led to some conclusions which are both unjustified and incompatible with the outcomes we are coming to value. For one thing, the remarkable progress of many children and adults who were previously thought to be incapable of learning has probably fostered the belief that, with enough time and effort, there are no limits to habilitation. Aside from the fact that this is simply not so, we need to acknowledge that people need to get on with life right now, not when some objective or goal in their plan has been achieved. For another, practitioners are increasingly called upon to make decisions on matters that are far from technical in nature, and which, in the case of persons who are not disabled, are simple issues that no one would ever think of consulting a professional about.

◇ **CHAPTER 33** ◇

Choices, Communication, and Control
A Call for Expanding Them in the Lives of People with Severe Disabilities

ROBERT WILLIAMS

United Cerebral Palsy Associations, Washington, D.C.

After languishing for 15 years on the back ward of an Australian institution, and having no speech, Anne McDonald wrote, in *Annie's Coming Out:* "To be imprisoned in one's body is dreadful. To be confined to an institution for the profoundly retarded does not crush you in the same way. It just removes all hope" (Crossley & McDonald, 1980, p. viii). Her statement and those made by other people who are unable to speak force us to ask ourselves what we can do to replace hopelessness with hope; boredom with curiousity; learned helplessness with initiative; speechlessness with meaningful expression; and confusion, anger, and resentment with choices that lead to a clearer sense of self-control and direction.

COMMUNICATION IMPERATIVE

Now that the Center on Human Policy (1979) has raised the consciousness of many people with their publication of *The Community Imperative,* we as never before need a *communication imperative.* Every person, regardless of the severity of his or her disabilities, has the right and ability to communicate with others, express everyday preferences, and exercise at least some control over his or her daily life. Each individual, therefore, should be given the chance, training, technology, respect, and encouragement to do so.

This imperative, when the need for it is fully recognized, can energize a fresh series of life-enhancing activities:

1.   It will help us to encourage people with severe disabilities to steadily increase the choices and communication in their daily lives.

2.   It will help us to recognize that people with severe disabilities, like all others, have personal preferences, likes, and dislikes that they can learn to express through a variety of effective means (Shevin & Klein, 1984).

3.   It will help us to see that individual preferences of persons with disabilities are often ignored because their expressions have been seen by others as "aberant," "off-task," "non-compliant," "inappropriate," "excessive," "challenging," "aggressive," "self-injurious," or "nonsensical," and are rarely seen as attempts to communicate to others their valid wants, needs, fears, wishes, or desires.

Houghton, Bronicki, and Guess (1987) found that classroom staff members respond at extremely low rates to students' expressions of choice or preference. The study showed that such staff members responded only 15% of the time to the expression of preference or choice during structured activities and 7% during unstructured times. On the positive side, when students were asked to express a preference or choice, they did so 99% of the time (Houghton et al., 1987).

4.   It will help us to identify the barriers faced by persons with severe multiple disabilities and increase everyday communication and choice making. These barriers include being: seen as too "low functioning" to communicate or to have likes and dislikes; unsure what a

An earlier version of this chapter appeared as "Communication, control, and choice" in the *TASH Newsletter* (1989, March), p. 10.

"choice" is since no one paid attention to such things before; improperly positioned; able to say only five words or less; unable to read or write; unwilling to try to communicate since no one listens anyhow; and dependent on unpredictable body movements for conveying needs, wants, fears, or desires.

5. It will help us to sense as never before the myriad ways that we all can communicate with each other, by: pointing, smiling or using other facial expressions, gesturing or hand signing, using picture boards, using an assistive device, looking directly at a desired object, selecting one kind of food over another, shaking or nodding our head for "no" or "yes," tuning in on a favorite radio or TV station, wearing our old faded jeans as often as possible, sleeping in, or doing our best at what we enjoy most.

6. It will help us to encourage a person to express as many preferences per day as possible, to decide: when to get up on weekends and holidays; when to go to bed; whether to shower before bed or in the morning; who helps with eating, bathing, getting dressed, and so on; what to wear; what to eat; what to do with free time and whom to do it with; or when it's time for a coffee break.

7. It will help us to allow ourselves to be guided by these expressions as much as possible. This helps the person make the connection between having likes and dislikes and making ac-tual choices in life (McDonald & Gillette, 1986). If necessary, structure can be added by: limiting the person's choices initially to one or two distinct options, presenting a set of real choices to the individual, and presenting a set of choices that would be socially and personally acceptable as well as age appropriate (Shevin & Klein, 1984).

8. It will help us to let technology be assistive and liberating—instead of forcing persons to be slaves to it—and to avoid overdependence on "high-tech" systems that tend to be too costly, too large and bulky, too impersonal, and too sophisticated for natural communication.

9. It will help us to concentrate instead on identifying, strengthening, and building upon the individual's existing communication and choice-making skills.

CONCLUSION

The time for expanding the choices—and the means to communicate them—in the lives of persons with severe disabilities has arrived. As Anne McDonald said, "unless someone makes a jump by going outside a . . . person's previous stage of communication there is no way the speechless person can do so. Failure is no crime. Failure to give someone the benefit of the doubt is" (Crossley & McDonald, 1980, p. 76).

REFERENCES

Center on Human Policy. (1979). *The community imperative.* Syracuse, NY: Author.

Crossley, R., & McDonald, A. (1980). *Annie's coming out.* New York: Penguin.

Houghton, J., Bronicki, B., & Guess, D. (1987). Opportunities to express preferences and make choices among students with severe disabilities in classroom settings. *Journal of The Association for Persons with Severe Handicaps, 12,* 18–27.

McDonald, J., & Gillette, Y. (1986). Communicating with persons with severe handicaps: Role of parents and professionals. *Journal of The Association for Persons with Severe Handicapps, 11,* 255–265.

Shevin, M., & Klein, N. (1984). The importance of choice-making skills for students with severe disabilities. *Journal of The Association for Persons for Severe Handicaps, 9,* 159–166.

Williams, R.R. (1989, March). Communication, control and choice. *TASH Newsletter,* p. 10.

◇ SECTION VI ◇

LIFE AND DEATH ISSUES

In 1981, TASH became the first of many national and international professional and disability rights associations that would subsequently pass a resolution condemning the use of aversives with persons with disabilities. Four years later, a young man with autism died while undergoing so-called "aversive therapy" in a specialized program for persons with severe behavior problems. This case drew national media attention as the state of Massachusetts tried unsuccessfully to halt the use of aversives such as: hits; pinches; water spray; ammonia spray; various forms of mechanical restraint; isolation time out; cold showers; food deprivation; muscle squeezes; rubber band; contingent physical excercise; taste aversive; a helmet with built-in water spray; social punisher (being tied to another, nonpreferred student); and a unique automatic vapor spray station that involved a visual screen helmet with white noise and built-in vapor spray, wrist and ankle restraint, standing barefoot on a corregated rubber mat, and finishing with an ice-cold bucket of water poured over the student's head. In the months and even years to follow, supporters for this school program would continue to argue that the students who were enrolled had such severe behavior problems that these were the only effective treatments available. Graphic pictures were shared with the media showing individuals with disabilities engaging in self-injury, and the school's director described the students as "animalistic" to justify his treatment practices. The media believed the stories, and area newspapers and national television news magazines were replete with coverage of the "persecution" of the school by the state agency and the advocates who were said to be biased or lacking in understanding regarding the needs of these individuals.

In 1987, a press conference was held in Baltimore, Maryland, to announce the development of a new, automated electric shock device that was being widely marketed for potential use with as many as 50,000 persons with mental retardation, said to engage in head banging, in the United States alone. In response, TASH and 12 other organizations joined together to protest the development and commercial sale of the device, demanding an investigation into its registration by the Food and Drug Administration and an immediate halt to its further use in the absence of any evidence regarding its safety and effectiveness (Document VI.5, this volume). In both this action and the original resolution on the more general use of aversives (Document VI.4, this volume), TASH emphasized the need for the development and validation of positive alternatives to treat severe self-injury and other serious challenging behaviors. Yet both statements provoked renewed attacks from those who defended the use of such aversives and the "right to effective treatment" for persons with disabilities that they argued would be denied if aversives were to be prohibited.

The chapters in this section detail the position taken by TASH that effective alternatives to aversives already exist, that aversives are no longer acceptable under any circumstances, and that what is needed is research on the development of positive alternatives rather than continued development and use of aversives. Another major issue addressed by the resolutions and chapters in this section involves judgments regarding the very lives of people with disabilities (see Documents VI.1 and VI.2, this volume). Again, wherever patterns of devaluing the possible lifestyles available to persons with severe disabilities are evident, decisions will be made that would never be acceptable for anyone else in our society. Thus, one baby born in America will be provided with standard surgical procedures to remedy a situation such as a blocked esophagus, while another baby will be starved to death because he or she also has Down syndrome or some other identifiable disability. In cases such as this, what would otherwise be a medical decision based upon likely outcomes associated with different types of medical interventions becomes instead an opportunity for prejudice to exercise a death sentence.

Perhaps the greatest irony of all is that the basis for such decisions most often rests upon the child's projected "quality of life" as now exemplified by the very institutions, segregated schools, sheltered workshops, social isolation, and lack of family supports that our society has created. Surely the quality of life for a person with severe disabilities is as dependent upon the opportunities provided to him or her as it is upon any individual characteristics that might be identified at birth or at any other time in his or her life.

Resolution on Infant Care

TASH opposes the withholding of medical treatment and/or sustenance to infants when the decision is based upon the diagnosis of, or prognosis for, retardation or any other disability. TASH affirms the right to equal medical treatment for all infants in accordance with the dignity and worth of these individuals, as protected by federal and state laws and regulations. TASH acknowledges the responsibilities of society and government to share with parents and other family members the support necessary for infants with disabilities. Finally, TASH acknowledges the obligation of society to provide for life-long medical, financial, and educational support to persons with disabilities extending to them opportunities offered to all members of society.

The rationale for this resolution is as follows.

- The right to life and liberty is guaranteed by our Constitution, Bill of Rights, and federal and state laws and regulations.
- The life and liberty of persons with disabilities are threatened by the prejudice which results from the ignorance generated by segregation and separation.
- This prejudice can only be overcome when the next generation of children born without disabilities grow up, play with, go to school with, and live and work with their peers with disabilities.
- TASH is extremely concerned with the practice of withholding medical treatment and/or sustenance from infants based upon the diagnosis of, or prognosis for, disability.

ORIGINALLY ADOPTED APRIL 1983
AMENDED APRIL 1989

*   *   *   *   *

Nutrition and Hydration Resolution

WHEREAS, There are an increasing number of decisions supporting the cessation of nutrition and hydration for individuals who are themselves unable to consent and have not with valid expression consented to such procedures; and

WHEREAS, The Association for Persons with Severe Handicaps is committed to the value of all people regardless of severity of disability;

THEREFORE BE IT RESOLVED, THAT The Association for Persons with Severe Handicaps strongly opposes any cessation of nutrition and hydration for people who are incapacitated and that The Association for Persons with Severe Handicaps will seek to involve itself in litigation and legislation judged to have potential for setting precedents that will affect the rights of individuals who are incapacitated and at risk of loss of life and health without provision of hydration, nutrition, and medical treatment; and

FURTHER BE IT RESOLVED, THAT The Association for Persons with Severe Handicaps strongly opposes approaches now advocated by many which authorize third parties exercising substitute judgment to decide "on behalf" of a person who has been labeled incapacitated that the person's life is no longer "worth" living, and strongly opposes any position that it would be in the best interests of a person to die rather than to live with a disability.

ORIGINALLY ADOPTED NOVEMBER 1986

* * * * *

Organ Transplant Unit

In response to the opening of the Loma Linda University Anencephaly Transplant Unit, transplants[1] of one or more vital organs should occur only when a donor patient is brain dead and proper consent has been obtained. The criteria for brain death must establish totality and irreversibility of cessation of brain functions. Anencephaly or any other disability alone does not meet the criteria of brain death. Determination of brain death should be made by physicians who are not on the transplant team, to minimize the possibility of conflict of interest.

ORIGINALLY ADOPTED MARCH 1988

* * * * *

---

[1]Non–life-threatening transplant of organs or donation of bodily parts or fluids is permissible with legally sufficient consent and upon reasonable medical judgment. The fact that a person from or to whom a transplant or donation is sought has a disability should not in and of itself prohibit or encourage the transplant or donation.

Resolution on the Cessation of Intrusive Interventions

WHEREAS, In order to realize the goals and objectives of The Association for Persons with Severe Handicaps, including the right of each person who has severe handicaps to grow, develop, and enjoy life in integrated and normalized community environments, the following resolution is adopted:

WHEREAS, Educational and other habilitative services must employ instructional and management strategies which are consistent with the right of each individual with severe handicaps to an effective treatment which does not compromise the equally important right to freedom from harm. This requires educational and habilitative procedures free from chemical restraint, aversive stimuli, environmental deprivation, or exclusion from services;

THEREFORE, TASH calls for the cessation of the use of any treatment option which exhibits some or all of the following characteristics: (1) obvious signs of physical pain experienced by the individual; (2) potential or actual side effects such as tissue damage, physical illness, severe physical or emotional stress, and/or death that would properly require the involvement of medical personnel; (3) dehumanization of persons with severe handicaps because the procedures are normally unacceptable for persons who do not have handicaps in community environments; (4) extreme ambivalence and discomfort by family, staff, and/or caregivers regarding the necessity of such extreme strategies or their own involvement in such interventions; and (5) obvious repulsion and/or stress felt by peers who do not have handicaps and community members who cannot reconcile extreme procedures with acceptable standard practice;

IT IS FURTHER RESOLVED, THAT The Association for Persons with Severe Handicaps' resources and expertise be dedicated to the development, implementation, evaluation, dissemination, and advocacy of educational and management practices which are appropriate for use in integrated environments and which are consistent with the commitment to a high quality of life for individuals with severe handicaps.

ORIGINALLY ADOPTED OCTOBER 1981
REVISED NOVEMBER 1986

* * * * *

DOCUMENT VI.5

SIBIS Resolution

Inasmuch as The Association for Persons with Severe Handicaps (TASH) has resolved to call for the cessation of the use of aversive and intrusive interventions, and it has come to the attention of the Association that an electro-shock device, the Self-Injurious Behavior Inhibiting System (SIBIS), that contravenes this resolution is being widely promoted both professionally and commercially by Human Technologies, Inc., and its associates;

WHEREAS, Information supplied to the press by the Applied Physics Laboratory at Johns Hopkins University and HTI promotional materials suggest widespread application of the device with thousands of persons with developmental disabilities in the U.S. alone, and emphasize the usefulness of this shock device without an attendant; and

WHEREAS, The use of electric shock to modify self-injurious behavior has virtually disappeared, with rare exception, from the professional literature over the past 5 years, while numerous positive and educative approaches have received increased emphasis in both the professional literature and professional community in services for persons with developmental disabilities; and

WHEREAS, The existing published literature on the use of shock does not include evidence of long-term effectiveness in the maintenance and generalization of behavior change, on the replacement of self-injurious behaviors with positive alternative behaviors, or meaningful improvements in lifestyle for persons treated for self-injury using shock, and does raise serious concerns regarding the safety of shock both in principle and in practice; and

WHEREAS, The evidence provided by Human Technologies, Inc., regarding clinical trials to date is equivocal and no published and/or peer-reviewed reports have been cited by HTI in promotional materials, the videotape report, or exhibits at professional conferences, nor have any such reports been made available to professionals requesting them to date; and

WHEREAS, It appears that various federal agencies and representatives of the professional community are being referred to in publicity and promotional materials as having supported the review, evaluation, and dissemination of the device;

THEREFORE BE IT RESOLVED, THAT TASH calls for the immediate cessation of any further use or sale of the SIBIS electro-shock device;

AND BE IT FURTHER RESOLVED, THAT TASH also calls for a formal investigation by all relevant parties, including the following:

- An immediate investigation by appropriate medical and behavioral professionals regarding the safety of the device and the potential for abuse in the use of the device with persons with disabilities, particularly in light of the self-activating features of the device and the explicit reference in promotional materials to its use "without an attendant" and in contrast to alternative treatments;
- An investigation into the accuracy and validity of claims made in promotional materials regarding potential applicability and potential use of this device to address the needs of large numbers of persons with developmental disabilities and the validity of claims made regarding clinical efficacy;
- Immediate disclosure of any data and other evidence regarding clinical trials submitted and utilized in any review of this or any similar device by the Food and Drug Administration, including the short- and long-term efficacy of use of the device as well as the pro-

fessional peer review procedures utilized to judge the validity of any clinical trial data;

- Explanation and justification of the absence of written professional standards for the review and registration of this and other medical devices listed as Class II medical devices under the 1976 Amendment to the Food, Drug, and Cosmetics Act;
- An explication and justification of the role of NASA and FDA involvement in view of media reports regarding such involvement;
- An explanation and justification of the role, if any, of the JHU–Applied Physics Laboratory, the Kennedy Institute, Georgetown University, Johns Hopkins University, and their affiliated units and faculty, and any federal funding support thereof, in the development and dissemination of the device;
- Exclusion of this and other such intrusive and aversive devices from use as a reimbursable expense under Title XIX of the Social Security Act, including the Medicaid Home and Community Quality Services Act of 1987.

ORIGINALLY ADOPTED MARCH 1988

*   *   *   *   *

CHAPTER 34

Medical Treatment

DAVID L. COULTER

Boston University and Boston City Hospital, Boston, Massachusetts

Treatment of medical disorders in people with severe disabilities should not be a "critical issue" at all. In an ideal world, medical treatment would be provided without any reference to the presence or absence of a severe developmental disability. The issues concerning treatment would be the same for all people with medical disorders. These issues may be summarized in the following guidelines:

1. Medical treatment that is in the best interest of the individual should always be provided.
2. Decision-making authority about what medical treatment should be provided belongs to the individual first and to the family or guardian second. Society and medicine have authority only to assure that guideline #1 is followed.
3. Resources should be provided to assure that guideline #1 is met. Access to these resources should be determined by medical necessity.

These guidelines, respectively, represent an application of the ethical principles of beneficence, autonomy, and justice to the problem of medical treatment.

Of course, we do not live in an ideal world. The right of people with severe disabilities to receive medical treatment according to these guidelines is threatened in diverse ways. This may result in inappropriate withholding or withdrawing of medical treatment, or in actions that seek to harm an individual with severe disabilities. This chapter explores the application of these guidelines to situations that occur in the real world from conception throughout the life cycle.

FRAMEWORK FOR DECISION MAKING

Jonsen, Siegler, and Winslade (1986) suggested that decisions about medical treatment require answers to four questions:

1. What are the indications for medical treatment, including the history, diagnosis, available treatment, and expected outcome?
2. What are the patient's preferences, including his or her goals, capabilities, and desired outcomes?
3. What is the patient's anticipated quality of life, including the range and degree of the patient's prospects for enjoying life?
4. Are there any relevant socioeconomic concerns, including burdens and benefits that may fall on other persons?

They suggested further that these questions are hierarchical and that answers to the first two questions are much more important than answers to the last two. The framework presented in this chapter incorporates the guidelines described above. Further, answers to each of these questions require three distinct types of information (Coulter, in press). We must have accurate and complete facts, we need to be aware of the values of all parties involved, and we must apply common sense to the analysis of these facts and values.

Using this framework for people with severe disabilities may be complicated in several ways. Analysis of the indications for medical treatment is often difficult because of the presence of considerable *uncertainty*. Recognition of the different types or sources of uncertainty may help indicate methods to reduce the uncertainty. Thus, uncertainty about the diagnosis may be reduced by obtaining more data or expert opinions. We must be careful, however, because data may be conflicting or confusing and experts may not be sufficiently knowledgeable. Uncertainty about the prognosis may be reduced by similar sources of information, but often we must simply wait to see what happens in order to clarify the prognosis. Certainly, when there is considerable residual uncertainty about the indications for medical treatment, and when the alternative to treatment is death, we should wait at least until the other questions in the framework are answered satisfactorily.

Many people with severe disabilities are unable to express a preference about medical treatment. This does not mean that the question should not be asked. Even a limited or immature preference should be taken into account. At the very least, we should assume that a person with severe disabilities would desire continued life, so long as there is an expectation of some quality to that life.

This raises the question of whether medically indicated treatment is ever not in the best interest of the patient. One such situation might be when the patient has expressed a clear and competent preference to forego such treatment. Another such situation might be when treatment cannot assure even a "minimal" quality of life. We must not impose our own feelings about quality of life on people with severe disabilities, however. The individual's personal satisfaction with life, seen from his or her point of view, is the best measure of the quality of that person's life.

From the point of view of a person with severe disabilities, medical treatment may not be desirable when any of the following cannot be assured (Coulter, Murray, & Cerreto, 1988):

1. Freedom from intractable pain and suffering, such as severe physical pain or shortness of breath that cannot be relieved by any treatment: The mere presence of a severe disability such as mental retardation is not "suffering" in this sense, however.
2. The capacity to experience and enjoy life, including the ability to enjoy such things as food, warmth, or the caring touch of another person: Anyone who is consciously aware of other people and the environment has this ability to experience and enjoy life. This capacity may be lacking in persons who are permanently unconscious or comatose, but great caution is needed in making this determination.
3. Expectation of continued life: If treatment cannot assure continued life, it may well be futile. One would not do a kidney transplant in a person with terminal cancer who has only a few months to live, for example. If

life may be expected to continue for even a few years, however, treatment to assure that life may well be worthwhile to the individual.

When this quality of life is present, we should assume (in the absence of a clear preference stated by a person with severe disabilities) that the medically indicated treatment is in the best interest of that individual.

When there is a question about the presence of this quality of life, significant moral uncertainty may exist regarding the proper course of action. This moral uncertainty may be reduced through external review by knowledgeable parties not involved in the decision, such as a properly constituted hospital ethics committee (Hastings Center, 1987). Advocates who affirm and seek to protect the individual's rights may be helpful in these ambiguous or "gray-zone" situations.

Treatment may be indicated and in the best interest of the individual, according to these considerations, yet its availability may be limited by socioeconomic concerns. The principle of justice may be interpreted to include the ideas that all persons are equal, that goods or resources belong to the community, and all persons should seek to distribute these resources to promote equality. Veatch (1986) argued that persons with severe disabilities have not only an equal claim on these resources, but also a claim on such resources as are needed and sufficient to restore equal opportunity to compete in society. Thus, when resources are limited, they should be allocated disproportionately to people with disabilities, up to the point that the allocation makes other people unable to compete with them. Advocates may be most effective in assuring that the resources of society are allocated according to this interpretation of justice.

With this understanding of the issues involved in making decisions about medical treatment, we may now consider their application to people with severe disabilities at various points during the life cycle.

ABORTION

Amniocentesis to determine if a fetus has Down syndrome is virtually a routine procedure and is often recommended when the woman is 35 years or older. The unstated implication of this recommendation is that the woman may choose to have an abortion if Down syndrome is present. This is sometimes described as a method for "prevention" of mental retardation. In fact, what is being prevented is the birth of a person who may have mental retardation. Yet, if that person is born, all indicated treatment is required. Does it make sense to allow destruction of a fetus solely because of the presence of a condition that, once the child is born, would require all appropriate treatment?

This issue hinges on the recognition of when a fetus becomes a human being or person. In a biological sense, any product of conception in a human being is human (that is, belonging to the species Homo sapiens and no other). One may make faith statements about when that human acquires the attribute of a "soul" or personhood, but these must be recognized as statements of faith and not verifiable fact. One may base personhood on the existence of "viability," but that implies a dependence on the changing capabilities of medical technology. If new technology were capable of sustaining a fetus born at 12 or 15 weeks gestation, would that mean the fetus was a person? If one requires existence independent of technological support, would that mean a full-term infant on a mechanical ventilator is not a person?

Until society and science come up with a reliable, verifiable, and universally accepted definition of personhood, the best definition may be the one that results in the greatest protection of human beings. In my opinion, at this point, recognizing that personhood begins at conception is the most logically consistent position that does not depend on faith or questionable philosophy alone. This means that decisions about medical treatment for human persons should follow the guidelines described above from the moment of conception.

A fetus with Down syndrome is likely to grow up and achieve at least the quality of life described above, so medically indicated treatment would be in the best interest of that person. A fetus with an irreversible, degenerative, and rapidly progressive disorder (such as Tay-Sachs disease) is unlikely to achieve this "minimal"

quality of life, however, and treatment would be futile in changing this outcome. The issues are the same for the fetus as for the child with either diagnosis. One is not justified in harming a fetus with Down syndrome (by abortion) if one would not be justified in harming a child with Down syndrome, since the issues are the same. This analysis may be extended to other situations when abortion is being considered solely because of the existence (or possible existence) of a severe disability if the child is born.

ANENCEPHALY

Anencephaly is a medical disorder in which most of the brain fails to develop, and the overlying skull and scalp also fails to develop. This absence of the skull and scalp distinguishes anencephaly from other severe brain disorders such as hydrocephalus. Infants with anencephaly usually do not survive for more than a few days and never for more than a few months. Since medical treatment cannot change this ultimately hopeless prognosis and would only prolong the act of dying, most physicians would not consider such treatment to be in the infant's best interest. Humane care, including nutrition and hydration (see later section of this chapter), should be provided however.

Because of the hopeless prognosis and the intactness of other organs, some have argued for allowing infants with anencephaly to serve as organ donors for heart or kidney transplantation (Holzgreve, Beller, Buchholz, Hansmann, & Kohler, 1987). Because these other organs may deteriorate while waiting for the infant to die, these authors have argued that the organs should be removed as soon as possible after birth, even while the infant is still breathing. This approach (which amounts to medical killing or euthanasia) cannot be justified (Coulter, 1988). Medical practice, law, and public policy only permit removal of living organs from individuals with brain death. The issues regarding brain death are the same for infants with anencephaly as for anyone else; namely, there must be irreversible cessation of all functions of the brain including the brainstem. Humane care must be continued until death occurs, either by cardiorespiratory arrest (somatic death) or cessation of all brain function (brain death). Organs may be removed for transplantation only after death has occurred. Strict adherence to this policy when anencephaly is present is essential to protect the rights of all infants with severe brain disorders.

INFANTS WITH DISABILITIES

In 1984, the American Academy of Pediatrics published a joint policy statement concerning infants with disabilities that was co-signed by many other organizations, including TASH. This statement (American Academy of Pediatrics, 1984) reflected the 1983 TASH Resolution on Infant Care (Document VI.1, this volume) in its call for provision of all "clearly beneficial" medical treatment, regardless of the individual's actual or potential disabilities, and in its demand for provision of those resources necessary to support the individual throughout life. Withholding treatment was only justified if the treatment was "clearly futile" and would only prolong the act of dying. Even in that event, sustenance and relief of pain and suffering were to be provided.

The United States Department of Health and Human Services (DHHS) developed two sets of rules to implement policy concerning infants with disabilities. The first (*Federal Register,* 1984) was based on the Rehabilitation Act and was subsequently overturned by the United States Supreme Court (*Otis R. Bowen, Secretary of Health and Human Services, Petitioner, v. American Hospital Association, et al.,* 1986). The second set of rules (*Federal Register,* 1985) was based on the Child Abuse and Neglect Prevention and Treatment Act and has not been overturned. These rules outline a process in which all medically indicated treatment must be provided, unless the infant is "chronically and irreversibly comatose" or the treatment would be futile and merely prolong the act of dying. DHHS called for the development of Infant Care Review Committees to oversee the application of these rules on a local basis.

This federal policy is consistent with the TASH resolution and with the framework for decision making described above. There are several limitations to it, however. One is the vague language that allows for various interpretations

of such concepts as virtual futility or reasonable medical judgment. Another is the difficulty of applying it to situations that do not fit neatly into those described in the rules. Most importantly, the provisions for enforcement are very weak, and consist only of withholding federal funds provided under the Child Abuse and Neglect Prevention and Treatment Act to states that do not implement these rules.

The consequence of these limitations is that, in practice, the rules have been all but forgotten. Infant Care Review Committees have either become inactive or have been incorporated into hospitalwide ethics committees. Actual decision making in intensive-care nurseries is generally left to discussions between parents and physicians, much as it was before 1984. The legacy of the rules is that there is now a presumption in favor of continued treatment in most cases. However, there is no process to assure that treatment decisions do in fact conform to the rules, and it is likely that inappropriate decisions are being made in situations remote from wider scrutiny. Perhaps it is time to reexamine the situation and to develop a new consensus that will more effectively protect and safeguard the rights of infants with disabilities to receive necessary medical treatment.

NUTRITION AND HYDRATION

Life in a permanent vegetative state is particularly tragic, since (by definition) there is no conscious awareness of the environment or social interaction with other people, and no expectation that this situation will ever change. We must affirm the inherent value, personhood, and immortal soul present in such persons, while acknowledging the tragedy of their complete isolation from social intercourse. No medical treatment presently available is likely to improve the situation, but spontaneous recovery from the vegetative state has occurred, however. Care that sustains life and prevents further deterioration is appropriate and respects the humanity of people in a permanent vegetative state. Treatment that may be harmful is not appropriate because it cannot be justified in terms of any expected benefit. Consideration of such potentially harmful treatment falls into a "gray zone" in which several possible courses of action may be permissible while none is morally necessary.

Providing nutrition and hydration, usually by some sort of tube feeding, is a form of care that sustains life and prevents further deterioration. Since it is not harmful, withholding or withdrawing it would not be appropriate. On the contrary, denying nutrition and hydration would be harmful and thus cannot be justified in terms of expected benefit. The only situation in which denying nutrition and hydration to a person in a permanent vegetative state might be justified would be when the person had previously stated a clear and competent desire not to receive such care.

In 1989, the American Academy of Neurology published a position statement on the care of patients in a permanent vegetative state. This statement (American Academy of Neurology, 1989) argued that nutrition and hydration may be withheld or withdrawn when the diagnosis of a permanent vegetative state has been made accurately, when it is clear that the patient would not want further treatment, and when the family agrees with the patient's desire in this regard. In an accompanying commentary, Munsat, Stuart, and Cranford (1989) stressed that the statement applies *only* to patients in this situation; namely, where the wishes of the patient are clearly known. They cite a number of legal precedents and statements by the American Medical Association and the President's Commission in support of the academy's position.

As a rule, people with severe disabilities have never had the opportunity to express a clear and competent desire regarding their care. Thus, the statement of the American Academy of Neurology (1989) does *not* apply to them, even if they are in a permanent vegetative state. Rather, the 1986 TASH Nutrition and Hydration Resolution (Document VI.2, this volume) provides a source of guidance for such considerations regarding people with severe disabilities. This resolution "strongly opposes" any cessation of nutrition or hydration and further opposes any attempt to allow other parties to exercise a "substituted judgment" on behalf of the person with severe disabilities to the effect that the person's life is not

worth living because of the disabilities. It should be noted that others have taken a different position on this issue, however (Hastings Center, 1987).

Munsat et al. (1989) recognized that there may be 5,000–10,000 patients in a permanent vegetative state in the United States. This is a fairly small number, and only a fraction of these patients have previously stated a clear desire to forego nutrition and hydration should they ever be in this condition. As shown above, this fraction represents the only individuals whose nutrition and hydration might legitimately be withheld or withdrawn. In all other cases, nutrition and hydration should be maintained. For the many other people with severe disabilities who are not in a permanent vegetative state, there would also be no justification for denying nutrition and hydration.

OTHER TREATMENTS

From time to time in the lives of people with severe disabilities, medical conditions arise that require decisions about treatment. Perhaps the best way to phrase the question is: "What medical treatment would be provided if the person did not have disabilities?" Usually that is precisely the treatment that should be provided to the person with disabilities.

As an example, consider a child with a disorder called septo-optic dysplasia. Such children have severe visual impairment and usually have severe mental retardation. In addition, they have deficiencies of most pituitary hormones, including those that control growth and sexual development. Some caregivers may find it convenient to keep them small and immature in order to prevent adult growth, puberty, menstruation, pregnancy, and adolescent aggressive behavior, which would be difficult to manage because of the presence of the other disabilities. These caregivers may not want the child to receive hormone replacement therapy for this reason. This preference cannot be justified. Clearly, the hormone replacement therapy would be provided if the child did not have these other disabilities. It is medically indicated to treat a medical condition, and thus it should be provided to children who do have these disabilities. The potential problems with menstruation, sexuality, and behavior should be managed appropriately, not "prevented" by neglectful denial of necessary medical treatment.

Similar considerations may be applied to other medical disorders such as infections, orthopedic conditions, heart disorders, or kidney problems. If treatment would be effective and would be provided if there were no disabilities, then it should be provided to people with severe disabilities.

CONCLUSIONS

In the real world, people with severe disabilities may not always receive appropriate medical treatment because of their disabilities. Correcting this situation requires adherence to the guidelines stated at the beginning of this chapter. Threats to the rights of people with severe disabilities to receive appropriate medical care, including deliberate harmful acts, may occur at any time during the life cycle from conception onward. This chapter has highlighted examples of several such threats. In some instances (such as abortion), we need to open debate and consider new policy. Existing policy deserves reexamination in other instances (such as treatment of infants with disabilities), to reinvigorate the protection of people with disabilities. And, in many situations (such as nutrition and hydration), we need to stand fast and defend our beliefs against an increasing threat to the rights of people with disabilities. Constant vigilance and informed advocacy are necessary to assure that all people with severe disabilities receive all necessary medical treatment.

REFERENCES

American Academy of Neurology. (1989). Position of the American Academy of Neurology on certain aspects of the care and management of the persistent vegetative state patient. *Neurology, 39,* 125–126.

American Academy of Pediatrics. (1984). Joint policy statement: Principles of treatment of disabled infants. *Pediatrics, 73,* 559–560.

Coulter, D.L. (1988). Beyond Baby Doe: Does infant transplantation justify euthanasia? *Journal of The Association for Persons with Severe Handicaps, 13,* 71–75.

Coulter, D.L. (in press). Approaches to ethics. In J.A. Mulick (Ed.), *Transitions in mental retardation: Vol. 5. The life cycle.* Durham, NH: American Association on Mental Retardation, Northeast Region 10.

Coulter, D.L., Murray, T.H., & Cerreto, M.C. (1988). Practical ethics in pediatrics. *Current Problems in Pediatrics, 18,* 137–195.

Federal Register. (1984). Nondiscrimination on the basis of handicap: procedures and guidelines relating to health care for handicapped infants: Final rules (45 CFR, part 84), *49,* 1622–1654.

Federal Register. (1985). Child abuse and neglect prevention and treatment program: Final rules (45 CFR, part 1340), *50,* 14878–14901.

Hastings Center. (1987). *Guidelines on the termination of life-sustaining treatment and the care of the dying.* Briarcliff Manor, NY: Author.

Holzgreve, W., Beller, F.K., Buchholz, B., Hansmann, M., & Kohler, K. (1987). Kidney transplantation from anencephalic donors. *New England Journal of Medicine, 316,* 1069–1070.

Jonsen, A.R., Siegler, M., & Winslade, W.J. (1986). *Clinical ethics* (2nd ed.). New York: Macmillan.

Munsat, T.L., Stuart, W.H., & Cranford, R.E. (1989). Guidelines on the vegetative state: Commentary on the American Academy of Neurology statement. *Neurology, 39,* 123–124.

Otis R. Bowen, Secretary of Health and Human Services, Petitioner, v. American Hospital Association, et al. United States Supreme Court, Case No. 84-1529, 1986.

Veatch, R.M. (1986). *The foundations of justice: Why the retarded and the rest of us have claims to equality.* New York: Oxford University Press.

◇ **CHAPTER 35** ◇

Nonaversive Interventions for Severe Behavior Problems

EDWIN HELMSTETTER
Washington State University, Pullman, Washington

V. MARK DURAND
State University of New York at Albany, Albany, New York

The TASH *Resolution on the Cessation of Intrusive Interventions* (Document VI.4, this volume) opposes the use of intrusive interventions and supports the development and implementation of practices that are appropriate for use in integrated environments, and that enhance an individual's quality of life. Intrusive interventions are defined in the resolution's third paragraph.

Several concerns appear to undergird recent recommendations, of which the aforementioned TASH resolution is but one example, to limit the use of intrusive interventions and to develop alternatives (Guess, Helmstetter, Turnbull, & Knowlton, 1986):

1. Although research has shown that some intrusive interventions effectively suppress behavior, the durability and generalizability of effects is questionable. Well-designed research that has addressed durability and generalization has achieved mixed results. It seems reasonable that researchers who use interventions that cause physical or psychological pain, dehumanize, are objectionable to others, and so on, be compelled to address these issues adequately before disseminating the technology.

2. Intrusive methods are being misused. They have been used to punish incorrect responses in skill acquisition, and with classes of behaviors and individuals for which they were never intended or validated.

3. Intrusive interventions can produce unpleasant side effects, such as fear, withdrawal, crying, and aggression. In other words, the "treatment" can generate a new set of problems.

4. Because the methods focus on decreasing the problem behavior, there is a danger that practitioners will ignore the human dimension, develop the attitude that the end (behavior reduction) justifies the means, and indiscriminately use whatever methods available to alter the behavior. This attitude also interferes with identification of personal (e.g., communication deficiencies) and setting factors (e.g, the instructional tasks) that may interact with the problem behavior.

5. Intrusive interventions are open to legal challenges because a person's constitutional rights to speech and privacy (and, therefore, autonomy) are violated by enforced behavioral conformity. Also at issue is the power relationship between the educator or therapist and the person with disabilities, a relationship that can interfere with voluntary consent for treatment. Legal challenge can also be based on failure to utilize the "least drastic means" of intervention, or provide adequate procedural safeguards to assure that a person is dealt with fairly.

In addition, no matter how aberrant the problem behaviors and how less skilled persons with severe disabilities may appear to be, these persons have the same rights as nondisabled persons, including the right to be integrated into society. This view, perhaps more intensely felt now than in the past, discourages the use of

The preparation of this manuscript was supported in part by U.S. Department of Education Grant #008630362 awarded to Washington State University. The content and opinions expressed herein do not necessarily reflect the position or policy of the U.S. Department of Education, and no official endorsement should be inferred. We gratefully acknowledge the assistance of Tina Baldwin, and Denise Argentine in completing this manuscript.

procedures that differ from those used with non-disabled persons because these practices communicate to peers, community members, families, and professionals that persons with disabilities are different and, therefore, can be deprived of the rights and privileges that are instrumental in supporting the development of nondisabled persons. Finally, it is arguably immoral to use intrusive procedures on persons who are so communicatively and otherwise behaviorally limited as to be unable to indicate their needs and concerns, or to adequately control their environments.

The remainder of this chapter reviews a number of promising practices that provide alternatives to intrusive interventions. In addition, these practices conform to the values expressed in the TASH *Resolution on the Cessation of Intrusive Interventions* (Document VI.4, this volume). To review, the most salient values contained in the resolution are: 1) integration with peers and other nondisabled persons; 2) access to normalized environments; 3) enjoyment of life; 4) individualized treatment; 5) effective treatments; 6) habilitation; and 7) freedom from harmful physical, psychological, or emotional effects on persons with disabilities, on their family, peers, or service providers, or on persons in the communities in which they function.

There are three major sections to the chapter: 1) a discussion of social validation, 2) a review of interventions, and 3) recommendations for future research.

SOCIAL VALIDATION

The TASH resolutions' values on integration with nondisabled peers and participation in normal environments argue for the involvement of peers and other community persons in the treatment of behavior problems of persons with disabilities. These values are congruent with the goal of many *applied* behavioral scientists: to treat behaviors that are important to individuals and to society, with outcomes that are of practical significance as judged by the individual undergoing treatment, or by other members of society (Baer, Wolf, & Risley, 1968). Social validation is one method for helping practitioners meet this challenge (Kazdin, 1977; Mal-

oney et al., 1976; Minkin et al., 1976; Wolfe, 1978).

Social validation can be applied at three points (Kazdin, 1977; Wolf, 1978):

1. *Focus of treatment:* Is it what the individual or society wants?
2. *Treatment procedure:* Is it acceptable when consideration is given to the individual involved, conditions, and desired outcomes?
3. *Outcomes:* Are the intended and unintended results satisfactory to the individual and society?

Kazdin (1977) described three social validation methods that can be used at each of the three points. First, *social comparison* involves the identification of the student's peer group. Then, either the peer group *and* the student are assessed in specific situations in order to determine whose behavior is extreme; or the level of behavior of peers who do not warrant treatment is assessed, and a normative level is established against which to compare a student's behavior. To illustrate the latter approach, Wilson, Reid, Phillips, and Burgio (1984) observed the family-style mealtime of group home residents with mild to moderate mental retardation in order to help identify important premeal, meal, and postmeal behaviors. Subsequently, this information was used in the development of a training program for institutionalized persons with profound disabilities.

Second, in *subjective evaluation,* persons who regularly interact with an individual or who are in a special position to judge behavior make an overall, qualitative judgment of performance. There is no overt reference to a normative group. For example, Rusch, Schutz, and Agran (1982) sent a 47-item questionnaire to 120 potential employers to identify the skills necessary for entry into competitive employment in the food, janitorial, or maid service occupations.

Third, a *combination* of social comparison and subjective evaluation methods can be used. An example of the combined approach, as applied to the validation of treatment outcomes, would be for peers to compare the individual's posttreatment behavior to the amount of behavior of similarly situated peers, and for parents and peers to subjectively evaluate whether the student's overall behavior had improved. (Because the combination method was not represented in the research literature, it is not included in the following discussion of social validation and problem behaviors.)

Application of Social Validation to Identification of Problem Behaviors

Social Comparison

Social comparison has been used in a number of studies of behavior problems. Patterson (1974) compared the home behavior of boys referred for treatment because of their disruptive behavior (e.g., teasing, whining, yelling) to the home behavior of a matched group of boys who were not referred for treatment. The preintervention behavior of the treatment group differed significantly from that of the comparison group. Azrin and Armstrong (1973) compared the inappropriate eating behaviors (e.g., throwing and spilling food) of institutionalized adults with mental retardation to a comparison group of nondisabled ward staff, and found significant discrepancies between the two groups at the pretreatment stage.

Subjective Evaluation

As part of their investigation into the social validation of the efficacy of treatment of children with autism, Schreibman, Koegel, Mills, and Burke (1981) asked undergraduate students to view pretreatment and posttreatment videotapes of the children and, using a rating scale, record their impressions of the children's behavior. The items in the rating scale were taken from essays on the children's characteristics written by 10 other undergraduates who had viewed the videotapes. Respondents indicated their agreement, on a scale of 1 to 7, with statements about behaviors (e.g., restless, talk to himself, tantrum, speak clearly), and indicated their willingness to interact with each child (e.g., Would you be willing to walk to the park with this child?). Results indicated that "certain behaviors (e.g., speech, self-stimulation, tantrums, play, and cooperation) seemed to heavily influence their global impressions of the children" (Schreibman et al., 1981, p. 622). Similar research with third-grade through seventh-grade students yielded similar results (Runco & Schreibman, 1988).

This approach, while utilized in research on the efficacy of treatment, could be adapted for use in identifying behaviors for treatment that non-disabled adults and children consider important.

Durand (1982a) polled a student's parents, teachers, and residential care staff about the desirability of behavior change goals. They were asked: "(1) 'Do you believe that there is a need to decrease the number of times Tim hits himself?' and (2) 'Do you believe Tim needs to increase or decrease the amount of time he plays with other people?'" (Durand, 1982a, p. 49).

Analysis

Social validation has been used at this stage to compare the pretreatment performance of a targeted individual or group to that of a nontargeted population, thereby establishing norms for behavior change. It has also been used in the form of analogues to identify important behavioral characteristics of children. However, social validation procedures could be utilized even more fully at this stage by having peers and community persons identify the adaptive and problem behaviors that need to be addressed in order to enhance the individual's social integration into community and school settings. The social comparison method is particularly useful here because persons who are, or will be, significant in an individual's life (e.g., an employer) observe the individual and peers as they participate in natural contexts, such as shopping in grocery stores or using public transportation. Observation in natural environments is important because of evidence that social and physical contexts can affect the behavior of persons with disabilities (Berkman & Meyer, 1988). Having peers and community persons observe the individual is important because it is difficult to predict accurately just what behaviors will be tolerated in any given situation. For example, what behaviors would teenage peers find offensive? Would the community be accepting of a young or petite individual who is aggressive, but be fearful of an older or larger aggressive person? Would occasional drooling be unacceptable in food service employment, but acceptable in an office job? Social comparison also permits data collection on how the ecological or service patterns might be reorganized to support individuals in integrated situations, instead of removing them for treatment.

Application of Social Validation to Intervention Procedures

Acceptability of treatment procedures refers "to the judgments about the treatment procedures by nonprofessionals, lay persons, clients, and other potential consumers of treatment" (Kazdin, 1980, p. 259). There are several reasons for evaluating the acceptability of treatments. First, treatments viewed as more acceptable, even though they may not be the most effective, are more likely to be used by consumers, and adhered to when implemented (Kazdin, 1980). Second, it guards against violation of client rights, and helps protect professionals from legal entanglements (Kazdin, 1980).

Social Comparison

Social comparison has not been extensively used to validate a behavioral intervention. This may be due to the difficulty in finding a comparison group, which would consist of nondisabled peers with similar behavior problems and in similar situations with which to develop normative levels for the use of various interventions. An alternative social comparison approach would be to have respondents assume that nondisabled peers had these problems, and project appropriate interventions for them in specific situations. This information would then be used in the selection of interventions for use with persons with disabilities. A method similar to this was used by Menchetti, Rusch, and Lamson (1981), who surveyed college and university food service professionals regarding, among other things, the behavior management strategies (e.g., ignore, yell at) that they would always, sometimes, or never allow for workers who were nonhandicapped and for those with handicaps.

Subjective Evaluation

Subjective evaluation has been frequently used to evaluate the acceptability of intervention procedures. The majority of this research, however, has been analogues in which respondents (e.g., teachers, parents) reviewed case studies and rated the social acceptability of various treatments. For example, Kazdin (1980) presented undergraduate students with audiotaped cases of children whose levels of behavior problems and disability varied in terms of severity. The undergraduates rated the acceptability of four procedures: differential reinforcement of incompatible behavior (DRI), time out, drugs, and electric shock. The DRI procedure was rated as most acceptable, followed by time out, drugs, and shock. This study evaluated the acceptability of procedures by potential consumers (students in an introductory psychology course) prior to any planned use of the procedures. (See Morgan, 1989, for a review of 20 studies that utilized analogues in evaluating treatment acceptability, and a discussion of the contextual variables that still need to be studied and the validity of analogues for making decisions about actual treatment situations.)

Subjective evaluation was used prior to treatment by Durand (1982a), who asked a subject's parents, teachers, physician, and residential staff, "Do you consider the use of the overcorrection procedure for Tim's behaviors as acceptable?" Prior to presenting this question, the individuals were given the results of an assessment of the influences on self-injurious behavior, and a detailed description of the proposed intervention procedures.

Subjective evaluation has also been used following actual implementation of treatments. Foxx and Shapiro (1978) included in their research on the use of a time-out ribbon a survey on the acceptability and practicality of the procedure. Respondents included special education teachers, students, classroom paraprofessionals, a principal, staff trainers, a chair of a human rights committee, institutional unit leaders and staff, graduate students, and program directors. Respondents rated the procedure based upon a two-page description of the technique. To further assess the practicality of the procedure, they evaluated whether teachers could properly implement the procedure based upon its brief description.

Porterfield, Herbert-Jackson, and Risley (1976) sent a questionnaire to service providers who implemented a contingent observation procedure with 1–2-year-olds in a day-care center. Respondents rated the procedure as easier to use than a procedure involving distracting the children and

redirecting them away from their disruptive behavior. Respondents also validated the outcomes, stating that the contingent observation
procedure taught students more than did the
comparison procedure.

Rosenbaum, O'Leary, and Jacob (1975) had
teachers rate individual and group reward systems in terms of side effects (negative and positive peer pressure) and practical concerns about
implementation. Kern, Koegel, Dyer, Blew, and
Fenton (1982), who examined the effects of jogging on the repetitive behavior of students with
autism, asked observers to rate the students' interest, happiness, and general behavior throughout all phases of the experiment. Observers rated
the students as disruptive, noncompliant, and
uninterested during nonjogging days, with opposite ratings for jogging days. The validation
procedures of Kern et al. (1982) addressed the
acceptability of outcomes, including side effects
(e.g., level of interest), and, indirectly, through
measures of happiness, the students' satisfaction
with the procedure.

Analysis

Most of the research on the social validation of
treatments has involved the use of analogues.
More work is needed under actual treatment conditions. Social validation must also be extended
to integrated work, leisure, living, and school
settings, and involve nondisabled persons in
those environments. In addition, methods must
be developed for ascertaining whether the person
being treated finds the intervention acceptable.

Application of Social
Validation to Treatment Outcomes

Social validation of treatment outcomes addresses the question of whether the intended and
unintended results are satisfactory to the individual, significant others, and society.

Social Comparison

This method is illustrated in a study by O'Brien
and Azrin (1972), who taught eating skills to institutionalized adults with mental retardation.
Their performance was compared to the number
of eating errors per meal displayed by nondisabled persons in a community restaurant, and
was found to be better than the norm.

Subjective Evaluation

Several studies used the subjective evaluation
approach. Kelly, Wildman, and Berler (1980)
had experienced personnel interviewers evaluate
the pretraining and posttraining job interview
skills of adolescents with mental retardation.
Schutz, Jostes, Rusch, and Lamson (1980) had
co-workers rate the acceptability of performance
of adults with mental retardation who had
learned how to sweep and mop. Rusch,
Weithers, Menchetti, and Schutz (1980) taught
co-workers how to decrease the topic repetitions
of a man with mental retardation. Co-workers
were asked at various stages of baseline and
treatment whether the individual repeated topics
too often, and whether he should repeat less.

Reid and Hurlbut (1977) taught adults with severe physical and communication disabilities to
use picture-word communication boards to request leisure activities. For social validation, 7
adults who had not previously interacted with
the individuals rated the subjects' responses to
the question "What would you like to do?" under
two conditions, with and without the communication boards. Wahler and Fox (1980), who
strengthened toy play in order to decrease oppositional behavior, had the parents of their nondisabled subjects provide global ratings of their
children's behavior. The ratings ranged from 1 to
7, where 1 represented good and 7 represented
bad. Durand (1982a) asked a subject's staff, parents, and teachers to compare the subject's self-
hitting, injuries, and play behavior before and after treatments.

Schreibman et al. (1981) had undergraduates
use a rating scale to record their impressions of
the pretreatment and posttreatment behavior of
children with autism as shown on videotapes
(the rating scale was described earlier in this
chapter). The results demonstrated that the naive
undergraduate observers saw changes in the
children's behavior from pretreatment to posttreatment. Their impressions corresponded to
objectively measured changes. The observers
also indicated greater willingness to interact
with students whose behavior had changed at the
posttreatment stage. Similar results were obtained when this line of research was conducted
with elementary school teachers, parents, and

third-grade through seventh-grade children (Runco & Schreibman, 1983, 1988; Schreibman, Runco, Mills, & Koegel, 1982).

Analysis

Much of the research on treatment outcomes has been concerned with teaching adaptive behavior, and has been conducted in segregated settings. Greater use of social validation in the treatment of behavior problems is needed, as well as application in integrated school and community settings, utilizing the judgment of nondisabled peers, co-workers, and other community persons. The definition of outcome should be expanded to include collateral effects, including the individual's overall quality of life. Furthermore, greater effort must go into determining whether the person with disabilities is satisfied with the outcomes.

REVIEW OF INTERVENTIONS

A discussion of positive interventions typically includes a review of differential reinforcement procedures—differential reinforcement of other behavior (or the omission of the target behavior) (DRO), of a low rate of behavior (DRL), and of incompatible behavior (DRI). These procedures are not covered in this chapter; the reader is referred, instead, to existing reviews of these procedures (Durand & Carr, 1989; LaGrow & Repp, 1984; LaVigna & Donnellan, 1986; Lennox, Miltenberger, Spengler, & Erfanian, 1988). Other interventions are not covered in this chapter because historically they have not been used in conjunction with a functional analysis in an effort to address the motivation of the problem behavior. These interventions include extinction (Lennox et al., 1988), satiation (Lennox et al., 1988), nonexclusionary time out (Lennox et al., 1988), response cost (Lennox et al., 1988), and teaching students to respond to certain commands (e.g., to comply to various "do" and "don't" commands) that result in generalized compliance (Neef, Shafer, Egel, Cataldo, & Parrish, 1983). Finally, other potentially useful interventions have not been included here because they lack a systematic research base with challenging behavior. This final group includes self-

management (Browder & Shapiro, 1985), gentle teaching (McGee, Menolascino, Hobbs, & Menousek, 1987), modifying emotional states (Meyer & Evans, 1989), and systematic densensitization (LaVigna & Donnellan, 1986; Meyer & Evans, 1989).

This chapter focuses, instead, upon several newly emerging practices that do incorporate information about the maintaining variables that are involved, or that look at how a person's behaviors relate to one another. The practices included are: 1) teaching functionally equivalent behavior; 2) altering setting events, including the physical environment, social environment, curricular and instructional practices, the individual's physiological condition, and lifestyle issues; 3) response covariation, altering target behaviors through covarying responses; and 4) systems change, addressing the needs of systems that support persons in integrated community and school settings. If a study utilized a combination of these approaches, then the research was placed in the category of the method judged to be the most pervasive. If a combination of approaches was utilized, but only one approach at a time was used, then the research was categorized according to the approach that proved to be the most effective. In some cases, an approach was combined with other methods, including aversive ones (e.g., time out, response cost). Because of the limited amount of information on some of the approaches, a review of these studies is also included here.

An article was selected for review if it was published between 1965 and 1989 in one of the journals listed in Table 35.1, and contained one of the interventions described above. In addition, it had to address a behavior problem that could be categorized as aggression-disruption (e.g., hitting others, throwing tantrums, yelling, interfering with other students), self-injury (e.g., pica, rumination, head hitting, biting self), or repetitive (e.g., rocking, gazing at own hand, vocalization). These labels should not be regarded as indicators of the functions of the behaviors. In other words, although behaviors produce self-injury or are disruptive, it should not be assumed that the primary purpose of the behavior is to self-harm or to be disruptive. The be-

Table 35.1. Journals reviewed for research related to practices

American Journal on Mental Retardation (formerly the American Journal of Mental Deficiency)

Behavior Modification

Behaviour Research and Therapy

Behavior Therapy

Behavioral Science

Child Development

Education and Training in Mental Retardation (formerly Education and Training of the Mentally Retarded)

Education and Treatment of Children

Journal of Abnormal Child Psychology

Journal of Applied Behavior Analysis

Journal of Autism and Developmental Disorders

Journal of Behavior Therapy and Experimental Psychiatry

Journal of Clinical Psychology

Journal of Consulting and Clinical Psychology

Journal of The Association for Persons with Severe Handicaps (formerly Journal of The Association for the Severely Handicapped and Association for the Education of the Severely and Profoundly Handicapped Review)

Journal of Experimental Child Psychology

Journal of Special Education

Journal of the Experimental Analysis of Behavior

Mental Retardation

Psychological Record

Psychological Reports

havioral categories are used solely to organize the research around common forms of problem behaviors.

Preference was given to articles that included at least one person who was categorized as having mental retardation, developmental disabilities, deafness-blindness, behavioral disorders, autism, childhood schizophrenia, hearing impairment or deafness, visual impairment or blindness, brain damage, or multiple disabilities. However, if a practice was not used with a member of one of these categories, then its use with other persons was reported in order to illustrate its application.

It should be noted that this section of this chapter does not constitute a comprehensive review of the literature. Selected articles were chosen to illustrate practices in each treatment category. The following is a summary and analysis of the selected review of the literature for three categories of problem behaviors that were

treated by: teaching functionally equivalent behavior, altering setting events, response covariation, or systems change.

Aggression-Disruption

Teaching Functionally Equivalent Behavior

Higher rates of behavior problems have been associated with greater communication difficulties in persons with mental retardation (Talkington, Hall, & Altman, 1971) and individuals with speech-language disorders (Baker, Cantwell, & Mattison, 1980; Mattison, Cantwell, & Baker, 1980). Researchers hypothesized that the frustration that resulted from the communication difficulties could lead to aggression or other inappropriate behaviors that functioned to gain attention (Talkington et al., 1971).

Only in recent years, however, has research begun to examine the attention getting and other functions of behavior problems in persons with severe disabilities. One recommendation that has emanated from this research is to capitalize on these communication opportunities by using them in the development of more appropriate, functionally equivalent, communicative responses (Carr & Durand, 1985a, 1985b; Donnellan, Mirenda, Mesaros, & Fassbender, 1984; Durand, 1982a, 1982b, 1986; Evans & Meyer, 1985; Meyer & Evans, 1989). This technology has continued to evolve, and includes a variety of well-documented assessment and intervention procedures (Durand, in press). This training should be incorporated into a larger agenda for communication training (Baumgart, Johnson, & Helmstetter, 1990) and overall lifestyle planning (Meyer & Evans, 1989). Developing specific behaviors to replace specific problem behaviors should not overlook the important issues of the individual's need for an adequate communication system, and an environment that adequately responds to attempts to communicate (Durand, in press).

Another approach in the category of teaching functionally equivalent behavior involves the provision of comparable sensory input (Durand, 1982a, in press). For example, if the purpose of a behavior, such as the repeated waving of one's fingers between a source of light and the eyes, is to obtain visual stimulation, then equivalent stimulation of the visual system might be provided by looking through a Viewmaster, an activity that would be more appropriate, yet provide the same sensory input.

Research with aggressive-disruptive behavior

A number of studies have demonstrated the value of teaching functionally equivalent behavior in reducing aggressive or disruptive behaviors (See Table 35.2). Durand and Kishi (1987) used the Motivation Assessment Scale (Durand & Crimmins, 1988) to assess the function of the severe behavior problems of 5 adults with multiple handicaps. Based upon individualized assessment results that indicated the behaviors were maintained by escape, social attention, and their tangible consequences, the individuals were taught to communicate nonverbally requests that were equivalent to the assessed functions of their behavior problems (e.g., requests for assistance, requests for attention, and requests for tangibles). This resulted in significant improvements in the problem behavior of 4 of the 5 adults.

Analysis

The strategy of teaching functionally equivalent alternative behavior holds much promise for contributing to an individual's overall development of a communication system, and reducing the need to use unusual behavior to communicate. It is particularly encouraging that the procedure has been successfully used with persons with severe disabilities and persons who are deaf-blind (Durand & Kishi, 1987). The presence of a severe behavior problem in these individuals can apparently signal the existence of strong motivation to support the acquisition of an alternative communication skill. In essence, teaching functionally equivalent behavior takes the reinforcer that maintains a problem behavior and uses it to teach communication as an appropriate alternative to engaging in aggression or disruption.

Identifying the function of problem behavior in otherwise minimally communicative students means that much more work needs to be done in the area of assessment, such as the development of observational systems, checklists, and for-

mulating and testing hypotheses. This work must also recognize that a single problem behavior may serve multiple functions for an individual, that more than one problem behavior can serve the same function, that the forms and functions of behavior may be highly inconsistent in an individual, and that similar behaviors may serve different functions for different persons. In those cases where it is difficult to identify a function, the effects of assigning a function and teaching an alternative communicative response must also be empirically tested.

Assessment practices must also provide means for pinpointing what causes the individual to need to engage in the behavior to obtain the desired function. In other words, if the function of the problem behavior is to escape a task, what is it about the task that elicits the problem behavior (e.g., boredom, task difficulty)? One troublesome side effect that has plagued behavior reduction research is the emergence or strengthening of other problem behaviors (Evans, Meyer, Kurkjian, & Kishi, 1988; Voeltz & Evans, 1982). One explanation of this phenomenon is that these other behaviors are members of the same response class or serve the same function as the original behavior. If this is the case, negative side effects should be minimized when functionally equivalent positive behaviors are taught. However, this issue has not yet been investigated.

Altering Setting Events

Another promising intervention model involves altering setting events. In fact, such changes might be long overdue in instances where the environment and experiences of the person are clearly deficient and deviant, so that they could hardly be expected to motivate positive and adaptive behavior. "The concept of setting events includes complex antecedent conditions, events, and stimulus-response interactions which overlap with or entirely preceded [*sic*] subsequent behaviors that they affect" (Wahler & Fox, 1981, p. 331). The concept subsumes what has traditionally been referred to as stimulus control procedures (Gaylord-Ross, 1980; LaVigna & Donnellan, 1986). Setting events include immediate stimulus conditions associated with a particular behavior (e.g., instructions), ongoing interac-

Table 35.2. Treating aggression-disruption by providing functionally equivalent behavior

Study	Subject		Behavior	Assessment procedure	Treatment	Outcome	Comments
	N	Diagnosis					
Carr & Durand (1985a) (Exps. 1 and 2)	1 2 1	Autism Brain damage DD/hearing impairment	Poking, hitting, pulling hair, striking objects, tantrums, SIB, oppositional, out of seat, stripping.	Exp. 1: Used ABACACABA-type designs to measure problem behavior in varying levels of adult attention and task difficulty. A = easy task, high level of adult attention; B = easy task, low level of attention; C = difficult task, high level of attention.	Exp. 2: Ss in Exp. 1 who exhibited high rates of problem behavior for difficult tasks were taught to request assistance verbally by saying, "I don't understand." Ss whose problem behaviors were maintained by attention were taught to request attention verbally by asking, "Am I doing good work?"	Problem behaviors declined to nearly zero after Ss were taught to request assistance or attention.	Also demonstrated that teaching an S to emit an irrelevant (i.e., not functionally equivalent) response was ineffective.
Carr, Newsom, & Binkoff (1980) (Exps. 1 and 3)	1	MR, autism	Scratching, hitting, biting, kicking.	Exp. 1: Used ABAB design to verify that problem behaviors were emitted to escape demands. A = high demand; B = low demand. Also found that aggression abruptly ceased when an event occurred that signaled the termination of demands (e.g., removal of materials).	Exp. 3: Task demands were terminated for either aggression or finger tapping (contact between index finger and back of other hand).	Aggression decreased as the nonaggressive act of finger tapping was strengthened by consequating it with termination of tasks.	Tapping and aggression were not physically incompatible, so tapping served the same function as aggression (i.e., escape).
Durand & Kishi (1987)	3 2	Severe MR/ Deafness-blindness Profound MR/ Deafness-blindness	Scratching, pinching, throwing objects, head banging and butting, hitting, hand biting, slapping.	Used Motivation Assessment Scale (Durand & Crimmins, 1988) to identify function and location of problem behavior, reinforcers, and alternative communicative responses. In all cases, function was to escape from tasks.	Ss taught to sign or present a token to request a break from a task.	Percentage of intervals with problem behaviors decreased for 4 of 5 students following training.	Results maintained during follow-up visits 9 months later. Positive changes in staff behavior appeared to correlate with positive change in Ss' behavior.

(continued)

Table 35.2. *(continued)*

Study	Subject		Behavior	Assessment procedure	Treatment	Outcome	Comments
	N	Diagnosis					
Horner & Budd (1985)	1	Autism	Grabbing, yelling.	Systematic observation linked problem behaviors with 5 stimulus conditions: presenting lunch meal, beginning of language session, beginning of 1-to-1 instruction, beginning of group sharing activity, offering a folder to take home.	Taught signs that were relevant for each of the 5 stimulus conditions: juice, timer, choose, bottle, folder. Identical procedure used to teach signs in natural and simulated conditions.	Problem behaviors decreased as use of signs increased.	Signing competency in simulation training did not affect use of signs in natural setting or frequency of problem behavior. Training in actual contexts was effective in eliciting use of signs.
Smith & Coleman (1986) (Case 1)	1	Autism	Tantrums: flapping hands, grabbing, bouncing, rapid verbalizations.	Antecedents and consequences of tantrums recorded for 1 month. Problem behaviors were associated with task difficulty.	Taught how to request assistance when having difficulty, and implementation of response cost in which 1 card representing a favorite activity was removed for each tantrum.	After 3 months tantrums decreased from 13 per month to 0 for 1 month, but remained at 1–6 per month for months 4–18, and 0 for month 19.	This is a case study (AB design) and a treatment package that included response cost.

DD = developmental delay; Exp. = experiment; MR = mental retardation; S = subject; SIB = self-injurious behavior.

tions between individuals and such factors as their history and condition (e.g., age, deprivation, satiation, health), and physical and social environmental factors (e.g., temperature, crowdedness, personal interactions). It also includes the person's lifestyle (Meyer & Evans, 1989; O'Brien, 1987). Is the lifestyle personally meaningful and motivating? Does the person have control over social relationships, work, and living situations? Are the activities in which a person engages meaningful? Does the person value his or her possessions? Does the individual have a valued social role, and is he or she afforded affection and approval?

If setting events related to problem behavior can be identified and changed, this would obviate the need for intensive punishment or reinforcement procedures to overpower the environmental stimuli that elicit the behavior. Controlling the setting events has obvious implications for programming for durable and generalized behavior change. For example, environmental factors associated with low rates of problem behavior could be initially used, then systematically modified to resemble naturally occurring conditions. Similarly, any setting events associated with the problem behavior could be temporarily eliminated, and appropriate events could be gradually reintroduced at a later stage. Even in cases where the precise stimuli for negative behavior cannot initially be identified, radical changes in the setting events can at least temporarily "interrupt" strong patterns of behavior, and provide a more positive context for more precise intervention strategies, such as skill instruction, that might require more time to generate positive behavior changes (Evans & Meyer, 1985; LaVigna & Donnellan, 1986; Meyer & Evans, 1989).

Research with aggressive-disruptive behavior

Table 35.3 describes the studies that reduced problem behavior by altering setting events. A number of studies manipulated *curricular or instructional factors*. For example, Carr and Newsom (1985) treated the escape-maintained tantrums in three persons with developmental disabilities. They provided strongly preferred reinforcers (i.e., special foods) contingent upon task compliance. The rationale for this interven-

tion was that the task setting was less aversive when these reinforcers were present, so the clients would not have to escape the situation through tantrums. These researchers found that escape-maintained tantrums were reduced to near-zero levels when highly preferred foods were introduced as task reinforcers.

Frederiksen and Frederiksen (1977) compared fixed and random schedules of classroom tasks and found that the majority of students, categorized as moderately mentally retarded, completed more tasks and displayed less disruptive behavior (noise, activity level) under the fixed-schedule condition. Plummer, Baer, and LeBlanc (1977) found that when instructions were presented at a pace of one per minute, or when paced instruction was combined with reinforcement, there was a significant reduction in the rate of problem behavior (e.g., grabbing, tantrums, hoarding play materials, echolalia) displayed by a student with autism. Paced instruction was more effective than a combination of time out and paced instruction.

Touchette, MacDonald, and Langer (1985) used their "scatter plot" data sheet to identify the situations and times of day in which an adolescent with autism was most likely to engage in aggression. After finding that high rates of aggression occurred during the afternoon classes and low rates were associated with morning instruction, they replaced the afternoon classes with conditions resembling the morning instruction. This simple activity change resulted in significant reductions in aggression. Over a 12-month period, the original afternoon classes were gradually reintroduced with no increases in problem behavior.

Weeks and Gaylord-Ross (1981) demonstrated that problem behavior was more frequent with difficult tasks. Unfortunately, attempts to control problem behavior by using erorrless learning procedures to lessen task difficulty were unsuccessful (see comments in Table 35.3). Winterling, Dunlap, and O'Neill (1987) found that varying the instructional tasks instead of presenting repeated trials of the same task resulted not only in higher rates of unprompted correct responses, but also much lower rates of problem behavior. Lastly, Singer, Singer, and Horner (1987) investigated the use of "pretask request-

Table 35.3. Treating aggression-disruption by altering setting events

Study	Subject		Behavior	Assessment procedure	Treatment	Outcome	Comments
	N	Diagnosis					
Curricular and instructional factors							
Carr & Newsom (1985) (Exps. 1 and 2)	2 1	Autism Childhood schizo- phrenia	Tantrums.	Exp. 1: Tantrums measured in ABAB design. A = demands; and B = no demands. Rate of tantrums was significantly higher in A, when a sig- nal was given that demands would be terminated, tantrums decreased immediately.	Exp. 2: In a multiple- baseline design across 3 Ss, demands plus verbal praise was compared to demands plus strongly preferred reinforcers (food) and verbal praise.	Tantrums decreased from a mean of 36% of observed intervals, to a mean of 2% under the strongly preferred reinforcer/ praise condition.	
Carr, Newsom, & Binkoff (1980) (Exps. 1 and 2)	1	MR, autism	Pinching, pulling hair, scratching.	Exp. 1: Same as Carr, Newsom & Binkoff (1980) in Table 35.2.	Exp. 2: Used ABAB design. A = de- mands plus praise; and B = demands plus praise, toys, and food. Introduction of strongly preferred reinforcers was used to mitigate the aver- siveness of the demand situation.	Mean number of aggressive acts was 61 and 73 in A condi- tions, and 12 and 9.8 in B conditions.	
Frederiksen & Frederiksen (1977)	11	Moderate MR	Disruption: interfering with other Ss by excessive noise, physical activity, dis- ruption of materials, physical interference.	No information on how class- room schedules were linked to disruptive behavior.	Behavior measured under a fixed, predict- able schedule, and a random, unpredict- able schedule. Appropriate behavior was verbally and non- verbally approved; inappropriate behavior resulted in verbal reprimand and nonverbal disap- proval.	Under fixed schedule, task completion was greater for 10 of 11 Ss and disruption less for 6 of 11 Ss, in comparison to ran- dom schedule condi- tion.	Two tasks were not involved in the schedule change. Completion of these tasks was better under the fixed- schedule condition.

Study	N	Diagnosis	Target behavior	Procedure	Design	Results	Notes
Mace et al. (1988) (Exp. 3)	1	Severe MR	Noncompliance.	Asked S to perform numerous tasks in order to identify low-p "do" and "don't" commands (complied 40% or less). Similar process used to identify high-p "do" commands (complied at least 80% of time).	Examined inter-prompt time (IPT) of 5 and 20 seconds. IPT was the time between the end of the high-p "do" command and onset of the low-p command. Used ABABAC design. A = 20-s IPT for low-p "do" and 5-s IPT for low-p "don't"; B = 20-s IPT for low-p "don't" and 5-s IPT for low-p "do"; C = 5-s IPT for both low-p commands.	Average compliance for 5-s IPT was 83%, 89%, 80%, 86%, 78% for phases ABABA, respectively. Compliance for 20-s IPT was 53%, 27%, 22%, 29%, 37% for phases ABABA, respectively. The procedure was more effective when the 5-s IPT was used.	Exp. 1 also demonstrated the effectiveness of using high-probability commands prior to low-probability commands. Exp. 2 showed that this procedure was more effective than providing neutral or positive statements prior to a low-probability command.
Mace et al. (1988) (Exp. 4)	2	Moderate MR	Extremely slow response to requests or to complete tasks.	High-p commands were determined empirically using a process similar to that used in Exp. 3 (see above).	Used multielement design (random order of treatment) to compare no high-p command prior to task request, use of high-p, and neutral or positive statements prior to task request.	Mean latency (time taken to initiate a task) was 156-s, 117-s, and 17-s for no high-p, high-p, and neutral/positive statements, respectively.	A 5th exp. showed that high-p procedure was more effective than contingency management and prompts when the dependent measure was time taken to complete a task.
Plummer, Baer, & LeBlanc (1977) (Exp. 1)	1	Autism	Disruption: hoarding materials, grabbing, leaving activities, echolalia, tantrums.	Observation indicated that disruptions usually followed requests to play appropriately with materials.	Used ABA within a multiple baseline across two teachers. A = attention, time-out, paced instruction; and B = attention and paced instruction.	Percentage of instructions followed by tantrums was greatest under A (0%–40%); and decreased to 0% in 6 sessions under B.	Paced instruction involved instruction every 2 minutes.
Plummer, Baer, & LeBlanc (1977) (Exp. 2)	1	Variously diagnosed as autism, MR, brain damage	Spitting and throwing food, rocking, playing with fingers.	Observation indicated that disruptions usually followed instructions to eat.	Used multiple baseline across 2 teachers. Examined effects on inappropriate eating of paced instruction (4 per minute), praise, and favorite food for proper behavior.	Problem behaviors occurred 50%–100% of the time during baseline; decreased to 0%–10% within 6 treatment sessions.	When time out was added for problem behavior, it was ineffective in decreasing the behaviors.

(continued)

Table 35.3. (continued)

Study	Subject N	Subject Diagnosis	Behavior	Assessment procedure	Treatment	Outcome	Comments
Singer, Singer, & Horner (1987)	4	Moderate to severe MR	Noncompliance, hitting, biting, scratching.	Prior implementation of pretask requesting was found to be effective with these Ss. Pretask requests involved presentation of a request which had a high-p of being followed (e.g., "Give me five") just prior to delivering a request with a low-p of being followed (e.g., "Go to group now").	Measured compliance to target request, "Go to group." Used ABA design with 2 Ss and BAB with 2 Ss. A = baseline (no pretask request); and B = pretask request. Compliance with target request was praised, noncompliance (within 3 minutes) resulted in physical assist.	The combined compliance to request scores for the 2 Ss in the ABA design were 17% (A), 97% (B), 17% (A). The combined scores for the other 2 Ss were 87% (B), 33% (A), 100% (B).	
Touchette, MacDonald, & Langer (1985) (Case 1)	1	Autism	Hitting, kicking, head butting, throwing objects.	Scatter plot: For each 30-minute period, recorded whether behavior occurred 0, 1–2, or 3 or more times. Results showed that behaviors occurred primarily during 1–4 P.M.	Made 1–4 P.M. resemble the morning: discontinued prevocational and community living classes, added informal activities (e.g., stories, play).	Aggression nearly eliminated (4 in 14 days).	Over 12 months, afternoon classes where reintroduced with no increase in aggression.
Weeks & Gaylord-Ross (1981) (Exp. 2)	1	Profound MR	Striking others, crying.	Observation indicated aggression was negatively reinforced by escape from demands.	Used ABACADA design. A = baseline; B = easy task; C = errorless task; and D = difficult task. Errorless programming to lessen task demands consisted of using oversize belt and buckle for putting belt on.	C and D conditions were comparable in terms of amount of problem behaviors. Lowest rates of problem behavior occurred in A and B.	There was a high rate of errors in the early stages, so the treatment was not errorless. Problem behaviors were associated with errors in tasks.

572

Study	N	Population	Target behaviors	Comments	Design/Conditions	Results	Conclusions
Winterling, Dunlap, & O'Neill (1987) (Exps. 1 and 2)	1 1 1	Autism Autism, MR Autism, severe MR	Aggression, crying, echolalia, grabbing therapist, throwing materials, flapping arms/hands, getting out of chair without permission.	No information on how constant or varied tasks were linked to problem behaviors.	Exp. 1: ABABAB design. A = constant task (presented repeatedly) and reinforcement; and B = varied task (task interspersed with 4 others) and reinforcement. Exp. 2: Same as Exp. 1 except for the use of alternating treatment design.	Aggression occurred 48% of time in constant, and 2% in varied-task condition.	A higher rate of correct unprompted responses and fewer trials to criterion also occurred under varied-task condition.

Physical environment

Study	N	Population	Target behaviors	Comments	Design/Conditions	Results	Conclusions
Boe (1977)	29	Severe to profound MR	Hitting, slapping, pushing, kicking, grabbing, pinching, biting, pulling hair, spitting, gouging, head banging.	No information on how it was determined that room size and toys might be related to problem behaviors.	Monitored problem behaviors under the following conditions: half room, half room with toys, full room, full room with toys, full room with noncontingent reinforcement.	Percentage of intervals with problem behaviors was highest under the half-room conditions (6%, 8%), and lowest under full room with reinforcement (0.8%).	Presence or absence of toys had no effect on the amount of aggression.
Horner (1980)	4 1	Profound MR MR	Hitting, pushing, kicking, pulling, clinging, throwing, tearing, and so forth, plus repetitive and SIB.	No information on how it was determined that room size and toys might be related to problem behaviors.	Monitored problem behaviors in the environmental conditions: austere, enriched, enriched with manipulative objects, enriched plus DRO, and enriched plus noncontingent reinforcement	Enriched environment resulted in increases in both adaptive and maladaptive behavior with objects, and decreases in self-directed maladaptive behavior.	Enriched plus DRO resulted in increases in adaptive behavior with adults and objects, and decreases in maladaptive behavior with self and objects. Object and self-direct maladaptive behavior may be incompatible.
McAfee (1987) (Descriptive study)	918	68% MR 27% behavior disorder, 5% multiple handicaps	Threats, calling names, swearing, yelling, damaging property, hitting, pushing, pinching, pulling hair, taking others' belongings, and so forth.	Correlated problem behaviors with amount of work space per student.	No treatment.	Low, but significant, correlation ($r = -.198$) between work space and target behaviors. Factors other than density can affect behavior (e.g., setting arrangements, classroom management practices).	

(continued)

Table 35.3. *(continued)*

Study	Subject N	Subject Diagnosis	Behavior	Assessment procedure	Treatment	Outcome	Comments
McAfee (1987) (Experimental study)	19	Moderate MR	(Same as McAfee, 1987, Descriptive study.)	No information on how work space (density) was linked to aggression by these subjects.	Alternating treatment design used to compare level of aggression of Ss in 2 special education classrooms under 2 conditions—low density and high density.	Frequency of aggression in low- and high-density conditions was 10.20 and 20.05 (classroom 1), and 19.95 and 35.65 for second classroom. Results significant at $p < .001$.	Room size did not affect aggression in linear fashion, only when room size was sufficiently large was a decrease in aggression observed.
Exercise							
Bachman & Fuqua (1983)	4	Moderate MR	Inappropriate vocals, repetitive, off task, inappropriate use of hands.	No information on how it was determined that jogging and target behaviors might be related.	Used alternating treatment within a multiple baseline across 2 S pairs to compare no exercise to warm-up exercises; jogging at moderate and vigorous rates; and short, moderate, and long distances.	Jogging resulted in 50% reduction in the rate of problem behaviors for 3 of 4 Ss as measured immediately after jogging, and 1 and 2 hours later.	There was an inverse relationship between level of exercise and amount of problem behavior. Caution: Ss' health and enjoyment must be monitored; procedure should be systematically implemented.
Jansma & Combs (1987)	5	MR/ED (mild to profound MR)	Aggression (e.g., hitting, biting), SIB (e.g., hitting, pinching), property destruction, non-compliance, disruption (e.g., whining, screaming), repetitive body movements.	No information on how it was determined that physical fitness would affect problem behaviors with these Ss.	Individualized fitness program (e.g., warm-up exercises, muscular endurance training, cardiovascular training) for 1 hour a day, 5 days a week; and reinforcement for activity completion. Used ABAB design. A = no training program; and B = training program.	The time period when problem behavior was most frequent for each S was selected. The training program took place 1 hour prior to the high-rate period. Problem behaviors occurred less when the 1-hour observation was preceded by fitness training. Mean rates for all 5 Ss were 84%, 28%, 73%, 27% for ABAB phases, respectively.	The rate at a 2-week follow up was 72%, indicating the need for continued monitoring of participation in the fitness program.

DRO = differential reinforcement of other behavior; ED = emotional disturbance; Exp. = experiment; high-p = high probability; low-p = low probability; MR = mental retardation; S = subject; SIB = self-injurious behavior; 5-s = 5-seconds (similar construction for other units of time).

574

ing" to increase the compliance of 4 students to the request "Go to group now." Noncompliant behavior of 2 of the students consisted of aggressive acts toward peers and staff. Pretask requesting consisted of the delivery of a request that had a high probability of being followed (e.g., "Give me five") immediately prior to the target request. Results showed a "functional relationship between pretask requesting and an increased probability that students will follow a directive that marks a transition from play to work" (Singer et al., 1987, p. 289).

Changing the *physical environment* is another approach to managing problem behavior by altering setting events. Horner (1980) found that enriching an institutional environment with toys and objects led to increases in both adaptive and maladaptive behavior involving objects, and decreases in self-directed maladaptive behavior. Adding a DRO procedure effectively reduced maladaptive behavior with objects. Boe (1977) and McAfee (1987) found that adequate amounts of physical space could reduce the amount of aggression by persons with mental retardation, behavior disorders, or multiple disabilities.

A third approach to altering setting events is to change the *condition of the individual*. One way in which this has been done is through *exercise*. For example, Bachman and Fuqua (1983) found that for 3 of their 4 subjects long and vigorous jogging sessions resulted in lower rates of problem behavior (off task, inappropriate vocalizations, repetitive movements) following the exercise period. The effects were evident as long as 2 hours later. Rather than viewing these results as evidence of the need for forced or contrived exercise events, we might hypothesize that certain problem behaviors occur because of the absence of typical physical activities. That is, perhaps some students would benefit from typical physical education, recess, and other efforts to encourage their active participation in the movement and play experiences enjoyed by other persons.

Analysis

The review of literature on altering setting events was dominated by the manipulation of curricular/instructional factors, the physical environment, and the condition of the individual. Areas

lacking in research included altering the social environment and changing the individual's lifestyle.

Although a conceptional framework for setting events exists within behavioral psychology, and the importance of its use has been acknowledged, the concept has not been extensively applied (Wahler & Fox 1981). The lack of application may be partly due to the complexity of identifying relevant setting events from the vast number of possible events, and understanding the interactional nature of person and setting variables. A major area for development, then, would be to expand upon the assessment practices for identifying relevant setting factors. A comprehensive approach would consider the behavior's immediate antecedents and consequences, as well as other setting events. It would highlight the factors that motivate the problem behavior, and contribute to an understanding of the function of the behavior. Ideally, intervention would involve a combination of changing environmental variables and teaching functionally equivalent behaviors. In addition, the influence of more distant events should be assessed (e.g., through interviews of persons in these settings, and collection of data), and the effects of altering these events should be empirically tested. Examples of distant events are disruptions in daily routines at home, changes in sleep patterns, ending of a social relationship, a stressful activity earlier in the day, and the individual's lifestyle.

Response Covariation

A person's behavioral repertoire may include interrelated responses so that when one response changes, one or more of the other responses vary (Kazdin, 1982; Voeltz & Evans, 1982; Wahler, 1975). This response covariation can consist of: 1) chains of responses in which each response cues the following response, and is a conditioned reinforcer for the previous response; 2) clusters of topographically similar or dissimilar responses that are functionally equivalent (i.e., they produce comparable outcomes); and 3) response hierarchies in which the subject has learned to engage in alternative responses whenever interference with another response occurs (Voeltz & Evans, 1982). This means that while specific behaviors can be controlled by setting events and consequences, they may also serve as independent variables for certain other behaviors (Staats, 1975).

Response covariation has important implications for treating problem behavior.

> If a child's behavior repertoire is indeed organized into functional "clusters," it is conceivable that his or her deviant actions might be modified indirectly. Thus, behaviors difficult to deal with directly, such as stealing, might be modified by the contingent management of behaviors more easily dealt with. (Wahler, 1975, p. 28)

This effectively increases the options for treating a problem behavior. It may also be true that some behaviors have greater effects than others. In this case, a behavior other than the target behavior might be selected because it positively affects a larger number of collateral behaviors.

The concept of response covariation may also help explain why effects do not always generalize when environmental events are altered. That is, perhaps one or more responses within the person's repertoire exerts greater control over the target response than does the environmental stimulus that is the usual focus of behavioral interventions. Similarly, response covariation may be responsible for increases in other problem behaviors when one target behavior is reduced by an intervention (Kazdin, 1982; Voeltz & Evans, 1982).

Much of the support for response interrelationships derives from both theory and specific research to increase a positive behavior or decrease a negative behavior that resulted in unintended positive collateral or negative side effects. For the most part, these studies did not systematically monitor such side effects as part of the research design, and were not trying to demonstrate response covariation. However, knowing about behavioral interrelationships can help practitioners avoid producing undesirable side effects. Reviews of the literature on side effects can be found in Evans et al. (1988), Guess et al. (1986), and Voeltz and Evans (1982). The response covariation literature that is most relevant here is that in which researchers sought to identify interrelated behaviors within or across subjects, or to alter target behaviors indirectly through response covariation.

Research with aggressive-disruptive behavior

The greatest challenge in using response covariation is how to identify the responses that covary in different situations in a manner that would be useful for practitioners. Strain and Ezzell (1978) used a 10-second-interval recording method to code 11 categories of disruptive or inappropriate behavior of 18 adolescents with behavior disorders (See Table 35.4). A series of sequential lag analyses indicated three patterns of disruptive-inappropriate behavior that did not vary across settings. They also found that the greatest proportion of problem behaviors occurred in one treatment setting.

Some researchers have gone beyond identification of covarying responses and attempted to alter a target behavior by manipulating a behavior that had been shown to covary with the target behavior (see Table 35.4). Wahler (1975) used a child-behavior coding system consisting of 19 categories and a 6-category social-environment coding system to measure the behaviors of a nondisabled child and a child who was labeled mildly mentally retarded. After a 2-month baseline, behavior categories were intercorrelated to identify behavior clusters for home and school for each child. For example, the first child demonstrated a behavior cluster at school, and a different cluster at home. The school cluster persisted across four different school settings. It consisted of schoolwork that was: 1) positively correlated with repetitive behavior, 2) negatively correlated with object fiddling, and 3) negatively correlated with staring into space. Response clusters maintained over a 2-year follow up. When reinforcement was used to strengthen a positive behavior in a cluster (e.g., social approval for schoolwork), and a negative behavior was weakened (e.g., time out as a consequence for object fiddling), the other behaviors in the cluster varied according to their correlation with the altered behaviors.

Wahler's (1975) study clearly illustrates the use of response covariation as an intervention. Typically, a behavior that covaries with the problem behavior is weakened, or an adaptive behavior that covaries inversely with the problem behavior is strengthened. The adaptive behavior does not have to be incompatible, and, in fact,

Table 35.4. Treating aggression-disruption by using response covariation

Study	Subject		Behavior	Assessment procedure	Treatment	Outcome	Comments
	N	Diagnosis					

Identifying covarying responses

Study	N	Diagnosis	Behavior	Assessment procedure	Treatment	Outcome	Comments
Strain & Ezzel (1978)	18	Behavior disorder	See assessment categories.	Eleven-category rating system used during classroom instruction, afternoon rap session, and transactional analysis: 1) SIB, 2) social isolation, 3) questioning and demanding, 4) physical aggression toward peers, 5) physical aggression toward adults, 6) verbal aggression toward peers, 7) verbal aggression toward adults, 8) encouraging inappropriate sexual, 9) encouraging inappropriate, 10) refusal, and 11) property destruction.	No treatment.	Three behavior patterns identified: 1) behaviors that occur as isolated events with no additional events (1, 5, 8, 11); 2) behaviors with a high probability of continuing to occur (2, 3); 3) behaviors that may persist, and other problem behaviors escalate (4, 6, 7, 9, 10).	Most problem behaviors occurred during transactional analysis (range 55%–100%), the lowest amount occurred in classroom instruction (range 0%–16%).

Altering behavior by response covariation

Study	N	Diagnosis	Behavior	Assessment procedure	Treatment	Outcome	Comments
Wahler (1975)	1	No disability	Refusal to work, fiddling with objects, distracting others, rule breaking, lack of peer interaction, repetitive.	Nineteen-category child behavior coding system and 6-category social environment coding system. Identified for the first S: 1) a school cluster that appeared across 4 settings in which schoolwork was correlated positively with repetitive behavior, and negatively with object fiddling and staring into space; and 2) a home cluster in which sustained toy play was negatively correlated with compliance, social interaction, and repetitive behavior. Identified for second S: 1) a school cluster in which repetitive behavior was negatively correlated with social interactions and schoolwork; and 2) a home cluster in which oppositional behavior was correlated positively with aversive opposition, and negatively with sustained toy play and social interaction.	Used ABAB design. A = baseline; and B (Subject 1) = time out for object fiddling plus social approval and tokens for schoolwork (treatment at school only for Subject 1). B (Subject 2) = time out for violating rules or noncompliance plus reinforcement for toy play (treatment at home only for Subject 2).	Subject 1: Slight increase in schoolwork and repetitive behavior, and slight decrease in object fiddling and staring. Increments in schoolwork associated with increments in repetitive behavior at home, and decrements in social interactions at home. Subject 2: decrease in oppositional and aversive opposition, and increase in social interaction and toy play. Change in oppositional behavior at home was inversely related to oppositional behavior and social interaction with peers at school.	Covarying responses were stable over 3 years. During this time, the treatment conditions were in effect. Manipulating a response in 1 environment (e.g., home) affected responses in other environments (e.g., school).
	1	Mild MR					

(continued)

577

Table 35.4. (continued)

Study	Subject		Behavior	Assessment procedure	Treatment	Outcome	Comments
	N	Diagnosis					
Strengthening an adaptive behavior							
Parrish, Cataldo, Kolko, Neef, & Egel (1986)	3 1	Moderate MR Mild MR	Noncompliance, pushing, hitting, pinching, biting, kicking, pulling hair, whining, crying, screaming, property destruction, pica, escaping.	No information on how it was determined that noncompliance covaried with other problem behaviors.	Used ABAB-type designs to compare treatments that focused on increasing compliance (reinforcement) or decreasing problem behaviors (DRO, social disapproval, contingent observation, extinction).	Compliance and problem behaviors were inversely related. This relationship held true both when compliance was manipulated and when the problem behaviors were the focus of treatment.	Compliance and problem behaviors were not incompatible (i.e., they could occur at the same time).
Russo, Cataldo, & Cushing (1981)	1 1 1	No diagnosis (age 3–6) scores on Bayley [1969] up to 18 mos.) No diagnosis (age 5–7, IQ 60) No diagnosis (age 3–7, scores on Bayley [1969] at 2 years)	Noncompliance, crying, SIB, hitting, kicking, biting, pulling hair, sucking thumb.	No information on how it was determined that noncompliance covaried with other problem behaviors.	Used ABAB-type and multiple-baseline designs to examine the effects of reinforcement of compliance or nagging (repeating the requests) on compliance and problem behaviors.	For all Ss, reinforcement of compliance resulted in an increase in compliance and a decrease in problem behavior to near zero in final treatment condition. Nagging the S to comply resulted in an increase in most problem behaviors and no change in compliance.	Results may have been due to presence of reinforcement because noncontingent reinforcement was not included in baseline. Problem behaviors were not physically incompatible with compliance.

DRO = differential reinforcement of other behavior; MR = mental retardation; S = subject; SIB = self-injurious behavior.

could occur simultaneously with the problem behavior. Behavioral interrelationships that have received the most attention with this approach are: 1) appropriate toy play and repetitive behavior (Meyer, Evans, Wuerch, & Brennan, 1985), 2) independent toy play and oppositional behavior, and 3) social skills and aggression (Voeltz & Evans, 1982). In the Russo, Cataldo, and Cushing (1981) study (see Table 35.4), researchers reinforced compliance to requests, and repeated their requests in instances of noncompliance, while monitoring crying, self-injury, hitting, kicking, and biting. They obtained reduced rates of problem behavior with increases in compliance. It may have been, however, that Russo et al's. subjects engaged in self-injurious behavior (SIB) because the activity was unpleasant. In this case, reinforcement may have made the situation more pleasant, and this could be interpreted as a case of altering the setting events. This would be similar to the Carr and Newsom (1985) study reported in Table 35.3.

Analysis

Response covariation research has mostly involved nondisabled persons (Harris, 1980; Kara & Wahler, 1977; Wahler & Fox, 1980; Wahler, Sperling, Thomas, & Teeter, 1970), or individuals with mild to moderate disabilities. It has seen limited use with persons with severe disabilities (for an exception, see the Meyer et al. [1985] study described later in the chapter). Most of the studies utilized a complex behavioral coding system over an extended time period. Simpler and more efficient observational methods for identifying covarying responses must be developed for use in applied research. In some cases, it is obvious why behaviors covary, such as with a response hierarchy in which the individual relies on an alternative response whenever interference with another response occurs. In other cases, however, the link between covarying responses is less clear, such as when the strengthening of an adaptive behavior produces change in a problem behavior.

Identification of covarying behaviors may be a useful adjunct in trying to decipher the function of problem behavior, particularly when students have multiple problem behaviors and no clear function can be identified for them. In other words, more sophisticated coding or observational techniques may be needed when a cluster or hierarchy of problem behaviors serve the same function. However, the sophisticated observational and coding systems that have been used in the studies must be refined if they are to be used by service providers.

Systems Change

Most research focuses upon changing a single target behavior under relatively artificial treatment conditions. In order for some individuals with behavior problems to participate in integrated school and community settings, the existing support systems must be changed, such as the addition of resources, staff training, and organizational restructuring.

Research with aggressive-disruptive behavior

Durand and Kishi (1987) used functional communication training to intervene successfully with the agressive and self-injurious behaviors of students with severe/profound retardation and deafness-blindness. They used a consultation model in which group home, school, and institutional ward staff were prepared to make curricular changes and conduct the functional communication training. Consultants implemented curricular changes and modeled functional communication training in the presence of the staff, and made videotapes of the procedures available for staff training. Results indicated that staff behavior change consistent with the consultants' recommendations was related to improvement in student behavior. More importantly, Durand and Kishi highlighted the importance of providing assistance not only at the program and implementation levels, but also at the administrative level. This includes seeing that the support mechanism for continued implementation is established, staff have the time to implement programs, new staff are trained, contingencies are established for staff implementation of programs, and someone is available to provide feedback and modify the program (Durand & Kishi, 1987).

Donnellan, LaVigna, Zambito, and Thvedt

(1985) utilized a program model to intervene with severe behavior problems that occurred in community settings. The 16 subjects were all diagnosed as having, among other things, either autism, mental retardation, or brain damage, or as being hyperactive. They also displayed aggressive-disruptive or self-injurious behavior. The general program model involved a modeling phase, during which an intervention specialist demonstrated the procedures to the mediators (family members, care providers, group home staff). The second phase involved the gradual transfer of the program to the mediators. The follow-up phase consisted of providing daily program reminders, maintenance contracts with mediators, monthly program meetings, and monthly follow-up telephone calls and consultations. In 15 of the 16 cases, behavior problems were significantly less at follow up in comparison to baseline levels.

Singer, Close, Irvin, Gersten, and Sailor (1984) described a group home utilized for intensive training for persons in transition from institutional to community residences (e.g., foster, natural, and group homes). The program served individuals with severe or profound disabilities who also displayed severe aggressive-disruptive or self-injurious behavior. The program addressed the personnel issues associated with rural services by providing ongoing staff training, and a career for employees. Staff members had to demonstrate new teaching skills and they were monitored to ensure implementation. The program included a community liaison who developed social support networks for the group home clients, coordinated home-school programming, and assisted in the transition of clients to subsequent residential settings. Observational data indicated a decrease in behavior problems for all 9 clients monitored for the study.

Analysis

The studies reflect the need for intensive and ongoing support to programs that provide services to persons with severe disabilities and behavior problems. They also point out the need for continued work that will identify the organizational variables that are most critical for the implementation and maintenance of such programs.

Self-Injury

Teaching Functionally Equivalent Behavior

Research with self-injury

Several studies used teaching functionally equivalent behavior as an intervention for SIB (Table 35.5). Durand (1982a) compared self-injury under four conditions: an easy task, a difficult task, continuous vibration and an easy task, and continuous vibration and a hard task. Continuous vibration nearly eliminated the problem behavior. Vibration may have provided comparable sensory input.

Favell, McGimsey, and Schell (1982) worked with individuals who engaged in SIB maintained by sensory consequences. These researchers taught their subjects to manipulate toys that provided equivalent sensory input, and found that self-injury was substantially reduced. Thus, providing these individuals with a more appropriate way of obtaining their preferred reinforcers (i.e., through toy play rather than through self-injury) resulted in clinically significant improvements in these dangerous behaviors.

SIB has also been found to be maintained by negative reinforcement (escape from difficult tasks) and been reduced through communication skill training. These studies are described in Table 35.2, where SIB was grouped with aggressive-disruptive behavior (Carr & Durand, 1985a; Durand & Kishi, 1987).

Analysis

The research described in Tables 35.2 and 35.5 indicates that providing comparable sensory input and communication skill training are effective approaches to reducing SIB. More research is needed in this area and, in particular, it must be demonstrated how the approach can be applied with extremely intense behaviors that must be interrupted in order to prevent immediate injury.

Altering Setting Events

Research with self-injury

Table 35.6 describes the studies that intervened upon self-injury by altering setting events. Curricular and instructional factors were investigated by Gaylord-Ross, Weeks, and Lipner

Table 35.5. Treating self-injurious behavior by providing functionally equivalent behavior

Study	Subject		Behavior	Assessment procedure	Treatment	Outcome	Comments
	N	Diagnosis					
Bird, Dores, Moniz, & Robinson (1989)	1	Autism, profound MR, blindness	Hitting face with fist, flicking chin/nose with finger, pulling hair, head banging.	Motivation Assessment Scale (Durand & Crimmins, 1988) and observation suggested that escape from requests to do tasks was motivating the SIB.	Communication training involved teaching the S to hand a token to his teacher as a signal for a break from demands. Prior to communication training, several other interventions were tried: DRI, DRI and response interruption, DRI and reprimand, DRO and response interruption.	Mean number of SIBs per request across interventions prior to communication training was 21. For communication training, the rate per request decreased in 12 weeks to 1 and remained at 1 for 14 weeks, and 0 for the last 6 weeks.	S began to initiate requests to work. Similar results obtained in a second study with an S who displayed SIB and aggression.
Durand (1982a) (Exp. 1)	1	Severe MR	Hitting head and face with hand, flicking nose with hand.	Used ABACADA design. A = easy task; B = difficult task; C = easy task plus vibration via vibrator attached to chair; and D = vibration plus no task demands. Social reinforcement also provided for independent responses in conditions A, B, C.	No treatment.	SIB hits were greatly reduced in C, and both hits and flicks were near zero in D. Hits increased under difficult tasks and may serve as escape/avoidance behavior. Both forms of SIB were influenced by sensory input (vibration).	Introduction of vibration reduced correct responding on easy task from 99.6% to 81.5%. No change in SIB in other settings.
Favell, McGimsey, & Schell (1982) (Exp. 1)	1	Profound MR, blindness	Chewing hand or wrist, mouthing toys.	Preferred toys were selected based upon staff reports. The sensory-fulfilling properties of the toys were evaluated based upon the S's interaction with them (i.e., mouthing them).	Used ABABCBC design. A = baseline (no toys); B = toys available; and C = reinforcement of toy play.	In A, mean rate of SIB was 60%. In B, 10%, but subject mouthed toys 80% of time. When playing with toys was reinforced, SIB remained at less that 10%, toy mouthing was 35%, and toy play was over 80%.	Mouthing of toys (a self-stimulatory behavior) replaced the SIB. When self-stimulation was reduced in C, there was no increase in SIB.

(continued)

581

Table 35.5. (continued)

Study	Subject N	Diagnosis	Behavior	Assessment procedure	Treatment	Outcome	Comments
Favell, McGimsey, & Schell (1982) (Exp. 2)	2	Profound MR, visual impairment	Eye poking	Toys selected based upon staff reports of Ss' toy preferences. All toys had "striking visual properties."	Used ABAB-type design. A = baseline (no toys); and B = toys available. For one S who did not spontaneously reach for toys, toys were handed to him. For other S, toys were handed to him only at the beginning of a session.	When toys were provided, both Ss' SIB decreased from 40% to 10% (mean scores).	SIB was lower with toys that elicited "visual" play. Toy play that is topographically similar to SIB may be more effective in reducing SIB than toy play dissimilar to SIB.
Favell, McGimsey, & Schell (1982) (Exp. 3)	3	Profound MR	Pica: placing inedible items in mouth (e.g., cloth, paper); toy chewing.	Gustatory reinforcement was suspected as maintaining the pica. Thus, popcorn, which was preferred by Ss, was selected as alternate means of providing gustatory stimulation.	Used alternating-treatment design. Treatment conditions were: no toys, toys available, popcorn, toys and popcorn, popcorn contingent on toy holding.	Pica decreased dramatically when toys were introduced, but toy chewing greatly increased for 2 Ss. Providing popcorn alone greatly reduced pica for 2 Ss, and popcorn plus toys resulted in low levels of pica and toy chewing for 2 Ss.	Popcorn contingent on toy holding effectively increased the toy holding in 2 Ss.

DRI = differential reinforcement of incompatible behavior; DRO = differential reinforcement of other behavior; Exp. = experiment; MR = mental retardation; S = subject; SIB = self-injurious behavior.

582

Table 35.6. Treating self-injurious behavior by altering setting events

Study	Subject N	Subject Diagnosis	Behavior	Assessment procedure	Treatment	Outcome	Comments
Curricular and instructional factors							
Gaylord-Ross, Weeks, & Lipner (1980)	1	Severe MR	Biting hands and arms.	Observation indicated SIB varied across tasks and was greatest in demand conditions. This was experimentally verified with an ABA design. A = baseline; and B = DRI-1. Each session consisted of a series of 3 8-minute subsessions: task 1, task 2, isolate (no demands).	No treatment.	SIB was most frequent for 1 task (16 occurrences), and lowest for the other task and isolate condition (2 occurrences).	SIB was highest when demands occurred more frequently. SIB correlated with loud vocalizations ($r = .88$, $p < .01$) and soft vocalizations ($r = .53$, $p < .01$). This is a case study. Conditions were presented in ABCD order.
Touchette, MacDonald, & Langer (1985) (Case 3)	1	Autism	Hitting face with fist and slamming head into walls, furniture, and objects (rate of 50–1,600 times a day).	Scatter plot: For each 30-minute interval, recorded whether behavior occurred 0, 1–4, or more than 4 times. No obvious pattern emerged.	Treatments were: A = loose schedule plus 5 minutes of mopping (punishment) for SIB, B = loose schedule plus water mist in face for SIB, C = altered schedule to include activities thought to be associated with low SIB rate, and D = rest of schedule altered to resemble C condition.	No change in SIB under A and B conditions; under C, SIB decreased and occurred mostly in P.M.; under D, SIB was zero for the last 5 days of the 27 days of the D condition.	
Weeks & Gaylord-Ross (1981) (Exp. 1)	1 1	Severe MR with autism Childhood schizophrenia	Biting fingers and wrist.	No information on how it was determined that SIB was related to task difficulty.	Used ABACADACAD design to compare: A = no task demands, B = easy task plus praise and edible for correct response, C = difficult task plus praise and edible, and D = difficult task taught with errorless procedure (stimulus shaping) plus praise edible.	For S 1, errors and SIB occurred almost entirely in C; for S 2, SIB occurred in all conditions but was highest in C.	If SIB is associated with task difficulty (e.g., to escape, frustration), it can be reduced by using errorless learning principles to reduce task difficulty.

(continued)

Table 35.6. *(continued)*

Study	Subject		Behavior	Assessment procedure	Treatment	Outcome	Comments
	N	Diagnosis					
Social environment							
Burke, Burke, & Forehand (1985)	8	Severe, profound MR	Banging chin, head, and ear; pica; hand wringing (resulting in tissue damage).	Recorded SIB and the following antecedents by staff: 1) negative physical interaction; 2) negative verbal interaction; 3) commands, directives, instruction; 4) positive physical or verbal interaction; and 5) no interaction.	No treatment.	SIB occurred less than chance levels ($p < .05$) for positive interaction, and more than chance levels ($p < .05$) when no interaction was the antecedent.	The implication is that SIB might be reduced by creating environments where positive interactions are prevalent.
Mace & Knight (1986)	1	Profound MR	Pica: ripping/shredding cloth, placing cloth between face and face shield of helmet, placing inedible object on lips/in mouth.	Used alternating treatment design to examine the effects of levels of interaction (none, limited, frequent) and helmet conditions (with face shield, without face shield, no helmet) on pica. Results indicated pica was less during frequent-interaction and no-helmet conditions.	Based upon assessment results, the treatment that was designed consisted of no helmet and limited interaction (a staff person, who remained 3–5 meters away, made eye contact on a variable 1-minute schedule, and spoke with S on a variable 3-minute schedule). Pica materials were removed from S's mouth with minimal interaction.	In an ABA design where A = no helmet and limited interaction, and B = baseline, the mean percentage of intervals with pica was 29%, 51%, 15% for phases ABA, respectively.	A helmet with shield had been prescribed by a physician for treatment of pica prior to this study.
Touchette, MacDonald, & Langer (1985) (Case 2)	1	Autism	Blows to body, striking body against objects.	Scatter plot: For each 30-minute interval, recorded whether SIB occurred 0, 1–2, or 3 or more times. Pattern showed majority of SIB occurred beginning at 3 P.M.	Afternoon/evening aide, who was associated with the S's high SIB rate, was switched to morning then back to afternoon shift.	Pattern of SIB shifted from P.M. to A.M. and back to P.M. and this coincided with staff pattern changes.	Investigators were unable to identify differences between aides that would account for differences in SIB.

584

Lifestyle change

Study	N	Diagnosis	Behavior	Assessment procedure	Treatment	Outcome	Comments
Berkman & Meyer (1988)	1	Moderate MR	Vomiting, threats to self-injure (e.g., to bang/hit head, poke eyes or nose), actual tissue damage to body.	Phase 1 (baseline): All activities on living unit, minimal demands, restraint for SIB. Phase 2: Activities included 10-minute walks off living unit, DRO for not engaging in restraint and time out for SIB. It was observed that time away from living unit and institution was associated with less self-injury, and that use of aversive procedures resulted in more frequent vomiting. These observations resulted in program changes (see Phases 3–5).	Phase 3: More activities off living unit; visits to community/family; avoided conditions associated with SIB, consistent use of verbal reprimand for SIB testing. Phase 4: More activities outside institution, skill instruction, decision making by S regarding daily/lifestyle choices, redirect and reprimand for SIB testing. Follow up (7 months): moved to community, full-time employment, community activities, contact with family, skill instruction, decision making by S, redirect and verbal reprimand.	Mean number of daily occurrences of SIB testing, tissue damage, and vomiting, respectively, were: Phase 1: 10, 5, 4. Phase 2: 3, 3, 5. Phase 3: 1.4, 1.4, 8. Phase 4: .3, .1, .9. Follow up (7 months): .3, .2, .1. Follow up (1 year): .07, .03, .0.	This is a case study.

DRI-1 = differential reinforcement of incompatible behavior each time the incompatible behavior occurs; DRO = differential reinforcement of other behavior; MR = mental retardation; S = subject; SIB = self-injurious behavior.

Table 35.7. Treating self-injurious behavior by using response covariation

Study	Subject		Behavior	Assessment procedure	Treatment	Outcome	Comments
	N	Diagnosis					

Identifying behavioral interrelationships

Study	N	Diagnosis	Behavior	Assessment procedure	Treatment	Outcome	Comments
Lovaas, Freitag, Gold, & Kassorla (1965) (Exps. 1–3)	1	Schizophrenia	Banging head and arms on walls, corners, furniture, and so forth.	Exp. 1: Used ABA design. A = extinction of appropriate music behavior; and B = reinforcement of appropriate music behavior (e.g., clapping to music). SIB varied inversely with music behavior across all phases. Exp. 2: Replication of Exp. 1, but with a different response and environment.	Exp. 3: Investigated effects of different types and amounts of attention, and a stimulus not associated with withdrawal of reinforcement (new songs in music class).	Attention for SIB produced slight increases in the behavior. Introduction of new songs results in a decrease in SIB to near zero level.	SIB may be a function of the reinforcement and subsequent extinction of another behavior (e.g., clapping to music).

Exp. = experiment; SIB = self-injurious behavior.

585

(1980), who found that SIB was highest for one task and positively correlated with the rate of demands. Weeks and Gaylord-Ross (1981) found that errors and SIB were much higher for difficult tasks.

The social environment can also be a factor in SIB, as illustrated by Burke, Burke, and Forehand (1985), who found that SIB occurred at less than chance levels when the antecedent was positive interaction, and at greater than chance levels when there were no antecedents. Touchette et al. (1985), using a scatter plot divided into 30-minute intervals to map the occurrence of SIB, found that it was highest during the afternoon. When an afternoon staff person was switched to the morning, then back to the afternoon, the daily period when SIB occurred the most also changed, and corresponded to the staff person's schedule change. When the afternoon staff person was no longer employed, the SIB stopped. The effects of altering the physical environment were shown in Table 35.2, where SIB was included in studies of aggression-disruption (Boe, 1977; Horner, 1980).

Berkman and Meyer (1988) presented a case study that illustrated how lifestyle changes produced dramatic, multiple positive outcomes for a man who had engaged in severe self-injurious behavior for over 40 years (see Table 35.6). Among the interventions that appeared to be associated with behavior change were movement to a community residence from an institution, skill instruction, decision making regarding daily and lifestyle choices, participation in the community, and employment training and placement.

Analysis

Much of the research with setting events and SIB has focused on identifying the factors associated with high rates of SIB. More work is needed on how to use this information to reduce SIB. Other areas needing study are altering the individual's physiological state (e.g., through exercise), and improving the individual's lifestyle.

Response Covariation

Research with self-injury

In the Gaylord-Ross et al. (1980) study, reported in Table 35.6, an additional finding was that SIB correlated positively with loud vocalizations,

and negatively with soft vocalizations. However, this information was not used to plan an intervention. Lovaas, Freitag, Gold, and Kassorla (1965) manipulated appropriate responses (e.g., clapping to music) and found that the level of SIB varied inversely with the amount of appropriate behavior (see Table 35.7, which appears on page 585).

Analysis

Response covariation has barely been tested with SIB. Obviously one cannot engage in a lengthy assessment to identify behavior patterns when the subject's health is at risk. An alternative would be to develop more efficient observational systems or assessment checklists completed by persons who are familiar with the individual, so that hypotheses about response covariation could be quickly generated and tested.

Systems Change

A handful of studies have investigated broader intervention strategies to reduce self-injurious behavior. Durand (1983) observed that a staff absenteeism policy affected problem behavior (including SIB) among the individuals living in one residential setting. He demonstrated that instituting a reward system for staff to reduce absenteeism, and the accompanying reduction in absenteeism, resulted in a concurrent reduction in problem behavior. This study suggests that changes such as staff/teacher management policies (e.g. absenteeism policies) can be an additional approach to dealing with problem behavior. Other studies have also addressed systems change issues as they relate to self-injury (e.g., Donnellan et al., 1985; Durand & Kishi, 1987), although such interventions in integrated school and community settings are only just appearing in the literature (e.g., Janney & Meyer, in press).

Repetitive Behavior

Teaching Functionally Equivalent Behavior

Research with repetitive behavior

Some individuals appear to engage in repetitive motor behavior for social reasons. For these individuals, functionally equivalent responses would include behavior that elicits specific social reactions by others. Following this reasoning, Durand and Carr (1987) assessed the rocking and hand flapping of 4 individuals and found that the behaviors were maintained by escape from unpleasant situations (see Table 35.8). The subjects were then taught assistance-seeking responses (e.g., saying the phrase "Help me") during difficult tasks. This resulted in significant reductions in repetitive motor behavior for all 4 individuals.

Rincover, Cook, Peoples, and Packard (1979) used a single-subject experimental design involving sensory extinction to assess the sensory input provided by repetitive behavior. Utilizing their assessment findings, they were able to reduce significantly the repetitive behavior of 3 of their 4 subjects with autism by providing toys that afforded the subjects with sensory input similar to that obtained through their repetitive behavior.

Analysis

A number of studies have found that teaching toy play can lead to reduced levels of repetitive behavior (Azrin, Kaplan, & Foxx, 1973; Eason, White, & Newsom, 1982; Favell, 1973). Because these studies provided no assessment of the function of the repetitive behavior exhibited by the subjects, as was done in the Rincover et al. (1979) research, it is unclear whether the purpose of the behaviors was to gain access to specific sensory input, and whether the toys these individuals were taught to play with provided equivalent sensory input. There is a need for further research in this area, as well as in the area of communicative functions of repetitive behavior.

Altering Setting Events

Research with repetitive behavior

The literature abounds with research on altering setting events in cases of repetitive behavior (Table 35.9). In the area of altering curricular and instructional factors, Dunlap, Dyer, and Koegel (1983) assessed intertrial interval duration and its relationship to repetitive behavior. They found that introducing short intertrial intervals (1–2 seconds) for students with autism resulted in much less repetitive behavior than long intertrial intervals (5 or more seconds).

Durand and Carr (1987) recently demonstrated that repetitive behaviors acquire social functions for some individuals, such as to escape academic demands. Providing objects to manip-

ulate may be equivalent to making academic demands on some students, thereby increasing their rate of repetitive behavior. Consistent with this explanation, Mace, Browder, and Lin (1987) observed that their subject engaged in more repetitive mouthing during difficult activities. When they introduced a prompt hierarchy to reduce the difficulty of the activity, they observed significant decreases in mouthing.

Research has also demonstrated that repetitive motor behavior can be significantly reduced by changing the physical and social environment (see Table 35.9). Specifically, repetitive behavior can be reduced by increasing the opportunities for individuals to manipulate objects. Guess and Rutherford (1967) found that, for persons with retardation and visual impairments, providing objects that produced a variety of sounds reduced repetitive responses by half. Other studies, however, have not obtained similar results. Hutt and Hutt (1965), for example, found that presenting toy blocks to their subjects produced higher rates of repetitive motor responses.

One factor that could account for these discrepant findings is that the provision of objects to manipulate may allow a person to receive the same or similar sensory input provided by the repetitive behavior (e.g., a toy that creates visual input may serve the same function as flapping one's hand in front of a light). In the Hutt and Hutt (1965) study, the blocks may not have provided sensory feedback equivalent to the subjects' repetitive behavior. A second factor is that just making objects available does not ensure that clients have the skills or the inclination to manipulate them properly. Research indicates that it may be necessary to provide instruction in toy play skills in order to obtain reductions in repetitive behaviors.

The effect of exercise on repetitive behavior has also been investigated (see Table 35.9). Generally, the results show that the rate of repetitive behaviors such as body rocking, hand flapping, and object spinning are moderately reduced following increased physical activity such as jogging (Kern et al., 1982; Watters & Watters, 1980).

Analysis

Most of the research with setting events has manipulated curricular and instructional variables,

Table 35.8. Treating repetitive behavior by providing functionally equivalent behavior

Study	Subject		Behavior	Assessment procedure	Treatment	Outcome	Comments
	N	Diagnosis					
Durand & Carr (1987) (Exps. 1–3)	2 2	Autism Developmental disabilities	Rocking, hand flapping.	Exp. 1: Used ABACACABA-type designs to identify condition in which repetitive behavior was most frequent. A = baseline; B = increased task difficulty; and C = decreased attention. Frequency of behavior was highest in B. Decreased attention had no effect on behavior. Exp. 2: Used ABABA-type design. A = baseline; and B = time out contingent on repetitive behavior (i.e., escape from task). Repetitive behavior was negatively reinforced by escape from task demands.	Exp. 3: Used multiple baseline across Ss design. Based upon results of Exps. 1 and 2, Ss taught communicative alternative to problem behavior (to say, "Help me" whenever an incorrect response was made to a task demand). Requests were responded to with assistance with the task.	Immediate reduction in repetitive behaviors for Ss 1, 2, 3 and 4 from 21% to 1%, 12% to 0.5%, 24.7% to 3.8%, and 14.8% to 0.4%, respectively.	Communication served same function as problem behaviors (i.e., to escape from an aversive situation [demands of a difficult task]).
Rincover, Cook, Peoples, & Packard (1979)	4	Autism	Flapping hands; twirling objects on hard surfaces; picking lint, small strings, feathers from clothing and throwing in air; finger flapping in front of eyes.	From observation, it appeared that the sensory consequences that reinforced behavior were proprioceptive (for flapping hands), auditory (for twirling objects), visual (for picking/throwing lint, etc.), and visual and proprioceptive (for finger flapping in front of eyes). Used ABAB design within a multiple baseline across Ss to verify reinforcing properties of sensory consequences. A = baseline; and B = sensory extinction. Problem behavior occurred much less in B (near zero for 3 of 4 Ss).	Based upon assessment information, toys were selected that provided equivalent sensory stimulation: music box or autoharp (auditory), interlocking blocks (proprioceptive), beads and string (proprioceptive), and bubble-blowing kit (visual). Baseline rate of playing with toys was 0% for all Ss. Ss were taught to use toys. Physical prompting, reinforcement, and sensory extinction were used during training.	After toy training, the rates of toy play and problem behaviors were assessed. Reinforcement and sensory extinction were not used in this phase. For 3 of 4 Ss, toy play was at a high rate (approximately 60%–100%). Problem behavior ranged from 0% to 20% for 3 of 4 Ss. At follow up, which varied from 1 to 13 months, toy play was 90%–100% for 3 of 4 Ss, and problem behavior 0% for 3 of 4 Ss.	Sensory consequences for hand flapping were eliminated by attaching vibrator to Ss' hand. Carpeting the table surface eliminated feedback for twirling objects; dimming the room lights was used for picking/throwing lint, and so on; blindfolding and a vibrator attached to the hand was used for finger flapping in front of eyes.

Exp. = experiment; S = subject.

588

Table 35.9. Treating repetitive behavior by altering setting events

Study	Subject		Behavior	Assessment procedure	Treatment	Outcome	Comments
	N	Diagnosis					

Curricular and instructional factors

Study	N	Diagnosis	Behavior	Assessment procedure	Treatment	Outcome	Comments
Dunlap, Dyer, & Koegel (1983)	4	Autism	Autistic self-stimulatory: vocalizations, hand gazing, staring, rubbing saliva, flinging and gazing at saliva, flapping hands, head shaking, echolalia. Other self-stimulatory behaviors: tapping and rubbing furniture, scratching or picking skin or clothing and so forth.	No information on how it was determined that ITI was related to problem behaviors.	Compared ITIs of less than 4 secs. (average 1–2 secs.) and long ITIs (greater than 5 secs.). Used ABA design. A = short ITI; and B = long ITI. Self-stimulatory behavior was ignored, except for infrequent use of brief physical restraint for disruptive or aggressive behaviors.	Short ITI resulted in an average of 66% fewer autistic behaviors and 51% more unprompted correct responses.	Other self-stimulatory behaviors were unaffected by ITI. ITI defined as the period between termination of verbal consequence for 1 trial, and the onset of instruction for the following trial.
Mace, Browder, & Lin (1987)	1	Moderate MR, SED, brain damage	Placing a portion of hand or fingers between lips, teeth, or tongue (repetitive nail biting, finger licking, hand biting).	Used a multiple-schedule design (both conditions conducted each day in a counterbalanced order) to compare repetitive behavior in tasks that required a low (snack) versus high (table game) rate of student response. Mean rate of stereotypy was 7% in low-, and 29% in high-response conditions. Next, a comparison was made of novel versus familiar snack activities, and avoidance versus partial avoidance table game activities. Stereotypy was highest in the novel snack (17% vs. 3%) and avoidance table games (32% vs. 19%) conditions.	Prompts and praise used to teach novel snack activities and table games that were associated with the highest levels of stereotypy. The procedure reduced task difficulty and did not permit stereotypy to delay instruction.	Prompts and reinforcement led to reduced levels of stereotypy for novel snack activities for 2 separate activities (means of 3%, 0%) and 3 separate avoidance table game activities (means of 3%, 0%, 0%).	In the avoidance condition, the S who was engaged in stereotypy did not have to do the task. In partial avoidance, a verbal cue to engage in the task was given. Stereotypy may be used to escape or avoid tasks that are difficult because of novelty or response requirements.

(continued)

589

Table 35.9. *(continued)*

Study	Subject		Behavior	Assessment procedure	Treatment	Outcome	Comments
	N	Diagnosis					

Physical and social environment

Study	N	Diagnosis	Behavior	Assessment procedure	Treatment	Outcome	Comments
Baumeister & Forehand (1970)	12	Severe MR (Exp. 1)	Body rocking.	Observation suggested some Ss rocked more when with others who rocked. Exp. 1: ABAB design replicated with 3 groups of 4 Ss each. A = S alone; and B = subject with 3 other rockers. Amount of rocking was greater (p ⅛ .01) in B. Exp. 2: AB design. A = S alone, and B = S with 3 other Ss who did not rock. Amount of rocking greatest in B. Rocking may be due to presence of others, rather than imitation of others' rocking activity.			Results imply that rocking activity could be reduced by manipulating the social environment.
	3	Severe MR (Exp. 2, Ss were also involved in Exp. 1)					
Brusca, Nieminen, Carter, & Repp (1989)	3	Severe MR, visual and hearing impairments	Biting/mouthing objects; contortions; repetitive limb, head, body movements; posturing; noise; touching objects/self; twirling; SIB.	Observed Ss 10 hours a day and recorded S behaviors, interaction conditions (e.g., interaction-task), type of activity (e.g., structured art), teacher presence.		Problem behaviors occurred less during interaction surrounding instructional events. Ss responded differently to various types of activities. Teacher presence, even when there was no contact, was associated with reduced rates of problem behavior.	Implications for treatment include restructuring environments to provide contacts and activities associated with low rates of problem behavior.
Guess & Rutherford (1967)	7	Profound MR	Stereotyped behavior.	Examined mean group rates of behavior under 5 conditions: A = no materials; B = materials; C = constant sound; D = objects that generated sounds when manipulated; and E on living unit. Level of stereotyped behavior highest in A, C, and E, and lowest in B and D.		Significant differences in rate were found between conditions E and B, E and D, A and B, and A and D.	
	4	Severe MR					
	2	Mild MR (All subjects also had severe visual impairment)					
Levy & McLeod (1977)	31	Severe and profound MR	Neutral and repetitive.	No information on how it was determined that an enriched environment would affect behavior.	Compared behavior in existing day room to the room after it	Ten categories were monitored under traditional and enriched	Significant positive change occurred in appropriate play,

Study	N	Population	Behaviors	Method	Results	Conclusions
				was enriched. In the enriched condition, the room was divided into a large group area for gross motor and crafts, and a small group/private area with booths containing lights, music, mirrors, punching bags, and so forth.	rooms (e.g., play, social, SIB, aggression). Neutral/repetitive behavior occurred 80% and 69% of the time in traditional and enriched rooms, respectively.	resident-resident social play, aide-resident social/training interaction, and resident-resident social play with toys.
Runco, Charlop, & Schreibman (1986)	6	Autism	Toe walking, mouthing objects, rocking, gazing, waving hands, flapping wrists, grimacing, slapping, tapping, bouncing, mouthing, panting, rolling head, snapping fingers.	Each S observed with familiar and unfamiliar therapists, in familiar and unfamiliar rooms, and during familiar and unfamiliar tasks. Ss also observed alone in unstructured situations with toys in familiar and unfamiliar rooms.	Self-stimulation occurred significantly more often with an unfamiliar rather than a familiar therapist ($p \leq .001$). Self-stimulation in the alone conditions was significantly greater than the therapist condition ($p \leq .01$).	Familiarity or unfamiliarity of settings and tasks had a negligible effect on self-stimulation.

Exercise

Study	N	Population	Behaviors	Method	Results	Conclusions
Kern, Koegel, Dyer, Blew, & Fenton (1982)	7	Autism	Vocalizations, rubbing and waving hands, shaking head, starting, twisting ears, rubbing clothes, tongue manipulation, hitting the body, tensing the body, eye rotation, yawning, and so forth.	A repeated ABA design was used with 4 Ss to measure the amount of repetitive behavior: A = before; B = after mildly strenuous jogging. No information on how it was determined that jogging and repetitive behavior were related.	Repetitive behavior slightly less immediately after jogging, with further reduction 15 minutes later. Sample data for 1S: problem behavior 75% of time prior to jogging, 65% immediately after, 35% 15 minutes later.	For 1 S, correct responding on 2 tasks was monitored and found to be greater following jogging. For 3 other Ss, on-task behavior was highest following recesses in which they jogged.
Watters & Watters (1980)	5	Autism	Configuring fingers, rocking, hand flapping, mouthing/biting hands, tapping fingers against things.	Percentage of correct answers and intervals with self-stimulation were recorded during language training sessions that were preceded by 1 of 3 conditions: academic training, watching TV for 10–15 minutes, 8–10 minutes of jogging. Observation indicated problem behaviors were less following gym periods, field trips, and outside excursions.	All Ss engaged in less self-stimulation following jogging as compared to the academic precondition. The difference was significant ($p \leq .05$). Results on correct answers were mixed, and not statistically significant.	No differences in correct responding and self-stimulation were found between academic training and TV preconditions.

ITI = intertrial interval; MR = mental retardation; S = subject; secs. = seconds; SED = severe emotional disturbance; SIB = self-injurious behavior.

the physical and social environment, and to a lesser extent, the person's physiological condition. Areas requiring study include the identification and manipulation of social variables and distant setting events, particularly changes in the individual's lifestyle. The research on the effects of exercise once more raises the issue that the results should not be viewed as supporting the need for contrived exercise sessions. Instead, it may indicate the need for a schedule of physical activities that is typical for persons of the same age.

Response Covariation

Research with repetitive behavior

Eason et al. (1982) found that *teaching* appropriate toy play skills resulted in significant reductions in repetitive motor behavior for their subjects (see Table 35.10). Similar results were obtained by Azrin et al. (1973) and Favell (1973).

Meyer et al. (1985) taught 4 leisure activities (e.g., TV video games, Simon, Pinball, Lego) to 4 adolescents with severe disabilities, while monitoring 10 behavior categories representing appropriate (e.g., independent play, exploration, attending) and inappropriate responses (e.g., self-stimulation with and without materials). For one student, self-stimulation with materials significantly increased following training on two games. To "discover what behavioral mediators these negative responses might be related to" (p. 132), correlation across training sessions was examined. This further analysis showed that self-stimulation with materials correlated negatively with independent play for one game but not the other. The authors presented evidence that these different patterns of self-stimulation were related to the individual's preferences for the various toys—thus emphasizing the importance of including preference assessments in the process of selecting leisure activities for training. Similar results were obtained with a second individual. A third subject's self-stimulation without materials decreased with commencement of training on one or two games. However, these negative responses were not correlated with independent play, so changes might have been a consequence of a specific intervention for the self-stimulation. The fourth subject's self-stim-

ulation without materials was significantly less during one game, but increased during a second activity.

Analysis

The research on the relationship between adaptive skills, and particularly object manipulation, and repetitive behavior is substantial. However, more research is needed that helps explain the relationship between the repetitive behavior and specific behavioral and training variables (cf. Meyer et al., 1985). For example, does the repetitive behavior change because the training procedure limits the opportunities to engage in the behavior, because during training newly acquired adaptive behavior occupies the time usually filled by the repetitive behavior, because adaptive behavior fills an equivalent sensory need, because new behavior fills a skill deficit that initially led to the repetitive behavior, or because the environment is more stimulating?

Systems Change

Research with repetitive behavior

There was no research on the systems-change approach to addressing behavior problems in integrated school and community settings.

RECOMMENDATIONS FOR FUTURE RESEARCH

There are certain assumptions in the following list of recommendations that should be made explicit. It will be assumed that any intervention procedure used with persons exhibiting severe behavior problems must be designed so that it can be successfully implemented in integrated community and school settings. It will also be assumed that interventions must be acceptable to consumers (i.e., the students themselves, parents, teachers, or other caregivers) and to prevailing community standards, and that the goals and outcomes of these treatments must also be regarded as meaningful by significant others.

There are also certain overriding concerns that should be highlighted. First, there appears to be a perception on the part of many professionals that the current technology as reported in the literature, if applied properly, is capable of

Table 35.10. Treating repetitive behavior by using response covariation

Study	Subject		Behavior	Assessment procedure	Treatment	Outcome	Comments
	N	Diagnosis					
Meyer, Evans, Wuerch, & Brennan (1985)	1 1 1 1	Moderate MR, SED Severe, multiple handicaps Autism Profound MR	See assessment procedure.	Ten behavioral categories were monitored during baseline and training of leisure activities: 1) independent play, 2) exploration, 3) attend, 4) self-stimulation with materials, 5) self-stimulation without materials, 6) destructiveness, 7) smiles, 8) vocalizations, 9) out of area, and 10) teacher presence.	Used multiple-baseline design across leisure activities.	For 1 S, independent play negatively correlated with self-stimulation with materials for 1 activity. For a second activity, self-stimulation with materials increased, but this may have been due to the greater proximity of toys. For S 2, self-stimulation with materials was negatively correlated with independent play. For S 3, self-stimulation without materials decreased greatly during training on 3 of 4 activities, but was not correlated with other behaviors. For S 4, self-stimulation without materials decreased for 1 activity and increased during a second activity.	

MR = mental retardation; SED = serious emotional disturbance.

593

successfully treating all problem behavior. We would argue that the current technology for treating all cases of severe behavior problems is still evolving, and that important work on assessment and intervention procedures remains to be conducted. Second, we would emphasize that the emerging assessment and treatment technologies should be developed and validated for practical use by both professionals and paraprofessionals who may not be highly skilled and who may not have extraordinary resources. It is not adequate to say that potentially successful treatments exist, but they cannot be carried out properly by existing staff and in typical settings. Behavioral technology needs to address the fact that less than optimal conditions might exist in many treatment environments. Finally, the techniques developed should be observable and quantifiable. Procedures that cannot be easily taught to others (e.g., certain approaches based upon philosophical beliefs but never clearly described) are not likely to be helpful for the field unless a more systematic effort is made to share their essential characteristics in terms of staff or caregiver behaviors and the programmatic changes involved.

With these underlying assumptions and expressed concerns in mind, the following recommendations are made for future research and practice related to the use of nonaversive intervention.

1. *Assessment of the function of behavior problems should be expanded.* Current efforts have identified functions related to escape, obtaining social attention, acquiring tangibles, and self-stimulation (Durand & Carr, 1985). These efforts should be expanded and refined. One approach to expanding this information might be to integrate research on social-communicative development. Guidelines for incorporating this information into an overall program of social and communicative development must be developed and tested.

2. *Response covariation research should be expanded, with one goal being the development of assessment systems of greater utility that can be used with minimal training and typical resources.* The response covariation concept has important implications for identifying target behaviors that affect multiple covarying behaviors and for minimizing negative side effects. Its contribution to the functional analysis of problem behavior must be explored, and practical applications should be validated for use in typical settings.

3. *The knowledge base regarding medical causes of problem behavior must be more widely disseminated, and guidelines developed for systematic consideration of possible medical factors.* Although medical factors should be the first consideration in all cases of problem behavior, very little information about how medical conditions can influence behavior is available to practitioners. Furthermore, there are few guidelines available that explain how to examine the problem behavior profile (e.g., sudden onset, topography, time of occurrence, accompanying behaviors that might signify pain), how to collect relevant data, and how to approach medical professionals about possible medical factors related to problem behavior.

4. *Assessment practices need to go beyond immediate events, and should include a consideration (where appropriate) of more distal events (e.g., illness, sleep disorders, environmental stimulation) and evaluation of the appropriateness of general setting events, especially lifestyle issues.* The majority of the work in assessment has focused on immediate events such as characteristics of the physical environment (population density, level of stimulation), frequency of demands, and scheduling. Assessment technology must be expanded in order to be capable of determining the role of such influences as illness, sleep, and general environmental considerations in a more formal manner (e.g., through reliable and valid devices or procedures). Evaluations of the person's lifestyle must also be included to validate that the general features of the environment are appropriate and motivating for the individual.

5. *Assessment technology must be improved, and the assessment devices and procedures that are developed must be usable, valid, reliable, and accessible to consumers.* It is clear that the admonition to "perform a functional analysis prior to designing treatments" is approaching the status of a cliché that is rarely being heeded, and when it is, the procedures used appear to be no

more valid than clinical intuition (Durand & Carr, 1989). In fact, the results of a recent exhaustive review of the intervention research with excess behavior reveal that only 21.6% of the studies reported that some form of a functional analysis had been performed (Scotti, Evans, Meyer, & Walker, 1990). A technology is needed that can guide the design of treatments, and that can be employed by consumers. Although this technology is developing (see Durand & Crimmins, 1988; O'Neill, Horner, Albin, Storey, & Sprague, 1989), more work is needed in this important area.

6. *Despite the prevalent assumption that "we know all we need to know about reinforcers," it is clear that the current understanding and technology concerning the selection of reinforcers must be expanded.* A large number of students continue to resist habilitation efforts. This may be due, in part, to an inability to find potent reinforcers, or the absence of any motivators in the individual's current lifestyle. To be successful in developing nonaversive behavior management procedures, greater effort must be directed at assessment procedures for identifying meaningful reinforcers and evaluating the individual's satisfaction with the circumstances of his or her daily life.

7. *The repertoire of behavioral interventions must be expanded to include validated adaptations of methods that have been used successfully with individuals with less severe disabilities and with nondisabled persons.* Some problem behaviors of persons with disabilities may result from difficulties in adjustment (Meyer & Evans, 1989). Certain treatment strategies that have been used with nondisabled persons with similar problems might be modified for use with persons with disabilities. Examples of interventions are mood induction, anger control, relaxation, and self-regulation (Meyer & Evans, (1989).

8. *Interventions must include a consideration of the individual's choice of treatment and control over change. Research should determine how we can provide persons with choices and more control over what happens to them, leading to successful interventions that are also acceptable to the individual with severe disabilities.* Efforts should be made to include the person with disabilities in decisions regarding the goals of treatment (i.e., Should you intervene?), the procedures used, and the outcomes. Current technology is sufficiently developed to allow choices and the expression of preferences. Although this may not always be achieved, it should clearly be a high priority of all intervention efforts. Such a consideration may lead to treatments that not only result in long-term reductions in problem behavior, but that also increase the individual's personal satisfaction with the procedures and the outcomes.

9. *The origins and course of severe behavior problems should be explored, and resources need to be provided at the earliest signs of a serious behavior problem.* It is obvious that the only true "cure" for severe behavior problems is to prevent them from developing into dangerous responses. Long-term follow-up research is needed that will explore the process by which such problems develop, and to examine procedures designed to prevent their occurrence, or to prevent them from becoming severe. The present pattern of providing expert consultation, rigorous clinical planning, human rights review, and extraordinary resources only at the point at which a request to use aversives is made must be replaced by the provision of such reviews and resources to support positive behavioral interventions at the first sign of serious behavioral needs.

10. *Social validity must play a larger part in the identification, treatment, and outcome stages of programs to alter behavior problems.* At the identification of the problem stage, the social comparison or subjective evaluation by consumers must be based upon observation of the person with disabilities in the integrated setting, and used as a basis for selecting target behaviors. At the treatment stage, decisions should be based upon observation of the intervention by significant others, and not upon analogues and respondents who are not associated with the individual. At the outcome stage, social validation must extend beyond specific behaviors to include changes in collateral behaviors and the individual's well-being. At all stages, much more work remains to be done in how to determine the preferences of the person with disabilities in terms of selection of target behaviors, acceptability of treatment, and satisfaction with outcomes.

11. *Greater emphasis is needed on develop-*

ing and evaluating systems change efforts to remediate behavior problems in integrated school and community settings. Current efforts focus on the involvement of a small number of practitioners who attempt to change a single behavior in relatively artificial environments. In contrast, a systems approach might include educating significant persons in the natural settings where the individual with disabilities will live, work, recreate, and attend school. By doing so, those significant persons will be better prepared to support the individual with disabilities in each environment through acceptance, advocacy, and accommodating rather than changing the individual's behavior. Systems change holds promise for significantly reducing the need for treatment by altering the systems in which the person functions, and in those cases where the behavior must be altered, for obtaining durable outcomes.

12. *New criteria for treatment effectiveness must be established—criteria that include both change in the target behavior in natural contexts*

and overall positive change in the individual's condition, with all outcomes validated both by the individual being treated and by the significant persons in his or her life. We end this chapter with one of the more important recommendations. Judgment of treatment effectiveness has traditionally been based upon the experimenter's data on the immediate change in a single target behavior in atypical contexts (e.g., clinics, self-contained classrooms). Consequently, this standard has led to the belief that aversive interventions are effective, in spite of evidence that effects are short lived, and that they are limited to specific treatment conditions (Guess et al., 1986; Murphy & Wilson, 1981). The repeated calls for further research on maintenance and generalization issues have not resulted in substantial attention to these issues in the research literature (Gannon, 1986; Guess et al., 1986). Maintenance and generalization may be less troublesome issues if, by effectiveness, we refer to meaningful, positive change in the person's life.

REFERENCES

Azrin, N.H., & Armstrong, P.M. (1973). The "minimeal"—A method for teaching eating skills to the profoundly retarded. *Mental Retardation, 11,* 9–13.

Azrin, N.H., Kaplan, S.J., & Foxx, R.M (1973). Autism reversal: Eliminating stereotypic self-stimulation of retarded individuals. *American Journal of Mental Deficiency, 78,* 241–248.

Bachman, J.E., & Fuqua, W. (1983). Management of inappropriate behaviors of trainable mentally impaired students using antecedent exercise. *Journal of Applied Behavior Analysis, 16,* 477–484.

Baer, D.M., Wolf, M.M., & Risley, T.R. (1968). Some current dimensions of applied behavior analysis. *Journal of Applied Behavior Analysis, 1,* 91–97.

Baker, L., Cantwell, D.P., & Mattison, R.E. (1980). Behavior problems in children with pure speech disorders and in children with combined speech and language disorders. *Journal of Abnormal Child Psychology, 8,* 245–256.

Baumeister, A.A., & Forehand, R. (1970). Social facilitation of body rocking in severely retarded patients. *Journal of Clinical Psychology, 26,* 303–305.

Baumgart, D., Johnson, J., & Helmstetter, E. (1990). *Augmentative and alternative communication systems for persons with moderate and severe disabilities.* Baltimore: Paul H. Brookes Publishing Co.

Bayley, N. (1969). *Bayley Scales of Infant Develop-*

ment: Birth to two years. New York: Psychological Corporation.

Berkman, K.A., & Meyer, L.H. (1988). Alternative strategies and multiple outcomes in the remediation of severe self-injury: Going "all out" nonaversively. *Journal of The Association for Persons with Severe Handicaps, 13,* 76–86.

Bird, F., Dores, P.A., Moniz, D., & Robinson, J. (1989). Reducing severe aggressive and self-injurious behaviors with functional communication training. *American Journal on Mental Retardation, 94,* 37–48.

Boe, R. (1977). Economical procedures for the reduction of agression in a residential setting. *Mental Retardation, 15*(5), 25–28.

Browder, D.M., & Shapiro, E.S. (1985). Applications of self-management to individuals with severe handicaps: A review. *Journal of The Association for Persons with Severe Handicaps, 10,* 200–208.

Brusca, R.M., Nieminen, G.S., Carter, R., & Repp, A.C. (1989). The relationship of staff contact and activity to the stereotypy of children with multiple disabilities. *Journal of The Association for Persons with Severe Handicaps, 14,* 127–136.

Burke, M.M., Burke, D., & Forehand, R. (1985). Interpersonal antecedents of self-injurious behavior in retarded children. *Education and Training of the Mentally Retarded, 20*(3), 204–208.

Carr, E.G., & Durand, V.M. (1985a). Reducing behavior problems through functional communication training. *Journal of Applied Behavior Analysis, 18,* 111–126.

Carr, E.G., & Durand, V.M. (1985b). The social-communicative basis of severe behavior problems in children. In S. Reiss & R.R. Bootzin (Eds.), *Theoretical issues in behavior therapy* (pp.219–254). New York: Academic Press.

Carr, E.G., & Newsom, C.D. (1985). Demand-related tantrums: Conceptualization and treatment. *Behavior Modification, 9,* 403–426.

Carr, E.G., Newsom, C.D., & Binkoff, J.A. (1980). Escape as a factor in the aggressive behavior of two retarded children. *Journal of Applied Behavior Analysis, 13,* 101–117.

Donnellan, A.M., LaVigna, G.W., Zambito, J., & Thvedt, J. (1985). A time-limited intensive intervention program model to support community placement for persons with severe behavior problems. *Journal of The Association for Persons with Severe Handicaps, 10,* 123–131.

Donnellan, A.M., Mirenda, P.L., Mesaros, R.A., & Fassbender, L.L. (1984). Analyzing the communicative functions of aberrant behavior. *Journal of The Association for Persons with Severe Handicaps, 9,* 201–212.

Dunlap, G., Dyer, K., & Koegel, R.L. (1983). Autistic self-stimulation and intertrial interval duration. *American Journal of Mental Deficiency, 88,* 194–202.

Durand, V.M. (1982a). Analysis and intervention of self-injurious behavior. *Journal of The Association for the Severely Handicapped, 7*(4), 44–53.

Durand, V.M. (1982b). A behavioral/pharmacological intervention for the treatment of severe self-injurious behavior. *Journal of Autism and Developmental Disorders, 12,* 243–251.

Durand, V.M. (1983). Behavioral ecology of a staff incentive program: Effects on absenteeism and resident disruptive behavior. *Behavior Modification, 7,* 165–181.

Durand, V.M. (1986). Self-injurious behavior as intentional communication. In K.D. Gadow (Ed.), *Advances in learning and behavioral disabilities* (Vol. 5, pp. 141–155). Greenwich, CT: JAI Press.

Durand, V.M. (in press). *Functional communication training: An intervention program for severe behavior problems.* New York: Guilford Press.

Durand, V.M., & Carr, E.G. (1985). Self-injurious behavior: Motivating conditions and guidelines for treatment. *School Psychology Review, 14,* 171–176.

Durand, V.M., & Carr, E.G. (1987). Social influences on "self-stimulatory" behavior: Analysis and treatment application. *Journal of Applied Behavior Analysis, 20,* 119–132.

Durand, V.M., & Carr, E.G. (1989). Operant learning methods with chronic schizophrenia and autism: Aberrant behavior. In J.L. Matson (Ed.), *Chronic*

schizophrenia and autism: Issues in diagnosis, assessment and treatment (pp. 231–273). New York: Springer.

Durand, V.M., & Crimmins, D.B. (1988). Identifying the variables maintaining self-injurious behavior. *Journal of Autism and Developmental Disorders, 18,* 99–117.

Durand, V.M., & Kishi, G. (1987). Reducing severe behavior problems among persons with dual sensory impairments: An evaluation of a technical assistance model. *Journal of The Association for Persons with Severe Handicaps, 12,* 2–10.

Eason, L.J., White, M.J., & Newsom, C. (1982). Generalized reduction of self-stimulatory behavior: An effect of teaching appropriate play to autistic children. *Analysis and Intervention in Developmental Disabilities, 2,* 157–169.

Evans, I.M., & Meyer, L.H. (1985). *An educative approach to behavior problems: A practical decision model for interventions with severely handicapped learners.* Baltimore: Paul H. Brookes Publishing Co.

Evans, I.M., Meyer, L.H., Kurkjian, J.A., & Kishi, G.S. (1988). An evaluation of behavioral interrelationships in child behavior therapy. In J.C. Witt, S.N. Elliot, & F.M. Gresham (Eds.), *Handbook of behavior therapy in education* (pp. 189–215). New York: Plenum.

Favell, J.E. (1973). Reduction of stereotypies by reinforcement of toy play. *Mental Retardation, 11,* 21–23.

Favell, J.E., McGimsey, J.F., & Schell, R.M. (1982). Treatment of self-injury by providing alternate sensory activities. *Analysis and Intervention in Developmental Disabilities, 2,* 83–104.

Foxx, R.M., & Shapiro, S.T. (1978). The timeout ribbon: A nonexclusionary timeout procedure. *Journal of Applied Behavior Analysis, 11*(1), 125–136.

Frederiksen, L.W., & Frederiksen, C.B. (1977). Experimental evaluation of classroom environments: Scheduling planned activities. *American Journal of Mental Deficiency, 81,* 421–427.

Gannon, P.M. (1986). Research with moderately, severely, profoundly retarded and autistic individuals (1975 to 1983): An evaluation of ecological validity. *Australia and New Zealand Journal of Developmental Disabilities, 12,* 33–53.

Gaylord-Ross, R. (1980). A decision model for the treatment of aberrant behavior in applied settings. In W. Sailor, B. Wilcox, & L. Brown (Eds.), *Methods of instruction for severely handicapped students* (pp.135–157). Baltimore: Paul H. Brookes Publishing Co.

Gaylord-Ross, R.J., Weeks, M., & Lipner, C. (1980). An analysis of antecedent, response, and consequence events in the treatment of self-injurious behavior. *Education and Treatment of the Mentally Retarded, 15*(1), 35–42.

Guess, D., Helmstetter, E., Turnbull, H.R., III, &

Knowlton, S. (1986). *Use of aversive procedures with persons who are disabled: A historical review and critical analysis* (TASH Monograph Series, No. 2). Seattle: The Association for Persons with Severe Handicaps.

Guess, D., & Rutherford, G. (1967). Experimental attempts to reduce stereotyping among blind retardates. *American Journal of Mental Deficiency, 71*, 984–986.

Harris, A. (1980). Response class: A Guttman scale analysis. *Journal of Abnormal Child Psychology, 8*, 213–220.

Horner, R.D. (1980). The effects of an environmental "enrichment" program on the behavior of institutionalized profoundly retarded children. *Journal of Applied Behavior Analysis, 13*, 473–492.

Horner, R.H., & Budd, C.M. (1985). Acquisition of manual sign use: Collateral reduction of maladaptive behavior, and factors limiting generalization. *Education and Training of the Mentally Retarded, 20*, 39–47.

Hutt, C., & Hutt, S. (1965). Effects of environmental complexity on stereotyped behavior of children. *Animal Behavior, 13*, 1–4.

Janney, R., & Meyer, L.H. (in press). A consultation model to support integrated educational services for students with severe disabilities and challenging behavior. *Journal of The Association for Persons with Severe Handicaps.*

Jansma, P., & Combs, C.S. (1987). The effects of fitness training and reinforcement on maladaptive behaviors of institutionalized adults, classified as mentally retarded/emotionally disturbed. *Education and Training in Mental Retardation, 22*, 268–279.

Kara, A., & Wahler, R.G. (1977). Organizational features of a young child's behaviors. *Journal of Experimental Child Psychology, 24*, 24–39.

Kazdin, A.E. (1977). Assessing the clinical or applied importance of behavior change through social validation. *Behavior Modification, 1*, 427–452.

Kazdin, A.E. (1980). Acceptability of alternative treatments for deviant child behavior. *Journal of Applied Behavior Analysis, 13*, 259–273.

Kazdin, A.E. (1982). Symptom substitution, generalization, and response covariation: Implications for psychotherapy outcome. *Psychological Bulletin, 91*(2), 349–365.

Kelly, J.A., Wildman, B.G., & Berler, E.S. (1980). Small group behavioral training to improve the job interview skills repertoire of mildly retarded adolescents. *Journal of Applied Behavior Analysis, 13*(3), 461–471.

Kern, L., Koegel, R.L., Dyer, K., Blew, P.A., & Fenton, L.R. (1982). The effects of physical exercise on self-stimulation and appropriate responding in autistic children. *Journal of Autism and Developmental Disorders, 12*, 399–419.

LaGrow, S.J., & Repp, A.C. (1984). Stereotypic responding: A review of intervention research. *American Journal of Mental Deficiency, 88*, 595–609.

LaVigna, G.W., & Donnellan, A.M. (1986). *Alternatives to punishment: Solving behavior problems with non-aversive strategies.* New York: Irvington.

Lennox, D.B., Miltenberger, R.G., Spengler, P., & Erfanian, N. (1988). Decelerative treatment practices with persons who have mental retardation: A review of five years of the literature. *American Journal on Mental Retardation, 92*, 492–501.

Levy, E., & McLeod, W. (1977). The effects of environmental design on adolescents in institutions. *Mental Retardation, 15*(2), 28–32.

Lovaas, O.I., Freitag, G., Gold, V.J., & Kassorla, I.C. (1965). Experimental studies in childhood schizophrenia: Analysis of self-destructive behavior. *Journal of Experimental Child Psychology, 2*, 67–84.

Mace, F.C., Browder, D.M., & Lin, Y. (1987). Analysis of demand conditions associated with stereotypy. *Journal of Behavior Therapy and Experimental Psychiatry, 18*, 25–31.

Mace, F.C., Hock, M.L., Lalli, J.S., West, B.J., Belfiore, P., Pinter, E., & Brown, D.K. (1988). Behavioral momentum in the treatment of noncompliance. *Journal of Applied Behavior Analysis, 21*, 123–141.

Mace, F.C., & Knight, D. (1986). Functional analysis and treatment of severe pica. *Journal of Applied Behavior Analysis, 19*, 411–416.

Maloney, D.M., Harper, T.M., Braukmann, C.J., Fixsen, D.L., Phillips, E.L., & Wolf, M.M. (1976). Teaching conversation-related skills to predelinquent girls. *Journal of Applied Behavior Analysis, 9*, 371.

Mattison, R.E., Cantwell, D.P., & Baker, L. (1980). Dimensions of behavior in children with speech and language disorders. *Journal of Abnormal Child Psychology, 8*, 323–338.

McAfee, J.K. (1987). Classroom density and the aggressive behavior of handicapped children. *Education and Treatment of Children, 10*, 134–145.

McGee, J.J., Menolascino, F.J., Hobbs, D.C., & Menousek, P.E. (1987). *Gentle teaching: A nonaversive approach to helping persons with mental retardation.* New York: Human Sciences Press.

Menchetti, B.M., Rusch, F.R., & Lamson, D.S. (1981). Social validation of behavioral training techniques: Assessing the normalizing qualities of competitive employment training procedures. *Journal of The Association for the Severely Handicapped, 6*(2), 6–16.

Meyer, L.H., & Evans, I.M. (1989). *Nonaversive intervention for behavior problems: A manual for home and community.* Baltimore: Paul H. Brookes Publishing Co.

Meyer, L.H., Evans, I.M., Wuerch, B.B., & Brennan, J.M. (1985). Monitoring the collateral effects of leisure skill instruction: A case study in multiple-baseline methodology. *Behaviour Research and Therapy, 23,* 127–138.

Minkin, N., Braukmann, C.J., Minkin, B.L., Timbers, G.D., Timbers, B.J., Fixsen, D.L., Phillips, E.L., & Wolf, M.M. (1976). The social validation and training of conversational skills. *Journal of Applied Behavior Analysis, 9,* 127–139.

Morgan, R.L. (1989). Judgments of restrictiveness, social acceptability, and usage: Review of research on procedures to decrease behavior. *American Journal on Mental Retardation, 94,* 121–133.

Murphy, G.H., & Wilson, B. (1981). Long term outcome of contingent shock treatment for self-injurious behavior. In P. Mittler (Ed.), *Frontiers of knowledge in mental retardation: Vol II. Biomedical aspects* (pp. 303–351). London: IASSMD.

Neef, N.A., Shafer, M.S., Egel, A.L., Cataldo, M.F., & Parrish, J.M. (1983). The class specific effects of compliance training with "do" and "don't" requests: Analogue analysis and classroom application. *Journal of Applied Behavior Analysis, 16,* 81–99.

O'Brien, F., & Azrin, N.H. (1972). Developing proper mealtime behaviors of the institutionalized retarded. *Journal of Applied Behavior Analysis, 5,* 389–399.

O'Brien, J. (1987). A guide to life-style planning: Using *The Activities Catalog* to integrate services and natural support systems. In B. Wilcox & G.T. Bellamy, *A comprehensive guide to* The Activities Catalog: An alternative curriculum for youth and adults with severe disabilities (pp.175–189). Baltimore: Paul H. Brookes Publishing Co.

O'Neill, R.E., Horner, R.H., Albin, R.W., Storey, K., & Sprague, J.R. (1989). *Functional analysis: A practical assessment guide.* Eugene: University of Oregon, Research and Training Center on Community-Referenced Nonaversive Behavior Management.

Parrish, J.M., Cataldo, M.F., Kolko, D.J., Neef, N.A., & Egel, A.L. (1986). Experimental analysis of response covariation among compliant and inappropriate behaviors. *Journal of Applied Behavior Analysis, 19,* 241–254.

Patterson, G.R. (1974). Interventions for boys with conduct problems: Multiple settings, treatments, and criteria. *Journal of Consulting and Clinical Psychology, 42,* 471–481.

Plummer, S., Baer, D.M., & LeBlanc, J.M. (1977). Functional considerations in the use of procedural time out and an effective alternative. *Journal of Applied Behavior Analysis, 10,* 689–705.

Porterfield, J.K., Herbert-Jackson, E., & Risley, T.R. (1976). Contingent observation: An effective and acceptable procedure for reducing disruptive behavior of young children in a group setting. *Journal of Applied Behavior Analysis, 9,* 55–64.

Reid, D.H., & Hurlbut, B. (1977). Teaching nonvocal communication skills to multihandicapped retarded adults. *Journal of Applied Behavior Analysis, 10,* 591–603.

Rincover, A., Cook, R., Peoples, A., & Packard, D. (1979). Sensory extinction and sensory reinforcement principles for programming multiple adaptive behavior change. *Journal of Applied Behavior Analysis, 12,* 221–233.

Rosenbaum, A., O'Leary, K.D., & Jacob, R.G. (1975). Behavioral intervention with hyperactive children: Group consequences as a supplement to individual contingencies. *Behavior Therapy, 6,* 315–323.

Runco, M.A., Charlop, M.H., & Schreibman, L. (1986). The occurrence of autistic children's self-stimulation as a function of familiar versus unfamiliar stimulus conditions. *Journal of Autism and Developmental Disorders, 16,* 31–44.

Runco, M.A., & Schreibman, L. (1983). Parental judgments of behavior therapy efficacy with autistic children: A social validation. *Journal of Autism and Developmental Disorders, 13,* 237–248.

Runco, M.A., & Schreibman, L. (1988). Children's judgments of autism and social validation of behavior therapy efficacy. *Behavior Therapy, 19,* 565–576.

Rusch, F.R., Schutz, R.P., & Agran, M. (1982). Validating entry-level survival skills for service occupations: Implications for curriculum development. *Journal of The Association for the Severely Handicapped, 7*(3), 32–41.

Rusch, F.R., Weithers, J.A., Menchetti, B.M., & Schutz, R.P. (1980). Social validation of a program to reduce topic repetitions in a non-sheltered setting. *Education and Training of the Mentally Retarded, 15,* 208–215.

Russo, D.C., Cataldo, M.F., & Cushing, P.J. (1981). Compliance training and behavioral covariation in the treatment of multiple behavior problems. *Journal of Applied Behavior Analysis, 14,* 209–222.

Schreibman, L., Koegel, R.L., Mills, J.I., & Burke, J.C. (1981). Social validation of behavior therapy with autistic children. *Behavior Therapy, 12,* 610–624.

Schreibman, L., Runco, M.A., Mills, J.I., & Koegel, R.L. (1982). Teachers' judgments of improvements in autistic children in behavior therapy: A social validation. In R.L. Koegel, A. Rincover, & A.W. Egel (Eds.), *Educating and understanding autistic children* (pp. 78–87). Houston, TX: College-Hill Press.

Schutz, R.P., Jostes, K.F., Rusch, F.R., & Lamson, D.S. (1980). Acquisition, transfer, and social validation of two vocational skills in a competitive employment setting. *Education and Training of the Mentally Retarded, 15,* 306–311.

Scotti, J., Evans, I.M., Meyer, L.H., & Walker, P. (1990). *A meta-analysis of intervention research with problem behavior: Treatment validity and standards of practice.* Paper submitted for publication.

Singer, G.H.S., Close, D.W., Irvin, L.K. Gersten, R., & Sailor, W. (1984). An alternative to the institution for young people with severely handicapping conditions in a rural community. *Journal of The Association for Persons with Severe Handicaps, 9,* 215–261.

Singer, G.H.S., Singer, J., & Horner, R.H. (1987). Using pretask requests to increase the probability of compliance for students with severe disabilities. *Journal of The Association for Persons with Severe Handicaps, 12,* 287–291.

Smith, M.D., & Coleman, D. (1986). Managing the behavior of adults in the job setting. *Journal of Autism and Developmental Disorders, 16,* 145–154.

Staats, A.W. (1975). *Social behaviorism.* Chicago: Dorsey Press.

Strain, P.S., & Ezzell, D. (1978). The sequence and distribution of behavioral disordered adolescents' disruptive/inappropriate behaviors: An observational study in a residential setting. *Behavior Modification, 2,* 403–425.

Talkington, L.W., Hall, S., & Altman, R. (1971). Communication deficits and aggression in the mentally retarded. *American Journal of Mental Deficiency, 76,* 235–237.

Touchette, P.E., MacDonald, R.F., & Langer, S.N. (1985). A scatter plot for identifying stimulus control of problem behavior. *Journal of Applied Behavior Analysis, 18,* 343–351.

Voeltz, L.M., & Evans, I.M. (1982). The assessment of behavioral interrelationships in child behavior therapy. *Behavioral Assessment, 4,* 131–165.

Wahler, R.G. (1975). Some structural aspects of deviant child behavior. *Journal of Applied Behavior Analysis, 8,* 27–42.

Wahler, R.G., & Fox, J.J. (1980). Solitary toy play and time out: A family treatment package for children with aggressive and oppositional behavior. *Journal of Applied Behavior Analysis, 13,* 23–39.

Wahler, R.G., & Fox, J.J. (1981). Setting events in applied behavior analysis: Toward a conceptual and methodological expansion. *Journal of Applied Behavior Analysis, 14,* 327–338.

Wahler, R.G., Sperling, K.A., Thomas, T.R., & Teeter, N.C. (1970). The modification of childhood stuttering: Some response-response relationships. *Journal of Experimental Child Psychology, 9,* 411–428.

Watters, R.G., & Watters, W.E. (1980). Decreasing self-stimulatory behavior with physical exercise in a group of autistic boys. *Journal of Autism and Developmental Disorders, 4,* 379–387.

Weeks, M., & Gaylord-Ross, R. (1981). Task difficulty and aberrant behavior in severely handicapped students. *Journal of Applied Behavior Analysis, 14,* 449–463.

Wilson, P.G., Reid, D.H., Phillips, J.F., & Burgio, L.D. (1984). Normalization of institutional mealtimes for profoundly retarded persons: Effects and noneffects of teaching family-style dining. *Journal of Applied Behavior Analysis, 17,* 189–201.

Winterling, V., Dunlap, G., & O'Neill, R.E. (1987). The influence of task variation on the aberrant behaviors of autistic students. *Education and Treatment of Children, 10,* 105–119.

Wolf, M.M. (1978). Social validity: The case for subjective measurement or how applied behavior analysis is finding its heart. *Journal of Applied Behavior Analysis, 11,* 203–214.

◇　**CHAPTER 36**　◇

A Dialogue on
Medical Responsibility

JAMES SCHAFFER
Bloomington, Indiana

DICK SOBSEY
University of Alberta, Edmonton, Alberta, Canada

Perhaps more than any other case in recent history, the 1982 Indiana *Baby Doe* case (see Horan & Balch, 1985; McMillan, Engelhardt, & Spicker, 1987) focused national attention on the practice of withholding care from infants with disabilities. Baby Doe was born with a tracheoesophogeal fistula, an opening between the separate passages to the lungs and stomach accompanied by a narrowing of the esophogus. This meant that feeding the baby would be very difficult and likely result in food or fluid entering the lungs. Although this defect is fatal if uncorrected, it is not uncommon and correctable by a surgical procedure with better than a 90% success rate when performed within the first 24 hours of life.

Baby Doe also exhibited characteristic signs of Down syndrome, and his parents chose to let their child die of starvation rather than prolong a life that they considered to be unworthy of living. The hospital administration and courts supported the parents' right to make this choice for their child. Testimony given to the court suggested that while Baby Doe's fistula was correctable, surgery would not correct the mental retardation that could be expected as a result of the child's Down syndrome. Judge C. Thomas Spencer's apparently paradoxical ruling recognized that without surgery the child would die due to failure to receive nourishment, but also found that the child's physical condition would not be endangered by his parents' refusal to provide medical care or food.

A small group of concerned individuals fought to save the child. James Schaffer, a practicing pediatrician and researcher in Bloomington, Indiana, was among the leaders of this group. His earlier work on the utilization of glucose in premature infants had been instrumental in reducing infant mortality and in reducing disability in the survivors of prematurity.

Dr. Schaffer views himself as a pediatrician and a researcher, not as a radical or activist; yet he chose to stand up for the rights of Baby Doe. The discussion that follows presents excerpts from a dialogue on medical responsibility between Dr. Schaffer and Dick Sobsey, a TASH member with a continuing interest in issues surrounding withholding care. It recounts some of the events that surrounded the short life of Indiana Baby Doe and helps to explain why Dr. Schaffer chose to confront his colleagues and the legal system to attempt to defend a child's rights.

Sobsey: The Indiana *Baby Doe* has received a lot of attention. In some ways it appears to be a sad, but simple story. A baby was born with a birth defect. The parents chose to withhold treatment. The child lived for 6 days, and then succumbed. In other ways, it's much more complicated. This particular baby had Down syndrome. There was a strong difference of opinion and ap-

---

Note from Dick Sobsey: Jim Schaffer, my coauthor for this chapter, passed away June 1, 1989. He was a dedicated pediatrician and an accomplished researcher. He was also a caring individual who recognized the value of all human beings and acted on his beliefs regardless of the personal consequences. His research in nutrition for premature infants saved many lives and prevented many disabilities. His actions in the Indiana Baby Doe case discussed in this chapter illustrate his commitment to the well-being of all children. I feel extremely fortunate to have had the opportunity to work with him on this chapter. His loss will be mourned by all who share his concerns and commitments.

parent confrontation among physicians about what constituted appropriate treatment. The court seemed to be ruling that failure to provide surgery would kill the baby, but would not necessarily be harmful to it. Can you tell us what really happened from your own perspective?

Schaffer: What happened here quite surprised me and I did not rush in and get myself involved in this. Essentially, a baby was born, the nurse tried to pass a nasogastric tube, but could not introduce the tube to the stomach. It was a full-term baby, around 6 or 7 pounds, from a rather prominent family in town. The mother and father were both active at one time in the management of youngsters who had mental handicaps, particularly among Down syndrome children, before they were married. They had one or two other children of their own, I think. I don't know the details because they weren't my patients. A classmate of mine who was a general practitioner in town would often go to some meetings of a state society and I would cover for him. This baby was his patient. Dr. Owens delivered the baby and I was called to see the infant right away because it was obvious that there was a tracheoesophageal fistula. It's important to get immediate treatment for those babies before pneumonia develops.

Owens told the parents that they really didn't have to treat the baby if they didn't want to, but that the baby should stay in the hospital. He suggested that because the baby had Down syndrome and might be handicapped in other ways, perhaps it might be best if the child received no treatment. The family was presented with this and decided to push it to the ultimate. At that particular time our hospital administrator was away, and the assistant administrator seemed very fearful that he might get into difficulty in the community if he took a strong stand. I don't know exactly what happened; I went in and made the recommendation that the baby be transferred to Indianapolis immediately. The parents said, "No, that's not necessary. You can wait."

I don't know what the parents discussed with Owens, but in the end they not only rejected transferring the baby for surgery, they even rejected the possibility that our hospital participate in the baby's care. That's when I first realized

that this was all about sacrificing the life of a child with Down syndrome.

I don't mind people having philosophical debates. I don't particularly mind if people are trying to change our laws, but I'm a little opposed to sacrificing children with disabilities to do it. I didn't feel that this child was severely impaired and I felt on the basis of my training that my primary responsibility was to maintain life. I couldn't be absolutely responsible for the quality of it, perhaps the Creator had more to do with it than I did, and on that basis I thought we should proceed to save this child's life. I thought that they might reconsider, but the mother didn't change her mind and the baby was still there. A judge had ruled that the baby did not have to be treated under the state law of Indiana (*Infant Doe v. Bloomington Hospital*, 1984). He ruled that the baby could be maintained without lifesaving treatment in a hospital and instructed the hospital to do this. At that point, I thought, "This is getting out of line. I'm not a judge, but he's not a physician. I don't judge this community and he doesn't determine medical care."

Sobsey: Since this wasn't your patient, it might have been an easy thing to stay out of this situation. Frankly, I think that is what most people would have done. Why did you decide to get involved?

Schaffer: If I was not called in to evaluate this baby, I might not have intruded any more than my other colleagues did. We tend to be conservative in our approach here and to let activists slug it out in the ring, but I was there and I saw what was happening. I came to the conclusion that this baby wasn't very well represented, and that was the sadness of it all. It began to bother me because this was completely contrary to everything I'd been taught and believed in both as a human being and as a physician. I couldn't believe it was happening here in Bloomington because it seemed senseless to me. There was nothing to be accomplished except a funeral.

The law in Indiana said that the parents do not have to allow treatment. In that case, I said, "Let them take the baby home." If they did that and the baby died, the parents might be charged with child neglect and prosecuted, but why is starving a baby in a hospital any better? The experience has marked me rather considerably, and it certainly disturbs me a bit that even the theological community in this area had very little to say on behalf of this child. It seemed like everyone stood back and said nothing.

Sobsey: Perhaps many theologists as well as many physicians, in that circumstance, are more concerned about the rights of the parents than the rights of their children. The parents are the ones who choose the services for their children and who pay the bills. Perhaps theologists and physicians who treat children see the parents as the consumers of their services, not the kids.

Schaffer: Of course they do, but there are times when we must recognize whose interests are really at stake and protect the child regardless of what the parents want. I think the biggest handicap that many children have is their parents, particularly in the first 1 or 2 years of life. I worked all my life as a pediatrician. My job is not to take care of the children; it's to educate the family so they can and will take care of them. Many good parents work incredibly hard to meet their responsibility, but unfortunately too many don't even try. I think there's something wrong with our society when we tolerate that and I believe that a change is due.

Sobsey: Social responsibility is an abstract concept for many of us, but your involvement was more direct and more personal. The translation of feelings of social responsibility to personal action is difficult for many of us. Because of the fact that you were there, because of the fact you had some interaction with this child, you felt a personal responsibility to take action.

Schaffer: He was my patient once; I saw him and I exercised my medical opinion, which was based upon pretty adequate training at the university and I think that judgment was reasonably good. Suddenly, that judgment was being ignored. It was ignored by Owens, the judge, and the hospital administration.

Sobsey: It wasn't your diagnosis or your treatment plan that was being questioned here. It was the fundamental premises upon which that treatment was based, the premise that the purpose of a hospital is to provide treatment, and that the role of a pediatrician is to maintain and restore

the health of children. Basically, the judge ruled that two courses of medical treatment were available: your plan to obtain surgical correction and Dr. Owens's plan to sedate the baby while it starved. He considered both plans to be reasonable medical treatment plans and recognized the parents' right to choose between these two plans. He viewed the two plans as equal alternatives. The fact that one was a plan to keep the child alive and the other was a plan to oversee the child's death didn't seem like an important difference to him.

Schaffer: We were suddenly in a game with new rules. The decisions had already been made at that point. It was a matter of finding out where this course would lead and what the future implications would be. I did not go outside the hospital; I did not purposely create any trouble. Suddenly a couple of lawyers showed up from the university with some affidavits for us to sign. They took this information to Indianapolis to try to get a stay order from the Supreme Court, but the Chief Justice of our Indiana Supreme Court closed the record.

Sobsey: As you said, it seems that everybody's interests were well represented except for Baby Doe's. By the time that it became apparent that none of the usual justice system checks and balances were going to save this baby, it might have already been too late to do anything, but you persisted. You saw Baby Doe again before he died and that final visit has been described as "one of the most bizarre episodes in the history of American medicine, an episode that saw one doctor guard a dying baby from another that was threatening to try to save his life" (Lyon, 1985, p.37). Your determination amazes me, but Dr. Owens's determination to prevent the saving of the baby's life is even more incredible. How did this incident come about?

Schaffer: Once I realized what was going on and we were mobilized, our lawyers got busy. A couple of my colleagues including my personal lawyer and lawyers of some patients of mine finally found a loophole in the law which indicated that if the hospital administration and the hospital staff concluded that a patient in the hospital structure was not being supplied adequate nutrition, that the hospital could immediately assume legal responsibility for that child and provide adequate nutrition. Once we found out that could be done, I went to see the baby along with a couple of my pediatric colleagues so there'd be a uniform approach to this. We went to the room where the dying baby was sedated with Demerol. I hate to describe it because it infuriates me. It was grotesque. When we entered the room, the baby was blue and cyanotic with blood running out of his mouth. The nurse reported, "Well, he hasn't been crying."

Sobsey: Between his respiratory problems, the Demerol, and his lack of nutrition, he probably couldn't get enough air in and out to cry. Was he beyond helping at this point?

Schaffer: He was unconscious and at that point it was just as well. These things happen. We have diseases that come along, respiratory distress, cystic fibrosis, that bring about the same kind of situation even when we do everything in our power to change the outcome. Even with mechanical ventilation and all the drugs we have, when children reach this state, they go right downhill and they die. That, as far as human efforts are concerned, is beyond our current capacity to change, but after spending a lifetime struggling against death, it is particularly devastating to watch a child die who might have easily been saved. Once I realized the baby's condition, there was no point in persisting and I left. There was nothing more to do of any practical value.

Sobsey: Are there lessons in this for all of us?

Schaffer: We do not as physicians go out and systematically begin to solve the problem of having "defective babies" in the world by trying to eliminate them. It's not really a new approach to social policy. Hitler tried that approach, but he didn't succeed. Stalin tried time after time, but he couldn't get it done either. After a while one would expect people to realize that the technique is not worthwhile. It's not very effective, it's not a rational human approach to any problem, and it can't be rationalized under any human ethics. It's got to be recognized as what it is and legal people particularly have no alternative except to interpret manslaughter as manslaughter.

Sobsey: In view of the failure of the legal system to protect the life of Baby Doe, do you feel that they have a place in making these decisions?

Schaffer: I think they do. There are some difficult decisions that must be made and advances in medical technology and life support force us to set limits, but these decisions must be made on the basis of an individual patient and that patient's current status. Decisions can't be made on a history of categories of patients or the kind of predictions we can base on them.

Sobsey: Are you saying that Baby Doe's individual status indicated a need for treatment, but that decisions were really based on his categorical labels of "Down syndrome" and "mentally retarded"?

Schaffer: Yes, I think that's true. If another child without those labels attached to him had the same fistula, he would never be allowed to die in that manner.

It has always worried me that people, who supposedly have so much feeling and caring for children with disabilities, would choose to end the life of such a child. Whose fault that is, I don't know; I don't think it's anybody's fault, but I think it is a problem that exists. I think we have to be very, very careful as physicians in the healing art and I think this is also true of judges, ministers, and of anyone who takes care of people who are under distress. We've got to be very, very careful that we don't present them with a quick and rather unfortunate solution to their problems.

Sobsey: One phrase that is commonly used in decisions about preserving life or withholding treatment is "quality of life." Everyone seems concerned about what the quality of life of this individual is going to be. Can anyone make quality of life judgments for another human being? Does this phrase have any real meaning or is it just a way of making killing someone sound like you're doing it in his or her best interest?

Schaffer: I think it's part of a salesmanship program. People are using a word and a concept they don't even understand. What is quality of life? To me it's one thing, to you it's another. It might have to do with your past experience and everything that's gone before you—probably even your ancestors 500 years ago have something to do with what your definition of quality of life is.

Sobsey: It seems to me in a lot of cases when people talk about quality of life really what they're talking about is expected IQ points, that really their supposition is that somehow if a baby is handicapped or potentially mentally retarded then he or she doesn't have quality of life.

Schaffer: I think that was the definition that was being used here, but that's ridiculous. There is no relationship between intelligence and quality of life; and besides, no one really knew anything about what that baby's intelligence would turn out to be. They just knew that he had Down syndrome (they never even tested to confirm that diagnosis although it seemed quite obvious). "Quality of life" just provides a good reason in place of the real one, and the real one was that they wanted to get rid of that baby. Freud (1924) even described this law of rationalization as giving good reasons for real ones. The real one in this case was that the poor youngster had Down syndrome.

Walter Owens did nothing more than offer these people an option and they took it. The parents of this baby decided nothing could be done except have a funeral. If these parents didn't want their child, thousands of people would have happily taken this baby. The court ruled that these parents had a right to let their baby die. It was okay for them to give up their baby to death, but not to another couple who would care for the child.

Sobsey: We also hear the terms "ordinary" and "extraordinary measures." Are the courts setting a double standard where ordinary treatment for a nonhandicapped child becomes an extraordinary measure for a child with cognitive impairment?

Schaffer: I think that is exactly the double standard that is being set when parents of handicapped children are allowed to let them die.

Sobsey: The law has often treated children as their parents' property. As property, the parent can do what they want with the child, even dispose of it.

Schaffer: If we want that as a law, we'll make that law, but the purpose of our laws should be to protect life, especially for those who can protect themselves the least. Judges and juries must make difficult decisions. In this case, if there had

been more time, the legal system might have worked.

I see no reason why that baby could not have been placed in a foster home, perhaps undergone the operation, and survived the tracheoesophageal fistula. On the basis of our government and the very rights that the parents had to make the decisions they made, that baby should have had an equal right to develop to the full potential— whatever that potential might have been. Maybe he would have become a newspaper boy or a magazine stand manager, or even an artist or a taxi driver. I have many patients with Down syndrome in my practice. There is nothing obviously wrong with their quality of life. Many of them are very verbal; some have been able to matriculate out of the eighth grade of school and their IQs are about normal.

This has been very difficult for me, and very confusing. I look around and to me it's very difficult on the basis of my upbringing; my mother was very religious in a fundamental religion. She taught me to follow the edicts of the Bible. It seems to me that our judicial system, based on Judean law, is there to protect the vulnerable, and I don't see how any judge could have made the decision that was made.

I don't think it will ever happen in this community again. Sometimes honest people can really be pushed around when something like this happens because they become very ambivalent; they do not want to be aggressive or abusive. They give the benefit of the doubt and assume that someone must have a reason for doing this. Perhaps, they don't really believe the worst is happening. They don't believe that everyone will just stand back and let a baby die. If they do realize it, it may be too late. That will not happen again here in Bloomington, Indiana. People have seen what can happen and they will not allow it to happen again. Very little good has come from this unhappy incident, but at least there is that.

Postscript

Baby Doe lived from April 9, 1982 to April 15, 1982, but the issues that this episode raised continue. On October 11, 1983, Baby Jane Doe was born in Port Jefferson, New York, and transferred to Stony Brook University Hospital. Her parents' refusal to allow surgical implantation of a shunt to relieve fluid pressure resulting from hydrocephalus again brought national attention and court involvement. Decisions were made and reversed and that case would have likely reached the Supreme Court except that it became moot when her parents reversed their decision, allowed surgery, and took her home to care for her in 1984.

The issues raised in withholding medical care continue to be difficult ones. They have not been easily resolved by changes in legislation and government regulations. The rights of parents to make difficult decisions regarding medical treatment for their children continue to merit consideration and the extent of parents' rights in these matters will require careful determination. The rights of children, however, must also be considered and no solution that creates a different set of standards for children with disabilities will ever be acceptable.

REFERENCES

Freud, S. (1924). *A general introduction to psycho-analysis*. New York: Boni and Liveright.

Horan, D.J., & Balch, B.J. (1985). Infant Doe and Baby Jane Doe: Medical treatment for the handicapped newborn. *Linacre Quarterly, 52,* 45–76.

Infant Doe v. Bloomington Hospital, 104 S.Ct. 394 (1984).

Lyon, J. (1985). *Playing God in the nursery*. New York: Norton.

McMillan, R.C., Engelhardt, H.T., Jr., & Spicker, S.F. (Eds.). (1987). *Euthanasia and the newborn*. Boston: Reidel.

CHAPTER 37

The Future of Applied Behavior Analysis for People with Severe Disabilities
Commentary I

ROBERT H. HORNER
University of Oregon, Eugene, Oregon

The chapters in this book: 1) define basic values that should guide support for people with severe disabilities, 2) provide empirical support for those values, and 3) discuss the gap between what currently exists and what the values imply should exist. This chapter addresses the interacting role between service values and applied behavior analysis in narrowing that gap. My objective is not to chronicle the substantive contributions made by applied behavior analysis to date, but rather to reflect on observed and anticipated developments that will be most useful for people with severe disabilities.

Applied behavior analysis is the application of behavioral principles to produce socially significant changes in behavior. The technology of applied behavior analysis is well named. It is a technology that deals with the description, prediction, and control of human *behavior*. It is an *applied* technology of tremendous value to people with severe disabilities because it is focused on socially important outcomes. In addition, it is a technology that is based upon systematic *analysis* of events. The emphasis on analysis reflects an expectation that the technology will result in specific strategies for achieving desired behavior change outcomes (see Baer, Wolf, & Risley, 1968, 1987, for a more complete discussion).

For persons with severe disabilities, three developments in applied behavior analysis seem particularly important: 1) the manner in which the outcomes (dependent variables) are being defined and measured, 2) an increase in the number and variety of variables included in behavioral analysis, and 3) renewed attention to the

need for a technology for implementing behavioral procedures in typical school and community settings.

REDEFINING OUTCOME MEASURES

In behavioral psychology you are what you measure. No decision has a more significant impact on the development of behavioral technology than the decisions associated with defining and measuring outcomes (Gilbert, 1978; Johnston & Pennypacker, 1980). Once the outcomes have been agreed upon, the behavioral approach to developing knowledge is to observe behavior under different environmental conditions until features of the environment (intervention procedures) are defined that reliably produce the desired outcomes. This approach to building a science of behavior is at once predicated on fundamental human values, measurement technology, and professional humility. Human values determine the outcomes that are worthy of study, our measurement technology determines the accuracy with which these values can be translated into operational outcomes, and a humble approach to learning allows one's professional behavior (and the definition of the technology) to be shaped by changes in these outcomes.

Values are changing the way outcomes are defined and measured in research and service settings, and these changes suggest important advances for people with severe disabilities. Perhaps the most relevant change is a renewed effort to build functional measures of lifestyle quality. Our traditional micro-analysis of behavior is irrelevant unless we demonstrate fundamental changes in the way people live. A clear value expressed in the TASH resolutions is that children and adults with severe disabilities should have the opportunity to live, learn, work, and enjoy life in their local communities. Students should learn skills because those skills change the way they live. Adults should gain employment and residential situations because those situations result in the social status, social integration, physical integration, physical comfort, and increased personal choices typical of their nondisabled peers. The message is that the purpose of behavior change should be change in the way people live. As such, the measures we use to assess our technology of support should be measures of how people live. While it is useful to show that behavioral procedures reliably result in the acquisition of skills or the reduction of specific undesirable behaviors, those demonstrations will stand as hollow gains unless we also document increased access to physical and social integration options. The TASH resolutions provide an important challenge to behavioral clinicians and researchers. The challenge is to make the technology relevant. We need the following:

1. *Development of lifestyle measures* Increasing effort should be focused on the development of valid indices of how people live (Baer, 1986). Terms and phrases such as "quality of life," "lifestyle," and "valued activities" are being used in efforts to operationalize the critical indices that should serve as broad outcome measures (Bellamy, Newton, LeBaron, & Horner, 1986; Emerson, 1985; Keith, Schalock, & Hoffman, 1986; Landesman, 1986). This movement is not a rejection of the traditional micro-analysis of behavior that has served us so well, but an addition that emphasizes the values of the technology (i.e., social validity) (Wolf, 1978). Behavioral psychologists have struggled to separate the stream of behavior into units of analysis that can be analyzed. The successes from that effort have been substantial, and have placed us in a position to begin to rebuild those units back into the complex stream of behavior that makes up daily living patterns.

This is an important time in both the history of

our science and our service technology. To date, we have done a better job of describing our values about how people live than we have done of translating those values into measures or technology. To the extent that the values discussions can be transformed into valid, reliable measures, the foundation will be established for shaping our professional behavior into building the needed applied technology for achieving the outcomes that are consistent with those values.

2. *Measuring multiple variables* Our knowledge of behavior has relied heavily upon observing the changes in single behaviors as we manipulate single variables. Human behavior, however, is a complex ecology. The behavior of one person seldom changes dramatically without affecting the behavior of others around him or her. Individual behavior patterns of one person seldom change without affecting other behavior patterns of that person. For example, most of us can recall the complex array of behavioral changes that occurred when a friend or companion made the noble transition from being a smoker to being a nonsmoker.

A feature of both our research and service efforts that reflects the ecology of behavior is the monitoring of multiple behaviors simultaneously. Although multiple-variable research has been reported and encouraged throughout the history of applied behavior analysis (Evans & Meyer, 1985; Patterson, 1982; Wahler & Fox, 1981), the importance of these efforts takes on renewed significance in light of the TASH resolutions. The resolutions call for building functional skills in complex settings that result in both specific behavior change and comprehensive lifestyle change. These criteria demand a much better understanding of how behaviors interrelate. Increased focus on response classes over single responses (Day & Horner, 1986; Durand & Carr, 1987; Johnston & Pennypacker, 1980), on the covariation of different behaviors (Carr & Durand, 1985; Parrish, Cataldo, Kolko, Neef, & Egel, 1986), and on clusters of behaviors that produce functional outcomes (Guess & Helmstetter, 1986; Wilcox & Bellamy, 1987) are examples of the types of work that will lead to a more comprehensive measurement system that will promote strategies consistent with TASH resolutions. Both the maturing of applied behavior analysis as a discipline and the applied demands established by the TASH resolutions encourage the accountability that can only come from measuring and analyzing the interrelatedness of behavior in community settings.

3. *Measuring behavior in real time*   Skinner (1976) frequently has chided applied behavior analysts for limiting their work to the counting of behavior frequencies. In part, his point has been that an effective technology of behavior analysis (one that allows us to make a difference) must go beyond comparatively crude measures of how often a behavior occurs to more specific and precise measures of duration, intensity, rate, and conditional probability. Recently, computer technology has increased the ease and feasibility of data collection procedures via small computers that allow: 1) the observation of multiple behaviors simultaneously, 2) data collection in "real time" that produces information on the rate and duration of individual responses, and 3) software packages that allow easy determination of interobserver agreement and inter-relationships (conditional probability) among behaviors. While these options have been used for many years by some researchers (Patterson, 1982), the new technology is making them much more economical and much more widely available.

The impact of these new data-collection options will make it possible for applied behavior analysts to monitor the relationships between behavior and environmental events with greater precision, and to be guided by the resulting data in the development of more effective support strategies. It is auspicious that as computer technology is improving our ability to conduct micro-analyses of behavior, our field is struggling with operationalizing the values that should guide application of such micro-analysis.

EXTENDING THE SCOPE OF BEHAVIORAL INTERVENTIONS

For too long special educators have viewed behavior analysis as the technology for manipulating consequences to increase and decrease behaviors. Applied behavior analysis is a rich

science with ramifications that go well beyond the powerful technology of manipulating consequences. As we look to the future, applied behavior analysis will be best used as a technology for creating competent environments (Gilbert, 1978). Such environments will produce discriminative stimuli for adaptive behavior and provide opportunities for a wide variety of activities that offer effective antecedent opportunities. Several trends exist that are encouraging for this view of a broadened scope to behavioral programming.

Integration of Instructional Procedures and "Behavior Management"

Within the texts and organizations that focus on people with severe disabilities, there often has been an implicit assumption that procedures to reduce negative behaviors were different from procedures to develop positive behaviors or to teach new skills. However, as a science, behavior analysis is based on the assumption that all behavior operates in response to the same lawful relationships. A comprehensive approach to changing behavior patterns must apply these common laws to teaching new skills and reducing old, undesirable behaviors. The incorporation of instruction within behavioral protocols is most clear in recent research documenting the reduction of undesirable responses through teaching functionally equivalent, desirable responses (Carr, 1988; Durand & Carr, 1987; Evans & Meyer, 1985; Horner & Billingsley, 1988; Parrish et al., 1986). The exciting implication is that our powerful technology of instruction is being meshed with functional analysis and behavior management procedures to produce behavioral programs that have tremendous potential for delivering valued, durable, generalizable changes in behavior.

Multielement Interventions

Applied behavior analysis is not a cookbook of tricks for modifying behavior. It is a technology that defines and predicts the complex interactions between the environment and behavior. As the technology becomes more sophisticated it should be more effective at defining and predicting behavior change. One piece of this sophistication will be an increase in the number of variables that are manipulated within individual interventions. Although intervention "packages" have been available for years (Walker, Hops, & Greenwood, 1981), I believe that future programming for people with severe disabilities will be characterized by a substantial increase in the use of multi-element interventions. It will not be uncommon to see programs that include recommendations such as: modification in the residential location of an individual; change in the activities that encompass a daily routine; increases in the base level of exercise; change in the noncontingent access to social contact, praise, and preferred events; and increases in the presentation of choice options. These elements will be combined with more traditional procedures for modifying specific antecedent events, and ensuring that consistent consequences are available.

We are learning more about behavior and the variables that affect behavior. People with severe disabilities present many of the most challenging behavioral conundrums. As behavioral technology develops, we should expect to witness less intrusive, more comprehensive strategies for supporting the learning and behavioral complexities that make life difficult for these individuals.

IMPLEMENTATION TECHNOLOGY

The technology of applied behavior analysis needs a companion technology for transferring behavioral skills to those who should use them. This is an often cited, and long-lamented, problem. A science of behavior will only have impact on the lives of people if the science is used by those who deliver behavioral support. People with severe disabilities receive support from their teachers, physicians, families, friends, and adult services staff. As with nondisabled people, each of these relationships affects the behavior of a person with disabilities. As our skills develop in understanding how to construct effective environments, we must continue to build a technology for transferring those skills to people in critical roles. The objective should not be to make everyone a teacher or clinician. A central feature of the TASH resolutions is recognition that people should have access to many different types of relationships. The effort should be to ensure that

the individuals who are responsible for systematic support have the skills to deliver the most effective support possible.

Implementing behavioral technology must become a more critical concern. I believe effective implementation will require the following: 1) teachers and staff must view the outcomes of implementing behavioral technology as valuable, 2) teachers and staff must have access to the training and material needed to acquire the technology, and 3) the economic and personal costs of technology implementation must not be so large as to inhibit implementation.

To the extent that behavior analysis documents valued changes in behavior, there will be a large number of individuals who wish to implement the technology. The TASH resolutions provide an excellent foundation for defining the outcomes that will serve as the criteria. The task remains, however, to translate these outcomes into valid measures.

The major implementation effort to date has been in designing books, manuals, videotapes, and instructional courses that teach behavioral technology. A great deal is known about the process for teaching individuals to use behavior analysis. As the technology matures, however, there will be an increasing need to extend this effort. We not only need preservice programs that teach behavioral skills to teachers, but simple strategies that those teachers can then use to teach their aides, residential staff, and staff in vocational settings.

A final concern that has received too little attention is the extent to which teachers and staff do not implement behavioral technology because the personal effort required or the existing economic barriers are too great. As behavioral procedures are developed, it should be incumbent upon the developers to include an index of "effort to implement" as part of the assessment of the procedure (or package of procedures). That is, how much teacher time is required to establish the procedure? What materials must be obtained? What time must be invested in data collection, summarization, and interpretation? An effective technology of applied behavior analysis must not only produce valued outcomes—it must be easy to use.

REFERENCES

Baer, D.M. (1986). Exemplary service to what outcome? [Review of *Education of learners with severe handicaps: Exemplary service strategies*]. *Journal of The Association for Persons with Severe Handicaps, 11,* 145–147.

Baer, D.M., Wolf, M.M., & Risley, T.R. (1968). Some current dimensions of applied behavior analysis. *Journal of Applied Behavior Analysis, 1,* 91–97.

Baer, D.M., Wolf, M.M., & Risley, T.R. (1987). Some still-current dimensions of applied behavior analysis. *Journal of Applied Behavior Analysis, 20*(4), 313–327.

Bellamy, G.T., Newton, J.S., LeBaron, N.M., & Horner, R.H. (1986). *Toward lifestyle accountability in residential services for persons with mental retardation.* Unpublished manuscript, University of Oregon, Specialized Training Program, Eugene.

Carr, E.G. (1988). Functional equivalence as a means of response generalization. In R.H. Horner, G. Dunlap, & R.L. Koegel (Eds.), *Generalization and maintenance: Life-style changes in applied settings* (pp. 221–241). Baltimore: Paul H. Brookes Publishing Co.

Carr, E.G., & Durand, V.M. (1985). Reducing behavior problems through functional communication training. *Journal of Applied Behavior Analysis, 18,* 111–126.

Day, H.M., & Horner, R.H., (1986). Response variation and the generalization of a dressing skill: Comparison of single instance and general case instruction. *Applied Research in Mental Retardation, 7,* 189–202.

Durand, V.M., & Carr, E.G. (1987). Social influences on "self-stimulatory" behavior: Analysis and treatment application. *Journal of Applied Behavior Analysis, 20,* 119–132.

Emerson, E.B. (1985). Evaluating the impact of deinstitutionalization on the lives of mentally retarded people. *American Journal of Mental Deficiency, 90,* 277–288.

Evans, I.M., & Meyer, L.H. (1985). *An educative approach to behavior problems: A practical decision model for interventions with severely handicapped learners.* Baltimore: Paul H. Brookes Publishing Co.

Gilbert, T.F. (1978). *Human competence: Engineering worthy performance.* New York: McGraw-Hill.

Guess, D., & Helmstetter, E. (1986). Skill cluster instruction and the individualized curriculum sequencing model. In R.H. Horner, L.H. Meyer, & H.D.B. Fredericks (Eds.), *Education of learners with severe handicaps: Exemplary service strategies* (pp. 221–250). Baltimore: Paul H. Brookes Publishing Co.

Horner, R.H., & Billingsley, F.F. (1988). The effect of competing behavior on the generalization and maintenance of adaptive behavior in applied settings. In R.H. Horner, G. Dunlap, & R.L. Koegel (Eds.), *Generalization and maintenance: Life-style changes in applied settings* (pp. 197–220). Baltimore: Paul H. Brookes Publishing Co.

Johnston, J.M., & Pennypacker, H.S. (1980). *Strategies and tactics of human behavioral research.* Hillsdale, NJ: Lawrence Erlbaum Associates.

Keith, K.D., Schalock, R.L., & Hoffman, K. (1986). *Quality of life: Measurement and programmatic implications.* Nebraska City, NE: Region V Mental Retardation Services.

Landesman, S. (1986). Quality of life and personal satisfaction: Definition and measurement issues. *Mental Retardation, 24*(3), 141–143.

Parrish, J.M., Cataldo, M.F., Kolko, D.J., Neef, N.A., & Egel, A.L. (1986). Experimental analysis of response covariation among compliant and inappropriate behaviors. *Journal of Applied Behavior Analysis, 19,* 241–254.

Patterson, G.R. (1982). *Coercive family process.* Eugene, OR: Castalia.

Skinner, B.F. (1976). Farewell, My LOVELY! *Journal of Experimental Analysis of Behavior, 25,* 218.

Wahler, R.G., & Fox, J.J. (1981). Setting events in applied behavior analysis: Toward a conceptual and methodological expansion. *Journal of Applied Behavior Analysis, 14*(3), 327–338.

Walker, H.M., Hops, H., & Greenwood, C.R. (1981). RECESS: Research and development of a behavior management package for remediating social aggression in the school setting. In P.S. Strain (Ed.), *The utilization of classroom peers as behavior change agents* (pp. 261–304). New York: Plenum.

Wilcox, B., & Bellamy, G.T. (1987). *The activities catalog: An alternative curriculum for youth and adults with severe disabilities.* Baltimore: Paul H. Brookes Publishing Co.

Wolf, M.M. (1978). Social validity: The case for subjective measurement, or how applied behavior analysis is finding its heart. *Journal of Applied Behavior Analysis, 11,* 203–214.

CHAPTER 38

The Future of Applied Behavior Analysis for People with Severe Disabilities
Commentary II

DONALD M. BAER
University of Kansas, Lawrence, Kansas

Robert Horner has written a superb prescription for the future role of applied behavior analysis in its interactions with the problems of people with severe handicaps (see Chapter 37, this volume). I can neither improve his statement nor add substantially to it. It will be no service to the readers of this book or to their clients if I use my invitation to fill this space only to state a little differently what he has already written with accuracy, clarity, and cogency. Rather, I will try here to look ahead in a different way—not prescriptively, but predictively, given what I can see of the character of applied behavior anaylsis and its typical role in our society.

That kind of prediction may be worth offering here, because applied behavior analysis has been and will be of great value in helping people with severe handicaps; yet it has not been and probably will not be of correspondingly great value to the society in which those people live and secure help. It may be worth commenting on that paradox in a way that might help to prevent it from being a handicap of its own. While I may not accomplish that here, clarifying the problem may cause many of us to think it through more thoroughly—and out of all that collective analysis we may improve the discipline's ability to help.

It would first be prudent to put this effort in its place. Prediction of behavior is a fool's errand. Our discipline is inherently good at the production of behavior, and inherently bad at its prediction: The more you know about how to produce behavior, the more you know that you could hardly know what the rest of the environment has done, is doing, and will do to produce the future

behavior of the organism under study. Prediction is an astronomer's game, not a behaviorist's. Perhaps everything to follow is idle—no more than a series of bets.

The safest bet (as usual) is that our future will be an extension of our present. Applied behavior analysis has a rather complex status in its society, and that status may nowhere be better than in its applications to the understanding and amelioration of severe handicaps. After all, it is a philosophy that leads us to explicitly and studiously separate the person from the organizations and disorganizations of that person's behaviors that constitute handicap. It lets us see that person as totally worthy, exactly because it lets us see the handicap as nothing more than an unfortunate organization or disorganization of some behaviors, most often as some crucial absent skills waiting to be seen as such and then to be taught. If we practice this discipline, we become moderately good at analyzing what skills are crucial to the amelioration of every form of handicap, and better than that at teaching those skills. In the field of severe handicaps, applied behavior analysis seems to be widely appreciated for just those characteristics.

However, the status of applied behavior analysis is not that good in most other areas. I suggest that this society contains a few hundred thousand psychologists, educational psychologists, special educators, speech pathologists, and other therapists and professionals who deal with people's problems, including severe handicaps—but I doubt if there are more than 5,000 applied behavior analysts just now, more than 50 years after the publication of Skinner's *The Be-havior of Organisms* (1938). We are clearly not the mainstream. Let me argue that we never will be, but please note that, ultimately, this is both an optimistic and a cheerful argument.

Applied behavior analysis is an exercise in behaviorism, and our recent history seems to show, as our long-term history has shown again and again, that behaviorism is not an attractive view of life for members of societies like ours—or, perhaps, for any of history's societies. The vast majority of us think of ourselves mentalistically, not behaviorally. Indeed, our stereotype of something called "behaviorism" is that it denies that we do anything resembling thinking, and so we prove that stereotype wrong every time we think about it.

It is difficult to replace that stereotype with an accurate one. I suspect that we all have a personal history of thinking through what to do about our problems and acting on our feelings. That kind of history seems to show us that we are mental organisms whose behavior merely testifies—poorly—to that mental activity. True, *shows* is not the same as *proves,* but the vast majority of us have not had the course in proof yet, and never will—and of those of us who do encounter it, few will generalize it enough to ask themselves what they mean when they attribute their behavior to what they think and feel.

Absent that course and a few more to follow, it is inevitable to think like that. As children, we learn our languages from people who think like that, and our language is full of stimulus controls and reinforcers for thinking like that. (Yes, I see the irony.) Consider the missing curricula: Unless we are taught to engage in constant, rigorous questions about what our languages can possibly mean when they attribute to our minds and feelings the cause of what we do; unless we are taught to consider the possibility that "mean" means only the environmental conditions under which those words are used and not used; unless we are shown that what we attribute to *mind* can also be attributed to *environment,* and that mind itself can be attributed to environment, and that how we talk about all of that can itself be attributed to environment; unless we are taught that case after case of those propositions can be put to empirical proof; and unless we are taught what

proof requires we shall remain generalized, practicing, uncritical mentalists.

As any teacher of behavior analysis knows, replacing that view with a more analytic one is difficult and tedious. It requires constant repetition of the essential questioning and argument in concept area after concept area. Just as breaking a smoking habit usually requires its explicit suppression in almost every stimulus situation in which it has ever systematically occurred, so the breaking of systematic mentalistic attribution requires effective counterargument in virtually every conceptual setting in which our language has ensconced it. Generalization in both those problems comes hard and very, very late.

So, an obvious bet is that the future of the discipline of applied behavior analysis is not to be adopted as such, but rather is to be stolen from, a concept at a time, a technique at a time. "Stealing" means that while the behavior-analytic system from which those concepts and techniques flow is ignored, some of its concepts and effective techniques will be used, after they are relabeled in everyday language—or in cognitive, pseudoneural, computer-electronic, and other dynamic analogues, all intrinsically surrogates for the mentalisms of everyday language. That will make the stealers more effective, but not more analytic; and even so, we should celebrate any increase in their effectiveness at dealing with problems, no matter how they came by it, no matter what they left behind. Like us, 'hey *deal* with problems; our task is to empower all of them as well as ourselves in that effort.

After all, they are not alone in that piecemeal application. At present, applied behavior analysis itself disseminates mainly half-analyzed programs as packages. It is possible to make a complete analysis of an effective package, and thus make the package optimally effective, but it is extraordinarily expensive in time, effort, and money to do so, and half-analyzed packages often work well enough. There is a great deal of punishment and almost no reinforcement for complete package analysis. Those costs and non-benefits will not change, so the practice will not change either.

Yet, we know that application is not application until it is effective at dissemination. So, we shall pursue dissemination nonanalytically for the most part, for the same reasons that we do not completely analyze most of our packages. Thus, dissemination will become increasingly a folklore rather than a system of principles and practices; and since dissemination requires packages to disseminate, and packages are rarely if ever analyzed thoroughly, our categorical imperative to disseminate is a trap luring us farther and farther away from knowing what we are doing at almost any truly analytic level. In that respect, we shall become increasingly like the people who steal from us.

I bet that this is what will happen, despite the fact that applied behavior analysis, as a system, will continue to be taught in the universities. The nature of universities is to preserve anything that once enters them, even if only in the library, and they will probably preserve us, too. But what we teach in the universities as an experimental system will be done outside the universities more and more unsystemically.

As a system, applied behavior analysis will continue not to be mainstream psychology. It has the wrong language, and its insistence on environmental causation is ruinous to psychology's bid for public acceptance with its various concepts of the autonomous person. But that may not be a long-term disadvantage for applied behavior analysis: Increasingly, there is no such thing as mainstream psychology; there is instead a collection of enterprises, too many of which are essentially show business to allow the collectivity to be considered as a scientific discipline. Sometime in the future, it may be to the advantage of a scientific system *not* to be part of that supposed mainstream.

Besides, would we really rather be mainstream in the stream that's main these days? Joseph V. Brady was quoted (accurately) in the *APA Monitor* as saying that behavior analysis was to psychology as astronomy was to astrol-ogy; in my opinion, apart from my belief that there is no one thing that can be called psychology, he is correct for too many of the parts of the conglomeration that nevertheless is called psychology. Do we want to be astrologers, even if that is what former President and Mrs. Reagan consulted? I trust that you are answering "No." (If you are answering "Yes," this is the wrong chapter for you.) Because of that, please note that astrology is much more our society's choice for making decisions than is behavior analysis. Consult the newspapers and the magazines any day, and see how easy it is to find your horoscope and some "Ann Landers/Dear Abby" mentalisms, and how unlikely it is to find any astronomy or any behavior analysis. Noting that, I can see that I *ought* to be nonmainstream.

But it is to psychology's advantage to be good show business, especially if too much of it has little but entertainment to sell. By contrast, applied behavior analysis is intrinsically not good show business, and displays no tendency to even attempt becoming better show business. If that does not change, the prediction of our continuing public insignificance despite sometimes having something effective to sell is obvious.

I bet that we shall continue to attract extraordinarily good people. They will have to be something special to choose us nonmainstreamers, and of the two kinds of "somethings special" that will apply, we had better learn to choose the heroes consistently over the charlatans.

We ought to be glad about that future. It includes, as does the present, a chance to learn and thus to understand, and out of that understanding a chance to serve, to help, and sometimes to solve. That opportunity is not at risk; rejoice in it and be glad. Obviously, we need not be mainstream to do what we do best, and very few people in this world knowingly get to do what they do best knowing what a good thing it is to do.

REFERENCE

Skinner, B.F. (1938). *The behavior of organisms.* New York: Appleton-Century-Crofts.

CHAPTER 39

A Dialogue on Power Relationships and Aversive Control

ANNE M. DONNELLAN
University of Wisconsin–Madison, Madison, Wisconsin

BARBARA C. CUTLER
Boston University, Boston, Massachusetts

Issues around behavior modification and its potential for controlling human behavior have been in the public eye since the publication of *A Clockwork Orange* (Burgess, 1962) in the '60s. Today, there is particular interest paid to the use of aversive control procedures in the name of treatment. Many advocates are concerned about the use of these procedures with disabled and dependent populations. In fact, some have argued that the use of punishment in behavioral treatment is confined almost totally to individuals with severe impairments at least in part because these individuals cannot speak out against what is being done to them. Others argue that these procedures are essentially for the effective treatment of problems such as severe self-injurious behavior and aggression often seen in these learner populations, and that the judgment of others is sufficient to justify their use with individuals who are not considered legally competent.

While vituperative, these arguments are typically limited to professional arenas and audiences. Occasionally, however, incidences occur that so outrage the consciousness of the professionals and the public that advocates for effective and respectful treatment of individuals challenged by severe behavior problems are able to find a forum outside the journals and professional meetings. Such is the situation in Massachusetts where, inside or outside the professional community, one voice that always speaks clearly, softly, but directly to the issues is that of Barbara Cutler. A parent, advocate, author, and

long-time professional educator, Ms. Cutler has been active on the local and national scene regarding aversive treatments. She talked with Anne Donnellan, a TASH member with her own longstanding interest in positive approaches to the education of all learners. The edited text of their dialogue follows.

Donnellan: Barbara, how has your experience shaped your present attitudes about behavior modification and behavioral technology?

Cutler: My son Rob is now 33 years old. That's a lot of time and experience with the services people with autism/challenging behaviors and their families receive. Too often the experience has been that one of us, or usually both Rob and I, have been put down by the people who are supposed to serve people like my son and me. However, there were a few years when we both experienced some degree of respect and hope. That was in the early 1970s when behavior modification was coming into vogue and there was for us a lot of emphasis on the positive: a belief in my son's ability, hope that he could do more, and some respect for me as a parent trying to work with professionals to help my son.

Donnellan: Of course, 30 years or so ago the official professional opinion was that parents—particularly mothers–caused autism.

Cutler: Indeed! So when he was little Rob and I went through the usual psychoanalytically oriented therapy. Rob was considered electively mute and I was, of course, the defective parent.

We had years of that treatment and it provided little help. But when behavior modification appeared he was seen as a learner and I was seen as someone who could become an effective teacher. And I did. We worked on speech, self-help, reading, and recreation, and he learned many things.

Donnellan: You must have really welcomed the behavioral approach after all that.

Cutler: More than welcomed! I became a major advocate of behavior modification in my state and developed one of the first behavioral education programs for people with autism and related challenging behaviors. Maybe I was lucky at that time to have those experiences. I had a special teacher at a critical time who believed in my son and me. We were partners in our efforts to help Rob.

Donnellan: Yet for the past few years you have been very active in promoting laws and regulations against the use of certain behavioral procedures. Have you changed your mind about the value of the technology as some would claim?

Cutler: Some people have forgotten that early on I was a force in supporting behavior modification in Massachusetts and nationally. Today, they consider me the enemy, mostly because I oppose the pain and dehumanization that some practitioners are employing—supposedly in the service of people with disabilities. Those people are wrong. I don't have to throw out the baby with the bath water. I can support the learning principles, the accountability, precision teaching (when needed), and the use of individualized reinforcement schedules (natural of course, but artificial when we don't know what else to do). I was trained to be a teacher using behavior modification in the SERVICE of the individual. But I'm now saying that we have to wonder what has happened to behavior modification. Why is it causing such physical and emotional pain to individuals with handicaps and their families? It's not just the terrible cases of injury and death that have occurred. It's the ordinary, everyday distortion of the technology into something that demeans through controls that is so scary.

Donnellan: Too often we forget that when we demean a child we can affect the family and its

relationship to that family member as well. Once my son, a typical child, was old enough to go to school, I began to face the experience of having a teacher tell me what was wrong with him and, by extension, with me as a parent. Of course, no one ever suggested some of the terrible things we suggest for and about learners with disabilities. Nonetheless, I began to think about what it would be like to be told that my child was so difficult that they wanted to put him in a dark, locked closet! Or so non-compliant that they would squirt him with water, or otherwise humiliate him. Buying into such notions, I believe, could begin to have a subtle negative effect on anyone's relationship with her child.

Cutler: I agree. We started out to serve and somewhere the behavioral approach got derailed. We stopped focusing on teaching and got off on control and suppression through any means available as long as we called it treatment. In my experience the effect on families and individuals has been horrendous. Families have been demeaned; and their children with handicaps have been both demeaned and dehumanized. Professionals must take responsibility for this condition.

Donnellan: We need to add your point to our social validity concerns. No matter how well meaning we may be as professionals, we have a responsibility to guard against words or actions that diminish a learner's value in anyone's eyes.

Cutler: One problem is that too many people who enter the field are well meaning but are programmed to treat their students/clients as less human than themselves. However good their intentions, they become the controllers, the holders of power; and parents who struggle for services become powerless.

Donnellan: For years now people have been calling for parent-professional partnerships and positive strategies—yet we still see so little of either. I believe that, at least in part, this emphasis on power and control is because we as professionals are shaped by the institutional pressures and the culture of the agencies and the settings in which we work. Unfortunately, many of us are working in models that are very hierarchical and very much into power and control.

Cutler: I'd say power and control over parent and child. And with what results? A friend of mine with a son in a segregated behavioral program in a local public school asked the staff to give her son some crayons or paper so he could be occupied while waiting his turn during a group activity, instead of waiting aimlessly 10 to 15 minutes at a time. Staff said that coloring to pass the time was not part of the program and that Alan [not his real name] needed to learn to wait. They saw him as a behavior problem—not as a kid—and his mom's suggestion as an interference with their right to control his behavior. It hurt his mother to think of his waiting and ultimately getting out of his seat and into "trouble." But her request and opinion were valueless; they had time-out procedures to deal with his out-of-seat behavior. Eventually, and not surprisingly, this boy required an out-of-home placement. The school, of course, blamed the family for this failure.

Donnellan: The story is so terrible because it is so familiar. Like you, I am distressed by this pervasive use of technology for control rather than to support people and their development. It's not so much the headline cases that frighten me. It's the banality of it, the everyday ordinariness of abuse and misuse to which some now claim these individuals have a "right" because it is based on treatment in the literature. Certainly there are plenty of examples of time out in the literature. But, the professionals could have taken a totally different approach with Alan and with his mother's suggestion. They needed to see him first and foremost as a child. They still could have decided that he could and should learn to wait. But they might have realized that as children develop they learn waiting very gradually, and that 15 minutes can seem an eternity, especially to a child who is not much interested in the behavior of the other kids around him. Even as adults, most of us use distractors to help us when the waiting gets too much. But, because this boy has a handicap that often includes behavior problems, the professionals concentrated on the "aberrant behavior." They stopped looking at ways to develop an incremental waiting program or for adaptations to help him. Instead, it became a power issue between the school and him and, then, between the school and his mom.

Cutler: But why the emphasis on power and control? Where does it come from?

Donnellan: There's no sure answer to that, of course, but I think in part it comes from the nature of the agencies in which we professionals work and in part from a misunderstanding of the real value of behavioral technology. Much of my own work is in school settings. In trying to understand better the power and control issues, I have gone back to the literature about the formation of present-day schools. The work of Willower (1969) and others suggests that the one universal value in American education is control of the students. Moreover, this emphasis on control is not surprising. Client control is a *given* in any mandated system whether the system is a church, a prison, the army, a 24-hour institution, or a school system. Certainly, in schools and institutions those in power decide who has access, who has information, and even the nature of that information. If a typical first grader doesn't learn to read because the teacher is incompetent the parents don't get that information. Instead they're told how their child failed to live up to the school's expectations of a child her age.

Cutler: Of course a certain level of control is essential in any group situation, even a family. But if, in fact, it's the one universal value it's not hard to see why there's conflict when special educators, advocates, and parents try to promote individualized programming based on individualized assessment and parental involvement.

Donnellan: Presently, I think the conflict is inevitable but not irresolvable. To start, however, we have to realize that it's not a "good guys-bad guys" issue. The least dangerous assumption is that most educators are doing their job the way they think it is supposed to be done. We can't continue to ignore the fact that the American education system was not designed to individualize or to allow meaningful input from the nonprofessional or parent or even the hands-on staff. As Callahan (1962) described in *Education and the Cult of Efficiency,* public schools were designed at the turn of the century to be maximally efficient along the lines of the state of the art in efficiency at the time, the assembly line. As the assembly line model was translated into education, all important decisions were to be made by management in the central office. Lay input was limited to the school boards, which were reduced in number and burdened with "administrivia," and the PTA-like groups typically controlled by administrators. Teachers were to follow orders in order to change large numbers of immigrants and native learners into needed workers in American factories. There were and are exceptions but one thing is still true: The end product of this effort was to reflect the mythical melting pot rather than individual development and diversity.

Cutler: So the best way to assure that the "product" looks the same at the end of schooling is to control access and activities, to maintain the power relationship over staff, parents, and kids.

Donnellan: Yes. And, for the most part the schools fulfilled their assigned function very well. For 50 years few questioned that the schools, the service providers, got to determine how and when learners got in and out and how success would be evaluated. The public schools did the job adequately enough to avoid any significant challenge until *Brown v. Board of Education* (1954). Since then, there have been changes but they come slowly. When I started as a professional in the early '70s it was *illegal* to educate students with autism in the California public schools, and no state routinely offered education to students with challenging behavior. Today, of course, special education is legally mandated and essentially nonexclusionary. However, special education is still part of and tied to the history and values of the larger educational system. Though there are laws such as PL 94-142 and certainly wonderful examples of programs in regular and special education that even go beyond the law, the institutional prejudices remain.

Cutler: Perhaps that helps to explain why, 15 years after PL 94-142 mandated individualized assessment, programming, and evaluation, there is so little real individualization.

Donnellan: What I typically see instead is that dozens of hours are spent on assessment just to learn the child is "autistic" or "TMR" and, therefore, belongs in the "autism classroom" or "the TMR Center." Then, his individualized education program (IEP) begins to look remark-

ably like the "individualized" program of everyone else in the class. More often that not, individualization is limited to the amount of help (or force) necessary to get him to comply with the routine and stay on task. And, if he is "off task," the assumption is made that he must be controlled by any means available to us. Too often that control comes through aversive technology.

Cutler: So, like Alan, if the activity requires waiting he must be made to wait. If what we require of him contributes to a behavior problem we can force him to obey and call it treatment.

Donnellan: It's not a pretty picture. But, I'm convinced that the fact that some core values of American education and other human services systems are about power relationships and control and are antithetical to individualized programming is not irreversible. There are so many good people in the educational community who want to see some needed changes. But first it is essential to understand the phenomena we are witnessing, including our own professional behavior within these systems. Santayana said it best: "Those who do not remember the past are condemned to relive it."

Cutler: I agree. Far better to know the issues and address them directly. I see a lot more interest in becoming part of regular education and working with the teaching training programs that bring new people into the system.

Donnellan: This should be a major focus of the regular education initiative. Moreover, our doctoral-level people have to be involved in regular, not just special education administration and vice versa. We can build upon what's best in regular education, and certainly that system has been good for millions of kids. But change is needed. We still have plenty of problems in typical classrooms and not just in the inner cities. In many communities we are not even able to individualize for the gifted and talented in regular classes. And there are many instances of aversive control and programs pushing out kids and calling them dropouts. Perhaps if those of us committed to individualization in education are clear in our values and strategies and present them in ways that work for broader educational change, ultimately we can influence the entire system and support individualization for typical learners as well.

Cutler: Might as well aim high. Maybe then the behavioral technology will be used to support and serve again. I still despair of this happening in the 24-hour segregated programs such as residential schools and institutions, however. There we have the double burden of the anti-individualization and control values as well as the history of devaluation of individuals with mental retardation that produced segregation and institutionalization in the first place.

Donnellan: Yes, Wolfensberger (1975) described this so well in *The Origin and Nature of the Institutional Model.*

Cutler: And like so many before them, Alan and his family lived out that history. Alan was placed in a residential school with a national reputation as a "strict behavior modification" program. His mother was in tears telling me of one visit. She went with the staff and Alan to the skating rink. As soon as he had the ice skates on he started laughing and flapping his hands. The staff pulled him back, took off his skates, and put him in time out. The mother protested but she was ignored (extinction?). It didn't matter to the staff that he was overjoyed at the prospect of skating. To me she said, "Alan was so happy! Why couldn't they just let him skate?" Unfortunately, the staff were trained and instructed to get rid of all of Alan's little "autisms" by timing him out for every event.

A year later Alan's mother told me what was happening to him at the residential school. He had lost 40 pounds and was grossly underweight. He had also torn out much of his hair and when approached by anybody he would cringe and try to crawl within himself. This last behavior was labeled his "contortions," which were undoubtedly tallied up on the data sheets. How was this allowed to happen? Isn't a child's 40-pound weight loss some sort of red flag? Why did Alan's mother put up with this treatment she did not want? I think it was because she was told to accept the program or take her son home. I instructed Alan's mother to take some pictures of him. I made this suggestion reluctantly, knowing how heartbreaking it would be for her to have a record of this handsome boy looking like a con-

centration camp victim. The pictures were used to file a complaint and the school was forced to change its policies on time out. But Alan was to be discharged.

Donnellan: I'll bet this didn't make Alan and his mother very popular with that program or any other that heard about it.

Cutler: Right! There was a frantic search for another school and the authorities considered sending him to a notoriously aversive program, which his parents resisted. During this stressful period, Alan's father died of a heart attack. Finally a program was found for Alan where they basically left Alan alone for the first year. It took 6 months for him to stop "contorting" and to begin to gain some of the weight back. The new school is also a behavioral program but one that relies less on punishment. Still the focus is on control; and Alan is not much better off 5 years after entering this program. My friend is a very caring parent but she has no clout. Most parents don't. We were somehow insidiously defective in the eyes of the psychoanalysts; we are now powerless in the hands of the behavioral controllers who tell us: "If you don't like our methods, take your child somewhere else."

Donnellan: Usually the child can't come home because there are almost no supports for families who have to face the challenges of hyperactivity, aggression, and/or self-abuse at home. So parents become compliant. They are not able to resist. They, too, are at risk.

Cutler: After a while, rather than live with the emotional pain (and some do live with that pain) many begin to believe that their child needs restrictive and punitive programming. To save their sanity they accept. But I know no parents who spontaneously ask for pain and degradation for their child.

Donnellan: Perhaps because some parents are constantly placed in a powerless position, they may come to doubt themselves and their sense of their own child. As in Alan's story, they may even begin to doubt their own eyes when they see a significant weight loss or other problems. Most of us remember that "power tends to corrupt." In our field it is equally appropriate to remember civil rights activist Flo Kennedy's words that "powerlessness also corrupts."

Cutler: And, if parents do notice problems, what can they do? These kinds of programs demand total compliance from parents as well as their students or clients. By disempowering the parents, professionals diminish the most important relationship the child with substantial disabilities has. This can have long-term effects on both families and the family member with disabilities. The disempowering inhibits the parents' advocacy capabilities for their children who need lifelong advocacy; the acceptance of the view of the family member as one who needs systematic punishment can affect the views of brothers and sisters who may take over for the parents one day; and such effects may leave the children with no one to pity or protect them. For those parents who know in their hearts this treatment is wrong and who cannot accept the program's degradation of their child, there is constant pain, frustration, and rage that their child is being mistreated and they are powerless to stop it.

Donnellan: It ought to be self-evident that the power paradigm in human services can negatively affect everyone involved. And we know what wonderful things can happen when there is a true parent-professional partnership.

Cutler: It seems to me that most of early interventions programs value that partnership notion. Maybe as more of those parents get into the regular service delivery systems their expectations about partnerships will begin to bring about a change. I hope so.

Donnellan: If we can just explode the myth about the effectiveness of punishment that both feeds into and is supported by the power paradigms in schools and human services we may begin to see real change. But the myth is so pervasive that it's going to be no easy task. Doug Guess and others (Guess, Helmstetter, Turnbull, & Knowlton, 1987) have done a nice job of describing the history back to the '60s where there were many examples of isolated interventions in back wards to demonstrate certain behavioral effects. I imagine that those early researchers know from the animal literature that the highly discriminable nature of aversive contingencies had inherent problems in terms of maintenance and generalization. Nonetheless, the use of aversive procedures then was probably justified on

the basis that so little was known about behavior modification at the time. And, though the procedures were seldom developed to make a significant positive contribution to any individual's life, they proliferated. Not surprising given the institutional need to control clients and the fact that they often contributed to dramatic (though not necessarily clinically or educationally significant) reductions in behavior. This was very reinforcing to institutional personnel and to researchers reinforced by publications. In the behavior reduction literature produced there was an enormous emphasis on aversive control with essentially no attention paid to functional analysis, to communicative needs or environmental causes, or to maintenance or generalization back then and there is little now. The prisoners and the patients in mental hospitals who were subjected to the aversive procedures eventually protested and these were stopped. But individuals with developmental disabilities, particularly in institutions, had no effective voice to protest.

Cutler: And there was no real protest from the lay or public community until recently when these procedures were being introduced in schools and community settings.

Donnellan: Exactly, but the problem is that whether or not these procedures made a meaningful change in the subject's life they often produced dramatic effects on data sheets. And, they got widely disseminated in books and workshops for 25 years so that lots of professionals believe that aversives are necessary to change some behavior—however illogical that may sound! Gary LaVigna and I (in press) have argued that this is a myth. If it can be demonstrated that an operant behavior comes under the control of aversive contingencies under the proper conditions then surely it must be true that under the proper conditions it will come under the control of nonaversive contingencies. Given the fact that the entire profession grew out of the early work with rats pushing bars and pigeons pecking keys it would seem that topography ought not to be more significant than all the other conditions and functions that would be determined by proper analysis. Tragically, there are now individuals suggesting that the least intrusive intervention be defined as that that has been demonstrated to be effective in the literature. They make no reference to the historical development of that literature or that effectiveness is defined therein only in terms of speed and degree of effects. It is really frightening.

Cutler: Because of Rob, what is most frightening to me is that some actually believe aversives will work for all behaviors—even those developing out of seizures and other neurological anomalies. This issue is very real to me because Rob developed some neurological problems in his 20s including noises and akinesia. He was labeled many things at the time including noncompliant when he couldn't move. Fortunately, I was able to find some competent diagnosticians who recognized a movement disorder when they saw it. Recognizing his difficulties meant that we could try to find ways to help him rather than punish him. I stood in awe and admiration of my son's efforts to deal with still another handicap. Yet I know that there is someone out there waiting with a *simple* solution when I am not able to protect my son. It seems to me that aversive behavioral technology is certainly not responsible for the shape of the various human services systems but it legitimizes many of the control tactics that endanger Rob and others like him.

Donnellan: You're right. What we have is an essentially neutral technology that will be shaped by the conditions in which it is used. If it is used in a power paradigm it will be used for control. We have power relationships of professionals over parents and over learners. Once we could reject those we did not like or who did not like what we offered. Now we use coercion.

Cutler: We need to stop even using words like "behavior management" or even "treatment" that connote hierarchical power relationships.

We don't develop treatment programs for our unhappy spouses or quarrelsome grandparents or friends nor do we typically choose to be "managed" by them. Maybe we need, instead, to think about our relationships with these learners and their families and how we can empower them all to be as successful as possible.

Donnellan: Well, it seems self-evident that in any successful relationship one tries to understand and respect the other's perspective. This is seldom easy as so many of these learners have limited communicative means. Sometimes we have to draw on everything we know about human development and communication, about curriculum and behavioral effects, and about neurology and biology. But even the most aversive model takes effort; you can't control anyone's behavior without allowing that person to control yours in return—even if it's only to make the aversive contingency available. How much more productive and positive, and more interesting, if every challenging behavior was assumed to be the individual learner's best effort to let us know what was wrong, including what was wrong with our behavior, from his or her perspective. We are not obliged to obey but at least it would give us the opportunity to give that person some control, to support and teach him or her to get needs met without our modeling aggression or causing pain to the learner or ourselves.

Cutler: Imagine encouraging and supporting professionals to develop partnership relationships with *both* the learner and his or her family as an alternative to the power relationships and power paradigms that require and promote aversive control.

Donnellan: *Imagine!*

REFERENCES

Brown v. Board of Education, 349 U.S. 294 (1954).

Burgess, A. (1962). *A clockwork orange*. New York: Norton.

Callahan, R.E. (1962). *Education and the cult of efficiency*. Chicago: University of Chicago Press.

Donnellan, A.M., & LaVigna, G.W. (in press). Myths about punishment. In A. Repp & N. Singh, *Current perspectives in the use of nonaversive and aversive interventions for persons with developmental disabilities*. Sycamore, IL: Sycamore Press.

Guess, D., Helmstetter, E., Turnbull, H.R., & Knowlton, S. (1987). *Use of aversive procedures with persons who are disabled: An historical review and critical analysis* (Monograph #2). Seattle: The Association for Persons with Severe Handicaps.

Iannaccone, L., & Button, H.W. (1967). *Functions of student teaching* (Research Project No. 1026, Report to Dept. of Health, Education, and Welfare). Unpublished manuscript, Washington University, St. Louis, MO.

Willower, D.J. (1969). The teacher subculture and rites of passage. *Urban Education,* 4, 103–113.

Wolfensberger, W. (1975). *The origin and nature of our institutional models.* Syracuse, NY: Human Policy Press.

SUGGESTED READINGS

Favell, J.E. (Chairperson), Azrin, N.H., Baumeister, A.A., Carr, E.G., Dorsey, M.F., Forehand, R., Foxx, R.M., Lovaas, O.I., Rincover, A., Risley, T.R., Romanczyk, R.G., Schroeder, S.R., & Solnick, J.V. (1982). The treatment of self-injurious behavior [Monograph]. *Behavior Therapy, 13,* 529–554.

Iwata, B.A. (1988). The development and adoption of controversial default technologies. *The Behavior Analyst, 11,* 149–159.

Lovett, H. (1985). *Cognitive counseling and persons with special needs.* New York: Praeger.

Martin, R. (1975). *Legal challenges to behavior modification: Trends in schools, corrections, and mental health.* Champaign, IL: Research Press.

Van Houten, R., Axelrod, S., Bailey, J.S., Favell, J.E., Foxx, R.M., Iwata, B.A., Lovaas, O.I. (1988). The right to effective behavioral treatment. *The Behavior Analyst, 11,* 111–114.

Vincent, L., Laten, S., Salisbury, C., Brown, P., & Baumgart, D. (1981). Family involvement in the educational process of severely handicapped students: State of the art and directions for the future. In B. Wilcox & R. York (Eds.), *Quality educational services for the severely handicapped: The federal perspective* (pp. 164–179). Washington, DC: U.S. Department of Education, Office of Special Education.

◇ **CHAPTER 40** ◇

Empowerment and Choices

HERBERT LOVETT

Boston, Massachusetts

The theme of "Empowerment: Choices and Change" for the 1988 TASH Conference came, it seems to me, at a particularly crucial moment in our work. We have, increasingly, a sense of what a community is and how it can support itself. At the same time, we have seen a sudden resurgence of the use of pain to control behavior. The debate about choosing between socially ordinary and socially unusual practices for people with behavioral difficulties has been argued largely in professional circles among people who practice psychology. The theme of *empowerment* introduces the idea, too long neglected and too easily overlooked, that the people themselves need to be included in this discussion.

One of my friends, a co-worker and collaborator, is a man who was labeled "retarded." Pat Worth has been clear that the institution most people with learning difficulties live in, and with, has been the label, the public perception of what a learning difference means. This has presented some difficulties for psychologists who have been trained to "diagnose" and to "treat" people with retardation. Many of them, well intentioned as they are, have a difficult time in seeing that their objectifying others is a type of oppression. People First, Speaking for Ourselves, and other groups around the world have become increasingly articulate and clear for us: We are a liberation movement; we are a people moving from being dependent and being spoken about to claiming our rights in society and speaking for our own lives.

People who used to be difficult to serve have been my collaborators in trying to put together a service that makes sense for them. I have found more and more that there are not so many people who are "behaviorally disordered," as there are people who have been systematically excluded and *inaccurately* served. I have stopped thinking about people as "clients" who need some extra measure of therapy so much as they are freedom fighters who have insisted, often at great personal cost, that what we have done is not what they need. Rather than struggle with people, I have learned it is far more sensible to work with them, to speculate, to guess; to ask the "what ifs . . . ?" we all need to ask as we work our lives to shape our selves.

Oddly, whether people use words to communicate seems not to be a critical variable so much as whether there are people of good will who stay around long enough to get it right. Sometimes, people are quite verbal and tell us directly, "This is what I need to get on with my life." Other times, people do not tell us and we need to make some tentative thoughtful guesses and see what works and what does not. I see my role not so much as someone who gets the best program written up so much as someone who "listens" to behavior. I have had, on occasion, ideas that I thought were quite inspired. Perhaps they were. But not for the person for whom I had them. So I have learned to make my attachments to people, and not to my "interventions."

As I am writing this, I am thinking of Christine, a woman who has had a horrific life. She found herself trooped from institution to institution, from program to program, all the while fighting for what she thought she was and what she deserved. She finally got connected with a service that built her "program" on the simple question "What do you want?" The people who provide her service are far too modest to be named and whenever I talk to them they are always admiring how strong this woman is and how much they still have to learn from her about life. This feels, to me, a lot like a community where we do not have the answers, necessarily, for any one person, but we stay together with them until we can learn to live cooperatively if not comfortably.

Christine has changed remarkably in the 2 years since she was last locked up. But just as she has changed, so too has the help she has gotten changed. It was not so much a matter of a new, "nicer" program that "fixed" her so much as it was a group of people who listened to her, took her seriously, and responded to her as a woman worthy of dignity and respect. Not surprisingly, she has grown to appreciate her own worth, that had of course always been there, but had never been called to. She is not "on a program for behavior" so much as she is involved in a life where what she does matters and has meaning. In institutions, no matter where they are located or in what form they appear, a few people take responsibility for a large number of other people. In communities, in competent communities, every person is responsible for and to every other person.

Some people, in response to troubling behavior, advocate "nonaversive" approaches. This is troubling in that it suggests the real power, the "real" approaches, are essentially painful. I have talked about "positive approaches" because this is what I think we really are about and also because it is sufficiently vague a term as to include a necessarily wide number of possibilities.

I have spent a great deal of time trying to impress upon people a few simple ideas: that the key variable in helping one another change is the mutuality of our relationships; how we cannot change others in a real way without ourselves in turn being changed; that difficult behaviors call us to listen to the person and to reflect what we need to change in our own lives and practices. Every now and again a well-meaning person will take me aside at the end of a workshop and say,

"That all sounds really nice. But what do you do about a head-banger?"

One of the fantasies we have inherited from institutions has been the idea that we can "fix" people. Some psychologists have tried to develop "positive" technologies just to do this. But these efforts have almost universally overlooked what function a behavior can serve. There can be no one "cure" for "self-injurious behavior" if one person hurts her head because she has an allergy, or another hurts his head because he is having a panic attack. Neither of them, I think, is much served by the use of painful interventions or even positive reinforcement programs to "control" the behavior. We need to learn to respond to rational and adaptive aspects of behavior and not simplistically, and often vainly, attempt to control it.

As we become more confident in listening to people in what they and their behavior have to say, we are going to be put to the test: Does our service serve or does it get in the way? We spend time asking ourselves that, professionally, a great deal as we look to quality assurance and team reviews. But the one group that we need for the answer is often not asked—the people themselves. And the one individual whose voice we need to listen to most closely is the *specific* person about whom we are concerned. Until people asked Christine her opinions and wishes and dreams for her own life, she had gone from one bad experience to another. The simple question "How can we help?" is a turning point. But the direction and course we follow from then on is set by our listening to people—by making certain that, as best we can, we provide what it takes to get them where they need to go.

◇ **SUMMARY** ◇

POLICY AND PRACTICES

CHAPTER 41

Advocacy, Research, and Typical Practices

A Call for the Reduction of Discrepancies Between What Is and What Ought To Be, and How To Get There

LUANNA H. MEYER

Syracuse University, Syracuse, New York

No doubt there are many examples in today's world of great discrepancies between what is achievable and what has been achieved. In some instances, these gaps exist because of very real, practical considerations: Thus, automobile travel powered by electricity rather than fossilized fuels has been technologically possible for nearly 100 years, but has continued to be impractical for several reasons. Despite the promise of a clean-running vehicle, the need for relatively frequent battery recharging as well as the lengthy time required for recharging places strict limitations upon range that are unacceptable for the demographics of most automobile travel. An "incomplete" technology could, of course, be at fault, and perhaps these limitations could be solved and make the electric vehicle commonplace. Continuing shortages of fossilized fuels and a growing sense of urgency regarding environmental pollution and depletion of the ozone layer should prompt major change in the manufacturing industry ending the production of vehicles that emit unacceptable hydrocarbons into the atmosphere (although electricity also must ultimately be powered by some alternative fuel source, which could merely distance the issue). Yet, this widespread recognition of the need for low-emission vehicles and decreased dependence upon fuels that pollute has thus far failed to generate major change in either the pro-

duction or use of such automobiles for personal travel.

In other instances, what is achievable is achieved by a very few wealthy individuals and never achieved by the vast majority of the population. Thus, supersonic air travel is available only to the very rich: Lack of more widespread access to this option is not generally regarded as a particularly troublesome discrepancy. (Environmental concerns about the effects of supersonic jets upon the atmosphere are even cited as a rationale for limited usage, though the basic principle has been sacrificed to enable a very small percentage of the population to enjoy a lifestyle convenience.) Purchase of consumer goods in a manner that might be referred to as "conspicuous consumption" provides yet another illustration of tremendous gaps—so much so, in fact, that on the very same street at the very same moment in any of America's major cities, for example, we could find a person from a "typical" family home, a person who has the financial resources to enjoy living in two or more very expensive homes, and a person who is homeless. Interestingly enough, the discrepancy between the first two individuals does not seem to bother our collective conscience as much as it has become a topic of curiosity—the "lifestyles of the rich and famous"—so that people who flaunt their wealth have become a source of en-

Portions of this chapter were prepared while I was the Roy MacKenzie Foundation Visiting Professor with the New Zealand Institute on Mental Retardation, University of Otago Medical School, Dunedin, New Zealand. I wish to express my gratitude for the support provided. Special thanks are also due to Ian Evans, Cap Peck, Anne Bray, Keith Ballard, Dennis Moore, and Ken Ryba for raising challenging questions and sharing their ideas with me in discussions of these issues.

tertainment for others. This is not unlike the manner in which, it was once charged, the majestic and massively rich cathedrals built during the Middle Ages were a distractor for the vast majority of the population who lived in abject poverty.

However, as a society we are greatly troubled by the discrepancies between having a home and *not* having a home. People who are homeless and families living in public shelters, cardboard boxes, and old automobiles are a highly visible source of discomfort. They are a blatant contradiction to the picture we like to have of our culture and our society. Thus, solutions to homelessness are constantly proposed and debated, and various "programs" are tried. As long as the discrepancies between the rich and the not-so-rich are confined to such nonessential issues as designer clothes, sports cars or limousines, and other extravagant spending that does not seem to offend as much as it models a fantasy world, there is a fair degree of tolerance and less in the way of arguments supporting a more equal distribution of wealth. But when the discrepancies between some people and others cross the line into poverty, homelessness, and chronic suffering, there is a continuous call to find solutions— or at least, there is much discussion about finding solutions. Again, however, solutions that would involve any major change—a redistribution of wealth, for example—are seldom taken seriously.

These more fundamental discrepancies represent global, very real, major sociological and economic challenges for all of us as we move into the 21st century. Do the resources exist to reduce these discrepancies at least to a level that would eliminate extreme poverty, homelessness, chronic illness, and even death due to failure to meet basic sustenance needs? One would think that they do. But those resources would presumably have to come from somewhere, and the most likely possibility is that the necessary redistribution would inevitably reduce the wealth of those who also have the power to control decisions on such issues in both subtle and very direct ways. Thus, major changes may be less likely than continuing the present pattern of charity, isolated and time-limited program efforts, and a great deal of public rhetoric. As an educa-

tor, I am, of course, merely a layperson in the social, political, and economic domains relevant to this issue, but the history of social movements and social reform in the 20th century is particularly marked by a proliferation of various interpretations of and apologies for the continuing failure to accomplish social justice and equality.

So how does all of this relate to people with severe disabilities? Throughout this volume, various authors have taken a close look at discrepancies in a particular area of interest to them. We could look very closely at issues such as supported employment or nonaversive behavioral intervention, and many questions can justifiably be asked regarding why we continue to fall short of achieving what is clearly achievable. We could also look more broadly—as many of our authors have done—at issues such as family services and special education; we could ask similar questions about why we continue, for the most part, to follow past practices that are widely acknowledged to restrict and handicap individuals and their families. On a values level, why should children continue to be expected to give up the opportunity for friendships in order to receive "special education"? And why should families be required either to give up their child altogether (through placement out of the home) or to sacrifice a normalized family life (through keeping the child at home without reasonable supports and services) through present patterns of services and respite? On an empirical level, we now know what families want. On an empirical level, we can now document unequivocally the benefits of integration done well for the children involved—both those with and without disabilities. And on a practical level, all of the things we call "most promising practices" have actually happened in at least some typical schools and communities without extraordinary resources, and in many different regions under various circumstances and contingencies. Furthermore, on perhaps the most practical level of all, the old ways of doing things are sufficiently costly that there is every reason to believe that the new way would not even require that we find additional resources in order to change.

Why, then, must people with severe disabilities continue to endure institutions, custodial care, and separation from their families and communities? Why, then, must children with severe disabilities be deprived of friends and fun and continue to be required to ride buses for long distances to go to a handicapped-only school that no other person in our society would agree to attend? Why, when we know better, do we continue to spend vast sums of money to support buildings and places and practices that have remained virtually unchanged in design and intent for as long as we can remember? What is the problem that keeps us from changing so that real people with severe disabilities can finally have their fair share?

We could examine each of the discrepancies, one at a time, at a micro level and derive some possible explanations for each. Because some of us like to view ourselves as empiricists, we might attribute discrepancies to technical issues such as systems change (on a broad scale), or dissemination and training (to different regions), or how to reorganize the classroom and modify intervention patterns (on the level of the individual). Discrepancies might also be attributed to failures to acknowledge the basic civil rights of all citizens and even to differences in values.

For the empiricists, however, answers are difficult because our science is still sufficiently imperfect to allow for various interpretations. Thus, those who refuse to change until all the proof is in can delay change indefinitely. There are many ways to accomplish this, including critiquing methodology, accusing the journal of bias in publication decisions, challenging the significance or importance of the outcome, and perhaps always refusing to acknowledge the generalizability of findings to one's own region, situation, conditions, and population. And for the advocates who emphasize values, other values can be advanced that have sufficient intuitive appeal that both the courts and the public are often convinced: Thus, those who wish to continue using aversives to intervene with problem behavior have persuasively argued that the person with self-injurious behavior has a "right to effective treatment," that his or her parents have a right to such services and a prior interest in their child's welfare, that a little pain from aversives is better than a lot of pain from self-injury, that aversive procedures are somehow no differ-

ent than lifesaving surgery, and so on. To a layperson or a judge who has never seen someone who injures himself but who has long since accepted the validity of cancer surgery, who is also a parent with a firm belief in the integrity of the family and the parent's right to discipline his or her child as he or she sees fit, and who may even believe that indeed, the "end justifies the means," a values-based argument may be doomed to fail. Values are indeed complex, and our society still struggles with the Kantian Categorical Imperative that the end *never* justifies the means: What do you believe?

So if neither science nor values can fully explain and resolve our dilemma, what can? A few potential solutions are offered, but first, a look at some of the discrepancies along with a discussion of solutions traditionally offered might help.

RELATIONSHIP BETWEEN RESEARCH AND PRACTICE

Baumeister's (1981) insightful critique of the general failure of mental retardation research to have an impact upon public policy ended with a caveat (see also Chapter 1, this volume):

> Research cannot be expected to solve problems that are substantially moral in character. The fundamental choices we face, as a society, in our efforts to come to terms with extremes of individual differences are not going to be resolved by more research. Having decided what it is we must do, then research is one means available that may tell us how to do it; that is all we can promise, nothing more. That is why research needs public policy. (p. 456)

Rather than holding service delivery agencies responsible for the continuing failure to translate research into practice, Baumeister largely faulted the research community. Research does *not* direct practice but must of necessity be secondary to economic, political, and social considerations. As evidence, he summarized clear policy directions that were widely advocated despite equivocal empirical support at the time (e.g., mainstreaming) as well as the "excruciatingly slow" evolution of public policy in other areas "where we do have relatively good data" (such as early education; Baumeister, 1981, p. 450).

Apparently, public policy is fickle in its relationship to science. And why not, Baumeister added, as "Science does not reveal truth; it sometimes reveals facts in certain restricted domains. Truth is ultimately a moral test, the outcome of the confrontation of values; truth does not depend on scientific methods" (1981, p. 451). If Baumeister is right, it should hardly surprise us to discover discrepancies between scientific knowledge and typical practices. This is not so much evidence that no one pays attention to science, but that science and practice are both being guided by other forces—perhaps those social, political, and economic forces that all of us ignore in our nearsighted devotion to what interests us.

Thus, the contrasts between what we *know* we can do ("most promising practices") and what we typically do in areas such as family support, education, employment, and behavior management—see Table 41.1 for examples—are simply illustrations of our continued delusions regarding the power of data to persuade and shape practices, and our naiveté that if "they" only knew what we know, things would change. When we assume positions of political power, of course, we can make some of the solutions listed in Table 41.2 happen and compel agencies to update their practices—albeit reluctantly and often ineffectively as a result. Alternatively, were researchers to develop increased sensitivity to the needs of the real world and the obstacles confronting practitioners, they would begin to change their own behavior along the lines suggested in Table 41.3. But is it as simple as leaving the laboratory and working in schools, then writing up the results in a newsletter, avoiding technical jargon? A good beginning, perhaps, but after all these years, why hasn't that worked either? And taking one's cues from policymakers regarding *what* to research hasn't resolved the controversy over how to treat self-injurious behavior (more on this later). What *is* the problem, and what is the solution?

PARADIGM TRAPS AND UNCONSCIOUS ASSUMPTIONS

Research and practice affecting the lives of people with severe disabilities has been dominated by positivist and behaviorist thinking throughout

Table 41.1. Some discrepancies between what we know is achievable versus what is typically achieved in practice

What we know we can achieve	What we most typically do achieve
Family Support	
• Family-scale living environments can be designed to enable persons with the most severe disabilities to live in the community.	• People with severe disabilities are still required to live in institutions all over the world.
• Families that report a balance between stressors and resources want to and do keep their minor child with severe disabilities at home.	• Services are not generally available to families with a child living at home to enable them to reach a better balance between stressors and resources.
Social and Educational Inclusion	
• The effects of social interactions between children with and without severe disabilities are *positive*.	• Children with severe disabilities attend separate schools and separate classes, isolated academically from their peers.
• There exist effective curricular and instructional strategies to educate students with and without severe disabilities in the regular classroom and program.	• Mainstreaming most often reflects "teacher deals" with minimal systems support and little curricular reform overall.
Vocational Training and Employment	
• Programs can be designed to provide employment training on actual job tasks in school and community settings.	• In school, students with severe disabilities do "pre" vocational training.
• A system of supported employment can enable persons with severe disabilities to do and be paid for meaningful work.	• As adults, persons with severe disabilities attend day activity centers and sheltered workshops.
Intervention with Challenging Behavior	
• Effective nonaversive behavioral intervention strategies exist to deal with even the most severe behavior problems.	• Aversive behavior management techniques continue to be promoted and used for both severe and mild behavior problems.
• Homogeneous grouping of persons with severe behavior problems is associated with long-term maintenance of problem behavior and high staff turnover and burnout.	• Persons with behavior problems are most likely to be segregated in places and programs with other persons who have behavior problems.

Table 41.2. Usual explanations and typical solutions proposed to guide services in adoption of most promising practices

Question: Why don't *services* adopt innovations supported by *research* findings?

Explanation	Solution
• Disinterest	• Agency licensing requirements for periodic retraining of staff • Administrative initiatives supporting curricular review
• Fiscal, economic, social-political constraints	• Redistribution of resources • Retraining incentives and support
• Incapability	• Availability of retraining and selective retention • Addition of professional resources

the adult life span of the majority of the readers of this book. Furthermore, efforts within this theoretical paradigm are themselves directed by several underlying unconscious assumptions, which were summarized by Bogdan and Kugelmass (1984) as follows:

(1) disability is a condition that individuals have;
(2) disabled/typical is a useful and objective distinction;
(3) special education is a rationally conceived and coordinated system of services that help children labeled disabled;
(4) progress in the field is made by improving diagnosis, intervention and technology. (p. 173)

The intervention literature does indeed focus almost exclusively upon the evaluation of various strategies designed to change the individual person with disabilities (Skrtic, 1986). Whether the goal is to teach a new skill or replace a problem behavior with a more appropri-

Table 41.3. Usual explanations and typical solutions proposed to guide research that addresses service delivery needs

Question: Why are *research* findings considered irrelevant to *service delivery* needs?

Explanation	Solution
• Wrong questions	• Research guided by public policy concerns
• Unrealistic methods	• Research conducted in the field, not the laboratory
• Silly language	• Research findings translated for practitioners

ate one, the person with disabilities is judged to have a deficient repertoire that must be enhanced through treatment and instruction. While it might perhaps be obvious that persons with severe disabilities have far fewer skills and positive social behaviors than those judged to be nondisabled, it does not necessarily follow that the solution to this need is the remediation of individual deficits. Lest this statement be misunderstood, I hasten to add my agreement that enhancing individual repertoires must be a good thing to do. But to set that goal as the *only* thing to do is problematic for several reasons. For example, attempting to accomplish desirable goals such as social integration, educational inclusion, employment, and family adjustment through an emphasis upon remedial instruction directed at the individual is doomed to fail. One day we might possess the professional knowledge and technology to override the cognitive, motoric, and other discrepancies that lead to a label such as severely disabled. It may indeed be theoretically possible, some day, to intervene so effectively that the people labeled as having severe disabilities become "typical" in the eyes of their society. But, in the meantime, while we work to develop the expertise to do that, generations of "partial successes" will continue to graduate from remedially oriented special education programs without the "cloak of competence" Edgerton (1967) wrote about that would enable them to move easily into the existing social structures of their communities.

At one level, we know this! Therefore, the major shifts in curriculum from a developmental to an enviromental reference and in vocational training from a transition service to a supported employment model both represent examples of how professional practices have acknowledged the fundamental flaw in approaches focusing upon the remediation of individual deficits. Thus, the special education remedial model represented by PL 94-142 is not likely to be replicated today in any new legislation for adults. Instead, the emphasis has unequivocally shifted to support models: The individual is indeed taught as many new (useful) skills as possible, but the system must also be designed to "fill in" for the absence of any critical skills through support models. Notice, however, that even the introduction of new concepts and terms such as "supported employment" and "supported education" does not necessarily imply a rejection of the deficit-remedial model. Rather, it could be viewed as a heuristic response to the practical reality or realization that teaching skills alone will not be sufficient to facilitate community acceptance and adjustment—supports must also be added to compensate.

Those who advocate strongly for support models clearly emphasize the individual's civil right to be part of his or her community and thus receive the support needed to be able to do this. What is less clear is whether this represents a fundamental challenge to the underlying unconscious assumptions that Bogdan and Kugelmass (1984) listed. Why does it matter? It matters because remediation is still focused sharply upon the person with disabilities: We now diagnose not only his or her skill deficits, but we add judgments about the special service supports that must be provided based upon predicted limitations to our ability to remediate all individual deficits. Keeping the focus upon the individual in this way could continue to absolve everyone and everything else from any responsibility to change *also*. Is it reasonable to challenge the underlying assumption that having severe disabilities is a fundamental distinction that calls for rationally ordered services and supports that are specially designed to reduce the gap between "disability" and "typical"? What if we were to argue that this is *not* the most useful nor is it a socially just solution to enabling people with severe disabilities to have their fair share? Suppose we were to maintain that disability is really yet another dimension of *diversity*, and that handicappism, sexism, racism, ethnocentrism, and so forth are actually reflections of a social structure with unrealistic "melting pot" expectations?

At a time when "minority" cultures have already become the "majority" population in many of America's urban centers, traditional educational models are being increasingly challenged for their failure to address this "demographic imperative" (Banks, 1989). The consequences of this failure are evident in the widespread concerns about school alienation and drop-out rates. And, it does seem rather pointless to continue to design more and more "remedial" programs for larger and larger subgroups. We are rapidly reaching the stage where America's schools seem ideally suited to meet the needs of only a few of its students. Do the students who don't fit—maybe the majority—need to change, or does the *system* need to change?

Positivist-Behavioral Research Paradigm

The domination of intervention research by the positivist-behavioral paradigm has had various positive and negative consequences for those in parenting and professional roles and for the people who become our subjects, clients, students, trainees, and employees. On the plus side, before applied behavior analysis entered the picture, the lives of people with severe disabilities such as autism, severe mental retardation, and dual sensory impairment were restrictive and, quite frankly, dismal. Prior to the work of those early behaviorists who first intervened with children with autism in their laboratories during the 1960s, for example, a label signifying a severe disability inevitably led to institutionalization and custodial care. Once these researchers and clinicians demonstrated that children who had been judged "ineducable" could indeed learn, expectations changed. An almost unlimited optimism swept the field about the possibilities of a better future for these young people and their families. Yet, a successful paradigm can also become a *paradigm trap,* and challenges to a paradigm can also generate paradigm wars rather than what might well be beneficial changes in professional behavior. Rather than continuing to view discrepancies in practice and major controversies regarding important issues in the field as relatively minor retooling of our predominant paradigms (according to a piecemeal social engineering model that was advanced by Karl Popper; see Miller, 1955), a more macro-level analysis of the problem and its solution is considered throughout the remainder of this chapter.

Intervention with the Individual

Despite the clear successes in the application of behavioral principles and practices in programs, a second, more critical look exposed a number of problems. First of all, something was amiss: Nearly 30 years after the first successful reports, research reports continue to appear in major professional journals demonstrating nothing more remarkable than eye contact, sitting in one's seat, and following one-step commands. For example, Matson et al. (1988) intervened to teach just such "target behaviors" to teenagers diagnosed as having a hearing impairment in addition to mental retardation. A report such as this could easily have appeared as early as the 1960s (see, for example, Risley & Wolf's 1968 overview of this early work and Kazdin, 1978, for a comprehensive history of parallel efforts with children with disabilities in Great Britain and the United States throughout the 1960s). Apparently, it was judged publishable because previous literature had involved demonstrations of acquisition by persons with slightly different disability combinations. Surely clinicians and teachers across America and elsewhere in the world have long since demonstrated that, given the use of operant conditioning procedures, such skills could be learned by virtually anyone provided with the necessary instruction (see, for example, the report by Ulicny, Thompson, Favell, & Thompson, 1985, as well as the evidence reported in the various review chapters in the present volume). Surely it would not require 30 years or more of continuing to teach simple operant responses to persons with all conceivable combinations of disabilities before we could move on to teaching more meaningful skills and behaviors and demonstrating their use in the real world rather than in institutions. In fact, Nelson and Evans (1968) had long since demonstrated that principles of behavior could be applied to teaching language (vocabulary items that they could indeed use) to children with autism and mental retardation. Why then would reports of the acquisition of simple responses in restrictive settings continue to be published—and apparently judged to be contributions to our knowledge base—decades later?

Further evidence that progress is a bit too slow has been documented by the growing concern about behavioral interrelationships—that is, evidence that planned interventions with particular target behaviors could result in unplanned effects on other behaviors as well. When these unplanned changes were good, they were labeled "collateral effects," and when they were negative, they were labeled "side effects." Behaviorist theory stood in obvious contrast to psycho-dynamic theory that had emphasized treating underlying causes rather than observable behaviors, including the warning that any intervention that failed to attend to those underlying causes would result in "symptom substitution" that could potentially be even more serious than the original target behaviors. Thus, the appearance of collateral and side effects was perhaps viewed as a theoretical threat, a fundamental challenge to the validity of a radical operant approach (Kazdin, 1982). Nevertheless, various behavioral psychologists have for many years considered the possibility of systematic behavioral interrelationships and offered explanatory theory for their existence: Voeltz and Evans (1982) provided a comprehensive overview of theoretical discussions of these issues, and in both the 1982 review and the 1988 update analyzed the empirical evidence of behavioral interrelationships in the published intervention literature (Evans, Meyer, Kurkjian, & Kishi, 1988). Thus, both behavioral theory and the data have indeed long predicted multiple effects as a function of the manipulation of behavior: Behaviors *must* be organized in a person's individual repertoire so that whenever one behavior is manipulated and changed, other behaviors could be expected to change as well. Yet, Voeltz and Evans (1982) and Evans et al. (1988) also documented the continuing narrow focus of the intervention literature upon single target behaviors, and showed that the percentage of studies systematically investigating multiple effects (as opposed to simply reporting anecdotal information in the discussion section) actually *declined* across the time period covered by the 1982 to the 1988 reviews.

Given the heuristic that persons with severe intellectual handicaps are likely to learn far fewer new behaviors and skills than other persons, it seems particularly unfortunate that more attention to the possibility of multiple effects and outcomes is not evident. Surely, the potential for maximizing positive outcomes and minimizing negative side effects would be a high priority in good programs—and published research—involving those persons with the most to gain, and lose, from our mistakes and errors in judgment.

Several years ago, Ian Evans and I were

sharply critical of this continuing failure to attempt more meaningful outcomes on behalf of persons with disabilities (Voeltz & Evans, 1983). We suggested that intervention research—which is almost exclusively behavioral in orientation—was still being guided primarily by notions of how to demonstrate experimental control rather than by values or goals regarding meaningful outcomes. In particular, an almost exclusive reliance upon one specific "way of knowing"—single-subject research designs—had become a paradigm trap, virtually demanding that we emphasize controlling behavior even at the expense of achieving multiple benefits and less restrictive lifestyles for the participants in our work. Behaviorist clinicians and researchers were not completely unaware of the problem, and the 1980s in particular were to see the emergence of major concerns regarding generalization and maintenance (cf. Horner, Dunlap, & Koegel, 1988). Test, Spooner, and Cooke (1987) responded directly to the aforementioned critique (Voeltz & Evans, 1983), and argued that this focus upon generalization provided an answer to the issues we had raised; they also discussed ways in which single-subject research designs were indeed adequate to the task of addressing such issues as part of their evaluation model. In reply, Ian Evans and I further elaborated the challenge to the continued reliance upon experimental designs that we maintained were fundamentally inadequate to meet the intervention goals now articulated as "most promising practices" (Evans & Meyer, 1987). We also charged that a failure to modify research practices was at least partly responsible for the restrictions placed upon the lives of people with disabilities as a direct consequence of the requirements to demonstrate "experimental control" as this was played out through existing research designs. To address the problem, we called for both the exploration of expanded within-subject designs (such as further use of case study and interrupted time series designs) and the discovery and utilization of alternative scientific paradigms—if need be—to ensure that opportunities made available to real people were driven by values, and not by methodologies and publication considerations.

Intervention with Systems

A more fundamental question that might be asked would be directed to "who needs to change?" Suppose we were to acknowledge that we have indeed demonstrated time and time again that children with severe disabilities can be taught the necessary social skills to interact with nondisabled peers and that adults with severe disabilities can live in family-scale homes with the provision of certain services and supports. Yet, children continue to be required to attend segregated schools and adults continue to be required to live in institutions, intermediate care facilities (ICFs), and group homes with as many as 8–12 roommates (who also have disabilities). Will these discrepancies be solved by more research directed to demonstrating yet one more time that people with disabilities can acquire the needed skills and learn to participate fully in their communities?

In an interesting report involving the remediation of self-injurious and other serious behaviors in 5 individuals, Durand and Kishi (1987) chose to focus their intervention upon the service delivery system as well as upon the persons who were self-injurious. In fact, they were able to relate the success of their behavior-change efforts to the behavior of staff. It may be axiomatic that an intervention won't work unless it is implemented. But a more profound concern might focus upon *why* staff would fail to implement a program designed to treat a behavior as serious as self-injury. Similarly, why would school districts continue to deliver only segregated services to students with severe disabilities once they are informed of the obvious benefits of integrated services for students? Why do state agencies continue to fund institutional care—and even pay staff in those institutions as much as two to three times the salary available to parallel staff in community homes—in view of the success of family-scale living arrangements?

Yet, in each of these instances (see Table 41.1), implementation of "most promising practices" is far more complicated than selecting a protypical journal article illustrating how to implement that intervention. Disability has become an industry, and changes on behalf of the individual or the population of people with disabilities may become secondary to the interests of an industry (Biklen, 1988). At the very least, we may need to acknowledge that *systems change* might be a process about which we know very little in comparison to what we know about changing the behavior of individuals: there are, for example, only a handful of published reports in the literature describing how major school systems made the shift from segregated to integrated services (Meyer & Kishi, 1985). Powers's (1988) book was an important effort to attempt to articulate systems-change issues and the need to expand our research and training models to address these issues. The disproportionate emphasis upon individual behavior change in the intervention literature in comparison to information available regarding how to change systems is no longer justifiable. We desperately need a cadre of researchers assisted by evaluation strategies that will allow us to identify the obstacles to change within static systems and how to overcome those obstacles effectively so that people are not unfairly deprived of opportunities to participate in best practices and are not expected to continue to tolerate outdated ones.

Summary

Despite the early successes, widespread use, and admittedly continuing technological superiority of applied behavior analysis in interventions with persons with severe disabilities, certain fundamental problems persist. First, the literature continues to report changes in single target behaviors in highly restrictive settings, and the majority of this research fails to systematically report evidence regarding collateral effects, side effects, generalization, and maintenance (see also Scotti, Evans, Meyer, & Walker, 1990, for further documentation of this claim). Second, there appears to be insufficient recognition of the limitations and implications of this situation among those who are operating within the behaviorist paradigm and publishing the majority of this research. Third, there may be substantive obstacles both within the research community and in service delivery environments that are responsible for this continuing problem and that, in turn, are directly responsible for the more

fundamental failures to translate "model" program outcomes into widespread practices for real people with disabilities in typical communities everywhere.

Quantitative-Qualitative Paradigm War

The challenge to the exclusive reliance upon single-subject research conventions palls in comparison to the almost acrimonious debate that has raged for more than a decade between the "quantitative" and "qualitative" methodologists (see Gage, 1989, for a futuristic look at various conceivable outcomes should this debate continue into the 21st century). Some of us have become so steeped in a particular research tradition that its methodological conventions may be regarded as hallowed tenets and universal principles, so that methodological disagreements include categorical rejection of alternative methodologies along with unquestioning adherence to the technical dimensions of one's preferred methodology. As action editor on two major journals (beginning in the mid-1980s to the present) that publish research on developmental disabilities, I have been surprised at the number of times that editorial board members will summarily dismiss the value of a research report because "the *n* is too small," a comment that apparently requires no further explanation as to *why* sample size is an issue and no recognition, in many instances, of the fact that the researcher was employing a methodology that approached concerns such as the generalizability of results in a different manner and with a different set of questions. In fact, the "quantitative-qualitative" debate is so clearly a false dichotomy in the context of scientific method and the history of science (see Jacob, 1989, for a discussion of this issue) that its very preeminence reveals the extent of our conventional rigidity as thinkers and scholars.

Quantitative Perspective

On the one hand, quantitative researchers accuse their qualitative colleagues of various methodological shortcomings, with a special emphasis perhaps upon subjectivity and, in quantitative terminology, a failure to demonstrate the reliability and generalizability of findings. Thus,

Mulick (1990) rejected the relevance of any scientific interest in introspection as opposed to the focus of behavioral science upon the "orderly and replicable interactions between individuals and their habitats, societies, cultures, affairs, and—in the case of psychology—between behavior and stimuli" (p. 7). Instead, he pronounced that "scientists look closely at physical properties of things and rely on quantitative descriptions of events" (Mulick, 1990, p. 7). Because quantitative scholars view the world of research through the positivist-colored lens of either a nomothetic or a single-subject research design perspective—and apply only their own semantic terminology to the issue—they tend to ignore the procedures to establish the "trustworthiness" of data (see, for example, Lincoln & Guba, 1985) by qualitative researchers. "Trustworthiness" is perhaps closest in construct to "reliability" but differs somewhat, as is appropriate to a different approach to what might even be a different question. And because quantitative traditionalists tend to dominate publication practices of the professional journals, qualitative traditionalists have historically been less able to communicate their methodology and observations to the field.

Qualitative Perspective

On the other hand, lest we view this tradition as the beleaguered underdog seeking only an opportunity to be heard and given a fair trial, qualitative researchers can be equally rejecting of other ways of knowing. At times, the very term "quantitative" has become a scholarly insult, and disparaging remarks have been made such as, "Well, I'm not interested in *numbers*; I want to understand the dynamics of people's lives."

Lincoln and Guba (1987) were unequivocal in their demand for a "shift in paradigms" due to what they labeled the "warrant to deceive in positivist inquiry [that] raises serious ethical difficulties in social research . . . " (p. 37). They elaborated on their criticisms of the ethical failure of quantitative research models: "The objectification of human beings in the process of searching for 'truth' (read: trying to discover the nature of 'reality') has led, as the feminist Keller has (1983) argued, to the depersonalization and

devaluing of human life" (Lincoln & Guba, 1987, p. 10). They further added:

> We have argued that a central failure of conventional, or positivistic, inquiry has been the inability to come to grips with the socially and morally repugnant fact of deception in research and its violation of societal ethics regarding dignity, self-determination and individual human agency. . . . Conventional inquiry acquires "permission" to engage in deceptive and injurious research by virtue of its focus upon a supposed single "reality" (Lincoln & Guba, 1987, pp. 35–36).

They provided the following examples:

> In theory, it sounds like good social science experimentation: group A gets the "treatment" (hardly a value-neutral term in itself), and group B gets "no treatment." . . . Social experiments conducted in this manner thus bring down harm on both target groups: the one for not having been asked what its perceived needs might be, the other for being denied what might have been an auspicious or gainful intervention. (Lincoln & Guba, 1987, pp. 16–17)

Finally, they asked, and concluded: " . . . how do we confront or sidestep the problems engendered by positivist social science? The simplest answer is to move to the contending alternative paradigm for social science research" (Lincoln & Guba, 1987, p. 24).

Thus, the unfortunate aftereffects of what might otherwise be a healthy challenge to an established paradigm could be the complete substitution of one methodology for the other. Would this be a good thing?

Summary

To answer the above question: Probably not, if we recognize that different methodologies represent alternative strategies to address different questions and even perform different—and sometimes quite complementary—functions in generating and testing theory, practice, and change in systems, programs, and people. It would not be appropriate to review the purposes of various research traditions here, but it would be helpful if those who are invested in the overall superiority of one or another method developed a better understanding of the purposes and capabilities of various "ways of knowing" (as Tharp, 1981, described it). Just as one example, Jacob (1989) noted:

. . . there are at least three major categories of generic research designs for understanding naturally-occurring human activity and thought: designs for describing variables or examining relationships among them (descriptive, correlational and causal-comparative designs), designs for examining a complex instance or instances (case study designs), and designs for developing theory (analytic induction and Glaser and Strauss' grounded theory method). (p. 36)

She elaborated in that paper and elsewhere regarding the potential usefulness and obvious appropriateness of different research designs and methodologies to address different issues or to complement one another in addressing the same issue (Jacob, 1987, 1988, 1989).

ANALYSIS AND APPLICATIONS

Skrtic (1986) summarized the "crisis in special education knowledge" that has evolved from the theory and practice of special education as an "insulated sub-culture of conventional knowledge . . . a way of seeing" (p. 6). He regarded this as the historical consequence of a professional community (in the field of special education) that has been trained primarily in psychology with certain underlying belief systems rooted in biology. Were this base to be broadened to include also the disciplinary perspectives of sociology, political science, and anthropology (as well as fields such as economics and history?), Skrtic suggested that:

> . . . the very notion of "disability" and the approach taken would be substantially different. Diagnosis, intervention, and technology would not be directed exclusively at the individual but would just as likely be directed at the conceptual and material structures, systems, and processes external to the individual. Things such as organization, institutions, and belief systems—not just children and youth—would be targets. (p. 6)

In this section, two "case study" examples are discussed to illustrate the need for what Guilford (1959) described many years ago as "divergent thinking" in order to achieve two generally accepted goals on behalf of persons with disabilities. One of these goals is broad, and applicable to all of us. The other is more specific and would be addressed to a particular need. But in both instances, stepping outside the conventional paradigms of research and practice currently dominating efforts to achieve those goals could direct us toward some constructive problem solving that might make a difference in the lives of the people involved.

Goal One: Achieving Social Integration

This goal might be stated in various ways, and the choice of the phrase "achieving social integration" is arbitrary. We could state the goal as "achieving full inclusion into the community," "increasing social support networks," "facilitating community acceptance and adjustment," and so on. Regardless of how we elect to describe the goal, an overarching principle of integration rather than segregation has become widely acknowledged and accepted as fair and just. Even those who continue to advocate for the need for intensive services that might be delivered to the individual in self-contained environments generally share the goal of community integration and differ primarily in their belief regarding the best strategies to achieve that goal. Even those who advocate long-term or even indefinite services for people with disabilities in handicapped-only environments base their position upon a belief that social acceptance is not achievable for certain individuals, so that isolation would be justified to protect them from negative consequences: Again, even this position ultimately acknowledges the *desirability* of social integration but differs in bias as to whether it is an achievable goal. (Those who would advocate for segregation based upon prejudice would obviously not share this goal—but achieving our goal might have an impact upon these beliefs as well.) Widespread acceptance of this goal has at the same time been accompanied by a major shift in attitudes toward persons with disabilities. Old attitudes of sympathy, protection and care have generally been replaced by a perspective valuing individual development, personal growth and self-determination, social interdependence, and full participation in society regardless of handicapping condition (Meyer & Putnam, 1988). The implications of this perspective for practice and service delivery have been fairly straightforward: People with disabilities, no matter how severe, are entitled to services that enable them to be a part of their natural communities.

There are, however, several different paths that might be taken to achieve this goal. Suppose, for example, that one's major interest is to enable children to be a part of their neighborhood school during the school years. Interestingly, special educators who embraced this goal never really questioned the best way to achieve it: While the procedural details have varied, the general process has consistently reflected a major emphasis upon the deficit-remedial model. Efforts to facilitate the social acceptance of students with disabilities in schools have largely stressed the need to teach them various social skills and other age-appropriate kinds of things that would make them more like their peers. Thus, teenagers might be taught how to play video games and the rules of "hanging out" to facilitate their social integration into the world of the high school. And perhaps because we are special educators and have become quite adept at teaching students the various skills traditionally found on individualized education programs (IEPs), it may have been inevitable that we would begin to teach "social competence" as well.

What happened next was perhaps also predictable given our successes as professional behavior-change agents: Even other children were recruited to help. Peers became peer tutors, students became teachers and teacher assistants, and potential friends became applied behavior analysts and even IEP planners. Because skill acquisition by the child with disabilities continued to be viewed as the major path to achieve social integration, virtually every social relationship experienced by that child was professionalized. (Parent training had, of course, long since co-opted various other traditional roles of the family, such as providing respite and unconditional positive regard or nurturance for its members.)

This professional intrusion into the lives of people with disabilities is also evident in the literature on community living and supported employment for adults. Is it appropriate or desirable to train co-workers to supervise people with disabilities on the job? Do staff assigned to family-scale homes in the community for people with severe disabilities need to be trained in behavior modification and data collection techniques to carry out their jobs well? Will the focus upon "lifestyle" become simply a larger life routine for task analysis and systematic instruction? In Chapter 31 in this volume, Smull and Bellamy rightly pointed out that it would *not* be appropriate to extend special education thinking into the design and control of adult lives. If we understand why this is not acceptable—regardless of the severity of the individual's disabilities—we must look again at our behavior in *every* domain, in *all* environments, and at *any* age.

Skill acquisition is clearly important, but few of us would allow our own lives to be defined by systematic, pervasive, and lifelong instruction and control by others. Now that we have satisfied ourselves and our society that everyone can learn, we must be more judicious about what and where we teach—and *who* should teach—to ensure that in our eagerness to achieve social integration we do not actually do serious damage to the integrity of the relationships experienced by people with disabilities. We have come to realize that friendships, family living, employment, and a community lifestyle are as important for people with severe disabilities as they are for everyone else. But it does not then follow that the way to attain these outcomes is to cast our various professional-disciplinary and remedial-technical nets over this new territory. On the contrary, it should be evident that we must not do so. What we should do may not be as clear, but will undoubtedly require divergent thinking (Guilford, 1959) along with respect for the integrity of each person's individuality and autonomy even as we rush to meet people's needs.

Goal Two: Remediation of Self-Injurious Behavior

Few needs seem as compelling as self-injurious behavior. Nearly everyone would agree that when an individual exhibits behaviors that jeopardize his or her life, remedial services are needed to solve the problem. The professional literature in developmental disabilities is replete with theory, description, and intervention research focused upon the remediation of serious behavior problems, with unanimous agreement that the presence of self-injurious behavior in particular is an urgent intervention priority. Furthermore, behavior therapy approaches in particular have been extensively applied to treat self-injurious behavior since the 1960s, and certain assumptions regarding principles of practice and treatment validity have become axiomatic in the field (see Scotti et al., 1990, for a review and meta-analytical evaluation of these issues). Yet, serious differences of opinion exist among professionals and experts in the treatment of self-injury regarding the use of aversive stimuli or control. In fact, even a National Institutes of Health Consensus Development Conference on the issue not only failed to achieve consensus but provoked increased debate and charges of bias in the conduct of the conference itself (Himelstein, 1990).

Those who support the use of aversives as contingent punishment for severe problem behavior argue that the major criterion for their use should be effectiveness: Particularly if the behavior problem itself is regarded as deplorable, painful, even life-threatening, the use of a painful aversive treatment is said to be defensible if there is evidence that its use will, in the long run, produce an overall decrease in pain experienced by the individual. Those who deplore the use of aversives argue that the use of dehumanizing and painful punishers is never justified, and add that their continued use has actually become an excuse for the absence of services to support appropriate lifestyles and a failure to utilize available, equally effective, positive treatments. No resolution of the controversy seems imminent and, in fact, the commercial marketing of a new electric shock device has introduced a new dimension into the picture and resulted in the filing of legal action demanding use of the device in a Michigan school district (Himelstein, 1990).

What is evident throughout this debate is that "effectiveness" is regarded as a central issue: Those who support aversives discuss the "right to effective treatment," and those who oppose their use have challenged their effectiveness, challenged the definition of effectiveness that has traditionally been used in this treatment research, and argued that positive alternatives have been demonstrated to be equally effective (see Chapter 35, this volume). Yet the published literature—whether dealing with the use of aversives or with the use of nonaversives to treat self-injury—continues to reveal the same nar-

row focus upon documenting a relatively short-term change in the target behavior, with little evidence of long-term maintenance of behavior change, generalization of behavior change to nontreatment settings and situations, or documentation that the individual's lifestyle has improved such that he or she now lives in a family, goes to a regular school, has friends, participates in the community, and so forth (Scotti et al., 1990). How, then, can the issue be resolved given our obvious complacence with such limited demonstration of "effectiveness"? It seems unlikely that the issue will be resolved through the continued proliferation of still more demonstrations of the kinds of research that are currently being reinforced through favorable publication decisions by major journals in the field.

Butterfield (1990) recently provided an interesting example of divergent thinking leading to his proposal for a "utilitarian ethics of the sort that are applied when deciding about any medical or behavioral treatment" (p. 11). I am citing his chapter not so much because I believe he has solved the problem, but because it illustrates something we need to do more often: Butterfield began by stating his questions and then documenting his thought processes in reaching his conclusions. There was no "hidden agenda" apparent in his contribution: rather, he told us what he was thinking as he evaluated each issue and reached each conclusion. This provides the opportunity to begin a sincere and open discussion whereby we could identify at which point the conflict begins. Yuskauskas (1990) did just that in her qualitative study of professionals who have strong and differing opinions on this issue—each of whom is involved in daily responsibilities to treat self-injury—with the intent of identifying shared values and a possible route to resolution of the conflict. She provided documentation that each of the professionals does share a primary interest in the welfare of the person with self-injurious behavior and the goal of community integration, and argued that these shared values and perspectives could be the basis for mediation to reach some understanding for the benefit of the person engaging in self-injury. In the interim, people with severe disabilities and serious behavioral needs such as the young man in the state of Michigan continue to engage in self-injurious behavior while the advocates and professionals and experts battle it out in the courts.

The Butterfield (1990) and Yuskauskaus (1990) papers have provided perhaps the only examples of a different perspective offering the possibility of solving a serious controversy in the field. Both authors succeeded in breaking away from their own biases and were able to propose alternative strategies for resolving the controversy that did not require—as the effectiveness strategy surely does—years and years of journal articles on self-injury with no consensus in sight. People who engage in self-injurious behavior persent us with a profound challenge; they should not become "subjects" for our research or our professional arguments. A modest alternative proposal might be to establish a national network of our best resources, along with the financial support to provide immediate services using those best resources, for the 5–10 most severe cases of self-injurious behavior in each state, for example. Surely, that would be more humane, more effective, and more responsive to real needs than continuing to apply obviously inadequate standards of behavior change evidence until—many years from now—we establish a "data base." And, in this instance, the solution to the problem might well be the systematic study of the controversy itself and the behavior of professionals and experts—not the behavior of the person with disabilities.

RECOMMENDATIONS

Researchers

Several recommendations can be offered, first of all, for professionals engaged in research and development activities intended to extend our knowledge on behalf of persons with severe disabilities:

1. *There is a need to expand our knowledge and use of alternative research methodologies.* This recommendation encompasses several issues. One is that researchers may well choose to develop substantial competence in the use of a particular methodology, but must nevertheless take on the responsibility of becoming at least an intelligent consumer of as many alternative

methodologies as is humanly possible. Unless they do so, their own ability to generate knowledge will become increasingly restricted as they fail to read and understand the work of others and must limit their own work to the kinds of questions for which their chosen methodology is well suited (Staats, 1988). The difficulties of communicating across multiple disciplines has long been acknowledged: The importance of nevertheless doing so receives virtually universal support (Skrtic, 1986). An intolerance of alternative research methodologies reflects a parallel threat to our abilities as professionals to work together—cooperatively—to address some far more important issues in the field than proving which version of science represents truth. Perhaps the very first measure of our own sophistication in becoming "intermethodologists" would be a review of the editorial criteria that are applied to make publication decisions about scientific reports. There are nearly two dozen professional journals that publish such research intended to expand knowledge, and, at present, the vast majority of these journals adhere to a particular methodology as a matter of publication policy. When reports are accepted for publication that employ alternative scientific approaches, lowered standards are implied through the use of a "lesser" format such as a brief report.

In general, the derogation of "other" approaches must stop. Methodologies are not in competition with one another, and those who believe that they are reveal their own lack of knowledge regarding the history of science and the restrictiveness of their own abilities to imagine new scientific developments that might well contribute to that history (for a discussion of how an integrated paradigm expands the domain of behavior therapy, see Eifert & Evans, 1990). Where adherents to particular methodologies succeed in communicating their intolerance to their students and to others in the field, they escalate a scientific ethnocentrism that will further limit the translation of innovations into typical practices. Furthermore, arguing among ourselves helps no one, rightly confuses and frustrates policymakers who might otherwise be interested in working with us, and fills our professional publications with scientific self-talk that makes it even less likely that anyone other than the "players" would be remotely interested in reading any of our journals at all.

To effect this recommendation, several sub-recommendations are offered. First, journal publication criteria should be expanded to recognize the variety of ways of knowing as valid approaches to knowledge production. Second, sponsored research and development efforts—particularly those supported by federal and state funding initiatives—should emphasize the intelligent articulation of research questions and require the use of more than one methodology to answer various questions. Third, university doctoral training programs might continue to require substantive competence in a particular methodology, but should also require at least consumer-level knowledge of more than one alternative methodology relevant to content interests. Finally, promotion and tenure decisions in higher education should be made based upon judgments regarding contributions to knowledge and scientific productivity, not whether someone has published certain kinds of research in certain journals hierarchically ranked according to how they match those biases.

2. *There is a need to augment traditional human subjects review criteria to protect the integrity of community lifestyles for persons with disabilities.* The traditional ideal of informed consent has always been subject to potential abuse where the "subject" cannot give informed consent, and alternative concepts such as substituted judgment have not completely eliminated this risk. The risk is most obvious whenever life and death decisions are made on behalf of persons with severe disabilities: Maybe (or maybe not) it is easy to say "If it were me, I would rather. . . ." However, it is *not* me, and our confidence that such notions solve the problem is undeserved. The risk is most pervasive at the present time, when persons with severe disabilities are finally being given their fair share and opportunities to join their communities and their culture. Our research practices are primarily highly intrusive ones: We observe people, with clipboards in hand; we count their behavior in the presence of others; we test them on a variety of tasks in both test and natural environments; and we drill them as well as their families and friends about what they've just done, thought, or said. In the past, when we imagined that people with severe disabilities were somehow so different that such intrusions didn't matter, informed consent from a guardian on behalf of the individual might have been good enough. But now we have come to recognize that every intrusion into the dignity of the individual further isolates and segregates that person from his or her community and culture. Every intrusion into the personal lives of people with disabilities and their families also stands as a stark reminder that professionals are still in control: Yes, we'll allow you into the community, but not alone and not without our supervision. Thus, even as we move to emphasize broader lifestyle issues to replace past obsessions with target behaviors such as eye contact and in-seat behavior, we insist on intruding in our data collection and evaluation procedures. This, too, has to stop. Would any of us accept the U.S. Census Bureau representative into our homes, neighborhoods, and places of employment on a weekly or even daily basis? Why, then, should people with disabilities have to continue to accept intrusions into their lives as the cost for finally having access to a reasonable "lifestyle"?

Obviously, we need evaluation strategies to ensure that program innovations are truly in the best interests of the people for whom they were designed. But if we believe that all we need do is transfer our laboratory research behaviors to family-scale homes in the community, to the regular education classroom, and to peer interactions and other social relationships around the clock, our own understanding of what living in the community really means still reflects "handicapped-only" visions and the protection of our own "professional-in-control" status.

Again, becoming more sophisticated and more tolerant of alternative ways of knowing would help us to discover strategies that won't intrude and ultimately institutionalize "lifestyles" as a second-class idea for people with handicaps. This would be a radical outcome consistent with a certain modest recognition that our status as professionals does not entitle some of us to stay in charge. Thus, our evaluation strategies will have to resemble more closely the kinds of things we have generally been able to do to monitor events in the lives of citizens who do not have disabilities. And any increased monitoring system required to document promised benefits and protect the individual from harm must be particularly vigilant in its commitment not to compromise the dignity of the individual in the process.

3. *There is a need to shift our thinking as scientists from the "experiment" to broader issues of credibility and integrity.* This may at first glance appear to contradict the first recommendation. However, the recommendation does not imply the rejection of the experiment as a method for hypothesis testing as much as it calls for an increased understanding of the purposes of the experiment to structure approaches to hypothesis testing. The controlled experiment as a scientific technique was intended to provide a demonstration of the effects of an independent variable—manipulated by the researcher—upon the dependent variable that is the desired outcome. This has been a reasonable way to demonstrate experimental control for independent variables that could be manipulated at will—particularly in the case of dependent variables that were apparently so transitory (or in such early stages of "acquisition") that they would come and go at the whim of the researcher's manipulations.

If we are serious about wanting meaningful outcomes for people with severe disabilities, our independent variables will change and our dependent variables will change. It is simply not reasonable to expect that severe self-injurious behavior that has been occurring for many years will be "cured" by a single treatment, whether that treatment is differential reinforcement of other behaviors (DRO) or teaching an alternative communicative response. People without disabilities who are motivated to change struggle with such relatively minor self-injurious but long-standing habits such as overeating and nailbiting, and both the population of our prisons and chemical dependency programs illustrate the magnitude of solving more serious behavior problems in our society. Furthermore, who would be impressed by evidence that someone who had been an alcoholic for years had not

taken a drink for several weeks? Why, then, do we allow "treatments" and "outcomes" for people with disabilities to be singular, simple, brief, and require virtually no information about what happens to these people years later?

A few subrecommendations for this issue are offered. First, acceptance of a package of multiple treatment (independent) variables should be contingent upon whether the recommended combination is both reasonable and powerful enough to be expected to have an impact. If the innovative treatment is so artificial, expensive, unnatural, or intrusive that typical environments could never use it, it makes little sense to continue expending major resources on such treatments at the expense of work on those that could ultimately be used in the real world. Thus, the relatively naive demand that "the" experimental variable be isolated in the experiment needs to be replaced by an appreciation for the dynamics of social science questions. Second, concern for demonstrating the internal validity of experimental treatments must be replaced by broader issues of documenting the credibility of the treatment as an explanation for behavior change. If, for example, we know virtually everything about what is happening to an individual and there is a long-standing pattern of behavior of many years duration, wouldn't an immediate shift in that pattern of behavior that correlates with the introduction of a new variable (the intervention package) be a credible demonstration of its effects? There are established standards for interrupted time series and case study research that do not require no-treatment control groups or treatment reversals to establish the credibility of the intervention (see, for example, Yin, 1989). The use of such alternative strategies will become increasingly critical as we move into the community and begin looking at more enduring dimensions of behavior change. Finally, the focus of the dependent variable in scientific research must shift from temporal changes in single target behaviors to meaningful outcomes that endure and have broader impact upon the quality of life of the individual. What are these meaningful outcomes? They might include things such as employment, friendships, living in the community with support, and being able to make various daily decisions that affect one's life. But they most certainly no longer include changing things such as eye contact, following one-step commands, sorting plastic objects by shape and color, and making one's bed, without any evidence that such "skills" make a difference in the individual's quality of life. Shifting to more meaningful outcomes will make even more urgent the need to develop and use alternative research methodologies that can do more than graph frequency data across time and treatment phase as the sole criterion of success.

4. *There is a need for researchers to* collaborate *with practitioners longitudinally and to learn to* communicate *with policymakers effectively.* Baumeister (1981) chastised researchers for failing to understand the needs and problems of service delivery agencies and policymakers, and suggested that we were mistaken in our assumption that scientific knowledge production contributed directly to innovations and practice and changes in social policy. Earlier in this chapter, Tables 41.2 and 41.3 listed a number of traditional solutions that have been proposed to narrow the gap between what we know and what we do. None of these has thus far solved the problem, but it is also true that implementation of such solutions has been imperfect at best. Nevertheless, it would seem fair to conclude that the traditional model of beginning with a pilot study under laboratory conditions and then attempting to gradually adapt the process for actual conditions and/or simply persuade policy-makers that the pilot study is indeed relevant regardless of artificial resources and circumstances *has not been successful.* My support for this radical claim is what Lindblom and Cohen (1979) called "ordinary knowledge"— something that we all know, that is not the result of formal hypothesis testing or systematic study, but is based upon common sense, clinical experience, and a realistic appraisal of the limited political power of research in the public policy arena.

So what should we do if we care about the relevance and usefulness of our work for public policy decisions? Again, using "ordinary knowledge" and common sense, the recommended tactic would be to establish and nurture long-standing relationships with service delivery agencies in one's region. If the collaboration is mutual and works well, there would eventually be daily and longitudinal demonstrations of the validity of "innovations" in practice in typical settings: Few research reports are as credible as those that are supported by actual demonstrations in practice in the real world. For their part, researchers would develop some significant skills in adapting experimental, scientific, and professional techniques for criterion environments, and their work would then presumably *have to* reflect the concerns of policymakers, practitioners, and consumers in their immediate environment.

This would mean, as Skrtic (1986) suggested, that research and clinical practices would be directed at changing the systems intended to support and serve persons with disabilities, as opposed to maintaining our current focus upon changing the individual to fit a system that clearly is not working well. Again: "Things such as organizations, institutions, and belief systems—not just children and youth—would be targets" (Skrtic, 1986, p. 6).

Through this process, a collateral effect would be the development of skills in translating scientific knowledge into ordinary knowledge through more effective communication and dissemination practices. Perhaps what we really need after all are more "regular people" who are in other avocations but who are interested in telling our stories to the public (because they went to school with people with severe disabilities from an early age?), and who will therefore make films such as *Rainman,* television serial dramas such as *Life Goes On,* and write best sellers that present people and decent practices positively.

Practitioners and Policymakers

Those of us who deliver services, make policy, and advocate for services and policy changes are also confronted with certain challenges if we are to reduce the discrepancies that now limit opportunities available to persons with severe disabilities.

1. *The predominant deficit-remedial and diagnostic-prescriptive approach to disability must be shifted to one that focuses upon structural as well as individual change to achieve our*

goals. Just for the sake of illustration, a critical look at the IEP process in America's post–PL 94-142 schools reveals that both placement and services are often dictated by available options and not by what is best for the individual. Within the range of those available options, the focus of the individual's education program then becomes primarily one of identifying instructional needs that take the shape of skill/behavioral deficits, and teaching things to that individual to remediate those deficits. While this is clearly an admirable and constructive process, it also signifies limited goals and commitments toward a more equitable and just society. Banks (1989) articulated a "demographic imperative" that mandates a structural, system-wide shift in the design of services to reflect more accurately and fairly the diverse nature of today's world and the students in today's schools. Just as students with severe disabilities are "knocking on the classroom door" (see Chapter 19, p. 382, this volume), large percentages of students in the mainstream are apparently headed the other way: Our schools are simply not coping well with diversity, and our traditional models of schooling are leaving unacceptable numbers of young people behind. This is not to deny that students with severe disabilities do indeed have important needs to learn new skills and behaviors and that instruction must be provided to meet those needs. It may also be that alienated "typical" students and students who are leaving school prior to graduation also have serious needs for instruction and support. But Banks's charge is that we have unnecessarily "handicapped" our youngsters by continuing to support schooling that requires a mythical image of a mainstream student in order to work and marginalizes all others as a result.

A serious alternative would be to take to heart Skrtic's (1986) challenge and become active participants in the general movement for education and system-wide reforms. Such reforms would address the structure of our systems even as we continue to meet the needs of individual students, and would be advanced on behalf of the majority of our students as well as those with severe disabilities. For every practitioner, this would entail a personal responsibility to begin at home: Regular class teachers must acquire the skills to provide instruction to heterogeneous groups of students; special educators must acquire the skills to become a resource service to the mainstream of education rather than deliver parallel services to various "special" groupings; administrators must create high expectations and provide the necessary supports for schools that will respond to the demographic imperative; and all of us must take on personal goals for making the necessary changes—one step at a time, perhaps, but immediately and not at some future, hypothetical time. For every demand we make that a person with severe disabilities must learn something new to participate more fully in his or her community, there should be a corresponding responsibility for systems to learn new information and make the necessary adaptations to ensure that those demands are reasonable ones.

2. *We need to reexamine the distribution of resources and funding to replace special interests and privileges with participation in achieving equity throughout services on behalf of all citizens.* After years of exclusion and even abuse, mandatory services and resources for persons with disabilities were long overdue. Unfortunately, many of these services and resources continue to be distributed according to various special interest categories where entitlement must be documented through selection and exclusion criteria. The consequence of such a system is a certain rigidity that does not accommodate individual needs as much as it models categorical myths and, further, the creation of new institutions of political power and privilege that compete against one another and, ultimately, themselves resist change and progress. Biklen (1988) eloquently described the "Myth of Clinical Judgment" whereby all of us believe that decisions are made on behalf of persons with disabilities based upon clinical expertise applied to deciding what is best for someone. In actuality, many if not most decisions are profoundly compromised by guild interests (what is best for the professional or the system), economic constraints (what our existing patterns of funding allow us to do), political influence (who's in charge), and other nonclinical criteria that have little to do with either the person's needs or clinical expertise to meet those needs.

Recognition of this reality as an inherent risk of any system would require that we, as practitioners, expand our role accordingly. We would continue to develop skills to teach and support people with disabilities directly, but we must also accept a responsibility to advocate for those things we cannot teach and supports we cannot provide—and this must be a nonextraordinary expectation for practitioners. In other words, as a culture of service delivery systems we need to move beyond doing business as usual until contradictions reach the "whistle blower" level; whistle blowers would not be needed in a professional culture where participants are expected to advocate as a matter of course.

3. *The nature of the relationship between those who deliver services and those who are the recipients of those services must be altered to correct the present imbalance of power.* Providing services to people with disabilities— including those with severe disabilities—does not then entitle us to be in charge of the lives of people with disabilities. The average citizen has in recent years rightfully demanded to be treated with respect by various service providers. For example, we now expect that physicians talk to us as "equals"; that they give us the information that is rightfully ours so that we can make our own, informed decisions; and that they cease making decisions on our behalf, "for our own good." Professionals have enjoyed a power status over others that has no real parallel in other domains of our lives: Thus, we may solicit and purchase services from an automobile dealer but regard dealers as unacceptably deceptive if they keep information from us, would hardly allow dealers to decide for us which car we shall buy, and expect to be treated with respect throughout our sales transaction. And we expect all of this despite the fact that most of us do not have the slightest idea of how our car really works or how to fix it when something goes wrong. Similarly, the relationship between the professional who provides services and the client who needs them should not intrude into decisions that should rightfully be made by the persons who must live with the consequences of those decisions. Furthermore, there is really no justification for a situation where professionals assume total charge over the very lives of people with disabilities—

simply because the one individual has a diagnosis and the other a degree.

An important first step to right this historical imbalance of power is to involve people with disabilities in decision making at all levels. Professional organizations, school boards, agency governing and advisory bodies, case conferences, and even weekly meetings of agency staff should be attended by persons with disabilities as full participants. Furthermore, our approach to staffing should be reevaluated: What does it mean to call someone a "paraprofessional"? At present, the designation seems to signify a preference to have fully trained professionals to carry out professional responsibilities, but as these resources are not available, we staff people with some of those qualifications ("para"). Recalling again Smull and Bellamy's admonition (see Chapter 31, this volume) that we not re-create the remedial model in our approach to non-school environments and across the life span, perhaps the roles now designated as paraprofessionals would best be redefined as something else entirely. Rather than teaching resident staff in family-scale homes in the community how to deliver rewards and keep observational data, perhaps we ought to regard them as live-in peer supports and take advantage of their potential as companions, community supports, and just ordinary people who will interact with people with disabilities in a natural and genuine way if we do not intrude by teaching them otherwise. This does not mean that standards would be eliminated or that such individuals would not be evaluated to ensure that jobs are done and people are protected and supported. But it would mean a major change in the way we approach various staffing and training issues, where what we do now is somehow viewed as "second best" in comparison to what professionals do.

POSTSCRIPT

It should be obvious that this book could not have been written as recently as 10 years ago. This is so not only because the research reported throughout its various chapters had not been done, but also because our thinking about disabilities and handicaps has changed dramatically. The research and development accomplishments mapped by the review chapters in each section of this volume are remarkable, and enable us to have a vision of what we could and can achieve for our society. Furthermore, as Peck stated in the very first chapter, the clarification of our values is a genuine cultural achievement as well. We couldn't be worried about discrepancies in the attainment of excellence and equity in our social systems had we not already developed this clear picture of social justice. It is a tribute to humanistic ideals that we want social justice for every person in today's world—including those with the most severe disabilities, with no exceptions. And it is a tribute to the efforts of advocates, families, people with disabilities, professionals, and the public that these ideals have been translated into practice through research showing us how to do it and services showing us that it can be done.

We have passed the first part of the test. It seems fair enough to feel a sense of accomplishment about our progress thus far. But the discrepancies described on paper throughout this book mean that for many people with severe disabilities, this progress has not yet made a difference in their lives. The next step is to achieve the second revolution that Laski wrote about in Chapter 23: It is the hope of the authors of this book—and the people with severe disabilities who have challenged our society to achieve the first revolution—that with energy, enthusiasm, constructive criticism, innovative practices, and continued knowledge production, the next decade will be both exciting and ordinary. Reaching goals and setting new ones signify growth: Achieving them for real people must now become an everyday occurrence.

REFERENCES

Banks, J.A. (1989, March). Teacher education and students of color: Conceptualizing the problem. Paper presented at the annual meeting of the American Educational Research Association, San Francisco.

Baumeister, A.A. (1981). Mental retardation policy and research: The unfulfilled promise. *American Journal of Mental Deficiency, 85,* 445–456.

Biklen, D. (1988). The myth of clinical judgment. *Journal of Social Issues, 44*(1), 127–140.

Bogdan, R., & Kugelmass, J. (1984). Case studies of mainstreaming: A symbolic interactionist approach to special schooling. In L. Barton & S. Tomlinson (Eds.), *Special education and social interests* (pp. 173–191). London: Croom-Helm.

Butterfield, E.C. (1990). *Serious self injury: The ethics of treatment and research.* In A.C. Repp & N.N. Singh (Eds.), *Current perspectives in the use of nonaversive and aversive interventions with developmentally disabled persons.* Sycamore, IL: Sycamore Publishing Co.

Durand, V.M., & Kishi, G.S. (1987). Reducing severe behavior problems among persons with dual sensory impairments: An evaluation of a technical assistance model. *Journal of The Association for Persons with Severe Handicaps, 12,* 2–10.

Edgerton, R. (1967). *The cloak of competence.* Berkeley: University of California Press.

Eifert, G.H., & Evans, I.M. (Eds.). (1990). *Unifying behavior therapy: Contributions of paradigmatic behaviorism.* New York: Springer.

Evans, I.M., & Meyer, L.H. (1987). Moving to educational validity: A reply to Test, Spooner, and

Cooke. *Journal of The Association for Persons with Severe Handicaps, 12,* 103–106.

Evans, I.M., Meyer, L.H., Kurkjian, J., & Kishi, G.S. (1988). An evaluation of behavioral interrelationships in child behavior therapy. In J.C. Witt, S.N. Elliott, & F.N. Gresham (Eds.), *Handbook of behavior therapy in education* (pp.189–215). New York: Plenum.

Gage, N.L. (1989). The paradigm wars and their aftermath: A "historical" sketch of research on teaching since 1989. *Educational Researcher, 18*(7), 4–10.

Guilford, J.P. (1959). Three faces of intellect. *American Psychologist, 14,* 469–479.

Himelstein, L. (1990). Taking aim at NIH's scientific methods: Critics say backers of controversial shock therapy stacked the deck. *Legal Times: Law and Lobbying in the Nation's Capitol, XII*(42), 1, 16–17.

Horner, R.H., Dunlap, G., & Koegel, R.L. (Eds.). (1988). *Generalization and maintenance: Life-style changes in applied settings.* Baltimore: Paul H. Brookes Publishing Co.

Jacob, E. (1987). Qualitative research traditions: A review. *Review of Educational Research, 57,* 1–50.

Jacob, E. (1988). Clarifying qualitative research: A focus on traditions. *Educational Researcher, 17*(1), 16–19, 22–24.

Jacob, E. (1989, July). Understanding and selecting designs for research in naturally-occurring situations. In *Proceedings, Research in Education of the Handicapped Project Directors' Meeting* (pp. 31–50). Reston, VA: Council for Exceptional Children.

Kazdin, A.E. (1978). *History of behavior modifica-*

tion: *Experimental foundations of contemporary research*. Baltimore: University Park Press.

Kazdin, A.E. (1982). Symptom substitution, generalization, and response covariation: Implications for psychotherapy outcomes. *Psychological Bulletin 91*, 349–365.

Keller, E.F. (1983). Feminism as an analytic tool for the study of science. *Academe, 69*, 15–22.

Lincoln, Y., & Guba, E. (1985). *Naturalistic inquiry*. Beverly Hills: Sage Publications.

Lincoln, Y.S., & Guba, E.G. (1987, April). *Ethics: The failure of positivist science*. Paper presented at the annual meeting of the American Educational Research Association, Washington, DC.

Lindblom, C.E., & Cohen, D.K. (1979). *Usable knowledge: Social science and social problem solving*. New Haven, CT: Yale University Press.

Matson, J.L., Manikam, R., Coe, D., Raymond, K., Taras, M., & Long, N. (1988). Training social skills to severely mentally retarded multiply handicapped adolescents. *Research in Developmental Disabilities, 9*, 195–208.

Meyer, L.H., & Kishi, G.S. (1985). School integration strategies. In K.C. Lakin & R.H. Bruininks (Eds.), *Strategies for achieving community integration of developmentally disabled citizens* (pp. 231–252). Baltimore: Paul H. Brookes Publishing Co.

Meyer, L.H., & Putnam, J. (1988). Social integration. In V.B. Van Hasselt, P.S. Strain, & M. Hersen (Eds.), *Handbook of developmental and physical disabilities* (pp. 107–133). New York: Pergamon Press.

Miller, D. (Ed.). (1955). *Popper selections*. Princeton, NJ: Princeton University Press.

Mulick, J. (1990). The ideology and science of punishment in mental retardation. *American Journal of Mental Retardation*.

Nelson, R.O., & Evans, I.M. (1968). The combination of learning principles and speech therapy techniques in the treatment of non-communicating children. *Journal of Child Psychology and Psychiatry, 9*, 111–124.

Powers, M.D. (Ed.) (1988). *Expanding systems of service delivery for persons with developmental disabilities*. Baltimore: Paul H. Brookes Publishing Co.

Risley, T., & Wolf, M. (1968). Establishing functional speech in echolalic children. In H.N. Sloane & B.D. MacAulay (Eds.), *Operant procedures in remedial speech and language training* (pp. 157–184). Boston: Houghton Mifflin.

Scotti, J.R., Evans, I.M., Meyer, L.H., & Walker, P. (1990). *A meta-analysis of intervention research with problem behavior: Treatment validity and standards of practice*. Paper submitted for publication.

Skrtic, T.M. (1986). The crisis in special education knowledge: A perspective on perspective. *Focus on Exceptional Children, 18*(7), 1–16.

Staats, A.W. (1988). Paradigmatic behaviorism, unified positivism, and paradigmatic behavior therapies. In D.B. Fishman, F. Rotger, & C.M. Franks (Eds.), *Paradigms in behavioral therapy: Present and Promise* (pp. 211–253). New York: Springer.

Test, D.W., Spooner, F., & Cooke, N.L. (1987). Educational validity revisited. *Journal of The Association for Persons with Severe Handicaps, 12*, 96–102.

Tharp, R.G. (1981). The metamethodology of research and development. *Educational Perspectives, 20*, 42–48.

Ulicny, G.R., Thompson, S.K., Favell, J.E., & Thompson, M.S. (1985). The active assessment of educability: A case study. *Journal of The Association for Persons with Severe Handicaps, 10*, 111–114.

Voeltz, L.M., & Evans, I.M. (1982). Behavioral interrelationships in child behavior therapy. *Behavioral Assessment, 4*, 131–165.

Voeltz, L.M., & Evans, I.M. (1983). Educational validity: Procedures to evaluate outcomes in programs for severely handicapped learners. *Journal of The Association of the Severely Handicapped, 8*(1), 3–15.

Yin, R. (1989). *Case study research: Design and methods* (rev. ed.). Beverly Hills: Sage Publications.

Yuskauskas, A. (1990). *Perspectives on a shifting treatment approach in Pennsylvania's community service system*. Unpublished paper. (Available from the author, Division of Special Education and Rehabilitation, 805 S. Crouse Ave., Syracuse University, Syracuse, NY 13244-2280)

Index

AAMD, *see* American Association on Mental
   Retardation
Abortion, 554–555
ABS, *see* Adaptive Behavior Scale
Academic skills, assessment of, 59
Accountability
  administrative, 532
  consumer, 491–492
  cooperative learning and, 255
  early intervention and, 482–483
Achievement, achievability and, discrepancies
   between, 629–631
Acquisition assessment, 60–61
Activities of daily living, *see* Self-care skills
Adaptation, family, *see* Family adaptation theory
Adaptive behavior
  community living and, 120–121
    in group homes, 123, 124
  competence and, 34–35
Adaptive Behavior Scale (ABS), 34, 35
Adaptive devices, 365–366
Adaptive instruction, 257–258
Adaptive Learning Environments Model (ALEM),
   258, 263, 415
Adjustment, supported employment and, 159
Administration, adult community services and,
   532–533
Administrators
  and community school, 383
  and regular education environments, 261
Adoption, special needs, 133–134
Adult(s)
  community services for, 527–535
    administration and, 532–533
    capacity development and, 534–535
    crisis in, 527–530
    local management and, 533–534
    need for new paradigm and, 528
    policy challenges and, 530–535
    resource allocation and, 531–532
    support paradigm and, 528–530
  federal programs for, 509–518
    see also Federal programs, for adults
  needs of, longitudinal research on, appropriate
    education and, 73
Adult service reform, 489
  TASH resolution on, 491–492
After-school programs
  friendships and, 208
  management needs related to, 252
Age, at start of early intervention, 442–444
Age-appropriate behaviors, leisure, community-
   based, 177–178
Agencies, coordination of, supported employment
   and, 148

Aggression-disruption, nonaversive intervention in,
   565–580
  by altering setting events, 566, 569–575
  by response covariation, 575–579
  by systems change, 579–580
  by teaching functionally equivalent behavior,
    565–566, 567–568
AIDD, see Analysis and Intervention in Develop-
   mental Disabilities
Alamo Heights Independent School District v. State
   Board of Education, 465
Alcohol, and fetal alcohol syndrome, 35
ALEM, *see* Adaptive Learning Environments Model
American Academy of Neurology, on vegetative
   state, 557
American Association on Mental Retardation
   (AAMR)
  Adaptive Behavior Scale of, 34, 35
  classification system of, 28
  mental retardation definition of, 26, 27
American Occupational Therapy Association
   (AOTA), 356
  consultation models of, 357
American Psychiatric Association (APA), classifica-
   tion system of, 28–29
American social policy, *see* Social policy
Analysis and Intervention in Developmental Disabil-
   ities (AIDD), 67
Anencephaly, 555–556
  organ transplants and, 549
AOTA, *see* American Occupational Therapy
   Association
APA, *see* American Psychiatric Association
Applied behavior analysis, future of, 607–610,
   613–615
Appraisals, coping and, in family, 283–286,
   297–299
Aptitude-treatment-interaction (ATI), 48, 263
Armstrong v. Kline, 464
Artificial supervision, 221
ASC, *see* Assessment of Social Competence
Assessment, 101–105
  context of, 104–105
  deficiency approach and, 101–102
  development and
    common beliefs about, 103
    reconsideration of, 103–104
  evaluation of, 93–100
    parents and, 98–100
  family, family empowerment and, 485–487
  functional, 45–63
    see also Functional assessment
  future directions for, 104–105
  historical considerations of, current practices and,
    101–103

Assessment—*continued*
  leisure, development of, 182–183
  of peer response patterns, 210–211
  psychometric model of, 102
  qualitative measures in, 105
  related services and, 370–371
  self-evaluation in, supported employment and,
      159
  of social networks, 211–212
  of sociometric status, 211
  see also Testing
Assessment of Social Competence (ASC), 50–51
Assistive devices, 365–366
Association for Persons with Severe Handicaps, *see*
      The Association for Persons with Severe
      Handicaps (TASH)
Assumptions, unconscious, paradigm traps and,
      632–639
ATI, *see* Aptitude-treatment-interaction
Attention, research needs involving, 81
Attitudes
  of children, 203–205, 210–211, 261
  of professionals, 325
Augmentative communication, 368
Aversive control, 545, 640–642
  power relationships and, 617–623
  SIBIS in, TASH resolution on, 551–552
  see also Nonaversive interventions
Avoidance coping styles, 285

Baby Doe case, 601–606
Balthazar Scales of Adaptive Behavior, 34
Bank Street Model of adaptive instruction, 258
Battle v. Commonwealth, 464
Beck Depression Inventory (BDI), 277
Behavior(s)
  adaptive
    community living and, 120–121, 123, 124
    competence and, 34–35
    assessment of, 46–48
    excess, reduction in, 79–80
    functions of, appropriate education and, 73–74
    leisure, age-appropriate, 177–178
    linguistic, social skills training and, 52–53
    measurement of, in real time, 609
    multiple, simultaneous measurement of, 608–609
  social
    assessment of, 50–53
    community integration and, 127
    context of, 199
Behavior analysis, applied, 607–610, 613–615
Behavior management, instructional procedures
      and, integration of, 609
Behavioral control
  aversive, *see* Aversive control
  need for, social skills use and, 197
Behavioral interventions
  nonaversive, *see* Nonaversive interventions
  scope of, extension of, 609–610

Behavioral marital therapy, 299
Behaviorism, education practices and, 392
Beliefs, research on, appropriate education and, 73
Benefit-cost analyses, wages and, supported em-
      ployment and, 149, 152–153, 162–163
Best practices, 316–331
  curricular content and, 317–319
    preservice, 333–334
    university, 337
  features of, 317
    preservice, 333–337
    university, 337–340
  implementation of, teachers and, 329–331
  outcomes of, 323–329
    community participation, 323–325
    ordinariness and invisibility, 325, 328–329
    preservice, 336–337
    social support networks, 325, 326–328
    university, 340
  processes of, 319–323
    family involvement, 319, 322
    instructional effectiveness, 322–323
    negotiation, 322
    preservice, 334–336
    supporting research for, 320–322
    team collaboration, 319
    university, 337–340
Beta Hostels, 129
*Board of Education of East Windsor Regional
      School v. Diamond*, 462, 463
Bonadaptation, salutogenesis and, pathogenesis/
      maladaptation versus, 274–275
Brain death, organ transplants and, 549
"Branching" task analyses, 206
Brown v. Board of Education, 412

CAI, *see* Computer-assisted instruction
Cain-Levine Social Competency Scale, 34
Campbell v. Talladega County Board of Education,
      413, 418
Capacity, development of, adult community services
      and, 534–535
CAPE scales, 50
Capital investment
  in institutional settings, 110
  in segregated settings, 113, 171–172
Caregiver stress, in family, 274–278
  chronic stressors and, 282–283
  as generic problem with generic solutions,
      275–278
  salutogenesis/bonadaptation versus pathogenesis/
      maladaptation and, 274–275
  see also Family *entries*
Case advocacy, Part H program and, 500–501
Case consultation, 357
*Cayuga-Onondaga Assessment for Children with
      Handicaps, Version 6.0*, 249
Centennial Development Services, 129
Center for Epidemiological Studies Depression

(CES-D) Scale, 277
Certification, teacher, 396–397
Change
  implementation of, values-based research on,
    10–11
  professionals and, 237
  service systems and, 237–238
  strategies for, education and, 264
Child Abuse and Neglect Prevention and Treatment
    Act, 556
Child-care services, 292–293
Child development, *see* Development
Children
  adoption of, 133–134
  families and, community and, 129–135, 236–237
  foster care for, 133
  out-of-home placement of, 130
  preschool, *see* Early intervention; Preschool
    integration
  school-age, federal programs for, 501–506
Choice-based approaches, diagnostic-prescriptive
    approaches versus, 529
Choices
  communication and, control and, 543–544
  empowerment and, 625–626
  TASH resolution on, 494
  see also Decision making
Civil rights, 409
  housing and transportation and, 514
  see also Right to services
CLAs, *see* Community living arrangements
Class size, community school and, 384
Classification
  definition and, testing and diagnosis and, 27–30
  education and, 68–69
  professional issues in, 38–39
Classmates, as resource, in regular education envi-
    ronments, 261
Classroom
  regular, *see* Regular education environments
  social relationships and, 199
Clustered placement, in supported employment, *see*
    Enclave model of supported employment
CMI, *see* Computer-managed instruction
Cognitive-behavioral interventions, for family,
    298–299
Cognitive coping, 283–285
Cognitive reframing, in family interventions,
    297–299
Cognitive retraining, 36
Cognitive theories of learning, 34
Collaboration
  core principles of, 358
  education and, 319, 320
  practice integration and, 354–355
  between researchers and practitioners, 645
  see also Team *entries*
Collaborative consultation, 358
Collaborative professional knowledge, support of,
    370

Collaborative team teaching, 259–260
Colleague consultation, 357
Communication
  augmentative, 368
  choices and, control and, 543–544
  between researchers and policymakers, 645
Communication imperative, 543–544
Communication skills
  assessment of, 58–59, 370
  teaching of, 75–77
    see also Language intervention
  see also Social skills
Communicative functioning, 48
Community, 236
  institutionalization in, 117
  movement into, 118–122
  participation in, best practices and, 323–325
  sense of, school and, 381–382
Community-based instruction, 57, 250
Community-based leisure behaviors, age-appropri-
    ate, 177–178
Community-based services
  for adults, 527–535
    see also Adult(s), community services for
  leisure, inadequacy of, 173–174
  Medicaid, absence of, 509–511
  TASH policy on, 109
Community goals, American social policy and, 497
Community integration, 126–127, 409–412
  assessment for, 57–58
  domains important to, 122
  recreation and, 173
  see also Integration
Community Intensive Instruction Model, 250
Community living, 115–137, 235–238, 491
  case studies of, 116–117
  for children and families, 129–135, 236–237
    federal support and, 132
    informal supports and networks and, 132–133
    out-of-home placement and, 130
    respite services and, 134–135
    special needs adoption/foster care and, 133–134
    state support and, 130–132
  community and, 236
  community integration and, 126–127
  concepts in, 238
  cost of, 121–122
  definition of, 117–118
  deinstitutionalization and, 235
  diversity and, 238
  geographic location and, 127
  government and, 238
  homes and, supports and, 237
  landlords and, 127–128
  meaningful life and, 237
  neighbors and, 127–128
  options for, 117, 118–119
    group homes, 122–126
    research on, 122–128
    supported living, 128–129

Community living—*continued*
  personal reports of, 116–117
  professionals and, change and, 237
  relationships and, 236
  research agendas for, 115–116
    future needs and, 135–137
  resident characteristics and, 120–121
  service systems and
    changing, 237–238
    limitations of, 235–236
  setting of, variables related to, 126–127
  shift from institution to, 118–119
  social behavior and, 127, 135–136
  supports versus facilities and, 236
Community living arrangements (CLAs), 119
Community living skills, teaching of, 79
Community Options program, 126
Community participation, personal futures and,
    537–541
Community resources, family adaptation and,
    288–291, 299–303
Community school, 379–385
  administration of, 383
  demise of specialization and, 379–381
  educational groupings in, 384
  funding of, 383
  monitoring in, 384
  nonteaching support services in, 383
  responsibility in, 384
  sense of community and, 381–382
  teacher training and, 383
Community surveys, supported employment and,
    148
Compensatory approach, in motor skills training, 79
Competence
  adaptive behavior and, 34–35
  context and, 104–105
  demonstration of, through choice/decision
    making, 175–177
  employee, extension of, 159–160
Competency-based personnel preparation, 331
"Competency/deviancy hypothesis," 210
Complete schools, 505–506
Component Model of Functional Competence, 72
Comprehensive integration, 355
Computer-assisted instruction (CAI), 263
Computer-managed instruction (CMI), 321, 323
Conservatism, science and, 3–4
Consultant teachers, 260
Consultation
  in related services provision, 357–359
  research on, 358–359
  strategies for, 357–358
  types of, 357
Consumer accountability, 491–492
Context(s)
  of assessment, 104–105
  natural, service provision in, 355–356
  of social relationships, 198–201

Continuing education, integrated related services
    and, 369
Continuum of services, 239
  problems with, metaphorical analysis of,
    229–234
  redefinition of, TASH resolution on, 241–242
Control
  aversive, *see* Aversive control
  communication and, choices and, 543–544
  locus of, coping and, 284
Conversation skills, direct instruction in, social rela-
    tionships and, 203
Cooperative activity, leisure education and, 178
Cooperative learning, 254–256
Coping
  appraisals and, in family, 283–286, 297–299
  cognitive, 283–285
Coping skills, 285–286
Cost(s)
  community living and, 121–122
  see also Financial stress; Funding
Cost-benefit analyses, wages and, supported em-
    ployment and, 149, 152–153, 162–163
Co-workers
  integrated work environment and, enclave option
    versus, 224–225
  supported employment and, 153–157
    ongoing support and, 160
Crawford v. Pittman, 464, 465
Credibility, in research, 644–645
Criterion of Ultimate Functioning, 196
Cultural sensitivity, TASH resolution on, 21
Culture
  values and
    early intervention and, 430–431
    science and, 7–8
  values-based research on, 11
Curriculum
  adaptations of
    for regular education environments, 256–258
    research recommendations for, 263
  Adaptive Learning Environments Model (ALEM),
    258, 263, 415
  content of, best practices and, 317–319,
    333–334, 337
  functional approach to, 318
  leisure skills, recommendations for, 183–185
  multilevel selection of, 256–257
  values-based research on, 10
Curriculum councils, community school and, 384
Curriculum development model, for resident advisor
    training, 126
Curriculum models, 73
Curriculum overlapping, 257

Daily hassles, family stress and, 281–282
Daily life, therapeutic interventions in, 355–356
Data-based decisions, 321, 322–323

Data-based instruction, 320–321
Day care, 293
Daytime options, 220–221
DD Act, *see* Developmental Disabilities and Bill of Rights Act
Death, life and, *see* Life and death issues
Decision making
    competence demonstration through, leisure education and, 175–177
    family participation in, early intervention and, 446
    about medical treatment, 553–554, 557–558
    supported employment and, 159
Decision models, in behavior management, 46–47
Decisions, data-based, 321, 322–323
Deficiency approach
    assessment and, 101–102
    shift from, 645–646
Dehumanization, federal disability policy and, 496
Deinstitutionalization, 107, 235
    cost of, 121–122
    court-ordered, 118
    skill changes resulting from, 119–120
    TASH policy on, 109
        leisure services delivery and, 171
Delay procedure, social responsiveness and, 200–201
Democracy, concept of, 8
Demographic trends, 271–273
Department of Education, State of Hawaii v. Katherine D., 251
Depression, in family caregivers, 277
Development
    common beliefs about, 105
    reconsideration of, 105–106
    theories of, early intervention and, 431, 442–443
Developmental Disabilities and Bill of Rights Act (DD Act), 410
Developmentally Disabled Assistance and Bill of Rights Act (PL 98-257), 508
Diagnosis, testing and, 25–40
    see also Testing
Diagnostic and Statistical Manual of Mental Disorders-III-Revised (DSM III-R), mental retardation classification of, 29
Diagnostic-prescriptive-remedial paradigm
    in individualized assessment and planning process, 529
    shift from, 645–646
    in special education, 392–393
Direct therapy, in related services provision, 356
Disability(ies)
    federal policy toward
        evolution of, 496
        see also Federal programs
    ideology about, 197
        shifting, 528–529
Disability Advisory Council, 507
Disease model, assessment and, 102

Disruptive behavior, aggressive behavior and, *see* Aggression-disruption
Diversity, 238
Divorce, 287
Doctoral training, 397
Down syndrome
    abortion and, 554–555
    early intervention and, age at start of, 446
Dressing skills, teaching of, 78
"Dual diagnosis," 36–38
Dynamic assessment, severe disabilities and, 59–62

Early intervention, 429–454
    axioms underlying, 432–450
        effectiveness, 433–442
        increased effectiveness with earlier age, 442–445
        increased effectiveness with family involvement, 445–450
        right to services, 432–433
    conventional wisdom and, 431–432
    cultural/political knowledge and values and, 430–431
    effectiveness of
        age at start and, 442–444
        empirical evidence of, 433–436
        family involvement and, 445–450
        research on, 436–442
    empirical base for, 429–432
    empirical knowledge and, 431
    federal programs of, effectiveness of, 498–501
    historical perspectives on, 429
    integration and, 417–418
    programmatic isolation in, reduction of, 501
    quality of, 479–483
        indicators of, 480–481
        institutionalization of, 481–483
        variance in, 479–480
    research recommendations for, 450–453
    see also Preschool integration
Eating skills
    teaching of, 77–78
    see also Oral-motor control
Ecobehavioral assessment
    social, 51
    vocational, 49
Economic stress, *see* Financial stress
Educability, 67
    research on, values and, 5
    Timothy W. v. Rochester, New Hampshire, School District and, 68
Education, 67–83
    appropriate, severe disabilities and, 69–74
    best-practices focus in, *see* Best practices
    community school and, *see* Community school
    continuing, integrated related services and, 369
    definition of, 70
    financing of, 388–389

Education—*continued*
  flexibility in, integrated related services and, 369
  inclusive, 399–407
    parameters of, 246–250
    see also Integration
  individualized program of, *see* Individualized
      education program (IEP)
  leisure, *see* Leisure education
  personnel preparation for, 313–341
    see also Professional(s), preparation of
  in regular education environments, 245–265
    see also Regular education environments
  relationships and, 399–407
  research on
    future needs in, 72–74, 80–83
    instructional formats in, 80–81
  social systems and, social policy and, 387–389
  state-of-the-art requirements in, 418–419
  strategies for, 74–83
    demonstrations of awareness and change,
        74–75
    teaching functional skills, 75–80
  supported, 383
    TASH resolution on, 244
  tracking in, 415
  values-based versus test-based, 379–380
Education Amendments of 1986 (PL 99-457),
    501–502
  early intervention and, 417–418
    Part H program and, 499–500
    right to services and, 432–433
  financing and, 502–503
  preschool integration and, 474
Education for All Handicapped Children Act of 1975
    (PL 94-142), 145, 460–464
  accomplishments of, 501–502
  educational benefit test and, 461–464
  extended year special education programming
      and, 459, 464–465
  extensions of, 423
  false assumptions and, 387
  integration and, 410
  least restrictive mandate of, 323–324
  problems impairing effectiveness of, 502–505
    financing inadequacy, 502–503
    school goals versus postschool demands,
        503–504
    unnecessary segregation within programs,
        504–505
  procedural requirements of, 460–461
  right to services and, 432
  state-of-the-art requirement in, 418
  substantive requirements of, 461
  teacher preparation and, 314
Education of the Handicapped Act (EHA), 111, 501
  amendments to, *see* Education Amendments of
      1986 (PL 99-457)
  Part B of, 497
  TASH resolution supporting, 425–426
Educational assistants, 260–261

Educational benefit test, PL 94-142 and, 461–464
Educational classifications, 29
Educational groupings, community school and, 384
Educational opportunity, right to, 432–433
Educational practice, myths about, 387–388
Educational reform, 314–316
Educational services
  and caregiver stress reduction, 293–294
  PL 94-142 extensions and, 423
Educational specialists, 260
Educational specialization, demise of, 379–381
Educational validity, 644–646
Educative approach to behavior problems, 80
Egalitarianism, concept of, 8
Electro-shock device, SIBIS, TASH resolution on,
    551–552
Eligibility, extended school year and, 467–468
Emotional disorders, mental retardation and, 20,
    36–38
Emotional support, intrafamily, 286–288
Emotions, research on, appropriate education and,
    73
Employee competence, extension of, 159–160
Employer incentives, 518
Employment, 491
  integration in, 219–227
    productivity and, 416–417
    see also Integrated work
  supported, *see* Supported employment
  unlawful practices of, legislation for prevention
      of, 518
  see also Job *entries*; Vocational *entries*; Work
      entries
Employment-related services, ongoing support and,
    supported employment and, 158–159
Empowerment, choices and, 625–626
Enclave model of supported employment, 50, 147
  definition of, 220
  integrated work environment versus, 221–226
Environment
  least restrictive, *see* Least restrictive environment
      (LRE)
  social relationships and, 198–201
Environmental assessment
  of leisure skills, 183
  of social behavior, 51
Espino v. Besteiro, 251
Ethnographic research, and social context, 199
Evaluation, *see* Assessment
Exceptional Children, 67
Excess behaviors
  reduction in, 79–80
  see also Problem behaviors
Experience(s)
  sequencing of, in communication skills
      instruction, 76
  values and, science and, 7–8
Expressive support, intrafamily, 286–288
Extended school year
  educational planning and, 467–470

eligibility and, 467–468
guide for, 470
program quality and, 469–470
service delivery and, 468–469
legal analysis of, 459–465
PL 94-142 and, 460–465
TASH resolution on, 427
Extracurricular activities, *see* After-school programs

Facilities, supports versus, 236
Family(ies), 271–305
caregiver stress in, 274–278
children and, community and, 129–135, 236–237
demographic trends and, 271–273
early intervention and, 445–450
family as interveners and, 446–449
planning and decision making and, 446
educational involvement of, 319, 320, 322
needs of, 279–280
policy trends and, 273–274
resources within, 286–288, 299
respite services for, 134–135, 292–293
special needs of, research needs involving, 82
see also Parent *entries*
Family adaptation theory, 280–291
community resources in, 288–291
strengthening of, 299–303
coping in, 283–286, 291
interventions centering on, 297–299
implications of, for family support interventions, 291–303
intrafamily resources in, 286–288
strengthening of, 299
stressors in, 281–283, 291
reduction of, 292–297
Family assessment, family empowerment and, 485–487
Family-implemented intervention, 446–449
child treatment gains and, maintenance and generalization of, 448–449
effectiveness of, 447–448
social interaction, 448
Family Support Services, Calvert County, Maryland, 132
Family supports
early intervention and, 449–450
family adaptation theory and, 280–291
see also Family adaptation theory
federal, 132
historical foundations of, 278–279
intrafamily, 286–288
strengthening of, 299
research recommendations for, 303–305
state, 130–132
stress and coping implications for, 291–303
interventions centering on appraisal and coping skills, 297–299
intrafamily support, 299
social ties outside family, 299–303

stress reduction, 292–297
Family systems theory, early intervention and, 445
Federal budget, Gramm Rudman resolution and, 111–112
Federal disability policy, evolution of, 496
Federal government
family support from, 132
integration and, 410
Federal programs, 495–519
for adults, 509–518
absence of community-based Medicaid services and, 509–511
access to health care and, 511–513
barriers in housing and transportation and, 513–514
income maintenance and rehabilitation programs in, 514–518
legislation for improvement of, 510–511, 513, 518
American social policy and, 495–498
effectiveness of, 498
for infants and toddlers, 498–501
legislation for improvement of, 500–501
overview of, 499
Part H program, 499–500
research activities and, 498–499
resources for, 521–525
for school-age children, 501–506
legislation for improvement of, 505–506
PL 94-142 program, 501–505
problems with, 502–505
transition, 506–508
legislation supporting, 508
outcomes of, 507
reasons for ineffectiveness of, 507–508
Feelings, *see* Emotional *entries*; Emotions
Fetal alcohol syndrome, 35
Fetus, abortion of, 554–555
Financial stress
family and, 281–282
fiscal assistance and, 295–297
Social Security Resolution and, 493
Financing, *see* Funding
Fine motor development
intervention strategies for, 363–365
see also Motor skills
Follow-up services, in supported employment, 148
Foster care, 133
Friendships
formation of, 206–209
supported employment and, 155
see also Relationships
Full inclusion, 245
research recommendations for, 261–262
Functional assessment, 45–63
academic, 59
behavioral, 46–48
characteristics of, 45
of communication skills, 58–59, 370
for community integration, 57–58

Functional assessment—*continued*
  dynamic, of persons with severe disabilities,
    59–62
  of home skills, 53–54, 55
  of leisure skills, 182
  motor, 58–59, 370–371
  parent-professional partnership for, 53–54
  related services and, 370–371
  for school integration, 56–57
  social, 50–53
  vocational, 48–50
  see also Assessment
Functional curricular approach, 318
Functional integration, 354
  adaptive devices and, 365
  language intervention and, 367–368
  oral-motor procedures and, 362–363
  social integration versus, 195–196
Functional skills
  assessment orientation toward, 104
    see also Functional assessment
  task analyses of, social skills within, 205–206
  teaching of, 75–80
    communication skills, 75–77
    community living skills, 79
    excess behavior reduction, 79–80
    motor skills, 78–79
    self-help skills, 77–78
Functionally equivalent behavior
  aggression-disruption and, 565–566, 567–568
  repetitive behavior and, 586–587, 588
  self-injury and, 580, 581–582
Funding
  distribution of, 646–647
  educational, 388–389
    community school, 383
  federal, of Part H program, 500
  personnel preparation, 506
  PL 94-142 program, inadequacy of, 502–503
  see also Cost(s)

Generalization
  early intervention and, family-implemented,
    448–449
  instructional effectiveness and, 322, 323
  language intervention and, 367
Generalization assessment, 61
*Georgia Association for Retarded Citizens v.
  McDaniel*, 464–465
Government
  community living and, 238
  see also Federal *entries*; State(s); *specific laws or
    programs*
Gramm Rudman resolution, 111–112
  leisure services delivery and, 172
Gross motor development
  intervention strategies for, 363–365
  see also Motor skills

Group(s)
  cooperative learning, 254–256
  educational, community school and, 384
  mutual assistance, 300–302
  social relationships and, 199
  supported employment placement in, *see* Enclave
    model of supported employment
Group homes, 122–126
  adaptive behavior and, 123, 124
  size of, impact of, 125–126
  social interaction in, 123, 125
  staff role in, 126

Halderman v. Pennhurst State School and Hospital,
  118
  changes resulting from, 119
Hall v. Vance City Board of Education, 462
Handicapped Children's Early Education Program,
  499, 521
Health care
  access to, 511–513
  see also Medical treatment
Health insurance
  private, access to, 512
  see also Medicaid *entries*; Medicare
Hilden v. Evans, 464
Home, supports and, 237
Home and Community Based Waivers program, 510
Home caregiving
  stress and, 274–278
  see also Family *entries*
Home school, 413–414
Home skills
  assessment of, 53–54, 55
  see also Self-care skills
*Homeward Bound, Inc. et al. v. Hissom Memorial
  Center et al.*, 279
Horizontal work enhancement, 223
House Subcommittee on Select Education, 497
Housing
  barriers in, 513–514
  see also Residential *entries*
Human resources, regular education environments
  and, 258–261
Hydration, nutrition and, 556–557
  TASH resolution on, 548
Hymes v. Harnett County Board of Education, 251

ICF/MR, *see* Intermediate Care Facility/Mental
  Retardation
ICS, *see* Individualized Curriculum Sequencing
IEP, *see* Individualized education program
Immigration, TASH resolution on, 23
IMPACT Curriculum, 62
Incidental teaching, 200–201
Inclusive education, parameters of, 246–250
Income maintenance programs, ineffectiveness of,
  514–518

Independent living, 506
Independent performance, supported employment and, 159
Individual, interventions with, positivist-behavioral research paradigm and, 634–636
Individual goals, American social policy and, 497
Individual placement, in supported employment, 50, 147
Individual Program Design Procedures Manual, 249
Individualized Curriculum Sequencing (ICS), 59
in early intervention, 439
Individualized education program (IEP), 69, 249
content of, 318
integrated programming team and, 361
objectives of, reevaluation of, 263–264
parental involvement in, 53–54
process of, appropriate education and, 73
Individualized service programs (ISPs), 506
Infants
anencephalic, 555–556
care of
medical responsibility and, 601–606
TASH resolution on, 547
developmental interventions and, 443
with disabilities, medical treatment of, 556
see also Early intervention
In-home respite services, 134–135
Initiation skills, social relationships and, 201–203
with peers, 203–205
Institutional issues, values-based research on, 10–11
Institutional settings
alternatives to, *see* Community *entries*; Deinstitutionalization
capital investment in, 110
shift to community living options from, 118–119
Institutionalization
in community, 117
community living versus, costs of, 121–122
see also Deinstitutionalization
Instruction
adaptive, 257–258
behavior management and, integration of, 609
community-based, 57, 250
computer-assisted, 263
computer-managed, 321, 323
data-based, 320–321
formats for, research needs involving, 80–81
functional skills, 75–80
integration and, 209–212
leisure skills, recommendations for, 183–185
modifications in
for regular education environments, 254–256
research recommendations for, 263
reinforcement-based, early intervention and, 439
values-based research on, 10
see also Education
Instructional design, social relationships and, 199
Instructional effectiveness, 320–323
Instructional methodology, social responsiveness and, 200–201

Instrumental support, intrafamily, 286
Insurance, health
private, 512
see also Medicaid *entries*; Medicare
Integrated programming teams, development of, 360–361
Integrated related services, 353–373
implications of
for philosophy, 370
for policy, 369–370
for practice, 370–371
for research, 371–373
intervention strategies for, 361–368
assistive and adaptive devices and, 365–366
effects of, 368
language and, 366–368
sensorimotor development and postural control and, 361–365
models of, 356–359
selection of, 359
multiple dimensions of integration and, 353–355
natural contexts and, 355–356
teamwork and, 359–361
Integrated therapy, *see* Integrated related services
Integrated work, 219–227
daytime options and, 220–221
enclave compared with, 221–226
personalized match with environment in, 225–226
social opportunities in, 224–225
supervision in, 221–222
transportation in, 222–223
work enhancement opportunities in, 223–224
see also Employment, integration in
Integration, 409–419
adult, 491
assessment for, 56–58
community, 409–412
domains important to, 122
into community, *see* Community *entries*
comprehensive, 355
construct of, centrality of social networks to, 196–198
current status of, 409–412
in education, 399–407, *see also* Regular education environments
full inclusion versus, 245
functional, 354
adaptive devices and, 365
language intervention and, 367–368
oral-motor procedures and, 362–363
social integration versus, 195–196
multiple dimensions of, 353–355
peer, 354
practice, 354–355
adaptive devices and, 365–366
combined interventions and, 368
preschool, 473–476
second revolution and, 412–419
early intervention and, 417–418

Integration—*continued*
    employment and, 416–417
    home school and, 413–414
    regular class and, 414–416
    state-of-the-art requirements and, 418–419
    shift toward, 529
    social, *see* Social integration
    supported employment and, 146, 153–157
        non-task-related interactions and, 155–157
        research suggestions for, 163–164
        task-related interactions and, 153–155
    see also Mainstreaming
Integrative reviews, of early interventions, 440–441
Integrity, in research, 644–645
Intelligence
    nature of, 32–34
    tests of, *see* IQ tests
Interagency coordination
    inadequacy of, PL 94-142 program and, 502–503
    supported employment and, 148
Interdependence, positive, 254–255
Interdisciplinary teams, 359
Intermediate Care Facility/Mental Retardation (ICF/
    MR) program, 509–510
Internal locus of control, coping and, 284
International Council for the Education of Excep-
    tional Children, 331
Interpersonal relationships, *see* Relationships
Intervention(s)
    early, *see* Early intervention
    intrusive, cessation of, TASH resolution on, 550,
        559
    strategies for, values-based research on, 11
    see also specific type
IQ tests
    mental retardation and, 26–27, 30
        AAMD classification of, 28
        APA classification of, 29
        educational classifications of, 29
    professional issues in, 38–39
    recommendations for, 40
    specific problems of, for people with severe
        disabilities, 30–32
    see also Intelligence
Irving Independent School District v. Tatro, 251
Isolated therapy model, integrated therapy versus,
    356
Isolation
    family, perceived support and, 288–289
    programmatic, in early years, 501
ISPs, *see* Individualized service programs

Job analyses, in supported employment, 148
Job match and placement, in supported
    employment, 148
Job separation, 160–161
Job-status change, supported employment and,
    160–161

Job training
    in supported employment, 148
    unavailability of, 515
Job Training and Partnership Act (JTPA), 515

Kaufman Assessment Battery for Children (K-ABC)
    mental retardation and, 31
    nature of intelligence and, 33
Knowledge, values and, science and, 7–8
Kruelle v. New Castle County School District, 460,
    463

Labeling, *see* Classification
Language intervention
    consultation and, 357
    early, 438–439
    natural contexts and, 355–356
    naturalistic, 367
        research on, 367–368
    strategies for, 366–368
    see also Communication skills; Related services
L'Arche program, 129
Law(s)
    appropriate education and, 73
    federal, integration and, 410
    to improve federal programs
        for adults, 510–511, 513, 518
        for infants and toddlers, 499–500
        for school-age children and youth, 505–506
        for transition, 508
    recommendations for, American social policy
        and, 497–498
    teacher preparation and, 314–315
    see also specific law
Learning
    cognitive theories of, 34
    common beliefs about, assessment and, 105
    cooperative, 254–256
    process of, 104
    response-contingent, early intervention and, 439
Least restrictive environment (LRE), 8
    flaws in, 413
    inclusive education and, 246
    PL 94-142 and, 323–324
Lee v. Clark, 464
Legal status, federal disability policy and, 496
Legislation, *see* Law(s); *specific legislation or sub-
    ject of legislation*
Leisure activities, community integration and, 173
Leisure assessments, development of, suggested
    protocols for, 182–183
Leisure education
    goals of, 175–181
        awareness of age-appropriate community-based
            behaviors, 177–178
        demonstration of competence, 175–177
        demonstration of social interaction skills,
            178–179

learning of skills, 180–181
  understanding of resource availability, 180
rationale for, 174–175
Leisure resources, availability of, education about,
  180
Leisure services, 171–186
  community-based, inadequacy of, 173–174
  current status of, 172–174
  development of, suggested protocols for, 183–185
  research recommendations for, 185–186
  TASH resolutions and, 171–172
    research supporting, 174–181, 185–186
Life and death issues, 545–546
  medical responsibility, 601–606
  medical treatment, 553–558
  see also Quality-of-life issues; specific issues
Life events, major, as stressors, 281
Lifestyle measures, development of, 608
Lifestyles, leisure, severe disabilities and, 172–173
Linguistic behaviors, social skills training and,
  52–53
Local management, adult community services and,
  533–534
Local schooling, 247–248, 413–414
Locus of control, coping and, 284
Loma Linda University Anencephaly Transplant
  Unit, 549
Longitudinal planning, meaningful outcomes and,
  education and, 249–250
LRE, see Least restrictive environment

Mainstreaming, see Integration
  social skills and, supporting research for,
    326–328
  see also Integration
Maintenance, generalization and, see Generalization
Maintenance assessment, 61
Major life events, as stressors, 281
Maladaptation, pathogenesis and, salutogenesis/
  bonadaptation versus, 274–275
Management, local, adult community services and,
  533–534
Management needs, instruction-related, 251–252
Marital distress, 287
Marital therapy, 299
Mastery, coping and, 283
McGill Action Planning System—MAPS, 249
Mealtime skills, teaching of, 77–78
Medicaid Home and Community Quality Services
  Act, 132, 510
Medicaid services, 511
  community-based, absence of, 509–511
Medicaid Waiver, 121
Medical management, instruction and, 251–252
Medical responsibility, 601–606
Medical treatment, 553–558
  abortion and, 554–555
  anencephaly and, 555–556

decision-making framework for, 553–554,
  557–558
for infants with disabilities, 556
nutrition and hydration in, 556–557
see also Health care
Medically fragile individuals, services for, 82
Medicare, 511
  access to appropriate health care under, 512
Mental illness, mental retardation and, 20, 36–38
Mental retardation
  classification of
    AAMD, 26, 27, 28
    APA, 28–29
    educational, 29
    validity of, 29
  IQ tests and, problems with, 30–32
  mental illness and, 20, 36–38
  neurological damage and, 35–36
  psychological testing and, 26–27
  see also Intelligence
Meta-analysis
  definition of, 440
  of early interventions, 441–442
Michigan Family Subsidy Act, 131
Michigan Specialized Adoption Program, 134
Microswitches, 81–82
  integration strategies and, 365–366
Milieu teaching, 200
Mills v. Board of Education of the District of
  Columbia, 460
Mobile work crews, 147, 220
  integrated work environment versus, 221–226
Monitoring
  in community schools, 384
  in related services provision, 356–357
Moore v. Roberts, 464
Motivation, research needs involving, 81
Motivation Assessment Scale, 48
Motor skills
  assessment of, 58–59, 370–371
  early intervention and, 437
  significant progress and, 72
  teaching of, 78–79
  see also Sensorimotor development
Movement, utilization of, in communication skills
  instruction, 76
Multidisciplinary teams, 359
Multilevel curriculum selection, 256–257
Multiple behaviors, simultaneous measurement of,
  608–609
Mutual assistance groups, 300–302

National Association for the Dually Diagnosed, 38
National Conference on the Transition of Profoundly/
  Multiply Handicapped Deaf-Blind Youth,
    recreation and leisure working group of, 185
National Council on Disabilities (NCD), 498
National Resource Center for Special Needs
  Adoption, 133, 134

Natural contexts, service provision in, 355–356
Natural match strategy, work environment and, 225
Natural proportion criterion, work environment and, 220–221
Natural supervision, 221
Naturalistic inquiry, 371
Naturalistic language intervention, 367
  research on, 367–368
NCD, see National Council on Disabilities
Negotiation, process of, 320, 322
Neighbors, community living and, 127–128
Neuromotor procedures, 361–362
Neuropsychological concepts of severe disability, 35–36
Nonaversive interventions, 559–596
  in aggression-disruption, 565–580
    by altering setting events, 566, 569–575
    by response covariation, 575–579
    by systems change, 579–580
    by teaching functionally equivalent behavior, 565–566, 567–568
  in repetitive behavior, 586–592
    by altering setting events, 587, 589–592
    by response covariation, 592, 593
    by teaching functionally equivalent behavior, 586–587, 588
  research recommendations for, 592, 594–596
  review of, 564–592, 593
  in self-injury, 580–586
    by altering setting events, 580, 583–586
    by response covariation, 586
    by systems change, 586
    by teaching functionally equivalent behavior, 580, 581–582
  social validation and, 560–564
  see also Aversive control
North Carolina, adoption project in, 134
Nutrition, hydration and, 556–557
  TASH resolution on, 548

Occupational therapy, see Related services
Office of Special Education and Rehabilitative Services, 497–498
Ongoing support, supported employment and, 157–162
  research suggestions for, 164–165
Options in Community Living, 129
Oral-motor control
  intervention strategies for, 362–363
  see also Eating skills
Ordinariness, invisibility and, best practices and, 325, 328–329
Organ transplant, 549
Otis R. Bowen, Secretary of Health and Human Services, Petitioner v. American Hospital Association, et al., 556
Outcome measures
  in community living research, 122, 136
  redefinition of, applied behavior analysis and, 607–609

science and, values and, 8
Out-of-home placement, for children, 130

Paradigm(s)
  definition of, 392
  diagnostic-prescriptive-remedial, 392–393, 529
    shift from, 645–646
  positivist-behavioral, 634–637
  quantitative versus qualitative perspective and, 637–639
  shifts in
    adult community services and, 527–528
    personnel preparation and, 393–395
    support, 528–530
    unconscious assumptions and, 632–639
Paraprofessionals, and regular education environment, 260–261
Parent(s)
  community school and, 384
  evaluation and, 98–100
  participation of, Part H program and, 500–501
  professionals and
    assessment and, 53–54
    relationships of, 289–291, 302–303
  single, 287
  see also Family *entries*
Parent-to-parent network, 301
Parent training
  early intervention and, 447–448
  and stress reduction, 294–295
Part H infant and toddler program, 499–500
  expanded federal financing of, 500
Participation skills, leisure education and, 180–181
PASS, see Program Assessment of Service Systems
Pathogenesis, maladaptation and, salutogenesis/bonadaptation versus, 274–275
PCMR, see President's Committee on Mental Retardation
Peer confederates, 204
Peer initiation interventions, 203–205
Peer integration, 354
Peer interactions, 639–640
  initiation skills and, 203–205
  research needs involving, 82
  supported, 206–209
  see also Social interaction
Peer nomination measures, in social network assessment, 211–212
Peer response patterns, a priori assessment of, 210–211
Peer training, in early intervention, 438
Peer tutoring, 204, 324
Peers, as resource, in regular education environments, 261
Pennsylvania Association for Retarded Citizens v. Commonwealth of Pennsylvania, 413, 460
Personalized matching, to work environment, 225–226
Personnel, see Professional(s); *specific type*

Philosophical issues
  and integrated related services, 370
  and social policy decisions, 2–4
Phobias, 37–38
Physical Environment Scale, 125
Physical therapy
  in natural contexts, 355
  see also Related services
Physicians, responsibility of, 601–606
PL 93-112, see Rehabilitation Act of 1973
PL 94-142, see Education for All Handicapped Children Act of 1975
PL 98-257, see Developmentally Disabled Assistance and Bill of Rights Act
PL 99-457, see Education Amendments of 1986
PL 99-506, see Rehabilitation Act Amendments of 1986
Planning guide, for extended school year services, 470
Planning process, family participation in, early intervention and, 446
Play, see Leisure entries
Policymakers
  recommendations for, 645–647
  researchers and, communication between, 645
  see also Social policy
Politics
  early intervention and, 430–431
  science and, 3
Polk v. Central Susquehanna Intermediate Unit 15, 462, 463–464
Portage Project, 447
Positive interdependence, 254–255
Positivist-behavioral research paradigm, 634–637
Postural control
  intervention strategies for, 361–365
  see also Motor skills
Power, imbalance of, between service providers and service recipients, 647
Power relationships, aversive control and, 617–623
Practice, research and, relationship between, 631–632
Practice integration, 354–355
  adaptive devices and, 365–366
  combined interventions and, 368
Practitioners
  recommendations for, 645–647
  researchers and, collaboration between, 645
  see also Professional(s)
Pregnancy, abortion of, 554–555
Preschool Grant Program, 474
Preschool integration, 473–476
  see also Early intervention
Preservice
  integrated related services and, 369
  personnel preparation and, 333–337
    best-practices teaching content and, 333–334
    best-practices teaching outcomes and, 336–337
    best-practices teaching processes and, 334–336
President's Committee on Mental Retardation (PCMR), 527

Prevention-intervention approach, in motor skills training, 79
Problem behaviors
  functional assessment of, 46–48
  nonaversive interventions for, 559–596
    see also Nonaversive interventions
  reduction in, 79–80
Problem-solving skills, coping and, stress and, 285
Production assessment, 61
Productivity, employment and, integration and, 416–417
Professional(s)
  attitudes of, 325
  change and, 237
  collaboration of, 354–355
    see also Integrated related services
  education and, 264
  parents and
    assessment and, 53–54
    relationships of, 289–291, 302–303
  preparation of, 313–341, 391–397
    best practices and, 316–331
    community school and, 383
    framework for reform in, 314–316
    funds for, 506
    model for, 333–340
    status of, 331–333
  in related services, see Related services personnel
  role of, in residential environments, 126
  service recipients and, balance of power between, 647
  staffing changes and, adult service programs and, 492
  see also Practitioners; specific type
Professional knowledge, collaborative, support of, 370
Professionalization, personnel preparation and, traditions of, 331–332
Profound disabilities, see Severe disability(ies)
Program Assessment of Service Systems (PASS), 123
Program evaluations, early intervention and, 439–440
Program paradigm, 531
Program quality, extended school year and, 469–470
Programmatic isolation, in early years, reduction of, 501
Progress, significant, definition of, 71–72
Project IMPACT, 134
Project SPAN, multilevel curriculum selection and, 257
Project S.T.A.R, 134
Psychiatric disorders, mental retardation and, 20, 36–38
Psychological testing
  family caregivers and, 277
  mental retardation and, 26–27
Psychometric model of assessment, 102
Psychosocial distress, in family, 282–283
Public, role of, shifting emphasis in, 529

Public Laws, *see* PL *entries*
Public policy, *see* Social policy
Public resources, allocation of, adult community
    services and, 531–532
Public settings, "blending" in, assessment of, 57–58

QRS, *see* Questionnaire on Resources and Stress
Qualitative assessment measures, 105
Qualitative-quantitative paradigm war, 637–639
Quality assurance, early intervention and, 479–483
Quality-of-life issues
    abortion and, 554–555
    appropriate education and, 74
    integration and, supported employment and, 163
    meaningful life, 237
    social relationships and, 197
    see also Medical responsibility; Medical treatment
Quantitative-qualitative paradigm war, 637–639
Questionnaire on Resources and Stress (QRS),
    respite care and, 292

Reciprocity, social support networks and, 52
Recreation and leisure, *see* Leisure *entries*
Reframing, cognitive, in family interventions,
    297–299
Regular education environments, 245–265, 414–416
    administrators in, 261
    curricular adaptations for, 256–258
    curricular practices in, 252–258
    human resources in, 258–261
    inclusive education parameters and, 246–250
    instruction in, management needs related to,
        251–252
    instructional modifications for, 254–256
    instructional practices in, 252–258
    need for, balance with special needs of, 262–263
    paraprofessionals in, 260–261
    peers in, 261
    related services personnel in, 260
    research recommendations for, 261–264
    structured social contact in, 253–254
    teachers in, 259–260
Regular Lives, 260
Rehabilitation Act Amendments of 1986 (PL
    99-506), 146, 149, 165
Rehabilitation Act of 1973 (PL 93-112), 145
    integration and, 410
    Section 504 of, TASH resolution supporting,
        425–426
Rehabilitation programs, ineffectiveness of,
    514–518
Reinforcement-based instruction, early intervention
    and, 439
Related services
    community school and, 383
    definition of, 501
    integrated, 353–373
        see also Integrated related services
    provision of, models of, 356–359

Related services personnel
    philosophy of, 370
    in regular education environments, 260
Relationships, 195–213, 236
    in community living, 135–136
        in group homes, 123, 125
    education and, 399–407
    functional versus social integration and, 195–196
    instruction and, integration outcomes and,
        209–212
    opportunities for, in integrated work environment
        versus enclave option, 224–225
    parent-professional, 289–291, 302–303
    power, aversive control and, 617–623
    between service providers and service recipients,
        647
    social networks and, 196–197
    supported, 206–209
    technologies for building of, 198–209
        contextual enhancement, 198–201
        direct social skills instruction, 201–206
        supported relationships, 206–209
    values-based research on, 9–10
    see also Peer interactions; Social interaction
Religion, in family support, 300
Repetitive behavior, nonaversive intervention in,
    586–592
    by altering setting events, 587, 589–592
    by response covariation, 592, 593
    by teaching functionally equivalent behavior,
        586–587, 588
Research
    best-practices, 316–331
        see also Best practices
    community living, 115–137
        future needs in, 135–137
        see also Community *entries*
    consultation, 358–359
    credibility in, 644–645
    early intervention, 436–442
        federal programs and, 498–499
        recommendations for, 450–453
    educational, future needs in, 72–74, 80–83,
        261–264
    ethnographic, and social context, 199
    family support, 303–305
    integrity in, 644–645
    language intervention, 367–368
    leisure education, 176–180, 181
        recommendations for, 185–186
    methodologies in, 642–643
    nonaversive intervention, 564–592, 593
        recommendations for, 592, 594–596
    practice and, relationship between, 631–632
    recommendations for, 642–645
    related services intervention, 361–368
        needs for, 371–373
    special needs adoption, 133–134
    supported employment, 148–165
    supporting mainstreaming and social skills,
        326–328

values and, social policy and, 4–6
values-based, 8–11
see also Science
Research paradigm(s), *see* Paradigm(s)
Researchers
collaboration of, with practitioners, 645
communication of, with policymakers, 645
Residential, Inc., 129
Residential options
for community living, 117, 118–119
see also Community living
see also Housing
Residential programs
size of, impact of, 125–126
staff role in, 126
Residualism, tradition of, family supports and, 278–279
Resources
community, family adaptation and, 288–291, 299–303
distribution of, 646–647
federal, 521–525
human, regular education environments and, 258–261
intrafamily, family adaptation and, 286–288, 299
leisure, education about, 180
public, allocation of, 531–532
Respite services, 134–135, 292–293
Response-contingent learning, early intervention and, 439
Response covariation
aggression-disruption and, 575–579
repetitive behavior and, 592, 593
self-injury and, 586
Rettig v. Kent City, 252
Right to services
early intervention and, 432–433
see also Civil rights
Rocky Mountain Adoption Exchange, 134
Romeo vs. Youngberg, 22
Roncker v. Walter, 246, 413, 418
Rotational assessment procedure, vocational training and, 49
Rowley v. Board of Education, 461–462, 463

St. Louis County, Missouri, Special School District of, 411
Salutogenesis, bonadaptation and, pathogenesis/maladaptation versus, 274–275
Scales of Independent Behavior (SIB), 35
Scheduling, in team development, 360
School(s)
community, 379–385
see also Community school
complete, 505–506
effective, characteristics of, 415–416
home, 413–414
School administrators
and community school, 383
and regular education environments, 261

School-age children, federal programs for, 501–506
School integration, assessment for, 56–57
School objectives, postschool demands versus, 503–504
School year, extended, *see* Extended school year
Schooling
local, 247–248, 413–414
see also Education
Science
philosophical views of, 2–4
values and
action and, 11–12
integration of, 6–8
see also Research
Seating devices, adaptive, 365
Second revolution, integration and, 412–419
see also Integration, second revolution and
Secondary analyses, of early interventions, 440–442
Secondary coping, 285–286
Segregated settings
capital investment in, 113, 171–172
educational, consequences of, 414–415
Segregation
within education programs, PL 94-142 and, 504–505
federal disability policy and, 496
Self-care skills
functional assessment of, 53–54, 55
teaching of, 77–78
Self-evaluation, supported employment and, 159
Self-injurious behavior
nonaversive intervention in, 580–586
by altering setting events, 580, 583–586
by response covariation, 586
by systems change, 586
by teaching functionally equivalent behavior, 580, 581–582
remediation of, goal of, 640–642
Self-Injurious Behavior Inhibiting System (SIBIS), TASH resolution on, 551–552
Senate Subcommittee on the Handicapped, 497
Sensitivity, enhancement of, communication skills and, 76
Sensorimotor development
intervention strategies for, 361–365
see also Motor skills
Sensory procedures, 361–362
Service continuum, *see* Continuum of services
Service delivery
planning of, extended school year and, 468–469
quality of, variance in, 479–480
Service providers, *see* Professional(s); *specific type*
Service provision
array of choices in, integrated related services and, 369–370
in natural contexts, 355–356
Service systems
changing, 237–238
limitations of, 235–23
Setting events
aggression-disruption and, 566, 569–575

Setting events—*continued*
  repetitive behavior and, 587, 589–592
  self-injury and, 580, 583–586
Seven Counties Services, 129
SIB, *see* Scales of Independent Behavior
SIBIS, *see* Self-Injurious Behavior Inhibiting
      System
Siblings, 287–288
  see also Family *entries*
Significant progress, definition of, 71–72
Simulation, in teacher preparation, 334–336
Single parents, 287
Site representation teams, community school and,
      384
Skill(s)
  changes in, resulting from deinstitutionalization,
      119–120
  coping, 285–286
  functional, teaching of, 75–80
  meaningful, definition of, 70–71
  for supported living, 129
  see also specific type
Skill screening, options for, home skills and, 54, 55
Social behavior
  assessment of, 50–53
  community integration and, 127
Social climate, relationships and, 199–200
Social comparison
  coping and, family and, 284–285
  social validation and, 560
    problem behaviors and, 561, 562, 563
Social integration, 354
  functional integration versus, 195–196
  goal of, 639–640
  implementation of, values-based research on, 11
  instruction and, 209–212
  research on, values and, 4–5, 9–10
Social interaction
  in community living, 135–136
    in group homes, 123, 125
  demonstration of skills in, leisure education and,
      178–179
  early intervention and, family-implemented, 448
  functional integration and, 197
  structured, in regular education environments,
      253–254
  supported employment and, 153–157
  see also Peer interactions; Relationships
Social networks, 132
  assessment of, 211–212
  centrality of, to construct of integration, 196–198
Social policy, 1–12, 495–498
  adult community services and, 530–535
  appropriate education and, 73
  decisions about, role of science in, 6–8
  federal disability policy, evolution of, 496
  implementation of, 8
  integrated related services and, 369–370
  legislative recommendations encompassing,
      497–498

  new, articulation of, 496–497
  philosophical issues and, 2–4
  research and, 631–632
  social systems and, educational practice and,
      387–389
  teacher preparation and, 314–315
  trends in, families and, 273–274
  values and, 1, 4–11
    integration of science with, 6–8
    research based on, 8–11
  see also Policymakers
Social responsiveness, relationships and, 200–201
Social Security Act
  Title XIX of, 509–510
  Title XVIII of, 511
Social Security Administration, vocational rehabili-
      tation system and, ineffectiveness of,
      516–517
Social Security Resolution, 493
Social skills
  leisure education and, 178–179
  within task analyses of functional skills, 205–206
  use of, behavioral control and, 197
Social skills training, 52–53
  direct instruction in, social relationships and,
      201–206
  in early intervention, 437–438
  integration and, 209–212
  supporting research for, 326–328
Social status, federal disability policy and, 496
Social support
  for family
    early intervention and, 449–450
    strengthening of, 299–303
    see also Family supports
  intrafamily, 286–288
    strengthening of, 299
  parent-professional relationships and, 289–291
  perceived, isolation and, 288–289
Social support networks, 51–52
  best practices and, 325, 326–328
Social systems, social policy and, educational prac-
      tice and, 387–389
Social validation, 560–564
  in problem behavior identification, 561–562
  in problem behavior intervention, 562–563
  and treatment outcomes, 563–564
Social validity, 47, 53, 210
Sociometric status, assessment of, 211
Special education
  definition of, PL 94-142 and, 461
  diagnostic-prescriptive-remedial paradigm in,
      392–393, 645–646
  myth of, 403–404
  traditions of, 331–332
  see also Education
Special education programming, extended year, *see*
      Extended school year
"Special Friends" approach, 208
Special needs adoption/foster care, 133–134

Special School District (SSD), St. Louis County, Missouri, 411
Specialization, demise of, 379–381
Specialized Adoption Program, in Michigan, 134
Speech and language intervention, *see* Language intervention; Related services
Stacy G. v. Pasadena Independent School District, 252
Staff, *see* Professional(s); *specific type*
State(s)
  educational financing by, 388
  family support from, 130–132
State-of-the-art requirements, in education, 418–419
State Protection and Advocacy Agency, 500
"Straight from the Heart," 134
Stress, caregiver, in family, 274–278
Stress and coping theory, families and, 280–303
  see also Family adaptation theory
Stressors
  family, 281–283
    early intervention and, 449
    reduction of, 292–297
  see also specific stressors
Subjective evaluation, social validation and, 560
  problem behaviors and, 561, 562–564
Subsidies, state, for family, 131
Supervised Apartments in Region V, 129
Supervision, in integrated work environment, enclave option versus, 221–222
Support(s)
  facilities versus, 236
  for families, 271–305
    see also Family supports
  formal versus informal, 529–530
  homes and, 237
  perceived, isolation and, 288–289
Support coordinator, role of, 533–534
Support networks
  best practices and, 325, 326–328
  informal, 132–133
  social behavior and, 51–52
Support paradigm, 528–530
  policy and, 530–535
Support services, nonteaching, *see* Related services *entries*
Supported education, 383
  TASH resolution on, 244
  see also Education
Supported employment, 145–166, 416–417, 506–507
  enclave model of, 50, 147, 220
    integrated work environment versus, 221–226
  individual placement model of, 50, 147
  integration and, 153–157
    non-task-related interactions, 155–157
    research suggestions for, 163–164
    task-related interactions, 153–155
  mobile work crews in, 147
  ongoing support and, 157–162
    co-worker involvement, 160

employment-related services, 158–159
  extension of employee competence, 159–160
  job-status change, 160–161
  research suggestions for, 164–165
placement approaches in, 147
  integration and, 163
program components of, 147–148
research on, 148–162
  recommendations for, 162–165
  values and, 5–6
unavailability of, 515
wages and, benefit-cost analyses and, 149, 152, 162–163
Supported Independence, 129
Supported living, 128–129
Supported relationships, 206–209
Supportive systems, needed development of, 83
Switch mechanisms, *see* Microswitches
Syracuse Community-Referenced Curriculum Guide, 249
System consultation, 357
Systems, interventions with, positivist-behavioral research paradigm and, 634–636
Systems change
  aggression-disruption and, 579–580
  self-injury and, 586

TASH, *see* The Association for Persons with Severe Handicaps
Task analysis
  of functional skills, social skills within, 205–206
  integrated team programming and, 360–361
Task domains, dynamic assessment and, 61–62
Task-related interactions, supported employment and, 153–155
Taxes, employer incentives and, 518
Teacher(s), 313–314
  preparation of, *see* Teacher preparation
  in regular education environments, 259–260
  see also Professional(s)
Teacher aides, 260–261
Teacher preparation, 391–397
  best practices and, 316–331
    see also Best practices
  at certification level, 396–397
  community school and, 383
  diagnostic-prescriptive-remedial paradigm and, 392–393
  doctoral training in, 397
  paradigm shifts and, 393–395
    need for, 395–396
  recommendations for, 396–397
  reform framework for, 314–316
Teaching, *see* Instruction
Teaching-Family Model, 126
Team(s)
  effective, development of, 360–361
  site representation, community school and, 384
  types of, 359

Team Assisted Individualization, 258
Team collaboration
    education and, 319, 320
    integrated related services and, 359–361
    see also Collaboration
Team functioning, issues affecting, 359–360
Team teaching, 259–260
Technology
    applied behavior analysis and, 607–610
    education and, 81–82
Template matching procedure, social skills training
        and, 209–210
Test-based education, values-based education
        versus, 379–380
Testing, 25–40
    of adaptive behavior, 34–35
    classification and, 27–30
    "dual diagnosis" and, 36–38
    IQ, *see* IQ tests
    professional issues in, 38–39
    psychological, mental retardation and, 26–27
    recommendations for, 39–41
    see also Assessment
The Association for Persons with Severe Handicaps
        (TASH), 1
    on adult service reform, 491–492
    deinstitutionalization policy of, 109
        leisure services delivery and, 171
    policy statement of, for cessation of capital invest-
        ment in segregated settings, 113, 171–172
    population served by, 19
    Related Services Subcommittee of Critical Issues
        Committee of, position statement of, 243
    resolutions of
        on cessation of intrusive interventions, 550,
            559
        on choices, 494
        on cultural sensitivity, 21
        on extended school year, 427
        on Gramm Rudman budget reduction pro-
            posals, 111–112, 172
        on immigration, 23
        on infant care, 547
        and leisure services delivery, 171–172,
            174–181, 185–186
        on nutrition and hydration, 548
        opposing capital investment in institutional set-
            tings in State of New York, 110
        on people with mental retardation also diag-
            nosed as mentally ill, 20
        on redefinition of continuum of services,
            241–242
        on *Romeo vs. Youngberg*, 22
        on SIBIS, 551–552
        on Social Security, 493
        on supported education, 244
        in support of EHA and Section 504 of Rehabili-
            tation Act, 425–426
Therapeutic services, *see* Related services
Time to Learn, 473

*Timothy W. v. Rochester, New Hampshire, School
        District*, 68, 69
Toddler Research and Intervention Project, 473
Toileting skills, teaching of, 78
Tokarcik v. Forest Hills School District, 251
Tracking, 415
Training School Bulletin, 331
Transactional Intervention Program (TRIP), 448
Transdisciplinary teams, 359
Transition programs, federal, effectiveness of,
        506–508
Transplants, 549
Transportation
    barriers in, 513–514
    integrated work environment and, enclave option
        versus, 222–223
Triarchic theory of intelligence, 33
TRIP, *see* Transactional Intervention Program
Tutors, peers as, 204, 324

Unconscious assumptions, paradigm traps and,
        632–639
Unemployment, 416
Ungraded, 331
Ungraded Class Teachers Association, 331
Unitary funding of education, 388–389
University of Kansas–Children's Rehabilitation
        Unit, 134
University structure
    best practices and
        curricular content and, 337
        outcomes of, 340
        processes of, 337–340
    preservice and, personnel preparation and,
        333–340
    see also Continuing education
U.S. Immigration and Naturalization Service, 23
U.S. Surgeon General's Report on Children with
        Special Health Care Needs, 132

Values
    concepts relating to, 8
    culture and, early intervention and, 430–431
    science and, 2–3
        action and, 11–12
        integration of, 6–8
    and social policy, 1
        research and, 4–6
Values-based education, test-based education versus,
        379–380
Values-based research, 8–11
Vegetative state, nutrition and hydration in,
        556–557
Vertical work enhancement, 223
Vineland Adaptive Behavior Scales, 35
Vineland Social Maturity Scale, 34, 50
Vocational assessment, 48–50
Vocational Assessment Curriculum Guide, 49

Vocational rehabilitation, 508
  current systems of, ineffectiveness of, 515–516
  Social Security system and, 516–517
  see also Employment
Vocational transition process, need for, 507

Wages, supported employment and, 146, 149,
  152–153
  research suggestions for, 162–163
Wechsler Adult Intelligence Scale (WAIS), mental
  retardation and, 30, 31–32
Wechsler Adult Intelligence Scale–Revised (WAIS-
  R), mental retardation and, 30, 31
Wechsler Intelligence Scale for Children–Revised
  (WISC-R), mental retardation and, 30, 31

Welsch v. Likins, 118
Wisconsin Family Support Program, 131–132
Work
  integrated, *see* Integrated work
  see also Employment
Work disincentives, 517–518
Work enhancement, opportunities for, in integrated
  work environment versus enclave option,
  223–224
Wyatt v. Stickney, 118

Yaris v. Special School District of St. Louis, 465
Year-round programming, *see* Extended school year
Youngberg vs. Romeo, 22